Integrative Medical Biochemistry Examination and Board Review

NOTICE

Medicine is an ever-changing science. As new research and clinical experience broaden our knowledge, changes in treatment and drug therapy are required. The authors and the publisher of this work have checked with sources believed to be reliable in their efforts to provide information that is complete and generally in accord with the standards accepted at the time of publication. However, in view of the possibility of human error or changes in medical sciences, neither the authors nor the publisher nor any other party who has been involved in the preparation or publication of this work warrants that the information contained herein is in every respect accurate or complete, and they disclaim all responsibility for any errors or omissions or for the results obtained from use of the information contained in this work. Readers are encouraged to confirm the information contained herein with other sources. For example and in particular, readers are advised to check the product information sheet included in the package of each drug they plan to administer to be certain that the information contained in this work is accurate and that changes have not been made in the recommended dose or in the contraindications for administration. This recommendation is of particular importance in connection with new or infrequently used drugs.

Integrative Medical Biochemistry Examination and Board Review

MICHAEL W. KING, PHD

Professor
Indiana University School of Medicine and
Center for Regenerative Biology and Medicine
Terre Haute, Indiana

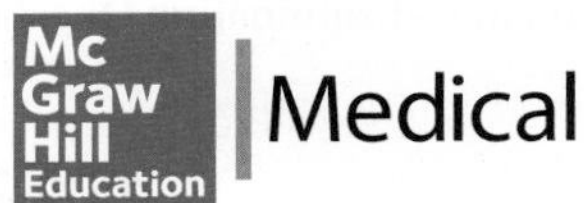

New York Chicago San Francisco Athens London Madrid Mexico City
Milan New Delhi Singapore Sydney Toronto

Integrative Medical Biochemistry
Examination and Board Review

1 2 3 4 5 6 7 8 9 0 CTP/CTP 18 17 16 15 14

ISBN 978-0-07-178612-6
MHID 0-07-178612-0

This book was set in Utopia Std by Cenveo® Publisher Services.
The editors were Michael Weitz and Karen G. Edmonson.
The production supervisor was Catherine H. Saggese.
Project management was provided by Anupriya Tyagi, Cenveo Publisher Services.
The cover designer was Thomas De Pierro.
China Translation & Printing Services, Ltd. was printer and binder.

This book is printed on acid-free paper.

Library of Congress Cataloging-in-Publication Data

King, Michael W. (Michael William), author.
Integrative medical biochemistry : examination and board review / Michael W. King.
p. ; cm.
Includes index.
ISBN 978-0-07-178612-6 (pbk. : alk. paper)—ISBN 0-07-178612-0 (pbk. : alk. paper)
I. Title.
[DNLM: 1. Biochemical Phenomena—Examination Questions. 2. Integrative Medicine—Examination Questions.
QU 18.2]
QP518.5
612'.015—dc23
2014007235

Contents

CHAPTER 36

Transcription: RNA Synthesis, Processing, and Regulation 512

CHAPTER 37

Translation: Protein Synthesis and Modification 532

CHAPTER 38

Glycoproteins 556

CHAPTER 39

Extracellular Matrix: Glycosaminoglycans and Proteoglycans 579

Preface

This book has been designed with the intention of preparing students, particularly those in medical school, for both regular course exams in biochemistry and medical biochemistry as well as medical board exams, namely the USMLE Step 1 exam taken by all US medical students at the completion of their second year of education. To accomplish this goal, there are 1100 multiple choice questions throughout all of the chapters with 50% being formatted in the current USMLE Step 1 format.

In addition to the general content and questions, a major focus of this book is on the integration of medical biochemistry with physiology, pathophysiology, pathology, and anatomy. This focus has been undertaken with this book to ensure that it serves that critical audience of current and future medical student, exposed to the shifting medical school curriculum, which is to use a more integrated content approach.

This review book is divided into four broad sections. The first section covers the basics of the major building blocks of all cells and tissues. The second section, and by far the major bulk of any medical biochemistry text, covers metabolic biochemistry with a strong emphasis on clinical correlations and clinical disorders related to these all-important pathways. The third section covers the cellular and molecular biology topics associated with medical biochemistry, physiology, and pathology. The fourth section includes 10 chapters dealing with high-yield integrative topics that are beneficial to not only medical students but to all students of the discipline.

Each chapter begins with an outline listing the major topics covered in the content. This is followed by a list of high-yield terms related to the included content. Each chapter includes numerous explanatory figures and tables aimed at allowing for increased understanding of and focus on the critical content. Most chapters include detailed Clinical Boxes that describe and discuss the high-yield information concerning diseases and disorders related to defects in the pathways being discussed. Although each chapter does not warrant one or more Clinical Boxes, there are over 90 such high-yield topics throughout the book. Each chapter content section is followed by a series of multiple choice questions, which also include explanatory answers for each and every question. Finally, at the end of each chapter is a Checklist designed to refocus the reader to the most important and high-yield concepts covered by each chapter. If a student finds concepts and/or content confusing or unclear when completing any chapter, it is highly recommended that for further detailed information they go to http://themedicalbiochemistrypage.org. This is the most complete resource for a more comprehensive study of the material reviewed in this book.

I would like to acknowledge the invaluable contributions provided by the McGraw-Hill editorial team of Michael Weitz, Karen Edmonson, Thomas DiPierro, Anthony Landi, and Laura Libretti. I give great thanks to the graphic design students, Matt Wilson, Janine Phelps, and Austin Woodall (at IUSM-Terre Haute host campus, Indiana State University) who were instrumental in preparing much of the artwork for this text. I would also like to acknowledge my students from the Indiana University School of Medicine-Terre Haute, class of 2017, for their willingness to serve as test subjects for many of the clinical vignette questions in this book. Finally, I would like to thank my colleagues for their support and encouragement throughout the process of completing this book.

PART I Biological Building Blocks of Cells and Tissues

CHAPTER 1 Amino Acids, Carbohydrates, Lipids, Nucleic Acids

CHAPTER OUTLINE

High-Yield Terms

pH: defined as the negative logarithm of the hydrogen ion (H^+) concentration of any given solution

pK_a: represents a relationship between pH and the equilibrium constant (K_a) for the dissociation of weak acids and bases in solution. Like pH, pK_a is the negative logarithm of K_a

Isoelectric point: defines the pH at which a molecule or substance carries no net electric charge

Hendersen-Hasselbalch equation: defines the relationship between pH and pK_a for any dissociation reaction of a weak acid or base such that when the concentration of any conjugate base (A^-) and its acid (HA) are equal, the pK_a for that dissociation is equivalent to the pH of the solution

Buffering: relates to the property that when the pH of a solution is close to the pK_a of a weak acid or base, the addition of more acid or base will not result in appreciable change in the pH

Amino Acids: Building Blocks for Protein

Chemical Nature of the Amino Acids

All peptides and polypeptides are polymers of α-amino acids. There are 20 α-amino acids relevant to the makeup of mammalian proteins (see later). Several other amino acids found in the body are in free or combined states (ie, not associated with peptides or proteins). These non–protein-associated amino acids perform specialized functions. Several of the amino acids found in proteins also serve functions distinct from the formation of peptides and proteins, for example, tyrosine in the formation of thyroid hormones or glutamate acting as a neurotransmitter.

The α-amino acids in peptides and proteins (excluding proline) consist of a carboxylic acid (–COOH) and an amino ($-NH_2$) functional group attached to the same tetrahedral carbon atom. This carbon is the α-carbon. Distinct R groups, that distinguish one amino acid from another, are also attached to the α-carbon (except in the case of glycine where the R group is hydrogen). The fourth substitution on the tetrahedral α-carbon of amino acids is hydrogen.

Classification of Amino Acids

Each of the 20 α-amino acids found in proteins can be distinguished by the R group substitution on the α-carbon atom. There are 2 broad classes of amino acids based upon whether the R group is hydrophobic or hydrophilic (Table 1-1).

The hydrophobic amino acids tend to repel the aqueous environment and, therefore, reside predominantly in the interior of proteins. This class of amino acids does not ionize nor participate in the formation of H-bonds. The hydrophilic amino acids tend to interact with the aqueous environment, are often involved

TABLE 1-1: L-α-Amino Acids Present in Proteins

Name	*Symbol*	*Structural Formula*	*pK_1* α-COOH	*pK_2* $\alpha\text{-}NH_3^+$	*pK_3* R Group
With Aliphatic Side Chains					
Glycine	Gly [G]	$H-CH-COO^-$ $\quad\;\; NH_3^+$	2.4	9.8	
Alanine	Ala [A]	$CH_3-CH-COO^-$ $\qquad\;\; NH_3^+$	2.4	9.9	
Valine	Val [V]	H_3C $\quad CH-CH-COO^-$ $H_3C \qquad NH_3^+$	2.2	9.7	
Leucine	Leu [L]	H_3C $\quad CH-CH_2-CH-COO^-$ $H_3C \qquad\qquad NH_3^+$	2.3	9.7	
Isoleucine	Ile [I]	CH_3 $\quad CH_2$ $\quad CH-CH-COO^-$ $\quad CH_3 \quad NH_3^+$	2.3	9.8	
With Side Chains Containing Hydroxylic (OH) Groups					
Serine	Ser [S]	$CH_2-CH-COO^-$ $OH \quad NH_3^+$	2.2	9.2	About 13
Threonine	Thr [T]	$CH_3-CH-CH-COO^-$ $\qquad OH \quad NH_3^+$	2.1	9.1	About 13
Tyrosine	Tyr [Y]	See below.			

(continued)

TABLE 1-1: L-α-Amino Acids Present in Proteins (*continued*)

Name	*Symbol*	*Structural Formula*	*pK₁* α-COOH	*pK₂* α-NH_3^+	*pK₃* R Group
With Side Chains Containing Sulfur Atoms					
Cysteine	Cys [C]	$\underset{SH}{CH_2}-\underset{NH_3^+}{CH}-COO^-$	1.9	10.8	8.3
Methionine	Met [M]	$\underset{S-CH_3}{CH_2}-CH_2-\underset{NH_3^+}{CH}-COO^-$	2.1	9.3	
With Side Chains Containing Acidic Groups or Their Amides					
Aspartic acid	Asp [D]	$^-OOC-CH_2-\underset{NH_3^+}{CH}-COO^-$	2.1	9.9	3.9
Asparagine	Asn [N]	$H_2N-\underset{O}{\underset{\|}{C}}-CH_2-\underset{NH_3^+}{CH}-COO^-$	2.1	8.8	
Glutamic acid	Glu [E]	$^-OOC-CH_2-CH_2-\underset{NH_3^+}{CH}-COO^-$	2.1	9.5	4.1
Glutamine	Gln [Q]	$H_2N-\underset{O}{\underset{\|}{C}}-CH_2-CH_2-\underset{NH_3^+}{CH}-COO^-$	2.2	9.1	
With Side Chains Containing Basic Groups					
Arginine	Arg [R]	$H-\underset{\underset{NH_2}{C=NH_2^+}}{N}-CH_2-CH_2-CH_2-\underset{NH_3^+}{CH}-COO^-$	1.8	9.0	12.5
Lysine	Lys [K]	$\underset{NH_3^+}{CH_2}-CH_2-CH_2-CH_2-\underset{NH_3^+}{CH}-COO^-$	2.2	9.2	10.8
Histidine	His [H]	(imidazole ring, HN, N)$-CH_2-\underset{NH_3^+}{CH}-COO^-$	1.8	9.3	6.0
Containing Aromatic Rings					
Histidine	His [H]	See above.			
Phenylalanine	Phe [F]	(benzene ring)$-CH_2-\underset{NH_3^+}{CH}-COO^-$	2.2	9.2	
Tyrosine	Tyr [Y]	$HO-$(benzene ring)$-CH_2-\underset{NH_3^+}{CH}-COO^-$	2.2	9.1	10.1
Tryptophan	Trp [W]	(indole ring, N–H)$-CH_2-\underset{NH_3^+}{CH}-COO^-$	2.4	9.4	
Imino Acid					
Proline	Pro [P]	(pyrrolidine ring, $\overset{+}{N}H_2$)$-COO^-$	2.0	10.6	

Source: Murray RK, Bender DA, Botham KM, Kennelly PJ, Rodwell VW, Weil PA. *Harper's Illustrated Biochemistry*, 29th ed. New York, NY: McGraw-Hill; 2012.

High-Yield Concept

An amino acid with no ionizable R group would be electrically neutral at this pH and is termed a *zwitterion*. The term zwitterion defines an electrically neutral molecule with one positive and one negative charge at different sites within that molecule.

in the formation of H-bonds, and are predominantly found on the exterior surfaces of proteins or in the reactive centers of enzymes.

Acid–Base Properties of the Amino Acids

The α-COOH and α-NH_2 groups in amino acids are capable of donating or accepting protons (as are the acidic and basic R groups of the amino acids). As a result of their ionizing, the following ionic equilibrium reactions may be written in the basic form:

$$HA \leftrightarrow H^+ + A^-$$

The equilibrium constant, K_a, for a reaction of this type is defined as:

$$K_a = \frac{[H^+][A^-]}{[HA]}$$

For the α-COOH and α-NH_2 groups of the amino acids, these equilibrium reactions would be:

$$R\text{-}COOH \leftrightarrow R\text{-}COO^- + H^+$$

$$R\text{-}NH_3^+ \leftrightarrow R\text{-}NH_2 + H^+$$

The equilibrium reactions, as written, demonstrate that amino acids contain at least 2 weakly acidic groups. However, the carboxyl group is a far stronger acid than the amino group. At physiological pH (~7.4) the carboxyl group will be unprotonated and the amino group will be protonated.

Like typical organic acids, the acidic strength of the carboxyl, amino, and ionizable R groups in amino acids can be defined by the association or equilibrium constant, K_a, or more commonly the negative logarithm of K_a ($-\log K_a$), the pK_a. This value is determined for any given acid or base from the Hendersen-Hasselbalch equation:

$$pH = pK_a + \log\frac{[A^-]}{[HA]}$$

The net charge (the algebraic sum of all the charged groups present) of any amino acid, peptide, or protein will depend upon the pH of the surrounding aqueous environment. As the pH of a solution of an amino acid or protein changes so too does the net charge. This phenomenon can be observed during the titration of any amino acid or protein (Figure 1-1). When the net charge of an amino acid or protein is zero, the pH will be equivalent to the isoelectric point (pI).

Functional Significance of Amino Acid R Groups

In solution, it is the nature of the amino acid R groups that dictate structure–function relationships of peptides and proteins. The hydrophobic amino acids will generally be encountered in the interior of proteins shielded from direct contact with water. Conversely, the hydrophilic amino acids are generally found on the exterior of proteins as well as in the active centers of enzymatically active proteins. Indeed, it is the very nature of certain amino acid R groups that allow enzyme reactions to occur.

The imidazole ring of histidine allows it to act as either a proton donor or acceptor at physiological pH. Hence, it is frequently found in the reactive center of enzymes. Equally important is the ability of histidines

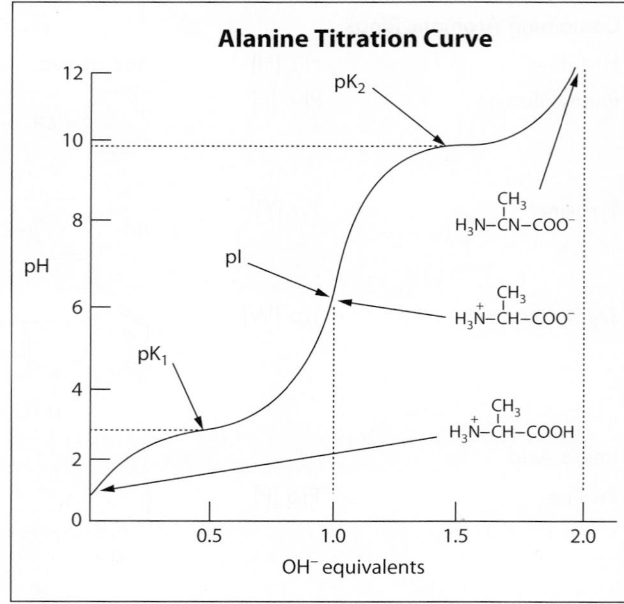

FIGURE 1-1: Titration of alanine. Reproduced with permission of themedicalbiochemistrypage, LLC.

in hemoglobin to buffer the H^+ ions from carbonic acid ionization in red blood cells. It is this property of hemoglobin that allows it to exchange O_2 and CO_2 at the tissues or lungs, respectively.

The primary alcohol of serine and threonine as well as the thiol (–SH) of cysteine allow these amino acids to act as nucleophiles during enzymatic catalysis. Additionally, the thiol of cysteine is able to form a disulfide bond with other cysteines:

Cysteine-SH + HS-Cysteine ↔ Cysteine-S-S-Cysteine

This simple disulfide is identified as *cystine*. The formation of disulfide bonds between cysteines present within proteins is important to the formation of active structural domains in a large number of proteins. Disulfide bonding between cysteines in different polypeptide chains of oligomeric proteins plays a crucial role in ordering the structure of complex proteins, for example, the insulin receptor.

Optical Properties of the Amino Acids

A tetrahedral carbon atom with 4 distinct constituents is said to be chiral. The one amino acid not exhibiting chirality is glycine since its R group is a hydrogen atom. **Chirality** describes the handedness of a molecule that is observable by the ability of a molecule to rotate the plane of polarized light either to the right (dextrorotatory) or to the left (levorotatory). All of the amino acids in proteins exhibit the same absolute steric configuration as L-glyceraldehyde. Therefore, they are all L-α-amino acids. D-amino acids are never found in proteins, although they exist in nature.

The aromatic R groups in amino acids absorb ultraviolet light with an absorbance maximum in the range of 280 nm. The ability of proteins to absorb ultraviolet light is predominantly due to the presence of the tryptophan, which strongly absorbs ultraviolet light.

FIGURE 1-2: Resonance stabilization forms of the peptide bond. Murray RK, Bender DA, Botham KM, Kennelly PJ, Rodwell VW, Weil PA. *Harper's Illustrated Biochemistry*, 29th ed. New York, NY: McGraw-Hill; 2012.

The Peptide Bond

Peptide bond formation is a condensation reaction leading to the polymerization of amino acids into peptides and proteins. *Peptide* is the term used to define a small compound consisting of only a few amino acids. A number of hormones and neurotransmitters are peptides. Additionally, several antibiotics and antitumor agents are peptides. Proteins are polypeptides of greatly divergent length. The simplest peptide, a dipeptide, contains a single peptide bond formed by the condensation of the carboxyl group of one amino acid with the amino group of the second with the concomitant elimination of water. The presence of the carbonyl group in a peptide bond allows electron resonance stabilization to occur such that the peptide bond exhibits rigidity not unlike the typical –C=C– double bond. The peptide bond is, therefore, said to have partial double-bond character (Figure 1-2).

REVIEW QUESTIONS

1. Which of the following correctly defines the term pK_a?

A. equilibrium constant for the dissociation of HA to A^- and H^+
B. ion constant of water
C. negative log of the concentration of H^+
D. pH at which a molecule is neutrally charged
E. pH at which an equivalent distribution of acid and conjugate base exist in solution

Answer E: The logarithmic measure of the acid dissociation constant of an acid or base, termed pK_a, is defined as the pH at which the protonated and unprotonated molecular species are at equal concentrations. With respect to this question the protonated species can be represented as HA while the unprotonated species would be A^-.

2. Which of the following correctly defines the isoelectric point (pI) of an amino acid or protein?

A. the equilibrium constant for the ionization of the substance
B. the ion constant of water
C. negative log of the concentration of H^+
D. pH at which a molecule is electrically neutral
E. pH at which an equivalent distribution of acid and conjugate base exists in solution

Answer D: The **isoelectric point** is that pH at which a substance exhibits no net charge. In other words, all the negative and positive charges, say for instance in a protein, are equal in number such that the molecule is electrically neutral.

3. The blood contains many compounds that serve to buffer the pH of the fluid such as bicarbonate and phosphate ions. Which of the following most correctly defines the meaning of the term buffering?

A. a solution containing a large concentration of a base such that the pH will not change significantly when an acid is added
B. a solution containing a large concentration of an acid such that the pH will not change significantly when more acid is added
C. a solution or substance which resists changes in pH when small quantities of an acid or base are added to it
D. pH at which a molecule or solution is neutrally charged
E. pH at which an equivalent distribution of acid and conjugate base exists in solution

Answer C: A *buffer* is a molecule that tends to either bind or release hydrogen ions in order to maintain a particular pH. More precisely, a **buffer** is defined as a mixture of a conjugate acid–base pair that can resist changes in pH when small amounts of strong acids or bases are added to it.

4. Which of the following best describes the characteristics of polar amino acids?

A. ionizable in water
B. more likely to be exposed to water than to be found in the interior of a folded protein
C. partially charged due to the oxygen atom in their carboxyl group
D. partially charged due to fairly consistent sharing of electrons among atoms in their R group
E. positively charged

Answer B: Polar amino acids are defined as those whose R groups are capable of forming hydrogen bonds with water. Due to this property they are also said to be hydrophilic (water loving) and, therefore, are most often found exposed to the aqueous environment on the surface of proteins as opposed to buried in the interior.

5. Which one of the following amino acids may be considered a hydrophobic amino acid at physiological pH of 7.4?

A. arginine
B. aspartic acid
C. glycine
D. isoleucine
E. threonine

Answer D: Hydrophobic amino acids are those with side chains that do not like to reside in an aqueous environment. For this reason, these amino acids are more often found buried within the hydrophobic core of a protein, or within the lipid portion of a membrane.

6. The greatest buffering capacity at physiological pH would be provided by a protein rich in which of the following amino acids?

A. alanine
B. cysteine
C. histidine
D. proline
E. tyrosine

Answer C: Histidine contains an imidazole ring as its R group. The nitrogen in this ring possesses a pK_a around 6.0, thus it is able to accept or donate a proton at physiological pH. This fact makes the amino acid an ideal buffering component of a protein containing several histidine residues.

Checklist

✓ All amino acids found in human proteins exist as L-α-amino acids, although D-amino acids are found in nature.

✓ All amino acids contain at least 2 weakly acidic groups, the α-NH_2 and the α-COOH groups. Many amino acids also contain weakly acidic function groups designated as the R group.

✓ The R groups of the amino acids determines their classification, for example, acidic or basic.

✓ The association constant, pK_a, can be determined for H^+ dissociation from any of the ionizable groups of each amino acid.

✓ As with all acids and bases, when titrating amino acids the pH at which the net charge on the molecule is neutral is referred to as the isoelectric point, pI.

✓ Amino acids form peptide bonds creating polymers called peptides and proteins. Due to resonance stabilization of electrons about the peptide bond, there is limited mobility leading to restricted protein conformations.

CHAPTER

2 Biological Building Blocks: Carbohydrates

CHAPTER OUTLINE

High-Yield Terms

Carbohydrate: any organic molecule composed exclusively of carbon, hydrogen, and oxygen where the hydrogen-to-oxygen ratio is usually 2:1, biological synonym is saccharide, commonly called sugars

Saccharide: synonym for carbohydrate in biological systems, lay terminology is sugar

Aldose: a monosaccharide that contains only one aldehyde (–CH=O) group per molecule

Ketose: a monosaccharide that contains only one ketone (–C=O) group per molecule

Enantiomer: one of 2 stereoisomers that are mirror images of each other, which cannot be superimposed

Anomeric carbon: the carbon of a carbohydrate bearing the reactive carbonyl about which free rotation into 2 distinct configurations (termed α and β) can occur when in the cyclic form

Glycosidic bond: any of the type of covalent bond that joins a carbohydrate molecule to another group

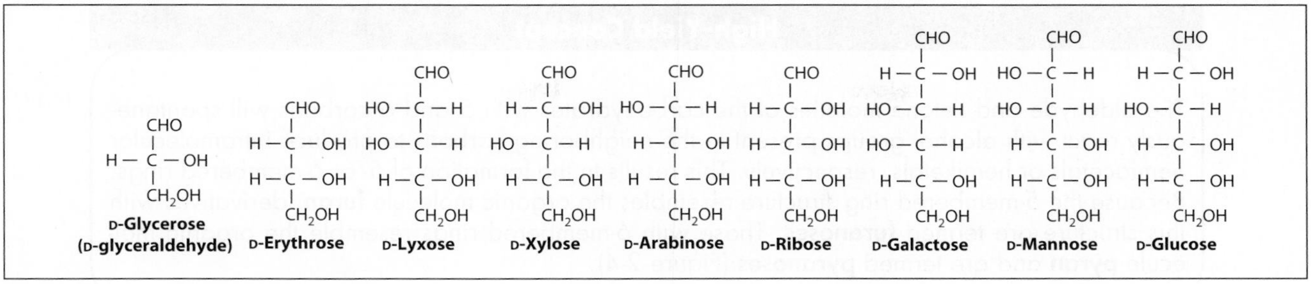

D-Glycerose (D-glyceraldehyde)	D-Erythrose	D-Lyxose	D-Xylose	D-Arabinose	D-Ribose	D-Galactose	D-Mannose	D-Glucose
CHO	CHO	CHO	CHO	CHO	CHO	CHO	CHO	CHO
H–C–OH	H–C–OH	HO–C–H	H–C–OH	HO–C–H	H–C–OH	H–C–OH	HO–C–H	H–C–OH
CH_2OH	H–C–OH	HO–C–H	HO–C–H	H–C–OH	H–C–OH	HO–C–H	HO–C–H	HO–C–H
	CH_2OH	H–C–OH	H–C–OH	H–C–OH	H–C–OH	HO–C–H	H–C–OH	H–C–OH
		CH_2OH	CH_2OH	CH_2OH	CH_2OH	H–C–OH	H–C–OH	H–C–OH
						CH_2OH	CH_2OH	CH_2OH

FIGURE 2-1: Examples of aldoses of physiologic significance. Murray RK, Bender DA, Botham KM, Kennelly PJ, Rodwell VW, Weil PA. *Harper's Illustrated Biochemistry*, 29th ed. New York, NY: McGraw-Hill; 2012.

Simple carbohydrates are biological compounds composed solely of carbon, oxygen, and hydrogen that generally contain large quantities of hydroxyl groups (-OH). In biochemistry, carbohydrate is synonymous with saccharide and the more common term, sugar. The simplest carbohydrates also contain either an aldehyde moiety and are termed *polyhydroxyaldehydes*, commonly called *aldoses* (Figure 2-1), or a ketone moiety and are termed *polyhydroxyketones*, commonly called *ketoses* (Figure 2-2).

All carbohydrates can be classified as either **monosaccharides**, **oligosaccharides**, or **polysaccharides**. Anywhere from 2 to 10 monosaccharide units, linked by glycosidic bonds, make up an oligosaccharide. Polysaccharides are much larger, generally containing hundreds of monosaccharide units. The presence of the hydroxyl groups allows carbohydrates to interact with the aqueous environment and to participate in hydrogen bonding, both within and between chains. Derivatives of the carbohydrates can contain nitrogen, phosphates, and sulfur compounds. Carbohydrates can also combine with lipid to form glycolipids (see Chapter 21) or with protein to form glycoproteins (see Chapter 38).

Carbohydrate Structure and Nomenclature

The predominant carbohydrates encountered in the body are structurally related to the aldotriose **glyceraldehyde** and to the ketotriose **dihydroxyacetone**. All carbohydrates contain at least one asymmetrical (chiral) carbon and are, therefore, optically active. In addition, carbohydrates can exist in either of the 2 conformations, as determined by the orientation of the hydroxyl group about the asymmetric carbon farthest from the carbonyl. With a few exceptions, those carbohydrates that are of physiological significance exist in the D-conformation. The mirror-image conformations, called **enantiomers**, are in the L-conformation (Figure 2-3).

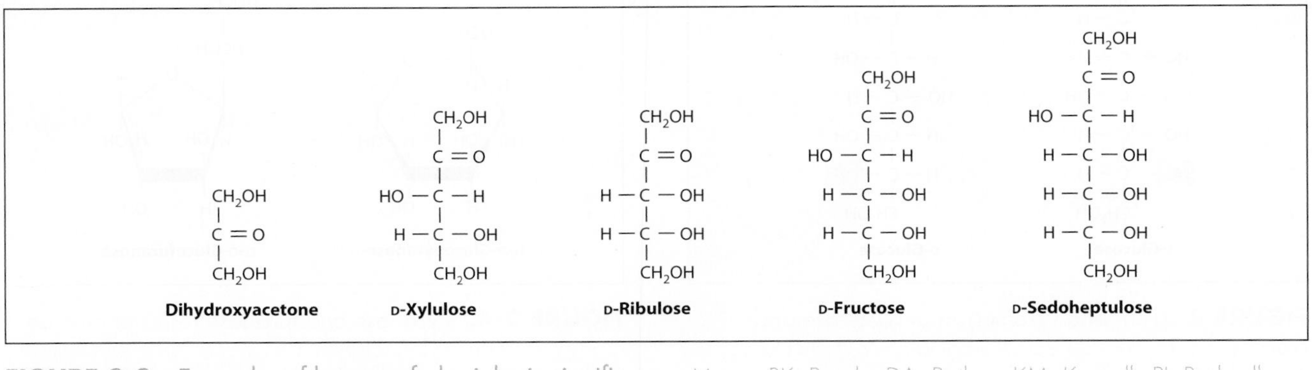

Dihydroxyacetone	D-Xylulose	D-Ribulose	D-Fructose	D-Sedoheptulose
CH_2OH	CH_2OH	CH_2OH	CH_2OH	CH_2OH
C=O	C=O	C=O	C=O	C=O
CH_2OH	HO–C–H	H–C–OH	HO–C–H	HO–C–H
	H–C–OH	H–C–OH	H–C–OH	H–C–OH
	CH_2OH	CH_2OH	H–C–OH	H–C–OH
			CH_2OH	H–C–OH
				CH_2OH

FIGURE 2-2: Examples of ketoses of physiologic significance. Murray RK, Bender DA, Botham KM, Kennelly PJ, Rodwell VW, Weil PA. *Harper's Illustrated Biochemistry*, 29th ed. New York, NY: McGraw-Hill; 2012.

High-Yield Concept

The aldehyde and ketone moieties of the carbohydrates with 5 and 6 carbons will spontaneously react with alcohol groups present in the neighboring carbons to produce intramolecular hemiacetals or hemiketals, respectively. This results in the formation of 5- or 6-membered rings. Because the 5-membered ring structure resembles the organic molecule **furan**, derivatives with this structure are termed **furanoses**. Those with 6-membered rings resemble the organic molecule **pyran** and are termed **pyranoses** (Figure 2-4).

The ring structures of the carbohydrates can be depicted by either **Fischer-** or **Haworth-** (also called the chair form) style diagrams (Figure 2-5). The numbering of the carbons in carbohydrates proceeds from the carbonyl carbon, for aldoses, or the carbon nearest the carbonyl, for ketoses. The rings can open and reclose, allowing rotation to occur about the carbon bearing the reactive carbonyl yielding 2 distinct configurations (α and β) of the hemiacetals and hemiketals (Figure 2-6). The carbon about which this rotation occurs is the **anomeric carbon** and the 2 forms are termed *anomers*. Carbohydrates can change spontaneously between the α- and β-configurations: a process known as **mutarotation**. When drawn in the Fischer projection, the α-configuration places the hydroxyl attached to the anomeric carbon to the right, toward the ring. When drawn in the Haworth projection, the α-configuration places the hydroxyl downward. Constituents of the ring that project above or below the plane of the ring are axial and those that project parallel to the plane are equatorial. In the chair conformation, the orientation of the hydroxyl group about the anomeric carbon of α-D-glucose is axial and equatorial in β-D-glucose.

Monosaccharides

The monosaccharides commonly found in humans are classified according to the number of carbons they contain in their backbone structures. The major monosaccharides,

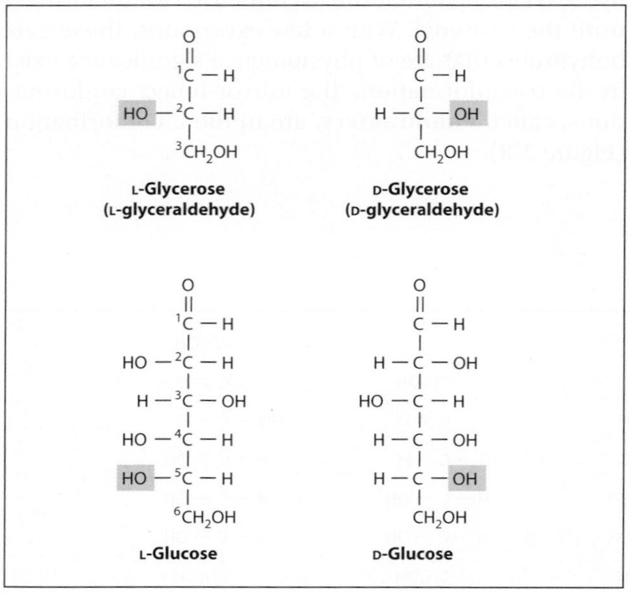

L-Glycerose (L-glyceraldehyde)

D-Glycerose (D-glyceraldehyde)

L-Glucose

D-Glucose

FIGURE 2-3: D- and L-isomerism of glycerose and glucose. Murray RK, Bender DA, Botham KM, Kennelly PJ, Rodwell VW, Weil PA. *Harper's Illustrated Biochemistry*, 29th ed. New York, NY: McGraw-Hill; 2012.

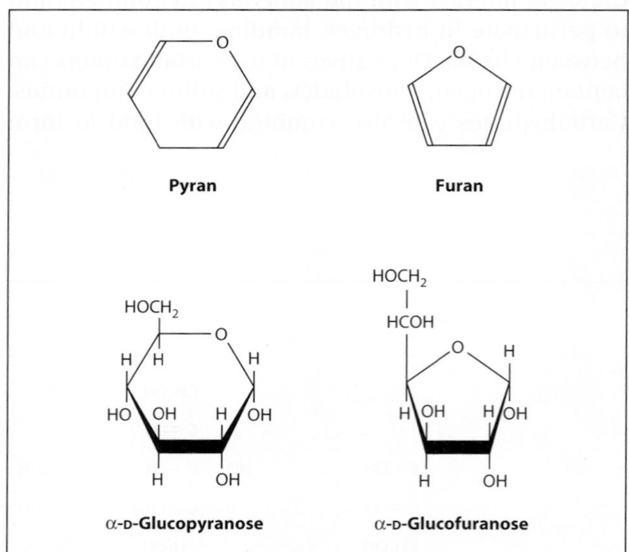

FIGURE 2-4: Pyranose and furanose forms of glucose. Murray RK, Bender DA, Botham KM, Kennelly PJ, Rodwell VW, Weil PA. *Harper's Illustrated Biochemistry*, 29th ed. New York, NY: McGraw-Hill; 2012.

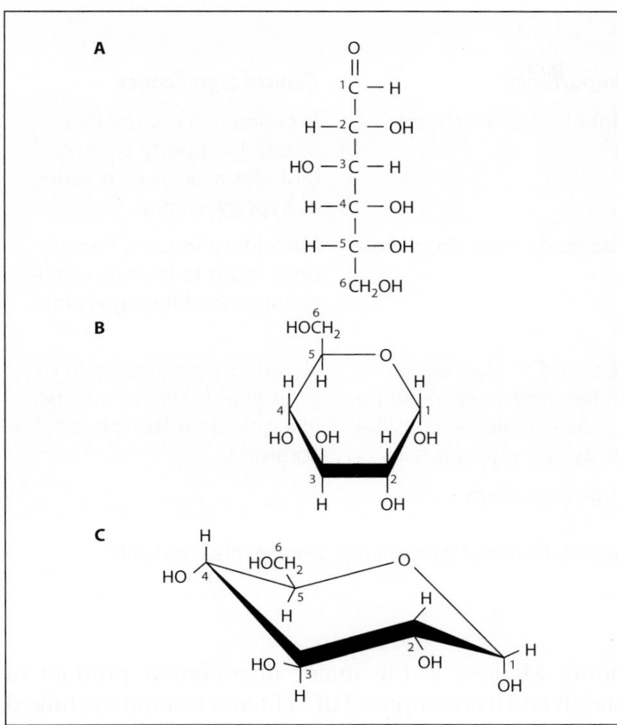

FIGURE 2-5: D-Glucose. (A) Straight-chain form. (B) α-D-glucose; Haworth projection. (C) α-D-glucose; chair form. Murray RK, Bender DA, Botham KM, Kennelly PJ, Rodwell VW, Weil PA. *Harper's Illustrated Biochemistry*, 29th ed. New York, NY: McGraw-Hill; 2012.

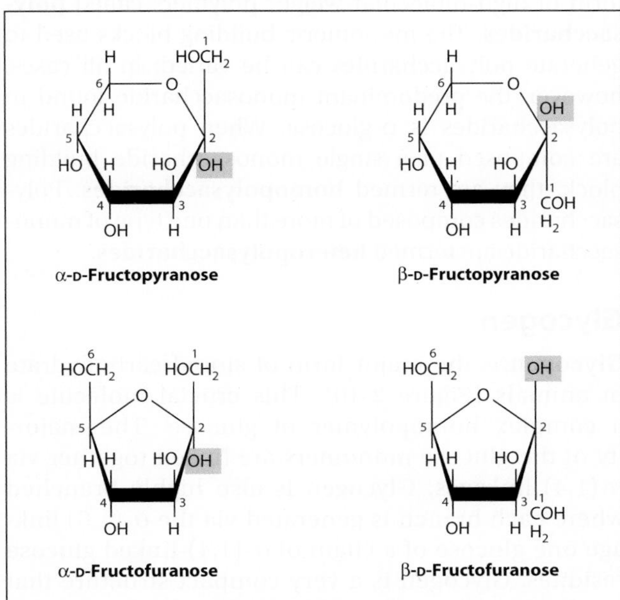

FIGURE 2-6: Pyranose and furanose forms of fructose. Murray RK, Bender DA, Botham KM, Kennelly PJ, Rodwell VW, Weil PA. *Harper's Illustrated Biochemistry*, 29th ed. New York, NY: McGraw-Hill; 2012.

TABLE 2-1: Classification of Important Sugars

	Aldoses	***Ketoses***
Trioses ($C_3H_6O_3$)	Glycerose (glyceraldehyde)	Dihydroxyacetone
Tetroses ($C_4H_8O_4$)	Erythrose	Erythrulose
Pentoses ($C_5H_{10}O_5$)	Ribose	Ribulose
Hexoses ($C_6H_{12}O_6$)	Glucose	Fructose
Heptoses ($C_7H_{14}O_7$)	—	Sedoheptulose

Murray RK, Bender DA, Botham KM, Kennelly PJ, Rodwell VW, Weil PA. *Harper's Illustrated Biochemistry*, 29th ed. New York, NY: McGraw-Hill; 2012.

used either for energy production, or as components in complex macromolecules, contain 3 to 6 carbon atoms (Table 2-1). The 5-carbon sugars (the pentoses, Table 2-2) and the 6-carbon sugars (the hexoses, Table 2-3) represent the largest groups of physiologically important carbohydrates in human metabolism. Sedoheptulose is an additional biologically important carbohydrate that contains 7-carbon atoms (see Figure 2-2). The amino sugars are another class of biologically significant carbohydrates that contain nitrogen. These include *N*-acetylglucosamine (GlcNAc: Figure 2-7), *N*-acetylgalactosamine (GalNAc), and *N*-acetylneuraminic acid (NANA; also known sialic acid, Sia: Figure 2-8).

TABLE 2-2: Pentoses of Physiologic Importance

Sugar	***Source***	***Biochemical and Clinical Importance***
D-Ribose	Nucleic acids and metabolic intermediate	Structural component of nucleic acids and coenzymes, including ATP, NAD(P), and flavin coenzymes
D-Ribulose	Metabolic intermediate	Intermediate in the pentose phosphate pathway
D-Arabinose	Plant gums	Constituent of glycoproteins
D-Xylose	Plant gums, proteoglycans, glycosaminoglycans	Constituent of glycoproteins
L-Xylulose	Metabolic intermediate	Excreted in the urine in essential pentosuria

Murray RK, Bender DA, Botham KM, Kennelly PJ, Rodwell VW, Weil PA. *Harper's Illustrated Biochemistry*, 29th ed. New York, NY: McGraw-Hill; 2012.

TABLE 2-3: Hexoses of Physiologic Importance

Sugar	*Source*	*Biochemical Importance*	*Clinical Significance*
D-Glucose	Fruit juices, hydrolysis of starch, cane or beet sugar, maltose and lactose	The main metabolic fuel for tissues; "blood sugar"	Excreted in the urine (glucosuria) in poorly controlled diabetes mellitus as a result of hyperglycemia
D-Fructose	Fruit juices, honey, hydrolysis of cane or beet sugar and inulin, enzymic isomerization of glucose syrups for food manufacture	Readily metabolized either via glucose or directly	Hereditary fructose intolerance leads to fructose accumulation and hypoglycemia
D-Galactose	Hydrolysis of lactose	Readily metabolized to glucose; synthesized in the mammary gland for synthesis of lactose in milk. A constituent of glycolipids and glycoproteins	Hereditary galactosemia as a result of failure to metabolize galactose leads to cataracts
D-Mannose	Hydrolysis of plant mannan gums	Constituent of glycoproteins	

Murray RK, Bender DA, Botham KM, Kennelly PJ, Rodwell VW, Weil PA. *Harper's Illustrated Biochemistry*, 29th ed. New York, NY: McGraw-Hill; 2012.

Disaccharides

Covalent bonds between the anomeric hydroxyl of a cyclic sugar and the hydroxyl of a second sugar (or another alcohol-containing compound) are termed **glycosidic bonds**, and the resultant molecules are **glycosides**. The linkage of 2 monosaccharides to form disaccharides involves a glycosidic bond (Figure 2-9). Several physiologically important disaccharides are sucrose, lactose, and maltose (Table 2-4).

Sucrose is the dominant carbohydrate in sugarcane and sugar beets and is composed of glucose and fructose linked via an α-(1,2)-β-glycosidic bond. Lactose is found exclusively in the milk of mammals and consists of galactose and glucose linked via a β-(1,4) glycosidic bond. Maltose is the major degradation product of starch and it is composed of 2 glucose monomers linked via an α-(1,4) glycosidic bond.

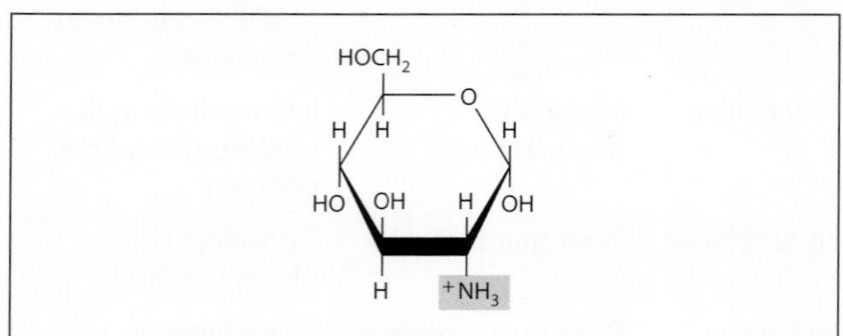

FIGURE 2-7: Glucosamine (2-amino-D-glucopyranose) (α form). Galactosamine is 2-amino-D-galactopyranose. Both glucosamine and galactosamine occur as *N*-acetyl derivatives in more complex carbohydrates, for example, glycoproteins. Murray RK, Bender DA, Botham KM, Kennelly PJ, Rodwell VW, Weil PA. *Harper's Illustrated Biochemistry*, 29th ed. New York, NY: McGraw-Hill; 2012.

Polysaccharides

Most of the carbohydrates found in nature occur in the form of high-molecular weight polymers called **polysaccharides**. The monomeric building blocks used to generate polysaccharides can be varied; in all cases, however, the predominant monosaccharide found in polysaccharides is D-glucose. When polysaccharides are composed of a single monosaccharide building block, they are termed **homopolysaccharides**. Polysaccharides composed of more than one type of monosaccharide are termed **heteropolysaccharides**.

Glycogen

Glycogen is the major form of stored carbohydrate in animals (Figure 2-10). This crucial molecule is a complex homopolymer of glucose. The majority of the glucose monomers are linked together via α-(1,4) linkages. Glycogen is also highly branched where each branch is generated via the α-(1,6) linkage one glucose of a chain of α-(1,4)-linked glucose residues. Glycogen is a very compact structure that results from the coiling of the polymer chains. This compactness allows large amounts of carbon energy to be stored in a small volume, with little effect on cellular osmolarity.

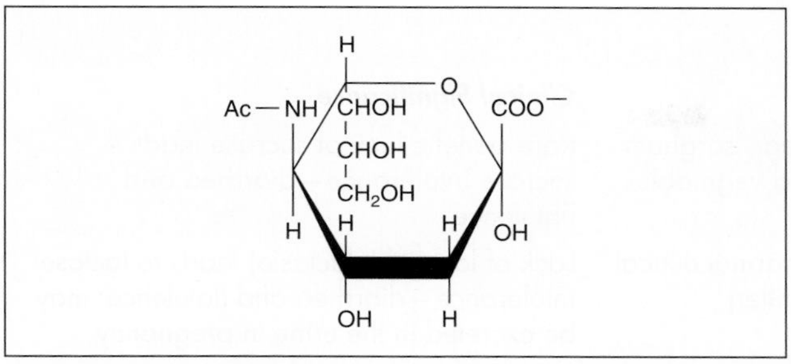

FIGURE 2-8: Structure of *N*-acetylneuraminic acid, a sialic acid (Ac = CH_3—CO—). Murray RK, Bender DA, Botham KM, Kennelly PJ, Rodwell VW, Weil PA. *Harper's Illustrated Biochemistry*, 29th ed. New York, NY: McGraw-Hill; 2012.

Starch

Starch is the major form of stored carbohydrate in plant cells. Its structure is identical to glycogen, except for a much lower degree of branching (about every 20-30 residues). Unbranched starch is called **amylose**; branched starch is called **amylopectin** (Figure 2-11).

Carbohydrates in complex structures

A variety of complex carbohydrate-containing compounds exist that are important both structurally and functionally. The major classes of these molecules are the glycoproteins (see Chapter 38), glycolipids and glycosaminoglycans (see Chapter 21), and the proteoglycans (see Chapter 39). Membrane-associated carbohydrate is exclusively in the form of oligosaccharides covalently attached to proteins forming glycoproteins, and to a lesser extent covalently attached to lipid forming the glycolipids. The physiological significance of protein glycosylation can be emphasized by the fact that approximately 50% of all proteins are known to be glycosylated and glycan biosynthesis genes represent at least 1% of the human genome. The distinction between proteoglycans and glycoproteins resides in the level and types of carbohydrate modification.

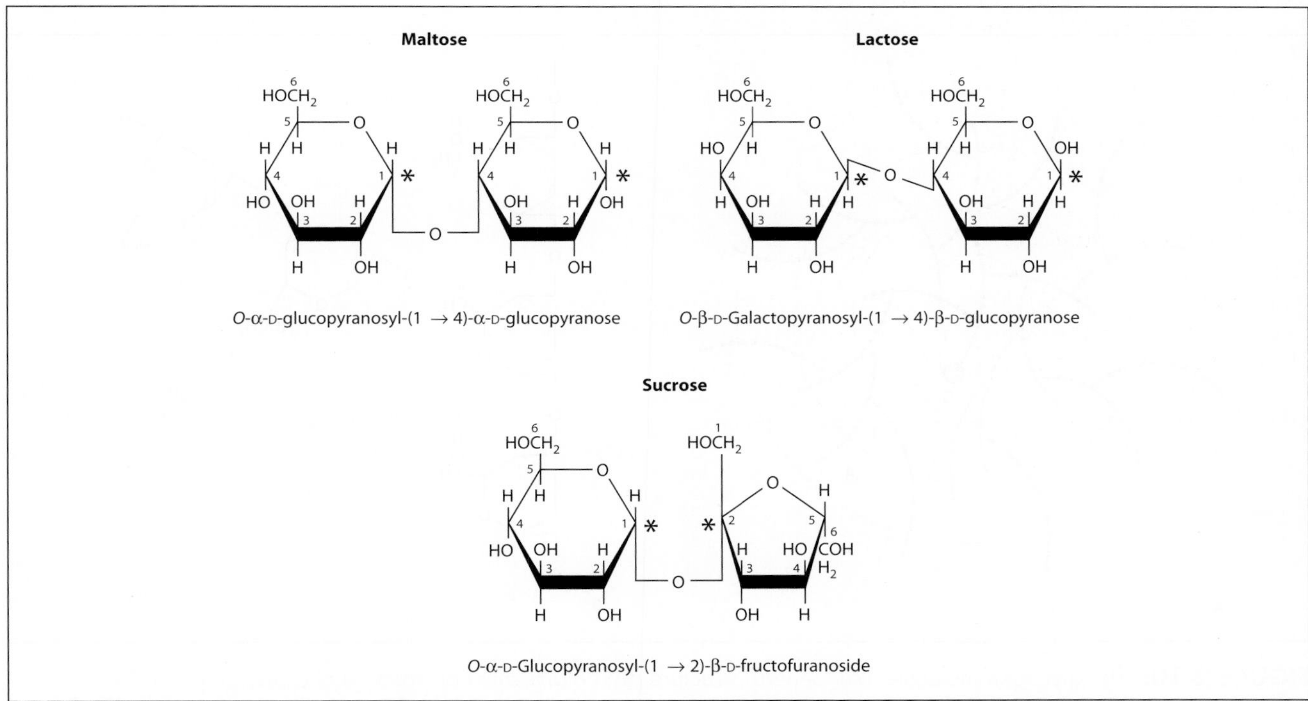

FIGURE 2-9: Structures of important disaccharides. α and β refer to the configuration at the anomeric carbon atom (*). When the anomeric carbon of the second residue takes part in the formation of the glycosidic bond, as in sucrose, the residue becomes a glycoside known as a furanoside or a pyranoside. As the disaccharide no longer has an anomeric carbon with a free potential aldehyde or ketone group, it no longer exhibits reducing properties. The configuration of the β-fructofuranose residue in sucrose results from turning the β-fructofuranose molecule depicted in Figure 14–4 through 180° and inverting it. (Murray RK, Bender DA, Botham KM, Kennelly PJ, Rodwell VW, Weil PA. *Harper's Illustrated Biochemistry*, 29th ed. New York, NY: McGraw-Hill; 2012.)

TABLE 2-4: Disaccharides of Physiologic Importance

Sugar	*Composition*	*Source*	*Clinical Significance*
Sucrose	O-α-D-glucopyranosyl-(1→2)-β-D-fructofuranoside	Cane and beet sugar, sorghum and some fruits and vegetables	Rare genetic lack of sucrase leads to sucrose intolerance—diarrhea and flatulence
Lactose	O-α-D-galactopyranosyl-(1→4)-β-D-glucopyranose	Milk (and many pharmaceutical preparations as a filler)	Lack of lactase (alactasia) leads to lactose intolerance—diarrhea and flatulence; may be excreted in the urine in pregnancy
Maltose	O-α-D-glucopyranosyl-(1→4)-α-D-glucopyranose	Enzymic hydrolysis of starch (amylase); germinating cereals and malt	
Isomaltose	O-α-D-glucopyranosyl-(1→6)-α-D-glucopyranose	Enzymic hydrolysis of starch (the branch points in amylopectin)	
Lactulose	O-α-D-galactopyranosyl-(1→4)-β-D-fructofuranose	Heated milk (small amounts), mainly synthetic	Not hydrolyzed by intestinal enzymes, but fermented by intestinal bacteria; used as a mild osmotic laxative
Trehalose	O-α-D-glucopyranosyl-(1→1)-α-D-glucopyranoside	Yeasts and fungi; the main sugar of insect hemolymph	

Murray RK, Bender DA, Botham KM, Kennelly PJ, Rodwell VW, Weil PA. *Harper's Illustrated Biochemistry*, 29th ed. New York, NY: McGraw-Hill; 2012.

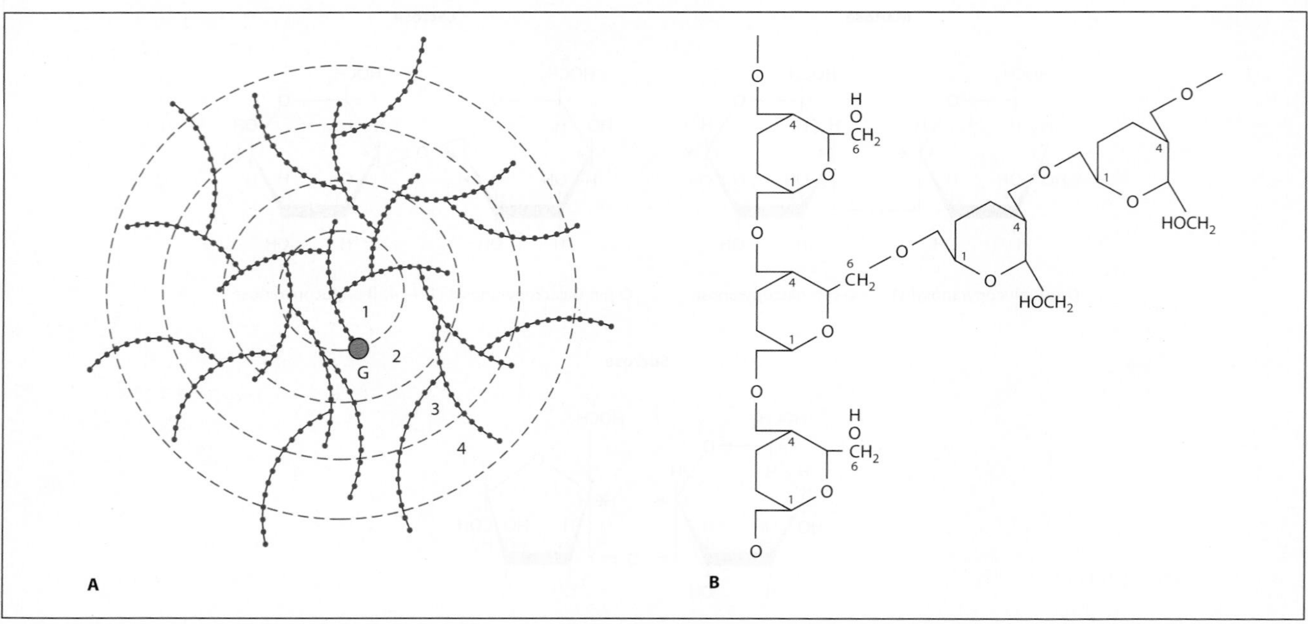

FIGURE 2-10: The glycogen molecule. (A) General structure. (B) Enlargement of structure at a branch point. The molecule is a sphere ~21 nm in diameter that can be seen in electron micrographs. It has a molecular mass of ~10^7 Da and consists of polysaccharide chains, each containing about 13 glucose residues. The chains are either branched or unbranched and are arranged in 12 concentric layers (only four are shown in the fi gure). The branched chains (each has two branches) are found in the inner layers and the unbranched chains in the outer layer. (G, glycogenin, the primer molecule for glycogen synthesis.) Murray RK, Bender DA, Botham KM, Kennelly PJ, Rodwell VW, Weil PA. *Harper's Illustrated Biochemistry*, 29th ed. New York, NY: McGraw-Hill; 2012.

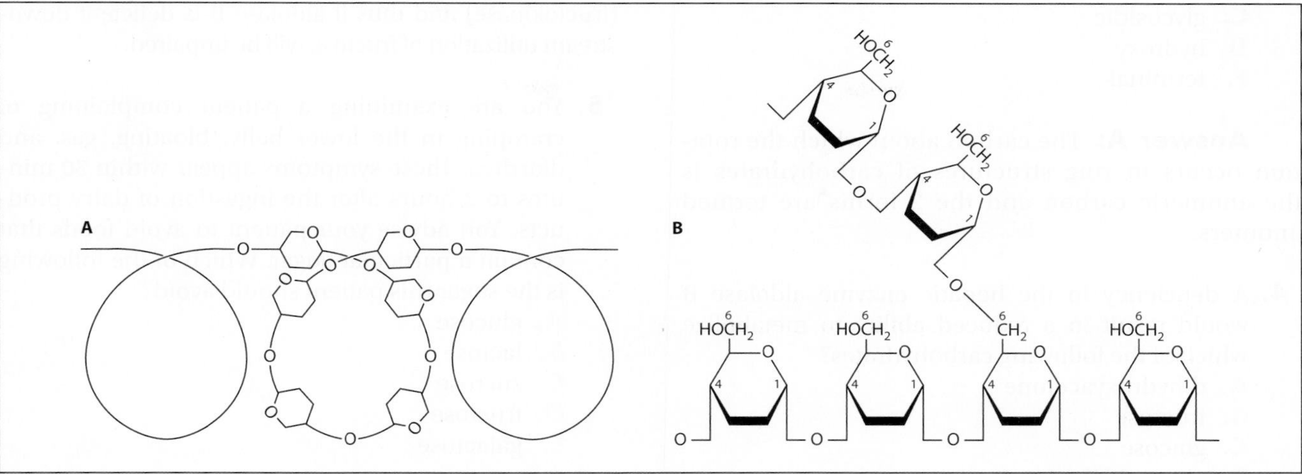

FIGURE 2-11: Structure of starch. (A) Amylose, showing helical coil structure. (B) Amylopectin, showing 1 → 6 branch point. Murray RK, Bender DA, Botham KM, Kennelly PJ, Rodwell VW, Weil PA. *Harper's Illustrated Biochemistry,* 29th ed. New York, NY: McGraw-Hill; 2012.

REVIEW QUESTIONS

1. The parents of a 7-month-old infant bring their son to the pediatrician because they have noticed that their child has a dull response to outside stimuli. In addition, they note that their child exhibits an exaggerated startle response (sudden extension of arms and legs) to sharp sounds and that he seems to be losing previously acquired motor and mental skills. His pediatrician makes a diagnosis of Tay-Sachs disease. Elevated intracellular levels of which of the following carbohydrate-containing compounds would provide useful information for confirmation of this diagnosis?

A. abnormal glycogen
B. aldohexoses
C. aldoketoses
D. gangliosides
E. glycosaminoglycans

Answer D: In the genetic disorder known as Tay-Sachs disease, ganglioside GM_2 is not catabolized. As a consequence, the ganglioside concentration is elevated many times higher than normal. The functionally absent lysosomal enzyme is β-*N*-acetyl hexosaminidase (more commonly called hexosaminidase A). The elevated GM_2 results in irreversible brain damage to infants, who usually die before the age of 3 years. Under normal conditions, this enzyme cleaves *N*-acetylgalactosamine from the oligosaccharide chain of this complex sphingolipid, allowing further catabolism to occur.

2. The parents of an 18-month-old girl are alarmed at the rapid deterioration in her motor skills and the appearance of an engorged belly. They note that when their daughter tries to follow the movement of an object she thrusts her head in the direction of movement as if she cannot move her eyes from side-to-side. Physical and laboratory examination reveals that the child is suffering from Gaucher disease. Which of the following carbohydrate-containing compounds would be expected to be elevated in macrophages from this patient?

A. abnormal glycogen
B. cerebrosides
C. glycosaminoglycans
D. GM_2 ganglioside
E. neuraminic acid

Answer B: Gaucher disease is characterized by the lysosomal accumulation of glucosylceramide (glucocerebroside) which is a normal intermediate in the catabolism of globosides and gangliosides. Gaucher disease results from defects in the gene encoding the lysosomal hydrolase: acid β-glucosidase, also called glucocerebrosidase. The hallmark feature of Gaucher disease is the presence of lipid-engorged cells of the monocyte/macrophage lineage with a characteristic appearance in a variety of tissues.

3. The aldehyde and ketone moieties of the carbohydrates with 5 and 6 carbons will spontaneously react with alcohol groups present in neighboring carbons to produce ring structures. The rings can open and close allowing for different configurations of the atoms in the ring. Which of the following represents the carbon about which this rotation occurs?

A. anomeric
B. chiral

C. glycosidic
D. hydroxy
E. terminal

Answer A: The carbon about which the rotation occurs in ring structures of carbohydrates is the anomeric carbon and the 2 forms are termed anomers.

4. A deficiency in the hepatic enzyme aldolase B would result in a reduced ability to metabolize which of the following carbohydrates?
   A. dihydroxyacetone
   B. fructose
   C. glucose
   D. glyceraldehyde
   E. sucrose

Answer B: Hepatic aldolase B is responsible for the hydrolysis of fructose-1-phosphate into dihydroxyacetone phosphate and glyceraldehyde. The fructose-1-phosphate is derived via the action of ketohexokinase (fructokinase) and thus if aldolase B is deficient downstream utilization of fructose will be impaired.

5. You are examining a patient complaining of cramping in the lower belly, bloating, gas, and diarrhea. These symptoms appear within 30 minutes to 2 hours after the ingestion of dairy products. You advise your patient to avoid foods that contain a particular sugar. Which of the following is the sugar this patient should avoid?
   A. glucose
   B. lactose
   C. sucrose
   D. fructose
   E. galactose

Answer B: The patient is most likely deficient in intestinal lactase and is thus, lactose intolerant. The signs and symptoms of lactose intolerance usually begin 30 minutes to 2 hours after eating or drinking foods that contain lactose and include nausea, vomiting, diarrhea, bloating, gas, and painful abdominal cramping.

Checklist

✓ Carbohydrates (saccharides) are major sources of energy for human tissues and they also represent major storage forms of energy in both plants and animals. Biologically significant carbohydrates contain different amounts of carbon (generally from 3 to 6 atoms) and can be found as monosaccharides, disaccharides, or polysaccharides.

✓ Glucose is the most important monosaccharide in humans. It is the storage form of carbohydrate, can be readily catabolized to generate energy even in the absence of oxygen, and most all other carbohydrates can be converted into glucose.

✓ Ribose is another physiologically significant monosaccharide as it serves as constituent of the nucleotides.

✓ Carbohydrates exist in different configurations and conformations in solution due to the presence of several asymmetric carbon atoms.

✓ The most significant disaccharides are sucrose (glucose and fructose) which is a major sweetener and dietary carbohydrate, maltose (2 glucose), which is an intermediate in the digestion of starch from plants, and lactose (glucose and galactose) which is the major carbohydrate of milk.

✓ Polymers of glucose found in plants are called starch and those in animals are called glycogen. Starch is a major source of dietary energy, whereas glycogen is a major form of intracellular stored energy.

✓ Complex carbohydrates are formed to serve both structural and functional roles in cells and tissues. These complex carbohydrates include the amino sugars, uronic acids, and sialic acids. Proteoglycans, glycosaminoglycans, glycoproteins, and glycolipids represent the major classes of complex carbohydrates in human tissues.

CHAPTER

3 Lipids of Biological Significance

CHAPTER OUTLINE

Major Roles of Biological Lipids
Fatty Acids
- Omega-3, and -6 PUFAs
- Triglycerides (Triacylglycerols)

Phospholipids
- Plasmalogens
- Sphingolipids

High-Yield Terms

Essential fatty acid: fatty acid required in the diet due to the inability of human cells to synthesize

Omega fatty acid: refers to the location of sites of unsaturation relative to the omega end (farthest from the carboxylic acid) of a fatty acid

Monounsaturated fatty acid (MUFA): a fatty acid with a single site of unsaturation, oleic acid, an omega-9 MUFA, is the most physiologically significant MUFA

Polyunsaturated fatty acid (PUFA): any fatty acid with multiple sites of unsaturation; omega-3 and omega-6 PUFA are the most significant clinically

Plasmalogen: any of a group of ether phospholipids

Sphingosine: an amino alcohol that serves as the backbone for the sphingolipid class of lipid, which includes the sphingomyelins and the glycosphingolipids

Ceramide: sphingosine containing a fatty *N*-acylation, serves as the backbone for the glycosphingolipids

Glycosphingolipid: any ceramide to which a carbohydrate or carbohydrates have been added, constitutes the cerebrosides, globosides, sulfatides, and gangliosides

High-Yield Concept

The melting point of fatty acids increases as the number of carbon atoms increases. In addition, the introduction of sites of unsaturation results in lower melting points when comparing a saturated and an unsaturated fatty acid of the same number of carbons. Saturated fatty acids of less than 8 carbon atoms are liquid at physiological temperature, whereas those containing more than 10 are solid.

Major Roles of Biological Lipids

Biological molecules that are insoluble in aqueous solutions and soluble in organic solvents are classified as *lipids*. The lipids of physiological importance for humans serve as structural components of biological membranes; provide energy reserves, predominantly in the form of triglycerides, serve as biologically active molecules exerting a wide range of regulatory functions, and the lipophilic bile acids aid in lipid emulsification during digestion of fats. The biologically relevant lipids consist of the fatty acids, triglycerides, phospholipids, sphingolipids, ceramides, cholesterol, bile acids, eicosanoids, omega fatty acid derivatives, and bioactive lipid derivatives, which also include the inflammation-modulating lipid derivatives.

Fatty Acids

Fatty acids are long-chain hydrocarbon molecules containing a carboxylic acid moiety at one end. The numbering of carbons in fatty acids begins with the carbon of the carboxylate group. At physiological pH, the carboxyl group is readily ionized, rendering a negative charge onto fatty acids in bodily fluids. Fatty acids play 3 major roles in the body: (1) they serve as components of more complex membrane lipids; (2) they are the major components of stored energy in the form of triglycerides; and (3) they serve as the precursors for the synthesis of the numerous types of bioactive lipids.

Fatty acids that do not contain carbon–carbon double bonds are termed *saturated fatty* acids; those that contain double bonds are unsaturated fatty acids. Fatty acids with multiple sites of unsaturation are termed *polyunsaturated fatty acids* (PUFAs). The numeric designations used for fatty acids come from the number of carbon atoms, followed by the number of sites of unsaturation (eg, palmitic acid is a 16-carbon fatty acid with no sites of unsaturation and is designated by 16:0; see Table 3-1).

As a general rule, oils from vegetables contain many more unsaturated fatty acids and are therefore, liquids at room temperature. In contrast, animal oils contain more saturated fatty acids. The steric geometry of unsaturated fatty acids can also vary such that the acyl groups can be oriented on the same side or on opposite sides of the double bond. When the acyl groups are on the same side of the double bond, it is referred to as a *cis* bond, such as is the case for oleic acid (18:1). When the acyl groups are on opposite sides, the bond is termed *trans* such as in elaidic acid, the *trans* isomer of oleic acid (Figure 3-1).

The majority of naturally occurring unsaturated fatty acids exist in the *cis*-conformation.

The site of unsaturation in a fatty acid is indicated by the symbol Δ and the number of the first carbon of the double bond relative to the carboxylic acid group (-COOH) carbon, which is designated carbon #1. For example, palmitoleic acid is a 16-carbon fatty acid with one site of unsaturation between carbons 9 and 10, and is designated by $16{:}1^{\Delta 9}$.

The majority of fatty acids found in the body are acquired in the diet. However, the lipid biosynthetic capacity of the body (fatty acid synthase and other fatty acid–modifying enzymes) can supply the body with all the various fatty acid structures needed. Two key exceptions to this are the PUFAs known as linoleic acid and α-linolenic acid, containing

High-Yield Concept

Trans fatty acids occur in some foods and as byproducts of the process of hydrogenating saturated fatty acids to make them solids at room temperature, such as in partially hydrogenated vegetable oils. Diets high in *trans* fatty acids have been associated with an increased risk of cardiovascular disease and development of the metabolic syndrome.

TABLE 3-1: Physiologically Relevant Fatty Acids

Numerical Symbol	*Common Name and Structure*	*Comments*
14:0	Myristic acid	Often found attached to the *N*-terminus of plasma membrane–associated cytoplasmic proteins
16:0	Palmitic acid	End-product of mammalian fatty acid synthesis
$16{:}1^{\Delta 9}$	Palmitoleic acid	
18:0	Stearic acid	
$18{:}1^{\Delta 9}$	Oleic acid	Physiologically most important omega-9 monounsaturated fatty acid (MUFA)
$18{:}2^{\Delta 9,12}$	Linoleic acid	Essential fatty acid, an omega-6 PUFA
$18{:}3^{\Delta 9,12,15}$	α-Linolenic acid (ALA)	Essential fatty acid, an omega-3 PUFA
$20{:}4^{\Delta 5,8,11,14}$	Arachidonic acid	An omega-6 PUFA, precursor for eicosanoid synthesis
$20{:}5^{\Delta 5,8,11,14,17}$	Eicosapentaenoic acid (EPA)	An omega-3 PUFA, enriched in krill and fish oils
$22{:}6^{\Delta 4,7,10,13,16,19}$	Docosahexaenoic acid (DHA)	An omega-3 PUFA, enriched in krill and fish oils

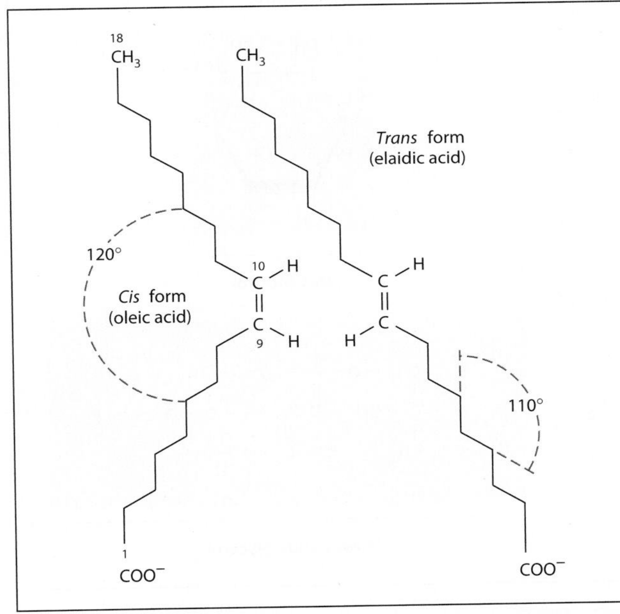

FIGURE 3-1: Geometric isomerism of Δ^9, 18:1 fatty acids (oleic and elaidic acids). Murray RK, Bender DA, Botham KM, Kennelly PJ, Rodwell VW, Weil PA. *Harper's Illustrated Biochemistry*, 29th ed. New York, NY: McGraw-Hill; 2012.

unsaturation sites beyond carbons 9 and 10 (relative to the α-COOH group). These 2 fatty acids cannot be synthesized from precursors in the body, and are thus considered the essential fatty acids; essential in the sense that they must be provided in the diet. Since plants are capable of synthesizing linoleic and α-linolenic acid, humans can acquire these fats by consuming a variety of plants or else by eating the meat of animals that have consumed these plant fats.

These 2 essential fatty acids are also referred to as omega fatty acids. The use of the Greek letter omega, ω, refers to the end of the fatty acid opposite to that of the -COOH group. Linoleic acid is an omega-6 PUFA and α-linolenic is an omega-3 PUFA. The role of PUFAs, such as linoleic and α-linolenic, in the synthesis of biologically important lipids is discussed in Chapter 20 (Table 3-1).

Omega-3, and -6 PUFAs

The term omega, as it relates to fatty acids, refers to the terminal carbon atom farthest from the carboxylic acid group (-COOH). The designation of a PUFA as an omega-3 fatty acid, for example, defines the position of the first site of unsaturation relative to the omega end of that fatty acid. Thus, an omega-3 fatty acid like α-linolenic acid (ALA), which harbors 3 sites of unsaturation (carbon–carbon double bonds), has a site of

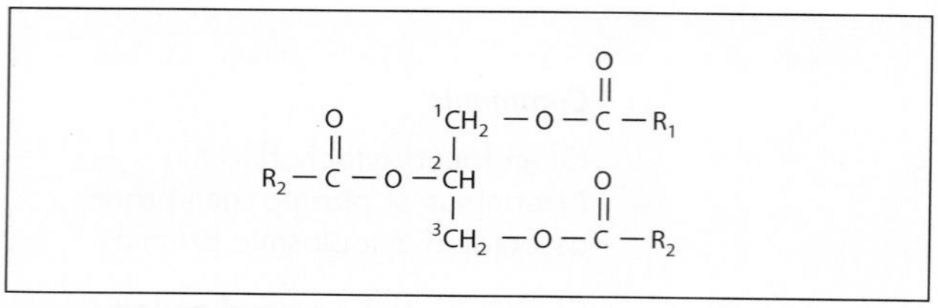

FIGURE 3-2: Triacylglycerol. Murray RK, Bender DA, Botham KM, Kennelly PJ, Rodwell VW, Weil PA. *Harper's Illustrated Biochemistry*, 29th ed. New York, NY: McGraw-Hill; 2012.

unsaturation between the third and fourth carbons from the omega end. There are 3 major omega-3 fatty acids that are ingested in foods and used by the body: ALA, eicosapentaenoic acid (EPA), and docosahexaenoic acid (DHA). Once eaten, the body converts ALA to EPA and DHA, the 2 omega-3 fatty acids, which serve as important precursors for lipid-derived modulators of cell signaling, gene expression, and inflammatory processes.

Most of the omega-6 PUFAs consumed in the diet are from vegetable oils and consist of linoleic acid. Linoleic acid is first converted to γ-linolenic acid (GLA), then to dihomo-γ-linolenic acid (DGLA), and finally to arachidonic acid (see Chapter 22). Due to the limited activity of human Δ^5-desaturase, most of the DGLA formed from GLA is inserted into membrane phospholipids at the same C-2 position as for arachidonic acid. GLA can be ingested from several plant-based oils including evening primrose oil, borage oil, and black currant seed oil.

Triglycerides (Triacylglycerols)

Triglycerides represent the storage form of fatty acids. In this form, the large amount of energy produced from the oxidation of fatty acids is readily available to the cell. All tissues store triglycerides but adipose tissue is by far the largest reservoir of this form of energy storage. Triglycerides are generated by the esterification of fatty acids to glycerol (Figure 3-2).

Phospholipids

The basic structure of phospholipids is very similar to that of the triglycerides except that C-3 (*sn*3) of the glycerol backbone is esterified to phosphoric acid. The other 2 hydroxyls of glycerol are esterified to fatty acids as in triglycerides. Phospholipids constitute major components of biological membranes. The different forms of phospholipids result from the esterification of various polar substituents to the phosphate of phosphatidic acid. These substitutions include ethanolamine (phosphatidylethanolamine: PE), choline (phosphatidylcholine: PC, also called lecithins), serine (phosphatidylserine: PS), glycerol (phosphatidylglycerol: PG), *myo*-inositol (phosphatidylinositol: PI), and phosphatidylglycerol (diphosphatidylglycerol more commonly known as cardiolipins). Phosphotidylinositols most often have one to several of the inositol hydroxyls esterified to phosphate-generating polyphosphatidylinositols (Figure 3-3).

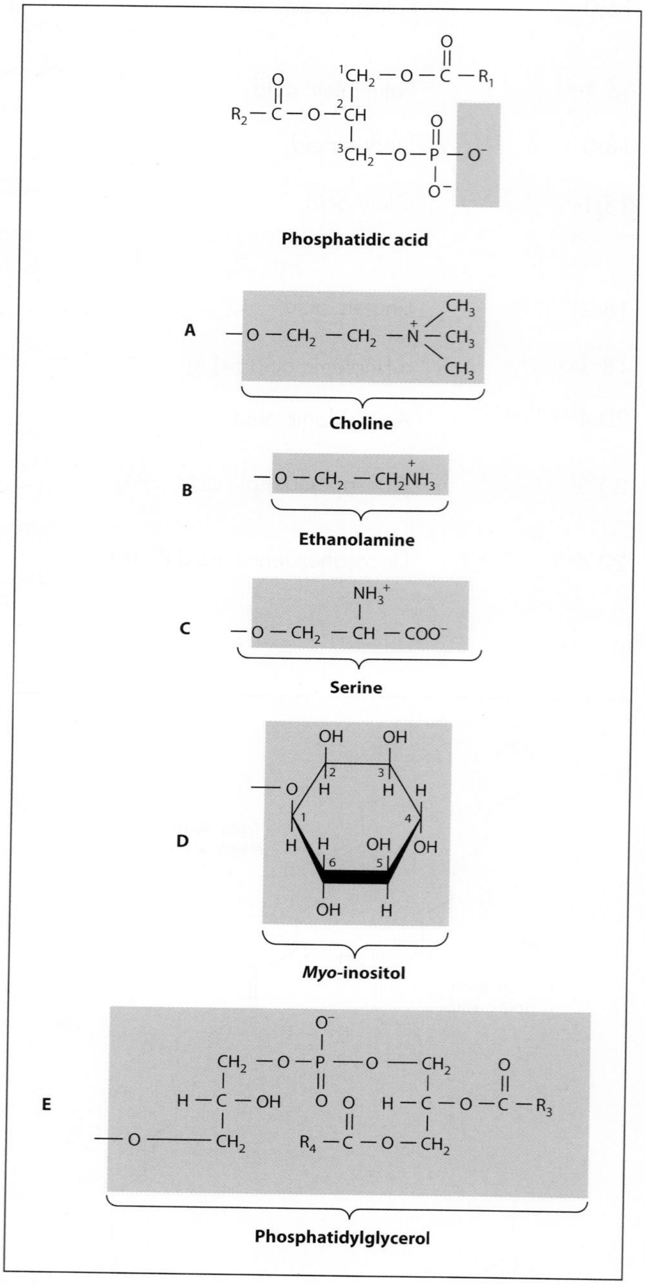

Phosphatidic acid

A Choline

B Ethanolamine

C Serine

D *Myo*-inositol

E Phosphatidylglycerol

FIGURE 3-3: Phosphatidic acid and its derivatives. The O– shown shaded in phosphatidic acid is substituted by the substituents shown to form in (A) 3-phosphatidylcholine, (B) 3-phosphatidylethanolamine, (C) 3-phosphatidylserine, (D) 3-phosphatidylinositol, and (E) cardiolipin (diphosphatidylglycerol). Murray RK, Bender DA, Botham KM, Kennelly PJ, Rodwell VW, Weil PA. *Harper's Illustrated Biochemistry*, 29th ed. New York, NY: McGraw-Hill; 2012.

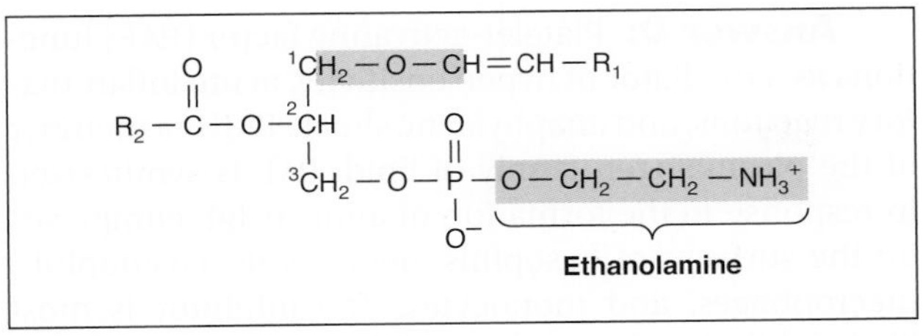

$$\begin{array}{l} \quad\quad\quad\quad\quad {}^{1}CH_2-O-CH=CH-R_1 \\ R_2-\overset{O}{\overset{\|}{C}}-O-\overset{2}{C}H \\ \quad\quad\quad\quad\quad {}^{3}CH_2-O-\overset{O}{\overset{\|}{P}}(O^-)-O-CH_2-CH_2-NH_3^+ \end{array}$$

Ethanolamine

FIGURE 3-4: Plasmalogen. Murray RK, Bender DA, Botham KM, Kennelly PJ, Rodwell VW, Weil PA. *Harper's Illustrated Biochemistry*, 29th ed. New York, NY: McGraw-Hill; 2012.

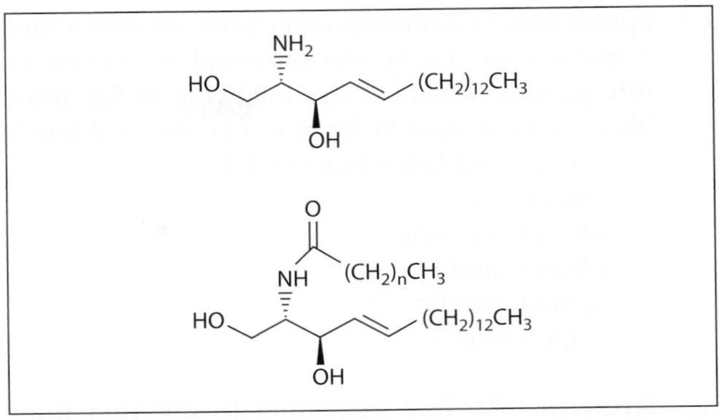

Plasmalogens

Plasmalogens are complex membrane lipids that resemble phospholipids, principally phosphatidylcholine. The major difference is that the fatty acid at C-1 (*sn*1) of glycerol contains either an *O*-alkyl (-O-CH_2-) or *O*-alkenyl ether (-O-CH=CH-) species. A basic *O*-alkenyl ether species is shown in the Figure 3-4.

One of the most potent plasmalogens is platelet-activating factor (PAF) which is a choline plasmalogen in which the C-2 (*sn*2) position of glycerol is esterified with an acetyl group instead of a long-chain fatty acid. PAF functions as a mediator of hypersensitivity, acute inflammatory reactions, and anaphylactic shock. PAF is synthesized in response to the formation of antigen-IgE complexes on the surfaces of basophils, neutrophils, eosinophils, macrophages, and monocytes. The synthesis and release of PAF from cells leads to platelet aggregation and the release of serotonin from platelets. PAF also produces responses in liver, heart, smooth muscle, and uterine and lung tissues (Figure 3-4).

Sphingolipids

Sphingolipids are composed of a backbone of sphingosine, which is derived from glycerol. Sphingosine is *N*-acetylated by a variety of fatty acids generating a family of molecules referred to as ceramides (see Chapter 21). Sphingolipids predominate in the myelin sheath of nerve fibers (Figure 3-5).

NH2 HO OH $(CH_2)_{12}CH_3$

O NH $(CH_2)_nCH_3$ HO OH $(CH_2)_{12}CH_3$

FIGURE 3-5: Structure of sphingosine and a basic ceramide.

Sphingomyelin is an abundant sphingolipid generated by transfer of the phosphocholine moiety of phosphatidylcholine to a ceramide, thus sphingomyelin is a unique form of a phospholipid. The other major class of sphingolipid (besides the sphingomyelins) is the glycosphingolipids generated by substitution of carbohydrates to the *sn*1 carbon of the sphingosine backbone of a ceramide. There are 4 major classes of glycosphingolipids:

Cerebrosides: contain a single moiety, principally galactose.

Sulfatides: sulfuric acid esters of galactocerebrosides.

Globosides: contain 2 or more sugars.

Gangliosides: similar to globosides, except also contain sialic acid (*N*-acetylneuraminic acid, NANA).

REVIEW QUESTIONS

1. An adult man suffered from stable angina pectoris for 15 years, during which time there was progressive heart failure and repeated pulmonary thromboembolism. On his death at age 63, autopsy disclosed enormous cardiomyopathy (1100 g), cardiac storage of globotriaosylceramide (11 mg lipid/g wet weight), and restricted cardiocytes. To which of the following lipid classes does globotriaosylceramide belong?

A. glycosphingolipid
B. phospholipid
C. saturated fatty acid
D. sphingomyelin
E. triglyceride

Answer A: This man was afflicted with Fabry disease, a disorder characterized by the lysosomal accumulation of glycosphingolipids with terminal α-galactosyl residues.

2. The parents of an 18-month-old girl are alarmed at the rapid deterioration in her motor skills and the appearance of an engorged belly. They note that when their daughter tries to follow the movement of an object she thrusts her head in the direction of movement as if she cannot move her eyes from side-to-side. Physical and laboratory examination reveals hepatosplenomegaly, skeletal lesions, dry scaly skin, and lipid-laden foam cells that have the appearance of wrinkled paper when viewed under a microscope. Given the observed symptoms in this patient, which of the following is the most likely class of lipid to be found at elevated levels within the lipid-laden foam cells?

A. ganglioside
B. omega fatty acid
C. phospholipid
D. sphingomyelin
E. triglyceride

Answer A: This individual is suffering from Gaucher disease, characterized by the lysosomal accumulation of glucosylceramide (glucocerebroside) which is a normal intermediate in the catabolism of globosides and gangliosides.

3. You are studying a cell line derived from a liver tumor. This cell line expresses a mutated form of glycerol kinase. Which of the following lipid classes is most likely to be found at reduced levels in this cell line due to this gene defect?

A. cholesterol
B. fatty acids
C. phospholipids
D. sphingolipids
E. triglycerides

Answer E: Triglycerides are composed of a backbone of glycerol to which 3 fatty acids are esterified. One of the pathways to triglyceride synthesis in hepatocytes is initiated by the phosphorylation of glycerol via the action of glycerol kinase. Therefore, a defect in glycerol kinase activity in these cells would result in reduced capacity to synthesize triglycerides.

4. You are doing experiments in cell culture with a novel inhibitor, of lipid metabolism. Your studies determine that in the presence of the inhibitor, the cells are unable to elicit a normal response to antigen addition to the culture. Which of the following lipid classes is likely to be reduced because of the addition of the inhibitor?

A. cholesterol
B. plasmalogen
C. phospholipids
D. sphingolipids
E. triglycerides

Answer D: Platelet-activating factor (PAF) functions as a mediator of hypersensitivity, acute inflammatory reactions, and anaphylactic shock. PAF is a member of the plasmalogen family of lipid. PAF is synthesized in response to the formation of antigen-IgE complexes on the surfaces of basophils, neutrophils, eosinophils, macrophages, and monocytes. The inhibitor is most likely inhibiting the synthesis of PAF in these cells thus, the lack of appropriate response to antigen addition.

5. Hypersensitive individuals have IgE to specific antigens (eg, pollen, bee venom) on the surface of their leukocytes (monocytes, macrophages, basophils, eosinophils). When these individuals are challenged with antigen, the antigen–IgE complexes induce synthesis and release of which of the following physiologically potent lipids?

A. arachidonic acid
B. leukotriene B_4
C. platelet-activating factor (PAF)
D. prostaglandin E_2
E. thromboxane A_2 (TXA_2)

Answer C: Platelet-activating factor (PAF) is a unique complex lipid of the plasmalogen family. PAF functions in hypersensitivity, acute inflammatory reactions, and anaphylactic shock by increased vasopermeability, vasodilation, and bronchoconstriction. Excess production of PAF production may be involved in the morbidity associated with toxic shock syndrome and strokes.

6. The omega-3 class of polyunsaturated fatty acids (PUFAs) has potent effects on cardiovascular function. The most active omega-3 PUFAs are docosahexaenoic acid (DHA) and eicosapentaenoic acid (EPA). These PUFAs are precursors for which of the following biologically active lipids?

A. gangliosides
B. leukotrienes
C. prostaglandins
D. resolvins
E. thromboxanes

Answer D: The resolvins are a class of lipid involved in the resolution of inflammatory responses, hence the derivation of their names. The D class resolvins are synthesized from DHA and the E class resolvins are derived from EPA.

Checklist

- ✓ The biologically relevant lipids consist of the fatty acids, triglycerides, phospholipids, sphingolipids, ceramides, cholesterol, bile acids, eicosanoids, omega fatty acid derivatives, and bioactive lipid derivatives which also include the inflammation-modulating lipid derivatives.
- ✓ Fatty acids are long-chain hydrocarbon molecules containing a carboxylic acid moiety at one end. Fatty acids that do not contain carbon–carbon double bonds are termed saturated fatty acids; those that contain double bonds are unsaturated fatty acids.
- ✓ The term omega, as it relates to fatty acids, refers to the terminal carbon atom farthest from the carboxylic acid group. The designation of a polyunsaturated fatty acid (PUFA) as an omega-3 fatty acid, for example, defines the position of the first site of unsaturation relative to the omega end of that fatty acid.
- ✓ Triglycerides are composed of 3 fatty acids esterified to a backbone of glycerol. These lipids represent the major storage form of fatty acids.
- ✓ Phospholipids have a structure similar to that of the triglycerides except that C–3 (*sn*3) of the glycerol backbone is esterified to phosphoric acid.
- ✓ The sphingolipids represent a complex class of lipid composed of a sphingosine backbone with the majority also containing carbohydrate forming the glycosphingolipids.

CHAPTER

4 Nucleic Acids

CHAPTER OUTLINE

Nucleoside and Nucleotide Structure and Nomenclature
Nucleotide Derivatives
Nucleotide Derivatives in tRNAs
Synthetic Nucleotide Analogs
Polynucleotides

High-Yield Terms

Nucleoside: refers to the complex of nonphosphorylate ribose sugar and a nucleobase such as purine or pyrimidine

Nucleotide: refers to the complex of phosphorylated ribose sugar and a nucleobase such as purine or pyrimidine

Phosphodiester bond: the bond formed when the phosphate of 1 nucleotide is esterified to the hydroxyls of 2 ribose sugars typical in polynucleotides

Phosphoanhydride bond: an anhydride is a bond formed between 2 acids, a phosphoanhydride is the bond formed from 2 phosphoric acids such as with the β and γ phosphates of di- and triphosphate nucleosides, respectively

High-Yield Concept

Chemically the nucleotides are basic compounds, which is the reason for the common term "bases" in the context of DNA and RNA. There are 5 major bases found in cells. The derivatives of purine are called adenine and guanine, and the derivatives of pyrimidine are called thymine, cytosine, and uracil. The common abbreviations used for these 5 bases are, A, G, T, C, and U, respectively.

As a class, the nucleotides may be considered one of the most important metabolites of the cell. Nucleotides are found primarily as the monomeric units comprising the major nucleic acids of the cell, RNA, and DNA. However, they also are required for numerous other important functions within the cell.

1. They serve as energy stores for future use in phosphate transfer reactions. ATP predominantly carries out these reactions.
2. They form a portion of several important coenzymes such as NAD^+, $NADP^+$, FAD, and coenzyme A.
3. They serve as mediators of numerous important cellular processes such as second messengers in signal transduction events. The predominant second messenger is cyclic-AMP (cAMP), a cyclic derivative of AMP formed from ATP.
4. They control numerous enzymatic reactions through allosteric effects on enzyme activity.
5. They serve as activated intermediates in numerous biosynthetic reactions. These activated intermediates include S-adenosylmethionine (S-AdoMet or SAM) involved in methyl transfer reactions as well as the many nucleotide-activated sugars involved in glycogen and glycoprotein synthesis.

Nucleoside and Nucleotide Structure and Nomenclature

The nucleotides found in cells are derivatives of the heterocyclic highly basic compounds, purine, and pyrimidine (Figure 4-1).

The purine and pyrimidine bases (Table 4-1) in cells are linked to carbohydrate and in this form are termed nucleosides. The nucleosides are coupled to D-ribose or 2′-deoxy-D-ribose through a β-*N*-glycosidic bond between the anomeric carbon of the ribose and the N^9 of a purine or N^1 of a pyrimidine. The carbon atoms of the ribose present in nucleotides are designated with a prime (′) mark to distinguish them from the backbone numbering in the bases. The base can exist in 2 distinct orientations about the *N*-glycosidic bond. These conformations are identified as *syn* and *anti* (Figure 4-2). The *anti*-conformation predominates in naturally occurring nucleotides.

Nucleosides are found in the cell primarily in their phosphorylated form and are called nucleotides. Nucleotides can exist in the mono-, di-, or tri-phosphorylated forms (Figure 4-3). Nucleotides are given distinct abbreviations to allow easy identification of their structure and state of phosphorylation. The monophosphorylated form of adenosine (adenosine-5-monophosphate) is written as AMP. The di- and tri-phosphorylated forms are written as, ADP and ATP, respectively.

The phosphate in a monophosphate nucleotide is linked via an ester bond to the ribose. The di- and tri-phosphates of nucleotides are linked by anhydride bonds. Acid anhydride bonds have a high $\Delta G^{0\prime}$ for hydrolysis imparting upon them a high potential to transfer the phosphates to other molecules. This property of the nucleotides results in their involvement in group transfer reactions in the cell.

The nucleotides found in the DNA are unique from those of the RNA in which the ribose exists in the 2′-deoxy form and the abbreviations of the deoxynucleotides contain a "d" designation. The monophosphorylated form of adenosine found in DNA (deoxyadenosine-5′-monophosphate) is written as dAMP (Figure 4-4).

The nucleotide uridine is never found in the DNA while thymine is almost exclusively found in the DNA. Thymine is found in tRNAs but not in rRNAs or mRNAs. There are several less common bases found in the DNA and RNA. The primary modified base in DNA is

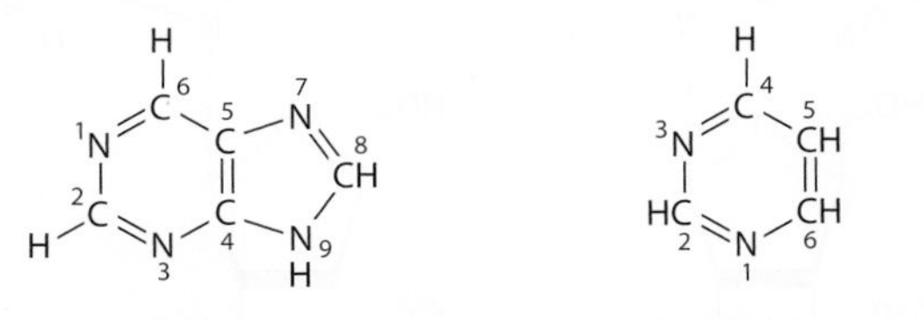

FIGURE 4-1: Purine and pyrimidine. The atoms are numbered according to the international system. Murray RK, Bender DA, Botham KM, Kennelly PJ, Rodwell VW, Weil PA. Harper's Illustrated Biochemistry, 29th Edition, Copyright 2012, New York: McGraw-Hill.

TABLE 4-1: Purine Bases, Ribonucleosides, and Ribonucleotides

Purine or Pyrimidine	*X = H*	*X = Ribose*	*X = Ribose Phosphate*
X	Adenine	Adenosine	Adenosine monophosphate (AMP)
X	Guanine	Guanosine	Guanosine monophosphate (GMP)
X	Cytosine	Cytidine	Cytidine monophosphate (CMP)
X	Uracil	Uridine	Uridine monophosphate (UMP)
dX	Thymine	Thymidine	Thymidine monophosphate (TMP)

Murray RK, Bender DA, Botham KM, Kennelly PJ, Rodwell VW, Weil PA. *Harper's Illustrated Biochemistry*, 29th ed. New York, NY: McGraw-Hill; 2012.

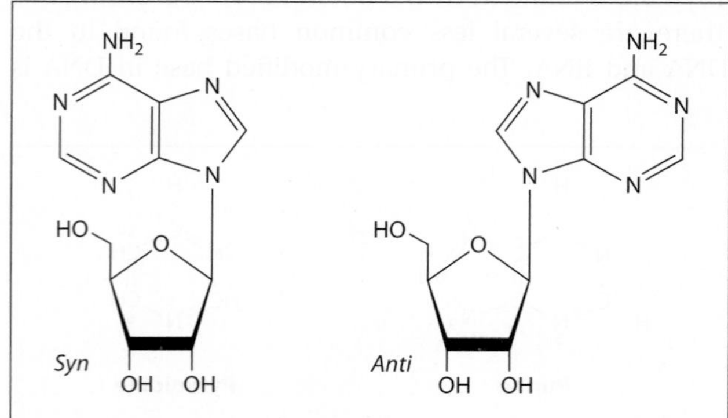

FIGURE 4-2: The *syn* and *anti* conformers of adenosine differ with respect to orientation about the *N*-glycosidic bond. Murray RK, Bender DA, Botham KM, Kennelly PJ, Rodwell VW, Weil PA. *Harper's Illustrated Biochemistry*, 29th ed. New York, NY: McGraw-Hill; 2012.

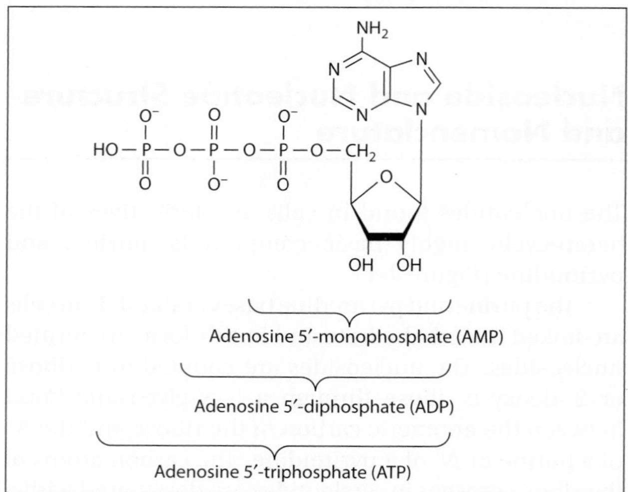

FIGURE 4-3: ATP, its diphosphate, and its monophosphate. Murray RK, Bender DA, Botham KM, Kennelly PJ, Rodwell VW, Weil PA. *Harper's Illustrated Biochemistry*, 29th ed. New York, NY: McGraw-Hill; 2012.

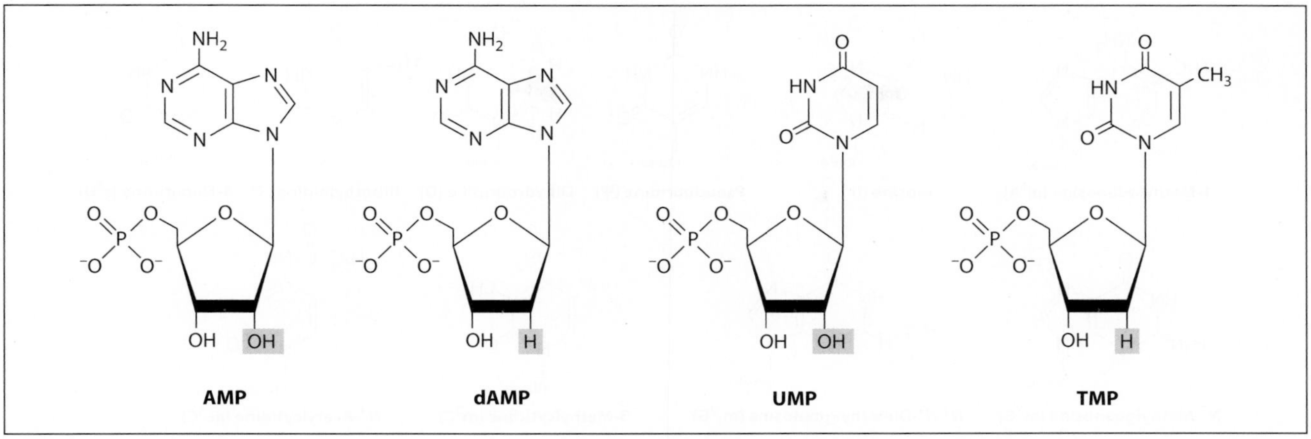

FIGURE 4-4: Structures of AMP, dAMP, UMP, and TMP. Murray RK, Bender DA, Botham KM, Kennelly PJ, Rodwell VW, Weil PA. *Harper's Illustrated Biochemistry*, 29th ed. New York, NY: McGraw-Hill; 2012.

5-methylcytosine (see Chapter 35). A variety of modified bases appears in the tRNAs. Many modified nucleotides are encountered outside of the context of DNA and RNA that serve important biological functions.

Nucleotide Derivatives

The most common adenosine derivative is the cyclic form, 3-5-cyclic adenosine monophosphate, cAMP. Formation of cAMP is catalyzed by adenylate cyclase. The activation of adenylate cyclase occurs in response to the ligand binding to membrane receptors of the type termed G-protein–coupled receptors, GPCR (see Chapter 40). Cyclic-AMP is a very powerful second messenger involved in passing signal transduction events from the cell surface to internal proteins primarily through the activation of cAMP-dependent protein kinase, PKA. Cyclic-AMP is also involved in the regulation of ion channels by direct interaction with the channel proteins such as in the activation of odorant receptors by odorant molecules.

A cyclic form of *guanosine* 5-monophosphate (cGMP) is also produced in cells and acts as a second messenger molecule (Figure 4-5). In many cases its role is to antagonize the effects of cAMP. Formation of cGMP occurs in response to receptor-mediated signals similar to those for activation of adenylate cyclase. However, in this case it is guanylate cyclase that is coupled to the receptor. One of most significant cGMP-coupled signal transduction cascades is the activation of photoreception (see Chapter 8). Another is its role in vascular tone via effects within arterial smooth muscle cells (see Chapter 31).

Another important adenosine derivative is S-adenosylmethionine (see Figure 30-8), a form of activated methionine which serves as a methyl donor in methylation reactions and as a source of propylamine in the synthesis of polyamines.

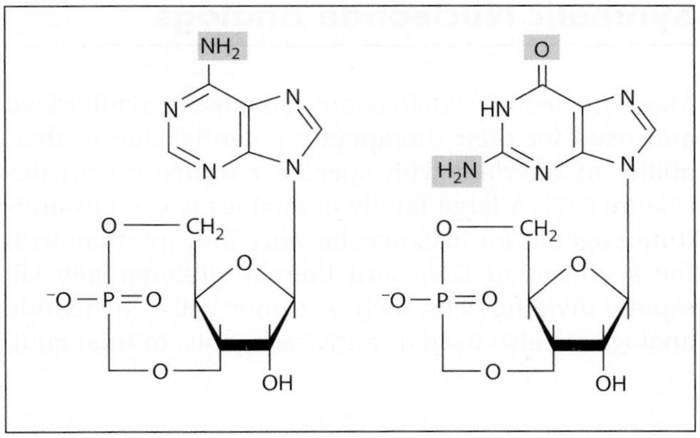

FIGURE 4-5: cAMP, 3′,5′-cyclic AMP, and cGMP, 3′, 5′-cyclic GMP. Murray RK, Bender DA, Botham KM, Kennelly PJ, Rodwell VW, Weil PA. *Harper's Illustrated Biochemistry*, 29th ed. New York, NY: McGraw-Hill; 2012.

Nucleotide Derivatives in tRNAs

As many as 25% of the nucleotides found in tRNAs (see Chapter 36) are modified posttranscriptionally. At least 80 different modified nucleotides have been identified at more than 60 different positions in various tRNAs. The 2 most commonly occurring modified nucleotides are dihydrouridine (abbreviated D) and pseudouridine (abbreviated ψ), each of which is found in a characteristic loop structure in tRNAs. Dihydrouridine is found in the D-loop (hence the name of the loop) and pseudouridine is found in the TΨC loop (hence the name of the loop) (Figure 4-6).

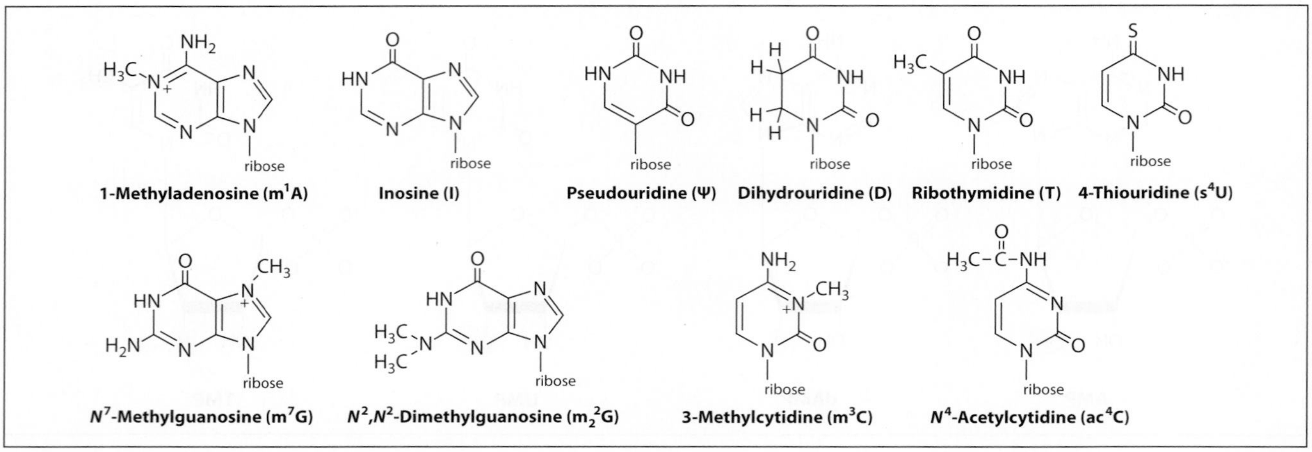

FIGURE 4-6: Modified purine and pyrimidine nucleotides commonly found in tRNAs. Murray RK, Bender DA, Botham KM, Kennelly PJ, Rodwell VW, Weil PA. *Harper's Illustrated Biochemistry,* 29th ed. New York, NY: McGraw-Hill; 2012.

Synthetic Nucleotide Analogs

Many nucleotide analogs are chemically synthesized and used for their therapeutic potential due to their ability to interfere with specific enzymatic activities (Figure 4-7). A large family of analogs is used as antitumor agents, for instance, because they interfere with the synthesis of DNA and thereby preferentially kill rapidly dividing cells such as tumor cells. Nucleotide analogs are also used as antiviral agents, to treat gout, and after organ transplantation in order to suppress the immune system and reduce the likelihood of transplant rejection by the host.

Polynucleotides

Polynucleotides are formed by the condensation of 2 or more nucleotides. The condensation most commonly occurs between the alcohol of a 5′-phosphate of one

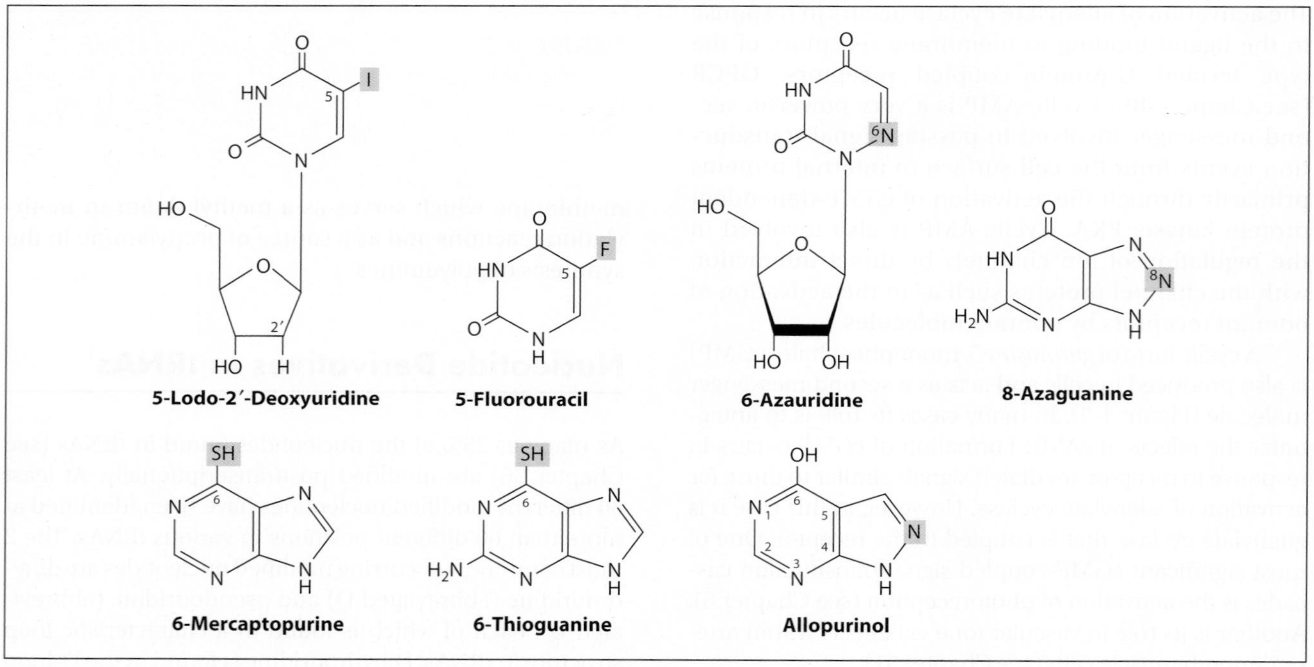

FIGURE 4-7: Selected synthetic pyrimidine and purine analogs. Murray RK, Bender DA, Botham KM, Kennelly PJ, Rodwell VW, Weil PA. *Harper's Illustrated Biochemistry,* 29th ed. New York, NY: McGraw-Hill; 2012.

nucleotide and the 3′-hydroxyl of a second, with the elimination of H_2O, forming a phosphodiester bond. The formation of phosphodiester bonds in DNA and RNA exhibits directionality. The primary structure of DNA and RNA (the linear arrangement of the nucleotides) proceeds in the 5′—>3′ direction. The common representation of the primary structure of DNA or RNA molecules is to write the nucleotide sequences from left to right synonymous with the 5′—>3′ direction as shown in the figure on the right:

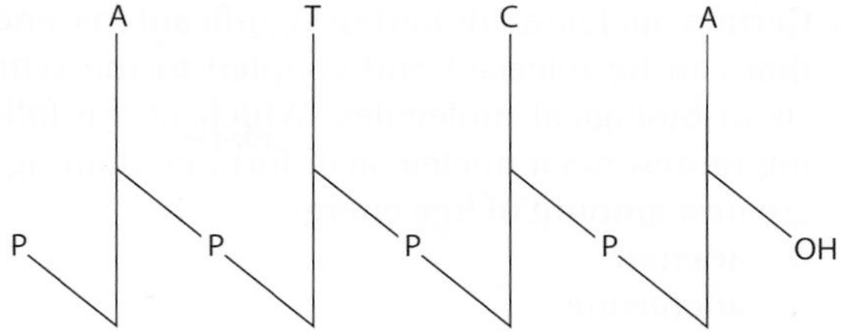

Murray RK, Bender DA, Botham KM, Kennelly PJ, Rodwell VW, Weil PA. *Harper's Illustrated Biochemistry*, 29th ed. New York, NY: McGraw-Hill; 2012.

REVIEW QUESTIONS

1. You are treating a 4-year-old child who has been afflicted with recurrent infections. The child exhibits retarded development, weakness, and weight loss. Physical examination also shows absent tonsils and blood work reveals a lack of lymphocytes. These signs and symptoms are typical of severe combined immunodeficiency syndrome. Which of the following compounds would be expected to be elevated in the blood of this patient?

A. bilirubin
B. cytosine
C. deoxyadenosine
D. deoxythymidine
E. xanthine

Answer C: Severe combined immunodeficiency disease (SCID) is a disorder related to defects in the activity of the purine nucleotide catabolism enzyme, adenosine deaminase (ADA). In ADA deficiency there is an elevation in the level of adenosine and 2′-deoxyadenosine in the blood and 2′-deoxyadenosine levels in the urine are also elevated. The consequences of the elevations in these two ADA substrates are impaired lymphocyte differentiation, function, and viability, which results in lymphopenia and severe immunodeficiency. Increases in 2′-deoxyadenosine, through the action of ubiquitous nucleoside phosphorylases, results in dramatic increases in cellular dATP pools. The consequences of increased dATP pools are an inhibition of ribonucleotide reductase (RR), the enzyme responsible for generating deoxyribonucleotides (necessary for DNA replication) from ribonucleotides.

2. You are examining a 7-year-old male child who exhibits delayed motor development, overexaggerated reflexes, and spasticity. In addition, the boy has a tendency to chew his lips and fingers often causing tissue damage and bleeding. He also has painful, swollen, and inflamed joints. The most likely diagnosis in this case is Lesch-Nyhan syndrome. Which of the following compounds would be expected to be elevated in the urine of this patient?

A. adenosine
B. guanine
C. hypoxanthine
D. uric acid
E. xanthine

Answer D: Lesch-Nyhan syndrome results from deficiencies in hypoxanthine-guanine phosphoribosyltransferase (HGPRT). HGPRT is a purine nucleotide salvage enzyme that converts guanine to GMP and hypoxanthine to inosine 5′-monophosphate (IMP). Loss of this salvage enzyme results in increased rates of purine nucleotide catabolism whose end product is uric acid.

3. You are examining a 5-year-old male child who has been exhibiting a tendency to bite his lower lip to the point of bleeding as well as chewing on his fingertips. Physical examination demonstrates swollen tender joints. These symptoms and lab results are indicative of a deficiency in HGPRT. Given this enzyme deficiency, which of the following compounds would be expected to be elevated in the serum of this patient?

A. bilirubin
B. cytosine
C. glycine
D. orotate
E. xanthine

Answer E: A deficiency in HGPRT is the cause of Lesch-Nyhan syndrome. HGPRT is a purine nucleotide salvage enzyme that converts guanine to GMP and hypoxanthine to IMP. Reduced activity of this enzyme results in increased rates of purine nucleotide catabolism due to the inability to effectively carry out purine salvage. The reduced rate of hypoxanthine salvage by HGPRT will result in increased production if xanthine catalyzed by the xanthine oxidase reaction.

4. Certain nucleic acids harbor significant free energy that can be released and coupled to the synthesis of biological molecules. Which of the following represents a nucleic acid form containing the greatest amount of free energy?

A. adenine
B. adenosine
C. adenosine monophosphate
D. adenosine diphosphate
E. adenosine triphosphate

Answer E: The high free energy in nucleic acids is imparted by the formation of phosphate bonds. The nucleobase and nucleosides do not contain sufficient energy to drive biosynthetic processes. The phosphate in a monophosphate nucleotide is linked via an ester bond to the ribose. The di- and tri-phosphates of nucleotides are linked by anhydride bonds. Acid anhydride bonds have a high $\Delta G^{0\prime}$ for hydrolysis imparting upon them a high potential to transfer the phosphates to other molecules. Since the triphosphate nucleotide contains 2 phosphoanhydride bonds, it is this form that has the greatest level of free energy.

5. When glucagon binds to its receptors on the surface of adipose tissue, it activates a signaling cascade leading to the release of free fatty acids that can be utilized by the liver and other peripheral tissues for energy production. Which of the following is the correct nucleic acid involved in the triggering of this cascade?

A. ATP
B. cAMP
C. cGMP
D. GTP
E. xanthine

Answer B: Glucagon binds to plasma membrane receptors coupled through a G-protein that activates adenylate cyclase. Adenylate cyclase generates cAMP from ATP and the resultant increases in cAMP in turn activate cAMP-dependent protein kinase, PKA. Activation of PKA leads to increased fatty acids release from triglycerides stored in adipose tissue.

Checklist

✓ The nucleotides found in cells are derivatives of the heterocyclic highly basic compounds, purine, and pyrimidine.

✓ Nucleosides are composed of a nucleobase (purine or pyrimidine) attached to ribose but containing no phosphate. Nucleotides are the result of phosphate addition to nucleosides and they can be either mono-, di- or triphosphate modified.

✓ The triphosphate and diphosphate groups of nucleotides are phosphoanhydride bonds imparting high transfer energy for participation in covalent bond synthesis, such as in the case of ATP.

✓ The nomenclature for the atoms in nucleosides and nucleotides includes a prime (′) designation to distinguish the atoms in the sugar from those in the base.

✓ Polynucleotides are composed of 2 or more nucleotides linked together via a phosphodiester bond between the 5′ phosphate of the sugar in one nucleotide and the 3′ hydroxyl of the sugar in another nucleotide. The common left-to-right nomenclature for polynucleotides is 5′ → 3′: eg, 5′-pApGpCpT-3′ or just 5′-AGCT-3′.

✓ Cyclic adenosine and guanine nucleotides act as second messengers in signal transduction events.

✓ Nucleotide analogs are used as antimicrobial and anticancer agents via their ability to interfere with nucleotide biosynthesis or DNA replication.

CHAPTER

5 Protein Structure and Function

CHAPTER OUTLINE

High-Yield Terms

Fibrous protein: any protein that is generally insoluble in water and exists in an elongated and rigid conformation; most structural proteins are fibrous

Globular protein: any protein that is generally soluble in water and exists in more compact spherical conformation; most functional proteins are globular

Primary Structure in Proteins

The primary structure of peptides and proteins refers to the linear number and order of the amino acids present. The convention for the designation of the order of amino acids is that the *N*-terminal end (ie, the end bearing the residue with the free α-amino group) is to the left (and the number 1 amino acid) and the *C*-terminal end (ie, the end with the residue containing a free α-carboxyl group) is to the right.

$^{+}H_3N$ … SH … O^-

Alanyl **Cysteinyl** **Valine**

Murray RK, Bender DA, Botham KM, Kennelly PJ, Rodwell VW, Weil PA. *Harper's Illustrated Biochemistry*, 29th ed. New York, NY: McGraw-Hill; 2012.

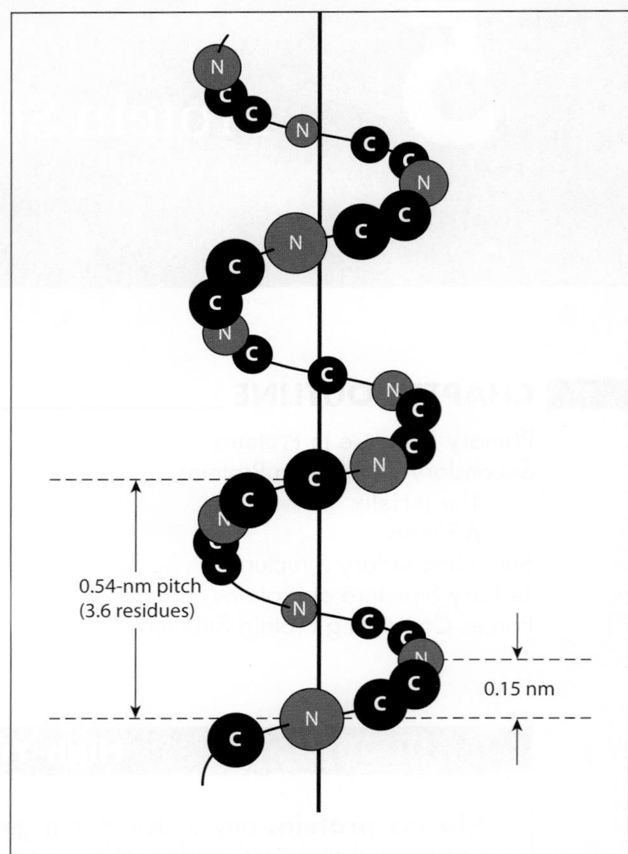

FIGURE 5-1: Orientation of the main chain atoms of a peptide about the axis of an α helix. Murray RK, Bender DA, Botham KM, Kennelly PJ, Rodwell VW, Weil PA. *Harper's Illustrated Biochemistry*, 29th ed. New York, NY: McGraw-Hill; 2012.

Secondary Structure in Proteins

The ordered array of amino acids in a protein confers regular conformational forms upon that protein. These conformations constitute the secondary structures of a protein. In general, proteins fold into 2 broad classes of structure termed *globular proteins* or *fibrous proteins*. Globular proteins are compactly folded and coiled, whereas, fibrous proteins are more filamentous or elongated. It is the partial double-bond character of the peptide bond that defines the conformations a polypeptide chain may assume. Within a single protein, different regions of the polypeptide chain may assume different conformations determined by the primary sequence of the amino acids.

The α-Helix

The α-helix is a common secondary structure encountered in proteins of the globular class. The formation of the α-helix is spontaneous and is stabilized by H-bonding between amide nitrogens and carbonyl carbons of peptide bonds spaced 4 residues apart. This orientation of H-bonding produces a helical coiling of the peptide backbone such that the R-groups lie on the exterior of the helix and perpendicular to its axis (Figure 5-1).

Not all amino acids favor the formation of the α-helix due to steric constraints of the R-groups. Amino acids, such as A, D, E, I, L, and M, favor the formation of α-helices, whereas, G and P favor disruption of the helix. This is particularly true for P since it is a pyrrolidine-based imino acid (HN=) whose structure significantly restricts movement about the peptide bond in which it is present, thereby, interfering with extension of the helix. The disruption of the helix is important as it introduces additional folding of the polypeptide backbone to allow the formation of globular proteins.

β-Sheets

An α-helix is composed of a single linear array of helically disposed amino acids, whereas β-sheets are composed of 2 or more different regions of stretches of at least 5 to 10 amino acids. The folding and alignment of stretches of the polypeptide backbone aside one another to form β-sheets is stabilized by H-bonding between amide nitrogens and carbonyl carbons. However, the H-bonding residues are present in adjacently opposed stretches of the polypeptide backbone as opposed to a linearly contiguous region of the backbone in the α-helix. β-sheets are said to be pleated. This is due to positioning of the α-carbons of the peptide bond, which alternates above and below the plane of the sheet. β-sheets are either parallel or antiparallel. In parallel sheets, adjacent peptide chains proceed in the same direction (ie, the direction of *N*-terminal to *C*-terminal ends is the same), whereas, in antiparallel sheets adjacent chains are aligned in opposite directions. β-sheets can be depicted in ball and stick format or as ribbons in certain protein formats (Figure 5-2).

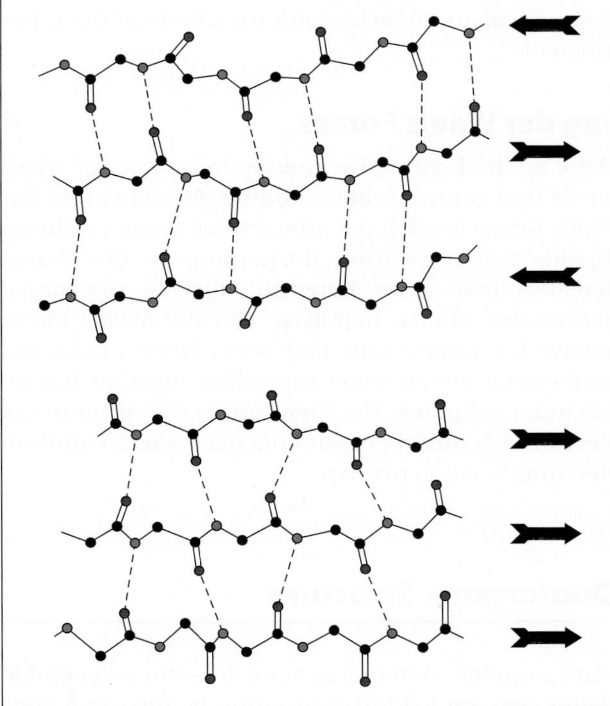

FIGURE 5-2: Spacing and bond angles of the hydrogen bonds of antiparallel and parallel pleated β sheets. Arrows indicate the direction of each strand. Hydrogen bonds are indicated by dotted lines with the participating α-nitrogen atoms (hydrogen donors) and oxygen atoms (hydrogen acceptors) shown in blue and red, respectively. Backbone carbon atoms are shown in black. For clarity in presentation, R groups and hydrogen atoms are omitted. Top: Antiparallel β sheet. Pairs of hydrogen bonds alternate between being close together and wide apart and are oriented approximately perpendicular to the polypeptide backbone. Bottom: Parallel β sheet. The hydrogen bonds are evenly spaced but slant in alternate directions. Murray RK, Bender DA, Botham KM, Kennelly PJ, Rodwell VW, Weil PA. *Harper's Illustrated Biochemistry*, 29th ed. New York, NY: McGraw-Hill; 2012.

Super-Secondary Structure

Some proteins contain an ordered organization of secondary structures that form distinct functional domains or structural motifs. Examples include the helix-turn-helix domain of bacterial proteins that regulate transcription and the leucine zipper, helix-loop-helix and zinc finger domains of eukaryotic transcriptional regulators. These domains are termed super-secondary structures.

Tertiary Structure of Proteins

Tertiary structure refers to the complete 3-dimensional structure of the polypeptide units of a given protein. Included in this description is the spatial relationship of different secondary structures to one another within a polypeptide chain and how these secondary structures themselves fold into the 3-dimensional form of the protein. Secondary structures of proteins often constitute distinct domains. Therefore, tertiary structure also describes the relationship of different domains to one another within a protein (Figure 5-3).

Forces Controlling Protein Structure

The interaction of different domains is governed by several forces: These include hydrogen bonding, hydrophobic interactions, electrostatic interactions, and van der Waals forces.

Hydrogen Bonding

Polypeptides contain numerous proton donors and acceptors both in their backbone and in the R-groups of the amino acids. The environment in which proteins are found also contains the ample H-bond donors and acceptors of the water molecule. H-bonding, therefore, occurs not only within and between polypeptide chains but with the surrounding aqueous medium.

Hydrophobic Forces

Proteins are composed of amino acids that contain either hydrophilic or hydrophobic R-groups. It is the nature of interaction of different R-groups with the aqueous environment that plays a major role in shaping protein structure. The spontaneous folded state of globular proteins is a reflection of a balance between the opposing energetics of H-bonding between hydrophilic R-groups

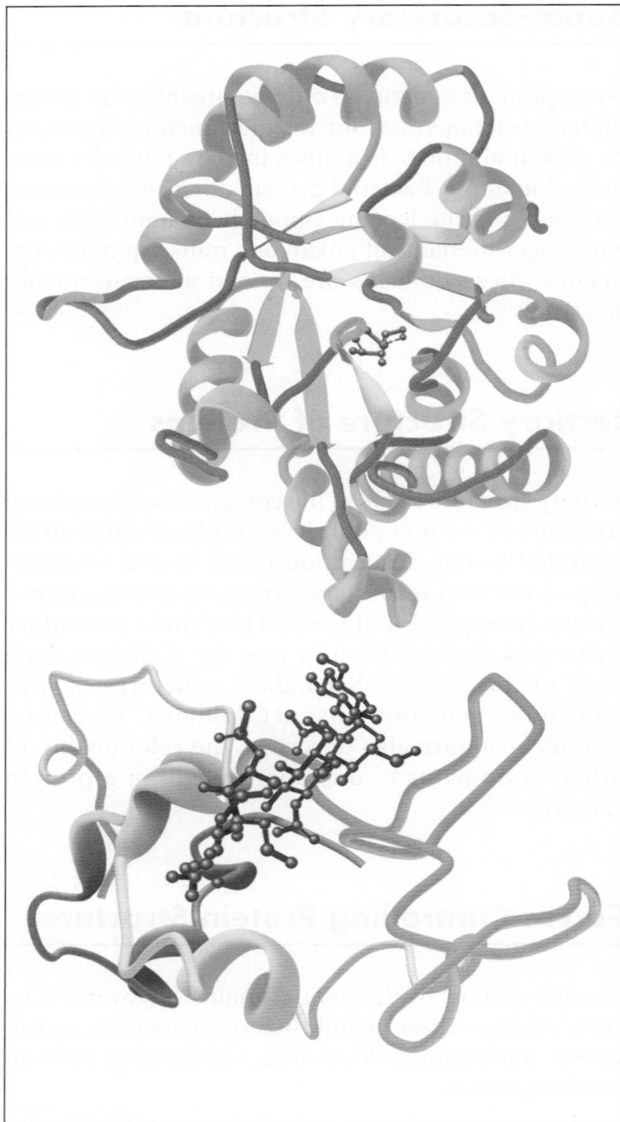

FIGURE 5-3: Examples of the tertiary structure of proteins. Top: The enzyme triose phosphate isomerase complexed with the substrate analog 2-phosphoglycerate (red). Note the elegant and symmetrical arrangement of alternating β sheets (light blue) and α helices (green), with the β sheets forming a β-barrel core surrounded by the helices. (Adapted from Protein Data Bank ID no. 1o5x.) Bottom: Lysozyme complexed with the substrate analog penta-N-acetyl chitopentaose (red). The color of the polypeptide chain is graded along the visible spectrum from purple (N-terminal) to tan (C-terminal). Notice how the concave shape of the domain forms a binding pocket for the pentasaccharide, the lack of β sheet, and the high proportion of loops and bends. (Adapted from Protein Data Bank ID no. 1sfb.) Murray RK, Bender DA, Botham KM, Kennelly PJ, Rodwell VW, Weil PA. *Harper's Illustrated Biochemistry,* 29th ed.New York, NY: McGraw-Hill; 2012.

and the aqueous environment and the repulsion from the aqueous environment by the hydrophobic R-groups. The hydrophobicity of certain amino acid R-groups tends to drive them away from the exterior of proteins and into the interior. This driving force restricts the available conformations into which a protein may fold.

Electrostatic Forces

Electrostatic forces are mainly of 3 types: charge-charge, charge-dipole, and dipole-dipole. Typical charge-charge interactions that favor protein folding are those between oppositely charged R-groups such as K or R and D or E. A substantial component of the energy involved in protein folding is charge-dipole interactions. This refers to the interaction of ionized R-groups of amino acids with the dipole of the water molecule.

van der Waals Forces

There are both attractive and repulsive van der Waals forces that control protein folding. Attractive van der Waals forces involve the interactions among induced dipoles that arise from fluctuations in the charge densities that occur between adjacent uncharged nonbonded atoms. Repulsive van der Waals forces involve the interactions that occur when uncharged nonbonded atoms come very close together but do not induce dipoles. The repulsion is the result of the electron-electron repulsion that occurs as 2 clouds of electrons begin to overlap.

Quaternary Structure

Many proteins contain 2 or more different polypeptide chains that are held in association by the same noncovalent forces that stabilize the tertiary structures of proteins. Proteins with multiple polypeptide chains are oligomeric proteins. The overall structure formed by the interaction of at least 2 protein subunits in an oligomeric protein is known as quaternary structure. Oligomeric proteins can be composed of multiple identical polypeptide chains or multiple distinct polypeptide chains. Proteins with identical subunits are termed *homo-oligomers*. Proteins containing several distinct polypeptide chains are termed *hetero-oligomers*. Hemoglobin, the oxygen-carrying protein of the blood, is a heterotetrameric protein that can be considered one of the most clinically significant oligomeric proteins in the body.

High-Yield Concept

Although van der Waals forces are extremely weak relative to other forces governing conformation, it is the huge number of such interactions that occur in large protein molecules that make them significant to the folding of proteins.

High-Yield Concept

In the broadest terms, fibrous proteins are involved in imparting structural characteristics to cellular constituents, whereas globular proteins represent the bulk of functional proteins in the cell, for example, the enzymes.

Major Protein Forms

All proteins in the human body can be grouped into one of 2 broad categories called fibrous or globular proteins.

Fibrous proteins are so called because they fold into long filamentous shapes and exhibit strong inflexible structural characteristics. In addition, fibrous proteins are generally insoluble in water. The predominant fibrous proteins are the collagens, keratins, and elastins which are used to construct connective tissues, muscle fibers, tendons, and the matrix of bones. As the name implies, globular proteins form spherical shapes and unlike fibrous proteins are more flexible and can more actively interact with the aqueous environment.

Collagens

In their various forms, the collagen proteins are the most abundant proteins in the body as well as representing one of the most clinically significant families of fibrous proteins (see Clinical Box 5-1). There are at least 28 different types of functional collagen protein whose subunits are encoded by 30 distinct collagen genes (see Table 39-1).

Each of the collagens contains a region of left-handed triple helix imparted by a high density of glycine and proline residues (Figure 5-4). In some collagens the entire molecule is composed of this triple helix, whereas, in other forms the triple helix represents only a small portion of the overall molecule. The glycine residues within the triple helical portion of the molecule are present in the repeating sequence: Gly-X-Y. The designation X and Y refers to the fact that any amino acid can occupy those positions. However, within the triple helix, proline (Pro) and hydroxyproline (Hyp) are present at high frequency. Hydroxyproline is a posttranslational modification that occurs to proline residues within collagen molecules via the action of a vitamin C–dependent prolyl hydroxylase. The presence of both proline and hydroxyproline induces rigidity into the triple helix of the collagen molecule. Another posttranslationally hydroxylated amino acid found in several types of collagen molecule is hydroxylysine (Hyl). Collagen molecules are also modified by glycosylation, specifically on Hyl residues in the molecule.

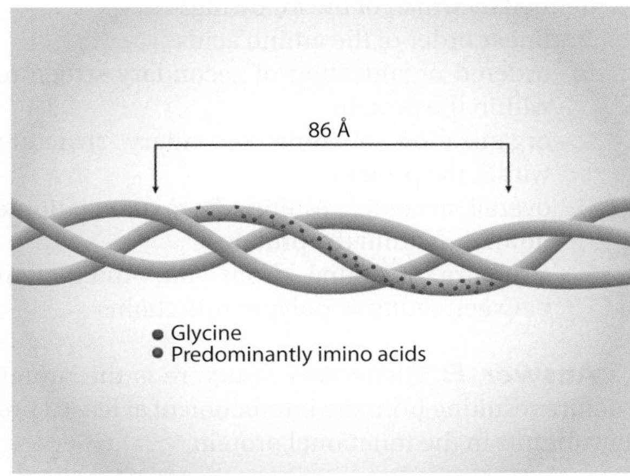

FIGURE 5-4: Triple helical structure of a typical collagen molecule. Reproduced with permission of themedicalbiochemistrypage, LLC.

CLINICAL BOX 5-1: CONNECTIVE TISSUE DISORDERS

Collagens are the most abundant proteins in the body. Alterations in collagen structure arising from abnormal genes or abnormal processing of collagen proteins results in numerous diseases, including Larsen syndrome, scurvy, osteogenesis imperfecta (OI), and Ehlers-Danlos syndrome (EDS).

Ehlers-Danlos syndrome is actually the name associated with at least 9 distinct disorders that are biochemically and clinically distinct yet all manifest structural weakness in connective tissue as a result of defective collagen structure. These 9 disorders are designated EDS I-XIII and X with EDS I and EDS II being referred to as classical EDS. The disorder that was originally designated as EDS IX is now more commonly called X-linked cutis laxa or occipital horn syndrome. The major manifestations of EDS are skin fragility and hyperextensibility and joint hypermobility. To date, mutations in 8 genes involved in collagen synthesis or processing have been identified as causing the EDS phenotypes. EDS I results from defects in the *COL5A1* and *COL5A2* genes. EDS II also results from mutations in *COL5A1*, but the symptoms of this form of the disease are less severe. EDS IV is called the arterial or vascular form of the disease and results from defects in the *COL3A1* gene. EDS VI is the ocular or kyphoscoliosis form of the disease. This form of EDS results from deficiencies in the activity of lysyl hydroxylase, which is responsible for proper posttranslational processing of certain collagen types. Lysyl hydroxylase is encoded by the *procollagen-lysine 2-oxoglutarate 5-dioxygenase 1 (PLOD1)* gene.

OI also encompasses more than one disorder. At least 4 biochemically and clinically distinguishable maladies have been identified as OI, all of which are characterized by bone fragility leading to multiple fractures and resultant bone deformities. All 4 forms of OI are due to defects in type I collagens. Type I OI is a mild form of the disease and also the most commonly encountered with a frequency of approximately 1 in 10,000 live births. Type I OI results from null mutations in the *COL1A1* gene. Type II OI is the most severe form and is referred to as the perinatal lethal form. These infants exhibit characteristic facial features that include dark sclera, a beaked nose, and an extremely soft calvarium. Type II OI results from mutations in both the *COL1A1* and *COL1A2* genes. The outlook for type II OI patients is grim with life spans of only minutes to a few months. Death is usually the result of congestive heart failure, pulmonary insufficiency, or infection.

REVIEW QUESTIONS

1. The quaternary structure of a given protein is defined by which of the following?
- **A.** linear order of the amino acids
- **B.** ordered organization of secondary structures within the protein
- **C.** organization of super-secondary structures within the protein
- **D.** overall structure resulting from association of domains within the protein
- **E.** structure resulting from the interactions between multiple polypeptide chains

Answer E: Quaternary structure is the protein structure resulting from the interaction of at least 2 protein subunits in the functional protein.

2. In an enzyme with a critical glutamic acid residue (Glu, E) in the active site, which of the following amino acid substitutions would be expected to have the least effect on enzyme activity?
- **A.** Arg
- **B.** Asp
- **C.** Lys
- **D.** Ser
- **E.** Tyr

Answer B: Since glutamic acid is a negatively charged amino acid at physiological pH, any other negatively charged amino acid, such as aspartic acid, could potentially be substituted without significant loss of enzyme activity.

3. A 12-year-old boy has suffered from chronic sinopulmonary disease including persistent infection of the airway with *Pseudomonas aeruginosa*. He has constant and chronic sputum production because of the airway infection. Additionally, he suffers from gastrointestinal (GI) and nutritional abnormalities that include biliary cirrhosis, meconium ileus, and pancreatic insufficiency. The symptoms are classical for which of the following disorders?
- **A.** congenital adrenal hyperplasia
- **B.** cystic fibrosis
- **C.** renal Fanconi syndrome

D. sickle cell anemia
E. Tay-Sachs disease

Answer B: Cystic fibrosis results from mutations in the gene encoding the cystic fibrosis transmembrane conductance regulator (CFTR). The disease is characterized by abnormal transport of chloride and sodium across an epithelium, leading to thick, viscous mucus secretions. This mucus builds up in the breathing passages of the lungs, as well as in the pancreas and intestines. Difficulty breathing is the most serious symptom and results from frequent lung infections, particularly with *P. aeruginosa*. The secretions in the pancreas block the exocrine movement of the digestive enzymes into the duodenum and result in irreversible damage to the pancreas. The lack of digestive enzymes leads to difficulty in absorbing nutrients with their subsequent excretion in the feces resulting in a malabsorption disorder.

4. You are examining the lipid-interaction characteristics of a particularly hydrophobic protein. Mutational studies with this protein have been designed to examine these lipid interaction properties. Addition of which of the following amino acids to the protein would most likely be expected to interfere with the lipid-interaction properties?
A. aspartate
B. glycine
C. isoleucine
D. leucine
E. valine

Answer A: Lipids would most likely interact with equally hydrophobic substances. Aspartic acid is an acidic amino acid and as such would be more likely to interact with an aqueous environment than a hydrophobic lipid one.

5. You are examining digestive enzymes and their processes of activation. You have isolated a mutant form of one particular enzyme and found that it remains inactive in a mixture of digestive juices. The wild-type enzyme is normally activated by hydrolysis on the *C*-terminal side of Arg and Lys residues and you determine that the mutant enzyme contains Ser residues at these critical positions. Which of the following digestive enzymes is most likely responsible for activation of the wild-type enzyme in your studies?
A. aminopeptidase
B. carboxypeptidase
C. chymotrypsin
D. enteropeptidase
E. lysozyme

Answer D: Trypsin is a pancreatic digestive enzyme derived from proteolytic cleavage of the precursor protein trypsinogen. Enteropeptidase is produced by cells of the duodenum. It is secreted from intestinal glands called the crypts of Lieberkühn following the entry of ingested food passing from the stomach. Enteropeptidase converts trypsinogen into its active form trypsin. Trypsin cleaves its target substrates on the *C*-terminal side of Arg and Lys residues.

6. You are studying the characteristics of membrane-associated proteins. You have isolated and characterized both wild-type and mutant forms of a particular protein. The mutant protein does not remain anchored in the plasma membrane. Which of the following properties results in membrane anchoring of the wild-type protein and is likely defective in the mutant version?
A. disulfide bond formation between the protein and its phosphatidylinositol anchor
B. extensive hydrogen bonding of the amino acid side chains of the protein and the membrane phospholipid tails
C. extensive hydrophobic interactions between the amino acid side chains of the protein and the membrane phospholipid tails
D. formation of ionic bonds between the amino acid side chains and the phospholipid tails
E. formation of β-pleated sheet structures to maximize protein interactions with the phospholipid head group

Answer C: Membranes are predominantly lipid and thus most likely to interact with hydrophobic amino acids. The interaction between the hydrophobic R-groups of amino acids and the hydrophobic lipid tails of membrane phospholipids anchors integral membrane proteins to the membrane.

7. You are examining the thermodynamically stable structures of proteins. In particular you are studying the α-helix and β-sheet conformations that form in the study proteins. These conformations correspond to which of the following?
A. native conformation
B. primary structure
C. secondary structure
D. tertiary structure
E. quaternary structure

Answer C: The formation of secondary structures in proteins is the result of the order folding of groups of amino acids into either α-helices or β-sheets.

8. In the β-sheet structure of proteins, the hydrogen bond on the peptide bond nitrogen of one of the peptides will most likely form a hydrogen bond with which of the following?

A. hydrophilic side chains in the adjacent sheet segment
B. hydrophobic side chains in the adjacent sheet segment
C. peptide bond carbonyl in the adjacent sheet segment
D. peptide bond carbonyl within 3 amino acids of the same segment
E. water in the surrounding medium

Answer C: The formation of both α-helices and β-sheets is the result of the hydrogen bonds formed between the hydrogen associated with the amide nitrogen of the peptide bond and the carbonyl oxygen of an adjacent peptide bond.

9. You have isolated a strain of cholera that does not induce the same symptoms in host organisms as the wild-type pathogen. The toxin from wild-type cholera is known to cause diarrhea only after its 2 polypeptide subunits dissociate from each other. This dissociation occurs when the toxin enters an acid environment. You find that the strain you have isolated is not localized to a particular cellular location, which likely explains the lack of activity. In which of the following cellular locations are the wild-type toxin subunits most likely to dissociate from each other, thereby becoming active?

A. coated vesicle
B. cytosol
C. endosome
D. mitochondrial matrix
E. nucleus

Answer C: Endosomes are membrane-bound compartments inside cells. They are compartments of the endocytic membrane transport pathway from the plasma membrane to the lysosome. For example, when low-density lipoprotein (LDL) binds the LDL receptor, the complex is internalized and fused to the endosomal membranes. Because of the slightly acidic environment of the endosome, ligands, such as LDL, dissociate.

10. During the normal processes of the cell cycle, specific types of DNA–protein complexes form and dissociate which allow condensation and decondensation of the chromosomes. Which of the following is the major attractive force between the DNA and the proteins, allowing these complexes to form?

A. disulfide linkages
B. electrostatic interactions
C. hydrogen bonds
D. hydrophobic interactions
E. van der Waals forces

Answer B: DNA is very highly negatively charged due to the phosphate backbone of the nucleotides. Therefore, DNA is most likely to interact with other molecules, such as proteins, via electrostatic interactions.

11. You are studying the relationships between protein structure and function. You are most interested in the characteristics of a family of proteins termed chaperones. Which of the following processes requires chaperone activity in order to facilitate correct biological function?

A. assembly of coated pits
B. correct folding of nascent proteins
C. formation of tight junctions
D. interaction between actin and myosin
E. processing of telomeres

Answer B: *Chaperones* are proteins that assist the noncovalent folding or unfolding and the assembly or disassembly of other macromolecular structures, but do not occur in these structures when the structures are performing their normal biological functions.

12. Digestive enzymes have been used in the study of protein structure. Which of the following explains the usefulness of trypsin and chymotrypsin in studies of protein structure?

A. efficiency as exopeptidases
B. high specificity for particular peptide bonds
C. high stability because of the presence of disulfide cross-links
D. high turnover rates
E. rapid digestion of proteins to yield amino acids and small oligopeptides

Answer B: Trypsin and chymotrypsin are enzymes of a class referred to as endoproteases. Both of these enzymes hydrolyze the peptide bond in substrate proteins at very specific sequences of amino acids. Trypsin cleaves the peptide bond that is *C*-terminal to a lysine or arginine residue. Chymotrypsin cleaves the peptide bond on the *C*-terminal side of tyrosine, tryptophan, or phenylalanine. Thus, the products of trypsin and chymotrypsin cleavage indicate the presence and number of these specific amino acids in a target protein.

13. The peptide bond of all proteins forms with highly specific orientation. This orientation contains atoms linked in which of the following ways?

A. C-N-C-C
B. C-N-H-C
C. C-O-N-C

D. C-C-O-N
E. C-S-S-C

Answer A: The peptide bond is formed between the α-carbon of one amino acid and the α-amino nitrogen of the adjacent amino acid, therefore the orientation of the atoms would be C-N. The second C in the correct orientation is α-carbon of the *C*-terminal amino acid and the last C atom of the correct answer represents the carbon of the carboxylic acid residue of the *C*-terminal amino acid in the peptide bond.

14. You are studying the characteristics of protein secondary structure. You find that the protein you are examining forms an α-helical structure more rapidly in an alcohol medium than it does in water. Which of the following is the best explanation for this difference?
A. competition for hydrogen bonding is lower for ethanol than for water
B. ethanol forms covalent interactions with the peptide
C. hydrophobic forces are greater in ethanol than in water
D. the peptide aggregates in water but not in ethanol
E. van der Waals interactions are lower in ethanol than in water

Answer A: The α-helix results due to the formation of hydrogen bonds between adjacent amino acids in the protein. Because these same atoms in the amino acids can form hydrogen bonds with water, there can be competition for the formation of the bonds required for the α-helix. In the presence of ethanol there would be less competition from the water molecules thus explaining the increased rate of α-helix formation in this medium.

15. You are studying the protein-folding characteristics of a particular protein. You find that under certain conditions the protein does not fold correctly and it precipitates within the cytosol. Which of the following processes is most directly responsible for aggregation and precipitation of the misfolded protein in the cytoplasm?
A. attachment of palmitate to the *C*-terminus
B. exposure of hydrophobic residues on the surface of the protein
C. formation of incorrect disulfide bonds between pairs of cysteine residues
D. nonenzymatic glycosylation of amino groups by free glucose
E. phosphorylation of threonine or serine side chains

Answer B: The correct folding of proteins involves several different forces. One of the strongest forces is hydrophobic interactions whereby, hydrophobic amino acids tend to be excluded from the aqueous surface of proteins. The exposure of hydrophobic amino acids to the surface of a protein due to improper folding could tend to lead to aggregation.

16. Mutational studies on collagen proteins demonstrate that substitution of one particular amino acid significantly affects the normal structure of the collagen molecules. Which of the following amino acids is absolutely required for the stable formation of the collagen triple helix?
A. alanine
B. cysteine
C. glycine
D. phenylalanine
E. tryptophan

Answer C: All collagens contain 3-stranded helical segments of similar structure. The unique properties of each type of collagen are due mainly to segments that interrupt the triple helix and that fold into other kinds of 3-dimensional structures. The triple-helical structure of collagen arises from an unusual abundance of 3 amino acids: glycine, proline, and hydroxyproline. These amino acids make up the characteristic repeating motif Gly-Pro-X, where X can be any amino acid. Each amino acid has a precise function. The side chain of glycine, an H atom, is the only one that can fit into the crowded center of a 3-stranded helix. Hydrogen bonds linking the peptide bond nitrogen of a glycine residue with a peptide carbonyl group in an adjacent polypeptide help hold the 3 chains together. It is because of this role of glycine in collagen that it is indispensable for normal collagen structure and function.

17. The parents of a 3-year-old boy bring him to the hospital following a fall as they are concerned he has broken his arm. His parents report that over the past year he has had several episodes of what they think is uncharacteristically easy fractures in his legs from minor falls. They indicate that there is no family history of bone disease. Physical examination shows bowing and deformities of the legs, and x-rays show evidence of previous fractures and osteopenia. The physician suspects a collagen defect and orders a skin biopsy. The results of the biopsy show unstable type I collagen that is due to a single-point mutation in one of the type I genes. This mutation is most likely caused by which of the following amino acid substitutions in this patient?

A. Ala → Asp
B. Glu → Gln
C. Gly → Leu
D. Tyr → Trp
E. Ser → Phe

Answer C: The triple-helical structure of collagen arises from an unusual abundance of 3 amino acids: glycine, proline, and hydroxyproline. These amino acids make up the characteristic repeating motif Gly-Pro-X, where X can be any amino acid. The side chain of glycine, an H atom, is the only one that can fit into the crowded center of a 3-stranded helix. Hydrogen bonds linking the peptide bond nitrogen of a glycine residue with a peptide carbonyl group in an adjacent polypeptide help hold the 3 chains together. It is because of this role of glycine in collagen that it is indispensable for normal collagen structure and function. Therefore, a mutation causing a substitution of glycine for leucine would result in the production of defective collagen.

18. A 28-year-old man sees his physician on a regular basis because he has suffered from bronchiectasis, chronic sinusitis, rhinitis, and secretory otitis media since childhood. He is currently being evaluated for infertility because he and his wife have been unable to conceive. His wife has been evaluated, and no abnormalities were found. The volume of his ejaculate and his sperm count are within reference ranges. Given his history and current findings, his infertility could best be explained by defective or absent production of which of the following cell structures?
A. Golgi complex
B. microtubules
C. mitochondria
D. peroxisomes
E. ribosomes

Answer B: *Microtubules* are filamentous intracellular structures that are responsible for various kinds of movements in all eukaryotic cells. Microtubules are involved in nuclear and cell division, organization of intracellular structures, and intracellular transport, as well as ciliary motility. The symptoms observed in this individual, bronchiectasis, sinusitis, rhinitis, and secretory otitis media are all the result of defective ciliary function.

19. Which of the following best describes how mitochondria reach the presynaptic endings of nerve cells?
A. ameboid migration down the axon from the neuronal cell body
B. assembly within the presynaptic ending from cytoplasmic lipids, amino acids, and other small molecules
C. assembly within the presynaptic ending using recycled presynaptic membranes
D. diffusion down the axon from the neuronal cell body
E. transport down the axon from the neuronal cell body along the microtubules

Answer E: Microtubules are filamentous intracellular structures that are responsible for various kinds of movements in all eukaryotic cells. Microtubules are involved in nuclear and cell division, organization of intracellular structures, and intracellular transport, as well as ciliary motility. Mitochondria have been shown to migrate inside cells, such as axonal movement, via the interaction with microtubules.

20. You are studying the activity of isolated anterior pituitary cells in culture. Specifically you are interested in the function of microtubules in these cells. Your studies involve the actions of the drug colchicine, which is a known inhibitor of microtubules function. Addition of colchicine to the culture medium will most likely result in which of the following in these pituitary cells?
A. induction of pseudopodia
B. inhibition of adenylate cyclase
C. inhibition of hormone secretion
D. stimulation of Ca^{2+} transport
E. stimulation of Na^+-K^+ transport

Answer C: Secretion of hormone requires migration and fusion of secretory vesicles with the plasma membrane. The migration of secretory vesicles is mediated via their interactions with the microtubule network inside the cell. Microtubules are filamentous intracellular structures that are responsible for various kinds of movements in all eukaryotic cells. Microtubules are involved in nuclear and cell division, organization of intracellular structures, and intracellular transport, as well as ciliary motility.

21. The movement and placement of organelles within animal cells is controlled by 2 ATP-binding motor proteins called kinesin and dynein. Mutations in either of these 2 proteins that interfere with these processes would most likely be associated with defective binding to which of the following structures?
A. actin filaments
B. ciliary doublets
C. intermediate filaments
D. microtubules
E. myosin fibrils

Answer D: Dynein and kinesin transport various cellular components by "walking" along cytoskeletal microtubules. Dyneins move toward the minus end of the microtubule, which is usually oriented toward the cell center. Thus, they are called minus end–directed motors. In contrast, kinesins are motor proteins that move toward the microtubules' plus end, are called plus end–directed motors. Microtubules are filamentous intracellular structures that are responsible for various kinds of movements in all eukaryotic cells. Microtubules are involved in nuclear and cell division, organization of intracellular structures, and intracellular transport, as well as ciliary motility.

22. An insoluble form of a prion protein accumulates in the brains of patients who have Creutzfeldt-Jakob disease, CJD. Conversion of the normal soluble form of the prion protein to the pathologic insoluble form is thought to involve conversion of α-helices to β-pleated sheets. In order for this structural transition to occur, which of the following is most likely disrupted and reformed?

A. disulfide bonds
B. hydrogen bonds
C. peptide bonds
D. salt bridges
E. zinc fingers

Answer B: The α-helix and β-sheet structures in proteins result from the formation of hydrogen bonds between the amide hydrogen of one peptide bond and an adjacent carbonyl oxygen in another peptide bond. For an α-helix to convert into a β-sheet it is required that the hydrogen bonds holding the structure together be broken and then a different series of hydrogen bonds need to form to generate the β-sheet structure.

23. Eukaryotic ribosomes consist of 2 subunits designated as 40*S* and 60*S*. The *S* value is most dependent on which of the following properties of the subunit?

A. composition of the RNA bases
B. interactions between the RNA and protein components
C. protein content
D. RNA content
E. shape and size of the subunit

Answer E: The "*S*" in 40*S* and 60*S* refers to the *Svedberg coefficient*, which is a unit of measure for sedimentation rate. The sedimentation rate is the rate at which particles of a given size and shape travel to the bottom of the tube under centrifugal force. The Svedberg coefficient is technically a measure of time and offers a measure of particle size based on its rate of travel in a tube subjected to high gravitational force.

Checklist

✓ Proteins are classified based upon numerous factors such as solubility, hydrophobicity, conformation, function, or the presence of specific types of prosthetic groups or cofactors.

✓ The structure and function of proteins are dictated, in part, by a combination of primary amino acid sequence and the forces that control the overall 3-dimensional conformation.

✓ Overall protein structure is a combination of primary, secondary, and tertiary structures. Quaternary structure represents an additional level of complexity imparted by multiple subunit proteins.

✓ Defects in protein structure, due primarily to mutations in the encoding gene, can have profound effects on function resulting in potentially debilitating disorders.

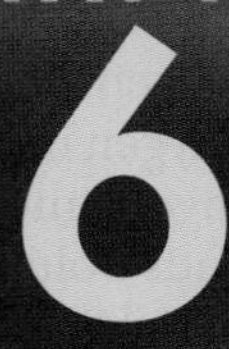

CHAPTER 6 Hemoglobin and Myoglobin

CHAPTER OUTLINE

Myoglobin
Hemoglobin
Oxygen-Binding Characteristics
Role of 2,3-Bisphosphoglycerate
The Hemoglobin Genes
The Hemoglobinopathies

High-Yield Terms

Heme: is formed when iron is inserted into the chemical compound protoporphyrin

Hemin: normal heme contains iron in the ferrous oxidation state (Fe^{2+}), whereas hemin contains iron in the ferric oxidation state (Fe^{3+})

Methemoglobin: the form of the hemoglobin protein that contains ferric iron (Fe^{3+}) in the heme prosthetic groups due to oxidation

Hemoglobinopathy: any disease resulting from either (or both) quantitative or qualitative defects in α-globin or β-globin proteins

Thalassemia: specifically refers to quantitative hemoglobinopathies due to either α-globin or β-globin protein defects

Sickle cell anemia: most commonly occurring qualitative hemoglobinopathy, results from a single amino acid substitution in the adult β-globin gene

Cooley anemia: is thalassemia major, which is either β^0– and β^+-thalassemia

Myoglobin and *hemoglobin* are hemeproteins whose physiological importance is principally related to their ability to bind molecular oxygen. *Hemoglobin* is a heterotetrameric oxygen transport protein found in red blood cells (erythrocytes), whereas myoglobin is a monomeric protein found mainly in muscle tissue where it serves as an intracellular storage site for oxygen. The oxygen carried by hemeproteins such as hemoglobin and myoglobin is bound directly to the ferrous iron (Fe^{2+}) atom of the heme prosthetic group. Oxidation of the iron to the ferric (Fe^{3+}) state renders the molecule incapable of normal oxygen binding. When the iron in heme is in the ferric state, the molecule is referred to as hemin.

Myoglobin

The tertiary structure of myoglobin is that of a typical water-soluble globular protein. Its secondary structure is unusual in which it contains a very high proportion (75%) of α-helical secondary structure. Each myoglobin molecule contains a single heme group inserted into a hydrophobic cleft in the protein. Hydrophobic interactions between the tetrapyrrole ring and hydrophobic amino acid R groups on the interior of the cleft in the protein strongly stabilize the heme–protein conjugate. In addition, a nitrogen atom from a histidine R group located above the plane of the heme ring is coordinated with the iron atom further stabilizing the interaction between the heme and the protein. In oxymyoglobin the remaining bonding site on the iron atom (the 6th coordinate position) is occupied by the oxygen, whose binding is stabilized by a second histidine residue.

Hemoglobin

Adult hemoglobin is a heterotetrameric [α(2):β(2)] hemeprotein (Figure 6-1) found in erythrocytes where it is responsible for binding oxygen in the lung and transporting the bound oxygen throughout the body, where it is used in aerobic metabolic pathways. Each subunit of a hemoglobin tetramer has a heme prosthetic group identical to that described for myoglobin. The quaternary structure of hemoglobin leads to physiologically important allosteric interactions between the subunits, a property lacking in monomeric myoglobin, which is otherwise very similar to the α-subunit of hemoglobin.

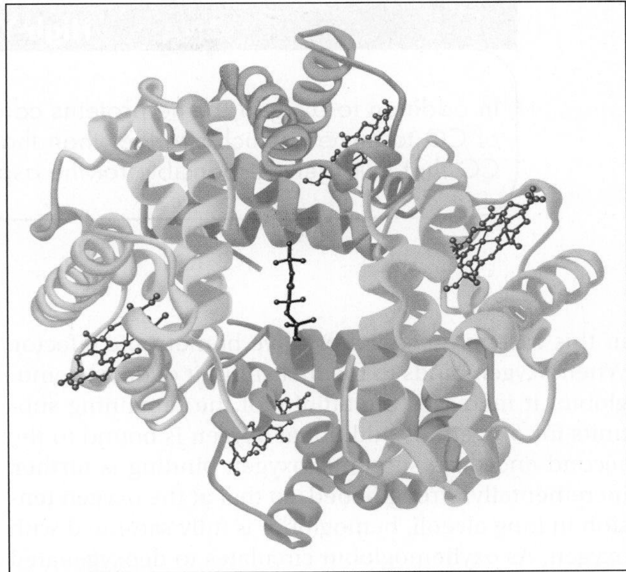

FIGURE 6-1: Hemoglobin. Shown is the three-dimensional structure of deoxyhemoglobin with a molecule of 2,3-bisphosphoglycerate (dark blue) bound. The two α subunits are colored in the darker shades of green and blue, the two β subunits in the lighter shades of green and blue, and the heme prosthetic groups in red. (Adapted from Protein Data Bank ID no. 1b86.) Murray RK, Bender DA, Botham KM, Kennelly PJ, Rodwell VW, Weil PA. *Harper's Illustrated Biochemistry,* 29th ed. New York, NY: McGraw-Hill; 2012.

Oxygen-Binding Characteristics

Comparison of the oxygen-binding properties of myoglobin and hemoglobin illustrates the allosteric properties of hemoglobin that result from its quaternary structure and differentiate hemoglobin's oxygen-binding properties from that of myoglobin (Figure 6-2). The curve of oxygen binding to hemoglobin is sigmoidal typical of allosteric proteins in which the substrate,

High-Yield Concept

In hemoglobin, when the iron is oxidized to the ferric state the resulting form of the protein is called methemoglobin. Methemoglobin, which is incapable of binding oxygen, generally represents less than 2% of the hemoglobin in the blood.

High-Yield Concept

In addition to oxygen, heme proteins can also bind carbon monoxide (CO). The binding of CO to heme is much stronger than that of oxygen and it is this preferential binding of CO that is largely responsible for the asphyxiation due to CO poisoning.

in this case oxygen, is a positive homotropic effector. When oxygen binds to the first subunit of deoxyhemoglobin, it increases the affinity of the remaining subunits for oxygen. As additional oxygen is bound to the second and third subunits, oxygen binding is further, incrementally, strengthened, so that at the oxygen tension in lung alveoli, hemoglobin is fully saturated with oxygen. As oxyhemoglobin circulates to deoxygenated tissue, oxygen is incrementally unloaded and the affinity of hemoglobin for oxygen is reduced. Thus at the lowest oxygen tensions found in very active tissues, the binding affinity of hemoglobin for oxygen is very low allowing maximal delivery of oxygen to the tissue. In contrast, the oxygen-binding curve for myoglobin is hyperbolic in character indicating the absence of allosteric interactions in this process.

The tertiary configuration of low-affinity, deoxygenated hemoglobin (Hb) is known as the *taut (T) state*. Conversely, the quaternary structure of the fully oxygenated high-affinity form of hemoglobin (HbO_2) is known as the *relaxed (R) state*.

In the context of the affinity of hemoglobin for oxygen there are 4 primary regulators, each of which exerts a negative effect. These regulators are CO_2, hydrogen ion (H^+), chloride ion (Cl^-), and 2,3-bisphosphoglycerate (2,3BPG, or also just BPG). Although they can influence O_2 binding independent of each other, CO_2, H^+, and Cl^- primarily function as a consequence of each other on the affinity of hemoglobin for O_2.

In the high O_2 environment (high Po_2) of the lungs, there is sufficient O_2 to overcome the inhibitory nature of the T state of hemoglobin to oxygen binding. During the O_2 binding–induced alteration from the T form to the R form, several amino acid side groups on the surface of hemoglobin subunits will dissociate protons as depicted in the following equation. This proton dissociation plays an important role in the expiration of the CO_2 that arrives from the tissues. However, because of the high Po_2, the pH of the blood in the lungs (≈7.4-7.5) is not sufficiently low enough to exert a negative influence on hemoglobin-binding O_2. When the oxyhemoglobin reaches the tissues, the Po_2 is sufficiently low, as well as the pH (≈7.2), that the T state is favored and the O_2 released.

$$4O_2 + Hb \leftrightarrow nH^+ + Hb(O_2)_4$$

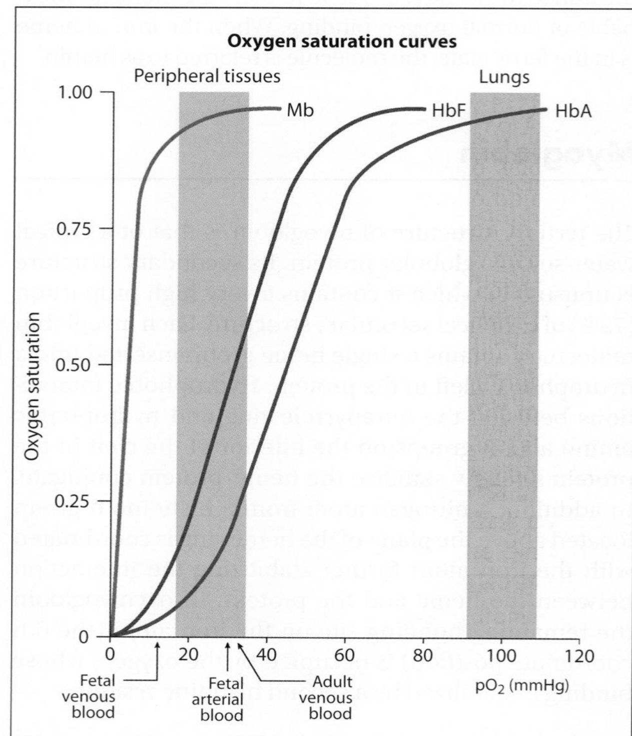

FIGURE 6-2: Oxygen saturation curves for myoglobin and hemoglobin. The saturation curve for myoglobin shows the typical rapid oxygen concentration–dependent saturation of this monomeric oxygen-binding protein. The other 2 curves show the typical sigmoidal saturation curves for cooperative oxygen binding exhibited by fetal hemoglobin (HbF) and adult hemoglobin (HbA). Also indicated in the diagram are the typical oxygen concentrations in peripheral tissues and the lungs. Note that whereas myoglobin can be fully oxygen saturated in the tissues, hemoglobin requires much higher oxygen tension to become fully saturated, which only occurs in the lungs. The position of HbF saturation to the left of HbA (ie, at lower oxygen tension) reflects the fact that fetal hemoglobin binds oxygen with higher affinity than adult hemoglobin and this is so that the fetus can acquire oxygen from the maternal circulation. Reproduced with permission of themedicalbiochemistrypage, LLC.

Within the tissues, metabolizing cells produce CO_2, which diffuses into the blood and enters the circulating erythrocytes. Within erythrocytes the CO_2 is rapidly converted to carbonic acid through the action of carbonic anhydrase. The carbonic acid then rapidly ionizes leading to increased production of H^+ and thus a reduction in the pH.

$$CO_2 + H_2O \rightarrow H_2CO_3 \rightarrow H^+ + HCO_3^-$$

The bicarbonate ion produced in this dissociation reaction diffuses out of the erythrocyte and is carried in the blood to the lungs. This effective CO_2 transport process is referred to as isohydric transport. Approximately 80% of the CO_2 produced in metabolizing cells is transported to the lungs in this way. A small percentage of CO_2 is transported in the blood as a dissolved gas.

In the tissues, the H^+ dissociated from carbonic acid is buffered by hemoglobin, which in turn exerts a negative influence on O_2 binding, forcing release of the O_2 which then diffuses into the tissues. As indicated earlier, within the lungs the high PO_2 allows for effective O_2 binding by hemoglobin leading to the T-to-R-state transition and the release of protons. The protons combine with the bicarbonate that arrived from the tissues forming carbonic acid, which then enters the erythrocytes. Through a reversal of the carbonic anhydrase reaction, CO_2 and H_2O are produced. The CO_2 diffuses out of the blood, into the lung alveoli, and is released on expiration. The effects of hydrogen ion concentration on the O_2-binding affinity of hemoglobin are referred to as the *Bohr effect* (Figure 6-3).

$$CO_2 + \text{Hb-NH}_2 \leftrightarrow H^+ + \text{Hb-NH-COO}^-$$

Formation of carbaminohemoglobin

Coupled to the diffusion of bicarbonate out of erythrocytes in the tissues, there must be ion movement into the erythrocytes to maintain electrical neutrality. This is the role of Cl^- and is referred to as the *chloride shift*. In this way, Cl^- plays an important role in bicarbonate production and diffusion and thus also negatively influences O_2 binding to hemoglobin.

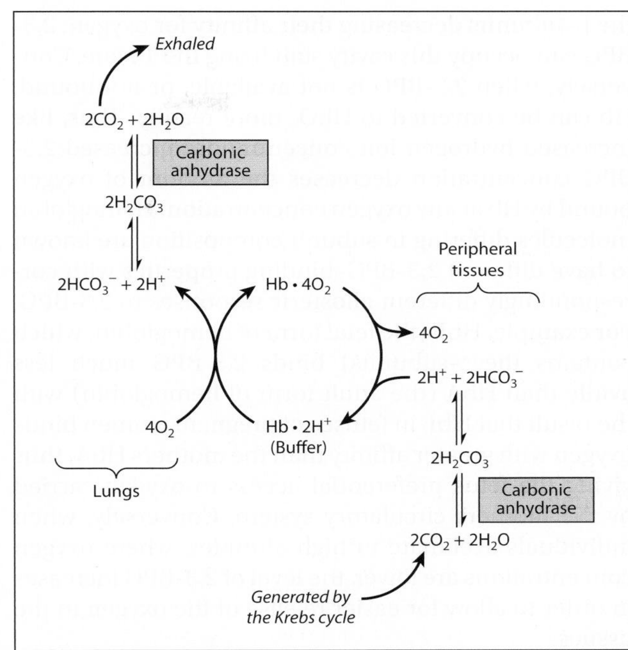

FIGURE 6-3: The Bohr effect. Carbon dioxide generated in peripheral tissues combines with water to form carbonic acid, which dissociates into protons and bicarbonate ions. Deoxyhemoglobin acts as a buffer by binding protons and delivering them to the lungs. In the lungs, the uptake of oxygen by hemoglobin releases protons that combine with bicarbonate ion, forming carbonic acid, which when dehydrated by carbonic anhydrase becomes carbon dioxide, which then is exhaled. Murray RK, Bender DA, Botham KM, Kennelly PJ, Rodwell VW, Weil PA. *Harper's Illustrated Biochemistry*, 29th ed. New York, NY: McGraw-Hill; 2012.

Role of 2,3-Bisphosphoglycerate

The compound 2,3-bisphosphoglycerate (2,3-BPG), derived from the glycolytic intermediate 1,3-bisphosphoglycerate, is a potent allosteric effector on the oxygen-binding properties of hemoglobin (Figure 6-4). In the dexoxygenated T state, a cavity forms in the center of the hemoglobin molecule allowing 2,3-BPG to bind to

High-Yield Concept

In addition to isohydric transport, as much as 15% of CO_2 is transported to the lungs bound to *N*-terminal amino groups of the T form of hemoglobin. This reaction forms what is called *carbaminohemoglobin*. The formation of H^+ via this reaction enhances the release of the bound O_2 to the surrounding tissues. Within the lungs, the high O_2 content results in O_2 binding to hemoglobin with the concomitant release of H^+. The released protons then promote the dissociation of the carbamino to form CO_2, which is then released with expiration.

the β-subunits decreasing their affinity for oxygen. 2,3-BPG can occupy this cavity stabilizing the T state. Conversely, when 2,3-BPG is not available, or not bound, Hb can be converted to HbO_2 more readily. Thus, like increased hydrogen ion concentration, increased 2,3-BPG concentration decreases the amount of oxygen bound by Hb at any oxygen concentration. Hemoglobin molecules differing in subunit composition are known to have different 2,3-BPG–binding properties with correspondingly different allosteric responses to 2,3-BPG. For example, HbF (the fetal form of hemoglobin, which contains the γ-subunits) binds 2,3-BPG much less avidly than HbA (the adult form of hemoglobin) with the result that HbF in fetuses of pregnant women binds oxygen with greater affinity than the mothers HbA, thus giving the fetus preferential access to oxygen carried by the mothers circulatory system. Conversely, when individuals acclimate to high altitudes, where oxygen concentrations are lower, the level of 2,3-BPG increases in order to allow for easier release of the oxygen to the tissues.

The Hemoglobin Genes

The α- and β-globin proteins contained in functional hemoglobin tetramers are derived from gene clusters. The *α-globin* genes are on chromosome 16 and the *β-globin* genes are on chromosome 11 (Figure 6-4). Both gene clusters contain not only the major adult genes, α and β, but other expressed sequences that are utilized at different stages of development. In addition to functional genes, both clusters contain nonfunctional pseudogenes.

Hemoglobin synthesis begins in the first few weeks of embryonic development within the yolk sac (Figure 6-5). The major hemoglobin at this stage of development is a tetramer composed of 2 zeta (ζ) chains encoded within the α-cluster and 2 epsilon (ε) chains from the β-cluster. By 6 to 8 weeks of gestation, the expression of this version of hemoglobin declines dramatically coinciding with the change in hemoglobin synthesis from the yolk sac to the liver. Expression from the α-cluster consists of identical proteins from the α_1 and α_2 genes and this cluster remains on throughout life.

Within the β-globin cluster there is an additional set of genes, the fetal *β-globin* genes identified as the *gamma* (γ) genes. The 2 fetal genes called *G*γ and *A*γ, the derivation of which stems from the single amino acid difference between the 2 fetal genes: glycine in Gγ and alanine in Aγ at position 136. These fetal γ genes are expressed as the embryonic genes are turned off. Shortly before birth there is a smooth switch from fetal *γ-globin* gene expression to adult *β-globin* gene expression. The switch from fetal γ- to adult *β-globin* does not directly coincide with the switch from hepatic synthesis to bone marrow synthesis since at birth it can be shown that both γ and β synthesis is occurring in the marrow.

The 2 predominant forms of hemoglobin are: (1) fetal, designated HbF, and (2) adult, designated HbA. Fetal hemoglobin consists of both $\alpha_2G\gamma_2$ and $\alpha_2A\gamma_2$ tetramers. Adult hemoglobin (more commonly HbA_1) is a tetramer of 2 α- and 2 β-chains. A minor adult hemoglobin, identified as HbA_2, is a tetramer of 2 α-chains and 2 δ-chains. The δ gene is expressed with a timing similar to the β gene, but because the promoter has acquired a number of mutations its efficiency of transcription is reduced. The overall hemoglobin composition in a normal adult is approximately 97.5% HbA_1, 2% HbA_2, and 0.5% HbF (Figure 6-6).

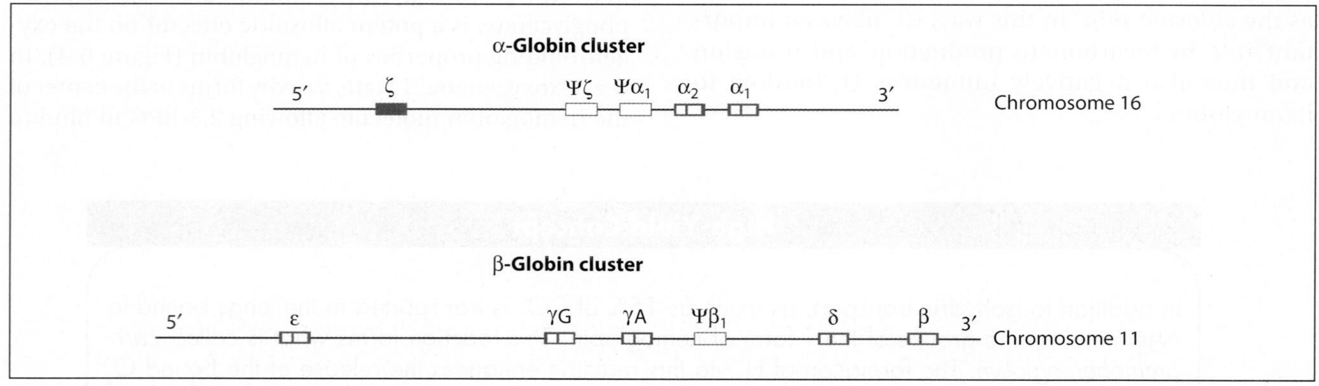

FIGURE 6-4: Chromosomal structure of the α- and β-*globin* gene clusters on chromosomes 16 and 11, respectively. The 5′ to 3′ orientation of the genes on each chromosome also reflects the developmental timing of their expression with the 5′-most genes expressed earliest. The ζ (zeta) and ε (epsilon) genes are the embryonic genes in each cluster. Genes with a Ψ (psi) designation represent pseudogenes. Reproduced with permission of themedicalbiochemistrypage, LLC.

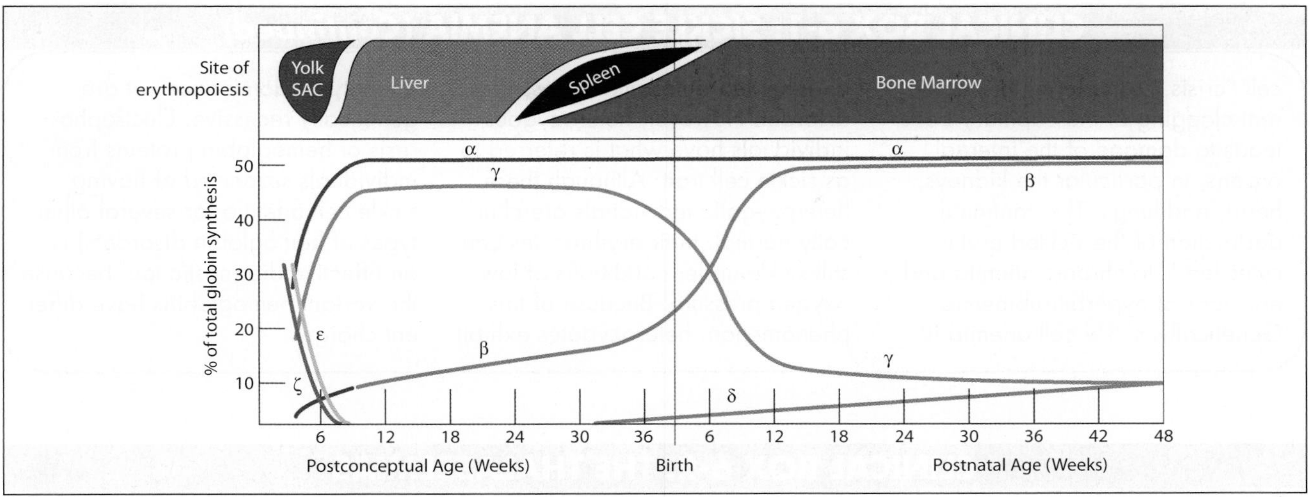

FIGURE 6-5: Developmental patterns of globin gene expression. Reproduced with permission of themedicalbiochemistrypage, LLC.

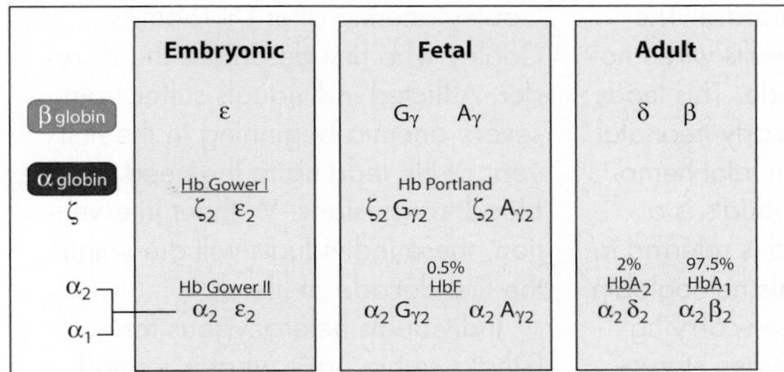

FIGURE 6-6: Major types of hemoglobins found during embryonic, fetal, and adult life. Reproduced with permission of themedicalbiochemistrypage, LLC.

The Hemoglobinopathies

The term hemoglobinopathy refers to any of several types of gene defect in the hemoglobin genes that result in the synthesis of abnormal or reduced levels of one of the globin chains of the hemoglobin molecule (see Clinical Boxes 6-1 and 6-2). Hemoglobinopathies are classified dependent upon whether the defect results in reduced (quantitative) or altered (qualitative) hemoglobin. More commonly, the term hemoglobinopathy is used to imply structural abnormalities in the globin proteins themselves. In contrast, the term thalassemia

CLINICAL BOX 6-1: SICKLE CELL ANEMIA

A large number of mutations have been described in the globin genes. These mutations can be divided into 2 distinct types: those that cause qualitative abnormalities (eg, sickle cell anemia) and those that cause quantitative abnormalities (the thalassemias). Taken together these disorders are referred to as the hemoglobinopathies. Of the mutations leading to qualitative alterations in hemoglobin, the missense mutation in the β-*globin* gene that causes sickle cell anemia is the most common. The mutation causing sickle cell anemia is a single-nucleotide substitution (A-T) in the codon for amino acid 6. The change converts a glutamic acid codon (GAG) to a valine codon (GTG). The form of hemoglobin in persons with sickle cell anemia is referred to as HbS. An additional relatively common mutation at codon 6 is the conversion to a lysine codon (AAG) which results in the generation of a variant hemoglobin called HbC.

The underlying problem in sickle cell anemia is that the valine for glutamic acid substitution results in hemoglobin tetramers that aggregate into arrays upon deoxygenation in the tissues. This aggregation leads to deformation of the erythrocyte into the characteristic sickle shape. The repeated cycles of oxygenation and deoxygenation lead to irreversible sickling of erythrocytes. These distorted erythrocytes are relatively inflexible and unable to traverse the capillary beds. The result is clogging of the fine capillaries such as those in the retina of the eye. In addition to their altered shape and poor capillary migration, sickled erythrocytes are weak and lyse very easily. Because bones are particularly affected by the reduced blood flow, frequent and severe bone pain results. This is the typical symptom during a sickle

CLINICAL BOX 6-1: SICKLE CELL ANEMIA (*Continued*)

cell "crisis." Long term, the recurrent clogging of the capillary beds leads to damage of the internal organs, in particular the kidneys, heart, and lungs. The continual destruction of the sickled erythrocytes leads to chronic anemia and episodes of hyperbilirubinemia. Genetically, sickle cell anemia is an inherited autosomal recessive disorder. However, heterozygous individuals have what is referred to as sickle cell trait. Although these heterozygotic individuals are clinically normal, their erythrocytes can still sickle under conditions of low oxygen pressure. Because of this phenomenon, heterozygotes exhibit phenotypic dominance yet are genetically recessive. Electrophoresis of hemoglobin proteins from individuals suspected of having sickle cell anemia (or several other types of hemoglobin disorders) is an effective diagnostic tool because the variant hemoglobins have different charges.

CLINICAL BOX 6-2: THE THALASSEMIAS

The thalassemias represent quantitative hemoglobinopathies resulting from abnormalities in the synthesis of either the a-globin or b-globin proteins. Deficiencies in β-globin synthesis result in the β-thalassemias and deficiencies in α-globin synthesis result in the α-thalassemias.

In the α-thalassemias, normal amounts of β-globin protein are made and they are capable of forming homotetramers ($β_4$). These tetramers are designated hemoglobin H, HbH. An excess of HbH in the erythrocytes leads to the formation of inclusion bodies commonly seen in patients with α-thalassemia. In addition, the HbH tetramers have a markedly reduced oxygen-carrying capacity. With the α-thalassemias, the level of α-globin production can range from none to very nearly normal levels. This is due in part to the fact that there are 2 identical *α-globin* genes on chromosome 16. Thus, the α-thalassemias involve inactivation of 1 to all 4 *α-globin* genes. If 3 of the 4 *α-globin* genes are functional, individuals are completely asymptomatic. This situation is identified as the "silent carrier" state or sometimes as α-thalassemia 2. If 2 of the 4 genes are inactivated, individuals are designated as α-thalassemia trait or as α-thalassemia 1. The phenotype of α-thalassemia 1 is relatively benign. The clinical situation becomes more severe if only 1 of the 4 *α-globin* genes is functional. In this latter circumstance, a high level of HbH results and the disorder is referred to as HbH disease. The most severe situation results when no α-globin chains are made. This leads to prenatal lethality or early neonatal death. The predominant fetal hemoglobin in afflicted individuals is a tetramer of γ-chains and is referred to as hemoglobin Bart. This hemoglobin has essentially no oxygen-carrying capacity resulting in oxygen starvation in the fetal tissues. Heart failure results as the heart tries to pump the unoxygenated blood to oxygen-starved tissues leading to marked edema defined as hydrops fetalis.

In β-thalassemia, where the *β-globins* are deficient, the α-globins are in excess and will form *α-globin* homotetramers. The α-globin homotetramers are extremely insoluble, which leads to premature erythrocyte destruction in the bone marrow and spleen. A large number of mutations have been identified leading to decreased or absent production of β-globin chains resulting in the β-thalassemias. In the most severe situation mutations in both the maternal and paternal *β-globin* genes leads to loss of normal amounts of β-globin protein. A complete lack of HbA is denoted as $β^0$-thalassemia. If one or the other mutations allows production of a small amount of functional β-globin then the disorder is denoted as $β^+$-thalassemia. Both $β^0$- and $β^+$-thalassemias are referred to as thalassemia major, also called Cooley anemia after Dr Thomas Cooley who first described the disorder. Afflicted individuals suffer from severe anemia beginning in the first year of life leading to the need for blood transfusions. Without intervention, these individuals will die within the first decade of life.

Individuals heterozygous for β-thalassemia have what is termed thalassemia minor. Afflicted individuals harbor one normal *β-globin* gene and one that harbors a mutation leading to production of reduced or no β-globin. Individuals that do not make any functional β-globin protein from one gene are termed $β^0$-heterozygotes. If β-globin production is reduced at one locus, the individuals are termed $β^+$-heterozygotes. Thalassemia minor individuals are generally asymptomatic. The term *thalassemia intermedia* is used to designate individuals with significant anemia but unlike thalassemia major do not require transfusions. This syndrome results in individuals where both *β-globin* genes express reduced amounts of protein or where one gene makes none and the other makes a mildly reduced amount. A person who is a compound heterozygote with α-thalassemia and $β^+$-thalassemia will also manifest as thalassemia intermedia.

is used to define hemoglobinopathies that are due to underproduction of normal globin proteins. The 2 conditions may overlap, however, since some conditions which cause abnormalities in globin proteins also affect their production which means that some hemoglobinopathies are also thalassemias.

REVIEW QUESTIONS

1. A 4-year-old patient is presented in the pediatric clinic with microcytic anemia. An analysis of his blood by non-denaturing electrophoresis reveals the following composition of hemoglobin isoforms: HbF = 75%, HbA_1 = 23%, HbA_2 = 2%, and HbS = 0%. Using these data, it is possible to determine that the infant is most likely homozygous for which of the following?
A. complete deletion of the α-globin locus
B. complete deletion of the β-globin locus
C. mutation in the promoter of the β-globin genes
D. nonsense mutation in the *α-globin* genes
E. nonsense mutation in the *β-globin* genes

Answer C: A mutation in the promoter region of the *β-globin* genes would result in reduced expression. This is evidenced by the lower than normal amount of HbA_1 in this child. Under these circumstances the body will tend to compensate by continuing to express the fetal hemoglobin genes at higher than normal levels resulting in potentially dramatic increases in measured HbF. Normal levels of HbF in a 4-year-old child would be around 0% to 2%, whereas, this child shows significant increase in HbF of 75%.

2. When the malarial parasite invades a red blood cell, its metabolic waste products result in the acidification of the cytoplasm. Which of the following best describes the consequences of this acidification on the activity of hemoglobin (Hb)?
A. formation of carbaminohemoglobin is enhanced
B. hemoglobin tetramers become less stable and the complex dissociates
C. there is a shift to a more R state conformation
D. there is a shift to a more T state conformation
E. there is no effect from the acidification

Answer D: The principal negative regulator of the affinity of hemoglobin for oxygen is proton, H^+. The acidification of the erythrocyte cytoplasm by malarial parasite metabolism would be reflected by a significant increase in [H^+] which would, in turn, result in a higher level of T state hemoglobin.

3. In one form of β-thalassemia, patients have significantly reduced levels of β-globin transcripts. Notably these β-globin transcripts are less than half the length of the normal β-globin mRNA. These patients exhibit elevated levels of HbF and no detectable HbA_1. Which of the following best explains the molecular reason for these observations?
A. addition of 7-methylguanosine to the β-globin mRNA
B. covalent modification of the β-globin protein
C. improper folding of the β-globin protein
D. promoter mutations in the β-globin gene
E. splicing alteration of the β-globin mRNA

Answer E: Numerous β-thalassemias result from mutations in the sequences that control proper splicing of the β-globin transcript. These mutations lead to β-globin mRNAs that are shorter or longer than the normal β-globin mRNA. Although mutations in the promoter region of the *β-globin* gene will lead to reduced levels of expression and thus, to reduced levels of β-globin mRNA, they generally do not result in mRNAs that are shorter than normal.

4. Although HbF represents fetal hemoglobin, some level of this form of hemoglobin persists in the adult. Which of the following represents the value for HbF in adults above which it would likely reflect some underlying pathophysiology?
A. 0.1%
B. 0.5%
C. 2.0%
D. 5.0%
E. 15%

Answer B: Normal levels of HbF in the adult are between 0% and 0.5%. An increase in HbF levels in the adult would result from circumstances where a decrease in the expression of the normal HbA_1 was evident. The increase in HbF results from a compensatory mechanism that is attempting to normalize the amount of oxygen carrying hemoglobin in the blood.

5. You are treating a patient who presents with microcytic anemia. Additional microscopic findings demonstrate the presence of inclusion bodies in the red blood cells. Electrophoresis of erythrocyte protein extracts shows a large excess of β-globins and a near complete lack of α-globins. Which of the following disorders most closely correlates to your findings?
A. hemoglobin H disease
B. hereditary persistence of fetal hemoglobin
C. hydrops fetalis
D. sickle cell anemia
E. β-thalassemia major

Answer A: The α-thalassemias result when there is reduced expression at one or both of the *α-globin* genes. In the α-thalassemias, normal amounts of β-globins are made. The β-globin proteins are capable of forming homotetramers (β_4) and these tetramers are called hemoglobin H, HbH. An excess of HbH in red blood cells leads to the formation of inclusion bodies commonly seen in patients with α-thalassemia. In addition, the HbH tetramers have a markedly reduced oxygen-carrying capacity. In β-thalassemia, where the β-globins are deficient, the α-globins are in excess and will form α-globin homotetramers. The α-globin homotetramers are extremely insoluble which leads to premature red cell destruction in the bone marrow and spleen. Clinically this is referred to as hemoglobin H disease.

6. You are studying the oxygen-binding characteristics of a synthetic oxygen transport compound. You want to design the compound so that it most closely mimics the oxygen affinity of native hemoglobin protein. If you are successful, addition of which of the following to a test solution would have the greatest negative effect on the ability of your compound to bind oxygen?

A. 2,3-BPG
B. bicarbonate ion
C. carbonic acid
D. phosphoric acid
E. water

Answer C: Addition of carbonic acid (H_2CO_3) to the solution would result in its ionization to bicarbonate (HCO_3^-) and proton (H^+). The increase in H^+ would, therefore, be expected to exert a large negative effect on oxygen binding by the synthetic hemoglobin construct just as is the case for the negative effect of increasing H^+ on the affinity of hemoglobin for oxygen.

7. Which of the following is referred to as a qualitative hemoglobinopathy?

A. hemoglobin H disease
B. hydrops fetalis
C. sickle cell anemia
D. α-thalassemia
E. β-thalassemia

Answer C: Sickle cell anemia results from a single nucleotide mutation in the *β-globin* gene resulting in a single amino acid change in the protein. There is no effect of this mutation on the amount (quantitative) of the mutant β-globin protein. The defect is manifest in a change in the character (qualitative) of the resultant β-globin protein. When in the deoxy state, this hemoglobin sticks together resulting in long polymers that distort the shape of the erythrocyte.

8. Aside from the obvious presence of HbS hemoglobin in individuals with sickle cell disease, which of the following hemoglobins is also found at high frequency in these individuals?

A. HbA_{1c}
B. HbA_2
C. HbC
D. HbF
E. HbH

Answer D: The presence of the HbS hemoglobin in the erythrocytes of sickle cell patients leads to reduced overall oxygen-carrying capacity. This results in a compensatory increase in the expression of fetal hemoglobin (HbF) in an attempt to increase oxygen capacity.

9. Which of the following is the primary source of the H^+ that leads to displacement of O_2 from hemoglobin in the tissues?

A. 2,3-BPG
B. bicarbonate ion
C. carbonic acid
D. phosphoric acid
E. water

Answer C: When the CO_2 from metabolism is released to the circulation, it enters the erythrocyte and is converted to carbonic acid via the actions of carbonic anhydrase. The carbonic acid then dissociates to H^+ and HCO_3^-. The resulting increase in H^+ inside the erythrocyte in the capillaries of the tissues reduces oxygen-binding affinity and the hemoglobin thus releases the bound oxygen to the tissues.

10. The "Bohr effect" is best described by which of the following statements?

A. binding of O_2
B. covalent attachment of CO_2 forming hemoglobin carbamate
C. release of O_2 from hemoglobin in response to the buffering of Cl^- by hemoglobin
D. release of CO_2 from erythrocytes when they enter the high O_2 concentration of the alveoli
E. release of O_2 from hemoglobin in response to the buffering of H^+ by hemoglobin

Answer E: The Bohr effect is the physiological phenomenon, first described by Christian Bohr, describing that the affinity of hemoglobin for oxygen is inversely related both to acidity and to the concentration of CO_2. A decrease in blood pH or an increase in blood CO_2 concentration will result in hemoglobin proteins releasing their oxygen and a decrease in carbon dioxide or increase in pH will result in hemoglobin picking up more oxygen. Since carbon dioxide reacts with water to form carbonic acid, an increase in CO_2 results in a decrease in blood pH.

11. Beta-thalassemias are genetic disorders in the synthesis of the β-globin chains in hemoglobin. Affected individuals usually begin to exhibit some degree of anemia at about 6 months of age. Therapy for severe anemia involves multiple transfusions. What is the most serious complication of transfusion therapy?

A. cardiac arrhythmias
B. copper overload
C. globin overload
D. increased blood viscosity
E. iron overload

Answer E: Iron is primarily absorbed from the diet, in the duodenum, as either organic or heme-bound forms. Inside the enterocyte the iron binds to cytoplasmic proteins, ferritin, and mobilferrin. Depending on total body iron stores, the iron is either transferred to the plasma, where it binds to plasma transferrin, or it remains in the enterocyte until it is lost with cell shedding. Once absorbed, iron is avidly retained by the body. An adult male excretes only about 0.03% of his total body stores per day (about 1 mg), while the loss in premenopausal women is still only about twice that amount. Blood normally contains 15 g of hemoglobin per 100 mL. The concentration of hemoglobin in blood is thus about 2.3 millimolar (mM). Since each molecule of hemoglobin contains 4 molecules of iron, the total blood iron concentration is almost 10 mM. A transfusion of 1 unit of packed red blood cells (about 500 mL) would thus add a total iron burden of about 250 mg. Given the body's limited excretory capacity, multiple transfusions can elevate iron to toxic levels. The liver is particularly susceptible to damage.

12. The thermodynamics of oxygen binding to hemoglobin are highly ordered. Which of the following reflects the physical characteristics relating the binding of O_2 to hemoglobin?

A. causes a large shift of the surrounding secondary structures leading to decreased affinity of the deoxy subunits for CO_2
B. is cooperative, meaning that after the first O_2 binds, the other subunits are more readily oxygenated
C. occurs with equal affinity at all 4 subunits
D. results in a release of the heme from the interior to the exterior of the α-subunits, leading to an increase in O_2 affinity of the β-subunits
E. results in a release of the heme from the interior to the exterior of the β-subunits leading to an increase in O_2 affinity of the α-subunits

Answer B: The binding of oxygen by hemoglobin exhibits a characteristic cooperative property. The first molecule of oxygen to bind requires a high partial pressure of oxygen. The binding of that oxygen changes the conformation of the hemoglobin molecule such that the second oxygen binds more easily, and so on. When the binding characteristics of hemoglobin are plotted one sees a typical sigmoidal curve, indicative of cooperativity.

13. Carbon monoxide (CO) poisoning is a significant cause of mortality in the United States. Which of the following statements about CO is correct?

A. competes with CO_2 for a common binding site on hemoglobin
B. competes with O_2 for a common binding site on hemoglobin
C. has a lower affinity for hemoglobin than does O_2
D. irreversibly binds to hemoglobin
E. is normally a perfusion-limited gas

Answer B: Carbon monoxide competes with oxygen binding to hemoglobin by binding in the same pocket of the protein. However, it forms such a strong bond with the iron in the heme that the binding is irreversible. Thus, high concentrations of CO rapidly use up the body's limited supply of hemoglobin molecules, and prevent them from binding to oxygen. Hemoglobin-binding affinity for CO is 200 times greater than its affinity for oxygen, meaning that small amounts of CO dramatically reduces hemoglobin's ability to transport oxygen.

14. A 35-year-old apparently healthy man undergoes a medical examination while applying for life insurance. He is not anemic. His hemoglobin electrophoresis is reported as: HbA_1, 62%; HbS, 35%; HbF, 1%; HbA_2, 1%; no variant C, D, G, or H bands are detected. The most likely diagnosis is which of the following?

A. sickle cell disease
B. sickle thalassemia minor
C. sickle trait
D. thalassemia major
E. thalassemia minor

Answer C: Individuals with sickle trait are healthy and not anemic. Hemoglobin electrophoresis demonstrates a minor proportion of hemoglobin

S (HbS) and a major proportion of hemoglobin A (HbA_1). Fetal hemoglobin (HbF) and HbA_2 are usually normal. Sickle trait confers the benefit of protecting erythrocytes from some forms of malarial infection. About 9% of African Americans in the United States have sickle trait. Conversely, in sickle cell disease almost all hemoglobin is HbS, no HbA_1 is detected, and patients have a clinical history of severe anemia. Sickle thalassemia minor presents as a chronic microcytic anemia with a major HbS component and elevated HbA_2.

15. You are a third-year emergency room (ER) resident tending to a 48-year-old woman who has come to the ER complaining of increasing fatigue and mild shortness of breath. Blood work reveals a hypochromic anemia with a hemoglobin of 10.4 g/dL, MCV of 76 μ/m^3, MCHC of 29 g/dL, and a decrease in the absolute reticulocyte count. WBC and platelet counts are within normal limits. Serum iron and ferritin levels are low and total iron-binding capacity is elevated. Which of the following conditions best accounts for these findings?

A. anemia of chronic disease
B. aplastic anemia
C. hypothyroidism
D. iron deficiency
E. pernicious anemia

Answer D: Laboratory findings of a hypochromic anemia with a decrease in MCV and MCHC indices and a decreased reticulocyte count suggest a hypoproliferative anemia. The various microcytic, hypochromic anemias belong to this category and a partial differential diagnosis for these includes iron deficiency anemia, anemia of chronic disease (ACD), thalassemias, and sideroblastic anemias. ACD can be distinguished from iron deficiency anemia by the additional iron studies that were performed in this case. While serum iron and ferritin levels are low and total iron-binding capacity (TIBC) is elevated in iron deficiency anemia, in ACD ferritin is typically normal or elevated, iron is low, and TIBC is low.

16. A 27-year-old female who is 5 months pregnant has come to her ob-gyn due to a fear that something wrong with her baby. Following her previous routine visit she noted that her baby was moving frequently but in the past 2 days she has not felt any movements. Her physician performs a routine physical exam and notes that the fetal heart rate is tachycardic. The physician orders an ultrasound and during this exam notes a significant pleural and pericardial effusion. A diagnosis of potential hydrops fetalis is made with additional diagnostic tests ordered. Which of the following is most closely associated with non-immune (Rh)-mediated hydrops fetalis?

A. Cooley's anemia
B. hemoglobin Barts
C. hemoglobin H disease
D. thalassemia major
E. thalassemia minor

Answer B: Hydrops fetalis is the result of the loss of expression of all four copies of the a-globin gene. This leads to a loss of any functional embryonic or fetal hemoglobin tetramers being synthesized. Instead, the fetus expresses only the gamma (γ) globin gene which forms homotetramers that are referred to as hemoglobin Barts. This hemoglobin has very high affinity for oxygen resulting in poor oxygen release and thus, oxygen starvation in the fetal tissues. Heart failure results as the heart tries to pump more oxygenated blood to oxygen starved tissues leading to marked edema evidence as pleural and pericardial effusions by ultrasound.

17. Hemoglobin and myoglobin are proteins composed primarily of which of the following types of secondary structures?

A. amide bond
B. disulfide bond
C. α-helix
D. β-pleated sheet
E. triple helix

Answer C: Both hemoglobin and myoglobin structure are determined by the high degree of α-helices present in these proteins. Indeed, most of the amino acids in hemoglobin form α-helixes, connected by short nonhelical segments.

18. Sickle cell disease is associated with a mutated form of hemoglobin (HbS) that aggregates to produce long rods within erythrocytes. Which of the following best explains how the mutation leads to aggregation of HbS?

A. creation of a hydrophobic area on the surface of the β-chain
B. creation of an abnormal ratio of α-chains to β-chains
C. prevention of assembly of β-chains with α-chains
D. prevention of β-chain from binding heme
E. production of a truncated β-chain

Answer A: HbS is the form of hemoglobin that results due to a missense mutation in the *β-globin* gene that causes sickle cell anemia. The mutation causing sickle cell anemia is a single nucleotide substitution (A-T) in the codon for amino acid 6. The change converts a glutamic acid codon (GAG) to a valine codon (GTG). Whereas, glutamate is an acidic and hydrophilic amino acid, leucine is hydrophobic. The presentation of this hydrophilic amino acid on the surface of the hemoglobin protein when in the deoxy state allows the proteins to aggregate via hydrophobic interactions. This aggregation leads to deformation of the erythrocyte, making it relatively inflexible and unable to traverse the capillary beds.

19. Which of the following types of bonds is primarily responsible for the aberrant aggregation of deoxy HbS molecules resulting from the glutamate to valine mutation in the sixth position of the β-globin chain?

A. amide
B. covalent
C. disulfide
D. hydrophobic
E. ionic

Answer D: HbS is the form of hemoglobin that results due to a missense mutation in the β-*globin* gene that causes sickle cell anemia. The mutation causing sickle cell anemia is a single nucleotide substitution (A-T) in the codon for amino acid 6. The change converts a glutamic acid codon (GAG) to a valine codon (GTG). Whereas, glutamate is an acidic and hydrophilic amino acid, leucine is hydrophobic. The presentation of this hydrophilic amino acid on the surface of the hemoglobin protein when in the deoxy state allows the proteins to aggregate via hydrophobic interactions. This aggregation leads to deformation of the erythrocyte making it relatively inflexible and unable to traverse the capillary beds.

20. During an experiment on hemoglobin function, knockout mice that are unable to synthesize globin proteins are created. Absence of which of the following globin proteins is most likely to be incompatible with life in these mice?

A. α
B. β
C. δ
D. γ

Answer A: The α-thalassemias result when there is reduced expression at one or both of the α-*globin* genes. In the α-thalassemias normal amounts of β-globin are made. The β-globin proteins are capable of forming homotetramers (β_4), and these tetramers are called hemoglobin H (HbH). An excess of HbH in red blood cells leads to the formation of inclusion bodies commonly seen in patients with α-thalassemia. In addition, the HbH tetramers have a markedly reduced oxygen-carrying capacity. High level of HbH results in the disorder known as HbH disease.

Checklist

✓ Myoglobin and hemoglobin are the oxygen-carrying proteins of the body. Myoglobin is a monomeric protein and hemoglobin is a heterotetrameric protein.

✓ Both myoglobin and hemoglobin contain the prosthetic group, heme, required for oxygen binding.

✓ Myoglobin binds oxygen with hyperbolic kinetics, whereas hemoglobin binds oxygen cooperatively and thus demonstrates sigmoidal-binding characteristics.

✓ Hemoglobin binds oxygen with reduced affinity in the low-oxygen environment of the tissues but with high affinity in the high oxygen pressures of the lungs.

✓ The affinity of hemoglobin for oxygen is controlled by several factors including hydrogen ion concentration, the partial pressure of CO_2, the level of chloride ion, and the concentration of bound 2,3-bisphosphoglycerate.

✓ Mutations in the genes encoding both the α-globin and β-globin proteins have been identified and these mutations are classified as to whether they result in decreased function (qualitative) or decreased amounts (quantitative) of hemoglobin tetramers.

✓ The most common qualitative hemoglobinopathy is sickle cell anemia, resulting from a single mutation in the adult β-*globin* gene.

✓ Quantitative hemoglobinopathies are referred to as the thalassemias and reflect defects in either the α-*globin* (α-thalassemias) or β-*globin* (β-thalassemias) genes.

CHAPTER

7 Biological Membranes and Membrane Transport

CHAPTER OUTLINE

High-Yield Terms

Lipid bilayer: a thin polar membrane made of 2 layers of lipid molecules

Integral membrane protein: a protein molecule that is permanently attached to the biological membrane

Peripheral membrane protein: a protein that adheres only temporarily to the biological membrane with which it is associated

Endoplasmic reticulum (ER): the ER functions as a packaging system working in concert with the Golgi apparatus, to create a network of membranes found throughout the whole cell

Golgi apparatus: the Golgi apparatus packages proteins inside the cell before they are sent to their destination; it is particularly important in the processing of proteins for secretion

Apical membrane: the layer of plasma membrane on the side toward the lumen of the epithelial cells

Basolateral membrane: the fraction of the plasma membrane at the basolateral side of the cell which faces adjacent cells and the underlying connective tissue

Gap junctions: intercellular channels designed for intercellular communication

Tight junctions: barriers that regulate the movement of solutes and water between various epithelial layers

Antiporter: protein or complex that couples the transport of 2 compounds across a membrane in opposite directions

Uniporter: protein or complex that transports 1 molecule of solute at a time down the solute gradient

Symporter: protein or complex that couples the transport of 2 compounds across a membrane in the same direction

Aquaporins: membrane water channels that facilitate rapid, highly selective water transport

Na^+/K^+-ATPases: membrane transporters that utilize the energy of ATP hydrolysis to transport sodium into and potassium out of a cell

Cardiotonic steroids: endogenous digitalis-like factors that inhibit the Na^+/K^+-ATPases

ABC family transporters: ATP-binding cassette transporters that couple the energy of ATP binding and hydrolysis to substrate transport

SLC family transporters: solute carrier transporters that include transporters that function by secondary active transport and facilitative diffusion

High-Yield Concept

The lipids that make up the components of membranes are of three major classes: glycerophospholipids, sphingolipids, and cholesterol.

Composition and Structure of Biological Membranes

Biological membranes are composed of lipid, protein, and carbohydrate that exist in a fluid state. Biological membranes are the structures that define and control the composition of the space that they enclose. All membranes exist as dynamic structures whose composition changes throughout the life of a cell. In addition to the outer membrane that results in the formation of a typical cell (this membrane is often referred to as the plasma membrane), cells contain intracellular membranes that serve distinct functions in the formation of the various intracellular organelles, for example, the nucleus and the mitochondria.

Sphingolipids and glycerophospholipids constitute the largest percentage of the lipid weight of biological membranes. The hydrocarbon tails of these two classes of lipid result in steric limitations to their packing such that they will form disk-like micelles. The structure of these micelles results from the interactions of the hydrophobic tails of the lipids and the exposure of the polar head groups to the aqueous environment. This orientation results in what is referred to as a lipid bilayer (Figure 7-1).

Lipid bilayers are essentially 2-dimensional fluids and the lipid components of the bilayer can diffuse laterally, and in fact evidence demonstrates that this lateral diffusion occurs readily. Lipids in the bilayer can also undergo transverse diffusion (also called a flip-flop) where the lipid diffuses from one surface to the other.

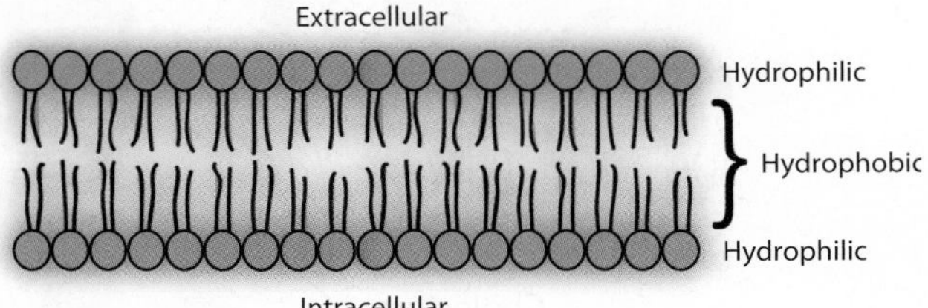

FIGURE 7-1: Diagrammatic representation of a section of a lipid bilayer composed of phospholipids. The hydrophobic fatty acids orient toward the middle of the bilayer, whereas the hydrophilic polar head groups orient toward the aqueous environment. Reproduced with permission of themedicalbiochemistrypage, LLC.

However, because the flip-flop requires the polar head group to pass through the hydrocarbon core of the bilayer, the process is extremely rare. Enzymes have been identified that facilitate the flip-flop process and these enzymes are referred to as flippases.

The carbohydrates of membranes are attached either to lipid, forming glycolipids of various classes, or to proteins forming glycoproteins. The lipid and protein compositions of membranes vary from cell type to cell type as well as within the various intracellular compartments that are defined by intracellular membranes. Protein concentrations can range from around 20% to as much as 70% of the total mass of a particular membrane.

Biological membranes also contain proteins, glycoproteins, and glycolipids.

High-Yield Concept

Proteins associated with membranes are of 2 general types: (1) integral and (2) peripheral (Figure 7-2). Integral membrane proteins (also called intrinsic proteins) are tightly bound to the membrane through hydrophobic interactions and are inserted into and/or penetrate the lipid bilayer. In contrast, peripheral membrane proteins (also called extrinsic proteins) are only loosely associated with the membrane either through interactions with the polar head groups of the lipids or through interactions with integral membrane proteins.

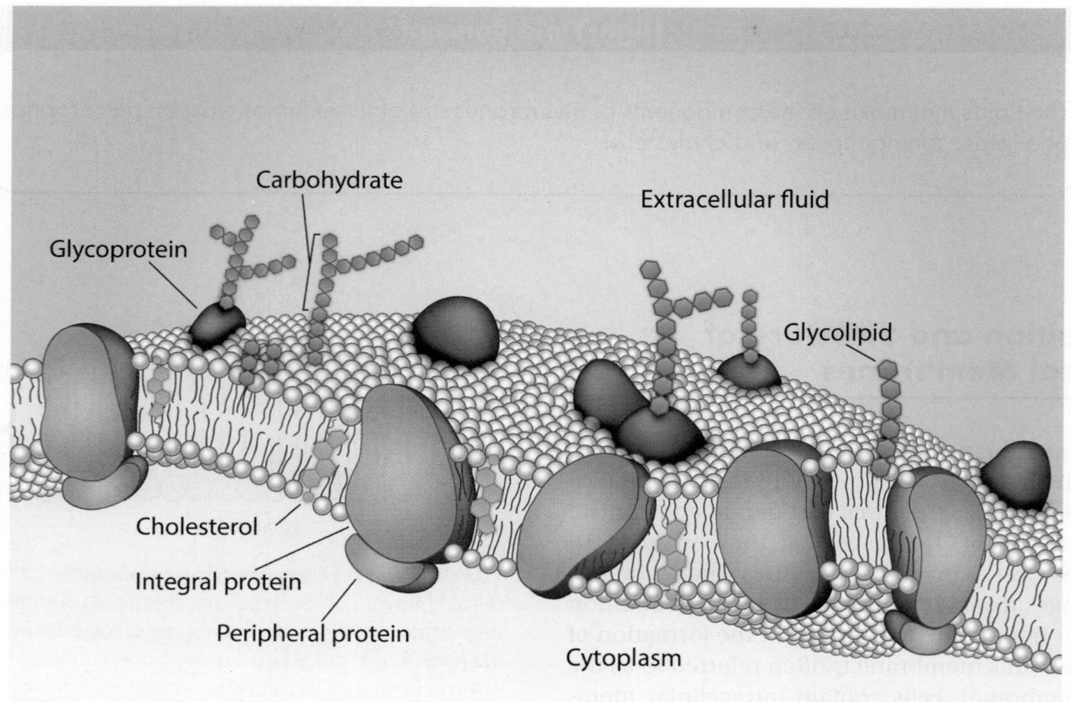

FIGURE 7-2: Structure of the typical lipid bilayer of the plasma membrane. Integral proteins are those that pass through the bilayer. Peripheral proteins are associated with the inner surface of the plasma membrane. Most integral proteins are modified by carbohydrate addition to their extracellular domains. Membranes also contain carbohydrate-modified lipids (glycolipids) in addition to the more common phospholipids and cholesterol that constitute the bulk of the lipid content of the membrane. Reproduced with permission of themedicalbiochemistrypage, LLC.

Peripheral membrane proteins are most often, if not exclusively, found on the cytosolic face of the plasma membrane or the luminal surface of subcellular organelle membranes.

Proteins that are found associated with membranes can also be modified by lipid attachment (lipoproteins). The lipid portion of a lipoprotein anchors the protein to the membrane either through interaction with the lipid bilayer directly or through interactions with integral membrane proteins. Lipoproteins associated with membranes contain 1 of 3 types of covalent lipid attachment. The lipids are isoprenoids such as farnesyl and geranylgeranyl residues (see Chapter 37 for the mechanism of protein prenylation), fatty acids such as myristic and palmitic acid, and glycosylphosphatidylinositol, GPI (termed glipiated proteins) (see Chapter 38 for details).

Activities of Biological Membranes

Although biological membranes contain various types of lipids and proteins, their distribution between the two different sides of the bilayer is asymmetric. As a general example, the outer surface of the bilayer is enriched in phosphatidylethanolamine (PE), whereas the intracellular surface is enriched in phosphatidylcholine (PC). Carbohydrates, whether attached to lipid or protein, are almost exclusively found on the external surfaces of membranes. The asymmetric distribution of lipids and proteins in membranes results in the generation of highly specialized subdomains within membranes. In addition, there are highly specialized membrane structures such as the endoplasmic reticulum (ER), the Golgi apparatus, and vesicles (eg, endosomes and lysosomes). The most important vesicles are those that contain secreted factors. Membrane-bound proteins (eg, growth factor receptors) are processed as they transit through the ER to the Golgi apparatus and finally to the plasma membrane. As these proteins transit to the surface of the cell, they undergo a series of processing events that include glycosylation.

The vesicles that pinch off from the Golgi apparatus are termed coated vesicles. The membranes of coated vesicles are surrounded by specialized scaffolding proteins that will interact with the extracellular environment. There are 3 major types of coated vesicles that are characterized by their protein coats.

High-Yield Concept

Clathrin-coated vesicles contain the protein clathrin and are involved in transmembrane protein, GPI-linked protein, and secreted protein transit to the plasma membrane.

High-Yield Concept

The membrane surface of cells that interacts with luminal contents is referred to as the apical surface or domain, the rest of the membrane is referred to as the basolateral surface or domain. The apical and basolateral domains do not intermix and contain different compositions of lipid and protein.

COPI (COP = **co**at **p**rotein) forms the surface of vesicles involved in the transfer of proteins between successive Golgi compartments. COPII forms the surface of vesicles that transfer proteins from the ER to the Golgi apparatus. Clathrin-coated vesicles are also involved in the process of endocytosis such as occurs when the LDL (low-density lipoprotein) receptor binds plasma LDL for uptake by the liver. The membrane location of these types of receptors is called a clathrin-coated pit.

In addition, certain cells have membrane compositions that are unique to one surface of the cell versus the other. For instance, epithelial cells have a membrane surface that interacts with the luminal cavity of the organ and another that interacts with the surrounding cells.

Most eukaryotic cells are in contact with their neighboring cells and these interactions are the basis of the formation of organs. Cells that are touching one another are in metabolic contact which is brought about by specialized tubular particles called junctions.

Gap junctions are intercellular channels designed for intercellular communication and their presence allows whole organs to be continuous from within. One major function of gap junctions is to ensure a supply of nutrients to cells of an organ that are not in direct contact with the blood supply. Gap junctions are formed from a type of protein called a connexin (Figure 7-3). Tight junctions are primarily found in the epithelia and are designed for occlusion. Tight junctions act as barriers that regulate the movement of solutes and water between various epithelial layers. At least 40 proteins have been found to be involved in the formation of the various tight junctions. These proteins are divided into 4 major categories: (1) scaffolding, (2) regulatory, (3) transmembrane, and (4) signaling. Adherens junctions are composed of transmembrane proteins that serve to anchor cells via interactions with the extracellular matrix. The proteins of adherens junctions are members of the various cadherin and integrin protein families. Related to the adherens junctions are the desmosomes and hemidesmosomes that are also involved in membrane-anchoring functions.

Given the predominant lipid nature of biological membranes, many types of molecules are restricted in their ability to diffuse across a membrane. This is especially true for charged ions, water, and hydrophilic compounds. The barrier to membrane translocation is overcome by the presence of specialized channels and transporters. Although channels and transporters are required to move many types of molecules and compounds across membranes, some substances can pass through from one side of a membrane to the other through a process of diffusion. Diffusion of gases such as O_2, CO_2, NO, and CO occurs at a rate that is solely dependent upon concentration gradients.

High-Yield Concept

Mammalian cells contain three major types of cell junctions called gap junctions, tight junctions, and adherens junctions.

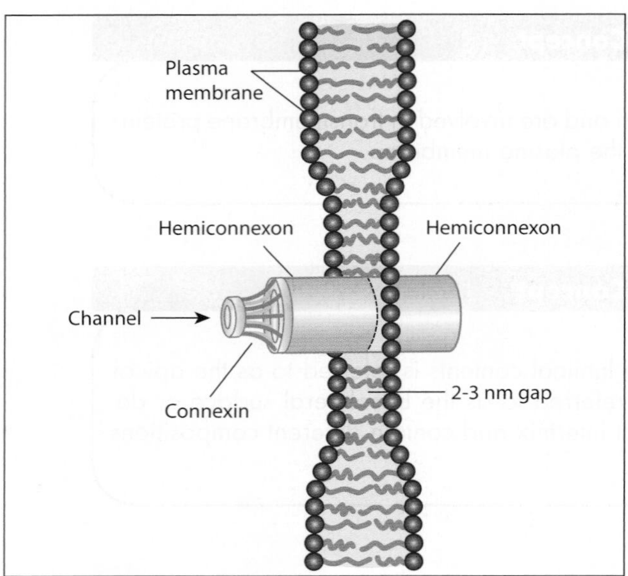

FIGURE 7-3: Schematic diagram of a gap junction. One connexon is made from 2 hemiconnexons. Each hemiconnexon is made from 6 connexin molecules. Small solutes are able to diffuse through the central channel, providing a direct mechanism of cell–cell communication. Murray RK, Bender DA, Botham KM, Kennelly PJ, Rodwell VW, Weil PA. *Harper's Illustrated Biochemistry,* 29th ed. New York, NY: McGraw-Hill; 2012.

Lipophilic molecules will also diffuse across membranes at a rate that is directly proportional to the solubility of the compound in the membrane.

Membrane Channels

The definition of a membrane channel (also called a pore) is that of a protein structure that facilitates the translocation of molecules or ions across the membrane through the creation of a central aqueous channel in the protein. Channel proteins do not bind or sequester the molecule or ion that is moving through the channel. Membrane channels facilitate diffusion in both directions dependent upon the direction of the concentration gradient. Specificity of channels for ions or molecules is a function of the size and charge of the substance. The flow of molecules through a channel can be regulated by various mechanisms that result in opening or closing of the passageway.

Membrane channels are of 3 distinct types: (1) α-type channels, (2) β-barrel channels, and (3) the pore-forming toxins. The α-type channels are homo- or hetero-oligomeric structures that in the latter case consist of several different proteins. The α-type class of channel protein has between 2 and 22 transmembrane α-helical domains, thus the derivation of the name of this type of channel. Molecules move through α-type channels down their concentration gradients and thus require no input of metabolic energy. The transport of molecules through α-type channels occurs by several different mechanisms. These mechanisms include changes in membrane potential (termed voltage-regulated or voltage-gated), phosphorylation of the channel protein, intracellular Ca^{2+}, G-proteins, and organic modulators. Some channels of this class are highly specific with respect to the molecule that moves across the membrane while others are not. In addition, there may be differences from tissue to tissue in the channel used to transport the same molecule. As an example, there are over 15 different K^+-specific voltage-regulated channels in humans.

The aquaporins assemble in the membrane as homotetramers with each monomer consisting of 6 transmembrane α-helical domains forming the distinct water pore. Probably the most significant location of aquaporin expression is in the kidney. Loss of function of the renal aquaporins is associated with several disease states such as nephrogenic diabetes insipidus (NDI), acquired hypokalemia, and hypercalcemia (Figure 7-4).

The β-barrel channels (also called porins) are so named because they have a transmembrane domain that consists of β-strands forming a β-barrel structure. Porins are found in the outer membranes of mitochondria. The mitochondrial porins are voltage-gated anion channels that are involved in mitochondrial homeostasis and apoptosis.

The pore-forming toxins family of channels is a large class of proteins first identified in bacteria. Subsequently several proteins of this class were identified in mammalian cells. The defensins are a family of small cysteine-rich antibiotic proteins that are pore-forming

High-Yield Concept

Aquaporins (AQP) are a family of α-type channels responsible for the transport of water across membranes.

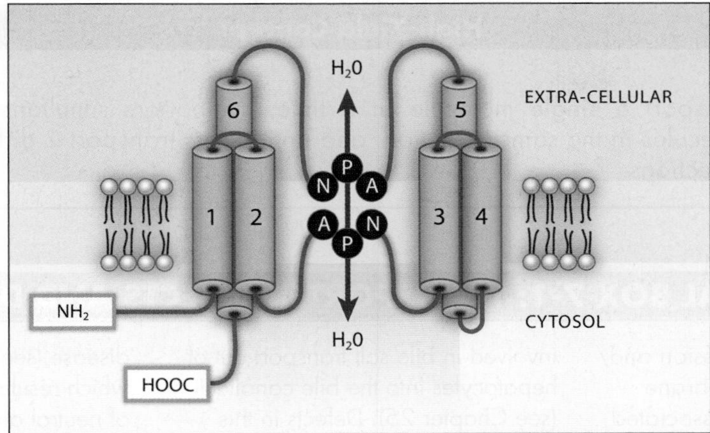

FIGURE 7-4: Diagrammatic representation of the structure of an aquaporin. The pores that form in the aquaporins are composed of 2 halves referred to as hemipores. Amino acids of the pore that are critical for water transport are the asparagine (N), proline (P), and alanine (A) residues indicated in each hemipore. Reproduced with permission of themedicalbiochemistrypage, LLC.

channels found in epithelial and hematopoietic cells. The defensins are involved in host defense against microbes (hence the derivation of their name) and may be involved in endocrine regulation during infection.

Membrane Transporters

Transporters are distinguished from channels because they catalyze (mediate) the movement of ions and molecules by physically binding to and moving the substance across the membrane. Transporter activity can be measured by the same kinetic parameters applied to the study of enzyme kinetics. Transporters exhibit specificity for the molecule being transported as well as show defined kinetics in the transport process. Transporters can also be affected by both competitive and noncompetitive inhibitors. Transporters are also known as carriers, permeases, translocators, translocases, and porters. Mediated transporters are classified based upon the stoichiometry of the transport process (Figure 7-5). Defects in many transporter-encoding genes are associated with the potential for severe clinical manifestation (see Clinical Box 7-1).

Facilitated diffusion involves the transport of specific molecules from an area of high concentration to one of low concentration which results in an equilibration of the concentration gradient. Glucose transporters are a good example of passive-mediated (facilitative diffusion) transporters. In contrast, active transporters

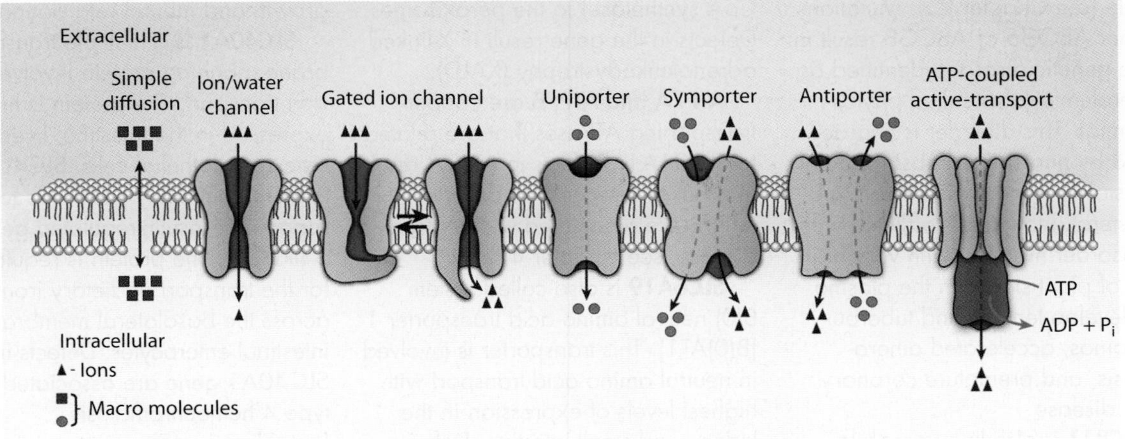

FIGURE 7-5: Representations of the various mechanisms for the passage/transport of ions and molecules across biological membranes. Reproduced with permission of themedicalbiochemistrypage, LLC.

High-Yield Concept

Uniporters transport a single molecule at a time, symporters simultaneously transport 2 different molecules in the same direction, and antiporters transport 2 different molecules in opposite directions.

CLINICAL BOX 7-1: TRANSPORTER DEFECTS AND DISEASE

Defects in the expression and/or function of membrane transporters have been associated with clinically significant diseases. Whereas, the total number is too numerous to mention, several important disorders are presented.

ABCA1 is involved in the transport of cholesterol out of cells when HDLs are bound to their cell surface receptor, SR-B1 (see Chapter 28). One important consequence of the activity of ABCA1 in macrophages is that the efflux of cholesterol results in a suppression of inflammatory responses triggered by macrophages that have become foam cells due to cholesterol uptake. Defects in ABCA1 result in Tangier disease which is characterized by 2 clinical hallmarks: (1) enlarged lipid-laden tonsils and (2) low serum HDL.

ABCG5 and ABCG8 form an obligate heterodimer pair that functions to limit plant sterol and cholesterol uptake by the gut and mediate cholesterol efflux from the liver into the bile (see Chapter 25). Mutations in either ABCG5 or ABCG8 result in a rare genetic disorder identified as sitosterolemia (also called phytosterolemia). This disorder is characterized by unrestricted absorption of plant sterols (such as sitosterol) and cholesterol. Individuals afflicted with this disorder manifest with very high levels of plant sterols in the plasma and develop tendon and tuberous xanthomas, accelerated atherosclerosis, and premature coronary artery disease.

ABCB11 is also known as bile salt export protein (BSEP) which is involved in bile salt transport out of hepatocytes into the bile canaliculi (see Chapter 25). Defects in this gene are associated with progressive familial intrahepatic cholestasis type 2 (PFIC2). The symptoms of PFIC2 usually present in early infancy as failure to thrive, jaundice, and severe pruritus (unpleasant sensation eliciting a desire to scratch). The symptoms of PFIC2 progress continuously, leading ultimately to liver failure and the need for liver transplantation in order to survive.

ABCC2 was first identified as the canalicular multispecific organic anion transporter (CMOAT) and is also called multidrug-resistance-associated protein 2 (MRP2). Defects in the gene encoding ABCC2 result in Dubin-Johnson syndrome (see Chapter 33), which is a form of conjugated hyperbilirubinemia.

ABCD1 is involved in the import and/or anchoring of very-long-chain fatty acid-CoA synthetase (VLCFA-CoA synthetase) to the peroxisomes. Defects in the gene result in X-linked adrenoleukodystrophy (XALD).

ATP7A and ATP7B are copper-transporting ATPases that are related to SLC31A1. Defects in ATP7A result in Menkes disease and defects in ATP7B are associated with Wilson disease (see Chapter 42).

SLC6A19 is also called system B(0) neutral amino acid transporter 1 [B(0)AT1]. This transporter is involved in neutral amino acid transport with highest levels of expression in the kidney and small intestine. Deficiency in SLC6A19 leads to Hartnup disease (see Clinical Box 30-1), which results from impaired transport of neutral amino acids across epithelial cells in renal proximal tubules and intestinal mucosa. Symptoms include transient manifestations of pellagra-like light-sensitive rash, cerebellar ataxia, and psychosis.

SLC35C1 is also known as the GDP-fucose transporter (gene symbol = FUCT1). Defects in the FUCT1 gene result in a congenital disorder of glycosylation (CDG) (see Chapter 38). Specifically the disorder is a type II CDG identified as CDGIIc. Type II CDGs result from defects in the processing of the carbohydrate structures on N-linked glycoproteins. CDGIIc is also called leukocyte adhesion deficiency syndrome II (LAD II). LAD II is a primary immunodeficiency syndrome which manifests due to leukocyte dysfunction. Symptoms of LAD II include unique facial features, recurrent infections, persistent leukocytosis, defective neutrophil chemotaxis, and severe growth and mental retardation.

SLC40A1 is a multiple transmembrane-spanning protein involved in iron transport. The protein is highly expressed in the intestine, liver, and reticuloendothelial cells. SLC40A1 is more commonly known as ferroportin or insulin-regulated gene 1 (IREG1). The protein is required for the transport of dietary iron across the basolateral membranes of intestinal enterocytes. Defects in the SLC40A1 gene are associated with type 4 hemochromatosis (see Chapter 42).

High-Yield Concept

The action of transporters is divided into 2 classifications: (1) passive-mediated transport (also called facilitated diffusion) and (2) active transport.

transport specific molecules from an area of low concentration to that of high concentration. Because this process is thermodynamically unfavorable, the process must be coupled to an exergonic process, for example, hydrolysis of ATP. There are many different classes of transporters that couple the hydrolysis of ATP to the transport of specific molecules. In general these transporters are referred to as ATPases. These ATPases are so named because they are autophosphorylated by ATP during the transport process. There are 4 different types of ATPases that function in eukaryotes.

1. **E-type ATPases:** Cell surface transporters that hydrolyze a range of nucleoside triphosphates that include extracellular ATP. The activity of the E-type ATPases is dependent on Ca^{2+} or Mg^{2+} and it is insensitive to specific inhibitors of P-type, F-type, and V-type ATPases.
2. **F-type ATPases:** Function in the translocation of H^+ in the mitochondria during the process of oxidative phosphorylation. F-type transporters contain rotary motors.
3. **P-type ATPases**: Mostly found in the plasma membrane and are involved in the transport of H^+, K^+, Na^+, Ca^{2+}, Cd^{2+}, Cu^{2+}, and Mg^{2+}. The P-type ATPases are so called because their activity is modified through phosphorylation. These transporters represent one of the largest families found in both prokaryotes and eukaryotes. The P-type ATPases are grouped into 5 classes designated P_1 to P_5 with several classes further divided into subclasses designated A, B, C, etc. For example, the P_2 class contains the A, B, C, and D subclasses. The P-type ATPases contain a core cytoplasmic domain structure that includes a phosphorylation domain (P domain), a nucleotide-binding domain (N domain), and an actuator domain (A domain). The P-type ATPases also possess 10 transmembrane helixes termed M1 to M10 where helixes M1 to M6 comprise the core of the membrane transport domain.
4. **V-type ATPases:** Located in acidic vesicles and lysosomes and have homology to the F-type ATPases and also contain rotary motors like F-type ATPases.

The Na^+/K^+-ATPases

One of the most thoroughly studied classes of ATPase is the Na^+/K^+-ATPase family found in plasma membranes. These transporters, sometimes called Na^+/K^+-pumps, are involved in the transport of Na^+ out of and K^+ into cells. Given that 3 moles of Na^+ are transported out and only 2 moles of K^+ are transported into the cell, an electrochemical gradient is established and is the basis for the electrochemical excitability of nerve cells. In fact, it is this transporter action that is the major requirement for ATP production from glucose oxidation in the central nervous system.

The Na^+/K^+-ATPases belong to the P_2 class and specifically to the P_{2C} subclass of ATPases. These ATPases are composed of 2 subunits (α and β). The α-subunit (≈113 kD) binds ATP and both Na^+ and K^+ ions and contains the phosphorylation sites typical of the P-type ATPases. The smaller β-subunit (≈35-kDa glycoprotein) is absolutely necessary for activity of the complex as it appears to be critical in facilitating the plasma membrane localization and activation of the α-subunit.

There are 4 α-subunit genes and 3 β-subunit genes in humans. The α_1-isoform is the predominant form and is ubiquitously expressed. The α_2 isoform is primarily expressed in muscle tissues (skeletal, smooth, and cardiac) as well as in adipose tissue, brain, and lung. The α_3-isoform is expressed primarily in the heart and neurons. The α_4-isoform is only expressed in the testes. The β_1-isoform is ubiquitously expressed and is associated with the α_1-subunit in the ubiquitously expressed $\alpha_1\beta_1$ Na^+/K^+-ATPase complex. The β_2-isoform is predominantly expressed in neurons and heart cells. The β_3-isoform is expressed in testes but has also been detected in early developing neurons.

In addition to the ability to form numerous complexes through the interactions of different α- and β-subunits, the Na^+/K^+-ATPases also associate with a family of small, single transmembrane-spanning protein termed the FXYD (*fix-id*) proteins. These proteins get their name from the fact that they all share a signature 35-amino-acid domain of homology that contains the conserved 4 amino acid motif: FXYD (F, phenylalanine; X, any amino acid; Y, tyrosine; D, aspartic acid). The human FXYD family of proteins is composed of at least 7 members identified as FXYD1 to FXYD7. FXYD2 is also known as the γ-subunit of the renal Na^+/K^+-ATPase (Figure 7-6).

When Na^+/K^+-ATPases have ATP bound, they can bind intracellular Na^+ ions. The hydrolysis of the ATP results in the phosphorylation of an aspartate residue in the P domain of the α-subunit of all P-type ATPases. The phosphorylation of the pump results in a conformational change which exposes the Na^+ ions to the outside of the cell and they are released. The pump then binds 2 extracellular K^+ ions which stimulate dephosphorylation of the α-subunit that in turn allows the pump to bind ATP again. In addition to the autophosphorylation site in the P domain of Na^+/K^+-ATPases, these pumps are subject to additional regulatory phosphorylation events catalyzed by PKA and PKC. Adrenergic, cholinergic, and dopaminergic receptor agonists result in PKA-mediated phosphorylation of the pumps (Clinical Box 7-2).

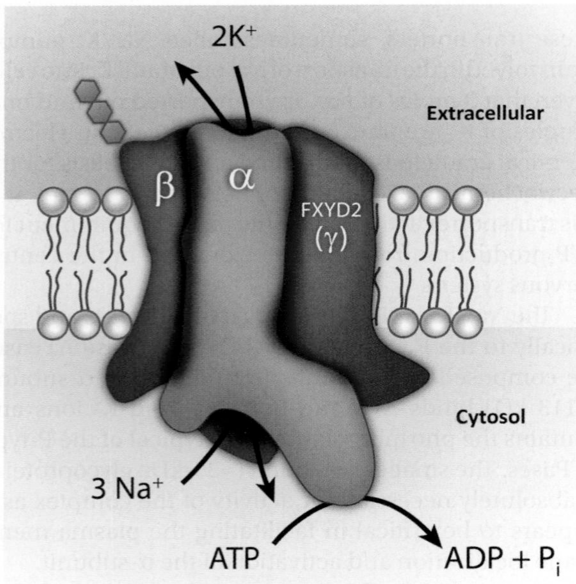

FIGURE 7-6: Functional organization of the α- and β-subunits of Na^+/K^+-ATPases, along with the FXYD2 subunit, in the plasma membrane. The movement of 2 moles of K^+ into the cell as 3 moles of Na^+ are transported out is shown. Associated with ion transport is the hydrolysis of ATP by the α-subunit which provides the energy to drive the process. Reproduced with permission of themedicalbiochemistrypage, LLC.

The ABC Family of Transporters

The ABC transporters comprise the ATP-binding cassette transporter superfamily. All members of this superfamily of membrane proteins contain a conserved ATP-binding domain and use the energy of ATP hydrolysis to drive the transport of various molecules across all cell membranes. There are 48 known genes of the ABC transporter superfamily and they are divided into 7 subfamilies based upon phylogenetic analyses. These 7 subfamilies are designated ABCA through ABCG. Each member of a given subfamily is distinguished with numbers (eg, ABCA1). (Table 7-1)

The Solute Carrier Family of Transporters

The solute carrier (SLC) family of transporters includes over 300 proteins functionally grouped into 51 gene families (Table 7-2). The SLC family of transporters includes facilitative transporters, primary and secondary active transporters, ion channels, and the aquaporins. The range of solutes transported by SLC family members includes both charged and uncharged organic molecules and numerous different inorganic ions (see Clinical Box 7-3). All members of the SLC family are integral transmembrane-spanning proteins.

CLINICAL BOX 7-2: CARDIOTONIC STEROIDS

The Na^+/K^+-ATPases are also receptors for the endogenous cardiotonic steroids as well as certain toxins from plants and amphibians. Binding of these various compounds to the pump results in activation of various kinases such as Src and PI3K resulting in modulation of cell adhesion and growth. Endogenous cardiotonic steroids (also referred to as cardiac glycosides) are specific inhibitors of Na^+/K^+-ATPases and have been isolated from adrenal glands, heart tissue, the hypothalamus, and cataractous lenses. Pregnenolone and progesterone are the precursors in the biosynthesis of endogenous ouabain (also identified as *g-strophanthin*) and endogenous digoxin. Ouabain and digoxin are referred to as cardenolides. Exogenous ouabain is a poisonous compound found in the ripe seeds of the African plant *Strophanthus gratus* and the bark of *Acokanthera ouabaio*. Another class of endogenous cardiotonic steroids is the bufadienolides, which includes marinobufagenin, marinobufotoxin (the C3-site arginine-suberoyl ester of marinobufagenin), telecinobufagin (the reduced form of marinobufagenin), and 19-norbufalin. Mevastatin (a statin drug that inhibits HMG-CoA reductase) treatment reduces the biosynthesis of marinobufagenin indicating that cholesterol is a precursor of bufadienolides in mammals. There are indications that many more endogenous cardiotonic steroids may exist in mammals.

TABLE 7-1: Representative ABC Transporters

Gene Symbol	*Other Names*	*Chromosome*	*Functions/Comments*
ABCA1	ABC1	9q31.1	Transfer of cellular cholesterol and phospholipids to HDLs (reverse cholesterol transport), defects in gene associated with development of Tangier disease
ABCB4	PGY3, MDR3	77q21.1	Class III multidrug resistance P-glycoprotein, canalicular phospholipid translocator, biliary phosphatidylcholine transport, defects in gene associated with 6 liver diseases: (1) progressive familial intrahepatic cholestasis type 3 (PFIC3), (2) adult biliary cirrhosis, (3) transient neonatal cholestasis, (4) drug-induced cholestasis, (5) intrahepatic cholestasis of pregnancy, and (6) low-phospholipid-associated cholelithiasis syndrome
ABCB11	BSEP, SPGP	2q24	Bile salt transport out of hepatocytes, gene defects associated with progressive familial intrahepatic cholestasis type 2 (PFIC2)
ABCC2	MRP2, CMOAT	10q24	Biliary excretion of many nonbile organic anions, gene defects result in Dubin-Johnson syndrome
ABCC8	SUR	11p15.1	Target of the type 2 diabetes drugs such as glipizide
ABCD1	ALD	Xq28	Involved in the import and/or anchoring of very-long-chain fatty acid-CoA synthetase (VLCFA-CoA synthetase) to the peroxisomes, gene defects result in X-linked adrenoleukodystrophy (XALD)
ABCD3	PMP70, PXMP1	1p21.3	70-kDa peroxisomal membrane protein, also called peroxisomal membrane protein 1, mutation associated with Zellweger syndrome 2 (ZWS2)
ABCG1	ABC8, White1	21q22.3	Involved in mobilization and efflux of intracellular cholesterol, responsible for approximately 20% of cholesterol efflux to HDLs (reverse cholesterol transport)
ABCG5	White3	2p21	Forms an obligate heterodimer with ABCG8, expressed in intestinal enterocytes and hepatocytes, functions to limit plant sterol and cholesterol absorption from the diet by facilitating efflux out of enterocytes into the intestinal lumen and out of hepatocytes into the bile
ABCG8	Sterolin 2	2p21	See above for ABCG5

BSEP, bile salt export protein; CMOAT, canalicular multispecific organic anion transporter; HDL, high-density lipoprotein; MDR3, multidrug resistance protein 3; MRP2, multidrug resistance–associated protein 2; PGY3, P-glycoprotein 3; SUR, sulfonylurea receptor.

TABLE 7-2: Representative SLC Transporters

SLC Family	*Functional Class*	*Member Names/Comments*
1	High-affinity glutamate and neutral amino acid transporters	SLC1A1-SLC1A7 SLC1A4 and SLC1A5 are the neutral amino acid transporters Decreased expression of SLC1A2 is associated with amyotrophic lateral sclerosis (ALS = Lou Gehrig disease)
2	Facilitative GLUT transporters	SLC2A1-SLC2A14 SLC2A1 is GLUT1: Ubiquitously expressed in various tissues but only at low levels in liver and skeletal muscle. This is the primary glucose transporter in erythrocytes SCL2A2 is GLUT2: Expressed predominantly in the liver, pancreatic β-cells, kidney, and intestines SCL2A3 is GLUT3: Found primarily in neurons and possesses the lowest K_m for glucose of any of the glucose transporters SLC2A4 is GLUT4: Expressed predominantly in insulin-responsive tissues such as skeletal muscle and adipose tissue SLC2A5 is GLUT5: Involved in fructose transport not glucose transport
5	sodium glucose cotransporters	SLC5A1-SLC5A12 SLC5A2 is also known as SGLT2 which is responsible for the majority of glucose reabsorption by the kidneys and as such is a current target of therapeutic intervention in the hyperglycemia associated with type 2 diabetes

(Continued)

TABLE 7-2: Representative SLC Transporters (*Continued*)

SLC Family	*Functional Class*	*Member Names/Comments*
6	Sodium- and chloride-dependent neurotransmitter transporters	SLC6A1-SLC6A20 SLC6A19 is involved in neutral amino acid transport, deficiency results in Hartnup disorder; protein also called system B^0 neutral amino acid transporter 1 (B^0AT1)
10	Sodium bile salt cotransporters	SLC10A1-SLC10A5, SLC10A7 SLC10A1: Also called NTCP for Na^+-taurocholate cotransporting polypeptide, NTCP is involved in hepatic uptake of bile acids through the sinusoidal/basolateral membrane
11	Proton-coupled metal ion transporters	SLC11A1, SLC11A2, SLC11A3 SLC11A2 is also known as the divalent metal-ion transporter-1 (DMT1) SLC11A3 is now referred to as SLC40A1; this protein is more commonly called ferroportin, but is also known as iron-regulated gene 1 (IREG1) and reticuloendothelial iron transporter (MPT1)
27	Fatty acid transporters (FATPs); see Chapter 25	SLC27A1-SLC27A6 FATP2 is also known as very-long-chain acyl-CoA synthetase (VLCS); FATP5 is also known as very-long-chain acyl-CoA synthetase-related protein (VLACSR) or very-long-chain acyl-CoA synthetase homolog 2 (VLCSH2); FATP6 is also known as very-long-chain acyl-CoA synthetase homolog 1 (VLCSH1)
28	Na^+-dependent concentrative nucleoside transport (CNTs)	SLC28A1, SLC28A2, SLC28A3
31	Copper transporters (CTRs)	SLC31A1, SLC31A2 ATP7A and ATP7B are related copper-transporting ATPases that mediate copper export ATP7A is defective in Menkes disease and ATP7B is defective in Wilson disease
35	Nucleoside sugar transporters	At least 17 family members divided into 5 subfamilies identified as A through E SLC35C1 is also identified as the GDP-fucose transporter (gene symbol = FUCT1)
37	Sugar-phosphate/phosphate exchangers (SPXs)	SLC37A1-SLC37A4 SLC37A4 is also known as glucose-6-phosphate transporter-1 (G6PT1), which is defective in glycogen storage disease type1b
40	basolateral iron transporter	SLC40A1 is more commonly known as ferroportin, but is also known as iron-regulated gene 1 (IREG1) or reticuloendothelial iron transporter (MTP1); was also identified as SLC11A3, which is no longer used

CLINICAL BOX 7-3: CYSTINURIA

As the name implies, cystinuria is a disorder associated with excess cystine in the urine. Cystine is the oxidized disulfide homodimer of 2 cysteines. Cystinuria is an autosomal recessive disorder that results from a failure of the renal proximal tubules to reabsorb cystine that was filtered by the glomerulus. The disorder results from defects in either of the 2 protein subunits of the cysteine transporter. In addition to excess cysteine in the urine, the disorder is also associated with increased urinary excretion of dibasic amino acids arginine, lysine, and ornithine. However, clinical consequences are only associated with the increased urinary cysteine and is due to the poor solubility of this homodimeric compound. Cystine will precipitate in the urine resulting in the formation of renal calculi (stones) that can lead to renal failure. The 2 subunits of the cystine transporter are encoded by the SLC3A1 and SCL7A9 genes that encode the basic amino acid transport protein (rBAT) and the functional subunit that transports neutral and basic amino acids ($b^{0,+}AT$), respectively. Common treatments for patients with cystinuria are to decrease protein and salt intake as well as to ensure increased hydration as this will dilute the cystine in the urine reducing the potential for crystal formation. In addition, patients are given drugs, such as acetazolamide, which alkalize the urine which reduces the potential for urinary precipitation of cystine.

REVIEW QUESTIONS

1. Digoxin is a member of the cardiac glycoside family of drugs. This drug can be used to treat patients with atrial fibrillation since it slows heart rate. Cardiac glycosides function by inhibiting which class of membrane transporter?

A. antiporters
B. facilitative diffusers
C. symporters
D. uniporters

Answer A: The cardiac glycosides function by inhibiting the action of Na^+/K^+-ATPases. These transporters transport Na^+ into the cell while simultaneously transporting K^+ out. Thus, they function as classical antiporters.

2. Aquaporins are a class of transporters that are involved in the transport of water across membranes. The aquaporins belong to which type of transporter family?

A. active
B. β-barrel channels (porins)
C. α-channels
D. facilitated
E. passive

Answer C: The aquaporin proteins are made up of 6 transmembrane α-helices arranged in a right-handed bundle. The a-type channels are homo- or hetero-oligomeric structures that in the latter case consist of several different proteins. The a-type class of channel protein has between 2 and 22 transmembrane α-helical domains, thus the derivation of the name of this type of channel.

3. You are treating a patient who complains of having an intense or uncontrollable thirst with a strong craving for ice water. The patient produces large amounts of urine (8-10 L per day). Additional symptoms include fatigue, headache, irritability, and muscle pains. Given the symptoms you suspect nephrogenic diabetes insipidus. If this diagnosis is correct, which of the following membrane transporter types would be defective in your patient?

A. aquaporin
B. F-type ATPase
C. Na^+/K^+-ATPase
D. P-type ATPase
E. SLC40A1 (ferroportin)

Answer A: Nephrogenic diabetes insipidus (NDI) is a disorder in which a defect in the tubules in the kidneys causes a person to pass a large amount of urine. This disorder is caused by an improper response of the kidney to antidiuretic hormone (ADH, also called vasopressin), leading to a decrease in the ability of the kidney to concentrate the urine by removing free water. The primary cause of NDI is a mutation in the ADH receptor in the kidney. However, NDI can also result from mutations in the aquaporin-2 gene.

4. A patient who presents with unique facial features, recurrent infections, persistent leukocytosis, defective neutrophil chemotaxis, and severe growth and mental retardation would likely be manifesting these symptoms due to a deficiency in which of the following transport proteins?

A. aquaporin
B. F-type ATPase
C. GDP-fucose transporter (FUCT1, SLC35C1)
D. Na^+/K^+-ATPase
E. P-type ATPase

Answer C: The symptoms seen in this patient are associated with leukocyte adhesion deficiency syndrome II (LAD II). LAD II belongs to the class of disorders referred to as primary immunodeficiency syndromes as the symptoms of the disease manifest due to defects in leukocyte function. Symptoms of LAD II are characterized by unique facial features, recurrent infections, persistent leukocytosis, defective neutrophil chemotaxis, and severe growth and mental retardation. The genetic defect resulting in LAD II is in the pathway of fucose utilization leading to loss of fucosylated glycans on the cell surface. Specifically, patients harbor mutations in the GDP-fucose transporter, FUCT1.

5. You have a patient presenting with neuropsychiatric symptoms, progressive chronic liver disease, Parkinsonian tremors, diminished facial expressions, and choreoathetosis. These symptoms are associated with a deficiency in which of the following?

A. aquaporin
B. ATP7A
C. ATP7B
D. Na^+/K^+-ATPase
E. SLC40A1 (ferroportin)

Answer C: These symptoms are indicative of the copper transport defect disease known as Wilson disease. Wilson disease is the result of defects in the P-type ATPase protein that is primarily responsible for copper homeostasis mediated by the liver. This protein is encoded by the ATPase, Cu^{2+}-transporting, β–polypeptide (ATP7B) gene. The majority of patients with Wilson disease present with hepatic or neuropsychiatric symptoms. Patients that manifest neurological symptoms of Wilson disease present in the second to third decade of life. In these patients there will be extrapyramidal, cerebellar, and cerebral-related symptoms such as Parkinsonian tremors, diminished facial expressions and movement, dystonia, and choreoathetosis. About 30% of Wilson disease patients will exhibit psychiatric disturbances that include changes in behavior, personality changes, depression, attention-deficit hyperactivity disorder, paranoid psychosis, suicidal tendencies, and impulsivity. The most significant sign in the diagnosis of Wilson disease results from the deposition of copper in Descemet's membrane of the cornea. These golden-brown deposits can be seen with a slit-lamp and are Kayser-Fleischer rings.

6. Deficiency in the copper transporter ATP7A would most likely be associated with which of the following symptoms?

A. excessive thirst, dry chapped skin
B. hemochromatosis
C. hepatic failure, movement disorder such as dystonia
D. recurrent infections, severe growth retardation
E. wiry brittle hair

Answer E: Defects in ATP7A result in the Menkes disease. The clinical spectrum associated with Menkes disease includes progressive neurodegeneration, connective tissue abnormalities, and wiry brittle hair.

7. Which of the following is involved in the simultaneous transport of 2 different molecules across a membrane in the same direction at the same time?

A. antiporter
B. α-channel
C. Na^+/K^+-ATPase
D. symporter
E. uniporter

Answer D: Symporters are so called because they transport 2 different molecules, or solutes, across a membrane in the same direction.

8. GLUT4 is the glucose transporter involved in insulin-stimulated glucose uptake into adipose tissue and skeletal muscle. The mechanism of glucose transport by GLUT4 is of which of the following types?

A. active transporter
B. facilitated diffusion
C. gated ion channel
D. simple diffusion

Answer B: Facilitated diffusion is the spontaneous passage of molecules or ions across a biological membrane passing through specific integral transmembrane proteins. The glucose transporters, of which GLUT4 is a member, carry out sugar transport via the mechanism of facilitated diffusion.

9. Cardiotonic steroids, produced by the adrenal glands, heart tissue, and hypothalamus are specific inhibitors of which of the following?

A. aquaporins
B. F-type ATPases
C. Na^+/K^+-ATPases
D. P-type ATPases
E. SLC type transporters

Answer C: The cardiotonic steroids (also called cardiac glycosides) function by inhibiting the action of Na^+/K^+-ATPases.

10. Ouabain is a poisonous compound found in the ripe seeds of the African plant *Strophanthus gratus.* This compound is poisonous due to the fact that it is a potent inhibitor of which of the following?

A. aquaporins
B. F-type ATPases
C. Na^+/K^+-ATPases
D. P-type ATPases
E. SLC type transporters

Answer C: The classic mechanism of action of ouabain involves its binding to and inhibition of plasma membrane Na^+/K^+-ATPases.

11. Intestinal epithelial cells possess 2 transport mechanisms to move glucose across the plasma membrane, a facilitated glucose carrier (GLUT2) as well as a sodium-dependent secondary active transporter (SGLT1). Which of the following attributes distinguishes these 2 transport modalities with respect to net glucose transport?

A. GLUT2 directly depends on ATP hydrolysis
B. GLUT2 is sensitive to competitive substrate inhibition
C. SGLT1 can transport glucose from a region of low to a region of high concentration
D. SGLT1 is carrier mediated
E. SGLT1 is saturable

Answer C: SGLT1 is a Na^+-dependent glucose cotransporter. Within the kidney tubule, the Na^+/K^+-ATPase pump on the basolateral membrane of the proximal tubule cell uses ATP to move Na^+ outward into the blood, while bringing in 2 K^+. This creates a downhill Na^+ gradient inside the proximal tubule cell in comparison to both the blood and the tubule. SGLT1 uses the energy from this downhill Na^+ gradient created by the ATPase pump to transport glucose across the apical membrane against an uphill glucose gradient.

12. Cardioactive steroids, like digoxin, exert a positive ionotropic effect on heart muscle cells. Because of this activity they can be used clinically to increase contraction of a failing heart. Which of the following proteins is important in the mechanism of action of digoxin on the cardiac muscle cell?

A. N-type calcium channels
B. Na^+/Ca^{2+} exchange protein (NCX)
C. plasma membrane calcium ATPase (PMCA)
D. potassium channels
E. sodium channels

Answer B: Cardioactive steroids inhibit the Na^+/K^+-ATPase present in the plasma membrane of the cardiac muscle cell. At the therapeutic dosages that are employed, there will be partial ATPase inhibition with decreased active sodium efflux from the myoplasm and a resultant increase in myoplasmic sodium ion concentration. Due to increased intracellular sodium concentration, the Na^+/Ca^{2+} exchange protein (NCX) can extrude less calcium from the cell and the intracellular concentration of calcium will increase. This increases force, since contractile force depends on calcium. Though calcium influx through N-type calcium channels is also an important source of calcium to regulate contraction, calcium channel activity is not regulated by the cardioactive steroids.

13. Which of the following proteins uses the sodium electrochemical gradient to actively transport a solute into the cell?

A. calcium-ATPase
B. GLUT2
C. Na^+/K^+-ATPase
D. Na^+/Ca^{2+} countertransport protein
E. SGLT1

Answer E: SGLT1 is a sodium-dependent cotransport protein that uses the sodium electrochemical gradient to actively move glucose into the cell.

14. A 3-day-old male neonate is diagnosed with meconium ileus. You should be concerned that he has which of the following conditions?

A. alkaptonuria
B. cystic fibrosis
C. hemophilia A
D. phenylketonuria
E. Wilson disease

Answer B: Meconium ileus is a very common early clinical expression of cystic fibrosis. Increased sodium chloride level in sweat confirms the diagnosis. About 70% of children with cystic fibrosis have a depletional abnormality of chromosome 7 which disrupts the expression of the *cystic fibrosis transmembrane conductance regulator (CFTR)* gene. CFTR is a member of the ATP-binding cassette (ABC) family of membrane transporters. Specifically, CFTR is a chloride channel expressed in numerous epithelial cell membranes. In addition to the classic pulmonary obstruction resulting from loss of CFTR function, cystic fibrosis is associated with pancreatic insufficiency, recurrent pulmonary infections, and biliary obstruction.

15. You are studying the electrophysiological characteristics of cardiac pacemaker cells. Which of the following is the primary determinant of the resting membrane potential in these cells?

A. background potassium conductance
B. background sodium conductance
C. delayed rectifier potassium current
D. sodium-calcium exchange current
E. transient outward current

Answer A: The resting membrane potential of cardiac cells is caused by the difference in ionic concentrations and conductances across the membrane of the cell during an action potential. This potential is determined by the selective permeability of the cell membrane to various ions. The membrane is most permeable to K^+ and relatively impermeable to other ions. The resting membrane potential is therefore dominated by the K^+ equilibrium potential according to the K^+ gradient across the cell membrane.

16. You are carrying out mutational studies on membrane-associated proteins. You are particularly interested in proteins that pass through the plasma membrane of cells. Alteration of which of the following properties of an integral membrane protein would most likely interfere with its ability to become membrane associated?

A. the ability to bind carbohydrates on both sides of the membrane
B. the ability to move laterally in the plane of the membrane
C. the ability to translocate across the bilayer of the membrane when the temperature is increased
D. flip-flopping across the bilayer of the membrane when the temperature is increased
E. high solubility in strong basic solutions

Answer B: Integral membrane proteins are permanently attached to a given biological membrane. The most common type of integral membrane protein is the transmembrane protein which spans the entire biological membrane. Integral membrane proteins possess a region of hydrophobic amino acids that allows interaction with the lipid interface of the membrane. For this reason, this class of protein can move laterally in the membrane, but cannot translocate across nor flip-flop within the membrane.

17. You are examining the characteristics of ion movement in cells in culture. You find that addition of a particular compound to the medium interferes with this movement. The compound you are using most likely interferes with the function of which of the following structures that allows ion and small molecule passage directly from the cytosol of one cell to another?
A. belt desmosome (zonula adherens)
B. chemical synapse
C. desmosome (macula adherens)
D. gap junction
E. tight junction (zonula occludens)

Answer D: Gap junctions do not seal membranes together, nor do they restrict the passage of material between membranes. Rather, gap junctions are composed of arrays of small channels that permit small molecules to shuttle from one cell to another and thus directly link the interior of adjacent cells. Importantly, gap junctions allow electrical and metabolic coupling among cells because signals initiated in one cell can readily propagate to neighboring cells.

18. Drugs that inhibit the plasma membrane Na^+/K^+ ATPase decrease which of the following cellular processes?
A. cell-to-cell communication via gap junctions
B. cellular uptake of iron by reticulocytes
C. endocytosis of low-density lipoproteins
D. export of calcium from cardiac muscle cells
E. transport of glucose into adipose tissue cells

Answer D: Inhibition of Na^+/K^+-ATPases present in the plasma membrane results in decreased active sodium efflux from the cell with a resultant increase in intracellular sodium ion concentration. Due to increased intracellular sodium concentration the Na^+/Ca^{2+} exchange protein (NCX) can extrude less calcium from the cell and the intracellular concentration of calcium will increase.

19. Acetylcholine exerts effects on several cell types. On certain cells, such as muscle, the activity of acetylcholine results in the opening of which of the following types of membrane channels?
A. Ca^{2+}-activated K^+ channel
B. transmitter-gated cation channel
C. transmitter-gated Cl^- channel
D. voltage-gated Ca^{2+} channel
E. voltage-gated Na^+ channel

Answer B: When acetylcholine binds to acetylcholine receptors on skeletal muscle fibers, it opens ligand-gated sodium channels in the cell membrane. Sodium ions then enter the muscle cell, initiating a sequence of steps that finally produce muscle contraction.

20. You are examining a 17-year-old adolescent girl presenting with decreased range of motion, redness, and swelling of the joints due to arthritis. The young woman also presents with xanthomas in the Achilles tendon and extensor tendons of the hand. Additional examination indicates splenomegaly. Analysis of serum shows very high levels of sitosterol, campesterol, stigmasterol, and avenosterol. You suspect the patient is suffering from sitosterolemia. Which of the following class of transport systems is likely to be defective in this patient?
A. ABC transporters
B. aquaporins
C. gap junctions
D. sodium-potassium ATPases
E. SLC transporters

Answer A: Sitosterolemia is a rare autosomal recessively inherited disorder characterized by hyperabsorption and decreased biliary excretion of dietary sterols leading to hypercholesterolemia, tendon and tuberous xanthomas, premature development of atherosclerosis, and abnormal hematological and liver function test results. The disorder is caused by mutations in either of the 2 ABC transporter proteins of the obligate heterodimer composed of ABCG5 and ABCG8.

21. Certain types of cell junctions render epithelial cells impermeable. Which of the following types of cell junction is responsible for impermeability, therefore requiring transcellular movement of substances from the apical surface to the basolateral surface of the epithelium?
A. desmosome (macula adherens)
B. belt desmosome (zonula adherens)
C. fascia adherens
D. gap junction
E. tight junction (zonula occludens)

Answer E: Tight junctions, or zonula occludens, are the closely associated areas of 2 cells whose membranes join together forming a virtually impermeable barrier to fluid.

Checklist

- ✓ Biological membranes consist of phospholipids, cholesterol, proteins, and carbohydrates.
- ✓ Biological membranes are composed of a lipid bilayer formed by 2 sheets of phospholipids whose hydrophobic tails interact and their polar head groups are presented on the outer surfaces where they interact with the aqueous environment.
- ✓ The structure of membranes is dynamic with lateral diffusion of lipids and proteins. In addition, lipids can flip-flop between the 2 faces of the membrane.
- ✓ Proteins that are associated with membranes can interact with the outer or inner surfaces or they can be embedded in, or through, the membrane. Integral membrane proteins are those that are firmly embedded in the membrane, whereas those that are attached by simple interaction are peripheral proteins.
- ✓ The various membranes of a cell have different compositions, which in turn defines the functional characteristics of the particular membrane. Within a given membrane, such as the plasma membrane, there can be highly specialized localized environments.
- ✓ Ions and molecules can move across membranes either by passive or active means. Ions are generally transported across membranes via the action of ligand-gated channels, whereas various types of transporter proteins are used to move solutes and other larger molecules across membranes.
- ✓ Membrane transporter classes are defined by the overall process of transport and also by whether or not energy is required for the process.
- ✓ There are several classes of ATP-driven membrane transporters including the ATP-binding cassette family (ABC), and the P-type (phosphorylated), F-type (energy factor), E-type (extracellular), and V-type (vacuolar).
- ✓ Numerous types of transporters are present in the membrane involved in transport of various solutes and are referred to as the solute carrier (SLC) family.
- ✓ Mutations that affect the structure and function of membrane proteins such as transporters, receptors, and ion channels can have profound effects leading to disease and disability.

PART II Metabolic Biochemistry

CHAPTER 8 Vitamins and Minerals

CHAPTER OUTLINE

High-Yield Terms

Beriberi: result of a diet that is carbohydrate rich and thiamin deficient; characterized by difficulty walking, loss of sensation in hands and feet, loss of muscle function of the lower legs, mental confusion/speech difficulties, nystagmus

Wernicke encephalopathy: manifests with symptoms similar to those of beriberi but not associated with carbohydrate-rich diet

Wernicke-Korsakoff syndrome: extreme consequence of chronic thiamin deficiency, resulting in loss of short-term memory and mild to severe psychosis

Pellagra: classically described by the 3 Ds: diarrhea, dermatitis, and dementia, caused by a chronic lack of niacin

Pernicious anemia: one of the many types of megaloblastic anemias, caused by loss of secretion of intrinsic factor, which is necessary for absorption of vitamin B_{12}

Megaloblastic anemia: a macrocytic anemia resulting from inhibition of DNA synthesis during erythrocyte production

Xerophthalmia: pathological dryness of the conjunctiva and cornea due to progressive keratinization of the cornea

Rickets: characterized by improper mineralization during the development of the bones resulting in soft bones

Osteomalacia: characterized by demineralization of previously formed bone leading to increased softness and susceptibility to fracture

High-Yield Concept

As is evident from its role in the activities of 3 TLCFN enzymes, thiamin plays a critical role in overall energy homeostasis and thus, a deficiency of this vitamin will lead to a severely reduced capacity of cells to generate energy (see Clinical Box 8-1).

Vitamins are organic molecules that function in a wide variety of capacities within the body. The most prominent function of the vitamins is to serve as cofactors (coenzymes) for enzymatic reactions. The distinguishing feature of the vitamins is that they generally cannot be synthesized by mammalian cells and, therefore, must be supplied in the diet. The vitamins are of 2 distinct types, water soluble and fat soluble.

The minerals that are considered of dietary significance are those that are necessary to support biochemical reactions by serving both functional and structural roles as well as those serving as electrolytes. The use of the term dietary mineral is considered archaic since the intent of the term *mineral* is to describe ions not actual minerals. The body requires both quantity elements and trace elements. The quantity elements are sodium, magnesium, phosphorous, sulfur, chlorine, potassium, and calcium. The essential trace elements are manganese, iron, cobalt, nickel, copper, zinc, selenium, molybdenum, and iodine. Additional trace elements (although not considered essential) are boron, chromium, fluoride, and silicon.

Water-Soluble Vitamins

Thiamin: Vitamin B_1

Thiamin (also written thiamine) is also known as vitamin B_1. Thiamin is derived from a substituted pyrimidine and a thiazole, which are coupled by a methylene bridge. Thiamin is rapidly converted to its active form, thiamin pyrophosphate (TPP), in the brain and liver by the enzyme thiamin diphosphotransferase (Figure 8-1).

TPP is necessary as a cofactor for a number of dehydrogenases, including pyruvate dehydrogenase (PDH) and α-ketoglutarate (2-oxoglutarate) dehydrogenase (α-KGDH). Both of these enzymes are critical to the functioning of the TCA (tricarboxylic acid) cycle (see Chapter 16). Additional important TPP-requiring

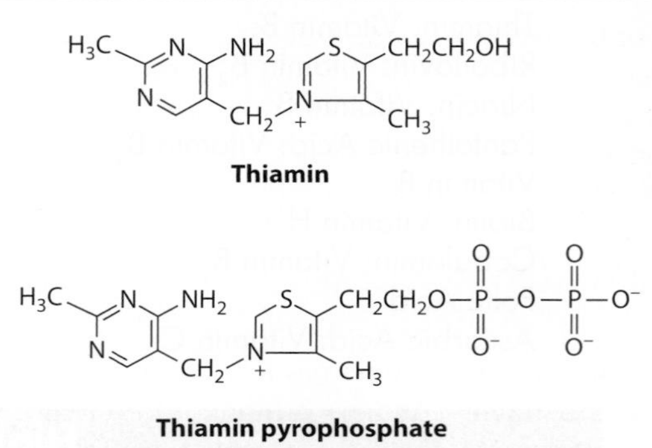

Thiamin

Thiamin pyrophosphate

FIGURE 8-1: Structures of thiamin and thiamin pyrophosphate. Reproduced with permission of themedicalbiochemistrypage, LLC.

CLINICAL BOX 8-1: THIAMIN DEFICIENCY

The earliest symptoms of thiamin deficiency include constipation, appetite suppression, nausea as well as mental depression, peripheral neuropathy, and fatigue. Chronic thiamin deficiency leads to more severe neurological symptoms including ataxia, mental confusion, and loss of eye coordination resulting in nystagmus. Other clinical symptoms of prolonged thiamin deficiency are related to cardiovascular and musculature defects.

The severe thiamin deficiency disease, known as Beriberi, is the result of a diet that is carbohydrate rich and thiamin deficient. An additional thiamin deficiency–related disease is known as Wernicke encephalopathy. This disease is most commonly found in chronic alcoholics due to their poor diet and has symptoms similar to those of beriberi. Wernicke-Korsakoff syndrome is an extreme manifestation of chronic deficiency of thiamin. It is characterized by acute encephalopathy followed by chronic impairment of short-term memory and mild-to-severe psychosis.

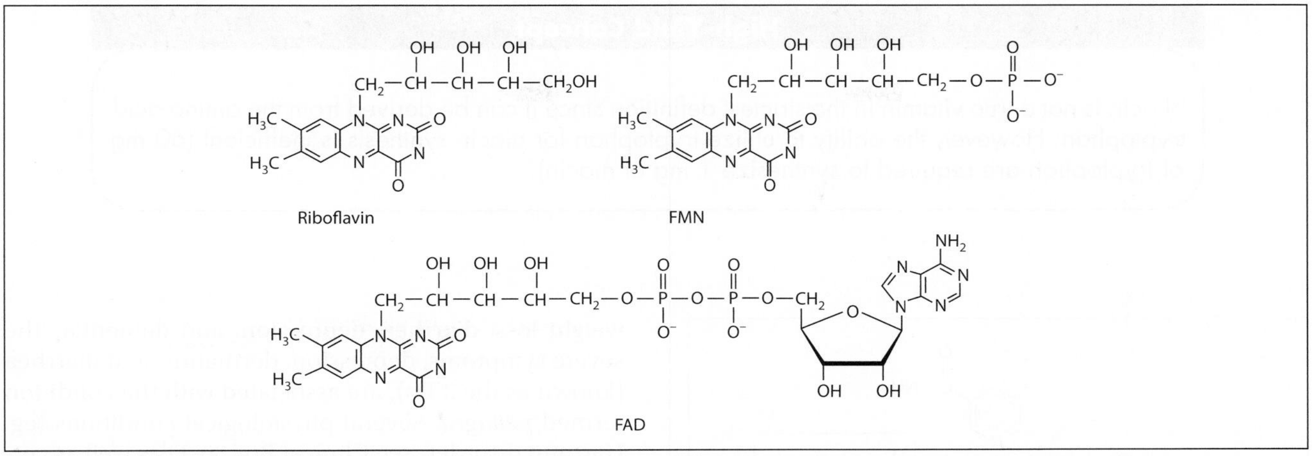

FIGURE 8-2: Riboflavin and the coenzymes flavin mononucleotide (FMN) and flavin adenine dinucleotide (FAD). Murray RK, Bender DA, Botham KM, Kennelly PJ, Rodwell VW, Weil PA. *Harper's Illustrated Biochemistry*, 29th ed. New York, NY: McGraw-Hill; 2012.

enzymes are transketolase of the pentose phosphate pathway (see Chapter 15) and branched-chain α-keto acid dehydrogenase (BCKD) involved in the catabolism of the branched-chain amino acids (see Chapter 30). The enzymes, PDH, α-KGDH, and BCKD are known as the *tender loving care for Nancy* (TLCFN) enzymes reflective of their requirement for thiamin, lipoic acid, coenzyme A, FAD, and NAD.

Riboflavin: Vitamin B_2

Riboflavin is also known as vitamin B_2. Riboflavin is the precursor for the coenzymes flavin mononucleotide (FMN) and flavin adenine dinucleotide (FAD). Synthesis of these 2 cofactors occurs in a 2-step process. FMN is synthesized from riboflavin via the ATP-dependent enzyme riboflavin kinase (RFK). FMN is then converted to FAD via the attachment of AMP (derived from ATP) through the action of FAD pyrophosphorylase, which is also known as FMN adenylyltransferase (FMNAT) (Figure 8-2).

The enzymes that require FMN or FAD as cofactors are termed *flavoproteins*. Several flavoproteins also contain metal ions and are termed metalloflavoproteins. Both classes of enzyme are involved in a wide range of redox reactions, for example, succinate dehydrogenase (of the TCA cycle, see Chapter 16) and xanthine oxidase (of purine nucleotide catabolism, see Chapter 32).

Riboflavin deficiencies are rare in the United States due to the presence of adequate amounts of the vitamin in eggs, milk, meat, and cereals. Riboflavin deficiency is often seen in chronic alcoholics due to their poor dietary habits. Symptoms associated with riboflavin deficiency include itching and burning eyes, angular stomatitis and cheilosis (cracks and sores in the mouth and lips), bloodshot eyes, glossitis (inflammation of the tongue leading to purplish discoloration), seborrhea (dandruff, flaking skin on scalp and face), trembling, sluggishness, and photophobia (excessive light sensitivity). Riboflavin decomposes when exposed to visible light. This characteristic can lead to riboflavin deficiencies in newborns treated for hyperbilirubinemia by phototherapy.

Niacin: Vitamin B_3

Niacin (nicotinic acid and nicotinamide) is also known as vitamin B_3. Both nicotinic acid and nicotinamide can serve as the dietary source of vitamin B_3. Niacin is required for the synthesis of the active forms of vitamin B_3, nicotinamide adenine dinucleotide (NAD^+), and nicotinamide adenine dinucleotide

High-Yield Concept

The redox reactions, involving the flavoproteins, generate the reduced forms of FMN and FAD, $FMNH_2$ and $FADH_2$, respectively.

High-Yield Concept

Niacin is not a true vitamin in the strictest definition since it can be derived from the amino acid tryptophan. However, the ability to utilize tryptophan for niacin synthesis is inefficient (60 mg of tryptophan are required to synthesize 1 mg of niacin).

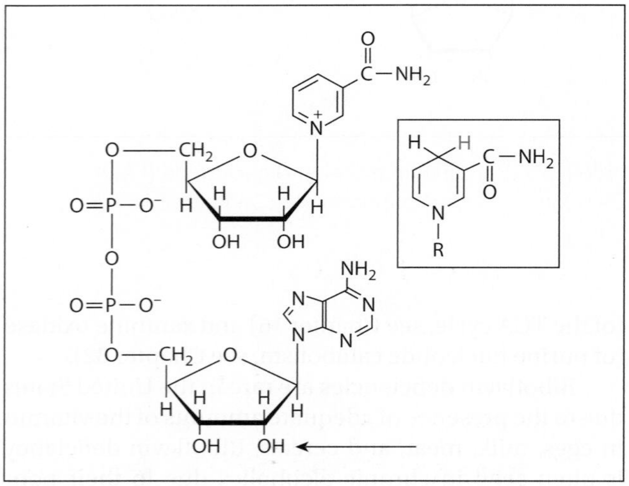

FIGURE 8-3: Structure of NAD^+. Inset box shows structure of the nicotinamide where the –R represents the adenine dinucleotide of NAD^+ or $NADP^+$. The arrow designates the location of the phosphate in $NADP^+$. The red H represents the hydrogen that is added during reduction of NAD^+ or $NADP^+$ to NADH or nicotinamide adenine dinucleotide phosphate (NADPH). Reproduced with permission of themedicalbiochemistrypage, LLC.

phosphate ($NADP^+$). Both NAD^+ and $NADP^+$ function as cofactors for several hundred different redox enzymes (Figure 8-3).

Also, synthesis of niacin from tryptophan requires vitamins B_1, B_2, and B_6 which would be limiting on a marginal diet.

A diet deficient in niacin (as well as tryptophan) leads to glossitis of the tongue (inflammation of the tongue leading to purplish discoloration), dermatitis, weight loss, diarrhea, depression, and dementia. The severe symptoms, depression, dermatitis, and diarrhea (known as the 3 Ds), are associated with the condition termed *pellagra*. Several physiological conditions (eg, Hartnup disorder: see Clinical Box 30-1) as well as certain drug therapies (eg, isoniazid) can lead to niacin deficiency. In Hartnup disease, tryptophan absorption from the gut is impaired.

The major action of nicotinic acid in this capacity is a reduction in fatty acid mobilization from adipose tissue. Although nicotinic acid therapy lowers blood cholesterol, it also causes a depletion of glycogen stores and fat reserves in skeletal and cardiac muscle. Additionally, there is an elevation in blood glucose and uric acid production. For these reasons, nicotinic acid therapy is not recommended for diabetics or persons who suffer from gout.

Pantothenic Acid: Vitamin B_5

Pantothenic acid is also known as vitamin B_5. Pantothenic acid is formed from β-alanine and pantoic acid. Pantothenate is required for synthesis of coenzyme A (CoA) and is a component of the acyl carrier protein (ACP) domain of fatty acid synthase (FAS). In the synthesis of CoA from pantothenate there are 5 reaction steps, Pantothenate is phosphorylated on the hydroxyl group via the action of pantothenate kinase. The reactive sulfhydryl group is added from cysteine via the action of phosphopantothenoylcysteine synthetase. After 3 more reactions, the molecule is decarboxylated and then the adenosine-5′-diphosphate (ADP) from ATP is added, forming the fully functional coenzyme A. Pantothenate is required for the metabolism of carbohydrate via the TCA cycle and all fats

High-Yield Concept

Nicotinic acid (but not nicotinamide), when administered in pharmacological doses of 2 to 4 g/d, lowers plasma cholesterol levels and has been shown to be a useful therapeutic agent for hypercholesterolemia (see Chapter 26).

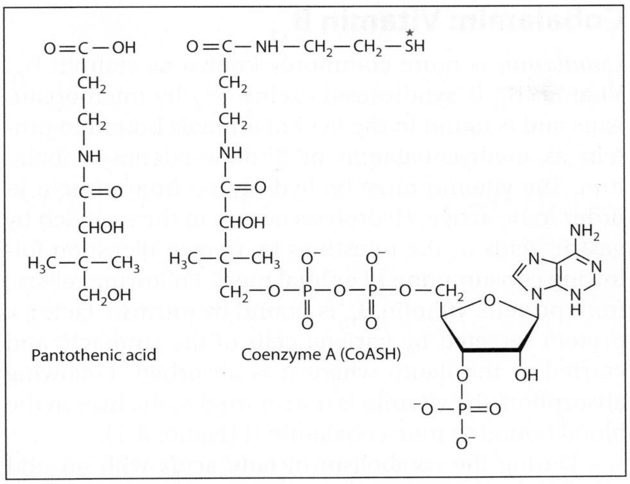

FIGURE 8-4: Pantothenic acid and coenzyme A. Asterisk shows site of acylation by fatty acids. Murray RK, Bender DA, Botham KM, Kennelly PJ, Rodwell VW, Weil PA. *Harper's Illustrated Biochemistry*, 29th ed. New York, NY: McGraw-Hill; 2012.

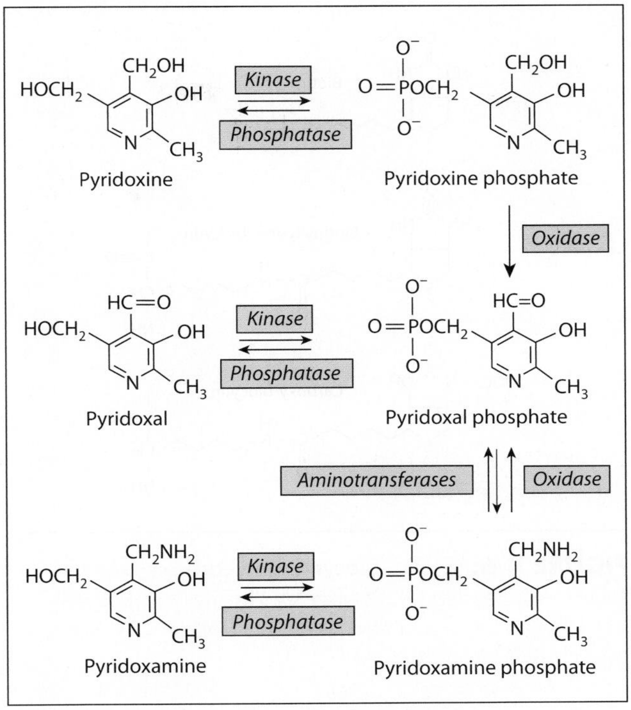

FIGURE 8-5: Interconversion of the vitamin B_6 vitamers. Murray RK, Bender DA, Botham KM, Kennelly PJ, Rodwell VW, Weil PA. *Harper's Illustrated Biochemistry*, 29th ed. New York, NY: McGraw-Hill; 2012.

and proteins. At least 70 enzymes have been identified as requiring CoA or ACP derivatives for their function (Figure 8-4).

Deficiency of pantothenic acid is extremely rare due to its widespread distribution in whole grain cereals, legumes, and meat. Symptoms specific to pantothenate deficiency are difficult to assess since they are subtle and resemble those of other vitamin B deficiencies. These symptoms include painful and burning feet, skin abnormalities, retarded growth, dizzy spells, digestive disturbances, vomiting, restlessness, stomach stress, and muscle cramps.

Vitamin B_6

Pyridoxal, pyridoxamine, and pyridoxine are collectively known as vitamin B_6. All 3 compounds are efficiently converted to the biologically active form of vitamin B_6, pyridoxal phosphate (PLP). This conversion is catalyzed by the ATP-requiring enzyme, pyridoxal kinase. Pyridoxal kinase requires zinc for full activity, thus making it a metalloenzyme (Figure 8-5).

Pyridoxal phosphate functions as a cofactor in enzymes involved in transamination reactions required for the synthesis and catabolism of the amino acids as well as in glycogenolysis as a cofactor for glycogen phosphorylase and as a cofactor for the synthesis of the inhibitory neurotransmitter γ-aminobutyric acid (GABA).

Deficiencies of vitamin B_6 are rare and usually related to an overall deficiency of all the B-complex vitamins. Isoniazid (see niacin deficiencies earlier) and penicillamine (used to treat rheumatoid arthritis and cystinurias) are 2 drugs that complex with pyridoxal and PLP resulting in a deficiency in this vitamin. Deficiencies in pyridoxal kinase result in reduced synthesis of PLP and are associated with seizure disorders related to a reduction in the synthesis of GABA. Other symptoms that may appear with deficiency of vitamin B_6 include nervousness, insomnia, skin eruptions, loss of muscular control, anemia, mouth disorders, muscular weakness, dermatitis, arm and leg cramps, loss of hair, slow learning, and water retention.

Biotin: Vitamin H

Biotin is the cofactor required of enzymes that are involved in carboxylation reactions, for example, acetyl-CoA carboxylase (ACC) (see Chapter 19) and pyruvate carboxylase (see Chapter 13). Biotin is found in numerous foods and is also synthesized by intestinal bacteria and as such deficiencies of the vitamin are rare. Deficiencies are generally seen only after long antibiotic therapies, which deplete the intestinal microbiota or following excessive consumption of raw eggs. The latter is due to the affinity of the egg white protein, avidin, for biotin, preventing intestinal

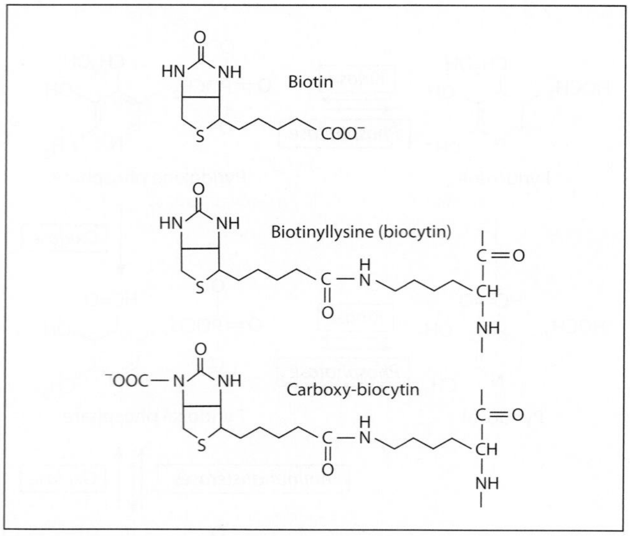

FIGURE 8-6: Biotin, biocytin, and carboxy-biocytin. Murray RK, Bender DA, Botham KM, Kennelly PJ, Rodwell VW, Weil PA. *Harper's Illustrated Biochemistry*, 29th ed. New York, NY: McGraw-Hill; 2012.

absorption of the vitamin. Symptoms that may appear if biotin is deficient are extreme exhaustion, drowsiness, muscle pain, loss of appetite, depression, and grayish skin color (Figure 8-6).

Cobalamin: Vitamin B_{12}

Cobalamin is more commonly known as vitamin B_{12}. Vitamin B_{12} is synthesized exclusively by microorganisms and is found in the liver of animals bound to protein as methycobalamin or 5′-deoxyadenosylcobalamin. The vitamin must be hydrolyzed from protein in order to be active. Hydrolysis occurs in the stomach by gastric acids or the intestines by trypsin digestion following consumption of animal meat. Following release from protein, vitamin B_{12} is bound by intrinsic factor, a protein secreted by parietal cells of the stomach, and carried to the ileum where it is absorbed. Following absorption, the vitamin is transported to the liver in the blood bound to transcobalamin II (Figure 8-7).

During the catabolism of fatty acids with an odd number of carbon atoms and the amino acids valine, isoleucine, and threonine the resultant propionyl-CoA is converted to succinyl-CoA for oxidation in the TCA cycle. One of the enzymes in this pathway, methylmalonyl-CoA mutase, requires vitamin B_{12} as a cofactor in the conversion of methylmalonyl-CoA to succinyl-CoA. The 5′-deoxyadenosine derivative of cobalamin is required for this reaction. The second reaction requiring vitamin B_{12} catalyzes the conversion of homocysteine to methionine and is catalyzed by methionine synthase (also called homocysteine methyltransferase). This reaction results

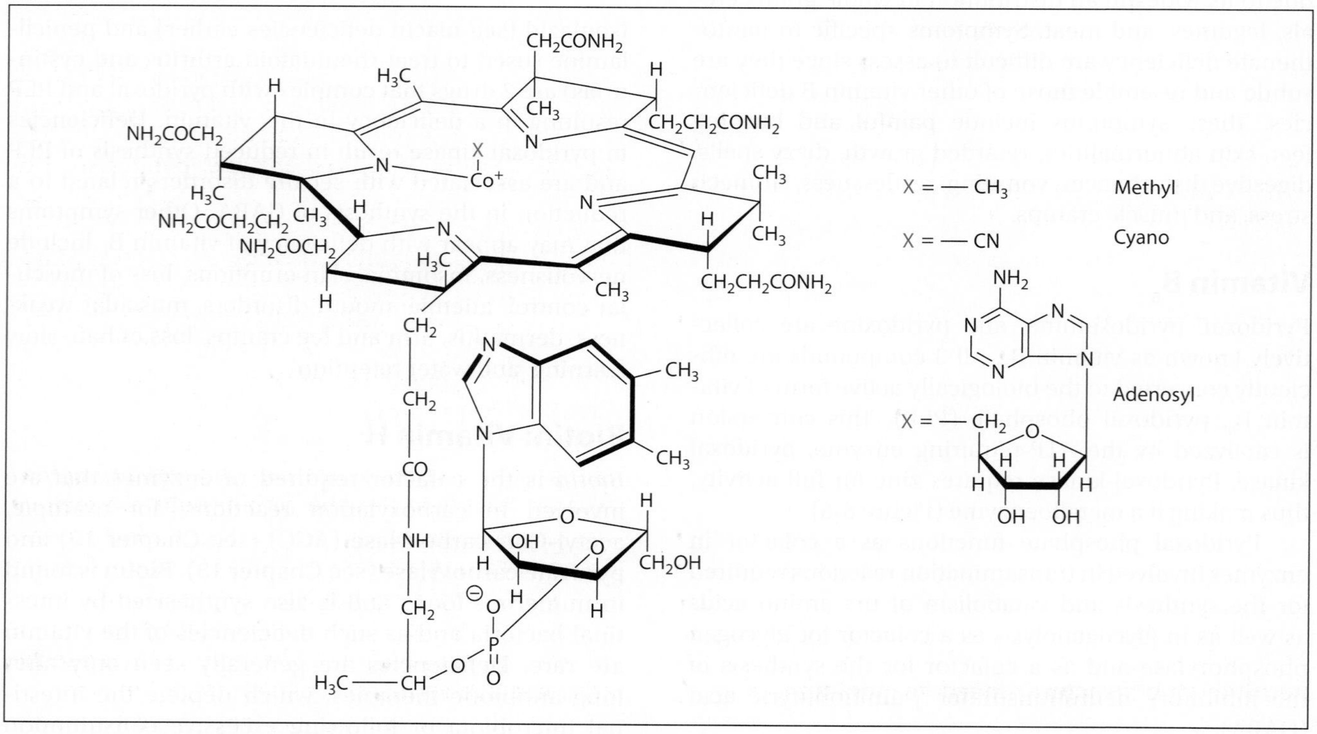

FIGURE 8-7: Structure of cobalamin. The red X indicates the position of the major substituents, methyl, cyano, or adenosyl, found in mammalian forms of vitamin B_{12}. Reproduced with permission of themedicalbiochemistrypage, LLC.

High-Yield Concept

Due to the lack of sufficient vitamin B_{12} in plant foods, it is added to breakfast cereals and this serves as a good source of the vitamin for vegetarians and vegans. Two plant sources that are useful for obtaining vitamin B_{12} are alfalfa and comfrey (also written comfry). However, to ensure adequate intake vegans should use a vitamin B_{12} supplement that contains at least 5 to 10 μg due to the low absorption rate of the vitamin in supplement form.

High Yield Concept

There are only 2 clinically significant reactions in the body that require vitamin B_{12} as a cofactor, methylmalonyl-CoA mutase and methionine synthase (see Clinical Box 8-2).

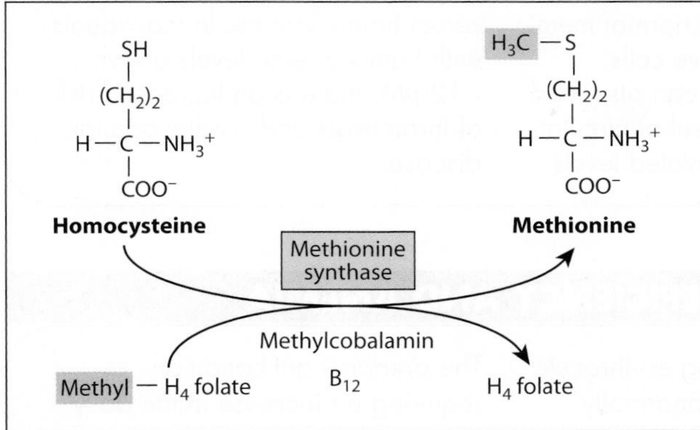

FIGURE 8-8: Homocysteine and the "folate trap." Vitamin B_{12} deficiency leads to impairment of methionine synthase, resulting in accumulation of homocysteine and trapping folate as methyltetrahydrofolate. Murray RK, Bender DA, Botham KM, Kennelly PJ, Rodwell VW, Weil PA. *Harper's Illustrated Biochemistry*, 29th ed. New York, NY: McGraw-Hill; 2012.

in the transfer of the methyl group from N^5-methyltetrahydrofolate to hydroxycobalamin generating tetrahydrofolate (THF) and methylcobalamin during the process of the conversion (Figure 8-8).

Folic Acid

Folic acid is a conjugated molecule consisting of a pteridine ring structure linked to para-aminobenzoic acid (PABA) that forms pteroic acid. Folic acid itself is then generated through the conjugation of glutamic acid residues to pteroic acid. Folic acid is obtained primarily from yeasts and leafy vegetables as well as animal liver. Animals cannot synthesize PABA nor attach glutamate residues to pteroic acid, thus, requiring folate intake in the diet. Folate itself is not biologically active, but in derivatives of the THF form, it participates in a number of one-carbon transfer reactions. THF, and the various derivatives, are formed from dihydrofolate (DHF) which is generated within the liver (Figure 8-9).

When stored in the liver or ingested, folic acid exists in a polyglutamate form. Intestinal mucosal cells remove some of the glutamate residues through the action of the lysosomal enzyme, conjugase. The removal of glutamate residues makes folate less negatively charged and therefore, more capable of passing through the basal lamina membrane of the epithelial cells of the intestine and into the bloodstream. Folic acid is reduced within cells (principally the liver where it is stored) to tetrahydrofolate (THF also H_4 folate) through the action of DHF reductase (DHFR), an NADPH-requiring enzyme.

The function of THF derivatives is to carry and transfer various forms of one-carbon units during biosynthetic reactions. The one-carbon units are methyl, methylene, methenyl, formyl, and formimino groups. These one-carbon transfer reactions are required in the biosynthesis of serine, methionine, glycine, choline, and the purine nucleotides and dTMP. The ability to acquire choline and amino acids from the diet and to salvage the purine nucleotides makes the role of N^5,N^{10}-methylene-THF in dTMP synthesis the most metabolically significant function for this vitamin (see Clinical Box 8-3). The role of vitamin B_{12} and N^5-methyl-THF in the conversion

CLINICAL BOX 8-2: B_{12} DEFICIENCY AND ANEMIA

Given the ability of the liver to store vitamin B_{12}, deficiencies in this vitamin are rare. *Pernicious anemia* is a megaloblastic anemia resulting from vitamin B_{12} deficiency that results from a lack of intrinsic factor in the stomach leading to malabsorption of the vitamin. The anemia results from impaired DNA synthesis due to a block in purine and thymidine biosynthesis. The block in nucleotide biosynthesis is a consequence of the effect of vitamin B_{12} on folate metabolism. When vitamin B_{12} is deficient, essentially all of the folate becomes trapped as the N^5-methyl-THF derivative as a result of the loss of functional methionine synthase. This trapping prevents the synthesis of other THF derivatives required for the purine and thymidine nucleotide biosynthesis pathways.

Neurological complications also are associated with vitamin B_{12} deficiency and result from a progressive demyelination of nerve cells. The demyelination is thought to result from the increase in methylmalonyl-CoA that results from vitamin B_{12} deficiency. Methylmalonyl-CoA is a competitive inhibitor of malonyl-CoA in fatty acid biosynthesis besides being able to substitute for malonyl-CoA in any fatty acid biosynthesis that may occur. Since the myelin sheath is in continual flux, the methylmalonyl-CoA–induced inhibition of fatty acid synthesis results in the eventual destruction of the sheath. The incorporation of methylmalonyl-CoA into fatty acid biosynthesis results in branched-chain fatty acids being produced that may severely alter the architecture of the normal membrane structure of nerve cells.

Deficiencies in B_{12} can also lead to elevations in the level of circulating homocysteine. Elevated levels of homocysteine are known to lead to cardiovascular dysfunction. Due to its high reactivity to proteins, homocysteine is almost always bound to proteins, thus thiolating them leading to their degradation. Homocysteine also binds to albumin and hemoglobin in the blood. The detrimental effects of homocysteine are thought to be due to its binding to lysyl oxidase, an enzyme responsible for proper maturation of the extracellular matrix proteins collagen and elastin. Production of defective collagen and elastin has a negative impact on arteries, bone, and skin and the effects on the arteries are believed to be the underlying cause for cardiac dysfunction associated with elevated serum homocysteine. In individuals with homocysteine levels above ≈12 μM, there is an increased risk of thrombosis and cardiovascular disease.

CLINICAL BOX 8-3: FOLATE DEFICIENCY AND ANEMIA

Folate deficiency results in complications nearly identical to those described for vitamin B_{12} deficiency. The most pronounced effect of folate deficiency on cellular processes is upon DNA synthesis. This is due to an impairment in dTMP synthesis, which leads to cell cycle arrest in S-phase of rapidly proliferating cells, in particular hematopoietic cells. The result is megaloblastic anemia as for vitamin B_{12} deficiency. The inability to synthesize DNA during erythrocyte maturation leads to abnormally large erythrocytes termed macrocytic anemia.

Folate deficiencies are rare due to the adequate presence of folate in food. Poor dietary habits as those of chronic alcoholics can lead to folate deficiency. The predominant causes of folate deficiency in nonalcoholics are impaired absorption or metabolism or an increased demand for the vitamin. The predominant condition requiring an increase in the daily intake of folate is pregnancy. This is due to an increased number of rapidly proliferating cells present in the blood. The need for folate will nearly double by the third trimester of pregnancy. Certain drugs such as anticonvulsants and oral contraceptives can impair the absorption of folate. Anticonvulsants also increase the rate of folate metabolism.

of homocysteine to methionine also can have a significant impact on the ability of cells to regenerate needed THF (Figure 8-10).

Ascorbic Acid: Vitamin C

Ascorbic acid is more commonly known as vitamin C. Ascorbic acid is derived from glucose via the uronic acid pathway, however, the enzyme L-gulonolactone oxidase, responsible for the conversion of gulonolactone to ascorbic acid, is absent in humans making ascorbic acid required in the diet (Figure 8-11).

The active form of vitamin C is ascorbic acid itself. The main function of ascorbate is as a reducing agent in a number of different reactions. Ascorbate is the

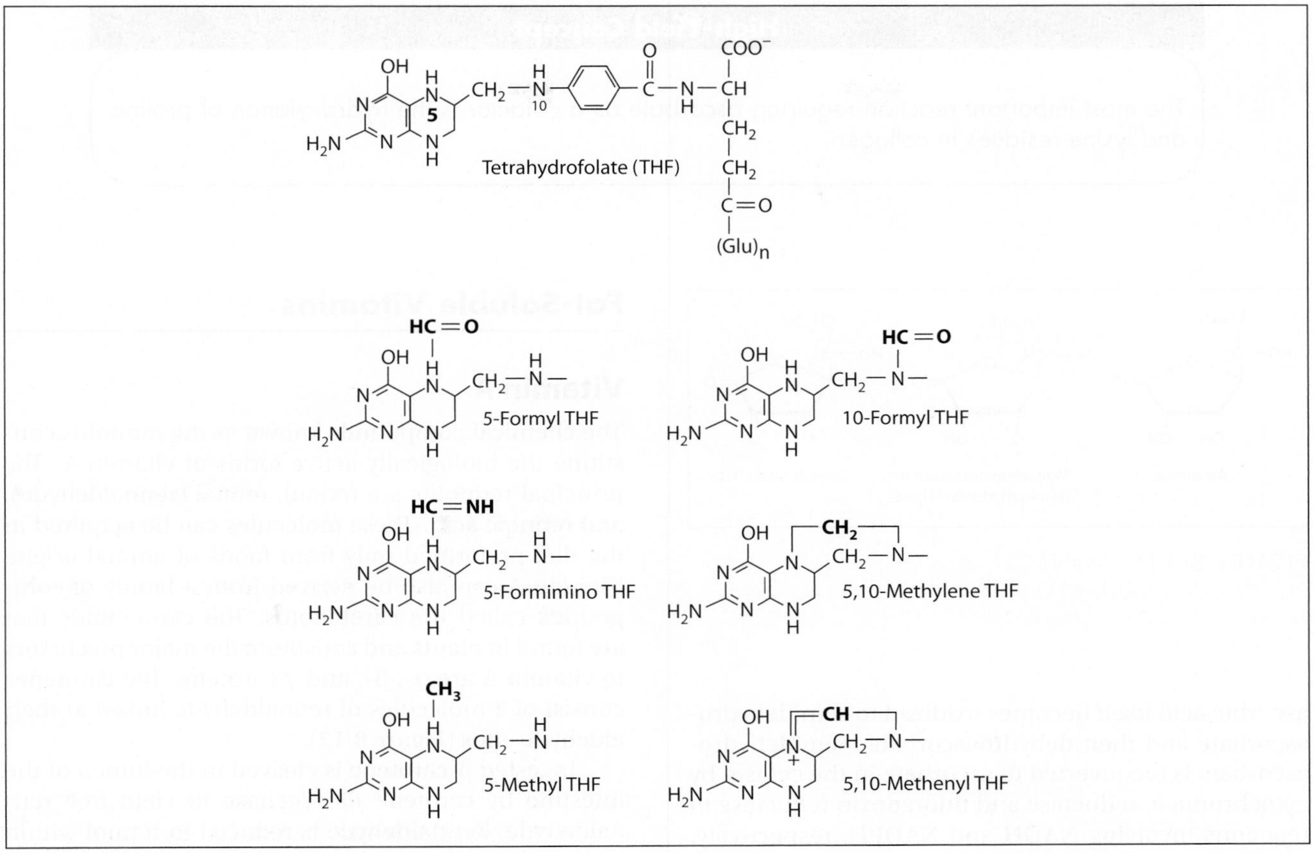

Tetrahydrofolate (THF)
5-Formyl THF
10-Formyl THF
5-Formimino THF
5,10-Methylene THF
5-Methyl THF
5,10-Methenyl THF

FIGURE 8-9: Tetrahydrofolic acid and the one-carbon substituted folates. Murray RK, Bender DA, Botham KM, Kennelly PJ, Rodwell VW, Weil PA. *Harper's Illustrated Biochemistry*, 29th ed. New York, NY: McGraw-Hill; 2012.

Sources of one-carbon units
Synthesis using one-carbon units
Serine
Glycine
Choline
Methylene-THF
Serine
Methyl-THF
Methionine
TMP + dihydrofolate
DNA
Histidine
Formimino-THF
Methenyl-THF
Formate
Formyl-THF
Formyl-methionine
Purines
CO2

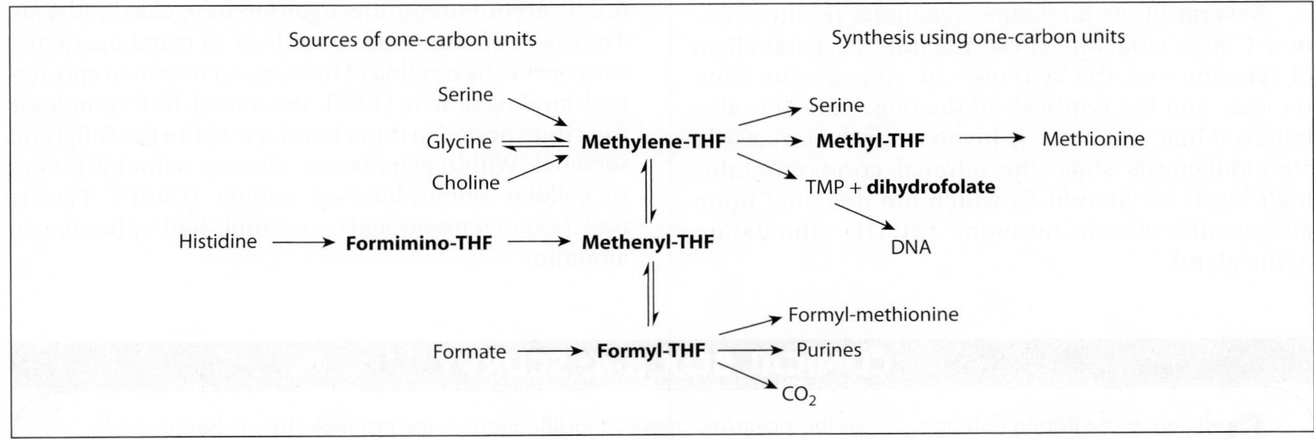

FIGURE 8-10: Sources and utilization of one-carbon substituted folates. Murray RK, Bender DA, Botham KM, Kennelly PJ, Rodwell VW, Weil PA. *Harper's Illustrated Biochemistry*, 29th ed. New York, NY: McGraw-Hill; 2012.

cofactor for Cu^{+}-dependent monooxygenases and Fe^{2+}-dependent dioxygenases. Ascorbate has the potential to reduce cytochromes *a* and *c* of the respiratory chain as well as molecular oxygen.

Vitamin C is, therefore, required for the maintenance of normal connective tissue as well as for wound healing since synthesis of connective tissue is the first event in wound tissue remodeling (see Clinical Box 8-4). Vitamin C also is necessary for bone remodeling due to the presence of collagen in the organic matrix of bones.

Ascorbic acid also serves as a reducing agent and an antioxidant. When functioning as an antioxidant,

High-Yield Concept

The most important reaction requiring ascorbate as a cofactor is the hydroxylation of proline and lysine residues in collagen.

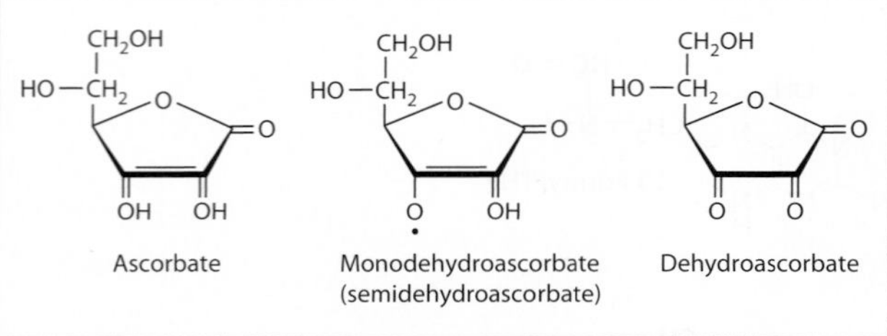

FIGURE 8-11: Vitamin C. Murray RK, Bender DA, Botham KM, Kennelly PJ, Rodwell VW, Weil PA. *Harper's Illustrated Biochemistry*, 29th ed. New York, NY: McGraw-Hill; 2012.

ascorbic acid itself becomes oxidized to semidehydroascorbate and then dehydroascorbate. Semidehydroascorbate is reconverted to ascorbate in the cytosol by cytochrome b_5 reductase and thioredoxin reductase in reactions involving NADH and NADPH, respectively. Dehydroascorbate, the fully oxidized form of vitamin C, is reduced spontaneously by glutathione, as well as enzymatically in reactions using glutathione or NADPH.

Several other metabolic reactions require vitamin C as a cofactor. These include the catabolism of tyrosine and the synthesis of epinephrine from tyrosine and the synthesis of the bile acids. It is also believed that vitamin C is involved in the process of steroidogenesis since the adrenal cortex contains high levels of vitamin C, which are depleted upon adrenocorticotropic hormone (ACTH) stimulation of the gland.

Fat-Soluble Vitamins

Vitamin A

The chemical compounds known as the retinoids constitute the biologically active forms of vitamin A. The principal retinoids are retinol, retinal (retinaldehyde), and retinoic acid. These molecules can be acquired in the diet preformed only from foods of animal origin. Vitamin A can also be derived from a family of compounds called the carotenoids. The carotenoids that are found in plants and constitute the major precursors to vitamin A are α-, β-, and γ-carotene. The carotenes consist of 2 molecules of retinaldehyde linked at their aldehyde ends (Figure 8-12).

Ingested β-carotene is cleaved in the lumen of the intestine by carotene dioxygenase to yield free retinaldehyde. Retinaldehyde is reduced to retinol within intestinal enterocytes by retinaldehyde reductase, an NADPH-requiring enzyme. Retinol is esterified to palmitic acid and delivered to the blood via chylomicrons. The uptake of chylomicron remnants by the liver results in delivery of retinol to this organ for storage as a lipid ester. Transport of retinol from the liver to extrahepatic tissues occurs by binding of hydrolyzed retinol to apo-retinol-binding protein (RBP). The retinol-RBP complex is then transported to the cell surface within the Golgi and secreted. Within extrahepatic tissues, retinol is bound to cellular retinol-binding protein (CRBP). Plasma transport of retinoic acid is accomplished by binding to albumin.

CLINICAL BOX 8-4: SCURVY

Deficiency of vitamin C leads to scurvy, a disease characterized by easily bruised skin, muscle fatigue, soft swollen gums, decreased wound healing and hemorrhaging, osteoporosis, an anemia. This happens because vitamin C plays an important role in the posttranslational modification of collagens. Vitamin C is readily absorbed and so the primary cause of vitamin C deficiency is poor diet and/or an increased requirement. The primary physiological state leading to an increased requirement for vitamin C is severe stress (or trauma). This is because of a rapid depletion in the adrenal stores of the vitamin. The reason for the decrease in adrenal vitamin C levels is unclear but may be due either to redistribution of the vitamin to areas that need it or an overall increased utilization.

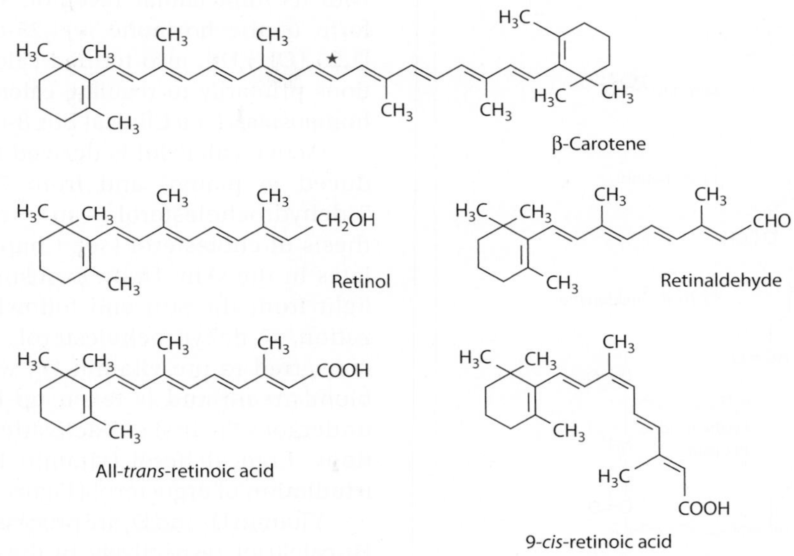

FIGURE 8-12: β-Carotene and the major vitamin A vitamers. Asterisk shows the site of cleavage of β-carotene by carotene dioxygenase, to yield retinaldehyde. Murray RK, Bender DA, Botham KM, Kennelly PJ, Rodwell VW, Weil PA. *Harper's Illustrated Biochemistry*, 29th ed. New York, NY: McGraw-Hill; 2012.

Gene Control Exerted by Retinoic Acid

Within cells, retinoic acid (as well as the related compound 9-*cis*-retinoic acid) bind to specific receptor proteins that are members of the nuclear receptor family of hormone receptors. Following binding, the receptor-retinoic acid complex interacts with specific sequences in several genes involved in growth and differentiation and affects expression of these genes. In this capacity, retinoic acid is considered a hormone of the steroid/thyroid hormone superfamily of proteins. The retinoic acid receptors are abbreviated RAR and the related retinoid X receptors (RXRs) bind 9-*cis*-retinoic acid. Several genes, whose patterns of expression are altered by retinoic acid, are involved in the earliest processes of embryogenesis including the differentiation of the 3 germ layers, organogenesis, and limb development. To date, there are at least 130 genes that have been shown to be directly regulated (either positive or negative) via interaction with RAR or RXR.

Vision and the Role of Vitamin A

Photoreception in the eye is the function of 2 specialized cell types located in the retina; the rod and cone cells. Both rod and cone cells contain a photoreceptor pigment in their membranes. The photosensitive compound of most mammalian eyes is a protein called opsin to which is covalently coupled an aldehyde of vitamin A. The opsin of rod cells is called scotopsin. The photoreceptor of rod cells is specifically called rhodopsin or visual purple. This compound is a complex between scotopsin and the 11-*cis*-retinal (also called 11-*cis*-retinene) form of vitamin A. Rhodopsin is a serpentine receptor embedded in the membrane of the rod cell. Coupling of 11-*cis*-retinal occurs at 3 of the transmembrane domains of rhodopsin. Within the membrane of visual cells, rhodopsin is coupled to a specific G-protein called transducin (Figure 8-13).

When the rhodopsin is exposed to light, it is bleached releasing the 11-*cis*-retinal from opsin. Absorption of photons by 11-*cis*-retinal triggers a series of conformational changes on the way to conversion to all-*trans*-retinal. One important conformational intermediate is metarhodopsin II. The release of opsin results in a conformational change in the photoreceptor. This conformational change activates transducin, leading to an increased GTP binding by the α-subunit of transducin. Binding of GTP releases the α-subunit from the inhibitory β- and γ-subunits. The GTP-activated α-subunit in turn activates an associated phosphodiesterase; an enzyme that hydrolyzes cyclic-GMP (cGMP) to GMP. Cyclic GMP is required to maintain the Na^+ channels of the rod cell in the open conformation. The drop in cGMP concentration results in complete closure of the Na^+ channels. Metarhodopsin II appears to be responsible for initiating the closure of the channels. The hyperpolarization causes the closure of calcium channels in the plasma membrane of the rod cell and since calcium ions are required for the release of glutamate from pre-synaptic vesicles, the release of glutamate is inhibited. The loss of glutamate release results less activation of the glutamate receptor on bipolar cells with the

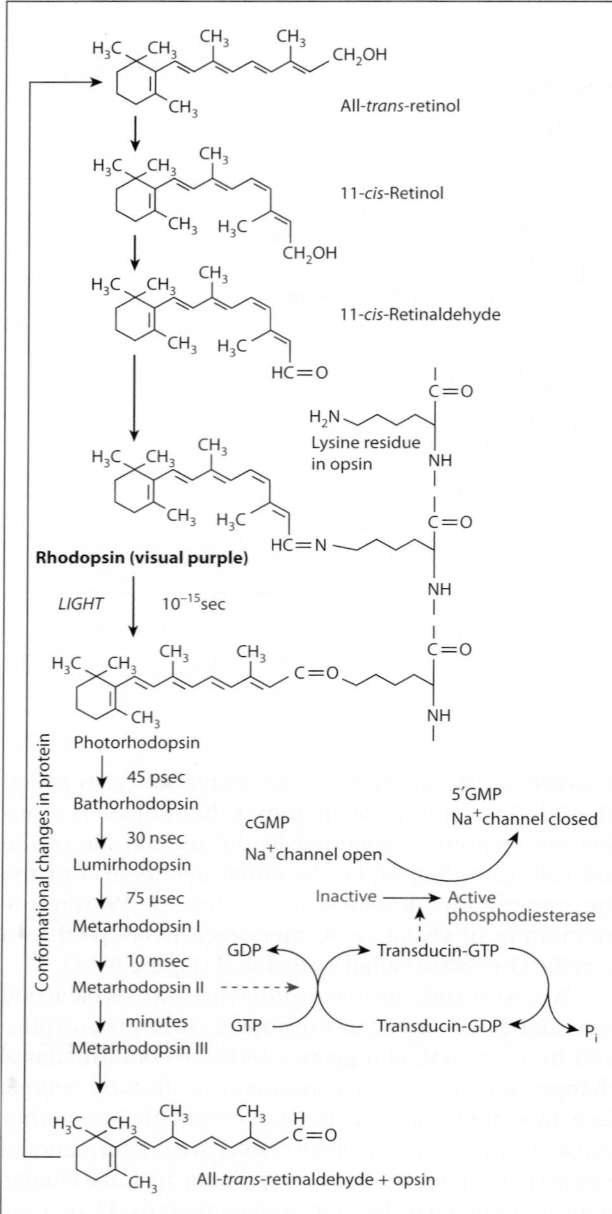

FIGURE 8-13: The role of retinaldehyde in the visual cycle. Murray RK, Bender DA, Botham KM, Kennelly PJ, Rodwell VW, Weil PA. *Harper's Illustrated Biochemistry*, 29th ed. New York, NY: McGraw-Hill; 2012.

consequences that these cells become depolarized and no longer release the inhibitory neurotransmitter, GABA. The result is that the optic nerve become disinhibited in the dark so that we can see with the limited light available at night (see Clinical Box 8-5).

Vitamin D

Vitamin D is a steroid hormone that functions to regulate specific gene expression following interaction with its intracellular receptor. The biologically active form of the hormone is 1,25-dihydroxy vitamin D_3 [1,25-$(OH)_2D_3$], also termed calcitriol. Calcitriol functions primarily to regulate calcium and phosphorous homeostasis (see Clinical Box 8-6).

Active calcitriol is derived from ergosterol (produced in plants) and from 7-dehydrocholesterol. 7-dehydrocholesterol is an intermediate in the synthesis of cholesterol (see Chapter 26) that accumulates in the skin. Upon exposure to ultraviolet (UV) light from the sun and following thermal isomerization, 7-dehydrocholesterol is nonenzymatically converted to pre-vitamin D_3, which then enters the bloodstream and is taken up by the liver where it undergoes the first of 2 activating hydroxylation reactions. Ergocalciferol (vitamin D_2) is formed by UV irradiation of ergosterol (Figures 8-14).

Vitamin D_2 and D_3 are processed to D_2-calcitriol and D_3-calcitriol, respectively, by the same enzymatic pathways in the body. Cholecalciferol (or ergocalciferol) are absorbed from the intestine and transported to the liver bound to a specific vitamin D–binding protein. In the liver, cholecalciferol is hydroxylated at the 25 position by a specific D_3-25-hydroxylase generating 25-hydroxy-D_3 [25-$(OH)D_3$], which is the major circulating form of vitamin D (see Figure 8-15). Conversion of 25-$(OH)D_3$ to its biologically active form, calcitriol, occurs through the activity of a specific D_3-1-hydroxylase present in the proximal convoluted tubules of the kidneys, and in bone and placenta. 25-$(OH)D_3$ can also be hydroxylated at the 24 position by a specific D_3-24-hydroxylase in the kidneys, intestine, placenta, and cartilage.

PTH is released in response to low serum calcium and induces the production of calcitriol. In contrast, reduced levels of PTH stimulate synthesis of the inactive 24,25-$(OH)_2D_3$. In the intestinal epithelium, calcitriol functions as a steroid hormone in inducing the expression of calbindinD_{28K}, a protein involved in intestinal calcium absorption. The steroid hormone action of vitamin D occurs via the action of calcitriol binding to a specific intracellular receptor that is a member of the nuclear receptor family of hormone receptors called the vitamin D receptor (VDR).

The increased absorption of calcium ions requires concomitant absorption of a negatively charged counter ion to maintain electrical neutrality. The predominant counter ion is phosphate. When plasma calcium levels fall, the major sites of action of calcitriol and PTH are bone, where they stimulate bone resorption, and the kidneys, where they inhibit calcium excretion by stimulating reabsorption by the distal tubules.

Vitamin E

Vitamin E is a mixture of several related compounds known as tocopherols and tocotrienols. The tocopherols

CLINICAL BOX 8-5: VITAMIN A DEFICIENCY AND BLINDNESS

Vitamin A is stored in the liver and deficiency of the vitamin occurs only after prolonged lack of dietary intake. The earliest symptoms of vitamin A deficiency are night blindness. Additional early symptoms include follicular hyperkeratosis, increased susceptibility to infection and cancer, and anemia equivalent to iron-deficient anemia. Prolonged lack of vitamin A leads to deterioration of the eye tissue through progressive keratinization of the cornea, a condition known as xerophthalmia.

The increased risk of cancer in vitamin deficiency is thought to be the result of a depletion in β-carotene. Beta-carotene is a very effective antioxidant and is suspected to reduce the risk of cancers known to be initiated by the production of free radicals. Of particular interest is the potential benefit of increased β-carotene intake to reduce the risk of lung cancer in smokers. However, caution needs to be taken when increasing the intake of any of the lipid-soluble vitamins. Excess accumulation of vitamin A in the liver can lead to toxicity, which manifests as bone pain, hepatosplenomegaly, nausea, and diarrhea.

CLINICAL BOX 8-6: VITAMIN D DEFICIENCY

As a result of the addition of vitamin D to milk, deficiencies of this vitamin are rare in this country. The main symptom of vitamin D deficiency in children is rickets and in adults is osteomalacia. Rickets is characterized by improper mineralization during the development of the bones resulting in soft bones. Rickets results from deficiency or impaired metabolism of vitamin D, phosphorus, or calcium. The most common treatment for rickets is the administration of vitamin D. Osteomalacia is defined as the softening of the bones caused by defective bone mineralization secondary to deficiency in available levels of phosphorus and calcium, or because of overactive resorption of calcium from the bone. Osteomalacia and osteoporosis do not describe the same bone defect. In osteoporosis, bone mineral density is reduced and the amount and variety of proteins in the bone are altered. Muscle weakness and achy bone pain are the major symptoms associated with osteomalacia. Treatment for osteomalacia involves replenishing low levels of vitamin D and calcium, and treating any underlying disorders that may be causing the deficiencies.

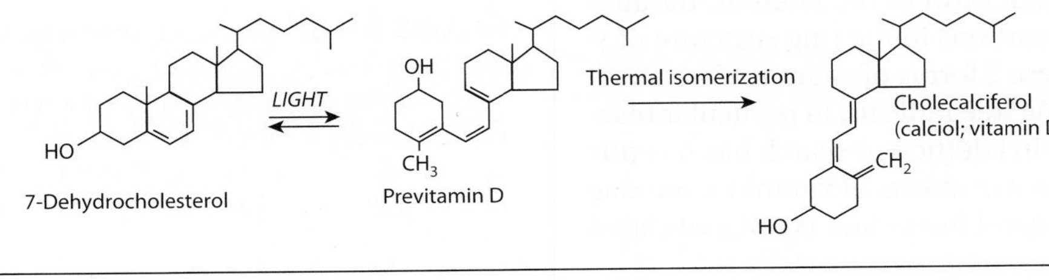

FIGURE 8-14: The synthesis of vitamin D in the skin. Murray RK, Bender DA, Botham KM, Kennelly PJ, Rodwell VW, Weil PA. *Harper's Illustrated Biochemistry*, 29th ed. New York, NY: McGraw-Hill; 2012.

are the major sources of vitamin E in the US diet. The tocopherols differ by the number and position of methyl ($-CH_3-$) groups present on the ring system of the chemical structure. The different tocopherols are designated α-, β-, γ-, and δ-tocopherol. Most vitamin E in US diets is in the form of γ-tocopherol from soybean, canola, corn, and other vegetable oils. All 4 tocopherols are able to act as free radical scavengers thus, they all have potent antioxidant properties. Vitamin E is absorbed from the intestines packaged in chylomicrons. It is delivered to the tissues via chylomicron transport and then to the liver through chylomicron remnant uptake. The liver can export vitamin E in very-low-density lipoproteins (VLDLs). Within the liver α-tocopherol transfer protein preferentially transfers α-tocopherol to VLDLs, thus α-tocopherol is the most abundant tocopherol in nonhepatic (liver) tissues. Due to its lipophilic nature, vitamin E accumulates in cellular membranes, fat deposits, and other circulating lipoproteins. The major site of vitamin E storage is in adipose tissue (Figure 8-16).

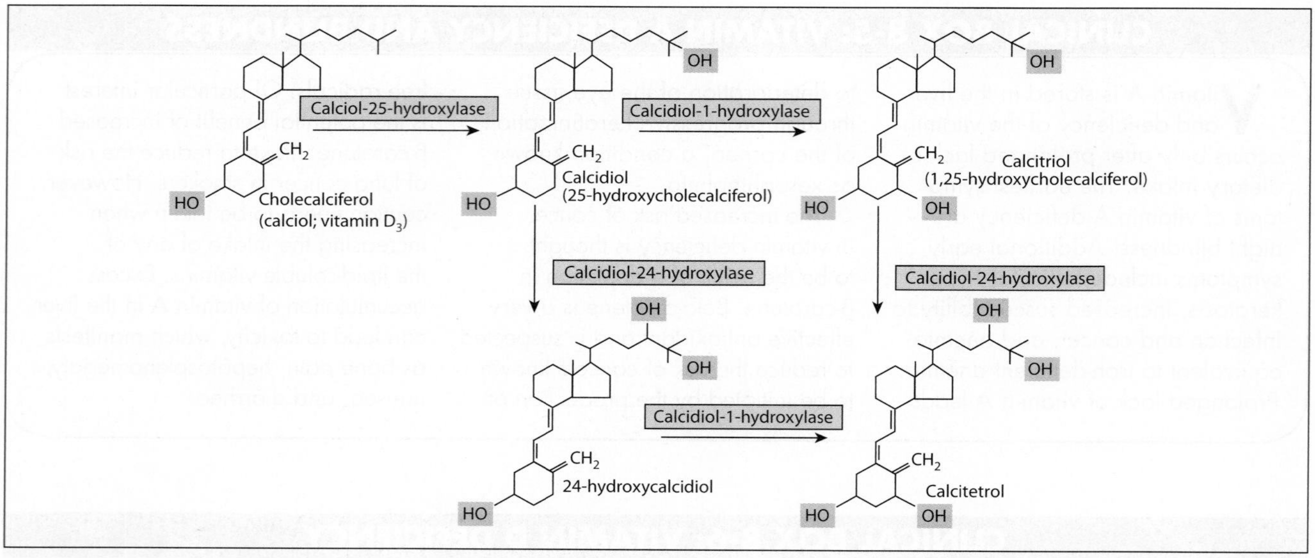

FIGURE 8-15: Metabolism of vitamin D. Murray RK, Bender DA, Botham KM, Kennelly PJ, Rodwell VW, Weil PA. *Harper's Illustrated Biochemistry*, 29th ed. New York, NY: McGraw-Hill; 2012.

In particular, vitamin E is important for preventing peroxidation of polyunsaturated membrane fatty acids. The vitamins E and C are interrelated in their antioxidant capabilities. Active α-tocopherol can be regenerated by interaction with vitamin C following scavenge of a peroxy free radical. Alternatively, α-tocopherol can scavenge 2 peroxy free radicals and then be conjugated to glucuronate for excretion in the bile.

Although α-tocopherol is the most abundant tocopherol in tissues outside of the liver, it is not the most potent antioxidant form of the vitamin. Because of the unmethylated carbons in the ring structure of γ- and δ-tocopherol, these 2 forms of vitamin E are much more active at trapping free radicals, in particular reactive nitrogen species. In addition, research has recently shown that the anticancer effects of vitamin E are due to the γ- and δ-tocopherol forms and is not associated with α-tocopherol.

No major disease states have been found to be associated with vitamin E deficiency due to adequate levels in the average American diet. The major symptom of vitamin E deficiency in humans is an increase in red blood cell fragility. Since vitamin E is absorbed from the intestines in chylomicrons, any disease associated with fat malabsorption can lead to deficiencies in vitamin E intake. Neurological dysfunction has been correlated to vitamin E deficiencies associated with fat malabsorptive disorders. Increased intake of vitamin E is recommended in premature infants fed formula milk that is low in the vitamin, as well as in persons consuming a diet high in polyunsaturated fatty acids. Polyunsaturated fatty acids tend to form free radicals upon exposure to oxygen and this may lead to an increased risk of certain cancers.

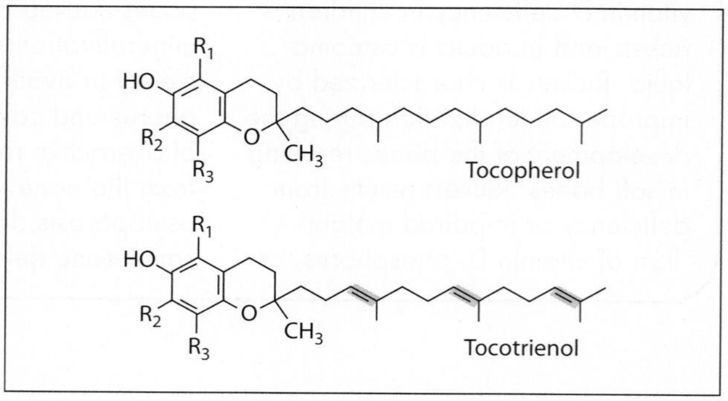

FIGURE 8-16: Vitamin E vitamers. In α-tocopherol and tocotrienol R_1, R_2, and R_3 are all $-CH_3$ groups. In the β-vitamers R_2 is H, in the γ-vitamers R_1 is H, and in the δ-vitamers R_1 and R_2 are both H. Murray RK, Bender DA, Botham KM, Kennelly PJ, Rodwell VW, Weil PA. *Harper's Illustrated Biochemistry*, 29th ed. New York, NY: McGraw-Hill; 2012.

Vitamin K

The K vitamins exist naturally as K_1 (phylloquinone) in green vegetables and K_2 (menaquinone) produced by intestinal bacteria and K_3 is synthetic menadione. When administered, vitamin K_3 is alkylated to one of the vitamin K_2 forms of menaquinone (Figure 8-17).

High-Yield Concept

The major function of vitamin E is to act as a natural antioxidant by scavenging free radicals and molecular oxygen.

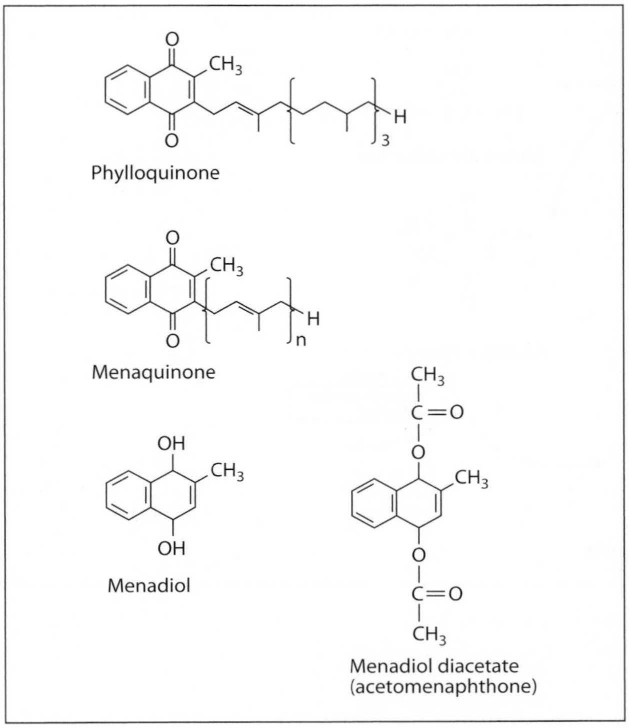

Phylloquinone

Menaquinone

Menadiol

Menadiol diacetate (acetomenaphthone)

FIGURE 8-17: The vitamin K vitamers. Menadiol (or menadione) and menadiol diacetate are synthetic compounds that are converted to menaquinone in the liver. Murray RK, Bender DA, Botham KM, Kennelly PJ, Rodwell VW, Weil PA. *Harper's Illustrated Biochemistry*, 29th ed. New York, NY: McGraw-Hill; 2012.

Conversion from inactive to active clotting factor requires a posttranslational modification of specific glutamate (E) residues. This modification is a carboxylation and the enzyme responsible requires vitamin K as a cofactor. The resultant modified E residues are γ-carboxyglutamate (*gla*). This process is most clearly understood for factor II, also called preprothrombin. Prothrombin is modified preprothrombin. The *gla* residues are effective calcium ion chelators. Upon chelation of calcium, prothrombin interacts with phospholipids in membranes and is proteolysed to thrombin through the action of activated factor X (Xa) (Figure 8-18).

During the carboxylation reaction, reduced hydroquinone form of vitamin K is converted to a 2,3-epoxide form. The regeneration of the hydroquinone form requires an uncharacterized reductase. This latter reaction is the site of action of the coumarin-based anticoagulants such as warfarin (trade name Coumadin).

Naturally occurring vitamin K is absorbed from the intestines only in the presence of bile salts and other lipids through interaction with chylomicrons. Therefore, fat malabsorptive diseases can result in vitamin K deficiency. The synthetic vitamin K_3 is water soluble and absorbed irrespective of the presence of intestinal lipids and bile. Since the vitamin K_2 form is synthesized by intestinal bacteria, deficiency of the vitamin in adults is rare. However, long-term antibiotic treatment can lead to deficiency in adults. The intestine of newborn infants is sterile, therefore, vitamin K deficiency in infants is possible if lacking from the early diet. The primary symptom of a deficiency in infants is a hemorrhagic syndrome.

α-Lipoic Acid

Alpha-lipoic acid (LA) is a naturally occurring dithiol compound synthesized enzymatically in the mitochondrion from the medium-chain fatty acid octanoic acid. Because LA can be synthesized in the body, it is not

High-Yield Concept

The major function of the K vitamins is in the maintenance of normal levels of the blood-clotting proteins, factors II, VII, IX, X, and protein C and protein S, which are synthesized in the liver as inactive precursor proteins.

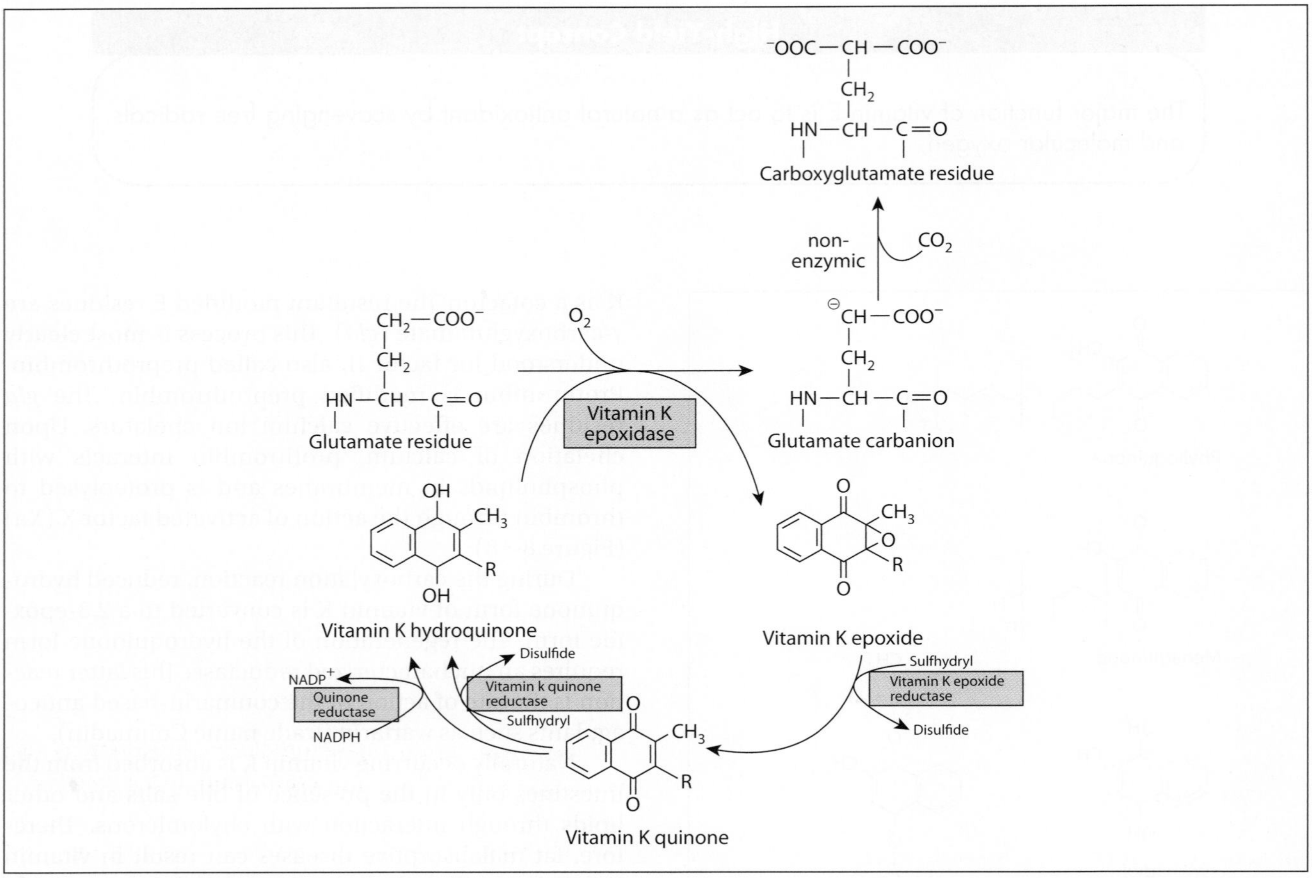

FIGURE 8-18: The role of vitamin K in the synthesis of γ-carboxyglutamate. Murray RK, Bender DA, Botham KM, Kennelly PJ, Rodwell VW, Weil PA. *Harper's Illustrated Biochemistry*, 29th ed. New York, NY: McGraw-Hill; 2012.

technically considered a vitamin but because of its vital role as an enzyme cofactor in overall cellular metabolism, it is considered as an important, but not necessary, dietary supplement. Lipoic acid has one chiral center and therefore exists in both *R*- and *S*-enantiomeric forms (Figure 8-19). However, only *R*-LA is conjugated to conserved lysine residues in an amide linkage (forming a lipoamide), thus making this isoform essential as a cofactor in biological systems. Enzymes containing lipoamide are typically mitochondrial multienzyme complexes that catalyze the oxidative decarboxylation of α-keto acids (eg, PDH and α-KGDH) (Figure 8-19).

Lipoic acid is an essential cofactor for the E2 component of α-ketoacid dehydrogenase complexes, exclusively located in mitochondria. These include the PDH, α-ketoglutarate dehydrogenase (KGDH), and branched chain α-ketoacid dehydrogenase (BCKDH) complexes. Thus, LA serves a critical role in mitochondrial energy metabolism.

Lipoic acid has been described as a potent biological antioxidant, a detoxification agent, and a diabetes medicine; it has been used to improve age-associated cardiovascular, cognitive, and neuromuscular deficits, and has been implicated as a modulator of various inflammatory signaling pathways. LA, either as a dietary supplement or as a therapeutic agent, modulates distinct redox circuits because of its ability to equilibrate between different subcellular compartments

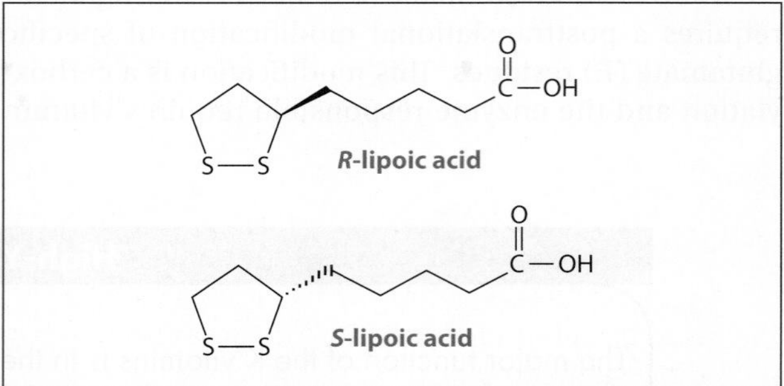

FIGURE 8-19: Enantiomeric forms of a-lipoic acid. Reproduced with permission of themedicalbiochemistrypage, LLC.

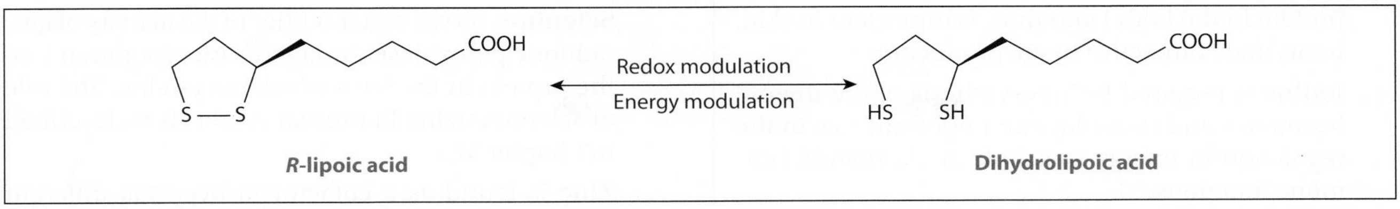

FIGURE 8-20: Redox interconversions α-lipoic acid (LA) and dihydrolipoic acid (DHLA). Reproduced with permission of themedicalbiochemistrypage, LLC.

and extracellularly. LA is a critical component of the antioxidant network and as such, it is important in the regeneration of other antioxidants, such as vitamins E and C. LA increases the intracellular levels of glutathione (GSH) and provides redox regulation of numerous proteins and transcription factors.

Lipoic acid may play an important role in the modulation of the extracellular redox state via the involvement of dihydrolipoic acid (DHLA) in the reduction of cystine to cysteine. This reduction facilitates a rapid uptake of cysteine into the cell, making it available to stimulate GSH synthesis. The cellular reduction of LA to DHLA (Figure 8-20) is accomplished by NAD(P)H-driven enzymes, thioredoxin reductase, lipoamide dehydrogenase, and glutathione reductase (Figure 8-20).

Extensive evidence suggests that LA may have therapeutic usefulness in lowering blood glucose levels in diabetic conditions and that the intracellular redox status plays a role in the modulation of insulin resistance. Lipoic acid has been shown to stimulate glucose uptake by affecting components of the insulin-signaling pathway (see Chapter 46).

Minerals

The functions of the "minerals" are numerous; either quite broad or highly specific. The minerals that are needed for normal cellular functioning can be divided into 2 broad categories termed macrominerals and trace minerals.

Calcium is required for bone mineralization, cardiac function, muscle contraction, and digestive system function. In addition, calcium is necessary for proper activity of a number of proteins involved in blood coagulation.

Chlorine (as chloride ion) is important to maintain the function of numerous cellular pumps and is used in the production of hydrochloric acid (HCl) in the stomach.

Iron, although considered a trace element, has a critical role in the transport of oxygen. Iron is the functional center of the heme moiety found in each of the protein subunit of hemoglobin. The function of iron is to coordinate the oxygen molecule into heme of hemoglobin so that it can be transported from the lungs to the tissues.

Magnesium is required for bone mineralization as well as for the proper functioning of ATP. In this latter function, essentially all of ATP in the cell has magnesium bound to the phosphates. This magnesium-ATP complex allows ATP to more readily release the terminal phosphate (the γ-phosphate) and while doing so to provide energy for cellular metabolism.

Phosphorous is the most important systemic electrolyte acting as a significant buffer in the blood in the form of phosphate ion: PO_4^{2-}. Phosphate is also required for bone mineralization and is necessary for energy utilization.

Potassium is a key circulating electrolyte involved in the regulation of ATP-dependent channels along with sodium. These channels are referred to as Na^+/K^+-ATPases and their primary function is the transmission of nerve impulses from the brain.

Sodium is a key circulating electrolyte also involved in the regulation of ATP-dependent channels with potassium. These channels are referred to as Na^+/K^+-ATPases and their primary function is the transmission of nerve impulses from the brain.

Sulfur has a primary function in amino acid metabolism but is also necessary for the modification of complex carbohydrates present in proteins and lipids, however, it should be noted that in this latter function the sulfur comes from the amino acid methionine.

The trace minerals function primarily as cofactors or regulators of enzyme function. The terminology of "trace" relates to the fact that these minerals are effective and necessary in only minute concentration.

Copper is involved in the formation of red bloods cells, the synthesis of hemoglobin, and the formation of bone. Additional functions of copper are energy production, wound healing, taste sensation, skin and hair color. Copper is also involved in the proper processing of collagen (the most abundant protein in the body) and thus, is important in skin, bone, and connective tissue production.

Iodine is required for the synthesis of the thyroid hormones and thus plays an important role in the regulation of energy metabolism via thyroid hormone functions.

Manganese is involved in reactions of protein and fat metabolism; promotes a healthy nervous system; and is necessary for digestive function, bone growth, and immune function. In addition, manganese is necessary for the proper function of super oxide dismutase (SOD) which is an enzyme required for preventing super oxide anions from damaging cells.

Molybdenum is primarily involved as a cofactor in several oxidases such as xanthine oxidase (see Chapter 32), aldehyde oxidase, and sulfite oxidase.

Selenium serves as a modifier of the activity of glutathione peroxidase through its incorporation into the protein in the form of selenocysteine. The role of selenocysteine in protein synthesis is described in Chapter 37.

Zinc is found as a cofactor in over 300 different enzymes and thus is involved in a wide variety of biochemical processes. Zinc interacts with the hormone insulin to ensure proper function and thus this trace mineral has an important role in regulation of blood glucose levels via insulin action. Zinc also promotes wound healing, regulates immune function, serves as a cofactor for numerous antioxidant enzymes, and is necessary for protein synthesis and the processing of collagen.

REVIEW QUESTIONS

1. You are tending to a patient in the emergency room (ER) who presents with the following symptoms: nystagmus, organic toxic psychosis, and ataxia. You notice that the patient is dirty and appears not to have bathed in several days or weeks. There is an odor of vomit and alcohol on his clothing. Given the outward appearance and observed symptoms, your diagnosis is indicative of a deficiency in which of the following vitamins?

A. biotin
B. folate
C. pantothenate
D. riboflavin
E. thiamin

Answer E: The symptoms observed in this patient are typical of Wernicke-Korsakoff syndrome. This disease is most commonly found in chronic alcoholics due to their poor dietetic lifestyles. Wernicke-Korsakoff syndrome is characterized by the symptoms described as well as acute encephalopathy followed by chronic impairment of short-term memory. Persons afflicted with Wernicke-Korsakoff syndrome appear to have an inborn error of metabolism that is clinically important only when the diet is inadequate in thiamin.

2. Wernicke encephalopathy results from a deficiency of vitamin B_1. Which of the following represents classical symptoms associated with this disorder?

A. megaloblastic anemia
B. nausea, peripheral neuropathy, mental depression, ophthalmoplegia
C. numbness, tingling, weakness, sore smooth tongue, anorexia, diarrhea, pallor of the skin and mucous membranes
D. seizure disorders
E. weight loss, diarrhea, dementia, and dermatitis

Answer B: Wernicke encephalopathy is most commonly found in chronic alcoholics due to their poor dietetic lifestyles. Wernicke encephalopathy is a syndrome characterized by ataxia, ophthalmoplegia, nystagmus, and confusion. If the disorder is left untreated, it will progress to Wernicke-Korsakoff syndrome which includes impairment of short-term memory, psychosis, coma, and eventually death.

3. A 60-year-old chronic smoker and alcoholic man suffering from odynophagia, insomnia, epigastric discomfort, and recurrent diarrhea presented to the outpatient department. Clinical examination revealed memory disorientation, stomatitis, glossitis, esophagitis, and exfoliative dermatitis with some vesicles on erythematous bases on photoexposed sites such as his hands shown in the attached image. These signs and symptoms are most likely the result of a deficiency in which of the following vitamins?

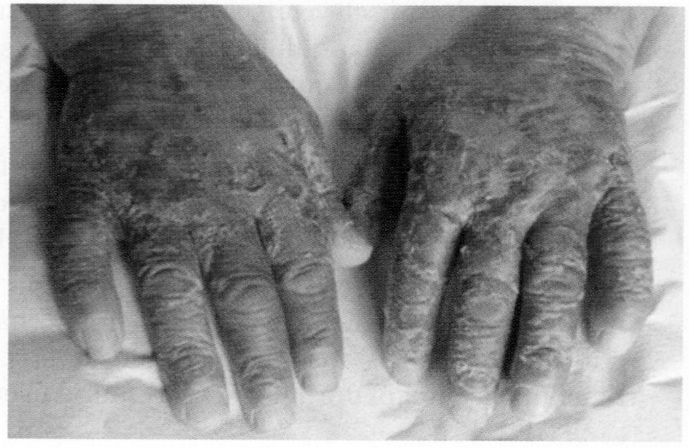

A. biotin
B. cobalamin
C. niacin
D. riboflavin
E. thiamin

Answer C: A diet deficient in niacin (as well as tryptophan) leads to glossitis of the tongue (inflammation of the tongue leading to purplish discoloration), dermatitis, weight loss, diarrhea, depression, and dementia. The severe symptoms, depression, dermatitis, and diarrhea, are associated with the condition known as pellagra and are sometimes referred to as the 3 Ds of niacin deficiency.

4. Deficiency in which of the following vitamins is associated with progressive keratinization of the cornea?
A. A
B. C
C. D
D. E
E. K

Answer A: The earliest symptoms of vitamin A deficiency are night blindness. Additional early symptoms include follicular hyperkeratosis, increased susceptibility to infection and cancer, and anemia equivalent to iron deficiency anemia. Prolonged lack of vitamin A leads to deterioration of the eye tissue through progressive keratinization of the cornea, a condition known as xerophthalmia.

5. The attached radiograph shows the typical bowed legs of an infant suffering from a deficiency in which of the following vitamins?

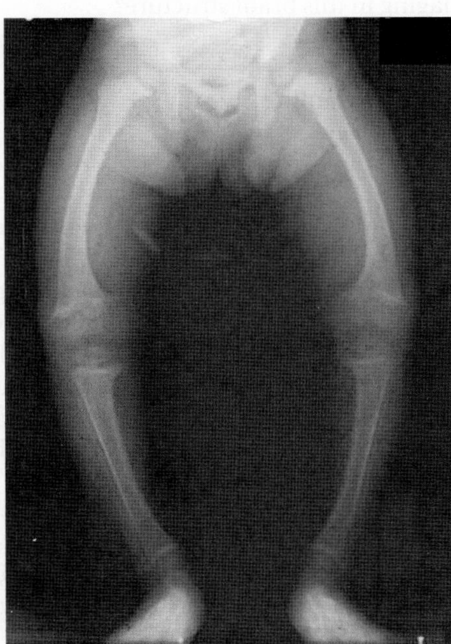

A. A
B. C
C. D
D. E
E. K

Answer C: The main symptom of vitamin D deficiency in children is rickets. Rickets is characterized by improper mineralization during the development of the bones resulting in soft bones, muscle weakness (rickety myopathy or "floppy baby syndrome,"), and increased tendency for fractures (especially greenstick fractures). In toddlers with rickets, a common skeletal deformity is bowed legs as depicted in the radiograph.

6. Although α-lipoic acid is not truly a vitamin, it is an essential cofactor for several important enzymes. An inability to maintain adequate levels of this lipid-derived molecule would result in which of the following consequences?
A. decreased insulin sensitivity
B. decreased production of reactive oxygen species, ROS
C. increased energy generation from carbohydrates
D. increased hepatic production of triglycerides
E. loss of the ability to clot blood

Answer A: Lipoic acid (LA) is an essential cofactor for the E2 component of α-ketoacid dehydrogenase complexes, exclusively located in mitochondria. These include the PDH, α-ketoglutarate dehydrogenase (KGDH), and branched chain α-ketoacid dehydrogenase (BCKDH) complexes. Extensive evidence suggests that LA may have therapeutic usefulness in lowering blood glucose levels in diabetic conditions and that the intracellular redox status plays a role in the modulation of insulin resistance. Lipoic acid has been shown to stimulate glucose uptake by affecting components of the insulin-signaling pathway.

7. Which of the following is associated with increased glucose uptake due to its ability to prevent phosphorylation of downstream effectors of the insulin-signaling cascade?
A. α-lipoic acid
B. vitamin A
C. vitamin D
D. vitamin E
E. vitamin K

Answer A: Lipoic acid (LA) is an essential cofactor for the E2 component of α-ketoacid dehydrogenase complexes, exclusively located in mitochondria. These include the PDH, α-ketoglutarate dehydrogenase (KGDH), and branched chain α-ketoacid dehydrogenase (BCKDH) complexes. Extensive evidence suggests that LA may have therapeutic usefulness in lowering blood glucose levels in diabetic conditions and that the intracellular redox status plays a role in the modulation of insulin resistance. Lipoic acid has been shown to stimulate glucose uptake by affecting components of the insulin-signaling pathway.

8. A deficiency in which of the following vitamins would most likely be associated with prolonged clotting times, hemorrhaging, and anemia?
A. α-lipoic acid
B. C
C. D
D. E
E. K

Answer E: The major role of the K vitamins is in the maintenance of normal levels of the blood-clotting proteins, factors II, VII, IX, X, and protein C and protein S, which are synthesized in the liver as inactive precursor proteins. Conversion from inactive to active clotting factor requires a posttranslational modification of specific glutamate (E) residues. This modification is a carboxylation and the enzyme responsible requires vitamin K as a cofactor. The resultant modified E residues are γ-carboxyglutamate (*gla*). Thus, a deficiency in vitamin K will result in prolonged bleeding and the potential for hemorrhage.

9. A 45-year-old man, a known alcoholic for at least the past 10 years, reported to a physician for consultation. He complained of burning of eyes, a sore tongue, reduced appetite, and mild abdominal discomfort. Physical examination revealed cracks on the lips and in the corners of the mouth; a red, fissured, and inflamed tongue; dull hair, oily skin, and split nails. A deficiency in which of the following vitamins would best explain the observed symptoms?
A. biotin
B. niacin
C. pantothenate
D. riboflavin
E. thiamin

Answer D: Although riboflavin deficiencies are rare in the United States, the common symptoms associated with deficiency include itching and burning eyes, angular stomatitis and cheilosis (cracks and sores in the mouth and lips), bloodshot eyes, glossitis (inflammation of the tongue leading to purplish discoloration), seborrhea (dandruff, flaking skin on scalp and face), trembling, sluggishness, and photophobia (excessive light sensitivity).

10. Not all water-soluble vitamins are strictly required in the diet since the human body has the capacity to synthesize at least one of this class of vitamin. However, the ability to do so is limiting and not of sufficient capacity to provide all the necessary coenzyme required for normal metabolic processes. Which of the following is this vitamin?
A. α-lipoic acid
B. folate
C. niacin
D. riboflavin
E. thiamin

Answer C: Niacin is not a true vitamin in the strictest definition since it can be derived from the amino acid tryptophan. However, the ability to utilize tryptophan for niacin synthesis is insufficient (60 mg of tryptophan are required to synthesize 1 mg of niacin). Also, synthesis of niacin from tryptophan requires vitamins B_1, B_2, and B_6 which would also likely be limiting on a marginal diet.

11. A 58-year-old male stumbles into a local soup kitchen mumbling about aliens and space craft. He is dirty, unshaven, wearing tattered clothing, and reeking of alcohol. He is discovered to have died in the alleyway during the night. At autopsy, a sagittal section through the brain shows severe pigmentation of the mammillary bodies due to apparent hemorrhage. A deficiency in which of the following vitamins would be expected to cause hemorrhaging in this brain structure?
A. biotin
B. folate
C. pyridoxamine
D. riboflavin
E. thiamin

Answer E: The mammillary bodies are a pair of small round bodies, located on the undersurface of the brain, and, as part of the diencephalon, form part of the limbic system. Damage to the mammillary bodies due to thiamine deficiency is implied in the pathogenesis of Wernicke-Korsakoff syndrome. Symptoms include impaired memory, also called anterograde amnesia, suggesting that the mammillary bodies may be important for memory.

12. A smear of your patients' blood is shown in the following picture demonstrating that the person suffers from a form of anemia. A deficiency in which of the following vitamins would lead to the anemia shown in the slide?

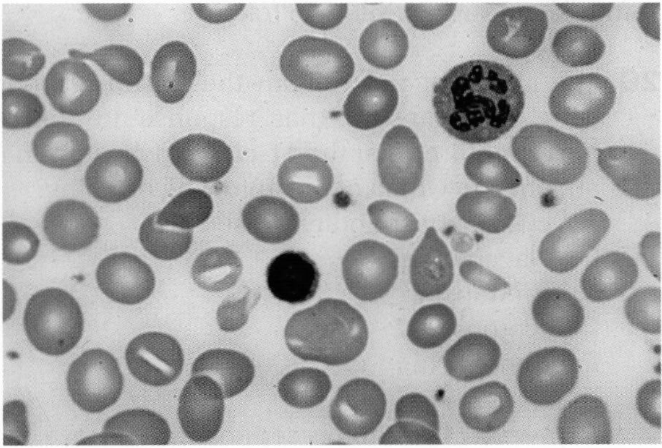

A. B_1 (thiamin)
B. B_6 (pyridoxal phosphate)
C. B_{12} (cobalamin)
D. biotin
E. K

Answer C: Pernicious anemia is a megaloblastic anemia resulting from vitamin B_{12} deficiency that develops as a result of a lack of intrinsic factor in the stomach, leading to malabsorption of the vitamin. The anemia results from impaired DNA synthesis due to a block in purine and thymidine nucleotide biosynthesis. The block in nucleotide biosynthesis is a consequence of the effect of vitamin B_{12} on folate metabolism. When vitamin B_{12} is deficient, essentially all of the folate becomes trapped as the N^5-methyl-THF derivative as a result of the loss of functional methionine synthase. This trapping prevents the synthesis of other THF derivatives required for the purine and thymidine nucleotide biosynthesis pathways.

13. A patient presents with pale skin, sunken eyes, sore gums, muscle pain, loose teeth, and corkscrew-shaped hair. A deficiency in which of the following vitamins would result in the observed symptoms?
A. ascorbic acid
B. biotin
C. pyridoxal
D. riboflavin
E. thiamin

Answer A: Deficiency in vitamin C leads to the disease scurvy due to the role of the vitamin in the post-translational modification of collagens. Scurvy is characterized by easily bruised skin, muscle fatigue, soft swollen gums, decreased wound healing and hemorrhaging, osteoporosis, and anemia.

14. The vitamin involved in biochemical reactions concerned with the transfer of methyl, methylene, or formyl groups is a derivative of which of the following vitamins?
A. α-lipoic acid
B. biotin
C. folic acid
D. pyridoxine
E. riboflavin

Answer C: The function of THF (synthesized from folic acid) derivatives is to carry and transfer various forms of one-carbon units during biosynthetic reactions. The one-carbon units are methyl, methylene, methenyl, formyl, or formimino groups.

15. Wernicke encephalopathy syndrome is caused by a deficiency of which of the following?
A. biotin
B. cobalamin
C. pyridoxal phosphate
D. riboflavin
E. thiamine

Answer E: Wernicke encephalopathy results from a dietary deficiency in thiamin. The disorder is most commonly found in chronic alcoholics due to their poor dietetic lifestyles. Wernicke encephalopathy is a syndrome characterized by ataxia, ophthalmoplegia, nystagmus, confusion, and impairment of short-term memory.

16. Scurvy is due to a dietary deficiency of which vitamin?
A. A
B. B_6 (pyridoxal phosphate)
C. B_{12} (cobalamin)
D. C
E. D

Answer D: Deficiency in vitamin C leads to the disease scurvy due to the role of the vitamin in the post-translational modification of collagens. Scurvy is characterized by easily bruised skin, muscle fatigue, soft swollen gums, decreased wound healing and hemorrhaging, osteoporosis, and anemia.

17. A deficiency of vitamin B_{12} in humans results in anemia primarily because it is which of the following?
A. a cofactor in the biosynthesis of purine nucleotides required for the synthesis of DNA
B. involved in the conversion of N^5-methyl-THF to THF
C. necessary for the absorption of folic acid from the gut

D. required for the conversion of cystathionine to cysteine
E. utilized as a cofactor in synthesis of thymidine nucleotides

Answer B: Pernicious anemia is a megaloblastic anemia resulting from vitamin B_{12} deficiency that develops as a result of a lack of intrinsic factor in the stomach, leading to malabsorption of the vitamin. The anemia results from impaired DNA synthesis due to a block in purine and thymidine nucleotide biosynthesis. The block in nucleotide biosynthesis is a consequence of the effect of vitamin B_{12} on folate metabolism. When vitamin B_{12} is deficient, essentially all of the folate becomes trapped as the N^5-methyl-THF derivative as a result of the loss of functional methionine synthase. This trapping prevents the synthesis of other THF derivatives required for the purine and thymidine nucleotide biosynthesis pathways.

18. Which of the following represents a significant biochemical role of vitamin C?
A. blood coagulation
B. calcium homeostasis
C. connective tissue production
D. metabolic functions of copper
E. steroid hydroxylation

Answer C: The active form of vitamin C is ascorbic acid itself. The main function of ascorbate is as a reducing agent in a number of different reactions. Ascorbate is the cofactor for Cu^+-dependent monooxygenases and Fe^{2+}-dependent dioxygenases. Ascorbate has the potential to reduce cytochromes *a* and *c* of the respiratory chain as well as molecular oxygen. The most important reaction requiring ascorbate as a cofactor is the hydroxylation of proline residues in collagen. Vitamin C is, therefore, required for the maintenance of normal connective tissue as well as for wound healing since synthesis of connective tissue is the first event in wound tissue remodeling.

19. When vitamin D is deficient, what 2 disorders occur most readily?
A. kidney failure and bent bones
B. megaloblastic anemia and Wernicke-Korsakoff syndrome
C. osteoporosis and diverticulosis
D. osteomalacia and xerophthalmia
E. rickets and osteomalacia

Answer E: The main symptom of vitamin D deficiency in children is rickets and in adults is osteomalacia. Rickets is characterized by improper mineralization during the development of the bones resulting in soft bones. Osteomalacia is characterized by demineralization of previously formed bone leading to increased softness and susceptibility to fracture.

20. The ability of rod cells in the eye to respond to light and transmit that response to the optic nerve requires that the 11-*cis* form of vitamin A be attached to which of the following proteins?
A. cGMP phosphodiesterase
B. Na^+ channel
C. rhodopsin
D. scotopsin
E. transducing

Answer D: Photoreception in the eye is the function of 2 specialized cell types located in the retina; the rod and cone cells. Both rod and cone cells contain a photoreceptor pigment in their membranes. The photosensitive compound of most mammalian eyes is a protein called opsin to which is covalently coupled an aldehyde of vitamin A. The opsin of rod cells is called scotopsin. The photoreceptor of rod cells is specifically called rhodopsin or visual purple. This compound is a complex between scotopsin and the 11-*cis*-retinal (also called 11-*cis*-retinene) form of vitamin A. Rhodopsin is a serpentine receptor imbedded in the membrane of the rod cell. Coupling of 11-*cis*-retinal occurs at 3 of the transmembrane domains of rhodopsin. Intracellularly, rhodopsin is coupled to a specific G-protein called transducin.

21. Vitamin K serves as a coenzyme in reactions that result in the modified activity of several enzymes of the blood coagulation cascade. Which of the following amino acid modifications requires the activity of vitamin K?
A aspartate to β-carboxyaspartate
B. glutamate to γ-carboxyglutamate
C. lysine to hydroxylysine
D. lysine to β-methyllysine
E. proline to hydroxyproline

Answer B: The major function of the K vitamins is in the maintenance of normal levels of the blood-clotting proteins, factors II, VII, IX, X, and protein C and protein S, which are synthesized in the liver as inactive precursor proteins. Conversion from inactive to active clotting factor requires a posttranslational modification of specific glutamate (E) residues. This modification is a carboxylation and the enzyme responsible requires vitamin K as a cofactor. The resultant modified E residues are γ-carboxyglutamate (*gla*).

22. The inability to rapidly synthesize DNA during the process of erythrocyte maturation leads to abnormally enlarged erythrocytes. This disorder is referred to as macrocytic anemia and is caused by a deficiency in which of the following vitamins?
A. ascorbate
B. biotin
C. folate
D. niacin
E. thiamine

Answer C: The most pronounced effect of folate deficiency on cellular processes is upon DNA synthesis. This is due to an impairment in dTMP synthesis, which leads to cell cycle arrest in S-phase of rapidly proliferating cells, in particular hematopoietic cells. The result is megaloblastic anemia as for vitamin B_{12} deficiency. The inability to synthesize DNA during erythrocyte maturation leads to abnormally large erythrocytes termed macrocytic anemia.

23. When fatty acids with odd numbers of carbon atoms are oxidized in the β-oxidation pathway, the final product is 1 mole of acetyl-CoA and 1 mole of the 3-carbon molecule, propionyl-CoA. In order to use the propionyl carbons, the molecule is carboxylated, converted ultimately to succinyl-CoA, and fed into the TCA cycle. Which of the following represents the vitamin cofactor required in one of the steps of this conversion?
A. cobalamin (B_{12})
B. pantothenic acid (B_5)
C. pyridoxine (B_6)
D. riboflavin (B_2)
E. thiamine (B_1)

Answer A: The conversion of propionyl-CoA to succinyl-CoA occurs through a series of 3 reactions. The terminal reaction is catalyzed by methylmalonyl-CoA mutase, which is dependent upon vitamin B_{12} (cobalamin) as a cofactor.

24. The terminal ileum was removed from a 50-year-old woman during excision of a tumor. About 3 years later, the patient was admitted to the hospital. She is very pale. Hemoglobin is 9 g/dL, MCV (mean corpuscular volume) has increased to 110 mm³ (110 fL). The provisional diagnosis is a vitamin deficiency. Which of the following vitamins is the most likely one causing the symptoms?
A. A
B. B_1
C. B_6
D. B_{12}
E. K

Answer D: Deficiency of vitamin B_{12} results in hematological, neurological, and gastrointestinal effects. The hematologic symptoms include a low red blood cell count with large-sized macrocytic red blood cells as described. Absorption of vitamin B_{12} is relatively complicated. The large and not very lipophilic molecule is released from food by the low pH of the stomach and pepsin digestion and binds to R protein (also called haptocorrin). Pancreatic proteases digest these complexes and the liberated cobalamin (vitamin B_{12}) now complexes with intrinsic factor (which is produced by gastric parietal cells) and is absorbed as such in the terminal ileum. Hence, vitamin B_{12} absorption will be low in this patient. Liver storage is thought to be sufficient for 3 to 6 years so that the 3-year latency of the anemia further supports a vitamin B_{12} deficiency. The water-soluble vitamins B_1 and B_6 (choices B and C) are absorbed in the duodenum by simple diffusion. Absorption of the lipid-soluble vitamins A and K (choices A and E) is supported by bile-acid-mixed micelles, although vitamin A and vitamin K_3 do not heavily rely on bile acids and can also enter the enterocytes by simple diffusion. Additionally, of the stated choices, only vitamin B_{12} deficiency is associated with anemia.

25. A patient is found to be deficient in folate. This patient is anemic, and a complete blood count indicates that the MCV is 105 fL (normal range: 80-96) and the mean corpuscular hemoglobin concentration (MCHC) is 34 g/dL (normal range: 32-36). The anemia is thus macrocytic and normochromic. In this patient, how would you predict that the MCH (mean corpuscular hemoglobin) would compare to the normal range?
A. MCH would be elevated with respect to the normal range
B. MCH would be depressed with respect to the normal range
C. MCH would be within the normal range
D. this cannot be determined based on the information provided

Answer A: These red blood cells are large (macrocytic) but have a normal hemoglobin concentration (normal MCHC). Since MCH is mean hemoglobin content per red cell, this value must be elevated since the cells are large and the concentration in the cell is normal.

26. The patient is a 43-year-old man. He is anemic, with a hemoglobin level of 12.2 g/dL (normal is 15.5 g/dL). The erythrocytes are microcytic (MCV = 70 fL, with normal MCV = 80-100 fL). Which of the following would most likely be present in this patient?

A. acute bleeding
B. folate deficiency
C. iron deficiency
D. vitamin B_{12} deficiency
E. vitamin K deficiency

Answer C: Microcytic anemia can often be associated with defective hemoglobin synthesis. In the case of iron deficiency, heme synthesis is impaired due to the lack of iron. Anemia due to B_{12} or folate deficiency is macrocytic.

27. A 14-month-old baby boy is brought to your office by his mother because he seems to be in pain whenever he tries to move. During your physical examination you note bowing of his legs, depression of the sternum with outward projection of the ends of the ribs, reluctance to move his limbs, and numerous bruises on his legs as well as gingival hemorrhages. These findings lead you to suspect that this child suffers from a dietary deficiency of which of the following vitamins?

A. A
B. B_1 (thiamine)
C. B_{12} (cyanocobalamin)
D. C (ascorbate)
E. D (calciferol)

Answer D: Deficiencies of vitamin C and vitamin D can produce similar skeletal abnormalities in young children such as those listed. However, a major difference is that vitamin C deficiency is accompanied by hemorrhages, as seen in this child. This also leads to hemarthrosis (bleeding into joints) that makes movement very painful.

28. As the ER physician you are tending to a 59-year-old female patient who has a broken left fibula. Upon physical exam you discover she also has multiple bruises on her arms, legs, and upper torso. She also complains of painful gums and significant bleeding whenever she brushes her teeth. She reports that she subsists on bouillon soup, tea, plain pasta, and dinner rolls. Blood work indicates that she is mildly anemic with microcytic erythrocytes. Given these signs and symptoms, this patient most likely is suffering from the effects of a deficiency in the activity of which of the following enzymes?

A. branched-chain ketoacid dehydrogenase
B. lysyl hydroxylase
C. methionine synthase
D. pyruvate dehydrogenase
E. transketolase

Answer B: The signs and symptoms exhibited by this patient are indicative of scurvy which results from a deficiency of vitamin C (ascorbate). Vitamin C is a critical co-factor for the enzymes lysyl hydroxylase and prolyl hydroxylase that are required for the correct post-translational modification of collagen. Loss of collagen processing leads to defective connective tissue synthesis and also results in poor platelet adhesion to exposed sub-endothelial extracellular matrix resulting prolonged bleeding time. Often times vitamin C deficient patients also exhibit mild anemia due to the role of vitamin C in the process of intestinal absorption of Fe2+ iron.

29. A 29-year-old female has just become pregnant and is at the doctor's office for her first pre-natal exam. This is the first time this patient has been seen by the ob-gyn. In reviewing the patients medical records the physician discovers that the woman takes Dilantin (phenytoin) to control her epileptic seizures. The physician recommends that the woman stop the Dilantin and switch to Carbatrol (carbamazepine). If the woman refuses to comply with the change in seizure medication which of the following is most likely to be defective in her newborn resulting in potentially fatal bleeding episodes?

A. γ-carboxylation of glutamate
B. hydroxylation of lysine
C. methylation of homocysteine
D. oxidation of lysine
E. synthesis of heme

Answer A: The hydantoin class (includes phenytoin) of anti-seizure medications interfere with the activity of vitamin K. Loss of vitamin K, as a co-factor, leads to reduced hepatic γ-carboxylation of glutamate residues in the coagulation factors II, VII, IX, X and also protein C and protein S. The net effect is defective, potentially fatal, bleeding disorder in a neonate.

30. A 23-year-old man has been consuming large quantities of raw egg whites as part of his current body-building routine. He has developed a rash and severe muscle pain. Blood work indicates he has anemia. His diet prevents intestinal absorption of a vitamin leading to inhibition in the synthesis of which of the following?

A. DNA
B. fatty acid
C. glycogen
D. protein
E. RNA

Answer B: The avidin in egg whites complexes with biotin preventing its absorption from the intestines. Biotin is a cofactor for enzymes involved in carboxylation reactions. Acetyl-CoA carboxylase (ACC) is the rate-limiting enzyme of de novo fatty acid synthesis. Therefore, a deficiency in biotin absorption from the gut would be expected to have a negative effect on fatty acid synthesis.

31. After metabolic conversion in the body, coenzyme forms of folate and vitamin B_{12} are both involved in methylation of which of the following?
- A. homocysteine
- B. norepinephrine
- C. pyridine
- D. serotonin
- E. uridylic acid

Answer A: Both folic and cobalamin (B_{12}) are involved in the function of methionine synthase. In the direction of methionine synthesis, the enzyme utilizes the methyl-group from N^5-methyl-THF in the methylation of homocysteine. During this reaction, the methyl group is initially transferred to hydroxycobalamin-generating methylcobalamin.

32. You are the attending physician in the ER. You are examining a 48-year-old man brought by his wife because of a recent change in his mental status. Physical examination shows horizontal and vertical nystagmus, bilateral facial nerve palsy, and truncal ataxia. The most likely explanation for these findings is a deficiency in which of the following vitamins?
- A. folate
- B. vitamin B_1
- C. vitamin B_6
- D. vitamin C
- E. vitamin D

Answer B: The patient is suffering from Wernicke encephalopathy. Wernicke encephalopathy is most commonly found in chronic alcoholics due to their poor dietetic lifestyles. Wernicke encephalopathy is a syndrome characterized by ataxia, ophthalmoplegia, nystagmus, and confusion. If the disorder is left untreated, it will progress to Wernicke-Korsakoff syndrome which includes impairment of short-term memory, psychosis, coma, and eventually death.

33. The activity of aspartate aminotransferase (AST) requires which of the following vitamins as a coenzyme?
- A. folate
- B. vitamin B_1
- C. vitamin B_2
- D. vitamin B_6
- E. vitamin B_{12}

Answer D: Numerous amino transferases, such as AST, utilize pyridoxal phosphate (PLP) as a cofactor. PLP is derived from vitamin B_6.

34. As an essential component of the nucleotide analog, FAD, which of the following vitamins plays a major role in the transfer of reducing equivalents?
- A. folate
- B. vitamin B_1
- C. vitamin B_2
- D. vitamin B_6
- E. vitamin B_{12}

Answer C: Flavin adenine dinucleotide is a derivative of the vitamin riboflavin (B_2).

35. The activity of which of the following enzymes in the erythrocyte will be decreased in patients with a deficiency of thiamin?
- A. adenosine deaminase
- B. aspartate aminotransferase (AST)
- C. pyruvate kinase
- D. transaldolase
- E. transketolase

Answer E: The pentose phosphate pathway (PPP) is a critical pathway of glucose oxidation within erythrocytes due to it being required for the generation of NADPH. The transketolase enzyme, involved in the nonoxidative reactions of the PPP, requires TPP as a cofactor.

36. Which of the following laboratory findings is most likely in a 37-year-old woman with a thiamin deficiency?
- A. decreased plasma concentration of alanine
- B. increased erythrocyte transketolase activity
- C. increased leukocyte α-ketoglutarate dehydrogenase activity
- D. increased plasma concentration of glucose
- E. increased plasma concentrations of pyruvate and lactate

Answer E: Thiamin serves as the precursor for TPP. TPP is necessary as a cofactor for the pyruvate dehydrogenase complex (PDHc) and, therefore, a deficiency thiamin results in impaired oxidation of pyruvate. This will lead to increased plasma concentrations of pyruvate. When lactate from erythrocyte and skeletal muscle metabolism reaches the liver, it will not be readily converted to pyruvate due to the reduced pyruvate oxidative capacity leading to elevated plasma lactate. In addition, the excess pyruvate will be a substrate for lactate dehydrogenase, resulting in additionally increased levels of pyruvate.

37. You are a physician working in a clinic, who sees many transient workers. You find that almost 30% of the patients you see are deficient in thiamin and their erythrocytes are markedly deficient in transketolase activity. Examination of liver function in these individuals would most likely show deficiency in which of the following metabolic processes?

A. biosynthesis of fatty acids from acetyl-CoA
B. biosynthesis of ketone bodies
C. conversion of glycerol to glucose during fasting
D. conversion of pyruvate to acetyl-CoA
E. incorporation of dietary glucose into hepatic glycogen

Answer D: Thiamin serves as the precursor for TPP. TPP is necessary as a cofactor for the PDHc and, therefore, a deficiency of thiamin results in impaired oxidation of pyruvate to acetyl-CoA.

38. You are an ER physician examining a 67-year-old woman. She was brought to the hospital by her neighbor because he found her passed out in the front yard. History reveals that she lives by herself and consumes a diet which consists primarily of lettuce and rice. She has not consumed any meat products for over 5 years and does not supplement her diet with vitamins. She reports that she is frequently quite tired. Blood work indicates she has severe megaloblastic anemia. Which of the following reaction pathways is most likely impaired in this patient?

A. branched-chain amino acid degradation
B. glucose 6-phosphate being converted to ribulose 5-phosphate and CO_2
C. glycolysis
D. heme synthesis
E. thymidine nucleotide biosynthesis

Answer E: This patient is suffering from a dietary deficiency in vitamin B_{12}. A deficiency in B_{12} leads to impairment in the methionine synthase–catalyzed reaction leading to trapping of folate as N^5-methyltetrahydrofolate. This trapping prevents the synthesis of other THF derivatives required for the purine and thymidine nucleotide biosynthesis pathways. The inability to synthesize DNA during erythrocyte maturation leads to abnormally large erythrocytes termed macrocytic or megaloblastic erythrocytes.

39. You are examining a 27-year-old pregnant woman who is at 32 weeks' gestation. Blood work indicates she is suffering from macrocytic anemia. Her diet consists mainly of starchy foods with little meat and green vegetables. Which of the following vitamins is most likely deficient in this woman?

A. folate
B. vitamin B_1
C. vitamin B_2
D. vitamin B_6
E. vitamin C

Answer A: Folate deficiency results in complications nearly identical to those of vitamin B_{12} deficiency. The most pronounced effect of folate deficiency on cellular processes is upon DNA synthesis. This is due to an impairment in dTMP synthesis, in particular in hematopoietic cells. The inability to synthesize DNA during erythrocyte maturation leads to abnormally large (macrocytic) erythrocytes and anemia.

40. A strict vegan diet restricts the intake of meat, eggs, milk, cheese, or other animal-derived foods. You are examining your patient who follows this particular dietary regimen. Urine analysis shows increased concentration of methylmalonic acid. This finding is indicative of which of the following?

A. excess methylmalonate in the diet
B. fatty acid deficiency
C. folate deficiency
D. protein deficiency
E. vitamin B_{12} (cobalamin) deficiency

Answer E: Vitamin B_{12} is a critical coenzyme in the methionine synthase and methylmalonyl-CoA mutase–catalyzed reactions. Therefore, a deficiency in B_{12} results in defective activity of these 2 enzymes. Methylmalonyl-CoA mutase is involved in the conversion of propionyl-CoA to the TCA cycle intermediate, succinyl-CoA, specifically the reaction whereby methylmalonyl-CoA is converted to succinyl-CoA. The inability to convert methylmalonyl-CoA to succinyl-CoA leads to excess excretion of the metabolite in the urine as well as increased concentrations in the blood.

41. A 45-year-old man is brought to the ER by his wife because he has exhibited confusion for the past few days. The attending physician asks him to follow his pen with his eyes. He notes that on extreme lateral motion his eyes exhibit an involuntary rhythmic movement toward the midline and then back to lateral gaze. The patient is unable to do finger-to-nose or heel-to-shin movements or walk in a straight line by placing the heel of one foot directly in front of the toes of the other foot. Given these signs and symptoms, which of the following vitamin deficiencies is most likely in this patient?

A. folate
B. vitamin B_1
C. vitamin B_2
D. vitamin B_6
E. vitamin B_{12}

Answer B: The patient is exhibiting symptoms of Wernicke encephalopathy resulting from deficiency in thiamin intake. Wernicke encephalopathy is a syndrome characterized by ataxia, ophthalmoplegia, nystagmus, and confusion.

42. An individual with pernicious anemia has an inability to metabolize which of the following compounds?

A. acetyl-CoA
B. butyryl-CoA
C. methylmalonyl-CoA
D. palmitoyl-CoA
E. stearoyl-CoA

Answer C: Pernicious anemia is one of many types of the larger family of megaloblastic anemias. It is caused by loss of secretion of intrinsic factor from the gut. Intrinsic factor is essential for subsequent absorption of vitamin B_{12} in the intestines. Vitamin B_{12} is a critical coenzyme in the methionine synthase and methylmalonyl-CoA–mutase catalyzed reactions. Methylmalonyl-CoA mutase is involved in the conversion of propionyl-CoA to the TCA cycle intermediate, succinyl-CoA, specifically the reaction whereby methylmalonyl-CoA is converted to succinyl-CoA.

43. Conversion of propionyl-CoA to succinyl-CoA requires which of the following pairs of vitamins?

A. vitamin B_1 (thiamin) and vitamin B_5 (pantothenate)
B. vitamin B_2 (riboflavin) and vitamin B_3 (niacin)
C. vitamin B_3 (niacin) and folate
D. vitamin B_6 (pyridoxine) and vitamin B_{12} (cobalamin)
E. vitamin B_{12} (cobalamin) and biotin

Answer E: The conversion of propionyl-CoA to succinyl-CoA requires 3 distinct enzymes. The first enzyme is the biotin-requiring enzyme propionyl-CoA carboxylase. Vitamin B_{12} is a critical coenzyme in the methylmalonyl-CoA–mutase catalyzed reaction, which is the third enzyme in this pathway.

44. Patients with scurvy are most likely to have a defect in which of the following reactions?

A. carboxylation
B. decarboxylation
C. hydroxylation
D. methyl group transfer
E. transamination

Answer C: The most important reaction requiring ascorbate (vitamin C) as a cofactor is the hydroxylation of proline residues in collagen. Deficiency in vitamin C leads to the disease scurvy. Scurvy is characterized by easily bruised skin, muscle fatigue, soft swollen gums, decreased wound healing, hemorrhaging, and osteoporosis.

45. You are examining a 57-year-old woman, who has complains that her teeth feel loose and that her gums bleed easily when she eats. In taking her history you find that her diet is restricted and includes no fresh citrus fruits or leafy green vegetables. Which of the following vitamins is most likely to be deficient in this patient?

A. A
B. B_1 (thiamin)
C. B_2 (riboflavin)
D. C
E. K

Answer D: This patient is showing the symptoms of scurvy caused by deficiency of vitamin C. The most important reaction requiring vitamin C as a cofactor is the hydroxylation of proline residues in collagen. Scurvy is characterized by easily bruised skin, muscle fatigue, soft swollen gums, decreased wound healing, hemorrhaging, and osteoporosis.

46. As a physician volunteer in a free clinic, you are examining a 52-year-old homeless man. You note that he has numerous petechiae and suspect impaired collagen production. Given his poor dietary habits, you determine that he lacks adequate intake of vitamin C. For which of the following steps of collagen synthesis is ascorbic acid required?

A. cross-linking lysine and hydroxylysine residues
B. glycosylation of hydroxylysine residues
C. hydroxylation of proline residues
D. removal of the signal peptide from preprocollagen
E. translocation of collagen peptides into the endoplasmic reticulum

Answer C: The most important reaction requiring ascorbate (vitamin C) as a cofactor is the hydroxylation of proline residues in collagen.

47. The active hormonal form of vitamin D requires several enzymatic steps. The final step in the synthesis of 1,25-dihydroxycholecalciferol occurs in which of the following tissues?

A. bone
B. intestine
C. kidney
D. liver
E. spleen

Answer C: Active calcitriol (1,25-dihydroxycholecalciferol) is derived from ergosterol (produced in plants) and from 7-dehydrocholesterol. Upon exposure to ultraviolet (UV) light from the sun and following thermal isomerization, 7-dehydrocholesterol is nonenzymatically converted to pre-vitamin D_3 (cholecalciferol) which then enters the bloodstream and is taken up by the liver. In the liver cholecalciferol is hydroxylated at the 25 position by a specific D_3-25-hydroxylase generating 25-hydroxy-D_3 [25-(OH)D_3]. Conversion of 25-(OH)D_3 to its biologically active form, calcitriol, occurs through the activity of a specific D_3-1-hydroxylase present in the proximal convoluted tubules of the kidneys.

48. A 50-year-old woman was diagnosed 2 years ago with primary biliary cirrhosis. Given her diagnosis, she is at greatest risk for becoming deficient in which of the following?

A. B_1 (thiamin)
B. B_{12} (cobalamin)
C. C
D. E
E. niacin

Answer D: Vitamin E is a fat-soluble vitamin. In order for the fat-soluble vitamins to be absorbed from the intestines, they must be emulsified along with all the other fatty molecules in the diet. The primary mechanism for fat emulsification is the release of bile salts from the gallbladder in response to food intake. The bile salts are synthesized from cholesterol within hepatocytes and then transported to the gallbladder via the bile canaliculi. Thus, cirrhosis of the biliary circulatory system will lead to impaired absorption of fats, including fat-soluble vitamins such as vitamin E.

49. A 10-year-old boy with cystic fibrosis is brought to the physician because his mother has noticed that it seems to take him significantly longer to stop bleeding when he has a cut. He had been prescribed pancreatic digestive enzyme supplements because his stools were bulky and large as well as malodorous. Being a child he admits that he does not take them regularly. Physical examination shows several bruises on his skin. A deficiency in which of the following nutrients is the most likely explanation for his bleeding disorder?

A. ascorbic acid
B. essential fatty acids
C. folate
D. iron
E. vitamin K

Answer E: Vitamin K is a fat-soluble vitamin. In order for the fat-soluble vitamins to be absorbed from the intestines, they must be emulsified along with all the other fatty molecules in the diet. The primary mechanism for fat emulsification is the release of bile salts from the gallbladder in response to food intake. The bile salts are synthesized from cholesterol within hepatocytes and then transported to the gallbladder via the bile canaliculi. Patients with cystic fibrosis exhibit abnormal transport of chloride and sodium across an epithelium, leading to thick, viscous secretions. In addition, there is a reduced or lack of pancreatic secretions into the gut leading to difficulty absorbing nutrients with their subsequent excretion in the feces. Individuals with cystic fibrosis also have difficulties absorbing the fat-soluble vitamins such as vitamin K.

50. A 50-year-old man is being examined by his physician due to complaints of frequent oily bowel movements. He indicates that his stools are also difficult to flush down the toilet. His history indicates chronic pancreatitis and a high level of alcohol consumption. Which of the following laboratory findings is most likely to be increased in this man?

A. erythrocyte count
B. eosinophil count
C. leukocyte count
D. platelet count
E. prothrombin time

Answer E: Vitamin K is a fat-soluble vitamin. In order for the fat-soluble vitamins to be absorbed from the intestines, they must be emulsified along with all the other fatty molecules in the diet. In addition, adequate nutrient absorption requires pancreatic secretion into the intestines to aid digestive processes. Due to the chronic pancreatitis in this patient, there is a reduced or lack of pancreatic secretions into the gut leading to difficulty absorbing nutrients with their subsequent excretion in the feces. Reduced intake of vitamin K will lead to defective modification of coagulation factors within the liver, resulting in prolonged bleeding times.

51. A dietary deficiency of vitamin C would result in a decrease in which of the following?

A. amount of THF available for one-carbon metabolism
B. conversion of norepinephrine to epinephrine
C. conversion of proline to hydroxyproline
D. production of creatine
E. supply of "active formaldehyde" units

Answer C: The active form of vitamin C is ascorbic acid itself. The main function of ascorbate is as a reducing agent in a number of different reactions. Ascorbate is the cofactor for Cu^{+}-dependent monooxygenases and Fe^{2+}-dependent dioxygenases. Ascorbate has the potential to reduce cytochromes *a* and *c* of the respiratory chain as well as molecular oxygen. The most important reaction requiring ascorbate as a cofactor is the hydroxylation of proline residues in collagen. Vitamin C is, therefore, required for the maintenance of normal connective tissue as well as for wound healing since synthesis of connective tissue is the first event in wound tissue remodeling.

52. Vitamin K is necessary for normal blood coagulation. Which of the following processes of hemostasis is dependent on the activity of this vitamin?

A. it complexes with platelets in the first wave of platelet aggregation
B. it induces the release of von Willebrand factor
C. it inhibits the activation of the fibrinolytic system
D. it initiates the contact phase by activating factor XI (plasma thromboplastin antecedent)
E. it is a required cofactor for the introduction of *gla*-residues into coagulation factors

Answer E: The major function of the K vitamins is in the maintenance of normal levels of the blood-clotting proteins, factors II, VII, IX, X, and protein C and protein S, which are synthesized in the liver as inactive precursor proteins. Conversion from inactive to active clotting factor requires a posttranslational modification of specific glutamate (E) residues. This modification is a carboxylation and the enzyme responsible requires vitamin K as a cofactor. The resultant modified E residues are g-carboxyglutamate (*gla*).

53. When increased in the serum, which of the following stimulates the synthesis of 1,25-dihydroxycholecalciferol?

A. calcitonin
B. calcium
C. 25-hydroxycholecalciferol
D. parathyroid hormone
E. phosphate

Answer D: Parathyroid hormone (PTH) is synthesized and secreted by chief cells of the parathyroid glands in response to systemic Ca^{2+} levels. PTH acts by binding to cAMP- and PLCγ-activating plasma membrane receptors, initiating a cascade of reactions that culminates in the biological response. There are 2 receptors that recognize PTH identified as the PTH-1 and PTH-2 receptors (PTH1R and PTH2R). The body response to PTH is complex but is aimed in all tissues at increasing Ca^{2+} levels in extracellular fluids. PTH induces the dissolution of bone by stimulating osteoclast activity, which leads to elevated plasma Ca^{2+} and phosphate. In the kidney, PTH reduces renal Ca^{2+} clearance by stimulating its reabsorption; at the same time, PTH reduces the reabsorption of phosphate and thereby increases its clearance. Finally, PTH acts on the liver, kidney, and intestine to stimulate the production of the steroid hormone 1,25-dihydroxycholecalciferol (calcitriol), which is responsible for Ca^{2+} absorption in the intestine.

Checklist

✓ Vitamins are organic nutrients that are generally required in the diet since they cannot be synthesized by human tissues.

✓ Vitamin derivatives play essential roles as cofactors for enzyme-catalyzed reactions critical to overall metabolic homeostasis.

✓ The B vitamins are water-soluble vitamins involved in important roles in cellular metabolism, these consist of thiamin (B_1), riboflavin (B_2), niacin (B_3), pantothenate (B_5), pyridoxal (B_6), and cobalamin (B_{12}); biotin and folic acid are sometimes also considered in the B vitamin class as B_7 and B_9, respectively.

- ✓ Vitamin C is a water-soluble antioxidant that is also critical as a cofactor for the modification of components of the extracellular matrix.
- ✓ Vitamin A is critical in the normal function of the visual processes; in the form of retinoic acid, vitamin A plays an essential role in the control of genes involved in embryonic patterning.
- ✓ Vitamin D is a prohormone that when converted to active calcitriol functions as a steroid hormone in the regulation of calcium and phosphorous homeostasis.
- ✓ Vitamin E is a potent antioxidant and as such serves as the most important lipid-derived antioxidant.
- ✓ Vitamin K functions as a cofactor in the enzymatic modification of numerous enzymes involved in the process of blood coagulation.
- ✓ The minerals are inorganic micronutrients that are necessary for the functions of numerous processes involved in whole body homeostasis.

CHAPTER

9 Enzymes and Enzyme Kinetics

CHAPTER OUTLINE

High-Yield Terms

Simple enzyme: binds only substrate and/or inhibitors

Holoenzyme: complex enzymes which are composed of protein plus a relatively small organic molecule

Apoenzyme: the protein component of a complex enzyme

Coenzymes: nonprotein components of enzymes

Isozyme: member of a set of enzymes sharing similar/same substrate specificity

Metalloenzyme: enzymes that require a metal in their composition

Ribozymes: RNA molecules that exhibit catalytic activity in the absence of any protein component

Reaction rate: described by the number of molecules of reactant(s) that are converted into product(s) in a specified time period

Chemical reaction order: relates to the number of molecules in a reaction complex that can proceed to product

Equilibrium constant: related to the ratio of product concentration to reactant concentration or rate constants for forward and reverse reactions

Michaelis-Menten constant (K_m): relates the maximum reaction velocity to substrate concentration such that K_m is the substrate concentration [*S*] at which a reaction has attained half the maximal velocity

Lineweaver-Burk plots: linear double reciprocal plots of substrate concentration versus reaction velocity

Allosteric enzymes: defined as any enzyme whose activity is altered by binding small molecule regulators referred to as effectors; plots of substrate concentration versus reaction velocity are sigmoidal instead of curvilinear

TABLE 9-1: International Union of Biochemistry (IUB) Classification of Enzymes

Number	*Classification*	*Biochemical Properties*
1	Oxidoreductases	Act on many chemical groupings to add or remove hydrogen atoms
2	Transferases	Transfer functional groups between donor and acceptor molecules. Kinases are specialized transferases that regulate metabolism by transferring phosphate from ATP to other molecules
3	Hydrolases	Add water across a bond, hydrolyzing it
4	Lyases	Add water, ammonia, or carbon dioxide across double bonds, or remove these elements to produce double bonds
5	Isomerases	Carry out many kinds of isomerization: L to D isomerizations, mutase reactions (shifts of chemical groups), and others
6	Ligases	Catalyze reactions in which 2 chemical groups are joined (or ligated) with the use of energy from ATP

Enzymes are biological catalysts responsible for supporting almost all of the chemical reactions that maintain animal homeostasis. Because of their role in maintaining life processes, the assay and pharmacological regulation of enzymes have become key elements in clinical diagnosis and therapeutics. The macromolecular components of almost all enzymes are composed of protein, except for a class of RNA-modifying catalysts known as ribozymes. Ribozymes are molecules of ribonucleic acid that catalyze reactions on the phosphodiester bond of other RNAs (see Chapter 35) (Table 9-1).

Enzyme Classifications

Enzymes are also classified on the basis of their composition. Enzymes composed wholly of protein are known as simple enzymes in contrast to complex enzymes, which are composed of protein plus a relatively small organic molecule. Complex enzymes are also known as holoenzymes. In this terminology the protein component is known as the apoenzyme, while the nonprotein component is known as the coenzyme or prosthetic group where prosthetic group describes a complex in which the small organic molecule is bound to the apoenzyme by covalent bonds; when the binding between the apoenzyme and nonprotein components is noncovalent, the small organic molecule is called a coenzyme. Many prosthetic groups and coenzymes are water-soluble derivatives of vitamins (Chapter 8). It should be noted that the main clinical symptoms of dietary vitamin insufficiency generally arise from the malfunction of enzymes, which lack sufficient cofactors derived from vitamins to maintain homeostasis.

The nonprotein component of an enzyme may be as simple as a metal ion or as complex as a small nonprotein organic molecule. Enzymes that require a metal in their composition are known as metalloenzymes if they bind and retain their metal atom(s) under all conditions with very high affinity. Enzymes that have a lower affinity for metal ion, but still require the metal ion for activity, are known as metal-activated enzymes.

Role of Coenzymes

The functional role of coenzymes is to act as transporters of chemical groups from one reactant to another. The chemical groups carried can be as simple as the hydride ion ($H^+ + 2e^-$) carried by NAD or the mole of hydrogen carried by FAD; or they can be even more complex such as the amine ($-NH_2$) carried by pyridoxal phosphate.

Since coenzymes are chemically changed as a consequence of enzyme action, it is often useful to consider coenzymes to be a special class of substrates, or second substrates, which are common to many different holoenzymes. In all cases, the coenzymes donate the carried chemical grouping to an acceptor molecule and are thus regenerated to their original form. This regeneration of coenzyme and holoenzyme fulfills the definition of an enzyme as a chemical catalyst, since (unlike the usual substrates, which are used up during the course of a reaction) coenzymes are generally regenerated.

Enzyme Relative to Substrate Type

Although enzymes are highly specific for the kind of reaction they catalyze, the same is not always true of substrates upon which they act. For example, while succinate dehydrogenase (SDH) always catalyzes an oxidation-reduction reaction and its substrate is invariably succinic acid, alcohol dehydrogenase (ADH) always catalyzes oxidation-reduction reactions but can act on a number of different alcohols, ranging from methanol to butanol. Generally, enzymes having broad substrate specificity are most active against one particular substrate. In the case of ADH, ethanol is the preferred substrate.

Enzymes also are generally specific for a particular steric configuration (optical isomer) of a substrate. For example, enzymes that hydrolyze D sugars will not recognize the corresponding L isomer. The enzymes known as racemases provide a striking exception to these generalities; in fact, the role of racemases is to convert D isomers to L isomers and *vice versa*.

As enzymes have a more or less broad range of substrate specificity, it follows that a given substrate may be acted on by a number of different enzymes, each of which uses the same substrate(s) and produces the same product(s). The individual members of a set of enzymes sharing such characteristics are known as isozymes. These are the products of genes that vary only slightly; often, various isozymes of a group are expressed in different tissues of the body.

Enzyme-Substrate Interactions

The favored model of enzyme-substrate interaction is known as the induced-fit model. This model proposes that the initial interaction between enzyme and substrate is relatively weak, but that these weak interactions rapidly induce conformational changes in the enzyme that strengthen binding and bring catalytic sites close to substrate bonds to be altered. After binding takes place, one or more mechanisms of catalysis generate transition-state complexes and reaction products. There are 4 possible mechanisms of enzyme-mediated catalysis.

1. **Catalysis by bond strain:** In this form of catalysis, the induced structural rearrangements that take place with the binding of substrate and enzyme ultimately produce strained substrate bonds, which more easily attain the transition state. The new conformation often forces substrate atoms and bulky catalytic groups, such as aspartate and glutamate, into conformations that strain existing substrate bonds.
2. **Catalysis by proximity and orientation:** Enzyme-substrate interactions orient reactive groups and bring them into proximity with one another. In addition to inducing strain, groups such as aspartate are frequently chemically reactive as well, and their proximity and orientation toward the substrate thus favors their participation in catalysis.
3. **Catalysis involving proton donors (acids) and acceptors (bases):** Other mechanisms also contribute significantly to the completion of catalytic events initiated by a strain mechanism, for example, the use of glutamate as a general acid catalyst (proton donor).
4. **Covalent catalysis:** In catalysis that takes place by covalent mechanisms, the substrate is oriented to active sites on the enzymes in such a way that a covalent intermediate forms between the enzyme or coenzyme and the substrate. One of the best-known examples of this mechanism is that involving proteolysis by serine proteases, which include both digestive enzymes (trypsin, chymotrypsin, and elastase) and several enzymes of the blood-clotting cascade. These proteases contain an active site serine whose R group hydroxyl forms a covalent bond with a carbonyl carbon of a peptide bond, thereby causing hydrolysis of the peptide bond.

Chemical Reactions and Rates

According to the conventions of biochemistry, the rate of a chemical reaction is described by the number of molecules of reactant(s) that are converted into product(s) in a specified time period. Reaction rate is always dependent on the concentration of the chemicals involved in the process and on rate constants that are characteristic of the reaction. For example, the reaction in which A is converted to B is written as follows:

$$A \rightarrow B \qquad (1)$$

The rate of this reaction is expressed algebraically as either a decrease in the concentration of reactant A as

$$-[A] = k[B] \qquad (2)$$

or an increase in the concentration of product B as:

$$[B] = k[A] \qquad (3)$$

In equation 2, the negative sign signifies a decrease in concentration of A as the reaction progresses, brackets define concentration in molarity, and the k is known as a rate constant. Rate constants are simply

High-Yield Concept

At equilibrium, the rate of the forward reaction is equal to the rate of the reverse reaction leading to the equilibrium constant of the reaction and is expressed by:

$$K_{eq} = \frac{K_{+1}}{K_{-1}} = \frac{[B]}{[A]} \quad (7)$$

proportionality constants that provide a quantitative connection between chemical concentrations and reaction rates. Each chemical reaction has characteristic values for its rate constants; these in turn directly relate to the equilibrium constant for that reaction. Thus, a reaction can be rewritten as an equilibrium expression in order to show the relationship between reaction rates, rate constants, and the equilibrium constant for this simple case. The rate constant for the forward reaction is defined as k_{+1} and the reverse as k_{-1}. At equilibrium the rate (v) of the forward reaction ($A \rightarrow B$) is, by definition, equal to that of the reverse or back reaction ($B \rightarrow A$), a relationship which is algebraically symbolized as

$$v_{forward} = v_{reverse} \quad (4)$$

where, for the forward reaction

$$v_{forward} = k_{+1}[A] \quad (5)$$

and for the reverse reaction

$$v_{reverse} = k_{-1}[B] \quad (6)$$

In the above equations, k_{+1} and k_{-1} represent rate constants for the forward and reverse reactions, respectively. The negative subscript refers only to a reverse reaction, not to an actual negative value for the constant. To put the relationships of the 2 equations into words, we state that the rate of the forward reaction [$v_{forward}$] is equal to the product of the forward rate constant k_{+1} and the molar concentration of A. The rate of the reverse reaction is equal to the product of the reverse rate constant k_{-1} and the molar concentration of B.

This equation demonstrates that the equilibrium constant for a chemical reaction is not only equal to the equilibrium ratio of product and reactant concentrations, but is also equal to the ratio of the characteristic rate constants of the reaction.

Chemical Reaction Order

Empirically, order is easily determined by summing the exponents of each concentration term in the rate equation for a reaction. A reaction characterized by the conversion of one molecule of A to one molecule of B with no influence from any other reactant or solvent is a first-order reaction. The exponent on the substrate concentration in the rate equation for this type of reaction is 1. A reaction with 2 substrates forming 2 products would form a second-order reaction. However, the reactants in second- and higher-order reactions need not be different chemical species. An example of a second-order reaction is the formation of ATP through the condensation of ADP with orthophosphate:

$$ADP + H_2PO_4^- \leftrightarrow ATP + H_2O \quad (8)$$

For this reaction the forward reaction rate would be written as:

$$v_{forward} = k_1[ADP][H_2PO_4^-] \quad (9)$$

Enzymes as Biological Catalysts

In cells and organisms most reactions are catalyzed by enzymes, which are regenerated during the course of a reaction. These biological catalysts are physiologically important because they speed up the rates of

High-Yield Concept

Reaction order refers to the number of molecules involved in forming a reaction complex that is competent to proceed to product(s).

reactions that would otherwise be too slow to support life. Enzymes increase reaction rates, sometimes by as much as 1-million fold, but more typically by about 1-thousand fold. Catalysts speed up the forward and reverse reactions proportionately so that, although the magnitude of the rate constants of the forward and reverse reactions is increased, the ratio of the rate constants remains the same in the presence or absence of enzymes. Since the equilibrium constant is equal to a ratio of rate constants, it is apparent that enzymes and other catalysts have no effect on the equilibrium constant of the reactions they catalyze.

Enzymes increase reaction rates by decreasing the amount of energy required to form a complex of reactants that are competent to produce reaction products. This complex is known as the activated state or transition state complex for the reaction. Enzymes and other catalysts accelerate reactions by lowering the energy of the transition state. The free energy required to form an activated complex is much lower in the catalyzed reaction. The amount of energy required to achieve the transition state is lowered; consequently, at any instant a greater proportion of the molecules in the population can achieve the transition state. The result is that the reaction rate is increased.

Michaelis-Menten Kinetics

In typical enzyme-catalyzed reactions, reactant and product concentrations are usually hundreds or thousands of times greater than the enzyme concentration. Consequently, each enzyme molecule catalyzes the conversion to product of many reactant molecules. In biochemical reactions, reactants are commonly known as substrates. The catalytic event that converts substrate to product involves the formation of a transition state, and it occurs most easily at a specific binding site on the enzyme. This site, called the catalytic site of the enzyme, has been evolutionarily structured to provide specific, high-affinity binding of substrate(s) and to provide an environment that favors the catalytic events. The complex that forms when substrates and enzymes combine is called the enzyme substrate (ES) complex. Reaction products arise when the ES complex breaks down releasing free enzyme.

Between the binding of substrate to enzyme, and the reappearance of free enzyme and product, a series of complex events must take place. At a minimum an ES complex must be formed; this complex must pass to the transition state (ES*); and the transition state complex must advance to an enzyme product complex (EP). The latter is finally competent to dissociate to product and free enzyme. The series of events can be shown thus:

$$\mathrm{E + S \leftrightarrow ES \leftrightarrow ES^* \leftrightarrow EP \leftrightarrow E + P} \qquad (10)$$

The kinetics of simple reactions like the above were first characterized by biochemists Michaelis and Menten. The concepts underlying their analysis of enzyme kinetics continue to provide the cornerstone for understanding metabolism today, and for the development and clinical use of drugs aimed at selectively altering rate constants and interfering with the progress of disease states. The Michaelis-Menten equation is a quantitative description of the relationship among the rate of an enzyme-catalyzed reaction [v_1], the concentration of substrate [S] and 2 constants, V_{max} and K_m (which are set by the particular equation). The symbols used in the Michaelis-Menten equation refer to the reaction rate [v_1], maximum reaction rate (V_{max}), substrate concentration [S], and the Michaelis-Menten constant (K_m).

$$V_1 = \frac{V_{max}[S]}{\{K_m + [S]\}} \qquad (11)$$

This fact provides a simple yet powerful bioanalytical tool that has been used to characterize both normal and altered enzymes, such as those that produce the symptoms of genetic diseases. Rearranging the Michaelis-Menten equation leads to:

$$K_m = [S]\left\{\left[\frac{V_{max}}{V_1}\right] - 1\right\} \qquad (12)$$

From this equation it should be apparent that when the substrate concentration is half that required to support the maximum rate of reaction, the observed rate, v_1, will, be equal to V_{max} divided by 2; in other words,

High-Yield Concept

The Michaelis-Menten equation (12) can be used to demonstrate that at the substrate concentration that produces exactly half of the maximum reaction rate, ie, ½V_{max}, the substrate concentration is numerically equal to K_m.

$v_1 = [V_{max}/2]$. At this substrate concentration V_{max}/v_1 will be exactly equal to 2, with the result that:

$$[S](1) = K_m \tag{13}$$

The latter is an algebraic statement of the fact that, for enzymes of the Michaelis-Menten type, when the observed reaction rate is half of the maximum possible reaction rate, the substrate concentration is numerically equal to the Michaelis-Menten constant. In this derivation, the units of K_m are those used to specify the concentration of S, usually molarity.

The Michaelis-Menten equation has the same form as the equation for a rectangular hyperbola; graphical analysis of reaction rate (v) versus substrate concentration [S] produces a hyperbolic rate plot (Figure 9-1).

The key features of the plot are marked by points A, B, and C. At high substrate concentrations, the rate of the reaction (the rate represented by point C) is almost equal to V_{max}, and the difference in rate at nearby concentrations of substrate is almost negligible. If the Michaelis-Menten plot is extrapolated to infinitely high substrate concentrations, the extrapolated rate is equal to V_{max}. When the reaction rate becomes independent of substrate concentration, or nearly so, the rate is said to be zero order. (Note that the reaction is zero order only with respect to this substrate. If the reaction has 2 substrates, it may or may not be zero order with respect to the second substrate). The very small differences in reaction velocity at substrate concentrations around point C (near V_{max}) reflect the fact that at these concentrations almost all the enzyme molecules are bound to substrate and the rate is virtually independent of substrate, hence zero order. At lower substrate concentrations, such as at points A and B, the lower reaction velocities indicate that at any moment only a portion of the enzyme molecules are bound to the substrate. In fact, at the substrate concentration denoted by point B, exactly half the enzyme molecules are in an ES complex at any instant and the rate is exactly one half of V_{max}. At substrate concentrations near point A the rate appears to be directly proportional to substrate concentration, and the reaction rate is said to be first order.

Inhibition of Enzyme-Catalyzed Reactions

To avoid dealing with curvilinear plots of enzyme-catalyzed reactions, biochemists Lineweaver and Burk introduced an analysis of enzyme kinetics based on double reciprocal rearrangement of the Michaelis-Menten equation such that straight line plots of $1/v$ versus $1/[S]$ are obtained where the slope reflects K_m/V_{max} and the y-intercept is $1/V_{max}$. (Figure 9-2)

$$\frac{1}{V_i} = \left(\frac{K_m}{V_{max}}\right)\frac{1}{[s]} + \frac{1}{V_{max}} \tag{14}$$

An alternative linear transformation of the Michaelis-Menten equation is the Eadie-Hofstee transformation

$$\frac{V}{[S]} = -V\left[\frac{1}{K_m}\right] + \left[\frac{V_{max}}{K_m}\right] \tag{15}$$

and when $v/[S]$ is plotted on the y-axis versus v on the x-axis, the result is a linear plot with a slope of $-1/K_m$ and the value V_{max}/K_m as the intercept on the y-axis and V_{max} as the intercept on the x-axis.

Enzyme inhibitors fall into 2 broad classes: those causing irreversible inactivation of enzymes and those

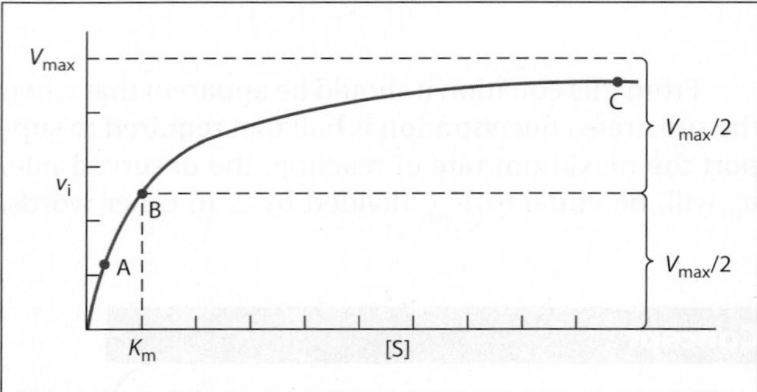

FIGURE 9-1: Effect of substrate concentration on the initial velocity of an enzyme-catalyzed reaction. Murray RK, Bender DA, Botham KM, Kennelly PJ, Rodwell VW, Weil PA. *Harper's Illustrated Biochemistry,* 29th ed. New York, NY: McGraw-Hill; 2012.

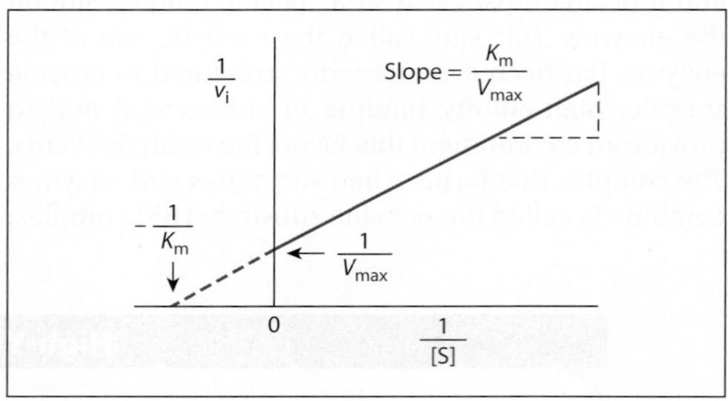

FIGURE 9-2: Double-reciprocal or Lineweaver–Burk plot of $1/v_i$ versus $1/[S]$ used to evaluate K_m and V_{max}. Murray RK, Bender DA, Botham KM, Kennelly PJ, Rodwell VW, Weil PA. *Harper's Illustrated Biochemistry,* 29th ed. New York, NY: McGraw-Hill; 2012.

High-Yield Concept

The hallmark of all the reversible inhibitors is that when the inhibitor concentration drops, enzyme activity is regenerated. Usually these inhibitors bind to enzymes by noncovalent forces and the inhibitor maintains a reversible equilibrium with the enzyme. The equilibrium constant for the dissociation of enzyme inhibitor complexes is known as K_i:

$$K_i = \frac{[E][I]}{[EI]} \tag{16}$$

whose inhibitory effects can be reversed. Irreversible inhibitors usually cause an inactivating, covalent modification of enzyme structure. The kinetic effect of irreversible inhibitors is to decrease the concentration of active enzyme, thus decreasing the maximum possible concentration of ES complex. Reversible inhibitors can be divided into 2 main categories: (1) competitive inhibitors and (2) noncompetitive inhibitors—with a third category, uncompetitive inhibitors, rarely encountered (Table 9-2).

The importance of K_I is that in all enzyme reactions where substrate, inhibitor, and enzyme interact, the normal K_m and/or V_{max} for substrate enzyme interaction appear to be altered. These changes are a consequence of the influence of K_i on the overall rate equation for the reaction. The effects of K_i are best observed in Lineweaver-Burk plots.

Competitive inhibitors always bind at the catalytic or active site of the enzyme. Most drugs that alter enzyme activity are of this type. Competitive inhibitors are especially attractive as clinical modulators of enzyme activity. A decreasing concentration of the inhibitor reverses the equilibrium restoring active-free enzyme. In addition, since substrate and competitive inhibitors both bind at the same site they compete with one another for binding. Raising the concentration of substrate, while holding the concentration of inhibitor constant, results in reversal of competitive inhibition.

Since high concentrations of substrate can displace virtually all competitive inhibitor bound to the active site of an enzyme, it becomes apparent that V_{max} is unchanged by competitive inhibitors. This characteristic of competitive inhibitors is reflected in the identical vertical-axis intercepts of Lineweaver-Burk plots, with and without inhibitor (Figure 9-3).

Since attaining V_{max} requires appreciably higher substrate concentrations in the presence of competitive inhibitor, K_m (the substrate concentration at half maximal velocity) is also higher, as demonstrated by the differing negative intercepts on the horizontal axis in panel B.

Analogously, panel C illustrates that noncompetitive inhibitors appear to have no effect on the intercept at the x-axis implying that noncompetitive inhibitors have no effect on the K_m of the enzymes they inhibit. Since noncompetitive inhibitors do not interfere in the equilibration of enzyme, substrate, and ES complexes, the K_m's of Michaelis-Menten type enzymes are not expected to be affected by noncompetitive inhibitors,

TABLE 9-2: Characteristics of Enzyme Inhibition

Inhibitor Type	*Binding Site on Enzyme*	*Kinetic Effect*
Competitive inhibitor	Specifically at the catalytic site, where it competes with substrate for binding in a dynamic equilibrium-like process. Inhibition is reversible by substrate	V_{max} is unchanged; K_m, as defined by [S] required for ½ maximal activity, is increased
Noncompetitive inhibitor	Binds E or ES complex other than at the catalytic site. Substrate binding unaltered, but ESI complex cannot form products. Inhibition cannot be reversed by substrate	K_m appears unaltered; V_{max} is decreased proportionately to inhibitor concentration
Uncompetitive inhibitor	Binds only to ES complexes at locations other than the catalytic site. Substrate binding modifies enzyme structure, making inhibitor-binding site available. Inhibition cannot be reversed by substrate	Apparent V_{max} decreased; K_m, as defined by [S] required for ½ maximal activity, is decreased

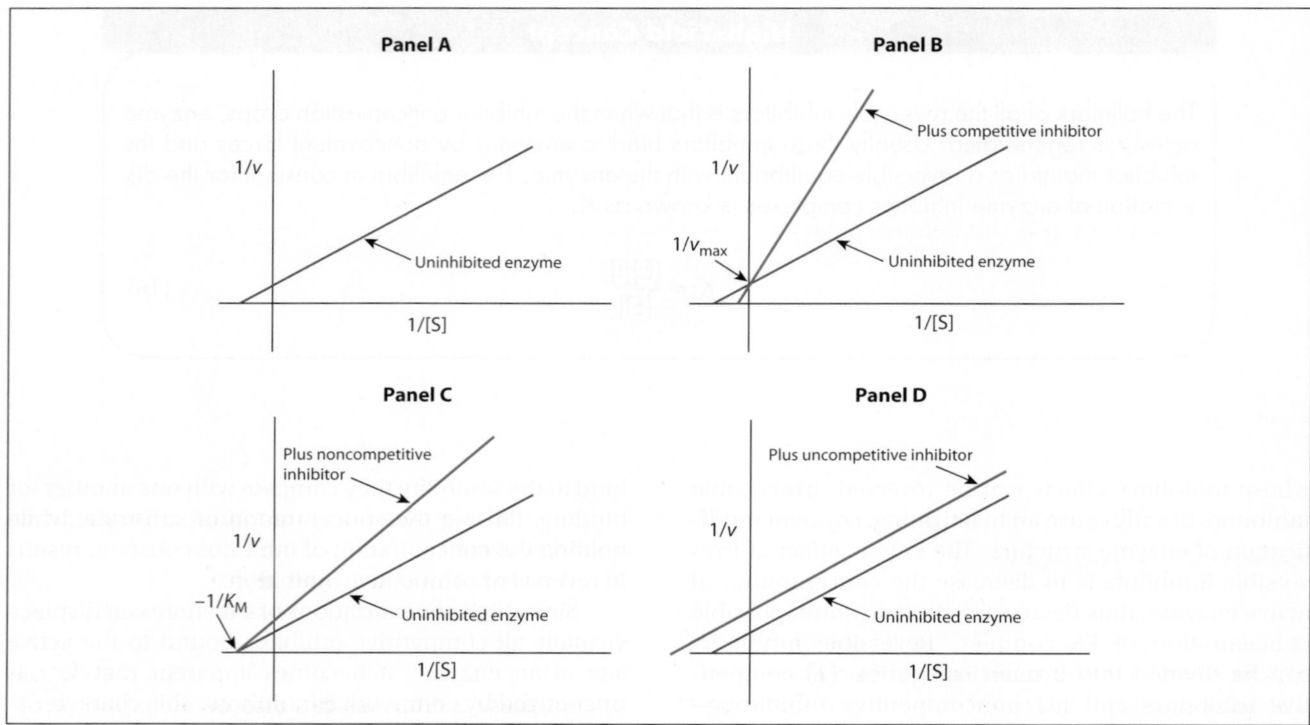

FIGURE 9-3: Lineweaver-Burk plots of inhibited enzymes. Reproduced with permission of themedicalbiochemistrypage, LLC.

as demonstrated by x-axis intercepts in panel C. However, because complexes that contain inhibitor (ESI) are incapable of progressing to reaction products, the effect of a noncompetitive inhibitor is to reduce the concentration of ES complexes that can advance to product. Since $V_{max} = k_2[E_{total}]$, and the concentration of competent E_{total} is diminished by the amount of ESI formed, noncompetitive inhibitors are expected to decrease V_{max}, as illustrated by the y-axis intercepts in panel C.

A corresponding analysis of uncompetitive inhibition leads to the expectation that these inhibitors should change the apparent values of K_m as well as V_{max}. Changing both constants leads to double reciprocal plots, in which intercepts on the x and y axes are proportionately changed; this leads to the production of parallel lines in inhibited and uninhibited reactions.

Regulation of Enzyme Activity

Enzyme concentration is continually modulated in response to physiological needs. Three principal mechanisms are known to regulate the concentration of active enzyme in tissues:

1. Regulation of gene expression controls the quantity and rate of enzyme synthesis.
2. Proteolytic enzyme activity determines the rate of enzyme degradation.
3. Covalent modification of preexisting pools of inactive proenzymes produces active enzymes.

Enzyme synthesis and proteolytic degradation are comparatively slow mechanisms for regulating enzyme concentration, with response times of hours, days, or even weeks. Proenzyme activation is a more rapid method of increasing enzyme activity, but, as a regulatory mechanism, it has the disadvantage of not being a reversible process. Proenzymes are generally synthesized in abundance, stored in secretory granules, and covalently activated upon release from their storage sites.

In contrast to regulatory mechanisms that alter enzyme concentration, there is an important group of regulatory mechanisms that do not affect enzyme concentration, are reversible, and are rapid in action, and actually carry out most of the moment-to-moment physiological regulation of enzyme activity. These mechanisms include allosteric regulation, regulation by reversible covalent modification, and regulation by control proteins such as calmodulin. Reversible covalent modification is a

High-Yield Concept

Allosteric effectors bring about catalytic modification by binding to the enzyme at distinct allosteric sites, well removed from the catalytic site, and causing conformational changes that are transmitted through the bulk of the protein to the catalytically active site(s). Effectors that increase catalytic activity are known as positive effectors and effectors that reduce or inhibit catalytic activity are negative effectors. Their single defining feature is that they are not identical to the substrate.

major mechanism for the rapid and transient regulation of enzyme activity.

Allosteric Enzymes

In addition to simple enzymes that interact only with substrates and inhibitors, there is a class of enzymes that bind small, physiologically important molecules and modulate activity in ways other than those already discussed. These are known as allosteric enzymes and the small regulatory molecules that bind to these enzymes are known as allosteric effectors.

There are 2 ways that enzymatic activity can be altered by effectors: the V_{max} can be increased or decreased, or the K_m can be raised or lowered. Enzymes whose K_m is altered by effectors are said to be K-type enzymes and the effector a K-type effector. If V_{max} is altered, the enzyme and effector are said to be V-type. Many allosteric enzymes respond to multiple effectors with V-type and K-type behavior.

Enzymes in the Diagnosis of Pathology

The measurement of the serum levels of numerous enzymes has been shown to be of diagnostic significance. This is because the presence of these enzymes in the serum indicates that tissue or cellular damage has occurred resulting in the release of intracellular components into the blood. Hence, when a physician indicates that he/she is going to assay for liver enzymes, the purpose is to ascertain the potential for liver cell damage. Commonly assayed enzymes in the blood are the amino transferases: alanine transaminase (ALT; sometimes still referred to as serum glutamate-pyruvate aminotransferase [SGPT]) and aspartate aminotransferase (AST; also referred to as serum glutamate-oxaloacetate aminotransferase [SGOT]). In addition, the enzymes cardiac troponin I (cTnI), lactate dehydrogenase (LDH), and creatine kinase (CK; also called creatine phosphokinase [CPK]) are commonly measured in the diagnosis of cardiac infarct.

The typical liver enzymes measured are AST and ALT. ALT is particularly diagnostic of liver involvement as this enzyme is found predominantly in hepatocytes. When assaying for both ALT and AST, the ratio of the level of these 2 enzymes can also be diagnostic. Normally in liver disease or damage that is not of viral origin the ratio of ALT to AST is less than 1. However, with viral hepatitis the ALT:AST ratio will be greater than 1. Measurement of AST is useful not only for liver involvement but also for heart disease or damage. The level of AST elevation in the serum is directly proportional to the number of cells involved as well as on the time following injury that the AST assay was performed. Following injury, levels of AST rise within 8 hours and peak 24 to 36 hours later. Within 3 to 7 days the level of AST should return to preinjury levels, provided a continuous insult is not present or further injury does not occur. Although measurement of AST is not, in and of itself, diagnostic for myocardial infarction (MI), taken together with LDH and CK measurements (see below) the level of AST is useful for timing of the infarct.

Troponins are complexes composed of 3 regulatory proteins (troponin C, I, and T) attached to tropomyosin and are found in the grooves between actin filaments in muscle tissue. The troponins are found in skeletal and cardiac muscle but not in smooth muscle. Cardiac troponins found in the serum, specifically troponin I and T, are excellent markers for MI as well as for any other type of heart muscle damage. The measurement of plasma troponin I levels is highly diagnostic of necrosis of cardiac muscle. Serum levels of troponin I rise within 4 to 8 hours after the onset of chest pain caused by MI. The levels peak within 12 to 16 hours after the onset of infarction and return to baseline within 5 to 9 days. Although measurement of serum LDH fractions was once considered the ideal marker for onset and severity of a heart attack, the high specificity of troponin I to heart muscle necrosis make this protein the preferred marker to measure in patients suspected of suffering an MI.

The measurement of plasma LDH is useful as a diagnostic indicator of MI because this enzyme exists in 5 closely related, but slightly different forms (isozymes). The 5 types and their normal distribution and levels in nondisease/injury are listed below:

1. LDH 1: Heart and red blood cells and is 17% to 27% of the normal serum total.
2. LDH 2: Heart and red blood cells and is 27% to 37% of the normal serum total.
3. LDH 3: Variety of organs and is 18% to 25% of the normal serum total.
4. LDH 4: Variety of organs and is 3% to 8% of the normal serum total.
5. LDH 5: Liver and skeletal muscle and is 0% to 5% of the normal serum total.

Following an MI the serum levels of LDH rise within 24 to 48 hours reaching a peak by 2 to 3 days and return to normal in 5 to 10 days. Especially diagnostic is a comparison of the LDH-1:LDH-2 ratio. Normally, this ratio is less than 1. A reversal of this ratio is referred to as a flipped LDH. Following an acute MI the flipped LDH ratio will appear in 12 to 24 hours and is definitely present by 48 hours in over 80% of patients. Also important is the fact that persons suffering chest pain due to angina only will not likely have altered LDH levels.

CPK is found primarily in heart and skeletal muscle as well as the brain. Therefore, measurement of serum CPK levels is a good diagnostic for injury to these tissues. The levels of CPK will rise within 6 hours of injury and peak by around 18 hours. If the injury is not persistent, the level of CK returns to normal within 2 to 3 days. Like LDH, there are tissue-specific isozymes of CPK and there designations are described below:

CPK3 (CPK-MM) is the predominant isozyme in muscle and is 100% of the normal serum total.

CPK2 (CPK-MB) accounts for about 35% of the CPK activity in cardiac muscle, but less than 5% in skeletal muscle and is 0% of the normal serum total.

CPK1 (CPK-BB) is the characteristic isozyme in brain and is in significant amounts in smooth muscle and is 0% of the normal serum total.

Since most of the released CPK after a myocardial infarction is CPK-MB, an increased ratio of CPK-MB to total CPK may help in diagnosis of an acute infarction, but an increase of total CPK in itself may not. CPK-MB levels rise 3 to 6 hours after an MI and peak 12 to 24 hours later if no further damage occurs and returns to normal 12 to 48 hours after the infarct.

REVIEW QUESTIONS

The interconversion of kJ/mol and kcal/mol in the following questions can be done with the formula: 1kcal/mol = 4.184kJ/mol.

1. You are studying the effects of a new drug on the activity of your favorite enzyme. The results of your assays indicate that the drug acts as a noncompetitive inhibitor. Which of the following changes to the K_m and V_{max} allowed that determination to be made regarding the drugs actions?

A. K_m decreased, V_{max} increased
B. K_m decreased, V_{max} unchanged
C. K_m increased, V_{max} decreased
D. K_m unchanged, V_{max} decreased
E. K_m unchanged, V_{max} unchanged

Answer D: Noncompetitive inhibitors bind to enzyme or ES complex other than at the catalytic site and thus have no effect on substrate binding. However, the resultant ESI complex cannot form products. This type of inhibition cannot be reversed by the addition of more substrate. Under these conditions K_m appears unaltered, while V_{max} is decreased proportionately to inhibitor concentration.

2. The drug acetazolamide is used in the treatment of glaucoma since it decreases the production of aqueous fluid, thereby reducing intraocular pressures. This drug is a noncompetitive inhibitor of carbonic anhydrase. Which of the following statements most accurately relates to the actions of this type of inhibitor?

A. decreases both V_{max} and apparent K_m
B. decreases apparent K_m
C. decreases V_{max}
D. increases apparent K_m
E. increases V_{max}

Answer C: Noncompetitive inhibitors bind to enzyme or ES complex other than at the catalytic site and thus have no effect on substrate binding. However, the resultant ESI complex cannot form products. This type of inhibition cannot be reversed by the addition of more substrate. Under these conditions K_m appears unaltered while V_{max} is decreased proportionately to inhibitor concentration.

3. Drugs that inhibit enzymes in a competitive manner will have which of the following effects on the Michaelis-Menten equation derived parameters: V_{max} and/or K_m?

A. decrease both V_{max} and K_m
B. decrease K_m but no effect on V_{max}
C. decrease V_{max} but no change on K_m
D. increase K_m but no change in V_{max}
E. increase V_{max} but no increase in K_m

Answer D: Competitive inhibitors bind enzyme at the catalytic site, thereby competing with substrate for binding in a dynamic equilibrium-like process. This type of inhibition is reversible by the addition of higher concentrations of substrate. With competitive inhibitors the maximum velocity (V_{max}) of the reaction is unchanged, while the apparent affinity of the substrate to the binding site is decreased. In other words, K_m, as defined by the substrate concentration required for half maximal activity, is increased.

4. Drugs that inhibit enzymes in a noncompetitive manner will have which of the following effects on the Michaelis-Menten equation derived parameters: V_{max} and/or K_m?
A. decrease both V_{max} and K_m
B. decrease K_m but no effect on V_{max}
C. decrease V_{max} but no change on K_m
D. increase K_m but no change in V_{max}
E. increase V_{max} but no increase in K_m

Answer C: Noncompetitive inhibitors bind to enzyme or ES complex other than at the catalytic site and thus have no effect on substrate binding. However, the resultant ESI complex cannot form products. This type of inhibition cannot be reversed by the addition of more substrate. Under these conditions K_m appears unaltered, while V_{max} is decreased proportionately to inhibitor concentration.

5. Drugs that inhibit enzymes in an uncompetitive manner will have which of the following effects on the Michaelis-Menten equation–derived parameters: V_{max} and/or K_m?
A. decrease both V_{max} and K_m
B. decrease K_m but no effect on V_{max}
C. decrease V_{max} but no change on K_m
D. increase K_m but no change in V_{max}
E. increase V_{max} but no increase in K_m

Answer A: Uncompetitive enzyme inhibition takes place when an enzyme inhibitor binds only to the complex formed between the enzyme and the substrate (the ES complex). This reduction in the effective concentration to the ES complex increases the enzyme's apparent affinity for the substrate (K_m is lowered) and decreases the maximum enzyme activity (V_{max}), as it takes longer for the substrate or product to leave the active site. Uncompetitive inhibition works best when substrate concentration is high.

6. Which of the following best explains why noncompetitive inhibitors of enzymes generally make better pharmaceuticals?
A. their inhibitory activity is unaffected by substrate concentration
B. they affect only K_m and not V_{max}
C. they bind to the same site as the substrate
D. they increase the rate of degradation of the target enzyme
E. they irreversibly inhibit the enzyme

Answer A: Pharmaceuticals that are designed to inhibit an enzyme in a noncompetitive manner are much more effective than inhibitors that function competitively because any increase in substrate will have no effect on the level of inhibition.

7. The standard free-energy change ($\Delta G^{0\prime}$) for the hydrolysis of phosphoenolpyruvate (PEP) is −14.8 kcal/mol.' The $\Delta G^{0\prime}$ for the hydrolysis of ATP is −7.3 kcal/mol. What is the $\Delta G^{0\prime}$ for the following reaction?

$$\text{Phosphoenolpyruvate} + \text{ADP} \rightarrow \text{pyruvate} + \text{ATP}$$

A. −22.1 kcal/mol
B. −14.8 kcal/mol
C. −7.5 kcal/mol
D. −7.3 kcal/mol
E. +7.3 kcal/mol

Answer C: The reaction, as written, actually represents the coupling of 2 distinct reactions. One is the hydrolysis of PEP to pyruvate and the other is the synthesis of ATP from ADP. Each of the 2 reactions has their own $\Delta G^{0\prime}$. To simplify, a coupled biochemical reaction is one where the free energy of a thermodynamically favorable reaction (PEP to pyruvate) is used to drive a thermodynamically unfavorable one (the formation of ATP from ADP) by coupling the 2 reactions. The coupling in this case is carried out by the enzyme pyruvate kinase. When 2 reactions are coupled, the resultant free-energy change is simply the mathematical sum of the 2 $\Delta G^{0\prime}$ values for each reaction. In the case of the formation of ATP from ADP, the $\Delta G^{0\prime}$ for the reaction in that direction is equal to, but mathematically opposite of, the reciprocal reaction.

8. Which of the following indicates whether the reaction, A → B, is thermodynamically favorable under standard state conditions at near physiological pH?
A. $\Delta G'$
B. $\Delta G^{0\prime}$
C. K_{eq}
D. K_m
E. V_{max}

Answer B: The Gibbs free-energy equation ($\Delta G = \Delta T - T\Delta S$) states the relationship between the change in fee energy (ΔG), the change in enthalpy (ΔH), the change in entropy (ΔS), and the temperature (T). When a reaction is carried out under standard state conditions of temperature and pressure, the values are denoted by the superscript 0, and the addition of the prime ($\Delta G^{0\prime}$) indicates that the reaction is carried out at pH 7.0. The spontaneity of a reaction is determined by comparing the free energy of the system before the reaction with the free energy of the system after reaction. If the system, after reaction, has less free energy than before the reaction (ie, the $\Delta G^{0\prime}$ value is negative), the reaction is thermodynamically favorable. One should also note that even if $\Delta G^{0\prime}$ is positive, the reaction can still become spontaneous due to coupling of the thermodynamically unfavorable reaction to a reaction (or reactions) that is favorable.

9. Which of the following relates to allosteric enzymes?

A. they are inactive on their substrates in the absence of accessory proteins
B. they can bind more than one substrate simultaneously
C. they can convert multiple different substrates to product
D. they possess binding sites for regulatory molecules in addition to substrate-binding sites
E. they require additional cofactor-binding sites for subsequent binding of substrate

Answer D: Allosteric enzymes are enzymes that change their conformational orientations upon binding of an effector which results in an apparent change in binding affinity at a different ligand-binding site. This action at a distance through binding of one ligand (or allosteric effector) affecting the binding of another at a distinctly different site is the essence of the allosteric concept.

10. Assessment of enzyme activity under standard condition and plotted as a linear Lineweaver-Burk plot gives the green line (x). The red line (y) was most likely obtained by addition of which of the following to this enzyme assay?

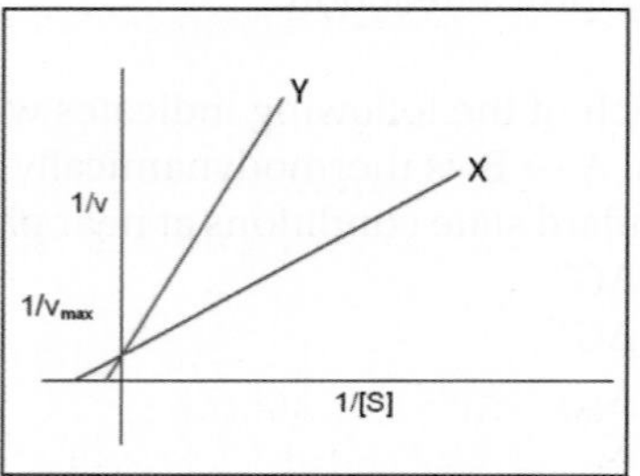

A. allosteric activator
B. competitive inhibitor
C. double the amount of enzyme
D. half the amount of enzyme
E. noncompetitive inhibitor

Answer B: Competitive inhibitors bind enzyme at the catalytic site, thereby competing with substrate for binding in a dynamic equilibrium-like process. This type of inhibition is reversible by the addition of higher concentrations of substrate. With competitive inhibitors the maximum velocity (V_{max}) of the reaction is unchanged, while the apparent affinity of the substrate to the binding site is decreased. In other words, K_m, as defined by the substrate concentration required for half maximal activity, is increased. These changes are visible in Lineweaver-Burk plots where the Y-axis intercept is unchanged, while the X-axis intercept is closer to the Y-axis. This is indicative of a larger value for K_m.

11. Kinases are a class of enzymes that incorporate a phosphate onto their substrates. The catalytic activity of kinases classifies them as members of which of the following enzyme families?

A. hydrolases
B. isomerases
C. ligases
D. oxidoreductases
E. transferases

Answer E: Kinases are any of the various enzymes that catalyze the transfer of a phosphate group from a donor, such as ADP or ATP, to an acceptor. As such, kinases represent a subfamily of the transferase class of enzyme.

12. You are studying the effects of the addition of a potential pharmaceutical compound on the activity of your enzyme of interest. You find that the addition of the compound results in an increase in the K_m of the reaction but does not affect the V_{max}. Which of the following defines the inhibitory action of the compound?

A. competitive
B. noncompetitive
C. suicide
D. uncompetitive

Answer A: Competitive inhibitors bind enzyme at the catalytic site, thereby competing with substrate for binding in a dynamic equilibrium-like process. This type of inhibition is reversible by the addition of higher concentrations of substrate. With competitive inhibitors the maximum velocity (V_{max}) of the reaction is unchanged, while the apparent affinity of the substrate to the binding site is decreased. In other words, K_m, as defined by the substrate concentration required for half maximal activity, is increased.

13. If the $\Delta G^{0\prime}$ of the reaction A → B is −40 kJ/mol, under standard conditions which of the following is correct?

A. the reaction is at equilibrium
B. $\Delta G^{0\prime}$ will never reach equilibrium
C. $\Delta G^{0\prime}$ will not occur spontaneously
D. $\Delta G^{0\prime}$ will proceed at a rapid rate
E. $\Delta G^{0\prime}$ will proceed spontaneously from left to right

Answer E: $\Delta G^{0\prime}$ is the Gibbs free energy value when a reaction is carried out under standard state conditions of temperature and pressure and at pH 7. The spontaneity of a reaction is determined by comparing the free energy of the system before the reaction with the free energy of the system after the reaction. If the system after reaction has less free energy than before the reaction (ie, the $\Delta G^{0\prime}$ value is negative), the reaction is thermodynamically favorable. Thus, since the reaction as written has a negative free-energy value, it will proceed favorably as written.

14. For the reaction A → B, $\Delta G^{0\prime}$ = −60 kJ/mol. The reaction is started with 10 mmol of A and no B is initially present. After 24 hours, analysis reveals the presence of 2 mmol of B and 8 mmol of A. Which of the following is the most likely explanation?

A. A and B have reached equilibrium concentrations
B. an enzyme has shifted the equilibrium toward A
C. B formation is kinetically slow; equilibrium has not been reached by 24 hours
D. formation of B is thermodynamically unfavorable
E. the result described is impossible, given the fact that $\Delta G^{0\prime}$ is −60 kJ/mol

Answer C: When this reaction is at equilibrium, the amount of product (B) would be greater than that of substrate (A) since the reaction proceeds favorably from A to B. Since the amount of B is still less than that of A, the reaction has not yet reached equilibrium even after 24 hours. The reaction is still thermodynamically favorable since the free-energy change for the reaction as written has a large negative value. In addition, since equilibrium has not yet been reached in the time frame of the analysis, it is implied that the reaction proceeds with slow kinetics.

15. When a mixture of 3-phosphoglycerate and 2-phosphoglycerate is incubated at 25°C with phosphoglycerate mutase until equilibrium is reached, the final mixture contains 6 times as much 2-phosphoglycerate as 3-phosphoglycerate. Which one of the following statements is most nearly correct, when applied to the reaction as written? (R = 8.315 J/mol·K; T = 298 K)

3-Phosphoglycerate → 2-phosphoglycerate

A. $\Delta G^{0\prime}$ is −4.44 kJ/mol
B. $\Delta G^{0\prime}$ is zero
C. $\Delta G^{0\prime}$ is +12.7 kJ/mol
D. $\Delta G^{0\prime}$ is incalculably large and positive
E. $\Delta G^{0\prime}$ cannot be calculated from the information given

Answer A: Since there is much more product than substrate when the reaction has reached equilibrium, the reaction can be assumed to be favorable when proceeding in the direction as written. Therefore, the free-energy change value for the reaction is most likely to be somewhat negative.

16. When a mixture of glucose 6-phosphate and fructose 6-phosphate is incubated with the enzyme phosphohexose isomerase (which catalyzes the interconversion of these 2 sugars) until equilibrium is reached, the final mixture contains twice as much glucose 6-phosphate as fructose 6-phosphate. Which one of the following statements is best applied to this reaction outlined below? (R = 8.315 J/mol·K; T = 298 K)

Glucose 6-phosphate → fructose 6-phosphate

A. $\Delta G^{0\prime}$ is incalculably large and negative
B. $\Delta G^{0\prime}$ is −1.72 kJ/mol
C. $\Delta G^{0\prime}$ is zero
D. $\Delta G^{0\prime}$ is +1.72 kJ/mol
E. $\Delta G^{0\prime}$ is incalculably large and positive

Answer D: Since there is more substrate than product when the reaction has reached equilibrium, the reaction can be assumed to be less than favorable when proceeding in the direction as written. Therefore, the free-energy change value for the reaction is most likely to be slightly positive.

17. Hydrolysis of 1 M glucose 6-phosphate catalyzed by glucose 6-phosphatase is 99% complete at equilibrium (ie, only 1% of the substrate remains). Which of the following statements is most nearly correct? (R = 8.315 J/mol·K; T = 298 K)

A. $\Delta G^{0\prime}$ = −11 kJ/mol
B. $\Delta G^{0\prime}$ = −5 kJ/mol
C. $\Delta G^{0\prime}$ = 0 kJ/mol
D. $\Delta G^{0\prime}$ = +11 kJ/mol
E. $\Delta G^{0\prime}$ cannot be determined from the information given

Answer A: At equilibrium, almost all of the substrate has been converted to product, therefore the reaction can be assumed to be highly favorable when proceeding in the direction of glucose production from glucose 6-phosphate, the direction catalyzed by glucose 6-phosphatase. Therefore, the most likely free-energy change value for the reaction can be expected to be quite negative.

18. The reaction $A + B \rightarrow C$ has a $\Delta G^{0\prime}$ of −20 kJ/mol at 25°C. Starting under standard conditions, one can predict which of the following?

A. at equilibrium, the concentration of B will exceed the concentration of A
B. at equilibrium, the concentration of C will be less than the concentration of A
C. at equilibrium, the concentration of C will be much greater than the concentration of A or B
D. C will rapidly break down to $A + B$
E. when A and B are mixed, the reaction will proceed rapidly toward formation of C

Answer C: Reactions with large negative free-energy changes are highly favorable. When these types of reactions reach equilibrium, it is expected that the concentration of product(s) would be much greater than that of substrate(s).

19. Which of the following reactions has the largest negative value for the standard free energy-change ($\Delta G^{0\prime}$)?

A. fructose 1,6-bisphosphate → fructose 6-phosphate
B. glucose 6-phosphate → fructose 6-phosphate
C. glycerol 3-phosphate → dihydroxyacetone phosphate
D. glycerol → glycerol 3-phosphate
E. phosphoenolpyruvate → pyruvate

Answer E: The standard free-energy change for the reaction catalyzed by pyruvate kinase (PK) is approximately −7.5kcal/mol. This reaction is 1 of the 2 reactions of glycolysis that releases enough energy such that it can be coupled to the synthesis of ATP.

20. For the following reaction, $\Delta G^{0\prime} = +29.7$ kJ/mol

L-Malate + NAD^+ → oxaloacetate + NADH + H^+

Which of the following correctly describes the characteristics of the reaction as written?

A. can never occur in a cell
B. can occur in a cell only if it is coupled to another reaction for which $\Delta G^{0\prime}$ is positive
C. can occur only in a cell in which NADH is converted to NAD^+ by electron transport
D. cannot occur because of its large activation energy
E. may occur in cells at some concentrations of substrate and product

Answer E: Although the reaction, as written, has a positive free-energy change and is thus thermodynamically favorable, it is known that within cells this reaction does indeed proceed in the forward direction. The means by which this TCA cycle (tricarboxylic acid cycle) reaction is driven in the forward direction, against the positive free-energy change, is by rapid removal of the product (OAA) via the enzyme catalyzing the next reaction in the cycle. Therefore, when certain reactions are coupled to subsequent favorable reactions that rapidly remove the product of the initial reaction, the less than favorable reaction can occur under these conditions.

21. In glycolysis, fructose 1,6-bisphosphate is converted to 2 products with a standard free-energy change ($\Delta G^{0\prime}$) of 23.8 kJ/mol. Under what conditions, encountered in a normal cell, will the free-energy change be negative, enabling the reaction to proceed spontaneously to the right?

A. under standard conditions, enough energy is released to drive the reaction to the right
B. the reaction will not go to the right spontaneously under any conditions because the $\Delta G^{0\prime}$ is positive
C. the reaction will proceed spontaneously to the right if there is a high concentration of products relative to the concentration of fructose 1,6-bisphosphate
D. the reaction will proceed spontaneously to the right if there is a high concentration of fructose 1,6-bisphosphate relative to the concentration of products

Answer A: Within the cell, under standard conditions, the 2 products of the hydrolysis of fructose 1,6-bisphosphate (F1,6BP) are rapidly removed by the subsequent reactions of glycolysis. This is, of course, assuming that the energy needs of the cell are high which would likely be the case since F1,6BP has been formed and would only be formed when the cell needs to oxidize glucose for energy.

22. During glycolysis, glucose 1-phosphate is converted to fructose 6-phosphate in 2 successive reactions:

Glucose 1-phosphate → glucose 6-phosphate $\Delta G^{0\prime} = -7.1$ kJ/mol

Glucose 6-phosphate → fructose 6-phosphate $\Delta G^{0\prime} = +1.7$ kJ/mol

For the overall reaction which of the following correctly identifies the free-energy change?

A. −8.8 kJ/mol
B. −7.1 kJ/mol
C. −5.4 kJ/mol

D. +5.4 kJ/mol
E. +8.8 kJ/mol

Answer C: When 2 reactions are coupled, the resultant free-energy change is the arithmetic sum of the $\Delta G^{0\prime}$ values for the coupled reactions. Therefore, the correct free-energy change for these 2 reactions is the sum of their individual free-energy change values.

23. The standard free-energy changes for the reactions below are given.

$$\text{Phosphocreatine} \rightarrow \text{creatine} + P_i \quad \Delta G^{0\prime} = -43.0 \text{ kJ/mol}$$

$$\text{ATP} \rightarrow \text{ADP} + P_i \quad \Delta G^{0\prime} = -30.5 \text{ kJ/mol}$$

What is the overall $\Delta G^{0\prime}$ for the following reaction?

$$\text{Phosphocreatine} + \text{ADP} \rightarrow \text{creatine} + \text{ATP}$$

A. −73.5 kJ/mol
B. −12.5 kJ/mol
C. +12.5 kJ/mol
D. +73.5 kJ/mol
E. $\Delta G^{0\prime}$ cannot be calculated without Keq′

Answer B: When 2 reactions are coupled, the resultant free-energy change is the arithmetic sum of the $\Delta G^{0\prime}$ values for the coupled reactions. In the case of the coupled reaction, instead of energy input from the hydrolysis of ATP the opposite reaction is being coupled. The $\Delta G^{0\prime}$ value for a given reaction is its reciprocal value when the reaction is running in the opposite direction to that for which the $\Delta G^{0\prime}$ value is denoted. Thus, for ATP synthesis from ADP, the $\Delta G^{0\prime}$ value would be +30.5kJ/mol. When the 2 reactions are coupled, there is sufficient energy released from the hydrolysis of phosphocreatine to drive the synthesis of ATP from ADP. The $\Delta G^{0\prime}$ value for the coupled reactions is the simple arithmetic sum of the $\Delta G^{0\prime}$ values for the individual reactions.

24. The $\Delta G^{0\prime}$ values for the 2 reactions shown below are given:

$$\text{Oxaloacetate} + \text{acetyl-CoA} + H_2O \rightarrow \text{citrate} + \text{CoASH} \quad \Delta G^{0\prime} = -32.2 \text{ kJ/mol}$$

$$\text{Oxaloacetate} + \text{acetate} \rightarrow \text{citrate} \quad \Delta G^{0\prime} = -1.9 \text{ kJ/mol}$$

What is the $\Delta G0'$ for the hydrolysis of acetyl-CoA?

$$\text{Acetyl-CoA} + H_2O \rightarrow \text{acetate} + \text{CoASH} + H^+$$

A. −34.1 kJ/mol
B. −32.2 kJ/mol
C. −30.3 kJ/mol
D. +61.9 kJ/mol
E. +34.1 kJ/mol

Answer C: When 2 reactions are coupled, the resultant free-energy change is the arithmetic sum of the $\Delta G^{0\prime}$ values for the coupled reactions. In the case of the coupled reaction, instead of energy input from the hydrolysis of ATP the opposite reaction is being coupled. The $\Delta G^{0\prime}$ value for a given reaction is its reciprocal value when the reaction is running in the opposite direction to that for which the $\Delta G^{0\prime}$ value is denoted. Thus, for ATP synthesis from ADP, the $\Delta G^{0\prime}$ value would be +30.5kJ/mol. When the 2 reactions are coupled, there is sufficient energy released from the hydrolysis of phosphocreatine to drive the synthesis of ATP from ADP. The $\Delta G^{0\prime}$ value for the coupled reactions is the simple arithmetic sum of the $\Delta G^{0\prime}$ values for the individual reactions.

25. Which one of the following compounds possesses the least negative free energy of hydrolysis?
A. 1,3-bisphosphoglycerate
B. 3-phosphoglycerate
C. ADP
D. phosphoenolpyruvate
E. thioesters (eg, acetyl-CoA)

Answer B: Only four of these molecules possess a negative ΔG of hydrolysis. The hydrolysis of 3-phosphoglycerate occurs with a free energy change of +1.1kcal/mol. However, within cells undergoing glycolysis, due to the rapid removal of products of one reaction to substrates of the next reaction the free energy released from 3-phosphoglycerate is an apparent −0.9kcal/mol. The free energy of 1,3-bisphosphoglycerate hydrolysis is −4.5kcal/mol, ADP is −7.3kcal/mol, phosphoenolpyruvate is -14.8kcal/mol, and acetyl-CoA is -8.5kcal/mol.

26. A 57-year-old man has just returned from an overseas trip and reports having had severe substernal chest pain 3 days ago. Which of the following is the most appropriate laboratory test to order for this patient?
A. aspartate aminotransferase
B. creatine kinase, MB fraction
C. creatine kinase, total
D. lactate dehydrogenase, LD_1 fraction
E. troponin I

Answer E: Troponin I is now the method of choice for the laboratory diagnosis of MI. There is a detectable increase within 4 to 8 hours of the infarction and the peak level is reached within 12 to 16 hours. Levels do not return to baseline for 3 to 10 days making it an appropriate test for this patient who was 3 days postinfarction. Aspartate aminotransferase was the first serum enzyme marker used for the diagnosis of MI, but it has poor specificity and sensitivity compared to newer markers and is no longer used for this purpose.

Creatine kinase total is not used for the diagnosis of MI since the cardiac fraction (MB) can be overwhelmed by the presence of the skeletal muscle fraction. Creatine kinase-MB is still being used in some institutions but it returns to baseline in 2 to 3 days and would not be useful for this patient. Lactate dehydrogenase (LD_1 fraction) returns to baseline later than creatine kinase but has been replaced by troponin I and is seldom used.

27. Enzymes are efficient catalysts because they can do which of the following?
- **A.** catalyze reactions that otherwise would not occur
- **B.** decrease the free energy of activation of reactants
- **C.** decrease the standard free-energy change ($\Delta G^{0\prime}$) of reactions
- **D.** prevent the conversion of product to substrate
- **E.** shift the equilibrium of reactions toward more complete conversion to product

Answer B: Like inorganic catalysts, enzymes are efficient catalysts because they are capable of lowering the energy of activation of the reactions in which they are active. A catalyst is a substance that increases the rate of a chemical reaction without itself being changed by the reaction. Enzymes affect the rate but not the equilibrium constant of a reaction. Catalysts, like enzymes, merely reduce the time that a thermodynamically favored reaction requires to reach equilibrium.

28. Which of the following is the mechanism by which allosteric effectors influence enzymatic activity?
- **A.** binding at the catalytic site
- **B.** changing the conformation of the enzyme
- **C.** forming high-energy complexes with substrate
- **D.** increasing hydration of the active site
- **E.** protecting against degradation of the enzyme

Answer B: Allosteric enzymes are enzymes whose conformation changes upon binding of an allosteric effector. This binding results in an apparent change in binding affinity in the enzyme at a different ligand-binding site. This action at a distance through binding of one ligand (or allosteric effector) affecting the binding of another at a distinctly different site is the essence of the allosteric concept.

29. Which of the following conditions is most likely if the reaction shown in the diagram is at equilibrium?

$$\mathrm{A} \underset{k_2}{\overset{k_1}{\rightleftharpoons}} \mathrm{B}$$

($K_1 = 500$/second, $K_2 = 5$/second)

- **A.** all of A is consumed
- **B.** all of B is consumed
- **C.** both A and B are present, but the concentration of A is greater than that of B
- **D.** both A and B are present, but the concentration of B is greater than that of A
- **E.** the concentrations of A and B are equal

Answer D: If the rate constant for the reaction in the direction of the formation of B is 100 times greater than for the reaction in the direction of A formation, the formation of B will be the favored direction. Therefore, when the reaction reaches equilibrium, there will be substantially more B than A present in the reaction vessel.

30. A newborn screening test for galactosemia is positive in your patient. Genetic studies demonstrate the infant harbors a particular mutation in the GALT gene that impairs the activity of galactose-1-phosphate uridyltransferase. The impaired enzyme cannot convert galactose 1-phosphate and UDP-glucose to UDP-galactose and glucose 1-phosphate. Galactose 1-phosphate accumulates and affects the activity of UTP-dependent glucose-1-phosphate pyrophosphorylase (UGP). Which of the following actions by galactose 1-phosphate proves that it is a competitive inhibitor of UGP?
- **A.** decreases the apparent K_m for glucose 1-phosphate
- **B.** decreases both the V_{max} and the apparent K_m for glucose 1-phosphate
- **C.** decreases the V_{max} for glucose 1-phosphate
- **D.** increases the apparent K_m for glucose 1-phosphate
- **E.** increases the V_{max} for glucose 1-phosphate

Answer D: Competitive inhibitors bind enzyme at the catalytic site, thereby competing with substrate for binding in a dynamic equilibrium-like process. With competitive inhibitors the maximum velocity (V_{max}) of the reaction is unchanged, while the apparent affinity of the substrate to the binding site is decreased. In other words, K_m, as defined by the substrate concentration required for half maximal activity, is increased.

31. You are studying the effects of compounds that inhibit the activity of succinate dehydrogenase, SDH. You demonstrate that malonate is a competitive inhibitor of this enzyme. Which of the following sets of findings would most likely provide ideal conditions for maximum inhibition of SDH by malonate?

	Succinate (mM)	K_m (mM)	Malonate (mM)	K_i (mM)
A.	1	1	1	1
B.	1	1	10	10
C.	1	10	1	10
D.	1	10	10	1

Answer D: Competitive inhibitors affect only the K_m because they displace the substrate by binding to the same site on the enzyme. Because competitive inhibitors bind to the substrate binding site they exhibit K_i values very similar, if not identical, to the K_m of the substrate. The addition of more substrate can compete with the inhibitor, therefore, in order to effectively inhibit the enzyme one needs to provide a higher concentration of the inhibitor. Given these facts only one of the choices is associated with increased K_m value, a similar K_i value to the substrate K_m, and provides excess inhibitor.

32. Given the table of values for the hydrolysis of some phosphorylated compounds, which of the following best describes the $\Delta G^{0\prime}$ for the following reaction?

phosphoenolpyruvate + ADP → pyruvate + ATP

Compound	*$\Delta G^{0\prime}$ of Hydrolysis (kcal/mol)*
Phosphoenolpyruvate	−14.8
Phosphocreatine	−10.3
ATP	−7.0
Glucose 1-phosphate	−5.0
Glucose 6-phosphate	−3.3

A. −22.1 kcal/mol
B. −14.8 kcal/mol
C. −7.8 kcal/mol
D. −7.0 kcal/mol
E. −5.0 kcal/mol

Answer C: When 2 reactions are coupled, the resultant free-energy change is the arithmetic sum of the $\Delta G^{0\prime}$ values for the coupled reactions. In the case of the coupled reaction, ATP is not being hydrolyzed but instead is being formed. In this case the $\Delta G^{0\prime}$ value for a given reaction is its reciprocal value when the reaction is running in the opposite direction to that for which the $\Delta G^{0\prime}$ value is denoted. Thus, for ATP synthesis from ADP, the $\Delta G^{0\prime}$ value would be +7.0kcal/mol. When the 2 reactions are coupled, there is sufficient energy released from the hydrolysis of phosphoenolpyruvate to drive the synthesis of ATP from ADP. The $\Delta G^{0\prime}$ value for the coupled reactions is the simple arithmetic sum of the $\Delta G^{0\prime}$ values for the individual reactions.

33. In the absence of an enzyme, the conversion of X → Y exhibits a $\Delta G^{0\prime}$ of +5.0 kJ/mol. Which of the following best describes the $\Delta G^{0\prime}$ of this reaction in the presence of an enzyme that accelerates the reaction 100 fold?
A. −500 kJ/mol
B. −50 kJ/mol
C. −5 kJ/mol
D. +5 kJ/mol
E. +50 kJ/mol

Answer D: Enzymes affect the rate but not the equilibrium constant of a chemical reaction. Thus, although the enzyme in this example may indeed accelerate the rate of the reaction 100 fold it has no effect on the equilibrium constant. The equilibrium constant is related to the free-energy change of a reaction via the equation: $\Delta G = \Delta G^0 + \mathrm{RT}\ln K_{eq}$.

34. The hydrolysis of ATP to ADP and inorganic phosphate proceeds with a $\Delta G^{0\prime}$ of −7kcal/mol. The hydrolysis of phosphocreatine has a $\Delta G^{0\prime}$ of −10kcal/mol. In the reaction catalyzed by creatine kinase (creatine phosphokinase), in the direction of phosphocreatine formation, which of the following is the overall $\Delta G^{0\prime}$ in kcal/mol?
A. −17
B. $17 \times T\Delta S$
C. −3
D. $-3 \times T\Delta S$
E. +3

Answer E: When 2 reactions are coupled, the resultant free-energy change is the arithmetic sum of the $\Delta G^{0\prime}$ values for the coupled reactions. In the case of the coupled reaction phosphocreatine is being formed not being hydrolyzed, therefore the $\Delta G^{0\prime}$ value for the reaction in that direction is the reciprocal value of that for phosphocreatine hydrolysis +10.0 kcal/mol. The $\Delta G^{0\prime}$ value for the coupled reactions is the simple arithmetic sum of the $\Delta G^{0\prime}$ values for the individual reactions.

35. Which of the following is most likely to increase as a result of the binding of an activating effector to the regulatory site of a multi-subunit, allosterically regulated enzyme?
A. $1/V_{max}$
B. acetylation of inactive subunits
C. K_m
D. proportion of subunits in an active conformation
E. ribosylation of inactive subunits

Answer D: Allosteric enzymes are enzymes whose conformation changes upon binding of an allosteric effector. This binding results in an apparent change in binding affinity in the enzyme at a different ligand-binding site. This action at a distance through binding of one ligand (or allosteric effector) affecting the binding of another at a distinctly different site is the essence of the allosteric concept.

Checklist

✓ Enzymes are biological catalysts that, like inorganic catalysts, decrease the energy required to drive a reaction forward without themselves being consumed or permanently altered in the process.

✓ Enzymes are specific for both the type of reaction catalyzed and the substrate, or a small subset of closely related substrates, acted upon.

✓ Enzymes are divided into 6 classifications based upon substrates involved and type of reaction catalyzed.

✓ Many enzymes are complexes consisting of both protein and organic or inorganic prosthetic groups, the latter being termed coenzymes. Many coenzymes are vitamins or vitamin derivatives.

✓ The study of enzyme kinetics allows for an understanding of the steps by which an enzyme can convert a substrate into product.

✓ The ratio of reaction rate constants is represented by the equilibrium constant, K_{eq}, which can be calculated from the concentration of substrates and products when a reaction has reached equilibrium.

✓ The rate of enzyme-catalyzed reactions is influenced by enzyme and substrate concentration, temperature, and pH, as well as the presence of inhibitors.

✓ The Michaelis-Menten equation illustrates the mathematical relationship between the initial reaction velocity and the substrate concentration.

✓ Linear forms of the Michaelis-Menten equation simplify the determination of K_m and V_{max} for a given enzyme-catalyzed reaction.

✓ The Michaelis-Menten constant, K_m, is defined as the concentration of substrate required for an enzyme-catalyzed reaction to attain half the maximal reaction velocity, V_{max}. Therefore, it becomes obvious that an enzyme with a lower K_m will carry out a reaction more efficiently than another enzyme with a higher K_m for the same substrate.

✓ Physiologically significant forms of enzyme inhibitor include competitive and noncompetitive inhibitors.

✓ Competitive inhibitors bind to the same site as substrate resulting in an increase in K_m while having no effect on V_{max}.

✓ Noncompetitive inhibitors bind to sites on the enzyme other than substrate resulting in a decrease in V_{max} with no change in K_m.

✓ Analysis of the inhibition of enzyme catalysis reveals potentially important clinically relevant information for use in the design of pharmaceutical compounds.

✓ Ribozymes are RNA-based enzymes that represent a unique class of nonprotein enzyme.

✓ Analysis of the changes of the levels of enzymes in the blood aids in the diagnosis of various diseases and disorders such as in the case of liver disease and MI.

CHAPTER

10 Carbohydrates: Glycolysis and Glucose Homeostasis

CHAPTER OUTLINE

High-Yield Terms

Hexokinase/Glucokinase: glucose phosphorylating enzymes, differential tissue expression and regulatory properties, humans express 4 distinct hexokinase/glucokinase genes

PFK1: 6-phosphofructo-1-kinase, major rate-limiting enzyme of glycolysis

PFK2: bifunctional enzyme that is responsible for the synthesis of the major allosteric regulator of glycolysis via PFK1 and gluconeogenesis via fructose-1,6-bisphophatase (F-1,6-BPase)

Pyruvate kinase: multiple forms with tissue-specific distribution and regulation

PKM2: isoform of pyruvate kinase expressed in proliferating and cancer cells, participates in the Warburg effect

Substrate-level phosphorylation: refers to the formation of ATP via the release of energy from a catabolic substrate as opposed to via oxidative phosphorylation

Glucose-fatty acid cycle: describes the interrelationship between how fatty acid metabolism results in inhibition of glucose metabolism and *vice versa*

Intestinal glucose homeostasis: in addition to regulating glucose uptake from the diet and delivery to the blood, in times of fasting or compromised liver function, the small intestine provides up to 20% of blood glucose via gluconeogenesis using glutamine and glycerol as substrates

Renal glucose homeostasis: kidneys regulate circulating glucose levels through efficient resorption of plasma glucose as well as by being able to carry out gluconeogenesis using glutamine as a carbon source

Importance of Glycolysis

Glycolysis represents a major metabolic pathway for the conversion of the carbons of carbohydrates into other forms of biomass and for the production of cellular energy in the form of ATP. The physiologically significant property of glycolysis is that the pathway can provide cellular energy whether or not oxygen is present, as discussed later. All tissues have varying needs for the glycolytic pathway with the brain being particularly dependent upon glycolysis for energy production. Red blood cells, which lack mitochondria, are totally dependent upon glucose oxidation in glycolysis for their energy needs. In the context of glycolysis, the major carbohydrate entering the pathway is glucose. However, other carbohydrates such as fructose (see Chapter 11) and galactose (see Chapter 12) are utilized for energy and biomass production by being oxidized within the glycolytic pathway. Entry of carbohydrates into glycolysis can occur either from dietary sources, which can include a wide variety of mono-, di-, and polysaccharides, or from carbohydrate stores in the form of glycogen (see Chapter 14).

Digestion and Uptake of Dietary Carbohydrate

The details of digestive processes are discussed in Chapter 43. Digestion and absorption of carbohydrates is covered here briefly. Dietary carbohydrates enter the body in complex forms, such as mono-, di-, and polysaccharides. Through the actions of various digestive enzymes, these complex sugars are broken down into monosaccharides consisting primarily of glucose, fructose, and galactose. Intestinal absorption of carbohydrates occurs via passive diffusion, facilitated diffusion, and active transport. The primary transporter involved in the uptake of glucose is the sodium-glucose transporter 1 (SGLT1). Galactose is also absorbed from the gut via the action of SGLT1. Fructose is absorbed from the intestine via GLUT5 uptake. Indeed, GLUT5 has a much higher affinity for fructose than for glucose.

Glucose Uptake and the Role of Sugar Transporters

Glucose transporters comprise a family of at least 14 members. The most well-characterized members of the family are **GLUT1, GLUT2, GLUT3, GLUT4,** and **GLUT5**. The glucose transporters are facilitative transporters that carry hexose sugars across the membrane without requiring energy. These transporters belong to a family of proteins called the solute carriers. Specifically, the official gene names for the GLUTs are solute carrier family 2 (facilitated glucose transporter) member. Thus, the *GLUT1* gene symbol is *SLC2A1*, *GLUT2* is *SLC2A2*, *GLUT3* is *SLC2A3*, *GLUT4* is *SLC2A4*, and *GLUT5* is *SLC2A5*.

The glucose transporters can be divided into 3 classes based upon primary amino acid sequence comparisons:

1. **Class I transporters:** GLUT1, GLUT2, GLUT3 (*GLUT14* represents a duplicated *GLUT3* gene), and GLUT4.
2. **Class II transporters:** GLUT5, GLUT7, GLUT9, and GLUT11.
3. **Class III transporters:** GLUT6, GLUT8, GLUT10, GLUT12, and HMIT (proton [H^+] myoinositol symporter: SLC2A13). HMIT is also known as GLUT13.

GLUT1 is ubiquitously distributed in various tissues with highest levels of expression seen in erythrocytes. In fact, in erythrocytes GLUT1 accounts for almost 5% of total protein. Although widely expressed, GLUT1 is not expressed in hepatocytes.

GLUT2 is found primarily in intestine, pancreatic β-cells, kidney, and liver. The K_m of GLUT2 for glucose (17 mM) is the highest of all the sugar transporters. The high K_m ensures a fast equilibrium of glucose between the cytosol and the extracellular space, ensuring that liver and pancreas do not metabolize glucose until its levels rise sufficiently in the blood. GLUT2 molecules can transport both glucose and fructose. When the concentration of blood glucose increases in response to food intake, pancreatic GLUT2 molecules mediate an increase in glucose uptake, which leads to increased insulin secretion. For this reason, GLUT2 is thought to be a "glucose sensor."

GLUT3 is found primarily in neurons and also in the intestine. GLUT3 binds glucose with high affinity (has the lowest K_m of the GLUTs), which allows neurons to have enhanced access to glucose especially under conditions of low blood glucose.

GLUT4 predominates in insulin-sensitive tissues, such as skeletal muscle and adipose tissue. Mobilization of GLUT4 to the plasma membrane is a major function of insulin in these tissues.

GLUT5 and the closely related transporter GLUT7 are involved in fructose transport. GLUT5 is expressed in intestine, kidney, testes, skeletal muscle, adipose tissue, and brain. Although GLUT2, -5, -7, 8, -9, -11, and -12 can all transport fructose, GLUT5 is the only transporter that exclusively transports fructose.

High-Yield Concept

Glycolysis is a major pathway for the utilization of carbohydrate carbons for redistribution into biomass as well as being oxidized for the production of ATP. The unique, and highly significant, feature of glycolysis is that it can occur in the presence (aerobic) or absence (anaerobic) of oxygen.

The Pathway of Glycolysis

The end product of glycolysis is pyruvate or lactate dependent upon the availability of oxygen. Although the reactions of glycolysis occur in the cytoplasm of all cells (Figure 10-1), the vast majority of ATP energy is generated by diversion of pyruvate into the mitochondria, where it undergoes oxidative decarboxylation and the carbons enter the TCA cycle (see Chapter 16). Under aerobic conditions, the dominant product in most tissues is pyruvate and the pathway is known as *aerobic glycolysis*. When oxygen is depleted, as for instance during prolonged vigorous exercise, the dominant glycolytic product in skeletal muscle is lactate and the process is known as *anaerobic glycolysis*. Since erythrocytes lack mitochondria, they can only carry out anaerobic glycolysis and, therefore, contribute the majority of lactate found in the blood.

The Individual Reactions of Glycolysis

The pathway of glycolysis can be seen as consisting of 2 separate phases. The first is the chemical priming phase requiring the input of energy in the form of ATP, and the second is considered the energy-yielding phase. In the first phase, 2 equivalents of ATP are used to convert glucose to fructose 1,6-bisphosphate (F1,6BP). In the second phase F1,6BP is sequentially oxidized to pyruvate, with the production of 4 equivalents of ATP and 2 equivalents of NADH.

The Hexokinase Reaction

The ATP-dependent phosphorylation of glucose to form glucose 6-phosphate (G6P) is the first reaction of glycolysis, and is catalyzed by tissue-specific isoenzymes known as *hexokinases*. The phosphorylation accomplishes 2 goals: first, the hexokinase reaction converts nonionic glucose into an anion that is trapped in the cell, since cells lack transport systems for phosphorylated sugars; second, the otherwise biologically inert glucose becomes activated into a labile form capable of being further metabolized.

Four mammalian isozymes of hexokinase are known (Types I-IV), with the Type IV isozyme often referred to as glucokinase. Glucokinase is the form of the enzyme found in hepatocytes and pancreatic β-cells. There are 2 major differences between hexokinases I, II, and III and glucokinase. Hexokinases have low K_m for glucose (20-130 μM), are allosterically inhibited by G6P, and can utilize other hexoses (eg, fructose, mannose, glucosamine) as substrate. In contrast, glucokinase has a high K_m for glucose (5-8 μM), is not feedback inhibited by G6P, and physiologically only recognizes glucose as a substrate. Glucokinase can phosphorylate other hexoses in vitro but is unable to do so at any physiologically relevant concentration of these other sugars. Although not product inhibited, hepatic glucokinase is allosterically inhibited by long-chain fatty acids (LCFA). In contrast, LCFAs do not inhibit the other forms of hexokinase. The ability of LCFAs to inhibit hepatic glucokinase is one of the mechanisms by which fatty acids inhibit glucose uptake into the liver (see discussion of Glucose-Fatty Acid Cycle later).

The kinetic properties of hepatic glucokinase allow the liver to effectively buffer blood glucose since most dietary glucose will pass through the liver and remain in the circulation for use by other tissues. After meals, when postprandial blood glucose levels are high, liver glucokinase is significantly active, which causes the liver to preferentially trap and store circulating glucose. When blood glucose falls to very low levels, since the liver is not highly dependent on glucose, it does not continue to use the meager glucose supplies that remain available.

Phosphohexose Isomerase

The second reaction of glycolysis is an isomerization, in which G6P is converted to fructose 6-phosphate, F6P. The enzyme catalyzing this reaction is phosphohexose isomerase (PHI) (also known as phosphoglucose isomerase). The reaction is freely reversible at normal cellular concentrations of the 2 hexose phosphates and thus catalyzes this interconversion during glycolysis and during gluconeogenesis.

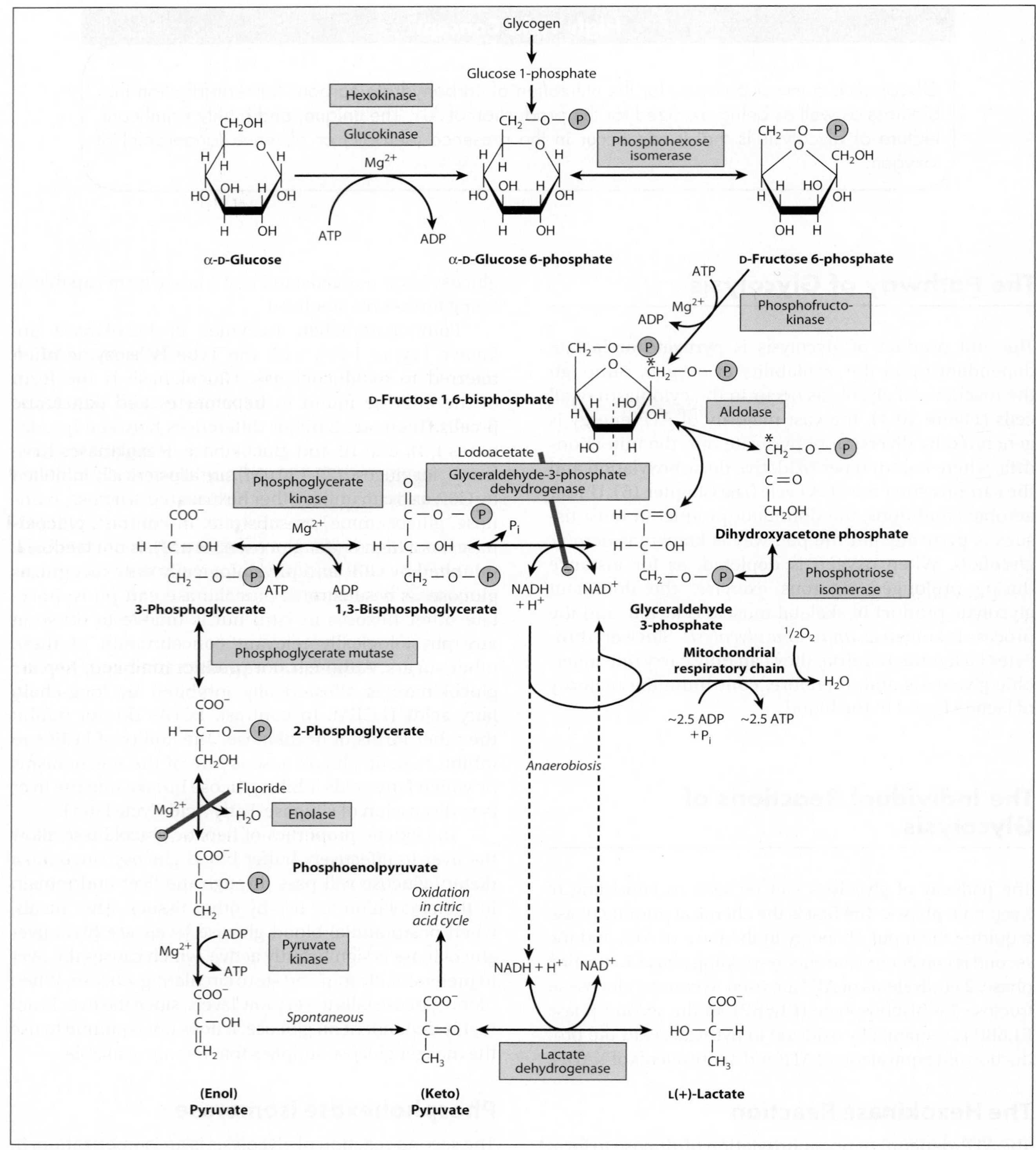

FIGURE 10-1: The pathway of glycolysis. (Ⓟ, $-PO_3^{2-}$; P_i, $HOPO_3^{2-}$; ⊖, inhibition.) *Carbons 1–3 of fructose bisphosphate form dihydroxyacetone phosphate, and carbons 4–6 form glyceraldehyde 3-phosphate. The term "bis-," as in bisphosphate, indicates that the phosphate groups are separated, whereas the term "di-," as in adenosine diphosphate, indicates that they are joined. Murray RK, Bender DA, Botham KM, Kennelly PJ, Rodwell VW, Weil PA. *Harper's Illustrated Biochemistry,* 29th ed. New York, NY: McGraw-Hill; 2012.

6-Phosphofructo-1-Kinase (Phosphofructokinase-1)

The next reaction of glycolysis involves the utilization of a second ATP to convert F6P to fructose 1,6-bisphosphate (F1,6BP). This reaction is catalyzed by 6-phosphofructo-1-kinase, better known as phosphofructokinase-1 or PFK1. This reaction is not readily reversible because of its large positive free energy ($\Delta G^{0\prime}$ = +5.4 kcal/mol) in the reverse direction. The activity of PFK1 is highly regulated and as such the enzyme is considered to be the rate-limiting enzyme of glycolysis.

Aldolase A

Aldolase A (also called fructose-1,6-bisphosphate aldolase) catalyses the hydrolysis of F1,6BP into two 3-carbon products: (1) dihydroxyacetone phosphate (DHAP) and (2) glyceraldehyde 3-phosphate (G3P). The aldolase reaction proceeds readily in the reverse direction, being utilized for both glycolysis and gluconeogenesis.

Triose Phosphate Isomerase

The 2 products of the aldolase reaction equilibrate readily in a reaction catalyzed by triose phosphate isomerase (TPI1). Succeeding reactions of glycolysis utilize G3P as a substrate.

Glyceraldehyde-3-Phosphate Dehydrogenase

The second phase of glucose catabolism features the energy-yielding glycolytic reactions that produce ATP and NADH. In the first of these reactions, glyceraldehyde-3-phosphate dehydrogenase (GAPDH) catalyzes the NAD^+-dependent oxidation of G3P to 1,3-bisphosphoglycerate (1,3BPG) and NADH. The GAPDH reaction is freely reversible.

Phosphoglycerate Kinase

The high-energy phosphate of 1,3-BPG is used to form ATP and 3-phosphoglycerate (3PG) by the enzyme phosphoglycerate kinase (PGK1). Note that this is the only reaction of glycolysis or gluconeogenesis that involves ATP and yet is reversible under normal physiological conditions.

Phosphoglycerate Mutase

Phosphoglycerate mutases (PGAM) represent a family of related enzymes where PGAM1 is the major glycolytic enzyme. PGAM is a heterodimer composed of a muscle (M) and/or a brain (B) isozyme, which generates MM, BB, and MB forms of the enzyme. The MM isoform predominates in muscle and the BB isoform is found at highest levels in liver, brain, and most other tissues. PGAM is responsible for converting the relatively low-energy phosphoacyl-ester of 3PG to a higher energy form, 2-phosphoglycerate, 2PG.

Enolase

Enolase (also known as phosphopyruvate hydratase) catalyzes the conversion of 2PG to phospho*enol*pyruvate, PEP. PEP represents the final high-energy intermediate in glycolysis.

Pyruvate Kinase

The final reaction of aerobic glycolysis is catalyzed by the highly regulated enzyme pyruvate kinase (PK). In this strongly exergonic reaction, the high-energy phosphate of PEP is transferred to ADP-yielding ATP.

There are 2 distinct genes encoding PK activity. One encodes the liver and erythrocyte PK proteins (identified as the *PKLR* gene) and the other encodes the PKM proteins. The *PKM* gene directs the synthesis of 2 isoforms of muscle PK termed PKM1 and PKM2. The *PKM* gene was originally identified as the *muscle pyruvate kinase* gene, hence the nomenclature PKM. However, it is now known that the PKM1 protein is expressed in many tissues, whereas the PKM2 protein is most highly expressed in proliferating cells and all types of cancer.

Anaerobic Glycolysis

Under aerobic conditions, pyruvate in most cells is further metabolized via the TCA cycle. Under anaerobic conditions and in erythrocytes, which lack mitochondria, pyruvate is converted to lactate by the enzyme lactate dehydrogenase (LDH), and the lactate is transported out of the cell into the circulation. The conversion of pyruvate to lactate, under anaerobic conditions, provides the cell with a mechanism for the oxidation of NADH (produced during the GAPDH reaction) to NAD^+, which occurs during the LDH-catalyzed reaction. This reduction is required since NAD^+ is a necessary substrate for GAPDH, without which glycolysis will cease. Normally, during aerobic glycolysis the electrons of cytoplasmic NADH are transferred to mitochondrial carriers of the oxidative phosphorylation pathway generating a continuous pool of cytoplasmic NAD^+.

The utility of anaerobic glycolysis, to a muscle cell during high physical exertion, stems from the fact that the rate of ATP production from glycolysis is approximately 100× faster than from oxidative phosphorylation.

During exertion, muscle cells do not need to energize anabolic reaction pathways. The requirement is to generate the maximum amount of ATP, for muscle contraction, in the shortest time frame. This is why muscle cells derive almost all of the ATP consumed during exertion from anaerobic glycolysis.

Cytoplasmic NADH

The NADH generated during glycolysis is used to fuel mitochondrial ATP synthesis via oxidative phosphorylation. Depending upon whether the malate-aspartate shuttle (Figure 10-2) or the glycerol phosphate shuttle (Figure 10-3) is used to transport the electrons from cytoplasmic NADH into the mitochondria , there will be approximately 4 or 6 moles of ATP generated for each mole of glucose oxidized to pyruvate.

Net Energy Yield from Glycolysis

The net yield from the oxidation of 1 mole of glucose to 2 moles of pyruvate is either 6 or 8 moles of ATP. This comprises 2 moles of ATP synthesized via substrate-level phosphorylation during the glycolytic reactions and 4 to 6 moles of ATP generated via oxidative phosphorylation from the reoxidation of cytoplasmic NADH, dependent upon which shuttle mechanism is utilized. Complete oxidation of the 2 moles of pyruvate, through the TCA cycle, yields an additional 30 moles of ATP; the total yield, therefore being either 36 or 38 moles of ATP from the complete oxidation of 1 mole of glucose to CO_2 and H_2O.

Lactate Metabolism

During anaerobic glycolysis the oxidation of NADH occurs through the reduction of an organic substrate. Erythrocytes and skeletal muscle (under conditions of exertion) derive all of their ATP needs through anaerobic glycolysis. The large quantity of NADH produced is oxidized by reducing pyruvate to lactate. This reaction is carried out by lactate dehydrogenase (LDH). The lactate produced during anaerobic glycolysis diffuses from the tissues and is transported to highly aerobic tissues, such as cardiac muscle and liver. The lactate is then oxidized to pyruvate in these cells by LDH and the pyruvate is further oxidized in the TCA cycle. In the liver, the pyruvate may be diverted into glucose biosynthesis via gluconeogenesis. Indeed, the connection between muscle lactate production and hepatic conversion of that lactate to glucose constitutes an important pathway referred to as the Cori cycle.

Mammalian cells contain 2 distinct types of LDH subunits, termed M and H. Combinations of these different subunits generate LDH isozymes with different characteristics. The H-type subunit predominates in aerobic tissues, such as heart muscle (as the H4 tetramer), while the M subunit predominates in anaerobic tissues, such as skeletal muscle (as the M4 tetramer). H4 LDH

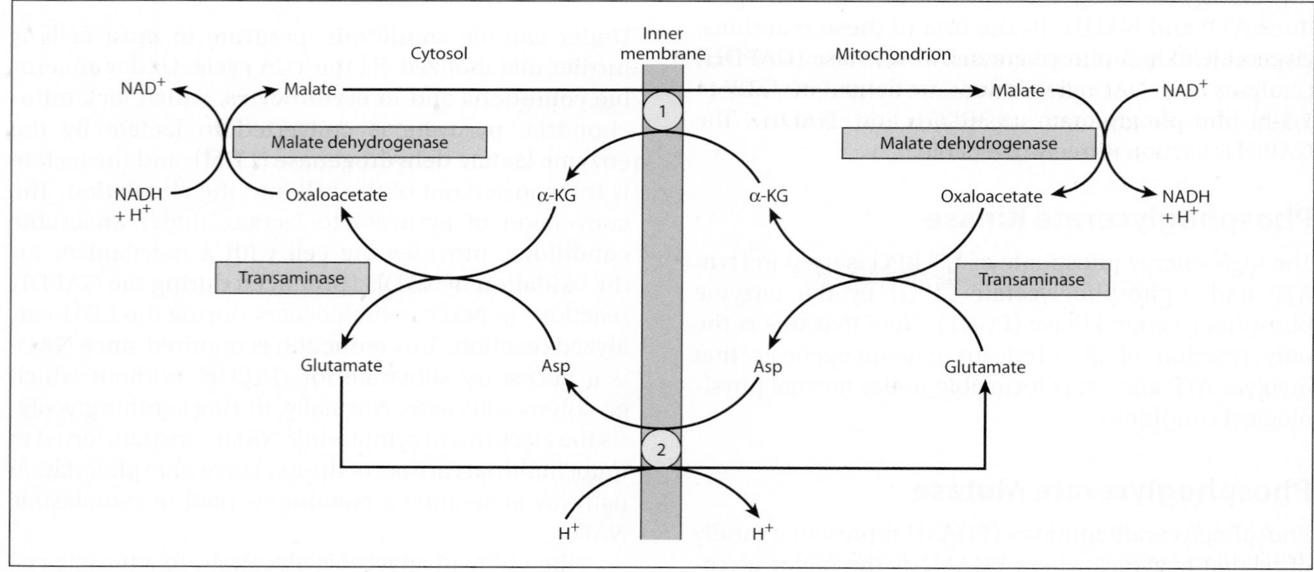

FIGURE 10-2: Malate shuttle for transfer of reducing equivalents from the cytosol into the mitochondrion. ① α-Ketoglutarate transporter and ② glutamate/aspartate transporter (note the proton symport with glutamate). Murray RK, Bender DA, Botham KM, Kennelly PJ, Rodwell VW, Weil PA. *Harper's Illustrated Biochemistry,* 29th ed. New York, NY: McGraw-Hill; 2012.

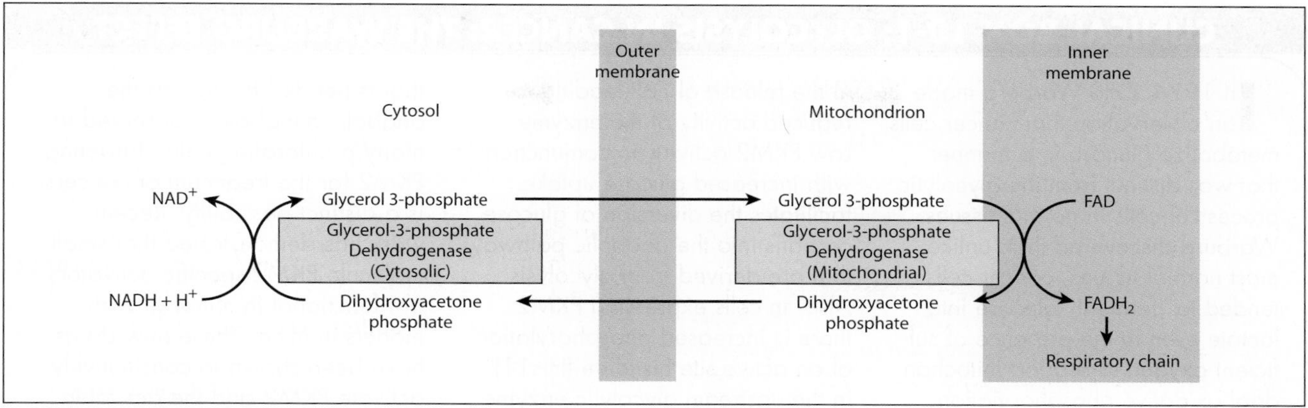

FIGURE 10-3: Glycerophosphate shuttle for transfer of reducing equivalents from the cytosol into the mitochondrion. Murray RK, Bender DA, Botham KM, Kennelly PJ, Rodwell VW, Weil PA. *Harper's Illustrated Biochemistry*, 29th ed. New York, NY: McGraw-Hill; 2012.

has a low K_m for pyruvate and is also inhibited by high levels of pyruvate. The M4 LDH enzyme has a high K_m for pyruvate and is not inhibited by pyruvate. This suggests that the H-type LDH is utilized for oxidizing lactate to pyruvate and the M-type the reverse.

Regulation of Glycolysis

The reactions catalyzed by hexokinase, PFK1, and PK all proceed with a relatively large free energy decrease. These nonequilibrium reactions of glycolysis would be ideal candidates for regulation of the flux through glycolysis. Indeed, all 3 enzymes are known to be allosterically controlled.

Regulation of hexokinase, however, is not the major control point in glycolysis. This is because large amounts of G6P are derived from the breakdown of glycogen (the predominant mechanism of carbohydrate entry into glycolysis in skeletal muscle) and, therefore, the hexokinase reaction is not necessary. Regulation of PK is important for reversing glycolysis when ATP levels are high in order to activate gluconeogenesis. As such, this enzyme-catalyzed reaction is not a major control point in glycolysis. However, different isoforms of PK are expressed in different tissues under different conditions and as such do have an impact on glycolysis. For example, see Clinical Box 10-1 discussing the Warburg Effect and proliferating cell glycolysis. The major rate-limiting step in glycolysis is the reaction catalyzed by PFK1 (Figure 10-4).

PFK1 is a tetrameric enzyme that exists in 2 conformational states termed R and T that are in equilibrium. ATP is both a substrate and an allosteric inhibitor of PFK1. Each subunit has 2 ATP-binding sites, a substrate site and an inhibitor site. The substrate site binds ATP equally well when the tetramer is in either conformation. The inhibitor site binds ATP essentially only when the enzyme is in the T state. F6P is the other substrate for PFK1 and it binds preferentially to the R state enzyme. At high concentrations of ATP, the inhibitor site becomes occupied and shifts the equilibrium of PFK1

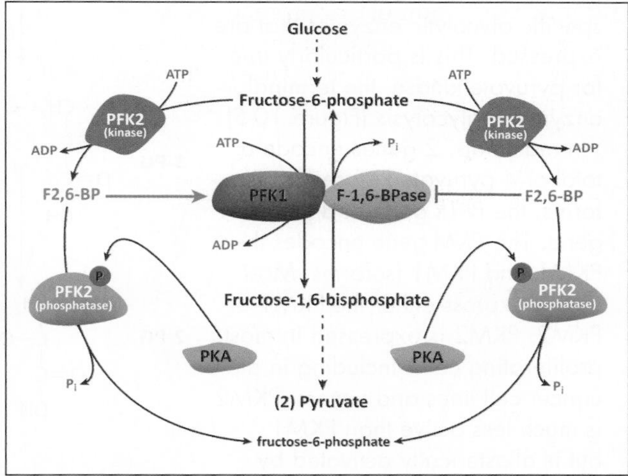

FIGURE 10-4: Regulation of glycolysis and gluconeogenesis by fructose 2,6-bisphosphate (F2,6BP). The major sites for regulation of glycolysis and gluconeogenesis are the phosphofructokinase-1 (PFK1)- and fructose-1,6-bisphosphatase (F-1,6-BPase)-catalyzed reactions. PFK2 is the kinase activity and F-2,6-BPase is the phosphatase activity of the bifunctional regulatory enzyme, phosphofructokinase-2/fructose-2,6-bisphosphatase (PFK2). PKA is cAMP-dependent protein kinase, which phosphorylates PFK2/F-2,6-BPase turning on the phosphatase activity. (+ve) and (−ve) refer to positive and negative activities, respectively. Reproduced with permission of themedicalbiochemistrypage, LLC.

CLINICAL BOX 10-1: GLYCOLYSIS IN CANCER: THE WARBURG EFFECT

In 1924, Otto Warburg made an observation that cancer cells metabolize glucose in a manner that was distinct from the glycolytic process of cells in normal tissues. Warburg discovered that, unlike most normal tissues, cancer cells tended to "ferment" glucose into lactate even in the presence of sufficient oxygen to support mitochondrial oxidative phosphorylation. This observation became known as the *Warburg Effect*. In the presence of oxygen, most differentiated cells primarily metabolize glucose to CO_2 and H_2O by oxidation of glycolytic pyruvate in the mitochondrial tricarboxylic acid (TCA) cycle. Proliferating cells, including cancer cells, require altered metabolism to efficiently incorporate nutrients such as glucose into biomass. The ultimate fate of glucose depends not only on the proliferative state of the cell but also on the activities of the specific glycolytic enzymes that are expressed. This is particularly true for pyruvate kinase, the terminal enzyme in glycolysis (Figure 10-5) . In mammals, 2 genes encode a total of 4 pyruvate kinase (PK) isoforms: the *PKLR* gene and the *PKM* gene. The *PKM* gene encodes the PKM1 and PKM1 isoforms. Most tissues express either the PKM1 or PKM2. PKM2 is expressed in most proliferating cells, including in all cancer cell lines and tumors. PKM2 is much less active than PKM1 but is allosterically activated by the upstream glycolytic metabolite fructose 1,6-bisphosphate (FBP). PKM2 is also unique in that it can interact with phosphotyrosine in tyrosine-phosphorylated proteins such as those resulting from growth factor stimulation of cells. The interaction of PKM2 with tyrosine-phosphorylated proteins results in the release of FBP leading to reduced activity of the enzyme. Low PKM2 activity, in conjunction with increased glucose uptake, facilitates the diversion of glucose carbons into the anabolic pathways that are derived from glycolysis. Also, in cells expressing PKM2 there is increased phosphorylation of an active site histidine (His11) in the upstream glycolytic enzyme phosphoglycerate mutase (PGAM1) which increases its mutase activity. The phosphate donor for His11 phosphorylation of PGAM1 is phospho*enol*pyruvate (PEP) which is the substrate for pyruvate kinases. Phosphate transfer from PEP to PGAM1 yields pyruvate without concomitant generation of ATP. This alternate pathway allows for a high rate of glycolysis that is needed to support the anabolic metabolism observed in many proliferating cells. Targeting PKM2 for the treatment of cancers is a distinct possibility. Recent work has demonstrated that small molecule PKM2-specific activators are functional in tumor growth models in mice. These new drugs have been shown to constitutively activate PKM2 and the activated enzyme is resistant to inhibition by tyrosine-phosphorylated proteins. PKM2-specific activators reduce the incorporation of glucose into lactate and lipids. In addition, PKM2 activation results in decreased pools of nucleotide, amino acid, and lipid precursors and these effects may account for the suppression of tumorigenesis observed with these drugs.

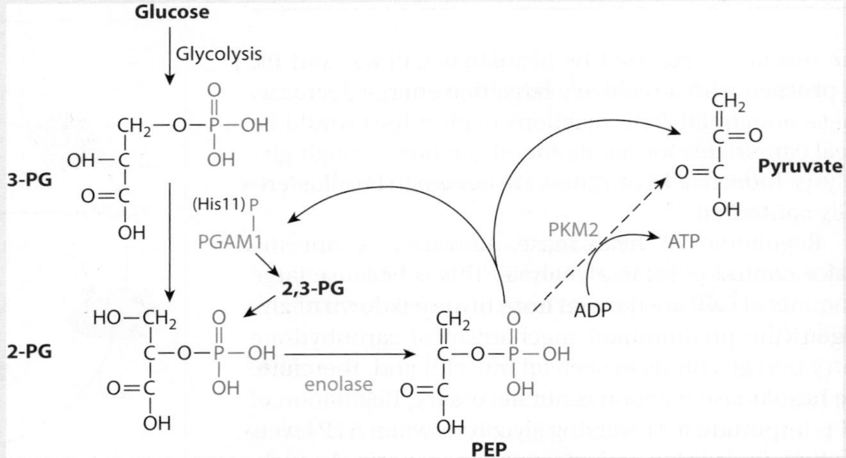

FIGURE 10-5: Alternative pathway of glycolysis is carried out in highly proliferative cells such as one observed in cancer cells. Cancer cells express the PKM2 isoform of pyruvate kinase, which is much less active than other isoforms and is also negatively regulated by binding to tyrosine-phosphorylated proteins. The dashed arrow for the PKM2 reaction is to demonstrate that this reaction is inefficient compared to the transfer of phosphate from PEP directly to PGAM1. PGAM1: phosphoglycerate mutase. PEP: phosphoenolpyruvate. 3-PG: 3-phosphoglycerate, 2-PG: 2-phosphoglycerate. 2,3-BPG: 2,3-bisphosphoglycerate. His11 refers to the catalytic site histidine that is phosphorylated by phosphate donation from PEP. Reproduced with permission of themedicalbiochemistrypage, LLC.

conformation to that of the T state, thereby decreasing the ability of PFK1 to bind F6P. The inhibition of PFK1 by ATP is overcome by AMP, which binds to the R state of the enzyme and, therefore, stabilizes the conformation of the enzyme capable of binding F6P. The most important allosteric regulator of both glycolysis and gluconeogenesis is fructose 2,6-bisphosphate, **F2,6BP**.

Regulation of Glycolytic Flux by PFK2

The synthesis of F2,6BP is catalyzed by the bifunctional enzyme 6-phosphofructo-2-kinase/fructose-2,6-bisphosphatase (simply abbreviated PFK2). The PFK2 enzyme in mammals exists as a homodimer. The PFK2 kinase domain is related to the catalytic domain of adenylate kinase. The F-2,6-BPase domain of the enzyme is structurally and functionally related to the histidine phosphatase family of enzymes. In the context of the active enzyme homodimer, the PFK2 domains function together in a head-to-head orientation, whereas the F-2,6-BPase domains can function as monomers. There are 4 *PFK2* genes in mammals that each generates several isoforms. These genes are identified as *PFKFB1* (liver isoform), *PFKFB2* (heart isoform), *PFKFB3* (brain/placenta isoform), and *PFKFB4* (testes isoform).

The *PFKFB1* gene expresses 3 mRNAs from 3 distinct promoters and the mRNAs and their respective promoters are called L, M, and F. The L mRNA is expressed in liver and white adipose tissue, the M mRNA is expressed in skeletal muscle and white adipose tissue, and the F mRNA is expressed in fibroblasts, proliferating cells, and fetal tissues.

The *PFKFB2* gene encodes 3 mRNAs (H1, H2, and H4), all 3 of which give rise to a single-enzyme isoform. A fourth mRNA (H3) has been identified that expresses a different-sized enzyme. Although the *PFKFB2* gene is referred to as the *heart PFK2*, none of the resultant mRNAs are strictly heart specific in their pattern of expression.

The 2 different isoforms of *PFKFB3* gene are called the ubiquitous (uPFK2; also called the constitutive form) and the inducible (iPFK2) isoforms, respectively. The inducible isoform is expressed at very low levels in adult tissues but its expression is induced in tumor cell lines and by pro-inflammatory stimuli. The uPFK2 isoform has the highest kinase:bisphosphatase activity ratio.

Rapid, short-term regulation of the kinase and phosphatase activities of PFK2 is exerted by phosphorylation/dephosphorylation events. The liver isozyme is phosphorylated in an *N*-terminal domain by PKA. This PKA-mediated phosphorylation results in inhibition of the kinase activity while at the same time leading to activation of the phosphatase activity of PFK2. In contrast, the heart isozyme is phosphorylated at the *C*-terminus by several protein kinases in different signaling pathways, resulting in enhancement of the kinase activity. One of these heart kinases is AMPK and this activity allows the heart to rapidly respond to stress conditions that include ischemia. Insulin action in the heart also results in phosphorylation and activation of the kinase activity of PFK2.

Under conditions where the kinase activity of PFK2 is high, fructose flow through the PFK1-catalyzed reaction is enhanced, with a net production of F1,6BP. Conversely, when PFK2 is phosphorylated, it no longer exhibits kinase activity, but the phosphatase activity hydrolyzes F2,6BP to F6P and inorganic phosphate. The result of this change in PFK2 activity is that allosteric stimulation of PFK1 ceases, whereas in the gluconeogenic direction, allosteric inhibition of F-1,6-BPase is eliminated, and net flow of fructose through these 2 enzymes is gluconeogenic, resulting in increased glucose production.

Regulation of Glycolytic Flux by PKA

The phosphorylation of PFK2 is catalyzed by cAMP-dependent protein kinase (PKA), whose activity is, in turn, regulated by circulating peptide hormones. When blood glucose levels drop, pancreatic insulin production falls, glucagon secretion is stimulated, and circulating glucagon is highly increased. Hormones such as glucagon bind to plasma membrane receptors on liver cells, activating membrane-localized adenylate cyclase, leading to an increase in the conversion of ATP to cAMP. This newly formed cAMP binds to the regulatory subunits of PKA resulting in release and activation of the catalytic subunits. PKA phosphorylates numerous enzymes, including the PFK2. Under these conditions, the liver stops consuming glucose and becomes metabolically gluconeogenic, producing glucose to reestablish normoglycemia.

Regulation of Glycolytic Flux by Pyruvate Kinase

Regulation of glycolysis also occurs at the step catalyzed by pyruvate kinase (PK). A number of PK isozymes have been described that are derived from 2 distinct genes. Each gene can undergo alternative promoter usage or alternative splicing resulting in 4 distinct types of PK. The *PKLR* gene encodes the liver (PKL or L-PK) and erythrocyte (PLR or R-PK) pyruvate kinase proteins. The *PKM* gene encodes 2 proteins identified as PKM1 and PKM2. The designation PKM reflects the fact that the enzyme was originally thought to be muscle specific in this expression. It is now known that most tissues express either the PKM1 of the PKM2 isoform. PKM1 is found in numerous normal differentiated tissues, whereas PKM2 is expressed in most proliferating cells (see Clinical Box 10-1).

The liver isozyme (L-PK) is regulated by phosphorylation, allosteric effectors, and modulation of gene expression. L-PK is inhibited by ATP and acetyl-CoA and is activated by F1,6BP. The inhibition of L-PK by ATP is similar to the effect of ATP on PFK1. The binding of ATP to the inhibitor site reduces its affinity for PEP. The liver enzyme is also controlled at the level of synthesis. Increased carbohydrate ingestion induces the synthesis of L-PK, resulting in elevated cellular levels of the enzyme. The activity of L-PK is regulated via PKA-mediated phosphorylation, whereas the M-type isozyme found in brain, muscle, and other glucose requiring tissue is unaffected by PKA. Because of these differences, blood glucose levels and associated hormones can regulate the balance of liver gluconeogenesis and glycolysis, while muscle metabolism remains unaffected. Expression of L-PK is strongly influenced by the quantity of carbohydrate in the diet, with high-carbohydrate diets inducing up to a 10-fold increase in L-PK concentration as compared to low carbohydrate diets. L-PK is phosphorylated and inhibited by PKA, and thus it is under hormonal control similar to that described earlier for PFK2. Muscle PK (M type) is not regulated by the same mechanisms as the liver enzyme. Extracellular conditions that lead to the phosphorylation and inhibition of L-PK, such as low blood glucose and high levels of circulating glucagon, do not inhibit the muscle enzyme. The result of this differential regulation is that hormones such as glucagon and epinephrine favor liver gluconeogenesis by inhibiting liver glycolysis, while at the same time muscle glycolysis can proceed in accord with the needs directed by intracellular conditions.

In erythrocytes, the fetal PK isozyme has much greater activity than the adult isozyme; as a result, fetal erythrocytes have comparatively low concentrations of glycolytic intermediates. Because of the low steady-state concentration of fetal 1,3BPG, the 2,3BPG shunt is greatly reduced in fetal cells and little 2,3BPG is formed (Figure 10-6). Since 2,3BPG is a negative effector of hemoglobin affinity for oxygen (see Chapter 6), fetal erythrocytes have a higher oxygen affinity than maternal erythrocytes. Therefore, transfer of oxygen from maternal hemoglobin to fetal hemoglobin is favored, assuring the fetal oxygen supply. In the newborn, an erythrocyte isozyme of the M type with comparatively low PK activity displaces the fetal type, resulting in an accumulation of glycolytic intermediates. The increased 1,3BPG levels activate the 2,3BPG shunt, producing 2,3BPG needed to regulate oxygen binding to hemoglobin. Genetic diseases of adult erythrocyte PK are known in which the kinase is virtually inactive. Pyruvate kinase deficiency is the most common cause of inherited nonspherocytic hemolytic anemia. This disorder is discussed in Clinical Box 10-2.

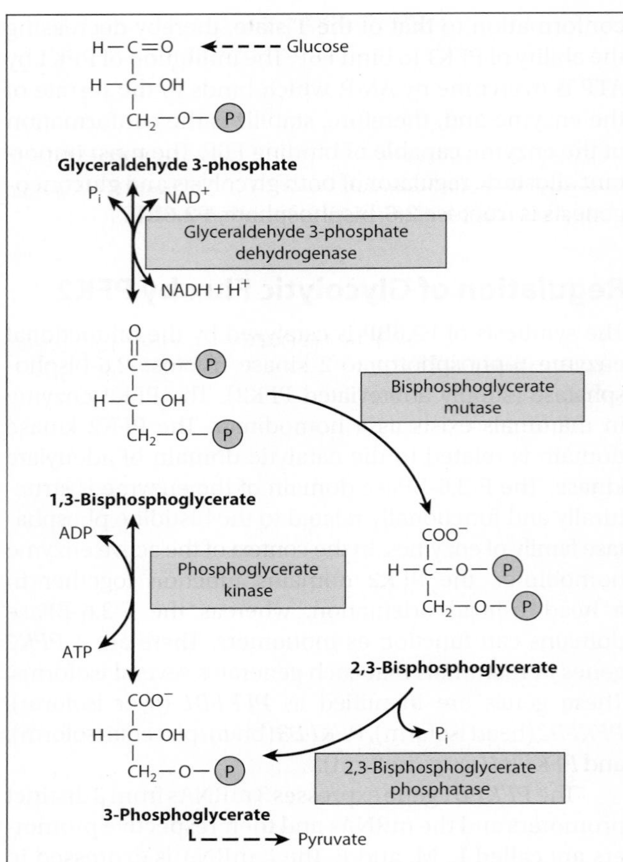

FIGURE 10-6: 2,3-Bisphosphoglycerate pathway in erythrocytes. Murray RK, Bender DA, Botham KM, Kennelly PJ, Rodwell VW, Weil PA. Harper's Illustrated Biochemistry. 29th ed. New York: McGraw-Hill; 2012.

The Glucose-Fatty Acid Cycle

The glucose-fatty acid cycle describes interrelationships of glucose and fatty acid oxidation as defined by fuel flux and fuel selection by various organs. The glucose-fatty acid cycle was first proposed by Philip Randle and coworkers in 1963 and is, therefore, sometimes referred to as the Randle cycle or Randle hypothesis. The cycle describes how nutrients in the diet can fine-tune metabolic processes on top of the more coarse control exerted by various peptide and steroid hormones. The underlying theme of the glucose-fatty acid cycle is that the utilization of one nutrient (eg, glucose) directly inhibits the use of the other (in this case, fatty acids) without hormonal mediation. The general interrelationships between glucose and fatty acid utilization, depicted in Figure 10-7, are most pronounced in skeletal muscle and adipose tissue.

When glucose levels are high, it is taken up by adipose tissue and skeletal muscle cells via the GLUT4

CLINICAL BOX 10-2: ERYTHROCYTE PK DEFICIENCY

Deficiency of pyruvate kinase is the most common enzyme deficiency resulting in inherited nonspherocytic hemolytic anemia. Pyruvate kinase deficiency is inherited as an autosomal recessive disorder and mutations in the *erythrocyte pyruvate kinase* gene occur with a frequency of 1 in 10,000. The disorder is characterized by lifelong chronic hemolysis of variable severity. Red blood cells from heterozygous individuals possess only 40% to 60% of the pyruvate kinase activity of normal individuals, yet these individuals are almost always clinically normal. The red blood cell pyruvate kinase protein is encoded by *PKLR* gene (pyruvate kinase, liver, and red blood cell).

Numerous mutations (130 to date) have been identified in the *PKLR* gene resulting in erythrocyte PK deficiency. In persons of European descent, over 50% of individuals with PK deficiency harbor a nucleotide change at position 1529 (encoding amino acid 510) that results in an Arg to Gln change in the protein and is identified as the R510Q mutation. The clinical severity of the anemia resulting from PKLR deficiencies varies from mild and fully compensated hemolysis to severe cases that require transfusions for survival. In the most severe cases an affected fetus will die in utero. Most PKLR-deficient patients are diagnosed in infancy or early childhood. Severely affected patients may require multiple transfusions or splenectomy. The requirement for transfusion in many infants will diminish during childhood or following splenectomy. There are many patients with mild PKLR deficiency who do not manifest symptoms until adulthood. In these individuals, the symptoms, that include mild to moderate splenomegaly, mild chronic hemolysis, and jaundice, often manifest incidental to an acute viral infection or during an evaluation in pregnancy. Clinical evaluation of blood from patients with PKLR deficiency will show normocytic anemia (sometimes macrocytic), which is reflective of the reticulocytosis that is invariably present. In normal individuals, reticulocytes comprise 0.5% to 1.7% of the total erythrocytes. An increase in the percentage of reticulocytes (reticulocytosis) is an important sign in any patient suffering from anemia. In PKLR deficiency, the level of reticulocytosis results in a reticulocyte level of 4% to 15%. In association with the reticulocytosis, there is a reduction in hematocrit (packed cell volume) to around 17% to 37% where it ranges from 41% to 50% in normal individuals. Hemoglobin measurement also shows a decrease to 6 to 12 g/dL, where normal ranges from 12 to 16.5 g/dL. Examination of bone marrow from PKLR-deficient patients will show normoblastic erythroid hyperplasia.

transporter and subsequently phosphorylated by hexokinase. The reactions of glycolysis drive the carbon atoms to pyruvate where they are oxidized to acetyl-CoA. The fate of the acetyl-CoA can be complete oxidation in the TCA cycle or return to the cytosol via citrate. In the cytosol, the citrate is hydrolyzed via ATP-citrate lyase (ACL), releasing acetyl-CoA. Within the cytosol, the acetyl-CoA can be a substrate for acetyl-CoA carboxylase (ACC), forming malonyl-CoA and ultimately long-chain fatty acid (LCFA) synthesis via fatty acid synthase (FAS). The synthesis of malonyl-CoA also results in the inhibition of long-chain fatty acyl-CoAs (LCFacyl-CoA) transport into the mitochondria via inhibition of carnitine palmitoyltransferase 1 (CPT-1). This effectively blocks the oxidation of fatty acids leading to increased triacylglycerol synthesis (TAG). The equilibrium between malonyl-CoA synthesis and breakdown back to acetyl-CoA is determined by the regulation of ACC and malonyl-CoA decarboxylase (MCD). As long as there is sufficient capacity to divert glucose carbons to TCA cycle oxidation and fatty acid synthesis, there will be limited acetyl-CoA-mediated inhibition of the pyruvate dehydrogenase complex (PDHc). On the other hand, when fatty acid levels are high, they enter the cell via one of several fatty acid transporter complexes (eg, fatty acid translocase [FAT]/CD36 which has a preference for LCFAs], and are then transported into the mitochondria to be oxidized. The large increase in fatty acid oxidation subsequently inhibits the utilization of glucose. This is the result of increased cytosolic citrate production from acetyl-CoA and the inhibition of phosphofructokinase-1 (PFK1). The increased acetyl-CoA derived from fat oxidation will in turn further inhibit glucose utilization via activation of PDH kinases (PDKs) that will phosphorylate and inhibit the PDHc. Under conditions where fat oxidation is favored, ACC will be inhibited and MCD will be activated, ensuring that LCFA that enter the cell will be transported into the mitochondria.

How do the dynamics of the glucose-fatty acid cycle play out under various physiological conditions and changing fuel substrate pools? In the fasted state,

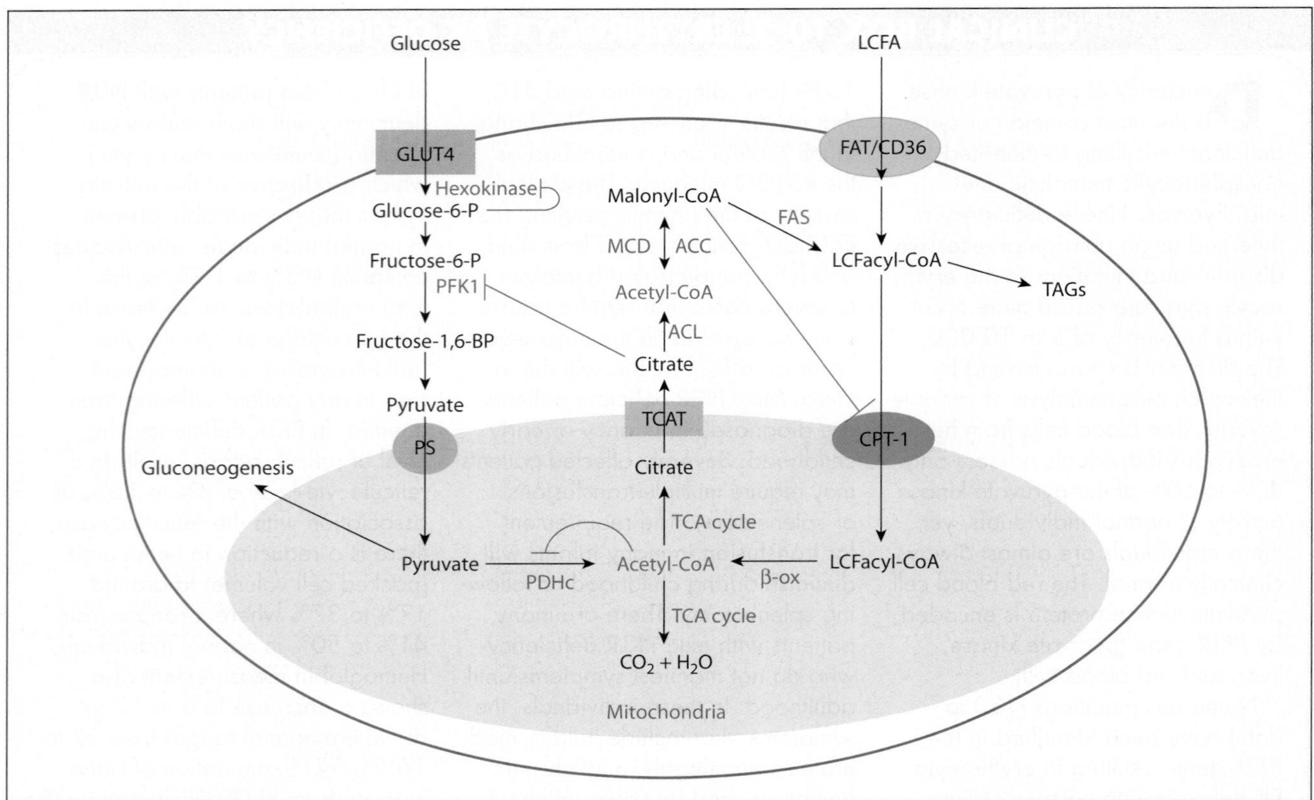

FIGURE 10-7: The glucose-fatty acid cycle represents the interactions between glucose uptake and metabolism and the consequent inhibition of fatty acid oxidation and the effects of fatty acid oxidation on the inhibition of glucose utilization. PS is pyruvate symporter responsible for mitochondrial uptake of pyruvate. TCAT is tricarboxylic acid transporter. Reproduced with permission of themedicalbiochemistrypage, LLC.

it is imperative that glucose be spared so that the brain can have adequate access to this vital fuel. Under these conditions, hormonal signals from the pancreas, in the form of glucagon, stimulate adipose tissue lipolysis releasing free fatty acids (FFAs) to the blood for use as a fuel by other peripheral tissues. When the released FFAs enter the liver, they are oxidized which results in inhibition of glucose oxidation as outlined in Figure 10-7. In addition to sparing glucose for the brain, fatty acid oxidation also preserves pyruvate and lactate, which are important gluconeogenesis substrates.

The inhibition of glucose utilization by fatty acid oxidation is mediated by short-term effects on several steps of overall glycolysis that include glucose uptake, glucose phosphorylation, and pyruvate oxidation. Acetyl-CoA that results from fatty acid oxidation can serve as an allosteric activator of PDKs that will phosphorylate and inhibit the PDHc. PDKs are also activated by increasing levels of NADH that will be the result of increased fatty acid oxidation. Thus, 2 products of fat oxidation result in inhibition of the PDHc. In addition, excess acetyl-CoA can be transported to the cytosol as citrate. Once in the cytosol, citrate serves as an allosteric inhibitor of PFK1 thus limiting entry of glucose into glycolysis. The increase in glucose 6-phosphate that results from inhibition of PFK1 leads to feedback inhibition of hexokinase, which in turn limits glucose uptake via GLUT4.

Regulation of Blood Glucose Levels

The maintenance of blood glucose homeostasis is of paramount importance to the survival of the human organism. The predominant tissue responding to signals that indicate reduced or elevated blood glucose levels is the liver. Indeed, one of the most important functions of the liver is to produce glucose for the circulation. Both elevated and reduced levels of blood glucose trigger hormonal responses to initiate pathways designed to restore glucose homeostasis. Low blood glucose triggers release of glucagon from pancreatic α-cells. High blood glucose triggers release of insulin from pancreatic β-cells. Additional signals, ACTH and growth hormone, released from the pituitary act to increase blood glucose by inhibiting uptake by extrahepatic tissues. Glucocorticoids also act to increase blood glucose levels by inhibiting glucose uptake. Cortisol, the major glucocorticoid released from the adrenal cortex, is secreted in response to increased circulating ACTH. The adrenal medullary hormone, epinephrine, stimulates production of glucose by activating glycogen breakdown in response to stressful stimuli.

Glucagon binding to its receptors on the surface of liver cells triggers an increase in cAMP production, leading to an increased rate of glycogenolysis by activating glycogen phosphorylase via the PKA-mediated cascade. The regulation of glycogen homeostasis by PKA is detailed in Chapter 11. Hepatocytes exhibit the response to epinephrine at the level of glycogen homeostasis. Stimulated glycogen breakdown results in increased levels of G6P in hepatocytes, which can be hydrolyzed to free glucose by glucose 6-phosphatase. The free glucose then diffuses out of hepatocytes into the blood. The glucose enters extrahepatic cells, where it is re-phosphorylated by hexokinase. Since muscle and brain cells lack glucose 6-phosphatase, the glucose-6-phosphate product of hexokinase is retained and oxidized by these tissues.

In opposition to the cellular responses to glucagon (and epinephrine on hepatocytes), insulin stimulates extrahepatic uptake of glucose from the blood and inhibits glycogenolysis in extrahepatic cells and conversely stimulates glycogen synthesis. As the glucose enters hepatocytes, it binds to and inhibits glycogen phosphorylase activity. The binding of free glucose stimulates the dephosphorylation of phosphorylase, thereby inactivating it. Why is it that the glucose that enters hepatocytes is not immediately phosphorylated and oxidized? Liver cells contain glucokinase, which has a much lower affinity for glucose than does hexokinase. Therefore, it is not fully active at the physiological ranges of blood glucose. Additionally, glucokinase is not inhibited by its product G6P, whereas, hexokinase is inhibited by G6P.

Hepatocytes, unlike most other cells, are essentially freely permeable to glucose and are, therefore, unaffected by the action of insulin at the level of increased glucose uptake. When blood glucose levels are low, the liver does not compete with other tissues for glucose since the extrahepatic uptake of glucose is stimulated in response to insulin. Conversely, when blood glucose levels are high, extrahepatic needs are satisfied and the liver takes up glucose for conversion into glycogen for future needs. Under conditions of high blood glucose, liver glucose levels will be high and the activity of glucokinase will be elevated. The G6P produced by glucokinase is rapidly converted to G1P by phosphoglucomutase, where it can then be incorporated into glycogen.

Role of the Kidney in Blood Glucose Control

Although the liver is the major site of glucose homeostasis, the kidneys do participate in the overall process of regulating blood glucose levels. The kidney carries out gluconeogenesis primarily using the carbon skeleton of glutamine and while so doing allows for the elimination of waste nitrogen and maintenance of plasma pH balance. In addition to carrying out gluconeogenesis, the kidney regulates blood glucose levels via its ability to excrete glucose via glomerular filtration as well as to reabsorb the filtered glucose in the proximal convoluted tubules. In the average adult, the kidneys will filter around 180 g of glucose per day. Of this amount, less than 1% is excreted in the urine due to efficient reabsorption. This reabsorption process is critical for maintaining blood glucose homeostasis and for retaining important calories for energy production.

Transport of glucose from the tubule into the tubular epithelial cells is carried out by specialized transport proteins termed sodium-glucose cotransporters (SGLTs). There are 2 SGLTs in the kidney involved in glucose reabsorption. SGLT1 is found primarily in the distal S2/S3 segment of the proximal tubule and SGLT2 is expressed exclusively in the S1 segment. The location of SGLT2 in the proximal tubule means that it is responsible for approximately 90% of renal glucose reabsorption. The reabsorbed glucose passively diffuses out of the tubule cell into the blood via the basolateral membrane-associated GLUT2. Because of the importance of SGLT2 in renal reabsorption of glucose, this transporter has become the target for therapeutic intervention of the hyperglycemia associated with type 2 diabetes. By specifically inhibiting SGLT2, there will be increased glucose excretion in the urine and thus a lowering of plasma glucose levels. Information on the SGLT2 inhibitors is covered in Chapter 47.

REVIEW QUESTIONS

1. You have a patient exhibiting severe episodes of hypoglycemia. Measurement of circulating insulin and glucagon levels indicate that they are normal and responsive to cycles of feeding and fasting. Which of the following enzyme defects would most likely explain the hypoglycemia?

A. a constitutively active glycogen synthase
B. glycogen synthase that lacks the phosphorylase kinase target site
C. hepatic glucokinase with a K_m equal to that of muscle hexokinase

D. pancreatic glucokinase with a K_m equal to that of hepatic glucokinase
E. PFK1 that is nonresponsive to the allosteric effects of fructose-2,6-bisphosphate

Answer C: The hepatic form of the glucose-phosphorylating enzyme is referred to as glucokinase, which is a hexokinase isoform. Humans express 4 distinct hexokinases that exhibit different patterns of expression and kinetic activities relative to substrates and catalytic rates. Hepatic glucokinase has a K_m significantly higher than that of the hexokinase that is expressed in skeletal muscle. This prevents the liver from trapping glucose, thereby ensuring that peripheral tissues such as the brain and muscle have easy access to dietary carbohydrate. In the case of this patient, the expression of a variant glucokinase with a K_m similar to that of muscle hexokinase would result in significant trapping of glucose inside hepatocytes. The outcome would be expected to be periods of hypoglycemia as described.

2. You are examining the effects of an experimental compound on the metabolic activities of primary hepatocytes in culture. You discover that addition of your compound to these cells activates changes in metabolic fluxes highly similar to those induced by addition of glucagon. Determination of phosphate incorporation shows that several proteins become hyperphosphorylated following addition of the compound. Which of the following statements would most accurately reflect these changes?
A. glycogen phosphorylase activity will be increased
B. PFK1 activity will be unaffected
C. PFK2 will exhibit an increased level of kinase activity
D. phosphorylase kinase activity will be decreased
E phosphoprotein phosphatase-1 activity will be increased

Answer A: Within hepatocytes, glucagon activation of its receptor results in activation of the kinase PKA. Activation of PKA will then lead to the phosphorylation of numerous substrates. One of the substrates for PKA is glycogen synthase/phosphorylase kinase (phosphorylase kinase) which results in activation of this PKA substrate. Activation of phosphorylase kinase results in the phosphorylation of both glycogen synthase and glycogen phosphorylase. When glycogen phosphorylase is phosphorylated its level of activity is increased.

3. You are treating an 11-year-old female type 1 diabetic patient who forgot to eat after she self-administered her afternoon insulin. Blood work demonstrates that her serum glucose level is 1 mM (18mg/dL). Which of the following statements correctly defines the metabolic situation in this patient?
A. a reversal of the muscle hexokinase reaction converts glucose 6-phosphate to glucose for oxidation in glycolysis
B. hepatic glycogen releases glucose in response to insulin-mediated dephosphorylation of glycogen phosphorylase
C. hepatic glycogen releases glucose through a reversal of the glycogen synthase reaction
D. phosphorylation of hepatic glycogen synthase prevents glucose incorporation into glycogen
E. the activity of muscle glycolysis is inhibited by the phosphorylation of PFK1

Answer D: As the level of blood glucose falls, the pancreas will secrete glucagon as a means to stimulate hepatic gluconeogenesis. Within hepatocytes, glucagon activation of its receptor results in activation of the kinase, PKA. Activation of PKA will then lead to the phosphorylation of numerous substrates. One of the substrates for PKA is glycogen synthase/phosphorylase kinase (phosphorylase kinase), which results in activation of this PKA substrate. Activation of phosphorylase kinase results in the phosphorylation of both glycogen synthase and glycogen phosphorylase. When glycogen synthase is phosphorylated, its level of activity is decreased resulting in reduced incorporation of glucose into glycogen.

4. You have been studying a cell line derived from a muscle tumor and comparing its activities, with respect to the effects of high levels of fatty acids on glucose oxidation, to those of normal skeletal muscle cells from the same individual. You find that exposing the normal cells to high levels of free fatty acids results in impaired levels of glucose oxidation. These results are expected based upon the interactions of the glucose-fatty acid cycle. However, the tumor-derived cells do not exhibit reduced glycolysis in the presence of high levels of free fatty acids. Which of the following best explains these observations?
A. the tumor cells contain a mutant form of acetyl-CoA carboxylase, which is insensitive to citrate resulting in reduced conversion of acetyl-CoA to malonyl-CoA and the acetyl-CoA then activates phosphoenolpyruvate carboxykinase
B. the tumor cells contain a mutant form of carnitine palmitoyltransferase 1, which restricts mitochondrial uptake of fatty acids which then build up in the cytosol leading to allosteric inhibition of PFK1
C. the tumor cells contain a mutant form of PFK1 which is insensitive to allosteric activation by fructose-2,6-bisphosphate

D. the tumor cells contain a mutant form of PFK1 which is insensitive to allosteric inhibition by citrate
E. the tumor cells contain a mutant more active form of ATP-citrate lyase, causing significant reductions in mitochondrial citrate resulting in loss of citrate-mediated inhibition of PFK1

Answer D: According to the glucose-fatty acid cycle, these 2 fuel sources reciprocally antagonize the utilization of each other. In other words, glucose oxidation can restrict fatty acid metabolism and fatty acid oxidation leads to reduced utilization of glucose. There are 2 major mechanisms by which fatty acid oxidation can restrict the flow of glucose through glycolysis. High levels of fat oxidation lead to generation of acetyl-CoA in excess of the cells' ability to fully oxidize it in the TCA cycle. Some of this acetyl-CoA is converted to citrate via the citrate synthase reaction of the TCA cycle, but the citrate cannot be further oxidized, so it is transported to the cytosol where it allosterically inhibits the PFK1 reaction. In addition, the acetyl-CoA allosterically activates pyruvate dehydrogenase complex (PDHc) kinases that, when activated, phosphorylate the PDHc. Phosporylated PDHc is less capable of oxidizing acetyl-CoA and leads to increased levels of pyruvate in the cytosol. The increased pyruvate restricts the ability of pyruvate kinase to oxidize phosphoenolpyruvate, resulting in reduced flow through glycolysis.

5. You are studying the effects of an experimental compound on the process of glucose metabolism in laboratory animals. Addition of the compound to the animal chow is associated with decreased glucose output by the liver of these animals. Analysis of liver biopsy cells isolated 2-days following compound addition indicates that citrate transport into the cytosol is impaired. The activity of which of the following glycolytic enzymes is most likely to be affected by your experimental compound?
A. glyceraldehyde-3-phosphate dehydrogenase
B. 6-phosphofructo-1 kinase, PFK1
C. 6-phosphofructo-2 kinase, PFK2
D. phosphoglycerate kinase
E. pyruvate kinase

Answer B: PFK1 represents the rate-limiting enzyme of glycolysis. This enzyme is subject to allosteric regulation, both positive and negative, by numerous effectors including citrate, which normally inhibits the enzyme allowing carbons to be diverted into glucose via gluconeogenesis.

6. Under conditions of anaerobic glycolysis, the NAD^+ required by glyceraldehyde-3-phosphate dehydrogenase is supplied by a reaction catalyzed by which of the following enzymes?
A. glycerol-3-phosphate dehydrogenase
B. α-ketoglutarate dehydrogenase
C. lactate dehydrogenase
D. malate dehydrogenase
E. pyruvate dehydrogenase

Answer C: During aerobic glycolysis, the NADH generated by the glyceraldehyde-3-phosphate dehydrogenase–catalyzed reaction is ultimately reoxidized to NAD^+ in the mitochondria via the oxidative phosphorylation pathway. The transfer of the electrons from cytoplasmic NADH to mitochondrial NADH occurs via 2 shuttles mechanism, resulting in the continued oxidation of NADH to NAD^+ keeping the glyceraldehyde-3-phosphate dehydrogenase reaction supplied with necessary NAD^+ for glycolysis. However, during anaerobic glycolysis pyruvate is not oxidized in the TCA cycle but is reduced to lactate via the action of lactate dehydrogenase, LDH. The reduction of pyruvate by LDH, within the cytosol, results in the oxidation of NADH to NAD^+, thus supplying the NAD^+ required for the glyceraldehyde-3-phosphate dehydrogenase and allowing glycolysis to continue.

7. You are examining the regulatory control of glycolysis by addition of a novel compound to a hepatocyte cell culture system. Your studies demonstrate that addition of the compound decreases the kinase activity of PFK2 while simultaneously increasing the phosphatase activity of the enzyme. This response most closely reflects which of the following naturally occurring controls exerted on PFK2?
A. allosteric inhibition by insulin
B. dephosphorylation by the appropriate protein phosphatase
C. increased AMP concentrations
D. increased glucose 6-phosphate concentrations
E. phosphorylation by cAMP-dependent protein kinase (PKA)

Answer E: When PFK2 is phosphorylated, via the action of PKA, its activity shifts from a kinase to a phosphatase. Within hepatocytes, this shift in catalytic activity of PFK2 results in less activation of the rate-limiting enzyme of glycolysis, PFK1, to ensure the liver produces glucose via gluconeogenesis instead of oxidizing the sugar.

8. You are examining the regulatory control of glycolysis by addition of a novel compound to a hepatocyte cell culture system. You discover that addition of the compound results in an increased rate of ATP production from glucose while simultaneously reducing glucose output into the culture medium. Your experimental compound is most likely mimicking which of the following?

A. fructose 1,6-bisphosphate
B. fructose 2,6-bisphosphate
C. fructose 1-bisphosphate
D. glucose 6-bisphosphate
E. phosphoenolpyruvate

Answer B: Fructose-2,6-bisphosphate (F2,6BP) is the most potent allosteric activator of PFK1, resulting in activation of glycolysis. Simultaneously, F2,6BP allosterically inhibits the gluconeogenic enzyme F-1,6-BPase.

9. You are examining the regulatory control of glycolysis by addition of a novel compound to a hepatocyte cell culture system. You discover that addition of the compound results in a decreased rate of ATP production from glucose while simultaneously increasing glucose output into the culture medium. Further studies demonstrate that the changes observed in your culture system with addition of the compound can be mimicked by altering the cytosolic levels of citrate. Your compound is most likely altering the rate of glycolysis by which of the following mechanisms?

A. inhibiting phosphodiesterase, PDE
B. inhibiting 6-phosphofructo-1-kinase (PFK1)
C. inhibiting pyruvate kinase
D. stimulating PEPCK
E. stimulating 6-phosphofructo-1-kinase (PFK1)

Answer B: Citrate, present in the cytosol, serves as a signal for a high-energy charge and inhibition of the TCA cycle. Under these conditions the rate of glucose oxidation via glycolysis needs to be reduced. Citrate serves as an allosteric inhibitor of the rate-limiting enzyme of glycolysis, PFK1.

10. Cytosolic reducing equivalents (NADH) generated by glycolysis in the liver, enter the mitochondria for generation of ATP by which of the following processes?

A. active transport of NADH into the mitochondrion
B. passive diffusion of NADH into the mitochondrion
C. transfer of electrons from NADH to NADH reductase at the mitochondrial surface
D. transfer of electrons to oxaloacetate with transport of malate into the mitochondrion
E. transfer of electrons to pyruvate with transport of lactate into the mitochondrion

Answer D: The electrons from reduced cytosolic NADH enter the mitochondria via either the malate-aspartate shuttle or the glycerol phosphate shuttle. In the context of the malate-aspartate shuttle, the electrons from cytosolic NADH are transferred to oxaloacetate, forming malate via the action of cytosolic malate dehydrogenase. The malate is then actively transported into the mitochondria, where it enters the TCA cycle.

11. You are examining the regulatory control of glycolysis by addition of a novel compound to a hepatocyte cell culture system. You discover that addition of the compound results in an increased rate of ATP production from glucose. Further studies demonstrate that the changes observed in your culture system with addition of the compound can be mimicked by a number of substances that activate the rate-limiting enzyme of glycolysis. Your compound is most likely altering the rate of glycolysis in a manner similar to all of which of the following?

A. AMP, citrate, and fructose 2,6-bisphosphate
B. AMP, inorganic phosphate, and fructose 2,6-bisphosphate
C. ATP, citrate, and inorganic phosphate
D. ATP, inorganic phosphate, and fructose 1,6-bisphosphate
E. inorganic phosphate, citrate, and fructose 2,6-bisphosphate

Answer B: Allosteric activation of PFK1 would be expected to occur under conditions of low-energy charge. Thus, as the level of ATP drops, there will be a concomitant rise in both AMP and inorganic phosphate levels. Both serve to allosterically activate PFK1. PFK1 is also allosterically activated by fructose-2,6-bisphosphate whose levels also rise in response to changing energy levels.

12. You are examining the effects of various oxygen concentrations on cultures of erythrocytes. You find that at low O_2 pressures there is rapid depletion of a necessary intermediate in the glycolytic pathway. Further analysis of the cells you are culturing indicates that the activity of the lactate dehydrogenase in these cells is extremely low relative to what is expected. Under these hypoxic conditions, which of the following is the most likely rapidly depleted intermediate?

A. ADP
B. citrate
C. FAD
D. glucose 6-phosphate
E. NAD^+

Answer E: Erythrocytes do not contain mitochondria and, therefore, only oxidize glucose via anaerobic metabolism. The end result of this oxidation is lactate. The coupling of NADH, produced by the glycolytic enzyme glyceraldehyde-3-phosphate dehydrogenase, and the reoxidation of the NADH to NAD^+ via lactate dehydrogenase is necessary for continued energy generation via this pathway of glucose oxidation. Therefore, a loss of lactate dehydrogenase activity would lead to rapid depletion of NAD^+ within the cell.

13. You are studying the effects of the addition of a novel compound to the chow of laboratory animals on the overall rate of flux through glycolysis. You discover that when the animals consume the compound containing chow, there is an increase in glycolytic flux to pyruvate. Examination of serum hormone levels in these animals indicates a change in the ratios of several key regulators of glucose homeostasis. The consumption of the test compound most likely causes an increase in which of the following hormone ratios, thus best explaining the observed changes in the rate of glycolysis?
A. cortisol to insulin
B. epinephrine to glucagon
C. glucagon to epinephrine
D. insulin to glucagon
E. insulin to cortisol

Answer D: As the level of insulin rises, there will be a concomitant increase in the activity of phosphodiesterase within responsive cells, such as the liver. The phosphodiesterase will hydrolyze cAMP leading to reduced activity of PKA. As the activity of PKA falls, the level of phosphorylation of 6-phosphofructo-2-kinase, PFK2 will fall which reduces its phosphatase activity. When functioning as a phosphatase, PFK2 hydrolyzes fructose-2,6-bisphosphate (F2,6BP) to fructose 6-phosphate. When PFK2 is not phosphorylated, it acts as a kinase and will, therefore lead to increased levels of F2,6BP. Conversely, as the level of glucagon increases, the activity of PKA increases leading to increased phosphorylation of PFK2. This in turn results in decreased F2,6BP levels due to the phosphatase activity of PFK2.

14. In the production of ATP during glucose metabolism in erythrocytes, which of the following is the immediate donor of the phosphoryl group to ADP?
A. 2,3-bisphosphoglycerate
B. fructose 1,6-bisphosphate
C. fructose 2,6-bisphosphate
D. glyceraldehyde 3-phosphate
E. phosphoenolpyruvate

Answer E: The phosphate donors during glycolysis are 1,3-bisphosphoglycerate and phosphoenolpyruvate. These high-energy intermediates of glycolysis function the same regardless of the cell in which glycolysis is occurring.

15. You are studying the effects of the addition of a novel compound to the chow of laboratory animals on the overall rate of flux through glycolysis. You discover that when the animals consume the compound containing chow, there is an increase in glycolytic flux to pyruvate. Examination of cells from the livers of these animals demonstrates that when the compound enters the cells, it causes a rapid decrease in the ATP:ADP ratio. This effect most likely results in which of the following?
A. decreased isocitrate dehydrogenase activity
B. decreased phosphofructokinase-1 activity
C. decreased rate of electron transport
D. increased glycogen synthase activity
E. increased glycolytic pathway flux

Answer E: As the level of ATP falls, the level of ADP and AMP will increase. AMP serves as an allosteric activator of the rate-limiting enzyme of glycolysis, PFK1. Thus, as the level of ATP falls, the rate of flux through glycolysis will increase.

16. A healthy 28-year-old woman exhibits a peak serum glucose concentration of 220 mg/dL within 30 minutes of the consumption of 75 g of glucose. Two hours after ingestion, her serum glucose concentration decreases to 100 mg/dL. The uptake and trapping of glucose within liver cells at high serum glucose concentrations is facilitated by which of the following enzymes?
A. galactokinase
B. glucokinase
C. phosphoenolpyruvate carboxykinase (PEPCK)
D. phosphofructokinase-1 (PFK1)
E. pyruvate dehydrogenase

Answer B: Hepatic glucokinase has a high K_m for glucose in order to ensure that the liver does not trap glucose before sufficient levels are obtained in the blood. As the level of blood glucose increases, glucokinase will become more active resulting in phosphorylation of more glucose thus, trapping it in the cell leading to a gradual reduction in blood glucose levels.

17. The hydrolysis of which of the following compounds is characterized by a standard free energy change ($\Delta G^{0\prime}$) that is more negative than that for the reaction: $ATP \rightarrow ADP + P_i$?
A. glucose 1-phopsphate
B. glucose 6-phosphate
C. glycerol 1-phosphate
D. phosphoenolpyruvate
E. 3-phosphoglycerate

Answer D: Only 2 compounds of glycolysis contain sufficient energy to drive the synthesis of ATP from ADP and thus, have $\Delta G^{0\prime}$ values more negative than the hydrolysis of ATP. These are 1,3-bisphosphoglycerate and phosphoenolpyruvate.

18. The Warburg effect states that cancer cells carry out glucose metabolism in a manner distinct from the glycolytic process of cells in normal tissues. Cancer cells tend to "ferment" glucose into lactate even in the presence of sufficient oxygen to support mitochondrial oxidative phosphorylation. Which of the following enzymes is most responsible for the observations accounting for the Warburg effect?
A. glucokinase
B. glyceraldehyde-3-phosphate dehydrogenase
C. PFK1
D. PFK2
E. pyruvate kinase

Answer E: In mammals, 2 genes encode a total of 4 pyruvate kinase (PK) isoforms. The *PKM* gene, so called originally due to initial characterization in muscle tissues, encodes the PKM1 and PKM1 isoforms. Most tissues express either the PKM1 or PKM2. PKM1 is found in many normal differentiated tissues, whereas PKM2 is expressed in most proliferating cells, including in all cancer cell lines and tumors tested to date. PKM2 is much less active than PKM1 but is allosterically activated by the upstream glycolytic metabolite fructose 1,6-bisphosphate (FBP). PKM2 is also unique in that, unlike other PK isoforms, it can interact with phosphotyrosine in tyrosine-phosphorylated proteins such as those resulting from growth factor stimulation of cells. The interaction of PKM2 with tyrosine-phosphorylated proteins results in the release of FBP leading to reduced activity of the enzyme. Low PKM2 activity, in conjunction with increased glucose uptake, facilitates the diversion of glucose carbons into the anabolic pathways that are derived from glycolysis. So, for proliferating cells such as cancers, even though it may seem counterproductive to prevent complete oxidation of glucose solely for ATP production, the demands for carbon incorporation into biomass clearly supersedes the needs for ATP production from glucose. Of metabolic significance to proliferating cells is that they must avoid ATP production in excess of demand to avoid allosteric inhibition of PFK1. Therefore, the inhibition of PKM2 by binding to tyrosine-phosphorylated proteins, following growth factor stimulation, may serve to uncouple the ability of cells to divert the carbons from nutrients (such as glucose) into biosynthetic pathways from the production of ATP. This may, in fact, be the underlying reason why PKM2 activity has evolved to be decreased in rapidly dividing cells.

19. You are studying the effects of the addition of a novel compound to the chow of laboratory animals on the overall rate of flux through glycolysis in skeletal muscle. You discover that when the animals consume the compound containing chow, there is a decrease in glycolytic flux to pyruvate while at the same time there is increased glucose output to the blood. Cells isolated from muscle biopsy tissue from these animals respond to addition of the compound with a dramatic rise in the levels of cAMP. Given this effect of the compound, which of the following will occur first?
A. binding to the regulatory subunits of cAMP-dependent protein kinase, PKA
B. desensitization of the catecholamine receptor
C. dissociation of the G protein into the a and bg components
D. increase in cytosolic Ca2+
E. inhibition of glycogen synthase

Answer A: The primary function of cAMP is to bind to the regulatory subunits of PKA, which leads to the release of the catalytic subunits.

20. A 9-month-old child is presented to the emergency room by his parents who report that he has been vomiting and has severe diarrhea. The episodes of vomiting began when the parents started feeding their child cow's milk. The infant exhibits signs of failure to thrive, weight loss, hepatomegaly, and jaundice. Laboratory tests show elevated blood galactose, hypergalactosuria, and metabolic acidosis with coagulation deficiency. These clinical and laboratory findings are most consistent with a deficiency in which of the following enzymes?
A. aldolase B
B. fructokinase
C. fructose-1,6-bisphosphatase
D. glucose-6-phosphate dehydrogenase
E. UDP-galactose uridyltransferase (GALT)

Answer E: This patient is suffering from classic (type 1) galactosemia. Type 1 galactosemia occurs as a consequence of mutations in the gene encoding GALT. Classic galactosemia manifests by a failure of neonates to thrive. Vomiting and diarrhea occur following ingestion of milk, hence individuals are termed lactose intolerant. Clinical findings include impaired liver function (which if left untreated leads to severe cirrhosis), elevated blood galactose, hypergalactosemia, hyperchloremic metabolic acidosis, urinary galactitol excretion, and hyperaminoaciduria. Unless controlled by exclusion of galactose from the diet, these patients can go on to develop blindness and fatal liver damage. Blindness is due to the conversion of circulating galactose to the sugar alcohol galacitol, by an NADPH-dependent aldose reductase that is present in neural tissue and in the lens of the eye.

21. Prolonged ethanol consumption and subsequent metabolism ultimately leads to a condition referred to as steatohepatitis or more commonly, "fatty liver syndrome." Ethanol metabolism results in alteration in the activity of which of the following enzymes, one of the consequences of which is excess lipid deposition in the liver?

A. fatty acyl-CoA oxidase
B. glucose-6-phosphate dehydrogenase
C. glycerol-3-phosphate dehydrogenase
D. lactate dehydrogenase
E. pyruvate dehydrogenase

Answer C: The metabolism of ethanol by the liver leads to a large increase in NADH. This increase in NADH disrupts the normal processes of metabolic regulation such as hepatic gluconeogenesis, TCA cycle function, and fatty acid oxidation. Concomitant with reduced fatty acid oxidation is enhanced fatty acid synthesis and increased triacylglyceride production by the liver. In the mitochondria, the production of acetate from acetaldehyde leads to increased levels of acetyl-CoA. Since the increased generation of NADH also reduces the activity of the TCA cycle, the acetyl-CoA is diverted to fatty acid synthesis. The reduction in cytosolic NAD^+ leads to reduced activity of glycerol-3-phosphate dehydrogenase (in the glycerol 3-phosphate to DHAP direction) resulting in increased levels of glycerol 3-phosphate which is the backbone for the synthesis of the triglycerides. Both of these 2 events lead to fatty acid deposition in the liver leading to fatty liver syndrome and excessive levels of lipids in the blood, referred to as hyperlipidemia.

22. You are tending to a teenage patient following a reported suicide attempt. The teen ingested rat poison and has diarrhea and severe vomiting which has resulted in hypovolemic shock. Outward signs include a strong odor of garlic on the patient's breath. Which of the following is the most likely action of the toxic substance in the rat poison resulting in the observed symptoms?

A. it activates pyruvate dehydrogenase
B. it enhances the rate of gluconeogenesis
C. it increases glutathione production
D. it inhibits pyruvate dehydrogenase
E. it reduces the concentration of pyruvate

Answer D: Rat poison often contains arsenic compounds as the toxic agents. The arsenic ingested by this patient accounts for the smell of garlic on his breath. Arsenic inhibits glycolysis and the TCA cycle, in particular at the pyruvate dehydrogenase-catalyzed reaction.

23. In patients with suspected metastatic cancer in the brain, a useful diagnostic is positron emission tomography, PET. This technique utilizes a radioactive form of glucose that cannot be metabolized but is rapidly taken up by cancer cells due to their high rates of metabolism. Which of the following is most responsible for the rapid uptake of this compound into the tumor cells in the brain?

A. GLUT2
B. GLUT3
C. GLUT4
D. insulin
E. PFK1

Answer B: When glucose is taken into cells, it is phosphorylated by one of the various hexokinases (called glucokinase in liver and pancreas), which trap it within the cell. Using a nonmetabolizable form of glucose that is tagged with a radioisotope allows for detection within cells via PET. Uptake of glucose into cells occurs via facilitated diffusion with one of several glucose transporters termed GLUTs. Within the brain, GLUT3 is the principal glucose transporter.

24. You are carrying out in vitro studies of skeletal muscle cell metabolism utilizing primary cultures of myocytes prepared from rectus femoris biopsies. Your studies involve the comparison of metabolic byproducts from carbohydrate metabolism under aerobic and anaerobic conditions. When your cell culture conditions allow for aerobic metabolism, which of the following compounds would be expected to be derived from any pyruvate generated from glycolysis?

A. acetyl-CoA
B. alanine
C. ethanol
D. lactate
E. oxaloacetate

Answer A: Under aerobic conditions, glucose can be completely oxidized to CO_2 and H_2O following the oxidative decarboxylation of pyruvate into acetyl-CoA, which then enters the TCA cycle for further oxidation. Although oxaloacetate is an intermediate in the TCA cycle and its formation requires continued input of acetyl-CoA, the 2 carbon atoms of pyruvate-derived acetyl-CoA are lost as CO_2 prior to oxaloacetate.

25. A 27-year-old man complains of intermittent right upper quadrant pain that extends to the inferior tip of his scapula. Analysis of blood reveals mild anemia with the presence of normocytic and normochromic nonsperical erythrocytes. Additional blood work shows elevated levels of glucose 6-phosphate (G6P) and 2,3-bisphosphoglycerate (2,3BPG). Ultrasonic examination of the abdomen shows cholelithiasis.

Following removal of her gallbladder, the stones are examined and shown to contain bilirubin. A deficiency in which of the following enzymes would most explain the signs and symptoms in this patient?

A. glucose 6-phosphate dehydrogenase
B. PFK1
C. pyruvate carboxylase
D. pyruvate dehydrogenase
E. pyruvate kinase

Answer E: Deficiency of pyruvate kinase is the most common enzyme deficiency resulting in inherited nonspherocytic hemolytic anemia. The disorder is characterized by lifelong chronic hemolysis of variable severity. Red blood cells from heterozygous individuals possess only 40% to 60% of the pyruvate kinase activity of normal individuals yet these individuals are almost always clinically normal. The clinical severity of the anemia resulting from PKLR deficiencies varies from mild and fully compensated hemolysis to severe cases that require transfusions for survival. Many patients with mild PKLR deficiency do not manifest symptoms until adulthood. In these individuals, the symptoms, that include mild to moderate splenomegaly, mild chronic hemolysis, and jaundice often manifest incidental to an acute viral infection or during an evaluation in pregnancy. Clinical evaluation of blood from patients with PKLR deficiency will show normocytic anemia (sometimes macrocytic) which is reflective of the reticulocytosis that is invariably present. The hemolysis results in increased heme metabolism in the liver generating bilirubin in excess, which then accumulates in the gallbladder resulting in the stones present in this patient. The presence of elevated levels of serum 2,3BPG and G6P is indicative of anemia due to erythrocyte PK deficiency as opposed to the more common cause due to glucose-6-phosphate dehydrogenase deficiency. The reduced PK leads to increased levels of PEP, which are diverted into the 2,3BPG pathway.

Checklist

- ✓ Glucose is activated for oxidation by hexokinase/glucokinase and PFK1 phosphorylation.
- ✓ Hexokinase, but not glucokinase can phosphorylate several 6-carbon sugars.
- ✓ K_m for glucose of glucokinase is high to prevent hepatic trapping of glucose, thus allowing for hepatic regulation of blood glucose.
- ✓ PFK1 is rate-limiting enzyme of glycolysis, regulated by multiple allosteric effectors.
- ✓ PFK2-critical bifunctional enzyme responsible for regulating levels of F2,6BP is a significant allosteric regulator of PFK1.
- ✓ PK isozymes control whether or not glucose oxidation proceeds from pyruvate into the TCA cycle or is reduced to lactate.
- ✓ Glucose oxidation can proceed aerobically whereby pyruvate is completely oxidized by entry into the TCA cycle or oxidation can occur anaerobically with the reduction of pyruvate to lactate.
- ✓ Insulin and glucagon are major counter-regulatory hormones influencing overall glucose storage and oxidation.
- ✓ Fatty acid oxidation interferes with glucose oxidation and can thus exacerbate the hyperglycemia typical of Type 2 diabetes.
- ✓ The interrelationship between glucose and fatty acid oxidation is referred to as the glucose-fatty acid cycle.
- ✓ Cancer cells are said to "ferment" glucose to lactate even under conditions of plentiful oxygen, referred to as the Warburg effect.
- ✓ Loss of PK-R activity is the leading cause of inherited nonspherocytic anemia.

CHAPTER

11

Carbohydrates: Fructose Metabolism and Feeding Behaviors

CHAPTER OUTLINE

High-Yield Terms

High-fructose corn syrup (HFCS): refers to the sugar syrup generated from corn starch by enzymatic conversion of a portion of the glucose to fructose. Commonly contains 55% fructose and identified as HFCS-55

HFCS and sucrose: represent the 2 primary sources of fructose in the human diet

GLUT5 and GLUT2: intestinal sugar transporters responsible for fructose uptake and then delivery to the blood, respectively

Ketohexokinase: two isoforms KHK-A and KHK-C catalyze phosphorylation of fructose to fructose 1-phosphate, also called fructokinase

Aldolase B: enzyme catalyzing hydrolysis of fructose 1-phosphate to glyceraldehyde and dihydroxyacetone phosphate (DHAP)

Fructose-induced feeding: metabolism of fructose within the brain results in suppression of anorexigenic signals while activating orexigenic signals

Hereditary fructose intolerance: potentially fatal infant disorder resulting from defect in the level of aldolase B activity

Dietary Fructose

Diets containing large amounts of sucrose (a disaccharide of glucose and fructose) can utilize the fructose as a major source of energy. The amount of fructose available from sucrose obtained from cane or beet sugars is not significantly less than that from corn syrup. Corn syrup is somewhat improperly identified as high-fructose corn syrup (HFCS), giving the impression that it contains a large amount of fructose. However, whereas the fructose content of sucrose is 50% (since it is a pure disaccharide of only glucose and fructose), the content in HFCS is only 55% (referred to as HFCS-55). The reason HFCS has more than 50% fructose is because the glucose extracted from corn starch is treated with glucose isomerase to convert most of the glucose to fructose yielding HFCS-90. The HFCS-90 is then mixed with glucose syrup to produce either HFCS-55 or HFCS-42, both of which are used in food preparations. Therefore, any disorder and/or dysfunction, attributed to the consumption of fructose, can be manifest whether one consumes cane or beet sugar or HFCS.

Following ingestion of sucrose or HFCS, it is degraded in the gut through the action of sucrose-isomaltase into its constituent monosaccharides, glucose, and fructose. As indicated in Chapter 7, glucose is absorbed from the lumen of the intestine via the action of SGLT1 and fructose is absorbed via GLUT5. Once in the intestinal enterocyte, the glucose and fructose can enter the blood via GLUT2-mediated transport. Fructose in the blood does not stimulate insulin secretion from the pancreas and its cellular uptake is insulin-independent.

Activation of Fructose

The pathway to utilization of fructose differs in muscle and liver due to the differential distribution of fructose-phosphorylating enzymes. Hexokinases are a family of enzymes that phosphorylate hexose sugars such as glucose and fructose. Four mammalian isozymes of hexokinase are known (Types I–IV), with the Type IV isozyme often referred to as glucokinase. Glucokinase is the form of the enzyme found in hepatocytes and pancreatic β-cells. In addition to hexokinases, fructose can be phosphorylated by fructokinases.

Although both KHK-C and KHK-A can metabolize fructose, KHK-C is considered to be the primary enzyme involved in fructose metabolism because its K_m for fructose is much lower than that of the KHK-A isoform.

Muscle, which contains 2 types of hexokinase (type I and type II), can phosphorylate fructose to F6P which is a direct glycolytic intermediate. However, the affinity of hexokinase for fructose is substantially less than that of fructokinase.

Entry of Fructose into Glycolysis

The liver contains mostly glucokinase (hexokinase type IV), which exhibits substrate specificity for glucose, and, thus, there is the requirement for KHK to utilize fructose in hepatic glycolysis. Hepatic KHK-C phosphorylates fructose on C-1 yielding fructose 1-phosphate (F1P). In liver (as well as in kidney and intestine), the form of aldolase that predominates (aldolase B, also called fructose-1,6-bisphosphate aldolase B) can utilize both F-1,6-BP and F1P as substrates. Therefore, when presented with F1P, the enzyme generates DHAP and glyceraldehyde. The DHAP is converted by triose phosphate isomerase to G3P and enters glycolysis. The glyceraldehyde can be phosphorylated to G3P by triose kinase or converted to DHAP through the concerted actions of alcohol dehydrogenase, glycerol kinase, and glycerol phosphate dehydrogenase.

Fructose Consumption and Feeding Behaviors

As pointed out in the Chapter 10, glucose is the primary fuel used for energy production in the brain. When glucose is metabolized within the hypothalamus, a

High-Yield Concept

Fructokinases are formally referred to as ketohexokinases (KHK). There are 2 forms of KHK in mammals that result from alternative splicing of the KHK gene. These 2 isoforms are called KHK-A and KHK-C. Expression of KHK-C is seen primarily in the liver, pancreas, kidney, and intestines. Expression of KHK-A is more ubiquitous and expressed at highest levels in skeletal muscle.

High-Yield Concept

Because hepatic fructose metabolism directly produces triose phosphates, its metabolism bypasses the hormonal regulation that is exerted on glucose metabolism at PFK1 (6-phosphofructo-1 kinase), and, in addition, there is no allosteric regulation of the process such as occurs at the PFK1 and hexokinase reactions (Figure 11-1).

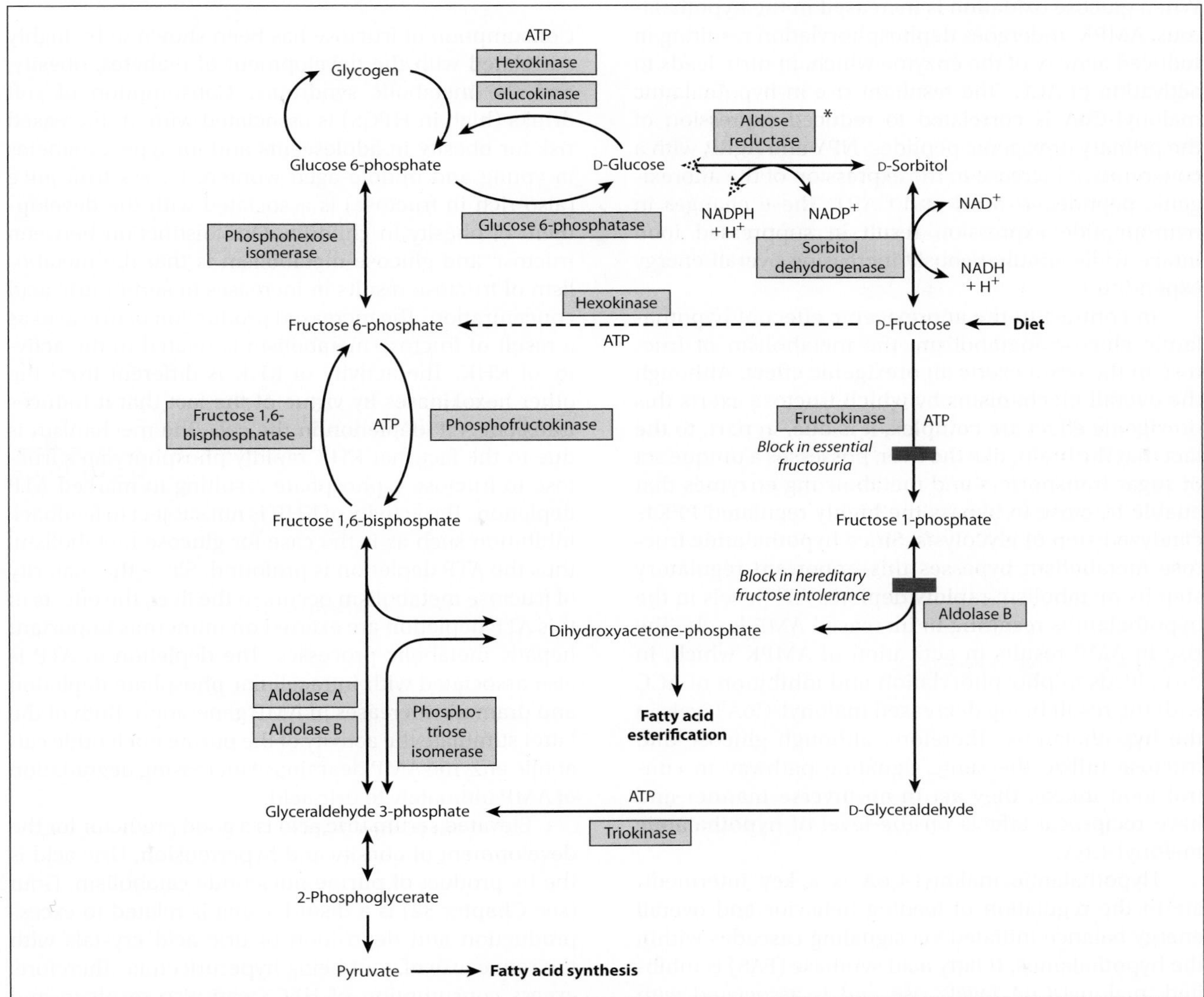

FIGURE 11-1: Metabolism of fructose. Aldolase A is found in all tissues, whereas aldolase B is the predominant form in liver. (*Not found in liver.) Murray RK, Bender DA, Botham KM, Kennelly PJ, Rodwell VW, Weil PA. *Harper's Illustrated Biochemistry*. 29th ed. New York, NY: McGraw-Hill; 2012.

signaling pathway is initiated that ultimately results in the suppression of food intake. Details on the role of the hypothalamus in the control of feeding behaviors are found in Chapter 44. The principal participants hypothalamic signaling cascade induced via glucose metabolism includes the enzymes AMPK and acetyl-CoA carboxylase (ACC) and the product of the ACC reaction, malonyl-CoA. Activation of AMPK results in the phosphorylation of ACC resulting in reduced activity of the latter enzyme. Conversely, when AMPK activity declines the phosphorylation state of ACC falls resulting in increased production of malonyl-CoA. When glucose oxidation is increased in the hypothalamus, AMPK undergoes dephosphorylation resulting in reduced activity of the enzyme which, in turn, leads to activation of ACC. The resultant rise in hypothalamic malonyl-CoA is correlated to reduced expression of the primary orexigenic peptides, NPY and AgRP, with a concomitant increase in the expression of the anorexigenic peptides, α-MSH and CART. These changes in neuropeptide expression result in suppressed food intake while simultaneously increasing overall energy expenditure.

In contrast to the anorexigenic effect of hypothalamic glucose metabolism, the metabolism of fructose in the brain exerts an orexigenic effect. Although the overall mechanisms by which fructose exerts this orexigenic effect are complex, it is due, in part, to the fact that the brain, like the liver, possesses a unique set of sugar transporters and metabolizing enzymes that enable fructose to bypass the highly regulated PFK1-catalyzed step of glycolysis. Since hypothalamic fructose metabolism bypasses this important regulatory step its metabolism rapidly depletes ATP levels in the hypothalamus resulting in increased AMP levels. The rise in AMP results in activation of AMPK which, in turn, leads to phosphorylation and inhibition of ACC with the result being decreased malonyl-CoA levels in the hypothalamus. Therefore, although glucose and fructose utilize the same signaling pathway to control food intake, they act in an inverse manner and have reciprocal effects on the level of hypothalamic malonyl-CoA.

Hypothalamic malonyl-CoA is a key intermediate in the regulation of feeding behavior and overall energy balance initiated via signaling cascades within the hypothalamus. If fatty acid synthase (FAS) is inhibited, malonyl-CoA levels rise and is associated with suppression of food intake. Conversely, if ACC activity is inhibited, suppression of feeding behavior with FAS inhibition is reversed. Overall malonyl-CoA levels in the hypothalamus correlate well with nutritional state. During periods when energy expenditure exceeds intake, such as during fasting, malonyl-CoA levels in the hypothalamus are low. Following food intake there is a rapid rise in hypothalamic malonyl-CoA levels. The changes in hypothalamic malonyl-CoA levels are followed quickly by changes in expression of orexigenic and anorexigenic peptides. In the fasting state NPY and AgRP levels are high, whereas α-MSH and CART levels are low. Upon refeeding this pattern immediately inverts.

Metabolic Disruption With Fructose Consumption

Consumption of fructose has been shown to be highly correlated with the development of diabetes, obesity, and the metabolic syndrome. Consumption of soft drinks (high in HFCS) is associated with an increased risk for obesity in adolescents and for type 2 diabetes in young and middle-aged women. Excess fruit juice (also rich in fructose) is associated with the development of obesity in children. One distinction between fructose and glucose metabolism is that the metabolism of fructose results in increases in serum uric acid concentration. The increased production of uric acid as a result of fructose metabolism is related to the activity of KHK. The activity of KHK is different from the other hexokinases by virtue of the fact that it induces transient ATP depletion in the cell. The mechanism is due to the fact that KHK rapidly phosphorylates fructose to fructose 1-phosphate resulting in marked ATP depletion. The activity of KHK is not subject to feedback inhibition such as is the case for glucose metabolism, thus the ATP depletion is profound. Since the majority of fructose metabolism occurs in the liver, the effects of this ATP depletion are exerted on numerous important hepatic metabolic processes. The depletion in ATP is also associated with intracellular phosphate depletion and dramatic increases in AMP generation. Both of the latter stimulate the activity of the purine nucleotide catabolic enzyme AMP deaminase increasing degradation of AMP ultimately to uric acid.

Elevated serum uric acid is a good predictor for the development of obesity and hypertension. Uric acid is the by-product of purine nucleotide catabolism. Gout (see Chapter 32) is a disorder that is related to excess production and deposition of uric acid crystals with the root cause of gout being hyperuricemia. Therefore, excess consumption of HFCS can also result in and exacerbate symptoms of gout.

Consumption of fructose by laboratory animals results in their developing several features of metabolic syndrome, including obesity, visceral fat accumulation, fatty liver, and elevated insulin and leptin levels. It is likely that the increase in leptin following fructose consumption represents leptin resistance, which could account for the increased food intake observed in fructose-fed animals. All of these phenomena associated with fructose consumption, including hyperuricemia, can be blocked in laboratory animals when both KHK-C and KHK-A isoforms are eliminated. The relationship between fructose metabolism-mediated hyperuricemia and development of the metabolic syndrome can also be demonstrated by the fact that treating animals with allopurinol, a drug used to lower uric acid levels in gout patients, partially prevents the fructose-induced metabolic syndrome.

Disorders of Fructose Metabolism

There are 3 primary inherited disorders in fructose metabolism: (1) essential fructosuria, (2) hereditary fructose-1,6-bisphosphatase deficiency, and (3) hereditary fructose intolerance.

Essential fructosuria is a relatively benign autosomal-recessive disorder resulting from defects in hepatic fructokinase (KHK-C). Hyperfructosemia and fructosuria are the principal signs associated with this metabolic defect.

Hereditary fructose-1,6-bisphosphatase deficiency is an autosomal-recessive disorder characterized by episodes of hypoglycemia, ketosis, lactic acidosis, and hyperventilation. The disorder can take a precipitous and often lethal course in the newborn infant. Later episodes are often triggered by fasting and febrile infections. Due to the enzyme defect, gluconeogenesis is severely impaired. Gluconeogenic precursors such as amino acids, lactate, and ketones accumulate as soon as liver glycogen stores are depleted. Patients past early childhood seem to develop normally.

Hereditary fructose intolerance (HFI) is the more severe form of inherited disorders in fructose metabolism which results from defects in the *aldolase B* gene. Details of this disease are contained in Clinical Box 11-1.

CLINICAL BOX 11-1: HEREDITARY FRUCTOSE INTOLERANCE

Hereditary fructose intolerance (HFI) is an autosomal-recessive disorder characterized by severe hypoglycemia and vomiting shortly after the intake of fructose. Aldolase B of liver, kidney cortex, and small intestine is deficient in these patients. Most of the *aldolase B* gene mutations are point mutations resulting in single amino acid changes that decrease stability or catalytic activity. The result is an inability to metabolize fructose, sucrose, and sorbitol correctly, manifesting as sugar toxicity that can lead to severe organ damage if untreated. The incidence of HFI is reportedly around 1 per 20,000 to 30,000 newborns and no cure is available. If appropriately diagnosed and treated, it constitutes a relatively benign disease, but without early intervention it can be lethal. Prolonged fructose ingestion in infants leads to poor feeding, vomiting, hepatomegaly, jaundice, hemorrhage, proximal renal tubular syndrome, and, finally, hepatic failure and death. Patients develop a strong distaste for noxious food. Hypoglycemia after fructose ingestion is caused by accumulation of F1P which simultaneously depletes phosphate pools, thereby inhibiting glycogenolysis at the level of glycogen phosphorylase which requires inorganic phosphate for activity. Aldolase B deficiency also impairs hepatic gluconeogenesis at the level of the DHAP and G3P condensation to F1,6BP. Patients remain healthy on a fructose-, sucrose-, and sorbitol-free diet. The need for sorbitol restriction is important since fructose can be derived endogenously from sorbitol. Additionally significant in the setting of HFI is that sorbitol can be synthesized in the body from glucose. Glucose is converted to sorbitol via the action of aldose reductase (also called aldehyde reductase 1). Sorbitol is then converted to fructose via sorbitol dehydrogenase. In the management of HFI this conversion has important clinical implications since sorbitol is found in numerous processed foods as a sweetener or conditioning agent and in the pharmaceutical industry as a bodying and emulsion agent.

REVIEW QUESTIONS

1. Which of the following represents the enzyme deficiency that leads to "essential fructosuria"?

A. fructose-1-phosphate aldolase (aldolase B)
B. fructose-1,6-bisphosphate aldolase (aldolase A)
C. fructokinase
D. hexokinase
E. 6-Phosphofructo-1 kinase, PFK1

Answer C: Essential fructosuria is a benign metabolic disorder caused by the lack of fructokinase which is normally present in the liver, pancreatic islets, and kidney cortex. The fructosuria of this disease depends on the time and amount of fructose and sucrose intake. Since the disorder is asymptomatic and harmless, it may go undiagnosed.

2. A child born and raised in Chicago planned to spend the summer on a relative's fruit farm and help with the harvest. The summer passed uneventfully, but several days after the harvest began, the child became jaundiced and very sick. On admission to the hospital the following clinical findings were recorded: in addition to the expected hyperbilirubinemia, the patient was hypoglycemic, had a markedly elevated rise in blood fructose concentration, and was hyperlactic acidemic. Further history taking revealed that during the harvest it was customary for the family to indulge in fruit-filled meals and to snack freely on fruit while carrying out the harvest. The elevated blood fructose in this child was most likely due to which of the following?

A. an allergic reaction to constituents in the fruit diet
B. defective hepatic aldolase B
C. defective hepatic fructokinase
D. defective hepatic fructose-1,6-bisphosphatase
E. defective hepatic glucokinase

Answer B: Hereditary fructose intolerance is a potentially lethal disorder resulting from a lack of aldolase B which is normally present in the liver, small intestine, and kidney cortex. The disorder is characterized by severe hypoglycemia and vomiting following fructose intake. Prolonged intake of fructose by infants with this defect leads to vomiting, poor feeding, jaundice, hepatomegaly, hemorrhage, and, eventually, hepatic failure and death. The hypoglycemia that results following fructose uptake is caused by fructose-1-phosphate inhibition of glycogenolysis, by interfering with the phosphorylase reaction, and inhibition of gluconeogenesis at the deficient aldolase step. Patients remain symptom free on a diet devoid of fructose and sucrose.

3. A 1-year-old girl is being examined by her physician because of a 3-month history of intermittent vomiting, shakiness, and a failure to thrive. The symptoms began when breast-feeding stopped and fruit and vegetables were added to her diet. Her current size is below the fifth percentile for length and weight. Upon physical examination the physician notes jaundice and hepatomegaly. Intravenous administration of fructose results in hypoglycemia and hypophosphatemia. Deficiency of which of the following hepatic enzymes is the most likely cause of the disorder in this patient?

A. aldolase B
B. fructokinase
C. galactose-1-phosphate uridyltransferase
D. glucose 6-phosphatase
E. glycogen phosphorylase

Answer A: Hereditary fructose intolerance is a potentially lethal disorder resulting from a lack of aldolase B which is normally present in the liver, small intestine, and kidney cortex. The disorder is characterized by severe hypoglycemia and vomiting following fructose intake. Prolonged intake of fructose by infants with this defect leads to vomiting, poor feeding, jaundice, hepatomegaly, hemorrhage, and, eventually, hepatic failure and death. The hypoglycemia that results following fructose uptake is caused by fructose-1-phosphate inhibition of glycogenolysis, by interfering with the phosphorylase reaction, and inhibition of gluconeogenesis at the deficient aldolase step. Patients remain symptom free on a diet devoid of fructose and sucrose.

4. Individuals harboring a mutation in the *aldolase B* gene are subject to severe hypoglycemia upon consumption of fructose. The hypoglycemia can be explained by an impairment in glycogen phosphorylase-mediated glucose release from glycogen in response to glucagon. This metabolic defect can best be explained by which of the following?

A. allosteric activation of glycogen synthase by fructose 1-phosphate
B. allosteric inhibition of phosphorylase by fructose 1-phosphate
C. depletion of the phosphate pool required by phosphorylase
D. the depletion in ATP leads to activation of AMPK which phosphorylates and inhibits phosphorylase
E. trapping of ATP in the form of fructose 1-phosphate

Answer C: Glycogen phosphorylase carries out a phosphorolysis reaction on glycogen utilizing inorganic phosphate in the process of this reaction. Hypoglycemia after fructose ingestion is caused by accumulation of fructose 1-phosphate which simultaneously depletes inorganic phosphate pools, thereby inhibiting glycogenolysis at the level of glycogen phosphorylase which requires inorganic phosphate for activity.

5. Patients with *aldolase B* gene mutations are required to avoid certain foods and products that contain fructose as their consumption can lead to significant hypoglycemia. In addition to fructose, consumption of which of the following carbohydrates must be avoided in these patients?
A. cellulose
B. glucose
C. lactose
D. maltose
E. sorbitol

Answer E: Sorbitol is a sugar often used in the pharmaceutical and food industries as a thickener or for the production of transparent gels such as in certain toothpastes. Sorbitol can be metabolized to fructose via the action of sorbitol dehydrogenase. Therefore, it is important that patients with hereditary fructose intolerance monitor food and pharmaceuticals for the presence of sorbitol as ingestion can lead to significant health complications.

6. Within the hypothalamus, metabolism of fructose results in a significant drop in the ATP:ADP ratio. The resulting increase in AMP results in altered metabolic pathways that in turn result in an increased desire for food intake. Which of the following metabolic changes is a contributing factor to the increased feeding behaviors associated with fructose consumption?
A. decreased fatty acid synthesis
B. decreased glycolysis
C. decreased fatty acid oxidation
D. increased fatty acid oxidation
E. increased gluconeogenesis

Answer D: Metabolism of fructose in the brain exerts an orexigenic (feeding desire) effect. Hypothalamic fructose metabolism rapidly depletes ATP levels in the hypothalamus resulting in increased AMP levels. The rise in AMP results in activation of AMPK which, in turn, leads to phosphorylation and inhibition of acetyl-CoA carboxylase (ACC [rate-limiting enzyme of fatty acid synthesis]) with the result being decreased malonyl-CoA levels in the hypothalamus. Decreased malonyl-CoA levels result in reduced inhibition of fatty acid uptake into the mitochondrial. Thus, when malonyl-CoA levels fall fat oxidation increases. This reduces the overall level of fatty acids and fatty acid esters within cells of the hypothalamus, triggering the synthesis and release of orexigenic peptides with an increased desire for food intake.

7. Hypothalamic fructose metabolism is associated with an increased desire for food intake. Altered feeding behaviors with fructose consumption are related to changing levels of which of the following metabolic intermediates?
A. acetyl-CoA
B. citrate
C. fructose 2,6-bisphosphate
D. malonyl-CoA
E. pyruvate

Answer D: Hypothalamic fructose metabolism bypasses rapidly depletes ATP levels resulting in increased AMP levels. The rise in AMP results in activation of AMPK which, in turn, leads to phosphorylation and inhibition of acetyl-CoA carboxylase (ACC) with the result being decreased malonyl-CoA levels in the hypothalamus. Hypothalamic malonyl-CoA is a key intermediate in the regulation of feeding behavior and overall energy balance initiated via signaling cascades within the hypothalamus. During periods when energy expenditure exceeds intake, such as during fasting, malonyl-CoA levels in the hypothalamus are low. Following food intake there is a rapid rise in hypothalamic malonyl-CoA levels. The changes in hypothalamic malonyl-CoA levels are followed quickly by changes in expression of orexigenic and anorexigenic peptides.

8. Although fructose-1,6-bisphosphatase (F1,6BPase) deficiency can lead to infant mortality due to severely impaired gluconeogenesis, beyond childhood afflicted individuals develop hypoglycemia usually only associated with fasting or febrile infections. Given the role of F1,6BPase in overall carbohydrate metabolism, which of the following metabolites would be expected to increase in the plasma of these patients following depletion of hepatic glycogen stores?
A. acetyl-CoA
B. cholesterol
C. free fatty acids
D. lactate
E. pyruvate

Answer D: During normal hepatic gluconeogenesis, the major substrates for glucose synthesis are alanine, pyruvate, and lactate. Defective F1,6BPase would restrict the flow of alanine and lactate conversion to pyruvate and the subsequent input of pyruvate into gluconeogenesis. The net effect would be a significant increase in circulating levels of lactate.

9. An advertisement promotes energy bars containing fructose as ideal food to take on extreme mountain-climbing expeditions. Which of the following statements concerning fructose absorption is true?

A. absorption of fructose into an intestinal epithelial cell is by facilitated transport and thus does not require energy
B. metabolism of fructose generates more energy than glucose
C. some fructose is already absorbed in the mouth and hence is the fastest way to get energy
D. the presence of fructose aids in absorption of vitamin A, C, and D
E. the presence of fructose inhibits reabsorption of glucose, which is then more readily available for muscle activity

Answer A: Carbohydrate absorption occurs at enterocytes of the upper region of small intestinal villi. Fructose absorption is via the facilitated transporters GLUT5 across the apical enterocyte membrane and GLUT2 across the basolateral enterocyte. Glucose and galactose on the other hand are transported into enterocytes on carriers in combination with a sodium ion. The energy for this secondary active transport is provided by the electrochemical sodium gradient that is created by Na/K-ATPases. Experimental conditions that collapse the sodium electrochemical gradient, hypoxia, or poisoning of the Na/K-ATPase by ouabain inhibit glucose, but not fructose absorption. Nevertheless, the physiological importance of "saving energy" under extreme conditions such as mountain climbing through the use of fructose as energy source is questionable.

Checklist

✓ Dietary fructose is absorbed by the intestine via GLUT5-mediated uptake.

✓ Metabolism of fructose in the intestine, liver, and kidneys involves fructokinase (ketohexokinase [KHK]).

✓ Fructose can be metabolized by most tissues but its utilization within the liver is most significant physiologically.

✓ Fructose metabolism in the glycolytic pathway, following fructokinase phosphorylation to fructose 1-phosphate, effectively bypasses all of the hormonal and allosteric regulations imposed on glucose metabolism.

✓ Fructose metabolism in the hypothalamus results in enhanced desire to consume food due to depletion of ATP with resultant activation of AMPK and subsequent altered metabolic processes.

✓ Defects in fructose metabolic genes can lead to a spectrum of disorders from relatively benign hyperfructosemia and fructosuria to neonatal fatal hypoglycemia and lactic acidemia.

CHAPTER 12

Carbohydrates: Galactose Metabolism

CHAPTER OUTLINE

High-Yield Terms

β-Galactosidase: intestinal enzyme complex involved in the hydrolysis of lactose to glucose and galactose. Commonly called lactase

Leloir pathway: primary pathway for the conversion of galactose to glucose

Galactosemia: results from defects in any of the 3 primary genes involved in conversion of galactose to glucose

Dietary Galactose

A major form of galactose found in these complex biomolecules is *N*-acetylgalactosamine (GalNAc). GalNAc is not acquired from the diet but is formed from dietary galactose. The major source of galactose in the human diet is from the disaccharide, lactose, found in dairy products. This sugar comprises around 2% to 8% of milk solids. Lactose is a disaccharide of glucose and galactose. Upon consumption of lactose, it is hydrolyzed to glucose and galactose via the action of the intestinal enzyme complex called β-galactosidase (lactase-glycosylceramidase). The enzyme complex is attached to the surface of intestinal brush border cells via a GPI linkage (see Chapter 38). There are 2 enzymatic activities associated with the β-galactosidase complex, one that hydrolyzes the β-glycosidic linkage in lactose (thereby releasing glucose and galactose), while the other activity hydrolyzes the β-glycosidic bond connecting galactose or glucose to ceramide in ingested glycolipids. Galactose is subsequently absorbed by intestinal enterocytes via the action of the same sodium (Na^+)-dependent glucose transporter (SGLT1) that is responsible for glucose absorption. Galactose enters the blood from intestinal enterocytes via GLUT2-mediated transport as for glucose and fructose.

Entry of Galactose Into Glycolysis

Although glucose is the form of sugar stored as glycogen within cells, galactose is utilized via conversion to glucose, which can then be oxidized in glycolysis or stored as glycogen. Indeed, up to 30% of ingested galactose is incorporated into glycogen. Galactose enters glycolysis by its conversion to glucose-1-phosphate (G1P). This occurs through a series of steps that is referred to as the Leloir pathway, named after Luis Federico Leloir who determined the overall process of galactose utilization. First, the galactose is phosphorylated by galactokinase to yield galactose-1-phosphate. The galactokinase protein is encoded by the *GALK1* gene. There is another gene identified as *GALK2* that was originally thought to encode a second galactokinase but was subsequently shown to be a GalNAc kinase. Epimerization of galactose-1-phosphate to G1P requires the transfer of UDP from uridine diphosphoglucose (UDP-glucose) catalyzed by galactose-1-phosphate uridyltransferase (GALT). The GALT-catalyzed reaction generates UDP-galactose and G1P. The UDP-galactose is epimerized to UDP-glucose by UDP-galactose-4 epimerase (GALE). The UDP portion is exchanged for phosphate-generating glucose-1-phosphate, which then is converted to G6P by phosphoglucose mutase. GALE catalyzes 2 distinct but analogous epimerization reactions, the epimerization of UDP-galactose to UDP-glucose and the epimerization of UDP-*N*-acetylgalactosamine to UDP-*N*-acetylglucosamine (Figure 12-1).

There are additional pathways of galactose metabolism in humans that do not involve all 3 of the enzymes of the classical Leloir pathway. Galactose can be converted to UDP-glucose by the sequential activities of GALK, UDP-glucose pyrophosphorylase (UGP2), and GALE. Galactose can also be reduced to galactitol by NADPH-dependent aldose reductase. This latter reaction becomes significant in the context of GALT and GALK1 deficiencies that result in galactosemias (Clinical Box 12-1). Finally, galactose can be oxidized to galactonate by galactose dehydrogenase. Under normal conditions, these alternative pathways are responsible for the metabolism of only trace quantities of galactose.

Disorders of Galactose Metabolism

Three inherited disorders of galactose metabolism have been delineated that all result in galactosemia of varying degrees. Classic galactosemia refers to a disorder arising from profound deficiency of the enzyme galactose-1-phosphate uridyltransferase (GALT) and is termed type 1 galactosemia (see Clinical Box 12-1).

High-Yield Concept

Galactose is an essential carbohydrate needed in the formation of glycolipids and glycoproteins that when present on the surfaces of cells enables cell–cell communication, immune recognition, growth factor-receptor interactions involved in signal transduction events, and many other critical cellular processes.

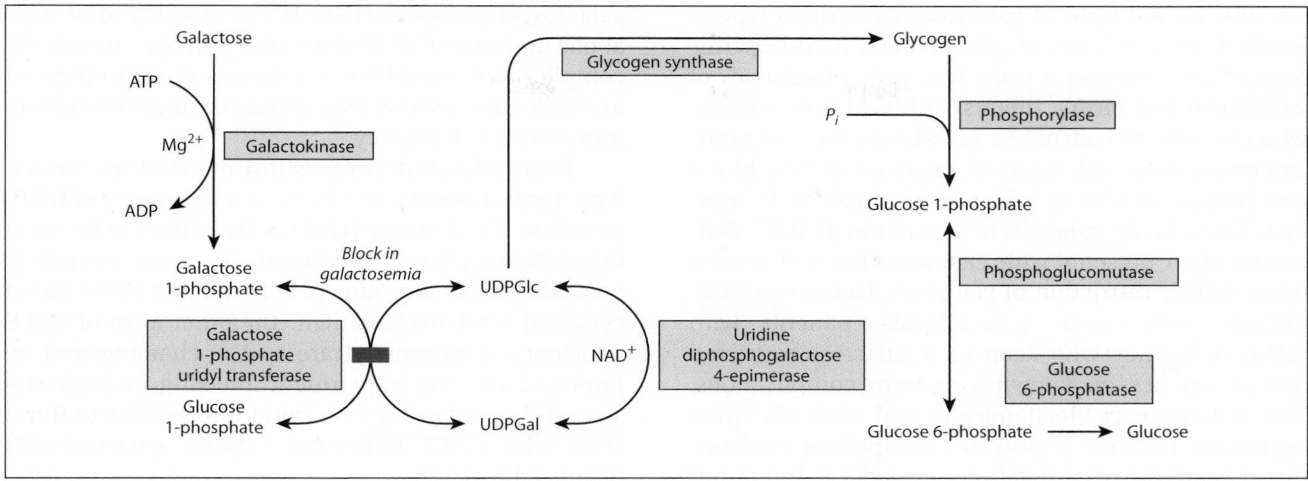

FIGURE 12-1: Pathway of conversion of (A) galactose to glucose in the liver. Murray RK, Bender DA, Botham KM, Kennelly PJ, Rodwell VW, Weil PA. *Harper's Illustrated Biochemistry,* 29th ed. New York, NY: McGraw-Hill; 2012.

CLINICAL BOX 12-1: GALACTOSEMIAS

Type 1 galactosemia (classic galactosemia) results from defects in the *galactose-1-phosphate uridyltransferase* (*GALT*) gene that leads to severe reductions in enzyme activity. The disease occurs with a frequency between 1:30,000 and 1:60,000 live births. Over 230 different mutations have been described in the gene encoding human *GALT*, resulting in type 1 galactosemia. The most commonly detected mutation in Caucasians results in the *Q188R* allele defined by the substitution of arginine (R) for glutamine (Q) at amino acid 188, which lies close to the active site of the enzyme. Homozygotes for the *Q188R* allele show very little to no GALT activity in their erythrocytes. The majority of heterozygotes are found to have no GALT activity, while others exhibit a low level of enzyme activity generally no more than 20% of the wild type. Whereas the Q188R allele is most common in Caucasians, the most commonly detected mutations in European populations are K285N, S135L, and N314D. The K285N mutation is associated with 0% and 50% *GALT* activity in homozygous and heterozygous individuals, respectively. Classic galactosemia most often presents within the first weeks after birth and manifests by a failure of neonates to thrive. Vomiting and diarrhea occur following ingestion of milk; hence individuals are termed lactose intolerant. Clinical findings of these disorders include impaired liver function (which if left untreated leads to severe cirrhosis), elevated blood galactose, hypergalactosemia, hyperchloremic metabolic acidosis, urinary galactitol excretion, and hyperaminoaciduria. Upon physical examination infants will be jaundiced and have hepatomegaly. Due to the involvement of the liver, patients will exhibit prolonged bleeding after venous or arterial sampling or will show excessive bruising. Unless controlled by exclusion of galactose from the diet, these galactosemias can go on to produce blindness and fatal liver damage. Blindness is due to the conversion of circulating galactose to the sugar alcohol galactitol, by an NADPH-dependent aldose reductase that is present in neural tissue and in the lens of the eye. At normal circulating levels of galactose, this enzyme activity causes no pathological effects. However, a high concentration of galactitol in the lens causes osmotic swelling, with the resultant formation of cataracts and other symptoms. The principal treatment of these disorders is to eliminate lactose from the diet. Even on a galactose-restricted diet, *GALT*-deficient individuals exhibit urinary galactitol excretion and persistently elevated erythrocyte galactose-1-phosphate levels. In addition, even with life long restriction of dietary galactose, many patients with classic galactosemia go on to develop serious long-term complications. These long-term complications include ovarian failure in female patients, cognitive impairment, and ataxic neurological disease.

The second form of galactosemia, termed type 2, results from deficiency of galactokinase (GALK1). This form of galactosemia is quite rare with a frequency of <1:100,000 live births. Infants with GALK deficiency, who continue to consume a milk-based diet, accumulate abnormally high levels of galactose in their blood and tissues, similar to infants with classic galactosemia. Like classic galactosemia patients, GALK1 deficiency often presents with cataracts that will resolve upon dietary restriction of galactose. However, unlike patients with classic galactosemia, patients with GALK deficiency who keep to a galactose-restricted diet experience no known long-term complications. This difference is biochemically and clinically quite significant because it provides compelling evidence that it is not the accumulation of galactose, but rather galactose-1-phosphate (Gal-1P), or possibly some metabolic derivative Gal-1P, that is the primary cause of the complications, in addition to cataracts, that are observed in classic galactosemia patients and the more rare severe form of GALE deficiency.

The third disorder of galactose metabolism, termed type 3 galactosemia, results from a deficiency of UDP-galactose-4-epimerase (GALE). Two different forms of this deficiency have been found. The more commonly occurring deficiency affects only red and white blood cells and is relatively benign. The other form of GALE deficiency is extremely rare and is characterized by profound enzyme impairment affecting multiple tissues and manifesting with symptoms similar to those seen with GALT deficiency (classic galactosemia) (Clinical Box 12-1).

REVIEW QUESTIONS

1. A 9-month-old child is presented to the emergency room by his parents who report that he has been vomiting and has severe diarrhea. The episodes of vomiting began when the parents started feeding their child cow's milk. The infant exhibits signs of failing to thrive. Laboratory tests show elevated blood galactose, hypergalactosuria, metabolic acidosis, albuminuria, and hyperaminoaciduria. These clinical and laboratory findings are most consistent with which of the following disorders?

A. alkaptonuria
B. essential fructosuria
C. hereditary galactosemia
D. Menkes disease
E. von Gierke disease

Answer C: This patient is suffering from classic (type 1) galactosemia. Type 1 galactosemia occurs as a consequence of mutations in the gene encoding *GALT*. Classic galactosemia manifests by a failure of neonates to thrive. Vomiting and diarrhea occur following ingestion of milk; hence individuals are termed lactose intolerant. Clinical findings include impaired liver function (which if left untreated leads to severe cirrhosis), elevated blood galactose, hypergalactosemia, hyperchloremic metabolic acidosis, urinary galactitol excretion and hyperaminoaciduria. Unless controlled by exclusion of galactose from the diet, these patients can go on to develop blindness and fatal liver damage. Blindness is due to the conversion of circulating galactose to the sugar alcohol galactitol, by an NADPH-dependent aldose reductase that is present in neural tissue and in the lens of the eye.

2. You are examining a patient who complains of gastric discomfort following the consumption of milk. Additional signs and symptoms include liver and kidney impairment as well as neural involvement. Blood work indicates an increased concentration of galactose-1-phosphate. This patient likely has a defect in which of the following enzymes?

A. fructose-1,6-bisphosphatase
B. galactokinase
C. galactose-1-phosphate uridyltransferase
D. glucokinase
E. ketohexokinase (fructokinase)

Answer C: This patient is suffering from classic (type 1) galactosemia. Type 1 galactosemia occurs as a consequence of mutations in the gene encoding *galactose-1-phosphate uridyltransferase* (*GALT*). Classic galactosemia manifests by a failure of neonates to thrive. Vomiting and diarrhea occur following ingestion of milk; hence individuals are termed lactose intolerant. Clinical findings include impaired liver function (which if left untreated leads to severe cirrhosis), elevated blood galactose, hypergalactosemia, hyperchloremic metabolic acidosis, urinary galactitol excretion, and hyperaminoaciduria.

3. A defect in which of the following enzymes of galactose metabolism would most likely be associated with hypoglycemia, hepatomegaly, and hyperaminoaciduria?

A. galactokinase
B. galactose-1-phosphate uridyltransferase
C. galactose-4-epimerase
D. phosphoglucomutase
E. UDP-glucose pyrophosphorylase

Answer B: Mutations in the gene encoding *galactose-1-phosphate uridyltransferase* (*GALT*) result in classic galactosemia. This disorder manifests by a failure of neonates to thrive. Vomiting and diarrhea occur following ingestion of milk; hence individuals are termed lactose intolerant. Clinical findings include impaired liver function (which if left untreated leads to severe cirrhosis), elevated blood galactose, and hyperaminoaciduria.

4. A 5-week-old girl, who appeared to be healthy at birth, develops diarrhea and vomiting a few days after birth. Your current examination reveals that she has hepatomegaly, jaundice, and early cataract formation and is not meeting developmental milestones. You suspect that she has which of the following conditions?
A. galactosemia
B. Hurler syndrome
C. pyloric stenosis
D Tay-Sachs disease
E. Type I glycogenosis (von Gierke disease)

Answer A: Galactosemia is an autosomal recessive disorder due (in this more common and more severe form of the disease) to a lack of galactose-1-phosphate uridyl transferase. This results in the formation and accumulation of galactose metabolites. If the infant's diet is not modified to exclude milk products, this will result in damage to the liver (fatty change, cholestasis, cirrhosis, liver failure), eyes (cataract formation), and brain (mental retardation).

5. Deficiencies in both galactokinase (GALK) and galactose-1-phosphate uridyltransferase (GALT) result in galactosemia. Which of the following additional symptoms would be useful in a differential diagnosis to confirm GALK deficiency from GALT deficiency?
A. hepatomegaly
B. hypotonia
C. lenticular cataracts
D. lethargy
E. urinary galactitol excretion

Answer C: Patients with GALK deficiency often present with cataracts that will resolve upon dietary restriction of galactose. However, although patients with classic galactosemia (GALT deficiency) also can develop cataracts, the prevalence among classic galactosemics is markedly less than among GALK-deficient patients due to the extremely high levels of galactitol found in the latter.

Checklist

✓ The primary source of galactose is milk sugar, lactose.

✓ Galactose is absorbed from the gut via the SGLT1 sugar transporter and enters the blood via the intestinal GLUT2 transporter.

✓ *N*-acetylgalactosamine (GalNAc) cannot be supplied in the diet and thus, humans require galactose in the diet to serve as a precursor for this amino sugar, which is a critical component of cellular function.

✓ Galactose carbons can be completely oxidized for ATP production following conversion to glucose or stored as glucose in glycogen polymers.

✓ Defects in galactose conversion to glucose result in galactosemias, with classic galactosemia, caused by defects in the *GALT* gene, being the most severe form.

CHAPTER 13 Carbohydrates: Gluconeogenesis, the Synthesis of New Glucose

CHAPTER OUTLINE

High-Yield Terms

Cori cycle: describes the interrelationship between lactate production during anaerobic glycolysis and the use of lactate carbons to produce glucose via hepatic gluconeogenesis

Endogenous glucose production: designated EGP, refers to the process of glucose production via gluconeogenesis

Glucose-alanine cycle: describes the interrelationship between pyruvate transamination and alanine during skeletal muscle glycolysis and delivery to the liver where the alanine is deaminated back to pyruvate, which is then diverted into hepatic gluconeogenesis

Critical Bypass Reactions of Gluconeogenesis

Gluconeogenesis is the biosynthesis of new glucose, (ie, not glucose from glycogen). The production of glucose from other carbon skeletons is necessary during periods of fasting and starvation. This is acutely true for the testes, erythrocytes, and kidney medullary cells since each is exclusively dependent upon glucose oxidation for ATP production. The brain, although not restricted solely to glucose, requires adequate rates of gluconeogenesis since it is the organ of highest daily glucose consumption. In addition to glucose, the brain can derive energy from ketone bodies (Chapter 25). The primary carbon skeletons used for gluconeogenesis are derived from pyruvate, lactate, glycerol, and the amino acids alanine and glutamine. The liver is the major site of gluconeogenesis; however, as discussed below, the kidney and the small intestine also have important roles to play in this pathway (Figure 13-1).

Pyruvate to Phosphoenolpyruvate, Bypass 1

Conversion of pyruvate to phosphoenolpyruvate (PEP) requires the action of 2 enzymes. The first is an ATP-requiring reaction catalyzed by pyruvate carboxylase (PC), which catalyzes the carboxylation of pyruvate to the TCA cycle intermediate, oxaloacetic acid (OAA). The second enzyme of bypass 1 is the GTP-dependent PEP carboxykinase (PEPCK), which converts OAA to PEP. Since PC incorporated CO_2 into pyruvate and it is subsequently released in the PEPCK reaction, no net fixation of carbon occurs. Human cells contain almost equal amounts of mitochondrial and cytosolic PEPCK (designated PEPCK-m and PEPCK-c, respectively), so this second reaction can occur in either cellular compartment.

If OAA is converted to PEP by PEPCK-m, it is transported to the cytosol where it is a direct substrate for gluconeogenesis and nothing further is required. However, the OAA produced by PC (or produced via the TCA cycle) can serve as a gluconeogenic substrate within the cytosol. This occurs by transamination of OAA to aspartate or reduction to malate and coupled transport via a pathway called the malate-aspartate shuttle (see Figure 10-2). The malate-aspartate shuttle is also a major mechanism for transferring electrons from cytosolic NADH into mitochondrial NADH where they can be shunted into oxidative phosphorylation (Chapter 17).

Transamination of OAA to aspartate allows the aspartate to be transported to the cytosol where the reverse transamination takes place yielding cytosolic OAA. This transamination reaction requires continuous transport of glutamate into, and α-ketoglutarate out of, the mitochondrion. Therefore, this process is limited by the availability of these other substrates. Either of these latter 2 reactions will predominate when the substrate for gluconeogenesis is lactate. The reduction of OAA to malate requires NADH, which will be accumulating in the mitochondrion as the energy charge increases. The increased energy charge will allow cells to carry out the ATP costly process of gluconeogenesis. The resultant malate is transported to the cytosol where it is oxidized to OAA by cytosolic malate dehydrogenase (MDH), which requires NAD^+ and yields NADH.

The NADH produced during the cytosolic oxidation of malate to OAA is utilized during the glyceraldehyde-3-phosphate dehydrogenase (GAPDH) reaction of glycolysis. The coupling of these 2 oxidation-reduction reactions is required to keep gluconeogenesis functional when pyruvate is the principal source of carbon atoms. The conversion of OAA to malate predominates when pyruvate (derived from glycolysis or amino acid catabolism) is the source of carbon atoms for gluconeogenesis. When in the cytoplasm, OAA is converted to PEP by PEPCK-c.

The net result of the PC and PEPCK reactions is:

$$\text{Pyruvate} + \text{ATP} + \text{GTP} + H_2O \rightarrow \text{PEP} + \text{ADP} + \text{GDP} + P_i + 2H^+$$

High-Yield Concept

The 3 reactions of glycolysis that proceed with a large negative free-energy change are bypassed during gluconeogenesis by using different enzymes. The bypass reactions represent the reversal of the pyruvate kinase, phosphofructokinase-1 (PFK1), and hexokinase/glucokinase-catalyzed reactions.

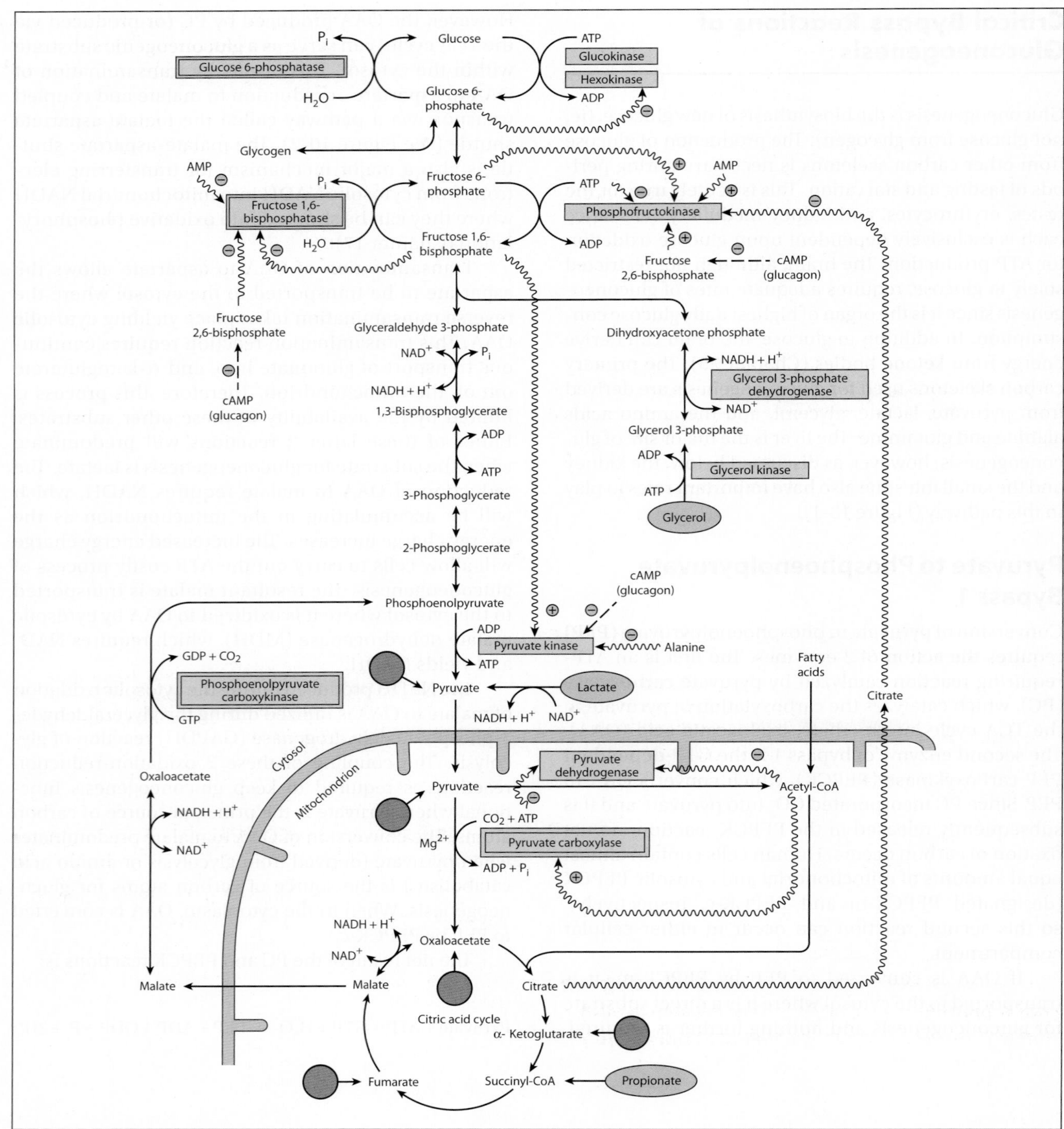

FIGURE 13-1: Major pathways and regulation of gluconeogenesis and glycolysis in the liver. Entry points of glucogenic amino acids after transamination are indicated by arrows extended from circles. The key gluconeogenic enzymes are enclosed in double-bordered boxes. The ATP required for gluconeogenesis is supplied by the oxidation of fatty acids. Propionate is of quantitative importance only in ruminants. Arrows with wavy shafts signify allosteric effects; dash-shafted arrows, covalent modification by reversible phosphorylation. High concentrations of alanine act as a "gluconeogenic signal" by inhibiting glycolysis at the pyruvate kinase step. Murray RK, Bender DA, Botham KM, Kennelly PJ, Rodwell VW, Weil PA. *Harper's Illustrated Biochemistry*, 29th ed. New York, NY: McGraw-Hill; 2012.

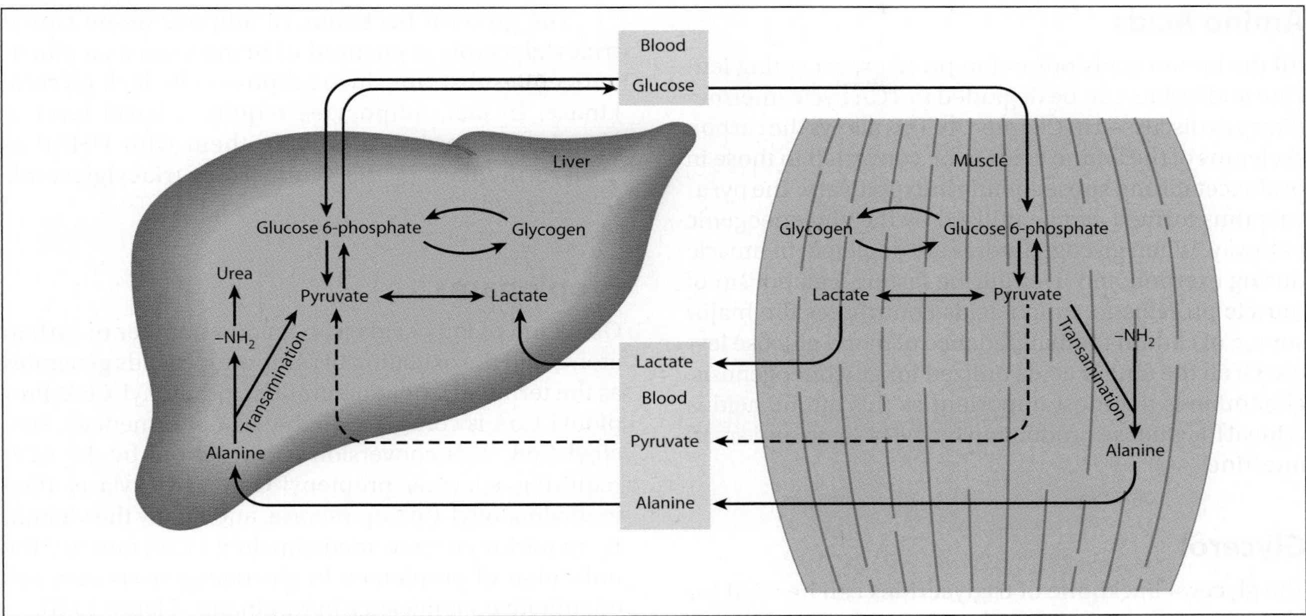

FIGURE 13-2: The lactic acid (Cori cycle) and glucose-alanine cycles. Murray RK, Bender DA, Botham KM, Kennelly PJ, Rodwell VW, Weil PA. *Harper's Illustrated Biochemistry*, 29th ed. New York, NY: McGraw-Hill; 2012.

Fructose 1,6-Bisphosphate to Fructose 6-Phosphate, Bypass 2

Fructose-1,6-bisphosphate (F1,6BP) conversion to fructose 6-phosphate (F6P) is the reverse of the rate-limiting step of glycolysis. The reaction, a simple hydrolysis, is catalyzed by fructose 1,6-bisphosphatase (F1,6BPase). Like the regulation of glycolysis occurring at the PFK1 reaction, the F1,6BPase reaction is a major point of control of gluconeogenesis (see Figure 10-4).

Glucose 6-Phosphate (G6P) to Glucose (or Glycogen), Bypass 3

G6P is converted to glucose through the action of glucose 6-phosphatase (G6Pase). This reaction is also a simple hydrolysis reaction like that of F1,6BPase. In the kidney, muscle, and, especially, the liver, G6P can be shunted toward glycogen if blood glucose levels are adequate. The reactions necessary for glycogen synthesis (Chapter 14) are an alternate bypass series of reactions.

Substrates for Gluconeogenesis

Lactate

Lactate is a major source of carbon atoms for glucose synthesis by gluconeogenesis in the liver. In erythrocytes and during anaerobic glycolysis in skeletal muscle, pyruvate is reduced to lactate by lactate dehydrogenase (LDH). This reaction serves 2 critical functions during anaerobic glycolysis. First, in the direction of lactate formation the LDH reaction requires NADH and yields NAD^+ which is then available for use by the GAPDH reaction of glycolysis. These 2 reactions are, therefore, intimately coupled during anaerobic glycolysis. Secondly, the lactate produced by the LDH reaction is released to the blood stream and transported to the liver where it is converted to glucose. The glucose is then returned to the blood for use by muscle as an energy source and to replenish glycogen stores. This cycle is termed the Cori cycle (Figure 13-2).

Pyruvate

Pyruvate, generated in muscle and other peripheral tissues, can be transaminated to alanine which is returned to the liver for gluconeogenesis. This pathway is termed the glucose-alanine cycle (see Figure 13-2). The glucose-alanine cycle serves a critical mechanism for muscle to eliminate waste nitrogen from amino acid catabolism while replenishing its energy supply as glucose. Within the liver the alanine is converted back to pyruvate and used as a gluconeogenic substrate or oxidized in the TCA cycle. The amino nitrogen is converted to urea in the urea cycle and excreted by the kidneys.

Amino Acids

All the amino acids present in proteins, excepting leucine and lysine, can be degraded to TCA cycle intermediates as discussed in Chapter 30. This allows the carbon skeletons of the amino acids to be converted to those in oxaloacetate and subsequently into pyruvate. The pyruvate thus formed can be utilized by the gluconeogenic pathway. When glycogen stores are depleted, in muscle during exertion and liver during fasting, catabolism of muscle proteins to amino acids contributes the major source of carbon for maintenance of blood glucose levels. Of all the amino acids utilized for gluconeogenesis, glutamine is the most important as this amino acid is critical for glucose production by the kidneys and small intestine.

Glycerol

The glycerol backbone of triglycerides can be used for gluconeogenesis. Indeed, the glycerol released from adipose tissue during periods of fasting provides a major source of carbon atom for hepatic gluconeogenesis. The glycerol is first phosphorylated to glycerol 3-phosphate by glycerol kinase followed by dehydrogenation to dihydroxyacetone phosphate (DHAP) by glycerol-3-phosphate dehydrogenase (GPD). The GPD reaction is the same as that used in the transport of cytosolic reducing equivalents into the mitochondrion for use in oxidative phosphorylation. This transport pathway is called the glycerol-phosphate shuttle (see Figure 10-3).

The glycerol backbone of adipose tissue stored triacylglycerols is ensured of being used as a gluconeogenic substrate since adipose cells lack glycerol kinase. In fact, adipocytes require a basal level of glycolysis in order to provide them with DHAP as an intermediate in the synthesis of triacylglycerols (Chapter 20).

Propionate

Oxidation of fatty acids with an odd number of carbon atoms and the oxidation of some amino acids generates as the terminal oxidation product, propionyl-CoA. Propionyl-CoA is converted to the TCA intermediate, succinyl-CoA. This conversion is carried out by the ATP-requiring enzyme, propionyl-CoA carboxylase, then methylmalonyl-CoA epimerase, and finally the vitamin B_{12} requiring enzyme, methylmalonyl-CoA mutase. The utilization of propionate in gluconeogenesis only has quantitative significance in ruminants (Figure 13-3).

Intestinal Gluconeogenesis: Glucose Homeostasis and Control of Feeding Behavior

The gut, in particular the small intestine, plays a critical role in the uptake and delivery of glucose from the diet. In addition, the small intestine participates in gluconeogenesis and thus, contributes to endogenous

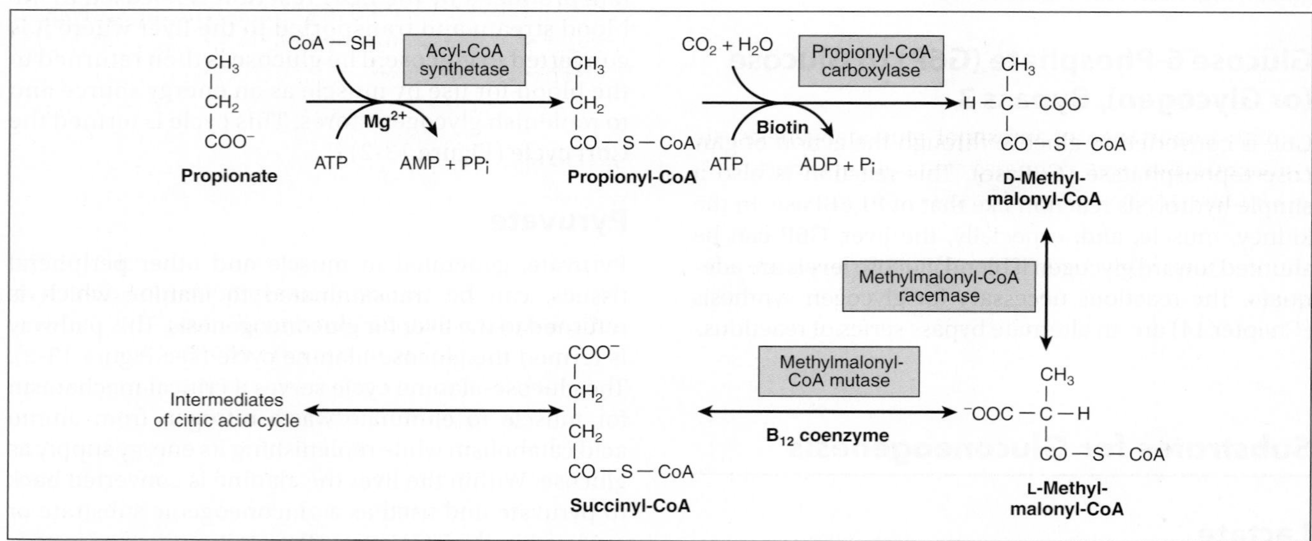

FIGURE 13-3: Metabolism of propionate. Murray RK, Bender DA, Botham KM, Kennelly PJ, Rodwell VW, Weil PA. *Harper's Illustrated Biochemistry*, 29th ed. New York: McGraw-Hill; 2012.

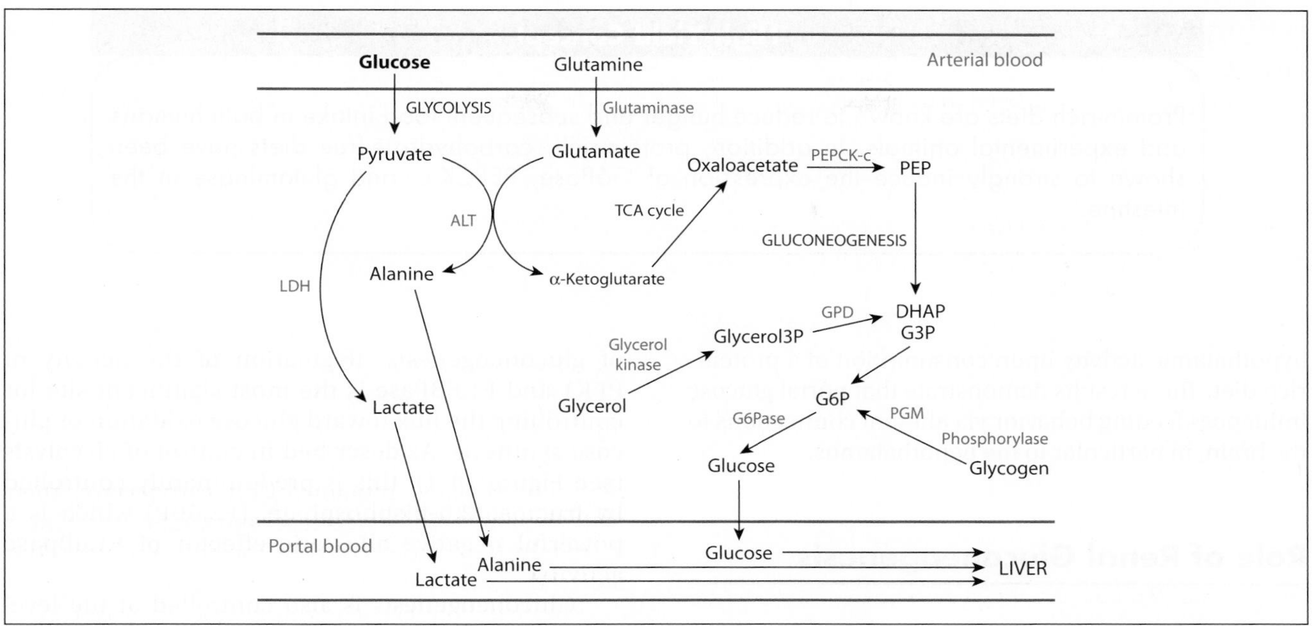

FIGURE 13-4: Pathways by which the small intestine contributes to maintenance of endogenous glucose production.
Reproduced with permission of themedicalbiochemistrypage, LLC.

glucose production, EGP (Figure 13-4). As such, the gut plays a central role in the overall regulation of glucose homeostasis. Only recently (a little more than 10 years ago) the expression of glucose 6-phosphatase (G6Pase) within enterocytes of the small intestine was characterized. Expression of G6Pase thus confers upon the intestine the ability to carry out gluconeogenesis. Glutamine serves as the major precursor of glucose formed within the small intestine. The genes for both G6Pase and the cytosolic form of phosphoenolpyruvate carboxykinase (PEPCK-c) are controlled by insulin in the small intestine, similarly to the regulation of these genes in the liver (Figure 13-4).

The importance of intestinal gluconeogenesis, to overall EGP, has been demonstrated both in experimental animals (mice with specific knockout of PEPCK-c in the liver) and in humans in the anhepatic phase during liver transplantation. Even with loss of hepatic PEPCK-c, there is an efficient adaptation to fasting conditions such that blood glucose levels decrease by only 30%. Simultaneously there occurs a significant increase in plasma glutamine concentration. These observations stressed the likely role of the kidney and/or intestine in glucose production, because glutamine is a major glucose precursor in the kidney and the small intestine, but not in the liver. The role of the intestine in plasma glucose control is demonstrated by the fact there are no observable differences in glucose concentration between arterial and portal blood. During periods of fasting, the small intestine accounts for approximately 20% of EGP by 48 hours and up to 35% by 72 hours.

In addition, the gut releases glucose to the portal circulation following the intake of a protein-rich, carbohydrate-free diet. The rate of glucose release by the gut can be 15% to 20% of total EGP when eating a protein-rich diet. Under these dietary conditions there is a demonstrable decrease in food intake in both humans and experimental animals. A similar decrease in food intake is observed in animals with an equivalent amount of glucose infusion directly into the portal vein. Under conditions where intestinal G6Pase is specifically abolished, protein-rich, carbohydrate-free diets do not lead to decreased. Chemical or surgical ablation of portal afferent nerve connections also results in loss of satiety induction by protein-rich diets or portal glucose infusion. Afferent nerves send nerve signals from various body locations to the brain. Brain areas involved in the control of feeding behaviors include the brain stem and the hypothalamus. Detailed discussion of the role of the hypothalamus in the control of feeding behaviors is presented in Chapter 44. Consuming a protein-rich diet (or glucose infusions into the portal vein in experimental animals) results in neuronal activation in several hypothalamic nuclei involved in feeding behavior including the arcuate nucleus (ARC), dorsomedial nucleus (DMN), ventromedial nucleus (VMN), and paraventricular nucleus (PVN). When intestinal afferent connections are destroyed, there is no increase in

High-Yield Concept

Protein-rich diets are known to reduce hunger and subsequent food intake in both humans and experimental animals. In addition, protein-rich, carbohydrate-free diets have been shown to strongly induce the expression of G6Pase, PEPCK-c, and glutaminase in the intestine.

hypothalamic activity upon consumption of a protein-rich diet. These results demonstrate that portal glucose influences feeding behavior via afferent connections to the brain, in particular to the hypothalamus.

Role of Renal Gluconeogenesis

Although the liver has the critical role of maintaining blood glucose homeostasis and therefore is the major site of gluconeogenesis, the kidney plays an important role. During periods of severe hypoglycemia that occur under conditions of hepatic failure, the kidney can provide glucose to the blood via renal gluconeogenesis. In the renal cortex, glutamine is the preferred substance for gluconeogenesis.

Glutamine is produced in high amounts by skeletal muscle during periods of fasting as a means to export the waste nitrogen resulting from amino acid catabolism. Through the actions of transaminases, a mole of waste ammonia is transferred to α-ketoglutarate via the glutamate dehydrogenase–catalyzed reaction yielding glutamate. Glutamate is then a substrate for glutamine synthetase which incorporates another mole of waste ammonia-generating glutamine (see Chapter 29). The glutamine is then transported to the kidneys where the reverse reactions occur liberating the ammonia and producing α-ketoglutarate which can enter the TCA cycle and the carbon atoms diverted to gluconeogenesis via oxaloacetate. This process serves 2 important functions. First, the ammonia (NH_3) that is liberated spontaneously ionizes to ammonium ion (NH_4^+) and is excreted in the urine effectively buffering the acids in the urine. Second, the glucose that is produced via gluconeogenesis provides the brain with critically needed energy.

Regulation of Gluconeogenesis

The regulation of gluconeogenesis is exerted in direct contrast to the regulation of glycolysis. In general, negative effectors of glycolysis are positive effectors of gluconeogenesis. Regulation of the activity of PFK1 and F1,6BPase is the most significant site for controlling the flux toward glucose oxidation or glucose synthesis. As described in control of glycolysis (see Figure 10-4), this is predominantly controlled by fructose 2,6-bisphosphate, (F2,6BP) which is a powerful negative allosteric effector of F1,6Bpase activity.

Gluconeogenesis is also controlled at the level of the pyruvate to PEP bypass. The hepatic signals elicited by glucagon or epinephrine lead to phosphorylation and inactivation of pyruvate kinase (PK) which will allow for an increase in the flux through gluconeogenesis. PK is also allosterically inhibited by ATP and alanine. The level of ATP signals adequate energy, while rising alanine levels indicate sufficient substrate for gluconeogenesis is available. Conversely, a reduction in energy levels as evidenced by increasing concentrations of ADP lead to inhibition of both PC and PEPCK. Allosteric activation of PC occurs through acetyl-CoA. Each of these regulations occurs on a short time scale, whereas long-term regulation can be effected at the level of PEPCK. The amount of this enzyme increases in response to prolonged glucagon stimulation. This situation would occur in a fasting individual or someone with an inadequate diet.

Whereas glucagon actions result in increased levels of cAMP and subsequent activation of gluconeogenesis, insulin action exerts the opposite effect. The mechanisms by which insulin turns off gluconeogenesis are complex but many of the mechanisms are coupled to alterations in cAMP levels. Insulin receptor activation results in increased phosphodiesterase which hydrolyses cAMP to AMP. At the level of the regulation of genes involved in gluconeogenesis, cAMP signaling also plays a role via regulation of the activity of the transcription factor, cAMP-response element-binding protein (CREB). Another mechanism by which insulin signaling antagonizes gluconeogenesis is through phosphorylation of the transcription factor FOXO1 which prevents it from migrating to the nucleus. FOXO1 is required for expression of the G6Pase and PEPCK genes.

REVIEW QUESTIONS

1. Acetyl-CoA enhances the rate of gluconeogenesis by acting as an obligate activator of which of the following enzymes?
A. phosphoenolpyruvate carboxykinase
B. phosphoglycerate kinase
C. phosphoglycerate mutase
D. pyruvate carboxylase
E. pyruvate kinase

Answer D: Unlike allosteric enzymes that function at some level in the absence on an allosteric effector, pyruvate carboxylase (PC) has no activity in the absence of acetyl-CoA. This property defines acetyl-CoA as an obligate activator of PC.

2. The purpose of the Cori cycle is to shift the metabolic burden in which of the following directions?
A. brain to liver
B. cardiac to skeletal muscle
C. liver to brain
D. liver to muscle
E. muscle to liver

Answer E: The Cori cycle represents a link between metabolic processes that occur in skeletal muscle and erythrocytes with those occurring in the liver. During anaerobic glycolysis in muscle the pyruvate is reduced to lactate. This pathway functions exclusively within erythrocytes because they lack mitochondria necessary for oxidation of NADH to NAD+. The lactate leaves these tissues, enters the blood, and is transported to the liver. Within the liver the lactate is oxidized to pyruvate and the pyruvate then serves as a substrate for glucose synthesis. The glucose leaves the liver and can be used by muscle and erythrocytes again.

3. The maximum capacity of the liver to carry out gluconeogenesis during starvation depends upon which of the following?
A. activation of glucose 6-phosphatase by insulin
B. activation of pyruvate kinase by insulin
C. induction of PEP carboxykinase synthesis by glucagon
D. inhibition of fructose 1,6-bisphosphatase by F1,6BP
E. inhibition of glucokinase by AMP

Answer C: When blood glucose levels fall, the pancreas releases glucagon to stimulate the liver to carry out gluconeogenesis. The effects of glucagon exerted on hepatic metabolism are both short term and long term. Prolonged fasting and starvation lead to long-term glucagon effects which are exerted at the level of gene expression. A major hepatic target of these long-term effects is the transcription of the *PEPCK* gene which is induced by glucagon.

4. A defect in lactate dehydrogenase would require the coupling of which enzyme reaction to that of glyceraldehyde-3-phosphate dehydrogenase in order for effective gluconeogenesis to proceed?
A. glucose-6-phosphate dehydrogenase
B. malate dehydrogenase
C. PEP carboxykinase
D. pyruvate carboxylase
E. pyruvate dehydrogenase

Answer B: In order for gluconeogenesis to occur, the NADH needed by the reversal of the glycolytic glyceraldehyde-3-phosphate dehydrogenase reaction must be supplied by either lactate dehydrogenase or the action of cytosolic malate dehydrogenase. In the latter reaction, the enzyme participates in the malate-aspartate shuttle.

5. You are studying a cell line in which gluconeogenesis is unaffected by changes in the level of acetyl-CoA. These cells most likely harbor an enzyme that has lost its allosteric binding site for acetyl-CoA. Which of the following enzymes is the candidate mutated-enzyme?
A. phosphoenolpyruvate carboxykinase
B. phosphoglycerate kinase
C. phosphoglycerate mutase
D. pyruvate carboxylase
E. pyruvate kinase

Answer D: Pyruvate carboxylase activity is absolutely dependent on allosteric activation by acetyl-CoA. Therefore, this must be the affected enzyme in these cells.

6. You are analyzing the activity of cells in culture following the introduction of a mutant form of lactate dehydrogenase exhibiting only 20% of normal activity. These cells continue to exhibit a deficit in gluconeogenesis when pyruvate instead of lactate is added as a substrate. Analysis of the NAD^+:NADH ratio indicates that it is elevated compared to normal cells. A defect in which of the following enzymes likely explains the observed results in these test cells?
A. glucose-6-phosphate dehydrogenase
B. malate dehydrogenase
C. PEP carboxykinase
D. pyruvate carboxylase
E. pyruvate dehydrogenase

Answer B: In order for gluconeogenesis to occur, the NADH needed by the reversal of the glycolytic glyceraldehyde-3-phosphate dehydrogenase reaction must be supplied by either lactate dehydrogenase or the action of cytosolic malate dehydrogenase. Since there is a deficit in the reduction of NAD^+ to NADH, the additional defective enzyme must be cytosolic malate dehydrogenase.

7. The ability of the liver to regulate the level of blood glucose is critical for survival. A number of sources of carbon atoms of nonhepatic origin are used by the liver for gluconeogenesis. However, the net conversion of carbons from fat into carbons of glucose cannot occur in humans because of which of the following?
- A. oxidation occurs in the mitochondria and gluconeogenesis occurs in the cytosol
- B. states of catabolism and anabolism are never concurrently active
- C. storage of fats occurs in adipose tissue and gluconeogenesis occurs in liver and kidney
- D. the carbons of acetyl-CoA from fat oxidation are lost as CO_2 in the TCA cycle
- E. the carbons of acetyl-CoA from fat oxidation inhibit conversion of pyruvate to oxaloacetate

Answer D: When the carbons of fatty acids are oxidized for energy production, the by-product of that process is the 2-carbon compound, acetyl-CoA. Acetyl-CoA can then enter the TCA cycle for complete oxidation. Although, several compounds of the TCA cycle can be directed into the gluconeogenic pathway of glucose synthesis, the carbons of acetyl-CoA cannot provide a net source of carbon in that latter pathway. This is due to the fact that, following entry of the 2 carbons of acetyl-CoA into the TCA cycle, 2 carbons are lost as CO_2 during the subsequent reactions of the cycle.

8. Shortly after birth, an infant presents with severe lactic acidemia, hyperammonemia, citrullinemia, and hyperlysinemia with the presence of α-ketoglurate in the urine. Definitive diagnoses of the causes of severe lactic acidemia are difficult and although these symptoms overlap with those seen with some of the urea cycle defect diseases, this is not the case with this neonate. A defect in which of the following enzymes would be expected to present with these findings?
- A. acetyl-CoA carboxylase
- B. electron transfer flavoproteinubiquinone oxidoreductase (EFT-QO)
- C. glutamic acid decarboxylase (GAD)
- D. phosphorylase
- E. pyruvate carboxylase

Answer E: Pyruvate carboxylase is the first enzyme in the gluconeogenic conversion of pyruvate carbons into glucose. A defect in pyruvate carboxylase would restrict the conversion of lactate into pyruvate and then subsequently to glucose. This would lead to severe lactic academia. The other symptoms are primarily the result of liver damage due to impaired gluconeogenesis.

9. During early fasting, glycogen is used as a source of glucose for the blood. After liver glycogen is depleted which of the following occurs?
- A. amino acids of muscle proteins are used to synthesize glucose in the liver
- B. blood glucose falls below 5mM until carbohydrate is eaten
- C. fatty acids of adipose tissue are converted into glucose in the liver
- D. liver fatty acids are degraded as precursors for blood glucose
- E. muscle glycogen is used as a source of glucose for the blood

Answer A: During periods of fasting and starvation, when liver glycogen levels are depleted, the major source of carbon atom for hepatic gluconeogenesis is from the amino acids released due to protein degradation within skeletal muscle.

10. When pyruvate is the substrate for gluconeogenesis, which of the following is the fate of oxaloacetate prior to traversing the mitochondrial membrane?
- A. conversion to phosphoenolpyruvate
- B. oxidation to malate
- C. reduction to malate
- D. transamination to aspartate
- E. transamination to glutamate

Answer C: The inner mitochondrial membrane is impermeable to oxaloacetate (OAA). In order for the carbon atoms of OAA to be transported out into the cytosol, where they can serve as precursors for glucose synthesis, OAA is reduced to malate. The malate is transported across the inner mitochondrial membrane where in the cytosol is oxidized to OAA.

11. Which of the following compounds would be utilized by a person on a carbohydrate-free diet as a source of carbon atoms for de novo glucose synthesis?
- A. palmitate
- B. β-hydroxybutyrate
- C. glycerol
- D. cholesterol
- E. acetoacetate

Answer C: In the absence of adequate carbohydrate the body will begin to divert stored fats into the metabolic pool in order to allow for adequate energy production. In addition, the liver will oxidize fatty acids to acetyl-CoA and then divert the acetyl-CoA into ketone synthesis to ensure the brain receives adequate amounts of an oxidizable energy source. When adipose tissue is stimulated to release fatty acids stored in triglycerides, the glycerol backbone diffuses into the blood and is delivered to the liver. Within the liver, glycerol is phosphorylated and converted to DHAP and then diverted into the glucose production via gluconeogenesis.

12. Deficiencies in the enzyme glucose 6-phosphatase are likely to lead to which of the following?
A. decreased glucagon production
B. decreased skeletal muscle glycogen accumulation
C. hyperglycemia
D. increased hepatic glycogen accumulation
E. increased accumulation of unbranched glycogen

Answer D: Deficiencies in glucose 6-phosphatase represent the causes of type 1 glycogen storage disease, more commonly called von Gierke disease. The hallmark features of this disease are hypoglycemia, lactic acidosis, hyperuricemia, and hyperlipidemia. When the liver is unable to release free glucose, it is diverted into excess glycogen storage which leads to hepatomegaly and consequent hepatic dysfunction.

13. A 44-year-old man is brought to the emergency room after he was rescued from being trapped under rubble in a building collapse for 4 days. Blood work shows that his serum glucose concentration is within the reference range. Which of the following processes is the most likely explanation for the maintenance of a normal serum glucose concentration in this patient?
A. decreased ketone body formation
B. gluconeogenesis
C. hepatic glycogen breakdown
D. increased hepatic glycogen storage
E. protein synthesis

Answer B: During periods of starvation and fasting the body will begin to divert stored fats into the metabolic pool in order to allow for adequate energy production. When adipose tissue is stimulated to release fatty acids stored in triglycerides, the glycerol backbone diffuses into the blood and is delivered to the liver. Within the liver glycerol is phosphorylated and converted to DHAP and then diverted into the glucose production via gluconeogenesis.

14. Plasma urea concentration is frequently up to 5-fold greater after a 5-day fast than after following a normal diet. This increase in urea concentration most likely reflects an increase in which of the following?
A. activity of carbamoyl phosphate synthetase I (CPS I)
B. rates of synthesis of ketone bodies
C. rates of transport of amino acids into skeletal muscle
D. rates of transport of fatty acids into skeletal muscle
E. use of amino acids for hepatic gluconeogenesis

Answer E: Protein breakdown into constituent amino acids provides an important source of carbon for oxidative energy production. When amino acids are oxidized, the nitrogen is first transferred to a suitable α-keto acid acceptor such as α-ketoglutarate. Eventually the waste nitrogen from hepatic amino acid metabolism is diverted into the urea cycle for excretion in a nontoxic form. This accounts for the increased plasma urea concentrations following fasting.

15. A normal subject fasts overnight. In the morning serum glucose concentrations are within the reference range. Which of the following is the best explanation for this result?
A. hepatic gluconeogenesis in response to insulin
B. hepatic gluconeogenesis in response to glucagon
C. hepatic ketogenesis in response to glucagon
D. muscle glycogenolysis in response to glucagon
E. muscle ketogenesis in response to insulin

Answer B: When blood glucose levels fall during the overnight period, the pancreas secretes glucagon. Glucagon binds to receptors on hepatocytes and triggers a series of metabolic changes that shift hepatic metabolism to glucose synthesis via gluconeogenesis.

16. A 2-year-old boy with weakness on exertion is found to have a pyruvate carboxylase deficiency. Which of the following compounds could this child use as a substrate for gluconeogenesis?
A. alanine
B. glycerol
C. lactate
D. proline
E. pyruvate

Answer B: A deficiency in pyruvate carboxylase would restrict the use of carbons from pyruvate, alanine, and lactate for glucose synthesis via gluconeogenesis.

Therefore, the burden is shifted to the use of the glycerol backbone of stored triglycerides. Glycerol is phosphorylated within hepatocytes to glycerol 3-phosphate and then converted to DHAP via the action of glycerol-3-phosphate dehydrogenase. The DHAP then can be used for glucose production via gluconeogenesis.

17. An obese 25-year-old woman starts following an extreme low-carbohydrate, high-fat diet. Which of the following components or immediate metabolites of her new diet can be used to help maintain adequate serum glucose concentration?

A. acetoacetate
B. cholesterol
C. glycerol
D. hydroxybutyrate
E. palmitate

Answer C: In the absence of adequate carbohydrate the body will begin to divert stored fats into the metabolic pool in order to allow for adequate energy production. In addition, the liver will oxidize fatty acids to acetyl-CoA and then divert the acetyl-CoA into ketone synthesis to ensure the brain receives adequate amounts of an oxidizable energy source. When adipose tissue is stimulated to release fatty acids stored in triglycerides, the glycerol backbone diffuses into the blood and is delivered to the liver. Within the liver glycerol is phosphorylated and converted to DHAP and then diverted into the glucose production via gluconeogenesis.

18. Although fructose-1,6-bisphosphatase (F1,6BPase) deficiency can lead to infant mortality due to severely impaired gluconeogenesis, beyond childhood afflicted individuals develop hypoglycemia usually only associated with fasting or febrile infections. Given the role of F1,6BPase in overall carbohydrate metabolism, which of the following metabolites would be expected to increase in the plasma of these patients following depletion of hepatic glycogen stores?

A. acetyl-CoA
B. cholesterol
C. free fatty acids
D. lactate
E. pyruvate

Answer D: During normal hepatic gluconeogenesis the major substrates for glucose synthesis are alanine, pyruvate, and lactate. Defective F1,6BPase would restrict the flow of alanine and lactate conversion to pyruvate and the subsequent input of pyruvate into gluconeogenesis. The net effect would be a significant increase in circulating levels of lactate.

Checklist

- ✓ Gluconeogenesis is carried out primarily within the liver as a means to ensure normal glucose homeostasis during periods of fasting.
- ✓ The primary sources of carbon for hepatic gluconeogenesis are lactate, pyruvate, and alanine.
- ✓ The primary source of carbon for intestinal and renal gluconeogenesis is glutamine.
- ✓ Gluconeogenesis is regulated at the level of pyruvate carboxylase (which is absolutely dependent upon acetyl-CoA as an allosteric activator), PEPCK, and F1,6-BPase.
- ✓ Regulation of gluconeogenesis at the level of F1,6-BPase represents a reciprocal regulation to that of the glycolytic enzyme PFK1.
- ✓ Delivery of lactate from the blood to the liver with the liver subsequently delivering glucose to the blood is referred to as the Cori cycle.
- ✓ Delivery of alanine, primarily from skeletal muscle, to the liver with subsequent delivery of glucose back to muscle via the blood is referred to as the glucose-alanine cycle.

- ✓ Intestinal gluconeogenesis contributes to overall endogenous glucose production.
- ✓ Intestinal glucose delivery to the portal circulation influences feeding behaviors via afferent circuits to the hypothalamus.
- ✓ Renal reabsorption of glucose and renal gluconeogenesis contribute to the maintenance of endogenous glucose production.

CHAPTER

14 Carbohydrates: Glycogen Metabolism

CHAPTER OUTLINE

High-Yield Terms

Glycosidic linkage: covalent bond that joins a carbohydrate (sugar) molecule to another group such as another sugar typical of the bonds between glucose molecules in glycogen

Glycogenin: protein with self-glycosylating activity that serves as the primer molecule for initiation of glycogen synthesis

Glycogen synthase-phosphorylase kinase: this enzyme is critical for the regulation of the flux of glucose into and out of glycogen as it reciprocally regulates the 2 key enzymes of glycogenolysis and glycogen synthesis

Glycogen storage disease: disorders that result from defects in genes encoding enzymes involved in the process of glycogen synthesis or breakdown, primarily affecting muscles and liver

Glycogen Composition

Stores of readily available glucose, used to supply the tissues with an oxidizable energy source, are found principally in the liver, as glycogen. Glycogen is a polymer of glucose residues linked by α-(1,4)- and α-(1,6)-glycosidic bonds. A second major source of stored glucose is the glycogen of skeletal muscle. However, muscle glycogen is not generally available to other tissues, because muscle lacks the enzyme glucose 6-phosphatase (Figure 14-1).

The major site of daily glucose consumption (75%) is within the brain. The remainder of it is utilized mostly by erythrocytes, skeletal muscle, and heart muscle. The body obtains glucose either directly from the diet or from amino acids and lactate via gluconeogenesis (see Chapter 13). Glucose obtained from these 2 primary sources either remains soluble in the body fluids or is stored as the glucose polymer, glycogen. Glycogen is considered the principal storage form of glucose and is found mainly in liver and muscle, with kidney and intestines adding minor storage sites. With up to 10% of its weight as glycogen, the liver has the highest specific content of any body tissue. Muscle has a much lower amount of glycogen per unit mass of tissue, but since the total mass of muscle is so much greater than that of liver, total glycogen stored in muscle is about twice that of liver. Stores of glycogen in the liver are considered the main buffer of blood glucose levels (Table 14-1).

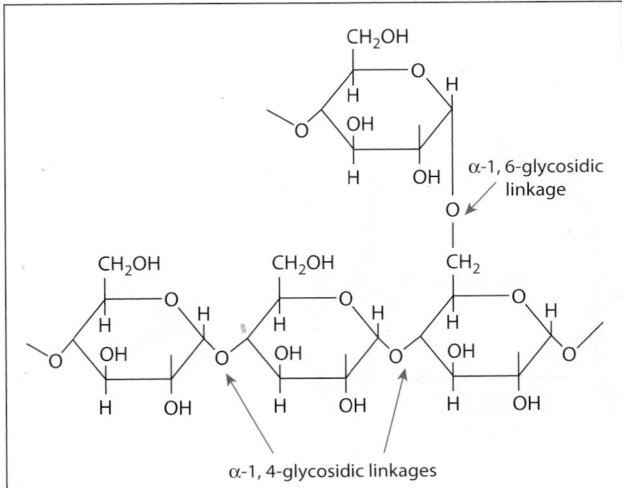

FIGURE 14-1: Section of glycogen showing α-1,4- and α-1,6-glycosidic linkages. Reproduced with permission of themedicalbiochemistrypage, LLC.

TABLE 14-1: Storage of Carbohydrate in a 70-kg Human Being

	Percentage of Tissue Weight	*Tissue Weight*	*Body Content (g)*
Liver glycogen	5.0	1.8 kg	90
Muscle glycogen	0.7	35 kg	245
Extracellular glucose	0.1	10 L	10

Murray RK, Bender DA, Botham KM, Kennelly PJ, Rodwell VW, Weil PA. *Harper's Illustrated Biochemistry*, 29th ed. New York, NY: McGraw-Hill; 2012.

Glycogen Synthesis (Glycogenesis)

De novo glycogen synthesis is initiated by the attachment of the first glucose residue to a protein known as *glycogenin*. Glycogenin has the unusual property of catalyzing its own glycosylation, attaching C-1 of a uridine diphosphate (UDP) glucose to a tyrosine residue on the enzyme. The attached glucose then serves as the primer required by glycogen synthase to attach additional glucose molecules.

Synthesis of glycogen from glucose is carried out by the enzyme glycogen synthase. This enzyme utilizes UDP glucose as one substrate and the nonreducing end of glycogen as another. The activation of glucose is carried out by the enzyme UDP glucose pyrophosphorylase. This enzyme exchanges the phosphate on C-1 of glucose 1-phosphate for UDP. The UDP is subsequently released during the glycogen synthase-mediated incorporation of glucose into glycogen. The α-1,6 branches in glucose are introduced by amylo-(1,4–1,6)-transglycosylase, more commonly just called branching enzyme. This enzyme transfers a terminal fragment of 6 to 7 glucose residues (from a polymer at least 11 glucose residues long) to an internal glucose residue at the C-6 hydroxyl position (Figures 14-2 and 14-3).

Regulation of Glycogen Synthesis

Glycogen synthase is a tetrameric enzyme consisting of 4 identical subunits. The liver and muscle glycogen synthase proteins are derived from different genes and share only 46% amino acid identity. The activity of glycogen synthase is influenced by phosphorylation of serine residues in the subunit proteins as well as via allosteric regulation. Phosphorylation of glycogen synthase reduces its activity toward UDP glucose.

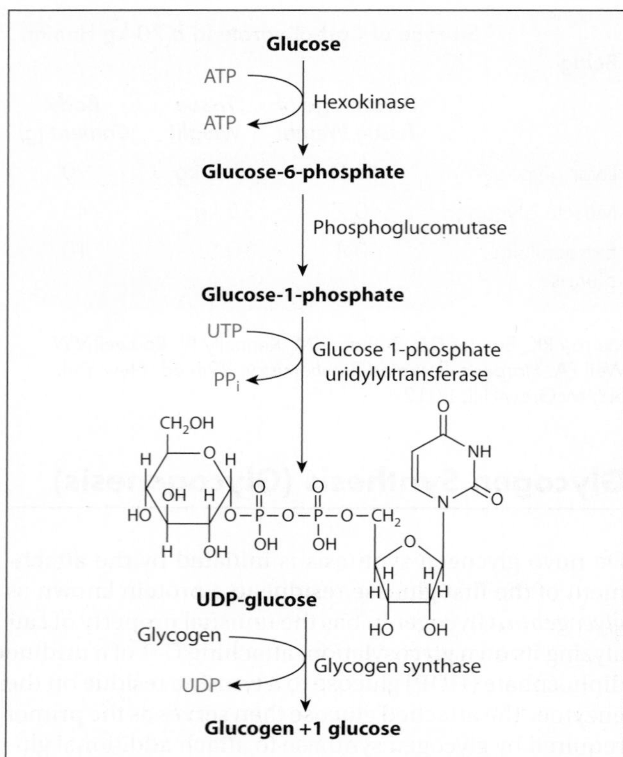

FIGURE 14-2: Enzymes necessary to activate glucose for incorporation into glycogen via glycogen synthase. Reproduced with permission of themedicalbiochemistrypage, LLC.

When phosphorylated, glycogen synthase activity can be increased by binding the allosteric activator, glucose 6-phosphate (G6P). Activation by G6P does not occur when glycogen synthase is not phosphorylated.

The 2 forms of glycogen synthase are identified by the use of "a" and "b" such that the nonphosphorylated, and most active form, is called synthase-*a* and the phosphorylated less active glucose-6-phosphate-dependent form is called synthase-*b*.

Numerous kinases have been shown to phosphorylate and regulate both hepatic and muscle forms of glycogen synthase (Figure 14-4). At least 5 sites of phosphorylation have been identified in hepatic glycogen synthase that are the targets of at least 7 different kinases. The 7 kinases that regulate glycogen synthase activity are glycogen synthase-phosphorylase kinase (commonly just called phosphorylase kinase, PhK), PKA, PKC, glycogen synthase kinase-3 (GSK-3), calmodulin-dependent protein kinase-II (CaMPK-II), casein kinase-I (CK-I), and casein kinase-II (CK-II). Phosphorylase kinase is a multi-subunit enzyme composed of α-, β-, γ-, and δ-subunits. The α- and β-subunits are the regulatory subunits that are subject to phosphorylation. The γ-subunit is the catalytic subunit and the δ-subunit is calmodulin.

When glucagon binds its receptor on hepatocytes, the receptor activates the enzyme adenylate cyclase. Activation of adenylate cyclase leads to a large increase in the formation of cAMP, which then binds to cAMP-dependent protein kinase, PKA. Binding of cAMP to the regulatory subunits of PKA leads to the release and subsequent activation of the catalytic subunits. The catalytic subunits then phosphorylate a number of target proteins such as glycogen synthase. PKA has been shown to phosphorylate glycogen synthase on at least 4 different sites. In addition, PKA activity results in an increase in the activity of phosphorylase kinase, which in turn phosphorylates glycogen synthase at one of the same sites as PKA. In addition, glucagon causes

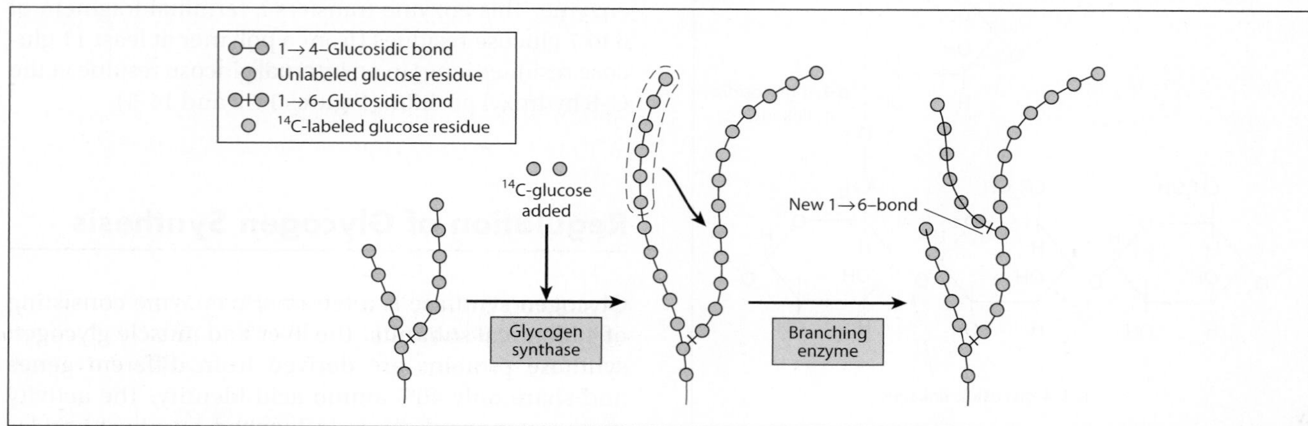

FIGURE 14-3: The biosynthesis of glycogen. The mechanism of branching as revealed by feeding 14C-labeled glucose and examining liver glycogen at intervals. Murray RK, Bender DA, Botham KM, Kennelly PJ, Rodwell VW, Weil PA. *Harper's Illustrated Biochemistry*, 29th ed. New York, NY: McGraw-Hill; 2012.

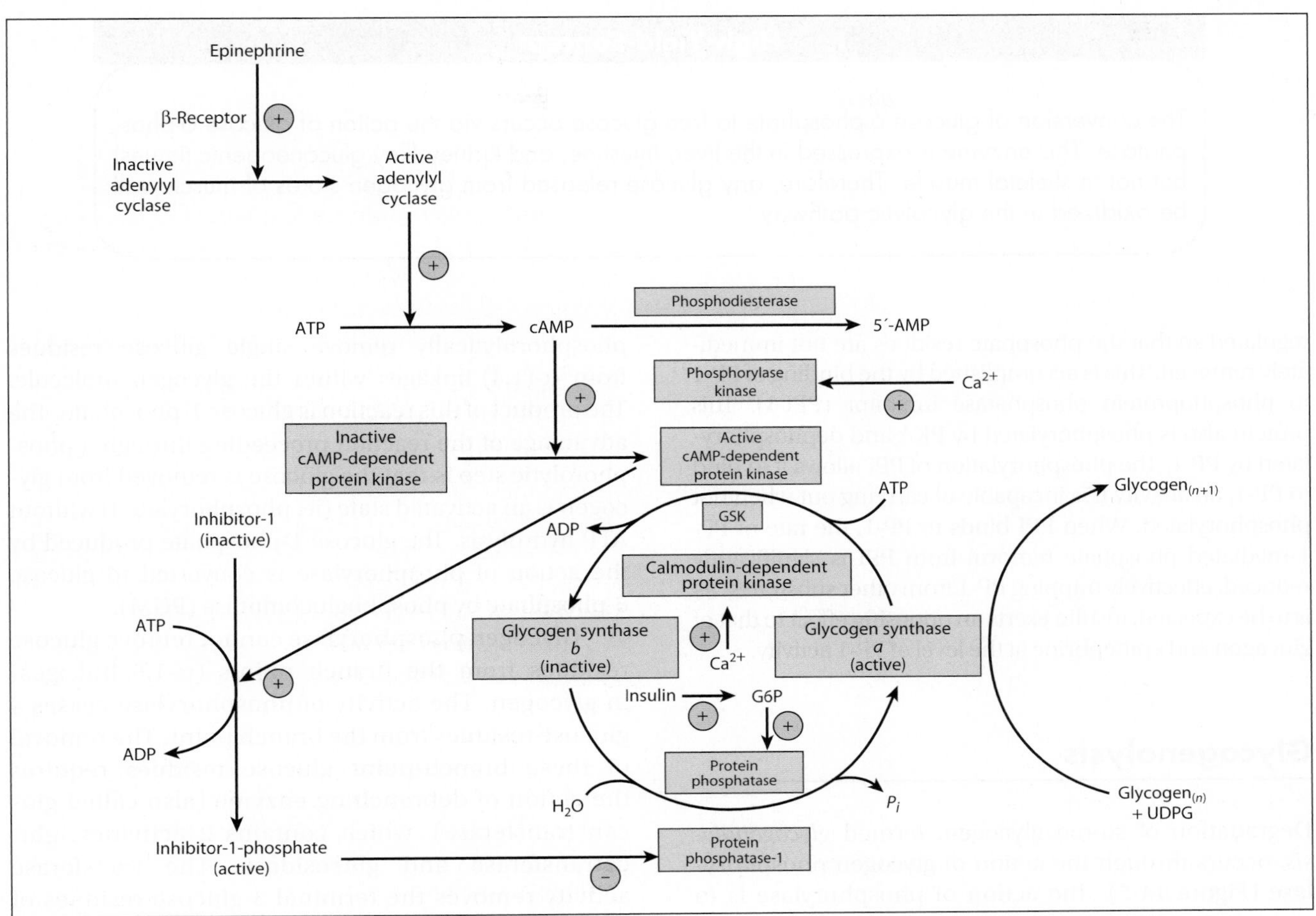

FIGURE 14-4: Control of glycogen synthase in muscle. (GSK, glycogen synthase kinase; G6P, glucose 6-phosphate; n, number of glucose residues.) Murray RK, Bender DA, Botham KM, Kennelly PJ, Rodwell VW, Weil PA. *Harper's Illustrated Biochemistry*, 29th ed. New York, NY: McGraw-Hill; 2012.

an increase in the activity of casein kinase-II (CK-II). Thus, the net effect of glucagon action on hepatocytes is activation of 3 distinct kinases that phosphorylate and thereby, inhibit glycogen synthase.

Since insulin and glucagon are counter-regulatory hormones, it should be clear that they will exert opposing effects on the rate and level of glycogen synthase phosphorylation. The action of insulin, at the level of PKA, is to increase the activity of phosphodiesterase, which hydrolyzes cAMP to AMP thereby reducing the level of active PKA. Insulin also exerts a negative effect on the activity of GSK-3 such that there is a reduced level of phosphorylation of glycogen synthase by this kinase.

Hormones and neurotransmitters that result in release of stored intracellular Ca^{2+} also affect negative regulation of glycogen synthase activity. The released Ca^{2+} ions bind to the calmodulin subunit of PhK and result in its activation leading to increased phosphorylation of glycogen synthase. Activation of α_1-adrenergic receptors in skeletal muscle results in activation of PLC-β, which hydrolyzes phosphatidylinositol 4,5-bisphosphate (PIP_2) releasing inositol trisphosphate (IP_3) and diacylglycerol (DAG). The action of IP_3 results in increased release of stored Ca^{2+} with the same net effect at the level of glycogen synthase. The released Ca^{2+} ions, in conjunction with DAG, in turn activate PKC, which phosphorylates glycogen synthase in the same domain of the enzyme that is one target for PKA and the site for CaMPK-II and CK-I phosphorylation. The overall effect of these various phosphorylation events, at the level of glycogen synthase activity, is decreased affinity for substrate (UDP glucose) and for the allosteric activator G6P.

Reactivation of glycogen synthase requires dephosphorylation, which is carried out predominately by the serine/threonine phosphatase identified as protein phosphatase-1 (PP-1). The activity of PP-1 must also be

High-Yield Concept

The conversion of glucose 6-phosphate to free glucose occurs via the action of glucose 6-phosphatase. This enzyme is expressed in the liver, intestine, and kidney (key gluconeogenic tissues) but not in skeletal muscle. Therefore, any glucose released from glycogen stores of muscle will be oxidized in the glycolytic pathway.

regulated so that the phosphate residues are not immediately removed. This is accomplished by the binding of PP-1 to phosphoprotein phosphatase inhibitor (PPI-1). This protein also is phosphorylated by PKA and dephosphorylated by PP-1. The phosphorylation of PPI allows it to bind to PP-1, an activity it is incapable of carrying out when not phosphorylated. When PPI binds to PP-1, the rate of PP-1-mediated phosphate removal from PPI is significantly reduced, effectively trapping PP-1 from other substrates. As is to be expected, insulin exerts an opposing effect to that of glucagon and epinephrine at the level of PP-1 activity.

Glycogenolysis

Degradation of stored glycogen, termed *glycogenolysis,* occurs through the action of glycogen phosphorylase (Figure 14-5). The action of phosphorylase is to phosphorolytically remove single glucose residues from α-(1,4)-linkages within the glycogen molecule. The product of this reaction is glucose 1-phosphate. The advantage of the reaction proceeding through a phosphorolytic step is that the glucose is removed from glycogen is an activated state (ie, phosphorylated) without ATP hydrolysis. The glucose 1-phosphate produced by the action of phosphorylase is converted to glucose 6-phosphate by phosphoglucomutase (PGM).

Glycogen phosphorylase cannot remove glucose residues from the branch points (α-1,6 linkages) in glycogen. The activity of phosphorylase ceases 4 glucose residues from the branch point. The removal of these branch-point glucose residues requires the action of debranching enzyme (also called glucan transferase), which contains 2 activities: glucotransferase and glucosidase. The transferase activity removes the terminal 3 glucose residues of

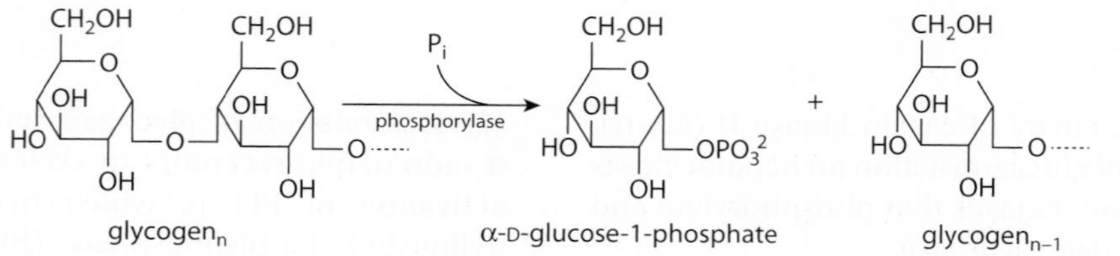

FIGURE 14-5: Phosphorylase-catalyzed reaction. Reproduced with permission of themedicalbiochemistrypage, LLC.

High-Yield Concept

The activity of hexokinase in muscle is so high that any free glucose is immediately phosphorylated and enters the glycolytic pathway. Indeed, the precise reason for the temporary appearance of the free glucose from glycogen is the need of the skeletal muscle cell to generate energy from glucose oxidation, thereby, precluding any chance of the glucose entering the blood.

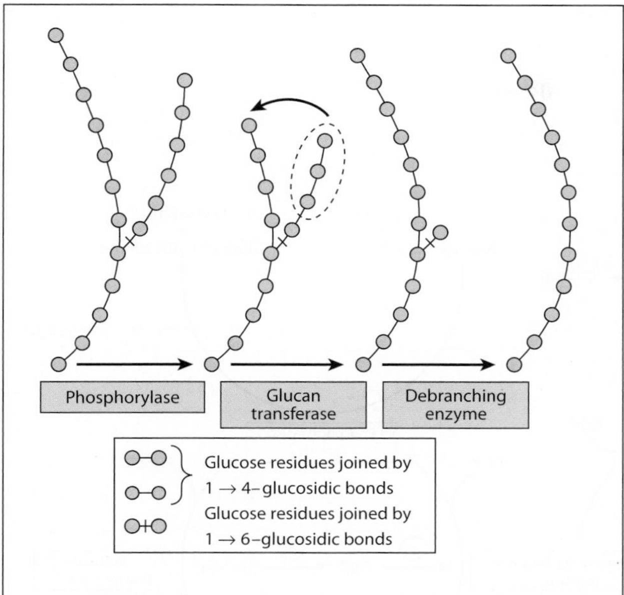

FIGURE 14-6: Steps in glycogenolysis. Murray RK, Bender DA, Botham KM, Kennelly PJ, Rodwell VW, Weil PA. *Harper's Illustrated Biochemistry,* 29th ed. New York, NY: McGraw-Hill; 2012.

one branch and attaches them to a free C-4 end of a second branch. The glucose in α-(1,6)-linkage at the branch is then removed by the action of glucosidase as free glucose (Figure 14-6).

Regulation of Glycogenolysis

Glycogen phosphorylase (most commonly just phosphorylase) is a homodimeric enzyme that exists in 2 distinct conformational states: a T (for tense, less active) and R (for relaxed, more active) state. Phosphorylase is capable of binding to glycogen when the enzyme is in the R state. This conformation is enhanced by binding the allosteric activator AMP and inhibited by binding the allosteric inhibitors ATP or glucose 6-phosphate. The activity of phosphorylase is also modulated by phosphorylation. The relative activity of the unmodified phosphorylase enzyme (phosphorylase-*b*) is sufficient to generate enough glucose 1-phosphate for entry into glycolysis for the production of adequate amounts of ATP to maintain the normal resting activity of the cell. This is true in both liver and muscle cells.

When blood glucose levels fall, the pancreas secretes glucagon, which binds to cell surface receptors. Liver cells are the primary target for the action of this hormone. The binding of glucagon to its cell surface receptor results in activation of PKA. Of significance to this discussion is the PKA-mediated phosphorylation of phosphorylase kinase (Figure 14-7). Phosphorylation of phosphorylase kinase activates the enzyme, which in turn phosphorylates the b form of phosphorylase. Phosphorylation of phosphorylase-*b* greatly enhances its activity toward glycogen breakdown. This modified enzyme is called phosphorylase-*a*. The net result is an extremely large induction of glycogen breakdown in response to glucagon binding to cell surface receptors.

This identical cascade of events occurs in skeletal muscle cells as well, even though these cells lack the glucagon receptor. In muscle, the induction of the cascade is the result of epinephrine binding to its receptors on these cells. Epinephrine is released from the adrenal glands in response to neural signals indicating an immediate need for enhanced glucose utilization in muscle, the so-called fight or flight response.

High-Yield Concept

Within skeletal muscle cells, calcium ions play a crucial role in the regulation of glycogenolysis. Calcium ions bind to the calmodulin subunit of phosphorylase kinase. Binding induces a conformational change in calmodulin, which in turn enhances the catalytic activity of the phosphorylase kinase toward its substrate, phosphorylase-*b*. This activity is crucial to the enhancement of glycogenolysis in muscle cells where muscle contraction is induced via acetylcholine stimulation at the neuromuscular junction.

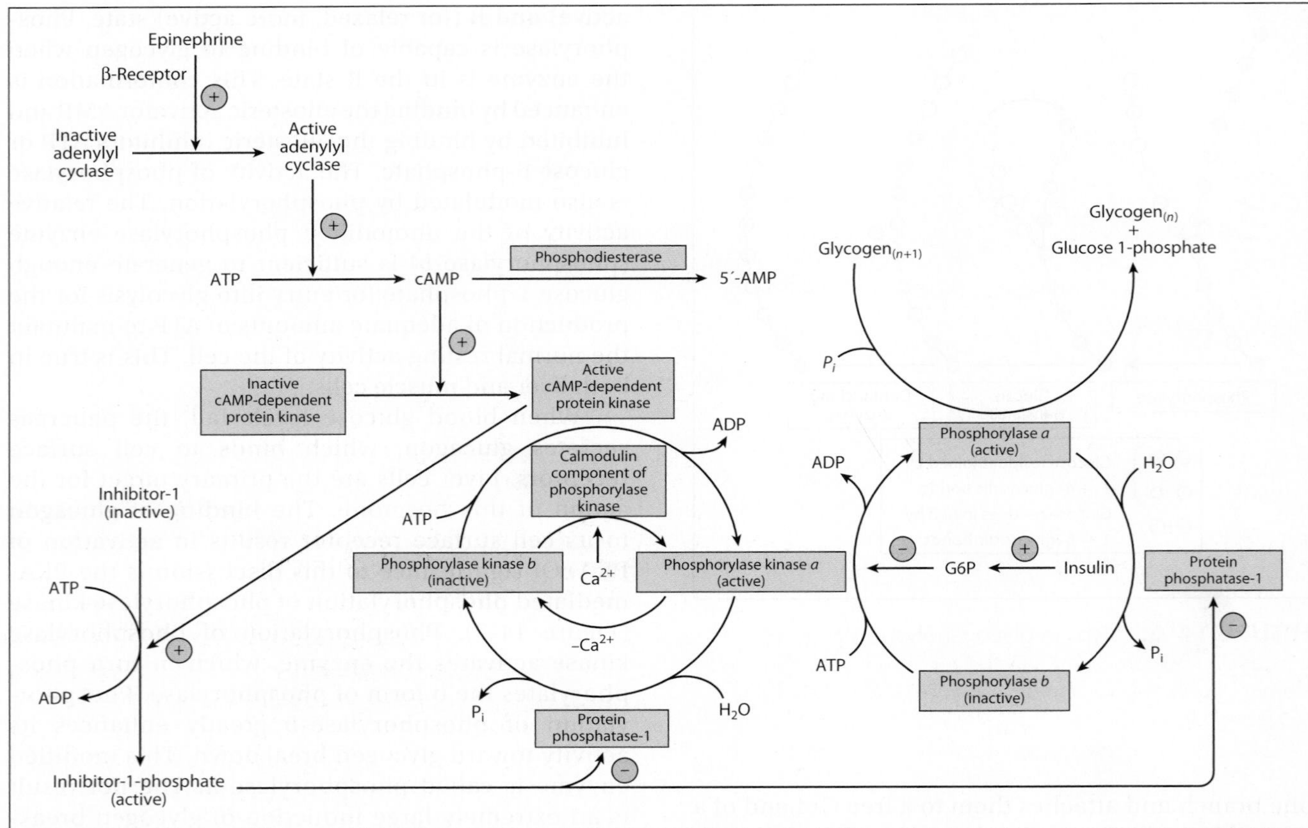

FIGURE 14-7: Control of phosphorylase in muscle. The sequence of reactions arranged as a cascade allows amplification of the hormonal signal at each step. (G6P, glucose 6-phosphate; *n*, number of glucose residues.) Murray RK, Bender DA, Botham KM, Kennelly PJ, Rodwell VW, Weil PA. *Harper's Illustrated Biochemistry*, 29th ed. New York, NY: McGraw-Hill; 2012.

The effect of acetylcholine release from nerve terminals at a neuromuscular junction is to depolarize the muscle cell leading to increased release of Ca^{2+} stored in the sarcoplasmic reticulum, thereby activating phosphorylase kinase.

Calcium ions are also involved in the ultimate response to activation of α-adrenergic receptors on skeletal muscle. α_1-adrenergic receptors are coupled to the activation of PLC-β. Activation of PLC-β leads to increased hydrolysis of membrane PIP_2 and release of IP_3 and DAG. IP_3 binds to receptors on the surface of the endoplasmic reticulum, leading to release of Ca^{2+} ions. The Ca^{2+} ions then interact with the calmodulin subunits of phosphorylase kinase resulting in its activation. Additionally, the Ca^{2+} ions activate PKC in conjunction with DAG.

As described earlier for glycogen synthase, once the signals that initiated the phosphorylation of phosphorylase have abated, the phosphates must be removed to return the enzyme to basal activity. The removal of the phosphates is catalyzed primarily by PP-1 as for glycogen synthase.

Glycogen Storage Diseases

Since glycogen molecules can become enormously large, an inability to degrade glycogen can cause cells to become pathologically engorged; it can also lead to the functional loss of glycogen as a source of cell energy and as a blood glucose buffer. Although glycogen storage diseases (GSDs) are quite rare, their effects can be most dramatic. The debilitating effect of many GSDs depends on the severity of the mutation causing the deficiency. In addition, although the GSDs are attributed to specific enzyme deficiencies, other events can cause the same characteristic symptoms.

The GSDs are divided into 2 primary categories: those that result principally from defects in liver glycogen homeostasis and those that represent defects in muscle glycogen homeostasis. The liver GSDs result in hepatomegaly and hypoglycemia or cirrhosis, whereas the muscle GSDs result in skeletal and cardiac myopathies and/or energy impairment (Table 14-2).

TABLE 14-2: Glycogen Storage Diseases

Type	*Name*	*Enzyme Deficiency*	*Clinical Features*
0	—	Glycogen synthase	Hypoglycemia; hyperketonemia; early death
Ia	von Gierke disease	Glucose 6-phosphatase	Glycogen accumulation in liver and renal tubule cells; hypoglycemia; lactic acidemia; ketosis; hyperlipemia (see Clinical Box14-1)
Ib	—	Endoplasmic reticulum glucose-6-phosphate transporter	As type Ia; neutropenia and impaired neutrophil function leading to recurrent infections
II	Pompe disease	Lysosomal $\alpha_1 \rightarrow 4$ and $\alpha_1 \rightarrow 6$ glucosidase (acid maltase)	Accumulation of glycogen in lysosomes: juvenile-onset variant, muscle hypotonia, death from heart failure by age 2; adult-onset variant, muscle dystrophy (see Clinical Box14-2)
IIIa	Limit dextrinosis, Forbe or Cori disease	Liver and muscle debranching enzyme	Fasting hypoglycemia; hepatomegaly in infancy; accumulation of characteristic branched polysaccharide (limit dextrin); muscle weakness
IIIb	Limit dextrinosis	Liver debranching enzyme	As type IIIa, but no muscle weakness
IV	Amylopectinosis, Andersen disease	Branching enzyme	Hepatosplenomegaly; accumulation of polysaccharide with few branch points; death from heart or liver failure before age 5
V	Myophosphorylase deficiency, McArdle syndrome	Muscle phosphorylase	Poor exercise tolerance; muscle glycogen abnormally high (2.5%-4%); blood lactate very low after exercise (see Clinical Box14-3)
VI	Hers disease	Liver phosphorylase	Hepatomegaly; accumulation of glycogen in liver; mild hypoglycemia; generally good prognosis
VII	Tarui disease	Muscle and erythrocyte phosphofructokinase 1	Poor exercise tolerance; muscle glycogen abnormally high (2.5%-4%); blood lactate very low after exercise; also hemolytic anemia
VIII		Liver phosphorylase kinase	Hepatomegaly; accumulation of glycogen in liver; mild hypoglycemia; generally good prognosis
IX		Liver and muscle phosphorylase kinase	Hepatomegaly; accumulation of glycogen in liver and muscle; mild hypoglycemia; generally good prognosis
X		cAMP-dependent protein kinase A	Hepatomegaly; accumulation of glycogen in liver

Murray RK, Bender DA, Botham KM, Kennelly PJ, Rodwell VW, Weil PA. *Harper's Illustrated Biochemistry,* 29th ed. New York, NY: McGraw-Hill; 2012.

CLINICAL BOX 14-1: von GIERKE DISEASE

Type I GSD was first described in 1929 by E. von Gierke as a "hepatonephromegalia glycogenica." For this reason, the disease is still more commonly referred to von Gierke disease. In 1952, G. Cori and C. Cori identified that the absence of glucose-6-phosphatase activity was the cause of von Gierke disease. This discovery was the first-ever identification of an enzyme defect in a metabolic disorder. Subsequent to the identification of the pathway of glucose release from glucose 6-phosphate, additional patients with similar clinical manifestations to von Gierke disease were identified. However, these patients were not deficient in glucose 6-phosphatase. These latter patients were identified as having type Ib GSD. Type Ia GSD is caused by a defect in the ER localized glucose 6-phosphatase. Type Ib disease results from defects in the glucose-6-phosphate transporter 1. Type Ic GSD was identified in 1983 and found to be the result of defects in the microsomal pyrophosphate transporter. This form of type I GSD has only been found in few cases. As shown in Figure 14-8, there are 4 enzyme activities that function in the release of free glucose in the cell, and as such there is the theoretical possibility that type Id GSD would be caused by defects in the microsomal glucose transporter. However, no individuals have been reported to exist with a defect in this latter enzyme activity. Type I GSD (von Gierke disease) is attributed to lack of glucose 6-phosphatase, G-6Pase. However, G-6Pase is localized to the luminal side of the endoplasmic reticulum (ER) membrane. In order to gain access to the phosphatase, glucose 6-phosphate must pass through a specific translocase in the ER membrane (Figure 14-8). Mutation of either the phosphatase or the translocase makes transfer of liver glycogen to the blood a very limited process. Thus, mutation of either gene leads to symptoms associated with von Gierke disease, which occurs at a rate of about 1 in 200,000 people (Figure 14-8).

The metabolic consequences of the hepatic glucose-6-phosphate deficiency of von Gierke disease extend well beyond just the obvious hypoglycemia that result from the deficiency in liver being able to deliver free glucose to the blood. The inability to release the phosphate from glucose 6-phopsphate results in diversion into glycolysis and production of pyruvate as well as increased diversion onto the pentose phosphate pathway. The production of excess pyruvate, at levels above the capacity of the TCA cycle to completely oxidize it, results in its reduction to lactate resulting in lactic acidemia. In addition, some of the pyruvate is transaminated to alanine, leading to hyperalaninemia. Some of the pyruvate will be oxidized to acetyl-CoA, which cannot be fully oxidized in the TCA cycle and so the acetyl-CoA will end up in the cytosol where it will serve as a substrate for triglyceride and cholesterol synthesis resulting in hyperlipidemia. The oxidation of glucose 6-phosphate

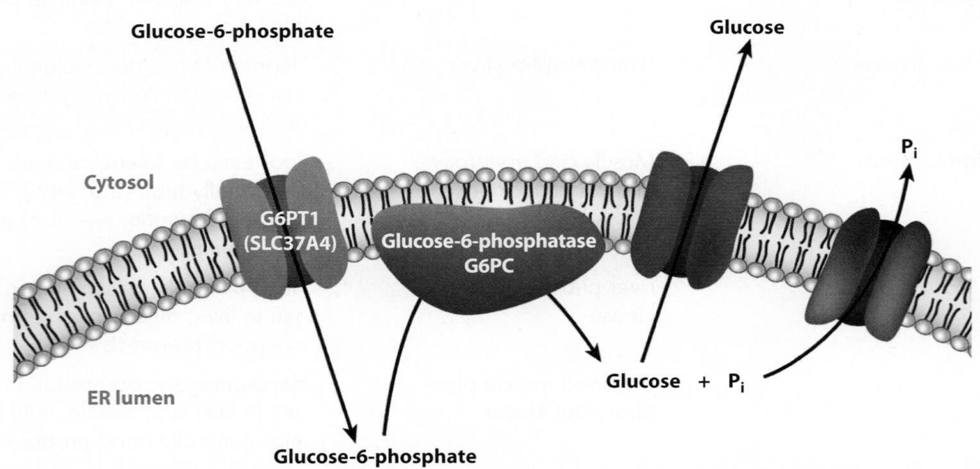

FIGURE 14-8: Multistep process for the removal of phosphate from glucose 6-phosphate so that free glucose can be relased from the cell. Reproduced with permission of themedicalbiochemistrypage, LLC.

CLINICAL BOX 14-1: von GIERKE DISEASE (*Continued*)

via the pentose phosphate pathway leads to increased production of ribose 5-phosphate, which then activates the de novo synthesis of the purine nucleotides. In excess of the need, these purine nucleotides will ultimately be catabolized to uric acid resulting in hyperuricemia and consequent symptoms of gout. The interrelationships of these metabolic pathways are shown in Figure 14-9.

Patients with type I GSD can present during the neonatal period with lactic acidosis and hypoglycemia. More commonly though, infants of 3 to 4 months of age will manifest with hepatomegaly and hypoglycemic seizures. The hallmark features of this disease are hypoglycemia, lactic acidosis, hyperuricemia, and hyperlipidemia. The severity of the hypoglycemia and lactic acidosis can be such that in the past affected individuals died in infancy. Infants often have a doll-like facial appearance due to excess adipose tissue in the cheeks. In addition, patients have thin extremities, a short stature, and protuberant abdomens (due to the severe hepatomegaly).

Long-term complications are usually seen now only in adults whose disease was poorly treated early on. The main problem is associated with liver function but multiple organ systems are also involved, in particular the intestines and kidneys. Growth continues to be impaired and puberty is often delayed. Affected female patients will have polycystic ovaries but none of the other symptoms of polycystic ovarian syndrome (PCOS) such as hirsutism.

The common treatment for type I GSD is to maintain normal blood glucose concentration. With normoglycemia will come reduced metabolic disruption and a reduced morbidity associated with the disease. To attain normoglycemia, patients are usually treated in infancy with nocturnal nasogastric infusion of glucose. Total parenteral nutrition or the oral feeding of uncooked cornstarch can also achieve the desired results. In the past the prognosis for type I GSD patients was poor. However, with proper nutritional intervention, growth will improve and the lactic acidosis, cholesterol, and lipidosis will decrease.

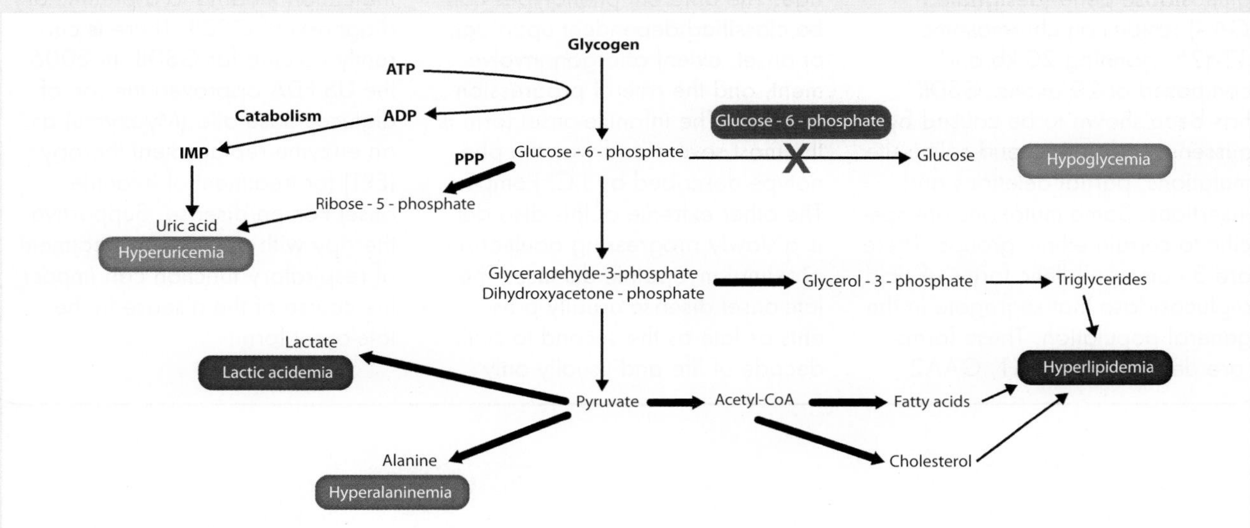

FIGURE 14-9: Interrelationships of metabolic pathway disruption in von Gierke disease. Reproduced with permission of themedicalbiochemistrypage, LLC.

CLINICAL BOX 14-2: POMPE DISEASE

Glycogen storage disease type II (GSDII) is also known as Pompe disease or acid maltase deficiency (AMD). This disease was originally referred to as Pompe disease since Joannes Cassianus Pompe (published in 1932) made the important observation of a massive accumulation of glycogen within the vacuoles of all tissues in a 7-month-old female infant who died suddenly from idiopathic hypertrophy of the heart. Through the investigations carried out by the Coris (Gerty T. Cori and Carl F. Cori), this disease was classified as GSD type II. GSDII is the most severe of all the GSDs. The excess storage of glycogen in the vacuoles is the consequence of defects in the lysosomal hydrolase, acid α-glucosidase, which removes glucose residues from glycogen in the lysosomes. The *acid α-glucosidase* gene (designated *GAA*) resides on chromosome 17q25 spanning 20 kb and composed of 20 exons. GSDII has been shown to be caused by missense, nonsense, and splice-site mutations, partial deletions and insertions. Some mutations are specific to certain ethnic groups. There are 3 common allelic forms of acid α-glucosidase that segregate in the general population. These forms are designated GAA1, GAA2, and GAA4. The normal function of acid α-glucosidase is to hydrolyze both α-1,4- and α-1,6-glucosidic linkages at acid pH. The activity of the enzyme leads to the complete hydrolysis of glycogen, which is its natural substrate. As would be expected from this activity, deficiency in acid α-glucosidase leads to the accumulation of structurally normal glycogen in numerous tissues, most notably in cardiac and skeletal muscle. The clinical presentation of GSDII encompasses a wide range of phenotypes but all include various degrees of cardiomegaly. Additional clinical manifestations associated with idiopathic cardiomegaly accompanied by storage of glycogen are indicative of Pompe disease. These symptoms included hepatomegaly, marked hypotonia, muscular weakness, and death before 1 year of age. The different phenotypes can be classified dependent upon age of onset, extent of organ involvement, and the rate of progression to death. The infantile-onset form is the most severe and was the phenotype described by J.C. Pompe. The other extreme of this disorder is a slowly progressing adult-onset proximal myopathic disease. The late-onset disease usually presents as late as the second to sixth decade of life and usually only involves the skeletal muscles. There is also a heterogeneous group of GSDII disorders that are classified generally by onset after early infancy and called the juvenile or childhood form. In addition to classical symptoms that can lead to a diagnosis of GSDII, analysis for the level and activity of acid α-glucosidase in muscle biopsies is used for confirmation. The infantile onset form of GSDII presents in the first few months of life. Symptoms include marked cardiomegaly, striking hypotonia (leading to the designation of "floppy baby syndrome"), and rapid progressive muscle weakness. Patients will usually exhibit difficulty with feeding and have respiratory problems that are frequently complicated by pulmonary infection. The prominent cardiomegaly that can be seen on chest x-ray is normally the first indication leading to a preliminary diagnosis of GSDII. There is currently no cure for GSDII. In 2006 the US FDA approved the use of alglucosidase alfa (Myozyme) as an enzyme replacement therapy (ERT) for treatment of infantile-onset Pompe disease. Supportive therapy with attention to treatment of respiratory function can impact the course of the disease in the late-onset form.

CLINICAL BOX 14-3: McARDLE DISEASE

Glycogen storage disease type V (GSDV) is also known as McArdle disease. This disease was originally described by B. McArdle in 1951, hence the association of his name with the disease. The disease was seen in a 30-year-old patient who was suffering from muscle weakness, pain, and stiffness following slight exercise. It was observed that blood lactate fell in this patient during exercise instead of the normal rise that would be seen. This indicated the patient had a defect in the ability to convert muscle glycogen to glucose and ultimately lactate. The identification that the deficiency causing these symptoms was the result of a muscle phosphorylase defect was not made until 1959. Glycogen phosphorylase (most commonly just called phosphorylase) exists in multiple tissue-specific isoforms. The muscle, brain, and liver forms are encoded by separate genes. The muscle form is the only isozyme found expressed in mature muscle. The clinical presentation of GSDV is usually seen in young adulthood and is characterized by exercise intolerance and muscle cramps following slight exercise. Attacks of myoglobinuria frequently accompany the muscle symptoms of GSDV. About half of GSDV patients will exhibit burgundy-colored urine after exercise. Diagnosis of muscle glycogenoses such as GSDV can be made by the observation of a lack of increased blood lactate upon ischemic exercise testing. In addition, there will be an associated large increase in blood ammonia levels. In order to distinguish GSDV from other muscle defects along the pathway from glycogen to glucose to lactate, an enzymatic evaluation of muscle phosphorylase must be done. In addition, molecular analysis for known mutations in the *muscle phosphorylase* gene can be accomplished using DNA extracted from leukocytes.

REVIEW QUESTIONS

1. You are examining the biochemical characteristics of the liver dysfunction in your patient who is exhibiting signs of a GSD. You have isolated the microsomal fraction (contains the endoplasmic reticulum) of a liver biopsy homogenate from your patient and a control individual for your studies. Incubation with radioactive phosphate–labeled glucose 6-phosphate results in an increase in isotope associated with the microsomes from your control sample but no increase in association with the microsomes from your patient. These results are best explained by a defect in which of the following?

A. glucose-6-phosphatase activity in the microsomes
B. microsomal glucose-6-phosphate transporter
C. cytosolic glucose 6-phosphatase
D. microsomal glucose transporter
E. microsomal phosphate transporter

Answer B: The patient is suffering from a form of type I glycogen storage disease (GSDI). The most common form of the disorder is referred to as von Gierke disease (also called type Ia) and results from a defect in the gene encoding glucose 6-phosphatase. However, some type I patients, although exhibiting identical symptoms turn out not to be deficient in glucose 6-phosphatase. These latter patients are identified as having type Ib GSD. The mechanism by which free glucose is released from glucose 6-phosphate involves several different steps. Glucose 6-phosphate must first be transported from the cytosol into the lumen of the endoplasmic reticulum, ER. Inside the ER, the phosphate is removed through the action of ER-localized glucose 6-phosphatase. Type Ib disease results from defects in the glucose-6-phosphate transporter 1. Thus, liver cells from type Ib patients will not accumulate glucose inside the membranes of the ER.

2. You are examining a 5-month-old infant who was brought to your office by distressed parents. Their infant has demonstrated progressive weakness and difficulty eating and appears to have a bulging abdomen. Upon examination, you find striking hypotonia and demonstrable palpable liver. Chest x-ray indicates prominent cardiomegaly. Before a correct diagnosis could be made, the infant lapses into a coma and dies. At autopsy, the heart was sectioned and stained with the result shown. Which of the following diseases is most likely given the symptoms and outcomes?

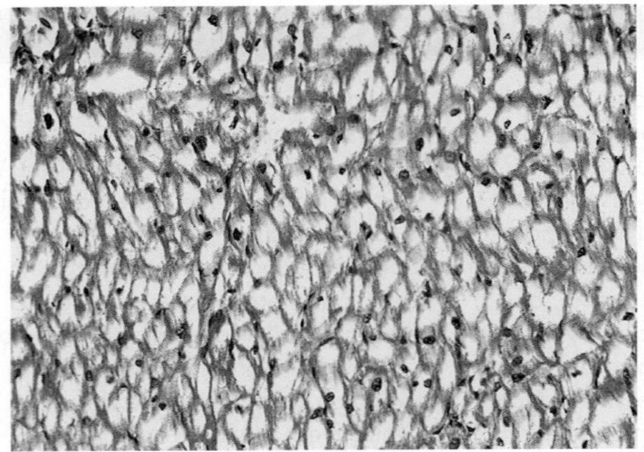

A. Andersen disease
B. Cori (Forbes) disease
C. McArdle disease
D. Pompe disease
E. von Gierke disease

Answer D: Glycogen storage disease type II (GSDII) is also known as Pompe disease and results from defects in the gene encoding lysosomal acid maltase. Thus, the disease is also referred to as or acid maltase deficiency (AMD). The clinical presentation of GSDII encompasses a wide range of phenotypes but all include various degrees of cardiomegaly. Additional clinical manifestations associated with idiopathic cardiomegaly accompanied by storage of glycogen are indicative of Pompe disease. These symptoms included hepatomegaly, marked hypotonia, muscular weakness, and death before 1 year of age. The different phenotypes can be classified dependent upon age of onset, extent of organ involvement, and the rate of progression to death.

3. Regulation of glycogen metabolism is tightly controlled at the level of the activity of glycogen phosphorylase. Which of the following is known to act as a negative effector of the phosphorylated (most active) form of glycogen phosphorylase?
A. AMP
B. cAMP
C. Ca^{2+}
D. glucose 6-phosphate
E. protein kinase A

Answer D: Glycogen homeostasis is controlled by regulating the rate of glycogen synthesis and breakdown. Release of glucose from stored glycogen is the role of glycogen phosphorylase (generally just called phosphorylase). The rate of glucose liberation from glycogen by phosphorylase is controlled primarily by short-term phosphorylation and dephosphorylation events. When phosphorylase is phosphorylated by glycogen synthase-phosphorylase kinase (generally just called phosphorylase kinase), it is more active in releasing glucose. This phosphorylation occurs in hepatocytes when stimulation by glucagon leads to increased activity of PKA, which in turn phosphorylates, and activates, phosphorylase kinase. Active phosphorylase liberates glucose 1-phosphate from glycogen which is converted to glucose 6-phosphate. The glucose 6-phosphate is either oxidized in the glycolytic pathway or the phosphate is removed by glucose 6-phosphatase and the free glucose flows into the blood. When glucose-6-phosphate levels rise in hepatocytes, due to reduced utilization, it acts as an allosteric inhibitor of the phosphorylated and active form of phosphorylase.

4. Cyclic AMP-independent activation of glycogen breakdown in hepatocytes occurs as a result of the binding of which of the following?
A. epinephrine to α_1-adrenergic receptors
B. epinephrine to β-adrenergic receptors
C. glucagon to its receptor
D. insulin to its receptor

Answer A: When epinephrine binds α-adrenergic receptors, there is an activation of the membrane-associated enzyme PLC-β. PLC-β hydrolyzes membrane PIP_2 into DAG and IP_3. The IP_3 then binds to receptors present in membranes of the endoplasmic reticulum (ER) resulting in release of stored calcium ion. The released calcium binds to the calmodulin subunit of glycogen synthase-phosphorylase kinase, resulting in activation of this regulatory enzyme. The net effect is enhanced activity of phosphorylase and inhibited activity of glycogen synthase.

5. An increase in the level of glucose 6-phosphate is expected to have which of the following effects on carbohydrate metabolism in hepatocytes?
A. activation of glycogen phosphorylase-*a*
B. activation of glycogen synthase-*a*
C. activation of glycogen synthase-*b*
D. inhibition of glycogen phosphorylase-*b*
E. inhibition of glycogen synthase-phosphorylase kinase

Answer C: Both covalent modification and allosteric effectors alter regulation of the activity of glycogen synthase. When glycogen synthase is phosphorylated by glycogen synthase-phosphorylase kinase, it is rendered less active (glycogen synthase-*b*). When in this less active state, the enzyme activity can be enhanced by the positive allosteric effector glucose 6-phosphate. The more active form, glycogen synthase-*a*, does not respond to changing levels of glucose 6-phosphate.

6. Epinephrine, released in response to exercise, will lead to phosphorylation events that will ultimately exert which of the following effects on hepatic glycogen metabolism?

A. activation of adenylate kinase
B. activation of glycogen synthase
C. activation of phosphorylase kinase
D. inhibition of glycogen phosphorylase
E. inhibition of glycogen synthase kinase-3 (GSK-3)

Answer C: Epinephrine can bind and activate both α-adrenergic and β-adrenergic receptors. When epinephrine binds α_1-adrenergic receptors, there is an activation of the membrane-associated enzyme PLC-β. PLC-β hydrolyzes membrane PIP_2 into DAG and IP_3. The IP_3 then binds to receptors present in membranes of the endoplasmic reticulum (ER), resulting in release of stored calcium ion. The released calcium binds to the calmodulin subunit of glycogen synthase-phophorylase kinase, resulting in activation of this regulatory enzyme. The net effect is enhanced activity of phosphorylase and inhibited activity of glycogen synthase. When epinephrine binds β-adrenergic receptors, there is activation of adenylate cyclase resulting in increased cAMP with consequent activation of PKA. PKA phosphorylates and activates glycogen synthase-phoshorylase kinase with the results being the same as for α_1-adrenergic receptor activation.

7. Muscle membrane will depolarize in response to acetylcholine binding its receptors at the neuromuscular junction. Associated with this depolarization are changes in glycogen metabolism in skeletal muscle cells. Which of the following represents the correct changes in enzyme activity seen in response to acetylcholine binding?

A. decreased glycogen phosphorylase kinase activity due to an increase in calcium binding to its calmodulin subunit
B. decreased phosphorylation of, and inhibited activity of, glycogen phosphorylase kinase
C. increased glycogen phosphorylase kinase activity due to an activation of phosphoprotein phosphatase
D. increased glycogen phosphorylase kinase activity due to an increase in calcium binding to its calmodulin subunit
E. increased phosphorylation of, and inhibited activity of, glycogen phosphorylase kinase

Answer D: Muscle contraction results in release of stored calcium ion from sarcoplasmic reticulum. The released calcium binds to the calmodulin subunit of glycogen synthase-phophorylase kinase resulting in activation of this regulatory enzyme. The net effect is enhanced activity of phosphorylase and inhibited activity of glycogen synthase.

8. An increase in the state of phosphorylation, in hepatocytes in response to glucagon action, will be most accurately reflected by which of the following statements?

A. glycogen phosphorylase activity will be increased
B. PFK-1 activity will be unaffected
C. PFK-2 will exhibit an increased level of kinase activity
D. phosphorylase kinase activity will be decreased
E. phosphoprotein phosphatase-1 activity will be increased

Answer A: When glucagon binds to its receptors on hepatocytes, there is activation of adenylate cyclase resulting in increased cAMP with consequent activation of PKA. PKA phosphorylates and activates glycogen synthase-phosphorylase kinase, which will phosphorylate and activate phosphorylase while also phosphorylating and inhibiting glycogen synthase.

9. Which of the following statements correctly defines the situation under conditions of low blood glucose?

A. a reversal of the muscle hexokinase reaction converts glucose 6-phosphate to glucose for oxidation in glycolysis
B. hepatic glycogen releases glucose in response to insulin-mediated dephosphorylation of glycogen phosphorylase
C. hepatic glycogen releases glucose through a reversal of the glycogen synthase reaction
D. phosphorylation of hepatic glycogen synthase prevents glucose incorporation into glycogen
E. the activity of muscle glycolysis is inhibited by the phosphorylation of PFK-1

Answer D: Conditions of low blood glucose result in glucagon release from the pancreas. When glucagon binds to its receptors on hepatocytes, there is activation of adenylate cyclase resulting in increased cAMP with consequent activation of PKA. PKA phosphorylates and activates glycogen synthase-phosphorylase kinase, which will phosphorylate and activate phosphorylase while also phosphorylating and inhibiting glycogen synthase.

10. A 7-year-old boy is examined by his pediatrician because of complaints of severe cramping pain in his legs whenever he rides his bike. In addition, he experiences nausea and vomiting during these attacks. The child has noted that the severity of the cramps is most intense after dinners that include baked potatoes or pasta and sometimes bread. Clinical studies undertaken following a treadmill test demonstrate myoglobinuria, hyperuricemia, and increased serum bilirubin. Which of the following enzyme deficiencies is associated with these clinical findings?

A. glucose 6-phosphatase
B. glycogen synthase
C. liver glycogen debranching enzyme
D. lysosomal acid maltase
E. muscle PFK1

Answer E: This patient is exhibiting symptoms of Tarui disease (GSD7) due to mutation in the gene encoding muscle and erythrocyte PFK1. The symptoms of this disease are very similar to those observed in patients suffering from McArdle disease (GSDV), in particular the presentation of exercise-induced pain and myoglobinuria. However, since Tarui disease also involves a defect in erythrocyte PFK1, there are associated mild forms of jaundice, resulting from accelerated destruction of erythrocytes.

11. A 6-month-old infant who is failing to thrive is brought to your clinic. Tests reveal hepatosplenomegaly, muscle weakness and atrophy, hypotonia, and decreased deep tendon reflexes. Blood tests reveal that the infant has normal glucose levels. Biopsy of the liver reveals initial stages of cirrhosis due to the accumulation of an abnormal glycogen with few branch points whose structure resembles amylopectin. The clinical and laboratory results presented are indicative of which GSD?

A. Andersen disease (type IV glycogen storage disease)
B. Cori or Forbes disease (type III glycogen storage disease)
C. McArdle disease (type V glycogen storage disease)
D. Tarui disease (type VII glycogen storage disease)
E. von Gierke disease (type I glycogen storage disease)

Answer A: Andersen disease, glycogen storage disease type IV (GSDIV), is also known as amylopectinosis. The disease results from defects in the gene encoding glycogen-branching enzyme, also called amylo-(1,4 to 1,6) transglycosylase. The disease manifests with progressive hepatosplenomegaly along with the storage of an abnormal glycogen that exhibits poor solubility in the liver. The abnormal glycogen is characterized by few branch points with long outer chains containing more α-1,4-linked glucose than normal glycogen. This resultant structure is similar to that of amylopectin (the structure of starch in plants), thus the associated name of amylopectinosis.

12. A 4-month-old White male infant with a temperature of 38.4°C is examined by his pediatrician. His mother indicates that he has had the fever for the past 4 days, been listless, vomiting, and has watery stools. Blood work indicates the infant is hypoglycemic but this condition does not respond to either epinephrine or glucose administration. In addition, his blood pH is slightly acidic and shows reduced bicarbonate. Other untoward blood chemistry includes elevated triglycerides, cholesterol, and liver enzymes. The child has a protuberant abdomen, thin extremities, and a doll-like face. The pediatrician suspects a specific condition and orders a liver biopsy to test for the activity of which of the following enzyme activities?

A. glucose 6-phosphatase
B. glycogen synthase
C. muscle phosphofructokinase
D. muscle phosphorylase
E. pyruvate kinase

Answer A: This child is manifesting the classic signs and symptoms of von Gierke disease (GSDI) which results from the absence of glucose-6-phosphatase activity. Patients with von Gierke disease can present during the neonatal period with lactic acidosis and hypoglycemia. The hallmark features of this disease are hypoglycemia, lactic acidosis, hyperuricemia, and hyperlipidemia. The severity of the hypoglycemia and lactic acidosis can be such that in the past the affected individuals died in infancy. Infants often have a doll-like facial appearance due to excess adipose tissue in the cheeks. The metabolic consequences of the hepatic glucose-6-phosphate deficiency of von Gierke disease extend well beyond just the obvious hypoglycemia that results from the deficiency in liver being able to deliver free glucose to the blood. The inability to release the phosphate from glucose 6-phopsphate results in diversion into glycolysis and production of pyruvate as well as increased diversion onto the pentose phosphate pathway. The production of excess pyruvate, at levels above of the capacity of the TCA cycle to completely oxidize it, results in its reduction to lactate leading to lactic acidemia. In addition, some of the pyruvate is transaminated to alanine leading to hyperalaninemia. Some of the pyruvate will be oxidized to acetyl-CoA, which cannot be fully oxidized in the TCA cycle and so the acetyl-CoA will end up in the cytosol where it will serve as a substrate for triglyceride and cholesterol synthesis resulting in hyperlipidemia. The oxidation of glucose 6-phosphate via the pentose phosphate pathway leads to increased production of ribose-5-phosphate which then activates the de novo synthesis of the purine nucleotides. In excess of the need, these purine nucleotides will ultimately be catabolized to uric acid, resulting in hyperuricemia and consequent symptoms of gout.

13. Synthesis of glycogen is inhibited in hepatocytes in response to glucagon stimulation primarily as a result of which of the following?
- A. a decrease in the level of phosphoprotein phosphatase
- B. a decrease in the level of phosphorylated phosphorylase kinase
- C. a decrease in the levels of phosphorylated phosphoprotein phosphatase inhibitor-1
- D. an increase in the level of the dephosphorylated form of glycogen synthase
- E. an increase in the level of the phosphorylated form of glycogen synthase

Answer E: Conditions of low blood glucose result in glucagon release from the pancreas. When glucagon binds to its receptors on hepatocytes, there is activation of adenylate cyclase resulting in increased cAMP with consequent activation of PKA. PKA phosphorylates and activates glycogen synthase-phosphorylase kinase, which will phosphorylate and activate phosphorylase while also phosphorylating and inhibiting glycogen synthase.

14. An 8-month-old female infant has died due to cardiorespiratory failure. Physical findings that were apparent prior to her death included feeding difficulties, cardiomegaly, macroglossia, mild hepatomegaly, hypotonia, and a rapidly progressing muscle weakness. Autopsy findings demonstrated marked intralysosomal accumulation of glycogen of normal structure in cardiac and skeletal muscle. These physical and clinical findings are consistent with which of the following glycogen storage diseases?
- A. Anderson disease
- B. Cori (or Forbes) disease
- C. McArdle disease
- D. Pompe disease
- E. Tarui disease

Answer D: Pompe disease, glycogen storage disease type II (GSDII), is the result of defective acid α-glucosidase (acid maltase) activity. Deficiency in acid maltase leads to intralysosomal accumulation of glycogen of normal structure in numerous tissues. Accumulation is most marked in cardiac, hepatic, and skeletal muscle tissues of infants with the generalized form of the disorder. The accumulation in skeletal muscle leads to hypotonia, and in the liver to hepatomegaly. The infantile form results in death due to cardiorespiratory failure usually before 2 years of age.

15. Which of the following shows the correct effects of hormones, when increased in serum, on liver glycogen content?

	Catecholamines	Glucocorticoids	Glucagon
A.	decreased	decreased	decreased
B.	decreased	decreased	increased
C.	decreased	increased	decreased
D.	increased	decreased	increased
E.	increased	increased	decreased

Answer C: Glucagon and catecholamines such as epinephrine stimulate the mobilization of glycogen by triggering the cAMP cascade. Hormones that increase liver cell cAMP promote glycogen breakdown, and hormones that decrease liver cell cAMP promote glycogen synthesis. Cortisol, the main glucocorticoid, regulates the metabolism of proteins, fats, and carbohydrates. It acts on most organs catabolically. However, on the liver it has anabolic effects, increasing glycogen synthesis and accumulation in the liver.

16. Which of the following enzymes is activated by dephosphorylation?
- A. glucose 6-phosphatase
- B. UDP-glucose pyrophosphorylase
- C. glycogen phosphorylase
- D. glycogen synthase
- E. phosphoglucomutase

Answer D: The activity of glycogen synthase is inhibited when the enzyme undergoes phosphorylation. There are a number of kinases that target this enzyme for inhibition including glycogen synthase-phosphorylase kinase, PKA, PKC, and GSK-3. Thus, removal of the phosphate added by any of these enzymes would result in increased glycogen synthase activity.

17. After fasting for 8 to 12 hours, the amount of glucose in the hepatic portal vein is markedly lower than the amount after a meal, but the amount in the systemic circulation remains near the normal level. Hepatocytes are able to maintain systemic glucose homeostasis in this situation primarily by gluconeogenesis and which of the following biochemical mechanisms?
- A. activation of lactase
- B. glycogenolysis
- C. glycolysis
- D. pentose phosphate pathway

Answer B: During periods of fasting, the pancreas releases glucagon to stimulate the liver to deliver glucose to the blood. When glucagon binds to its receptors on hepatocytes, there is activation of adenylate cyclase resulting in increased cAMP with consequent activation of PKA. PKA phosphorylates and activates glycogen synthase-phosphorylase kinase, which will phosphorylate and activate phosphorylase while also phosphorylating and inhibiting glycogen synthase. The increased activity of phosphorylase results in increased release of glucose from glycogen and its subsequent release to the blood.

18. During the past 3 years, a 20-year-old man has had increasing fatigue and muscle pain in his legs after jogging. Following exercise of his left upper arm, the lactate concentration remains decreased in blood obtained from a vein draining the exercised muscle. A deficiency is most likely in which of the following enzyme activities in the muscle?

A. fructose 1,6-bisphosphatase
B. fructose 1-phosphate aldolase
C. glucose 6-phosphatase
D. glycogen phosphorylase
E. pyruvate carboxylase

Answer D: Deficiency in muscle phosphorylase activity is associated with the development of McArdle disease (glycogen storage disease type V [GSDV]). The clinical presentation of GSDV is usually seen in young adulthood and is characterized by exercise intolerance and muscle cramps following slight exercise. Attacks of myoglobinuria frequently accompany the muscle symptoms of GSDV. About half of GSDV patients will exhibit burgundy-colored urine after exercise.

19. A 28-year-old man who recently received an injection of epinephrine following a bee sting now has hyperglycemia. The most likely cause is an increase in which of the following processes?

A. absorption of carbohydrate from the digestive tract
B. hepatic glycogenesis
C. hepatic glycogenolysis
D. proteolysis in muscle and release of amino acids
E. synthesis of glucose from fat

Answer C: Epinephrine can bind and activate both α-adrenergic and β-adrenergic receptors. When epinephrine binds α_1-adrenergic receptors, there is an activation of the membrane-associated enzyme PLC-β. PLC-β hydrolyzes membrane PIP_2 into DAG and IP_3. The IP_3 then binds to receptors present in membranes of the endoplasmic reticulum (ER) resulting in release of stored calcium ion. The released calcium binds to the calmodulin subunit of glycogen synthase-phosphorylase kinase, resulting in activation of this regulatory enzyme. The net effect is enhanced activity of phosphorylase and inhibited activity of glycogen synthase. When epinephrine binds β-adrenergic receptors, there is activation of adenylate cyclase resulting in increased cAMP with consequent activation of PKA. PKA phosphorylates and activates glycogen synthase-phosphorylase kinase with the results being the same as for α-adrenergic receptor activation.

20. Patients with an inherited deficiency of phosphorylase in skeletal muscle (McArdle disease) have decreased ability to derive energy from which of the following?

A. glucose
B. glycerol
C. glycogen
D. lactate
E. pyruvate

Answer C: McArdle disease is a glycogen storage disease of the muscle glycogenoses family. A deficiency in muscle phosphorylase results in defective release of glucose from glycogen stores preventing energy production from glucose oxidation during periods of fasting and exertion.

21. A 27-year-old man has an 11-year history of intermittent muscle pain, weakness, and stiffness following exercise. During exercise, serum lactate concentration does not increase. The most likely explanation for these findings is a deficiency of which of the following in muscle?

A. adenosine
B. calcium
C. glucose-6-phosphatase activity
D. inorganic phosphate
E. phosphorylase activity

Answer E: Deficiency in muscle phosphorylase activity is associated with the development of McArdle disease (glycogen storage disease type V [GSDV]). The clinical presentation of GSDV is usually seen in young adulthood and is characterized by exercise intolerance and muscle cramps following slight exercise. Attacks of myoglobinuria frequently accompany the muscle symptoms of GSDV. About half of GSDV patients will exhibit burgundy-colored urine after exercise.

22. Which of the following is most likely to result from an increased concentration of intracellular cAMP in skeletal muscle?

A. decreased activity of the TCA cycle
B. increased rate of glycogenolysis

C. increased synthesis of glycogen
D. inhibition of phosphofructokinase (PFK1)
E. rapid gluconeogenesis

Answer B: Increased intracellular cAMP results in the activation of PKA. PKA phosphorylates and activates glycogen synthase-phosphorylase kinase, which will phosphorylate and activate phosphorylase while also phosphorylating and inhibiting glycogen synthase. The increased activity of phosphorylase results in increased release of glucose from glycogen and its subsequent release to the blood.

23. The following reaction (where *n* represents the number of glucosyl residues), catalyzed by an enzyme activated by AMP, is essential for the mobilization of hepatic glycogen. In the equation, *X* and *Y* correspond to which of the following?

$$\text{Glycogen}_{(n)} + X \rightarrow \text{Glycogen}_{(n-1)} + Y$$

A. AMP and glucose
B. ATP and ADP
C. ATP and glucose 6-phosphate
D. H_2O and glucose
E. inorganic phosphate and glucose 1-phosphate

Answer E: The reaction is that catalyzed by glycogen phosphorylase, which catalyzes the phosphorolytic release of glucose from glycogen. The phosphorolysis reaction utilizes inorganic phosphate and the products are glucose 1-phosphate and glycogen with one less glucose.

24. A 24-year-old man comes to his doctor because of a 3-month history of pain in the arms and legs after strenuous exercise. He also had severe cramps and passed red urine after digging out several bushes from his front yard. Physical examination now shows abnormalities. This patient most likely has an inherited deficiency in which of the following enzymes?

A. glucocerebrosidase
B. glucose 6-phosphatase
C. hexosaminidase A
D. muscle phosphorylase
E. sphingomyelinase

Answer D: Deficiency in muscle phosphorylase activity is associated with the development of McArdle disease (glycogen storage disease type V [GSDV]). The clinical presentation of GSDV is usually seen in young adulthood and is characterized by exercise intolerance and muscle cramps following slight exercise. Attacks of myoglobinuria frequently accompany the muscle symptoms of GSDV. About half of GSDV patients will exhibit burgundy-colored urine after exercise.

25. A 25-year-old woman has just finished 30 minutes of vigorous weight lifting, which included several sets of squats. Which of the following substances has decreased most significantly in muscle cells of her thighs?

A. calcium
B. carbon dioxide
C. glycogen
D. lactate
E. myoglobin

Answer C: Vigorous exercise can lead to anaerobic metabolism in skeletal muscle cells. Under these conditions, the cells break down stored glycogen to release glucose for oxidation and energy production. Thus, the level of glycogen would decrease by the largest percentage. Conversely, lactate and carbon dioxide would increase under these conditions.

26. When glucose is incorporated into liver glycogen, which of the following is required as the direct glucosyl donor?

A. ADP glucose
B. CDP glucose
C. glucose 1-phosphate
D. sucrose
E. UDP glucose

Answer E: Glycogen synthase is the enzyme responsible for the incorporation of glucose into glycogen. The active form of glucose used as a substrate by glycogen synthase is UDP glucose.

27. A healthy 25-year-old man participates in a clinical study to determine glycogen stores after an 8-hour overnight fast. In preparation for the study, he follows a high-carbohydrate diet for 3 days. In the morning, he receives an injection of glucagon, which results in a significant increase in his serum glucose concentration. Which of the following best describes a reaction that would occur during the breakdown of hepatic glycogen to glucose in this patient?

A. debranching enzyme catalyzes the transfer of an oligomeric sugar unit from one glycogen branch to another
B. glucose 6-phosphate is converted to glucose 1-phosphate
C. glucose 6-phosphate plus ADP yields glucose plus ATP by hexokinase
D. α-1,6-glucosidase catalyzes the cleavage of glucose 1,6-bisphosphate

Answer A: During glucagon-stimulated glycogen breakdown, phosphorylase is activated and glucose present in α-1,4-glycosidic linkages is phosphorylytically released. Phosphorylase cannot remove glucose residues from the branch points (α-1,6 linkages) in glycogen. The activity of phosphorylase ceases 4 glucose residues from the branch point. The removal of these branch point glucose residues requires the action of debranching enzyme, which contains 2 activities: glucotransferase and glucosidase. The transferase activity removes the terminal 3 glucose residues of one branch and attaches them to a free C–4 end of a second branch. The glucose in α-(1,6)-linkage at the branch is then removed by the action of the glucosidase activity.

28. A 20-year-old man comes to the physician because of progressive, painful muscle cramps and intolerance to exercise during the past 3 months. On one occasion, he passed burgundy-colored urine. His serum lactate concentration does not increase in blood from the vein proximal to an exercised right forearm. A biopsy specimen of muscle shows an increased concentration of glycogen. Which of the following enzymes is most likely deficient in this patient's muscle?

A. debrancher enzyme
B. glucose 6-phosphatase
C. α-1,4-glucosidase
D. glycogen phosphorylase
E. UTP-dependent pyrophosphorylase

Answer D: Deficiency in muscle phosphorylase activity is associated with the development of McArdle disease (glycogen storage disease type V [GSDV]). The clinical presentation of GSDV is usually seen in young adulthood and is characterized by exercise intolerance and muscle cramps following slight exercise. Attacks of myoglobinuria frequently accompany the muscle symptoms of GSDV. About half of GSDV patients will exhibit burgundy-colored urine after exercise.

29. A 27-year-old man has been preparing for a marathon. As part of his normal prerace routine, he consumes a large meal consisting of pasta and mashed potatoes the night before the race. Which of the following enzymes is most likely to be stimulated in his hepatocytes, resulting in increased glycogen stores in this man?

A. glucokinase
B. glucose 6-phosphatase
C. glycogen phosphorylase
D. hexokinase
E. lactate dehydrogenase

Answer A: High carbohydrate loading, as is typical for distance runners, results in an increased level of insulin release from the pancreas. Insulin effects on the liver include changes in the activities of several enzymes, such as that of glucokinase. Glucokinase is the hepatic form of the glucose-phosphorylating enzymes.

30. A 9-month-old infant has a 6-month history of progressive muscle weakness and congestive heart failure with a markedly enlarged heart. She can no longer roll over, is flaccid, and her head flops back when she is lifted. She remains alert and interested in her environment. A muscle biopsy shows increased glycogen particles in lysosomes. The most likely cause of these symptoms is a deficiency of which of the following enzymes?

A. acid maltase
B. glucose 6-phopshatase
C. α-glucosidase
D. muscle PFK1
E. muscle phosphorylase

Answer A: Glycogen storage disease type II (GSDII) is also known as Pompe disease and results from defects in the gene encoding lysosomal acid maltase. Thus, the disease is also referred to as acid maltase deficiency (AMD). The clinical presentation of GSDII encompasses a wide range of phenotypes, but all include various degrees of cardiomegaly. Additional clinical manifestations associated with idiopathic cardiomegaly accompanied by storage of glycogen are indicative of Pompe disease. These symptoms included hepatomegaly, marked hypotonia, muscular weakness, and death before 1 year of age. The different phenotypes can be classified dependent upon age of onset, extent of organ involvement, and the rate of progression to death.

31. A 19-year-old man comes to the physician because of muscle cramping that began after he participated in a race 24 hours ago. He has had similar but mild symptoms since adolescence that have progressed in severity since he joined a college track team. Physical examination shows no abnormalities. No significant lactate concentration increase is observed in blood obtained distal to an exercised ischemic right arm. A deficiency of which of the following in muscle is the most likely cause of this patient's symptoms?

A. acid maltase
B. carnitine
C. debranching enzyme
D. glucose 6-phosphatase
E. glycogen phosphorylase

Answer E: Deficiency in muscle phosphorylase activity is associated with the development of McArdle disease (glycogen storage disease type V [GSDV]).

The clinical presentation of GSDV is usually seen in young adulthood and is characterized by exercise intolerance and muscle cramps following slight exercise. Attacks of myoglobinuria frequently accompany the muscle symptoms of GSDV. About half of GSDV patients will exhibit burgundy-colored urine after exercise.

32. A 2-year-old girl is brought to the physician because of irritability and failure to thrive. Physical examination shows hepatomegaly. Laboratory studies show mild fasting hypoglycemia. A high-protein diet or intravenous administration of fructose results in an increased serum glucose concentration. Biopsy of hepatic tissue shows increased amounts of glycogen with short outer branches. The most likely cause of her condition is a defect in which of the following?

A. debranching enzyme
B. glucokinase
C. glucose 6-phosphatase
D. glycogen phosphorylase
E. glycogen synthase

Answer A: The child is suffering from glycogen storage disease type III (GSDIII), which is also known as Cori disease, Forbes disease, or limit dextrinosis. This GSD results from defects in the gene encoding glycogen debrancher enzyme, also known as amylo-1,6-glucosidase. Deficiency in glycogen-debranching activity causes hepatomegaly, ketotic hypoglycemia, hyperlipidemia, variable skeletal myopathy, and cardiomyopathy and results in short stature. Patients with both liver and muscle involvement have GSDIIIa and those with only liver involvement (~15% of GSDIII patients) are classified as GSDIIIb. Because hepatomegaly, hypoglycemia, hyperlipidemia, and growth retardation are common symptoms in both GSDI and GSDIII, it is difficult to initially determine from which disease an infant is suffering. Definitive diagnosis is made only by examining the structure of the glycogen in patients as well as assaying for the level of activity of the debranching enzyme.

33. A healthy subject who fasts for 24 hours is most likely to have a decrease in which of the following?

A. hepatic glycogenesis
B. ketone body formation
C. plasma cortisol concentration
D. plasma glucagon concentration
E. renal gluconeogenesis

Answer A: During periods of fasting, the pancreas releases glucagon to stimulate the liver to deliver glucose to the blood. When glucagon binds to its receptors on hepatocytes, there is activation of adenylate cyclase resulting in increased cAMP with consequent activation of PKA. PKA phosphorylates and activates glycogen synthase-phosphorylase kinase, which will phosphorylate and activate phosphorylase while also phosphorylating and inhibiting glycogen synthase. The increased activity of phosphorylase results in increased release of glucose from glycogen while the inhibited glycogen synthase reduces glycogenesis.

34. Analysis of a tissue sample obtained on biopsy of the liver in a patient with GSD shows normal activities of glycogen phosphorylase, glycogen debranching enzyme, and glucose 6-phosphatase. A defect in the signal transduction pathway for glycogen metabolism is suspected. Which of the following enzymes is most likely to be defective?

A. glycogen branching enzyme
B glycogen synthase
C hexokinase
D phosphorylase phosphatase
E phosphorylase kinase

Answer E: A deficiency in the activity of phosphorylase kinase results in a glycogen storage disease (GSD9) whose symptoms include hepatomegaly, mild hypoglycemia, hyperlipidemia, and ketosis. These symptoms are similar to those exhibited by GSDVI, also known as Hers disease.

35. When serum glucose concentrations are decreased, glucagon is released from the pancreas and binds to a receptor on hepatic cell membranes. As a result, hepatic glycogen synthesis is inhibited. By which of the following mechanisms is glycogen synthase modified to cause this inhibition?

A. allosteric inhibition by bound AMP
B. binding of intracellular glucose 1-phosphate with a lower K_m
C. dephosphorylation by a glucagon-dependent phosphatase
D. increased amounts of the enzyme due to the CREB protein
E. phosphorylation on serine residues

Answer E: During periods of fasting, the pancreas releases glucagon to stimulate the liver to deliver glucose to the blood. When glucagon binds to its receptors on hepatocytes, there is activation of adenylate cyclase resulting in increased cAMP with consequent activation of the serine/threonine kinase, PKA. PKA phosphorylates and activates glycogen synthase-phosphorylase kinase, which will phosphorylate and activate phosphorylase while also phosphorylating and inhibiting glycogen synthase.

36. A 4-month-old girl with a 1-month history of poor head control and progressive muscle weakness is brought to the physician for a follow-up examination. Physical signs show a large tongue, hepatomegaly, and severe generalized hypotonia. A chest x-ray shows cardiomegaly. She dies of cardiac failure at the age of 10 months. Autopsy shows a markedly enlarged globular heart, hepatomegaly, and glycogen in the skeletal muscle, heart, and liver. This patient most likely had a deficiency in which of the following?

A. acid α-glucosidase
B. branching enzyme
C. debranching enzyme
D. glucose 6-phosphatase
E. hepatic phosphorylase

Answer C: The infant is suffering from glycogen storage disease type III (GSDIII), which is also known as Cori disease, Forbes disease, or limit dextrinosis. This GSD results from defects in the gene encoding glycogen debrancher enzyme, also known as amylo-1,6-glucosidase. Deficiency in glycogen debranching activity causes hepatomegaly, ketotic hypoglycemia, hyperlipidemia, variable skeletal myopathy, cardiomyopathy, and results in short stature. Patients with both liver and muscle involvement have GSDIIIa and those with only liver involvement (~15% of GSDIII patients) are classified as GSDIIIb. Because heptomegaly, hypoglycemia, hyperlipidemia, and growth retardation are common symptoms in both GSDI and GSDIII, it is difficult to initially determine from which disease an infant is suffering. Definitive diagnosis is only made by examining the structure of the glycogen in patients as well as assaying for the level of activity of the debranching enzyme.

Checklist

✓ Glycogen constitutes the primary storage form of carbohydrate from which glucose can be released during periods of fasting, starvation, and aerobic metabolism particularly within skeletal muscle.

✓ The 2 major sites for glycogen storage are the liver and skeletal muscle. Hepatic glycogen allows the liver to respond to low blood glucose levels and readily release its stored glucose to the blood for use by extra hepatic tissues. Within skeletal muscle, glycogen allows this tissue to respond to periods of aerobic metabolism by readily releasing the glucose into the glycolytic pool.

✓ Release of glucose from glycogen does not require the input of energy since the release is a phosphorylytic reaction catalyzed by phosphorylase.

✓ The primary hormone-mediated regulator of glycogen synthesis and breakdown is cAMP, which activates PKA. Glucagon stimulates cAMP production leading to inhibition of glycogen synthesis and activation of glycogenolysis. Conversely, insulin stimulates the hydrolysis of cAMP, reversing the effects of glucagon.

✓ Epinephrine also stimulates glycogenolysis via the activation of β-adrenergic receptors that result in increased cAMP production.

✓ Skeletal muscle twitch leads to release of stored calcium from the sarcoplasmic reticulum. The calcium then activates phosphorylase kinase, resulting in phosphorylation and inhibition of glycogen synthase while simultaneously phosphorylating and activating phosphorylase.

✓ Deficiencies in many of the enzymes of glycogen synthesis and breakdown result in mild to severe disorders. These disorders primarily affect the liver and/or skeletal muscle and therefore, manifest with symptoms associated with defects in metabolic functions in these 2 tissues.

CHAPTER

15 Carbohydrates: Pentose Phosphate Pathway

CHAPTER OUTLINE

High-Yield Terms

Glucose-6-phosphate dehydrogenase (G6PDH): primary rate-limiting, oxidative enzyme of the PPP; mutations in this gene are the most common causes of hemolytic anemia worldwide, yet protect individuals from malaria

Transketolase: thiamine-requiring enzyme, enzyme of the nonoxidative stage of the PPP that transfers 2-carbon units

Transaldolase: thiamine-requiring enzyme, enzyme of the nonoxidative stage of the PPP that transfers 3-carbon units

Oxygen burst: phagocytic cells of the immune system utilize NADPH generated via the PPP to generate superoxide radicals to kill phagocytized microorganisms. This requires a dramatic increase in O_2 consumption referred to as the oxygen burst

Chronic granulomatous disease: results in individuals harboring defects in the NADPH oxidase system of phagocytic cells, results in frequent pneumonia, abscesses of the skin, tissues, and organs, suppurative arthritis, and osteomyelitis. Defects occur in both the NADPH oxidase complex itself and the enzymes of the PPP that yield the required NADPH, particularly G6PDH

The Pentose Phosphate Pathway

The pentose phosphate pathway (PPP) (also called hexose monophosphate shunt, HMS) consists of series of interconnected reactions that serve as an alternate route for the metabolism of glucose. The pathway is primarily an anabolic pathway that utilizes the 6 carbons of glucose to generate 5-carbon sugars and reducing equivalents in the form of NADPH. However, this pathway does play a role in the oxidation of glucose and under certain conditions can completely oxidize glucose to CO_2 and water. The 2 primary functions of this pathway are (1) the generation of NADPH for use in other reductive biosynthetic (anabolic) pathways and (2) to convert glucose carbons into ribose 5-phosphate (R5P) for the synthesis of the nucleotides and nucleic acids. Although not a significant function of the PPP, it can operate to metabolize dietary pentose sugars derived from the digestion of nucleic acids as well as to rearrange the carbon skeletons of dietary carbohydrates into glycolytic/gluconeogenic intermediates (Figure 15-1).

Enzymes that function primarily in the reductive direction utilize the $NADP^+$/NADPH cofactor pair as cofactors as opposed to oxidative enzymes that utilize the NAD^+/NADH cofactor pair. The reactions of fatty acid biosynthesis and steroid biosynthesis utilize large amounts of NADPH. As a consequence, cells of the liver, adipose tissue, adrenal cortex, testis, and lactating mammary gland have high levels of the PPP enzymes. In fact 30% of the oxidation of glucose in the liver occurs via the PPP. Additionally, erythrocytes utilize the reactions of the PPP to generate large amounts of NADPH used in the reduction of glutathione (see below). The conversion of ribonucleotides to deoxyribonucleotides, through the action of ribonucleotide reductase, requires NADPH, therefore any rapidly proliferating cell needs large quantities of NADPH.

Although the PPP operates in all cells, with high levels of expression in the above indicated tissues, the highest levels of PPP enzymes (in particular glucose 6-phosphate dehydrogenase) are found in neutrophils and macrophages. These leukocytes are the phagocytic cells of the immune system and they utilize NADPH to generate superoxide radicals from molecular oxygen in a reaction catalyzed by NADPH oxidase. Superoxide anion, in turn, serves to generate other reactive oxygen species (ROS) that kill the phagocytized microorganisms.

Reactions of the Pentose Phosphate Pathway

The reactions of the PPP operate exclusively in the cytoplasm. The PPP is composed of both oxidative and nonoxidative reactions. The oxidation steps, utilizing glucose 6-phosphate (G6P) as the substrate, occur at the beginning of the pathway and are the reactions that generate NADPH. The reactions catalyzed by G6PDH and 6-phosphogluconate dehydrogenase each generate 1 mole of NADPH for every mole of glucose 6-phosphate (G6P) that enters the PPP. The net yield from both of these oxidative reactions is 2 moles of NADPH per mole of G6P (Figure 15-2).

The nonoxidative reactions of the PPP are primarily designed to generate R5P. Equally important reactions of the PPP are to convert dietary 5-carbon sugars into both 6- and 3-carbon sugars (fructose 6-phosphate and glyceraldehydes 3-phosphate, respectively) which can then be utilized by the pathways of glycolysis or gluconeogenesis. The primary enzymes involved in the nonoxidative steps of the PPP are transaldolase and transketolase. Transketolase functions to transfer 2-carbon groups from substrates of the PPP, thus rearranging the carbon atoms that enter this pathway. Like other enzymes that transfer 2-carbon groups, transketolase requires thiamine pyrophosphate (TPP) as a cofactor. Transaldolase transfers 3-carbon groups, and thus is also involved in a rearrangement of the carbon skeletons of the substrates of the PPP.

The net result of the PPP is the oxidation of 3 moles of G6P into 3 moles of 5-carbon sugars and 3 moles of CO_2. Following rearrangement of the 5-carbon sugars in the nonoxidative reactions 2 moles of G6P are regenerated along with 1 mole of glyceraldehydes 3-phosphate. The G6P can be recycled into the oxidative reactions of the PPP, generating more NADPH. The glyceraldehydes

High-Yield Concept

Following exposure to bacteria and other foreign substances there is a dramatic increase in O_2 consumption by phagocytes in a phenomenon referred to as the oxygen burst.

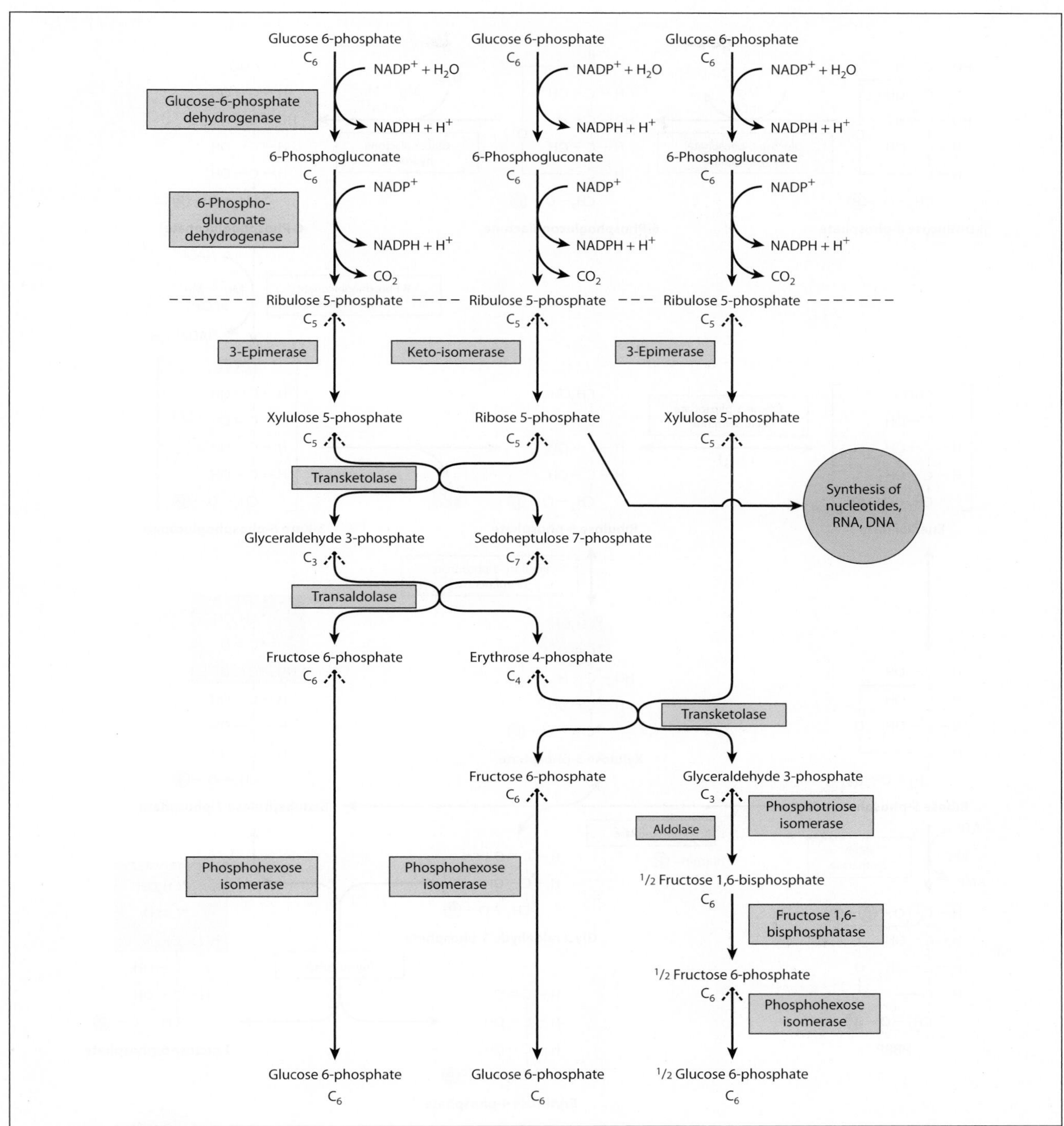

FIGURE 15-1: Flow chart of pentose phosphate pathway and its connections with the pathway of glycolysis. The full pathway, as indicated, consists of three interconnected cycles in which glucose 6-phosphate is both substrate and end product. The reactions above the broken line are nonreversible, whereas all reactions under that line are freely reversible apart from that catalyzed by fructose 1,6-bisphosphatase. Murray RK, Bender DA, Botham KM, Kennelly PJ, Rodwell VW, Weil PA. *Harper's Illustrated Biochemistry*, 29th ed. New York, NY: McGraw-Hill; 2012.

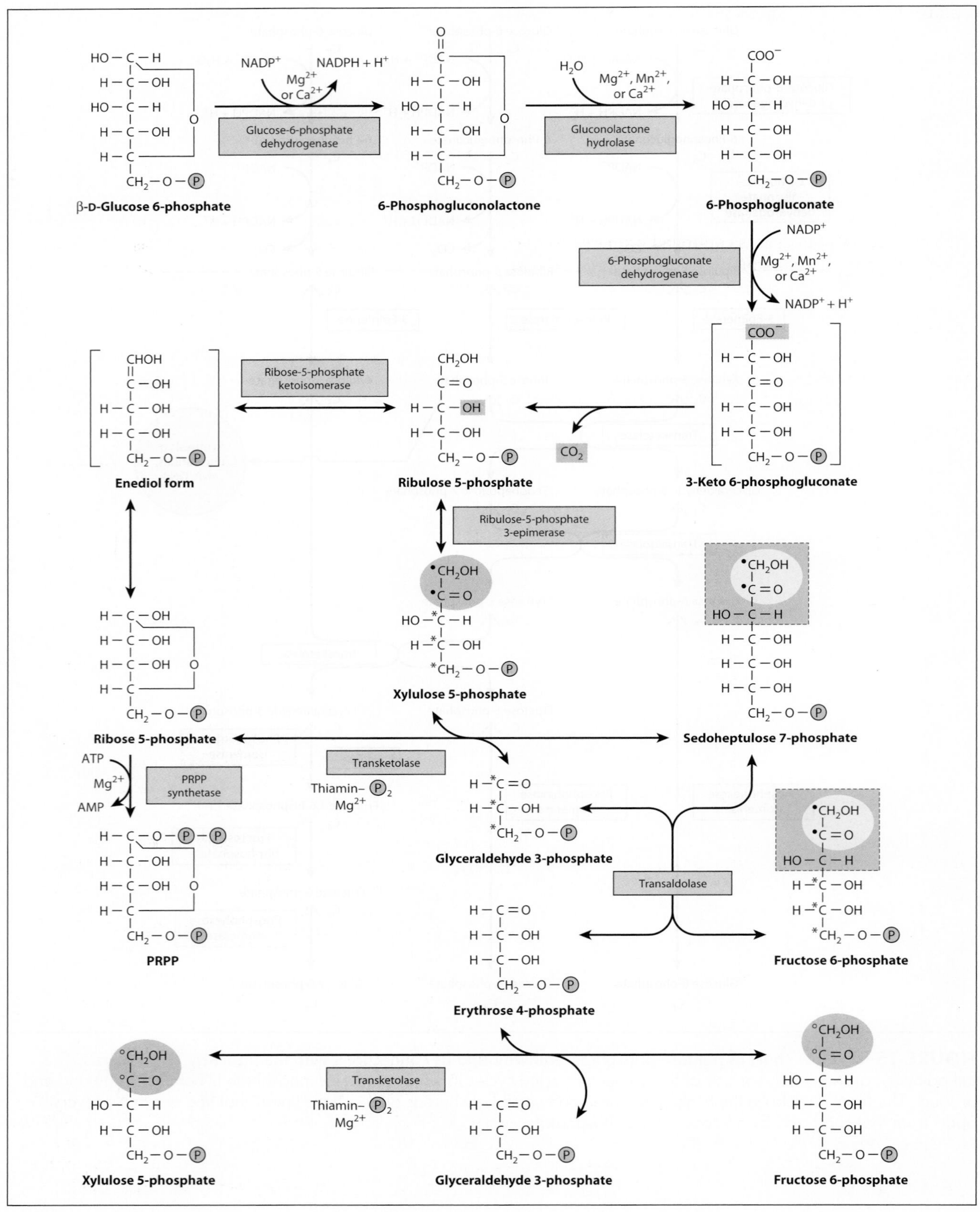

FIGURE 15-2: The pentose phosphate pathway. (P, $-PO_3^{2-}$; PRPP, 5-phosphoribosyl 1-pyrophosphate.) Murray RK, Bender DA, Botham KM, Kennelly PJ, Rodwell VW, Weil PA. *Harper's Illustrated Biochemistry*, 29th ed. New York, NY: McGraw-Hill; 2012.

3-phosphate can be shunted into glycolysis and oxidized to pyruvate or alternatively; it can be utilized by the gluconeogenic enzymes to generate more 6-carbon sugars (fructose 6-phosphate or G6P).

The PPP and the Control of Oxidative Stress

Oxidative stress within cells is controlled primarily by the action of the peptide, glutathione (GSH). GSH is a tripeptide composed of γ-glutamate, cysteine, and glycine. The sulfhydryl side chains of the cysteine residues of 2 glutathione molecules form a disulfide bond (GSSG) during the course of being oxidized in reactions with various oxides and lipid hydroperoxides (LOOH) in cells (Figure 15-3).

Oxidative stress also generates peroxides that in turn can be reduced by glutathione to generate water and an alcohol, or two waters if the peroxide is hydrogen peroxide. Regeneration of reduced glutathione (GSH) is carried out by the enzymes glutathione reductase (requiring NADPH) and glutathione peroxidase.

There are at least 3 inborn errors in the PPP that have been identified. The most common being the result of mutations in G6PDH. Extremely rare occurrences of ribose-5-phosphate isomerase and transaldolase deficiency have also been documented. In the transaldolase deficiency individuals with liver problems are the principal symptom in neonates. Any disruption in the level of NADPH production may have a profound effect upon the ability of a cell to deal with oxidative stress (Clinical Box 15-1).

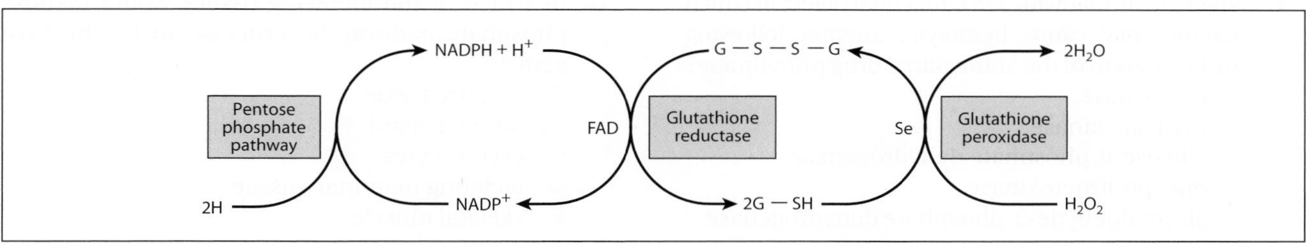

FIGURE 15-3: Role of the pentose phosphate pathway in the glutathione peroxidase reaction of erythrocytes. (G-SH, reduced glutathione; G-S-S-G, oxidized glutathione; Se, selenium-containing enzyme.) Murray RK, Bender DA, Botham KM, Kennelly PJ, Rodwell VW, Weil PA. *Harper's Illustrated Biochemistry*, 29th ed. New York, NY: McGraw-Hill; 2012.

CLINICAL BOX 15-1: CHRONIC GRANULOMATOUS DISEASE

Because of the need for NADPH in phagocytic cells, by the NADPH oxidase system, any defect in enzymes in this process can result in impaired killing of infectious organisms. Chronic granulomatous disease (CGD) is a syndrome that results in individuals harboring defects in the NADPH oxidase system. There are several forms of CGD involving defects in various components of the NADPH oxidase system. Individuals with CGD are at increased risk for specific recurrent infections. The most common are pneumonia; abscesses of the skin, tissues, and organs; suppurative arthritis (invasion of the joints by infectious agent leading to generation of pus); and osteomyelitis (infection of the bone). The majority of patients with CGD harbor mutations in an *X-chromosome* gene that encodes a component of the NADPH oxidase system. The encoded protein is the β-subunit of cytochrome b_{245} (gene symbol *CYBB*), also called p91-PHOX or NOX2. This form of the disorder is referred to as cytochrome *b*-negative X-linked CGD. There is an autosomal recessive cytochrome *b*-negative form of CGD due to defects in the α-subunit of cytochrome b_{245} (gene symbol *CYBA*), also called p22-PHOX or NOX1. There are also 2 autosomal recessive cytochrome *b*-positive forms of CGD identified as cytochrome *b*-positive CGD type I and type II. The type I form is caused by mutation in the neutrophil cytosolic factor 1 (NCF1) gene, which encodes the p47-PHOX (phagocyte oxidase) protein. The type II form is caused by mutation in the NFC2 gene which encodes the p67-PHOX (phagocyte oxidase) protein. Given the role of NADPH in the process of phagocytic killing, it should be clear that individuals with reduced ability to produce NADPH (such as those with G6PDH deficiencies) may also manifest with symptoms of CGD.

The Role of the PPP in the Erythrocyte

The predominant pathways of carbohydrate metabolism in the erythrocyte are glycolysis, the PPP, and 2,3-bisphosphoglycerate (2,3-BPG) metabolism. Glycolysis provides ATP for membrane ion pumps and NADH for reoxidation of methemoglobin (Chapter 6), while the PPP supplies the erythrocyte with NADPH to maintain the reduced state of glutathione. The inability to maintain reduced glutathione in erythrocytes leads to increased accumulation of peroxides, predominantly H_2O_2, that in turn results in a weakening of the cell wall and concomitant hemolysis. Accumulation of H_2O_2 also leads to increased rates of oxidation of hemoglobin to methemoglobin that also weakens the cell wall. Glutathione removes peroxides via the action of glutathione peroxidase. The PPP in erythrocytes is essentially the only pathway for these cells to produce NADPH. Any defect in the production of NADPH could, therefore, have profound effects on erythrocyte survival.

Deficiency in the level of activity of G6PDH is the basis of favism, primaquine (an antimalarial drug) sensitivity, and several other drug-sensitive hemolytic anemias, anemia and jaundice in the newborn, and chronic nonspherocytic hemolytic anemia. In addition, G6PDH deficiencies are associated with resistance to the malarial parasite, *Plasmodium falciparum*, among individuals of Mediterranean and African descent. The basis for this resistance is the weakening of the erythrocyte membrane such that it cannot sustain the parasitic life cycle long enough for productive growth.

REVIEW QUESTIONS

1. Which of the following is a congenital defect in which enzyme may cause hemolytic anemia following administration of the antimalarial drug primaquine?
- **A.** hexokinase
- **B.** pyruvate kinase
- **C.** glucose-6-phosphate dehydrogenase
- **D.** phosphofructokinase
- **E.** glyceraldehyde-3-phosphate dehydrogenase

Answer C: Primaquine is used to treat malaria since it causes lysis of erythrocytes that have been weakened by the presence of the parasite. When administered to humans, primaquine is metabolized into an arylhydroxylamine metabolite that exerts the hemotoxi effects. Primaquine causes methemoglobinemia in all patients. However, dangerous levels of methemoglobinemia only occur in patients with glucose-6-phosphate dehydrogenase (G6PDH) deficiency and, thus, this drug should not be administered to anyone with a deficiency in this enzyme.

2. The transketolase enzyme of the pentose phosphate pathway requires which of the the following for maximal activity?
- **A.** biotin
- **B.** calcium ions
- **C.** coenzyme A
- **D.** tetrahydrofolate
- **E.** TPP

Answer E: Transketolase functions to transfer 2-carbon groups from substrates of the PPP, thus rearranging the carbon atoms that enter this pathway. Like other enzymes that transfer 2-carbon groups, transketolase requires TPP as a cofactor in the transfer reaction.

3. In which of the following tissues would pentose phosphate pathway be expected to be the least active?
- **A.** adipose tissue
- **B.** adrenal gland
- **C.** erythrocytes
- **D.** lactating mammary tissue
- **E.** skeletal muscle

Answer E: The reactions of fatty acid biosynthesis and steroid biosynthesis utilize large amounts of NADPH. As a consequence, cells of the liver, adipose tissue, adrenal cortex, testis, and lactating mammary gland have high levels of the PPP enzymes. Skeletal muscle, although active at de novo fatty acid synthesis, have the lowest levels of expression of enzymes of the PPP.

4. Your patient is suffering from chronic granulomatous disease (CGD) which results in recurrent bouts of infection. CGD is characterized by an inability of phagocytic cells to kill invading microbes that they have engulfed because these cells lack the ability to generate reactive oxygen species such as H_2O_2. A defect in which of the following enzymes is most likely the cause of the phagocytic cell dysfunction?
- **A.** G6PDH
- **B.** glyceraldehyde-3-phosphate dehydrogenase
- **C.** glycerol-3-phosphate dehydrogenase
- **D.** α-ketoglutarate dehydrogenase
- **E.** pyruvate dehydrogenase

Answer A: The highest levels of PPP enzymes (in particular G6PDH) are found in neutrophils and macrophages. These leukocytes are the phagocytic cells of the immune system and they utilize NADPH to generate superoxide radicals from molecular oxygen in a reaction catalyzed by NADPH oxidase. Therefore, deficiency in the activity of G6PDH can result in defective function in the NADPH oxidase system in these cells.

5. A 22-year-old black male was given the antimalaria drug primaquine to take while on an expedition on the Amazon River. After taking the drug, he developed an acute anemia. The anemia was secondary to an intravascular hemolytic crisis. This crisis was reversed when he discontinued taking the primaquine. This drug-induced hemolytic anemia arises in persons who have a deficiency in which of the following enzymes?

A. glyceraldehyde-3-phosphate dehydrogenase
B. glycerol-3-phosphate dehydrogenase
C. G6PDH
D. pyruvate dehydrogenase
E. succinate dehydrogenase

Answer C: Primaquine is used to treat malaria since it causes lysis of erythrocytes that have been weakened by the presence of the parasite. When administered to humans, primaquine is metabolized into an arylhydroxylamine metabolite that exerts the hemotoxi effects. Primaquine causes methemoglobinemia in all patients. However, dangerous levels of methemoglobinemia only occur in patients with G6PDH deficiency and, thus, this drug should not be administered to anyone with a deficiency of this enzyme.

6. Oxidative breakdown of glucose can occur in certain mammalian cells by mechanisms other than classic glycolysis. In most of these cells, G6P is oxidized to 6-phosphogluconate. Which of the following represents the next intermediate in this alternative glucose oxidation pathway?

A. an aldolase-type split to form glyceric acid and glyceraldehyde 3-phosphate
B. an aldolase-type split to form glycolic acid and erythrose 4-phosphate
C. conversion to 1,6-bisphosphogluconate
D. decarboxylation to produce an aldopentose
E oxidation to a 6-carbon dicarboxylic acid

Answer D: The next reaction in the PPP, catalyzed by 6-phosphogluconate dehydrogenase, oxidatively decarboxylates 6-phosphogluconate to the 5-carbon aldose sugar, ribulose 5-phopshate.

7. A 2-year-old child who is a native of East Africa has been diagnosed with a deficiency in G6PDH. Following consumption of fava beans the child experiences a mild hemolytic anemia. Which of the following symptoms would also likely be present in this child?

A. coarse facial features and bulging forehead
B. dermatitis, diarrhea, and dementia
C. hypoglycemia and galactosemia
D. ocular stomatitis
E. splenomegaly and jaundice

Answer A: Favism is the term associated with the hemolytic anemia that results from the consumption of fava beans in individuals with deficiencies in G6PDH. The deficiency prevents erythrocytes from coping with the oxidative stress induced by metabolism of substances in fava beans. The continued hemolysis leads to hyperbilirubinemia, splenomegaly, and skeletal abnormalities in infants. The facial anomalies associated with favism are due to repeated episodes of intracranial hemorrhage.

8. Which of the following represents the main function of the pentose phosphate pathway?

A. provides a mechanism for the utilization of the carbon skeletons of excess amino acids
B. provides an alternative pathway for energy production should glycolysis fail
C. provides an alternative pathway for oxidation of excess fructose
D. supplies the cell with hexose sugars and NADH
E. supplies the cell with pentose sugars and NADPH

Answer E: The 2 major functions of the PPP are (1) the generation of reducing equivalents, in the form of NADPH, for reductive biosynthesis reactions within cells and (2) to provide the cell with ribose 5-phosphate (R5P) for the synthesis of the nucleotides and nucleic acids.

9. The reactions of the PPP using glucose 6-phosphate as the initial substrate are best described by which of the following statements?

A. they are not required for the production of NADPH in the mature erythrocyte
B. they are required for the metabolism of glucose in the muscles
C. they generate 2 moles of adenosine triphosphate per mole of G6P metabolized to ribulose 5-phosphate.
D. they occur in the matrix of mitochondria
E. they produce 2 moles of NADPH for each mole of CO_2 released

Answer E: During the oxidative reactions of the PPP, the enzymes G6PDH and 6-phosphoglucinate dehydrogenase each generate a mole of NADPH. The latter reaction is an oxidative decarboxylation reaction generating the mole of CO_2 produced via the PPP.

10. A 50-year-old alcoholic male presents with pain, numbness, tingling, and weakness in his feet. He is diagnosed with thiamine deficiency. Thiamine is required as a cofactor for which of the following enzymes?
- **A.** gluconolactone hydrolase
- **B.** G6PDH
- **C.** 6-phosphogluconate dehydrogenase
- **D.** transaldolase
- **E.** transketolase

Answer D: Transketolase functions to transfer 2-carbon groups from substrates of the PPP, thus rearranging the carbon atoms that enter this pathway. Like other enzymes that transfer 2-carbon groups, transketolase requires TPP as a cofactor in the transfer reaction.

11. Which of the following enzymes represents a key regulated enzyme of the PPP?
- **A.** gluconolactone hydrolase
- **B.** G6PDH
- **C.** 6-phosphogluconate dehydrogenase
- **D.** transaldolase
- **E.** transketolase

Answer B: The key regulated enzyme of the PPP, G6PDH, catalyzes the initial oxidation reaction of the pathway.

12. Xylulose 5-phosphate can be formed from ribulose 5-phosphate via the action of which of the following enzymes?
- **A.** G6PDH
- **B.** phosphopentose epimerase
- **C.** phosphopentose isomerase
- **D.** transaldolase
- **E.** transketolase

Answer B: The conversion of ribulose 5-phosphate to xylulose 5-phosphate is an epimerization reaction. This reaction is catalyzed by the phosphopentose epimerase more commonly called ribulose 5-phosphate epimerase.

13. The PPP is active in liver, adipose tissue, adrenal cortex, thyroid, erythrocytes, testis, and lactating mammary gland. Why is the pathway less active in skeletal muscle?
- **A.** muscle tissue contains very small amounts of the enzymes of the nonoxidative phase of the PPP
- **B.** muscle tissue contains very small amounts of the dehydrogenases of the PPP
- **C.** muscle tissues do not require NADPH
- **D.** the pentose sugars generated by the PPP are not required by muscle tissue

Answer B: The enzymes of the PPP are expressed at highest levels in tissues that carry out high rates of lipid biosynthesis. Skeletal muscle, although active at de novo fatty acid synthesis, does not require high rates of fatty acid synthesis because it can acquire them readily from the blood. Therefore, expression of the oxidative enzymes of the PPP is at low levels in this tissue.

14. While training for a triathlon, a 25-year-old female follows a high-carbohydrate diet that provides for adequate glycogen and fat synthesis. When she begins the competition, fatty acid synthesis stops. The best explanation for this is a decrease in which of the following?
- **A.** gluconeogenesis
- **B.** glycogenolysis
- **C.** oxidative phosphorylation
- **D.** PPP
- **E.** TCA cycle

Answer D: Fatty acid synthesis requires NADPH derived from the PPP via the oxidation of G6P. During strenuous exercise the vast majority of the glucose is shunted into glycolysis for complete oxidation. Therefore, little G6P is available for the PPP.

15. A 32-year-old man of Mediterranean descent is brought to the physician because of a 2-day history of fatigue and shortness of breath. He recently had a urinary tract infection treated with trimethoprim-sulfamethoxazole. His pulse is 100/minute. Physical examination shows pallor and scleral icterus. Laboratory studies show a decreased erythrocyte count and an increased serum bilirubin concentration that is mainly indirect. This patient's anemia is most likely due to failure of which of the following?
- **A.** bone marrow production of reticulocytes
- **B.** erythrocyte production of lactic acid
- **C.** erythrocyte protection against membrane oxidation
- **D.** reticulocyte maturation
- **E.** reticulocyte synthesis of heme

Answer C: Erythrocytes require a continuous source for NADPH to ensure that oxidized glutathione can be reduced by the glutathione peroxidase system. Glutathione is oxidized when it scavenges reactive oxygen species and by reducing oxidized membrane lipids. Administration of oxidizing drugs such as those of the sulfa class can lead to weakening of erythrocyte plasma membranes due to rapid depletion of reduced glutathione levels and inadequate NADPH-dependent reduction of the oxidized form.

Checklist

✓ The PPP reactions occur in the cytosol and oxidize glucose while producing NADPH and CO_2 but they do not generate ATP energy.

✓ The oxidative reactions of the PPP are irreversible, whereas the nonoxidative reactions are reversible.

✓ Major tissues utilizing the reactions of the PPP have a high need for NADPH for reductive biosynthesis pathways or a high need for ribose 5-phosphate for nucleic acid synthesis.

✓ Erythrocytes have a critical need for the oxidative reactions of the PPP to generate NADPH for use in the regeneration of oxidized glutathione (GSH), via the glutathione peroxidase reaction, in order that it can be used to continuously repair oxidized membrane lipids.

✓ Generation of NADPH via the PPP is critical for the function of phagocytic cells. Mutations in G6PDH can lead to chronic granulomatous disease, whose symptoms are reflective of the lack of phagocytic killing of pathogens.

✓ Inherited mutations in G6PDH can cause hemolytic anemia in afflicted individuals who are exposed to high oxidizing conditions in the blood or following the ingestion of certain pharmaceuticals. However, G6PDH deficiencies also protect afflicted individuals from the harmful effects of the malarial parasite.

CHAPTER

16 Pyruvate Dehydrogenase Complex and the TCA Cycle

CHAPTER OUTLINE

High-Yield Terms

PDH kinases: allosteric regulated family of kinases that modify the activity of the PDHc

Malate-aspartate shuttle: principal mechanism for the movement of reducing equivalents (in the form of NADH) from the cytoplasm to the mitochondria

Substrate-level phosphorylation: the succinyl-CoA synthetase–catalyzed reaction involves the use of the high-energy thioester of succinyl-CoA to drive synthesis of a high-energy nucleotide phosphate (GTP). This process is referred to as *substrate-level phosphorylation*

The bulk of ATP used by many cells to maintain homeostasis is produced by the oxidation of pyruvate in the TCA cycle. During this oxidation process, NADH and $FADH_2$ are generated. The NADH and $FADH_2$ are principally used to drive mitochondrial oxidative phosphorylation, a process for converting the reducing potential of NADH and $FADH_2$ into the synthesis of high-energy phosphate in ATP.

Oxidative Decarboxylation of Pyruvate

The fate of pyruvate depends on the cell energy charge. In liver, intestine, and kidney under conditions of high-energy charge, pyruvate is directed toward gluconeogenesis. However, when the energy charge is low, pyruvate is preferentially oxidized to CO_2 and H_2O in the TCA cycle. The oxidation of the carbon atoms of pyruvate results in the generation of 15 equivalents of ATP per pyruvate. The enzymatic activities of the TCA cycle (and of oxidative phosphorylation) are located in the mitochondrion. When transported into the mitochondrion, pyruvate encounters 2 principal metabolizing enzymes: pyruvate carboxylase (PC) and the pyruvate dehydrogenase complex (PDHc).

With a high cell-energy charge, coenzyme A (CoA) is highly acylated, principally as acetyl-CoA, and able to allosterically activate PC, directing pyruvate toward gluconeogenesis (see Chapter 13). When the energy charge is low, CoA is not acylated and PC is inactive. Under these conditions, pyruvate is preferentially metabolized to CO_2 and H_2O via the PDHc and the enzymes of the TCA. Reduced NADH and $FADH_2$ generated during the oxidative reactions can then be used to drive ATP synthesis via oxidative phosphorylation.

The Pyruvate Dehydrogenase Complex

The **Pyruvate Dehydrogenase Complex** (PDHc) is composed of multiple copies of 3 separate enzymes: pyruvate dehydrogenase (PDH, E1: 20-30 copies), dihydrolipoamide S-acetyltransferase (DLAT, E2: 60 copies), and dihydrolipoamide dehydrogenase (DLD, E3: 6 copies). The complex also requires 5 different coenzymes: CoA, NAD^+, FAD^+, lipoic acid, and thiamine pyrophosphate (TPP). The factors required for the function of the PDHc can be remembered by the mnemonic: Tender (thiamine) Loving (lipoate) Care (coenzyme A) For (flavin) Nancy (nicotinamide), TLCFN. Three of the coenzymes of the complex are tightly bound to enzymes of the complex (TPP, lipoic acid, and FAD^+) and 2 are employed as carriers of the products of PDHc activity (CoA and NAD^+) (Figure 16-1).

The first enzyme of the PDHc is PDH itself (E1) which oxidatively decarboxylates pyruvate. The resulting acetyl group is initially bound to TPP then to the lipoic acid coenzyme of DLAT. The acetyl group is then transferred to CoA, forming acetyl-CoA. In the process, the electrons released during the oxidation pass from pyruvate to FAD (forming $FADH_2$) and ultimately to NAD^+ (forming NADH). The formation of NADH is catalyzed via the DLD enzymes of the PDHc. The fate of the NADH is oxidation via mitochondrial electron transport to produce 3 equivalents of ATP. The net result of the reactions of the PDHc is:

$$\text{Pyruvate} + \text{CoA} + \text{NAD}^+ \rightarrow \text{CO}_2 + \text{acetyl-CoA} + \text{NADH} + \text{H}^+$$

Regulation of the PDH Complex

The reactions of the PDHc serve to interconnect the metabolic pathways of glycolysis, gluconeogenesis, and fatty acid oxidation to the TCA cycle. The activity of the PDHc is also important in regulating the flux from glucose to malonyl-CoA, which is required for the *de novo* synthesis of fatty acids (see Chapter 19). The activity of the PDHc is highly regulated by a variety of allosteric effectors and by covalent modification. The importance of the PDHc to the maintenance of homeostasis is evident from the fact that although diseases associated with deficiencies of the PDHc have been observed, affected individuals often do not survive to maturity. Since metabolism in highly aerobic tissues such as the brain, skeletal muscle, and the heart is dependent on normal conversion of pyruvate to acetyl-CoA, aerobic tissues are most sensitive to deficiencies in components of the PDHc. Most genetic diseases associated with PDHc deficiency are due to mutations in PDH. The main pathologic result of such mutations is moderate-to-severe cerebral lactic acidosis and encephalopathies.

Acetyl-CoA, produced in the mitochondria via the action of the PDHc, will be transported out into the cytosol in the form of citrate when the energy charge of the cell rises. In the cytosol the citrate is hydrolyzed by ATP citrate lyase, yielding oxaloacetate and acetyl-CoA. In the cytosol the acetyl-CoA can be converted to malonyl-CoA via the action of acetyl-CoA carboxylase (ACC). This malonyl-CoA serves as the precursor for the synthesis of fatty acids. Accumulation of cytosolic malonyl-CoA, as will happen in energy-rich conditions, partitions cytosolic fatty acids away from the oxidizing machinery of the mitochondria by inhibiting carnitine palmitoyltransferase I (CPT I). This effect of malonyl-CoA, derived from acetyl-CoA, couples increased rates of glucose oxidation to inhibition of fatty acid oxidation (Figure 16-2).

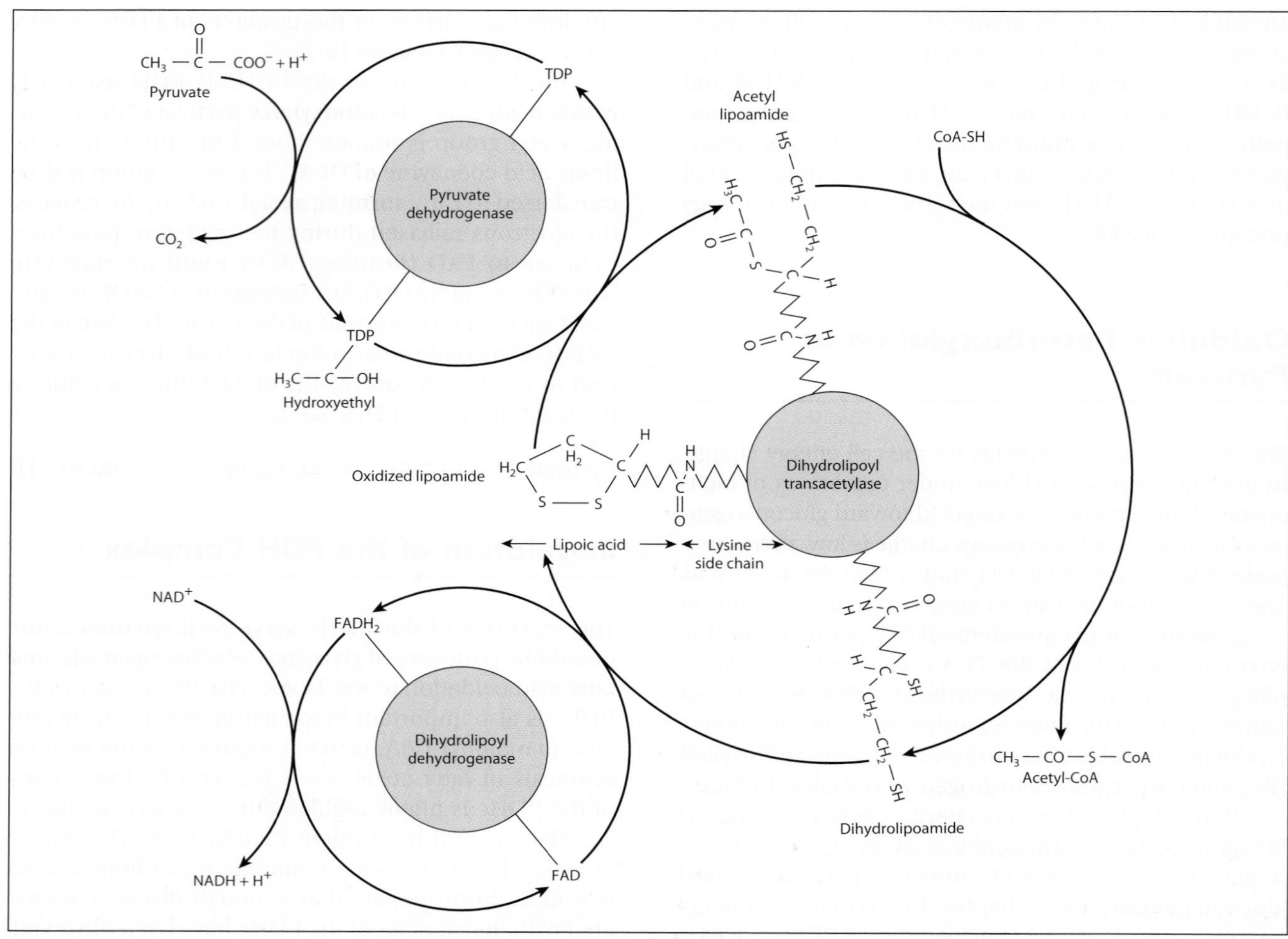

FIGURE 16-1: Oxidative decarboxylation of pyruvate by the pyruvate dehydrogenase complex. Lipoic acid is joined by an amide link to a lysine residue of the transacetylase component of the enzyme complex. It forms a long flexible arm, allowing the lipoic acid prosthetic group to rotate sequentially between the active sites of each of the enzymes of the complex. (FAD, flavin adenine dinucleotide; NAD^+, nicotinamide adenine dinucleotide; TDP, thiamin diphosphate.) Murray RK, Bender DA, Botham KM, Kennelly PJ, Rodwell VW, Weil PA. *Harper's Illustrated Biochemistry*, 29th ed. New York, NY: McGraw-Hill; 2012.

The activity of PDH (E1) is rapidly regulated by phosphorylation and dephosphorylation events that are catalyzed by PDH kinases (PDKs) and PDH phosphatases (PDPs), respectively. Phosphorylation of PDH results in inhibition of activity, whereas, dephosphorylation increases it. Four PDK isozymes have been identified in humans: PDK1, PDK2, PDK3, and PDK4. Analysis of the patterns of expression of the PDKs shows that PDK2 is the most widely expressed with the highest levels of expression seen in heart, liver, and kidney. PDK1 expression is highest in the heart and is not seen in the liver. PDK4 expression is high in heart, liver, pancreatic islets, and kidney.

Regulation of the activity of the various PDKs exhibits isoform specificity. PDK2 is most sensitive to inhibition by pyruvate, whereas, PDK4 is relatively insensitive. Energy charge, reflected in ATP:ADP and NADH:NAD ratios, influence the activity of the PDKs. High ATP levels result in allosteric activation of the PDKs to ensure the excess carbon atoms can be diverted into anabolic synthesis pathways instead of into the TCA cycle. Conversely, as the ATP:ADP ratio falls, the increasing ADP will exert an allosteric inhibition on the activity of the PDKs. ADP exerts its allosteric inhibition of PDKs both independently and in synergy with pyruvate inhibition. In contrast to inhibition of PDKs by pyruvate, products of the PDHc, namely acetyl-CoA and NADH, allosterically activate the PDKs. PDK2 is the most sensitive to increases in the level of acetyl-CoA in comparison to the other PDK isoforms. The ratio of NADH to NAD^+ also exert isoform-specific allosteric regulation of PDKs. PDK4 is highly activated by an increased $NADH/NAD^+$, whereas, PDK2 is much less sensitive to this activation. NADH and acetyl-CoA are also negative

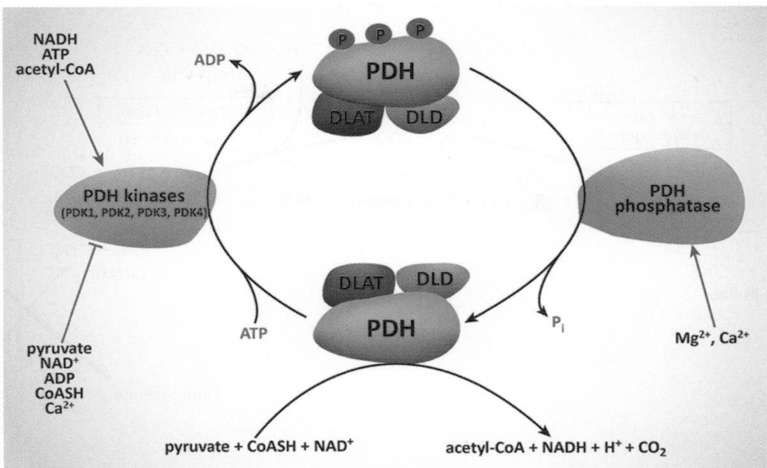

FIGURE 16-2: Factors regulating the activity of the PDHc. PDH activity is regulated by its state of phosphorylation; being most active in the dephosphorylated state. Phosphorylation of PDH is catalyzed by 4 specific PDH kinases, designated PDK1, PDK2, PDK3, and PDK4. The activity of these kinases is enhanced when cellular energy charge is high, which is reflected by an increase in the level of ATP, NADH, and acetyl-CoA. Conversely, an increase in pyruvate strongly inhibits PDH kinases. Additional negative effectors of PDH kinases are ADP, NAD^+, and CoASH, the levels of which increase when energy levels fall. The regulation of PDH phosphatases (PDPs) is less well understood but it is known that Mg^{2+} and Ca^{2+} activate the enzymes and that they are targets of insulin action. In adipose tissue, insulin increases PDH activity and in cardiac muscle PDH activity is increased by catecholamines.

allosteric effectors, the nonphosphorylated and active form of the PDHc. Both effectors reduce the affinity of the enzyme for pyruvate, thus limiting the flow of carbon through the PDHc. Note, however, that pyruvate is a potent negative effector on all PDKs, with the result that when pyruvate levels rise, active PDH will be favored even with high levels of NADH and acetyl-CoA.

Phosphate removal from the PDHc is catalyzed by 2 genetically and biochemically distinct PDP isoforms, PDP1 and PDP2. PDP1 is an Mg^{2+}-dependent and Ca^{2+}-stimulated protein serine phosphatase of the protein phosphatase-2C (PP-2C) superfamily (see Chapter 40) composed of a catalytic subunit (PDPc) and a regulatory subunit (PDPr). PDP1 is considered a major regulator of PDHc activity. The role of Ca^{2+} in stimulating the phosphatase activity of PDP1 toward the PDHc is by increasing its interaction with the PDHc. Calcium ion also increases the association of PDPc with the phosphorylated E1α subunit of PDH. Both PDP1 subunits are targeted by reactions of the TCA cycle (Figure 16-3).

Citrate Synthase (Condensing Enzyme)

The first reaction of the cycle is the condensation of acetyl-CoA with oxaloacetate (OAA). The standard free energy of the reaction, –8.0 kcal/mol, propels reaction in the forward direction. Since the formation of OAA from malate is thermodynamically unfavorable, the highly exergonic nature of the citrate synthase reaction is of central importance in keeping the entire cycle going in the forward direction, since it drives oxaloacetate formation by mass action principals.

When the cellular energy charge increases, the rate of flux through the TCA cycle will decline leading to a buildup of citrate. Excess citrate is used to transport acetyl-CoA carbons from the mitochondrion to the cytoplasm, where they can be used for fatty acid and cholesterol biosynthesis. Additionally, the increased levels of citrate in the cytoplasm activate the key regulatory enzyme of fatty acid biosynthesis, acetyl-CoA carboxylase (ACC), while also inhibiting the rate-limiting enzyme of glycolysis, PFK-1.

Aconitase

The isomerization of citrate to isocitrate by aconitase is stereospecific. The stereospecific nature of the isomerization determines that the CO_2 lost, as isocitrate is oxidized to succinyl-CoA, is derived from the oxaloacetate used in citrate synthesis. Aconitase is one of several mitochondrial enzymes known as non-heme iron proteins. These proteins contain inorganic iron and sulfur, known as iron sulfur centers, in a coordination complex with cysteine sulfurs of the protein.

Isocitrate Dehydrogenase

Isocitrate is oxidatively decarboxylated to α-ketoglutarate (2-oxoglutarate) by isocitrate dehydrogenase, IDH. IDH catalyzes the rate-limiting step, as well as the first NADH-yielding reaction of the TCA cycle. Control of carbon flow through the TCA cycle is regulated at IDH by the

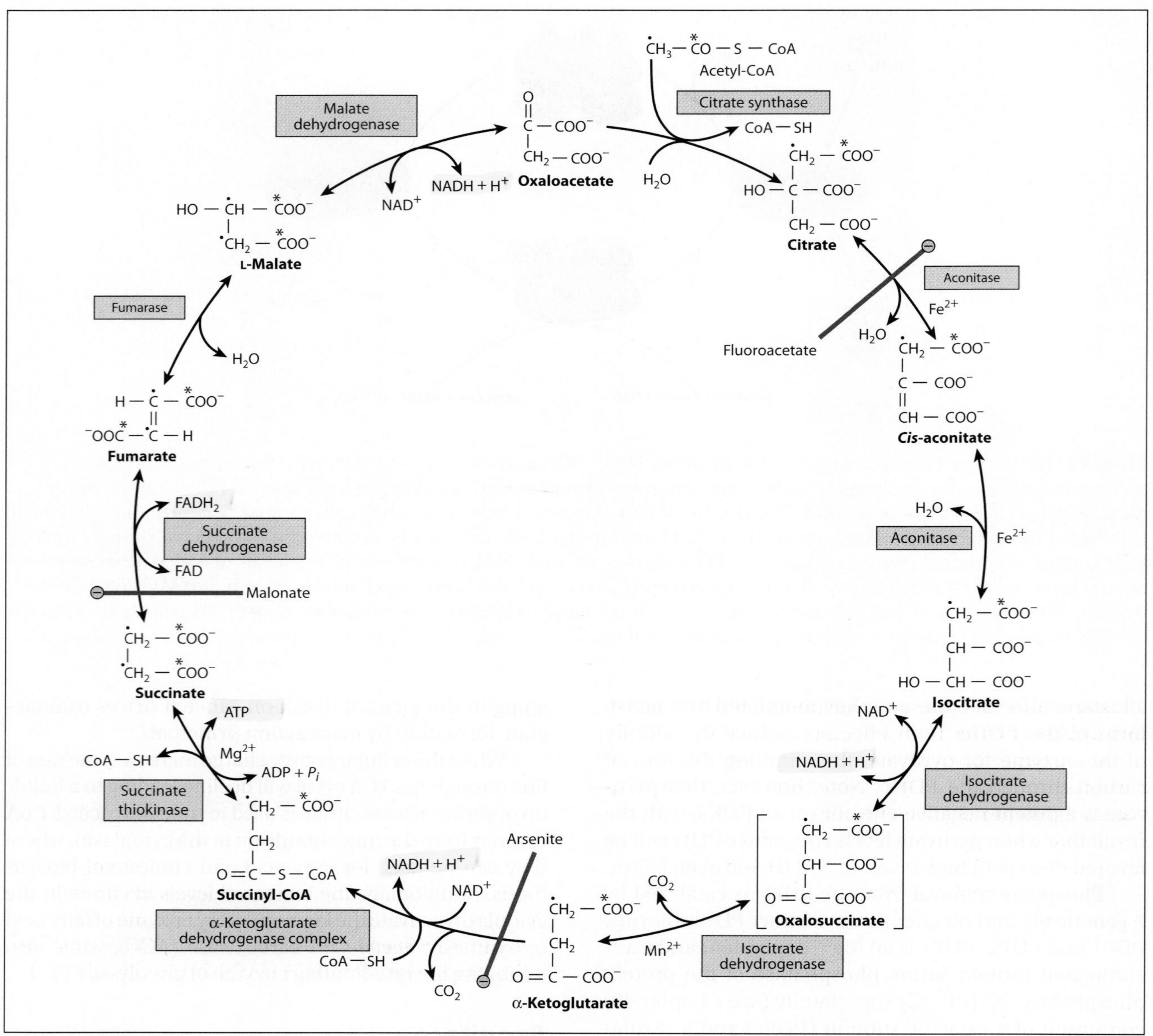

FIGURE 16-3: The citric acid (Krebs) cycle. Oxidation of NADH and $FADH_2$ in the respiratory chain leads to the formation of ATP via oxidative phosphorylation. In order to follow the passage of acetyl-CoA through the cycle, the 2 carbon atoms of the acetyl radical are shown labeled on the carboxyl carbon (*) and on the methyl carbon (•). Although 2 carbon atoms are lost as CO_2 in 1 turn of the cycle, these atoms are not derived from the acetyl-CoA that has immediately entered the cycle, but from that portion of the citrate molecule that was derived from oxaloacetate. However, on completion of a single turn of the cycle, the oxaloacetate that is regenerated is now labeled, which leads to labeled CO_2 being evolved during the second turn of the cycle. Because succinate is a symmetric compound, "randomization" of label occurs at this step so that all 4 carbon atoms of oxaloacetate appear to be labeled after 1 turn of the cycle. During gluconeogenesis, some of the label in oxaloacetate is incorporated into glucose and glycogen. The sites of inhibition (⊖) by fluoroacetate, malonate, and arsenite are indicated. Murray RK, Bender DA, Botham KM, Kennelly PJ, Rodwell VW, Weil PA. *Harper's Illustrated Biochemistry,* 29th ed. New York, NY: McGraw-Hill; 2012.

powerful negative allosteric effectors NADH and ATP and by the potent positive effectors, isocitrate, ADP, and AMP. From this fact, it should be clear that cell energy charge is a key component in regulating carbon flow through the TCA cycle.

α-Ketoglutarate Dehydrogenase Complex

α-ketoglutarate (also called 2-oxoglutarate) is oxidatively decarboxylated to succinyl-CoA by the α-ketoglutarate dehydrogenase (AKGDH) complex. The AKGDH complex is also called 2-oxoglutarate dehydrogenase (OGDH). This reaction generates the second TCA cycle equivalent of CO_2 and NADH. This multienzyme complex is very similar to the PDHc in the intricacy of its protein makeup, cofactors (TLCFN), and its mechanism of action. Also, as with the PDHc, the reactions of the AKGDH complex proceed with a large negative-standard free-energy change. Although the AKGDH complex is not subject to covalent modification, allosteric regulation is quite complex, with activity being controlled by energy charge, the NADH/NAD^+ ratio, and effector activity of substrates and products.

Succinyl-CoA and α-ketoglutarate are also important metabolites outside the TCA cycle. In particular, α-ketoglutarate represents a key anaplerotic metabolite linking the entry and exit of carbon atoms from the TCA cycle to pathways involved in amino acid metabolism. α-ketoglutarate is also important for driving the malate-aspartate shuttle (see Figure 13-2). Succinyl-CoA (along with glycine) contributes all the carbon and nitrogen atoms required for heme synthesis (see Chapter 33) and for nonhepatic tissue utilization of ketone bodies (see Chapter 25).

Succinyl-CoA Synthetase (succinate-CoA ligase, succinate thiokinase)

Mitochondrial GTP (guanosine triphosphate) is used in a *trans*-phosphorylation reaction catalyzed by the mitochondrial enzyme nucleoside diphosphokinase to phosphorylate ADP, producing ATP and regenerating GDP for the continued operation of succinyl-CoA synthetase.

Succinate Dehydrogenase

Succinate dehydrogenase (SDH) catalyzes the oxidation of succinate to fumarate with the sequential reduction of enzyme-bound FAD to $FADH_2$. In mammalian cells, the final electron acceptor in this reaction is coenzyme Q (CoQ) of the oxidative phosphorylation machinery.

Fumarase (Fumarate Hydratase)

The fumarase-catalyzed reaction is specific for the *trans* form of fumarate. The result is that the hydration of fumarate proceeds stereospecifically with the production of L-malate.

Malate Dehydrogenase

L-malate is the specific substrate for malate dehydrogenase (MDH), the final enzyme of the TCA cycle. The oxidation of malate to oxaloacetate (OAA) has a standard free energy of approximately $^+7$ kcal/mol. This indicates that the reaction, in the TCA cycle direction, is thermodynamically unfavorable. However, as noted earlier, the citrate synthase reaction that condenses OAA with acetyl-CoA has a standard free energy of about −8 kcal/mol and is responsible for pulling the MDH reaction in the forward direction.

TCA Cycle Stoichiometry

The overall stoichiometry of the TCA cycle, beginning and ending with acetyl-CoA, can be written as:

$$\text{acetyl-CoA} + 3NAD^+ + FAD + GDP + P_i + 2H_2O \rightarrow 2CO_2 + 3NADH + FADH_2 + GTP + 2H^+ + HSCoA$$

Regulation of the TCA Cycle

Regulation of the TCA cycle, like that of glycolysis, occurs at both the level of entry of substrates into the cycle as well as at the key reactions of the cycle.

High-Yield Concept

The conversion of succinyl-CoA to succinate, by succinyl-CoA synthetase, drives synthesis of a high-energy nucleotide phosphate (GTP) in a process known as substrate-level phosphorylation.

High-Yield Concept

Numerous by-products of amino acid oxidation can be shunted into the TCA cycle to ensure that the intermediates do not become limiting to the processes of the cycle. This latter process is referred to as anaplerosis (Figure 16-4).

Fuel enters the TCA cycle primarily as acetyl-CoA. The generation of acetyl-CoA from carbohydrates is, therefore, a major control point of the cycle. This is the reaction catalyzed by the PDHc with regulation being effected as described earlier.

Since 3 reactions of the TCA cycle, as well as the PDHc, utilize NAD^+ as cofactor, it is not difficult to understand why the cellular ratio of NADH to NAD^+ has a major impact on the flux of carbon through the TCA cycle. Substrate availability can also regulate TCA flux. This occurs at the citrate synthase reaction as a result of reduced availability of OAA. Product inhibition also controls the TCA flux, for example, citrate inhibits citrate synthase and α-KGDH is inhibited by NADH and succinyl-CoA. The key enzymes of the TCA cycle are also regulated allosterically by Ca^{2+}, ATP, and ADP.

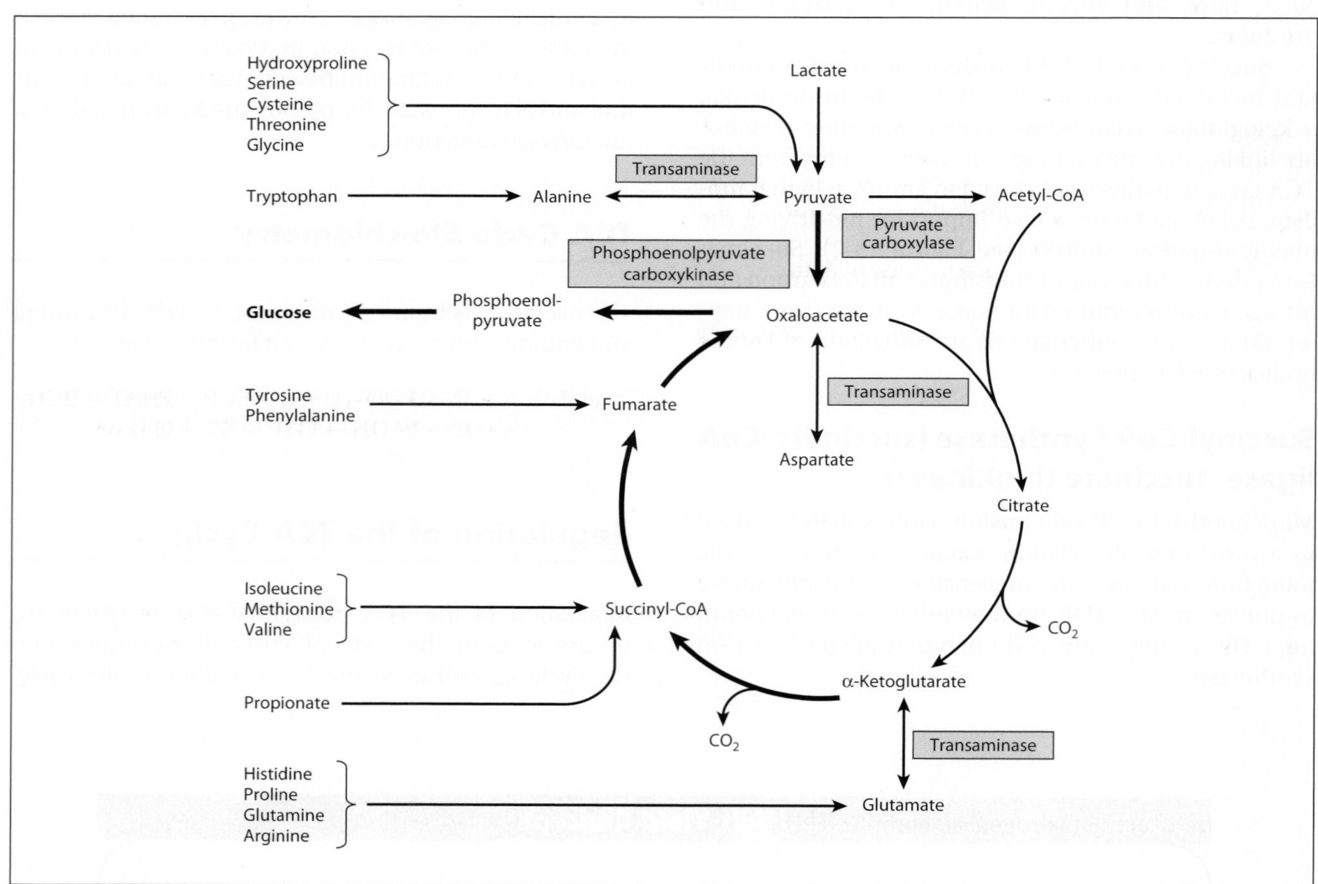

FIGURE 16-4: Involvement of the citric acid cycle in transamination and gluconeogenesis. The bold arrows indicate the main pathway of gluconeogenesis. Murray RK, Bender DA, Botham KM, Kennelly PJ, Rodwell VW, Weil PA. *Harper's Illustrated Biochemistry*, 29th ed. New York, NY: McGraw-Hill; 2012.

TCA Cycle Involvement in Overall Metabolism

The TCA cycle is principally designed to completely oxidize the carbons of acetyl-CoA to CO_2 and H_2O while simultaneously generating large amounts of the reduced electron carriers, NADH and $FADH_2$. However, numerous important metabolites are generated via the diversion of intermediates of the cycle into other biosynthetic pathways. For example, the carbons in POAA represent major building blocks for glucose synthesis via gluconeogenesis (see Chapter 13).

The TCA cycle is also an important metabolic pathway contributing to the synthesis of fatty acids. The acetyl-CoA derived from glucose oxidation, or from amino acid oxidation, can be diverted from the mitochondria to the cytosol in the form of citrate. When citrate is transported into the cytosol, it is converted to acetyl-CoA and OAA via the action of ATP-citrate lyase (see Figure 16-2). There the acetyl-CoA serves as a substrate for fatty acid and cholesterol biosynthesis (Figure 16-5).

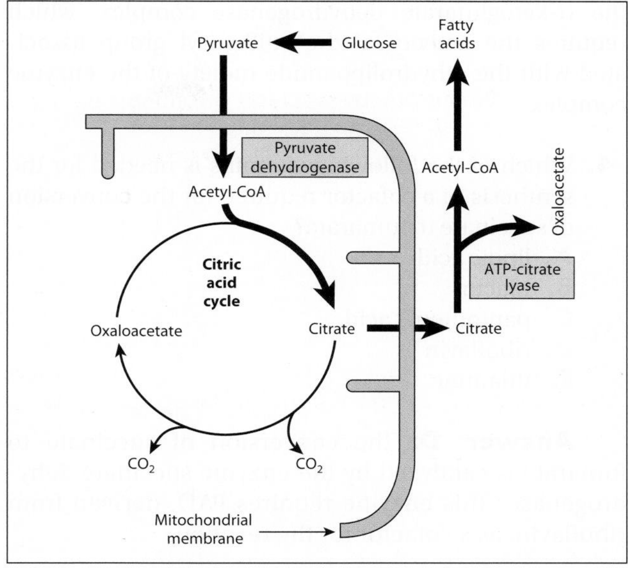

FIGURE 16-5: Participation of the citric acid cycle in fatty acid synthesis from glucose. Murray RK, Bender DA, Botham KM, Kennelly PJ, Rodwell VW, Weil PA. *Harper's Illustrated Biochemistry*, 29th ed. New York, NY: McGraw-Hill; 2012.

REVIEW QUESTIONS

1. In exercising skeletal muscles, pyruvate oxidation in the TCA cycle is stimulated by which of the following?

A. allosteric activation of isocitrate dehydrogenase by NADH
B. allosteric activation of malate dehydrogenase by NAD^+
C. increased product inhibition of citrate synthase by oxaloacetate
D. phosphorylation of α-ketoglutarate dehydrogenase to an inactive form
E. stimulation of pyruvate dehydrogenase activity by Ca^{2+}

Answer E: Muscle contraction results in release of stored calcium ion from sarcoplasmic reticulum. The released calcium allosterically inhibits the activity of the PDH kinases. Reduced activity of PDH kinases results in reduced phosphorylation of the PDHc thus, allowing for greater oxidation of pyruvate.

2. The pyruvate dehydrogenase complex (PDHc) is a multi-subunit enzyme whose activity is regulated by both allosteric effectors and covalent modification. Which of the following exerts a positive influence on the activity of PDHc toward pyruvate?

A. acetyl-CoA
B. ATP
C. dephosphorylation
D. NADH
E. phosphorylation

Answer C: The level of active PDHc is controlled by its state of phosphorylation. A family of enzymes called the PDH kinases phosphorylates the PDHc. In order to return the PDHc to full activity following PDH kinase-mediated phosphorylation, the phosphates are removed by PDH phosphatase.

3. A 24-year-old woman presents with diarrhea, dysphagia, jaundice, and white transverse lines on the fingernails (Mees lines). The patient is diagnosed with arsenic poisoning. Arsenic is known to inhibit which of the following enzymes of TCA cycle?

A. aconitase
B. citrate synthase
C. α-ketoglutarate dehydrogenase
D. malate dehydrogenase
E. succinate dehydrogenase

Answer C: Arsenic is toxic at many levels due to its broad specificity of enzyme inhibition. The mode of action of arsenic-containing compounds, primarily arsenic trioxide, is via it reacting with biological ligands that possess available sulfur groups. Arsenic interferes with the activity of the TCA cycle by inhibiting the α-ketoglutarate dehydrogenase complex, which requires the activity of the sulfhydryl group associated with the dihydrolipoamide moiety of the enzyme complex.

4. Which of the following vitamins is needed for the synthesis of a cofactor required for the conversion of succinate to fumarate?
A. lipoic acid
B. niacin
C. pantothenic acid
D. riboflavin
E. thiamine

Answer D: The conversion of succinate to fumarate is catalyzed by the enzyme succinate dehydrogenase. This enzyme requires FAD, derived from riboflavin, as a cofactor for the reaction.

5. Pyruvate dehydrogenase complex (PDHc) deficiency is an autosomal recessive disorder and leads to anion gap metabolic acidosis. Which of the following accumulates to cause metabolic acidosis?
A. acetoacetate
B. fumarate
C. β-hydroxy butyrate
D. hydrochloric acid
E. lactate

Answer E: Inhibition of 3 PDHc results in impaired oxidation of pyruvate. As the level of pyruvate increases in the cytosol, it is reduced to lactate which can diffuse out of the cell into the blood resulting in lactic acidosis.

6. A 3-year-old child presents with a history of recurrent rash upon sun exposure and passage of purple-colored urine. The child is diagnosed with congenital erythropoietic porphyria (CEP), a disorder associated with the pathway of heme biosynthesis. Which of the following intermediates of TCA cycle is used as a precursor for heme biosynthesis?
A. acetyl-CoA
B. malate
C. pyruvate
D. succinate
E. succinyl-CoA

Answer E: The initiation of heme biosynthesis requires glycine and the TCA cycle intermediate, succinyl-CoA.

7. A 2-year-old child was brought to pediatric emergency with convulsions. The child was diagnosed with ammonia intoxication due to some urea cycle disorder. Reduced formation of GABA, due to depletion of glutamate, which serves as the precursor for its synthesis, is considered to be the most important cause of the convulsions. Which of the following intermediates of TCA cycle is involved in the formation of glutamate?
A. isocitrate
B. α-ketoglutarate
C. malate
D. pyruvate
E. succinate

Answer B: The enzyme glutamate dehydrogenase is an important metabolic regulatory enzyme. It catalyzes the interconversion of α-ketoglutarate to glutamate under conditions of high-energy charge. When energy charge is low, the reverse reaction allows for glutamate to serve an anaplerotic role in the TCA cycle.

8. In the TCA cycle, GTP is produced via a process referred to as substrate-level phosphorylation. Which of the following enzymes is involved in this process of formation of GTP from GDP?
A. citrate synthase
B. isocitrate dehydrogenase
C. malate dehydrogenase
D. succinate-CoA synthetase
E. succinate dehydrogenase

Answer D: Succinyl-CoA synthetase catalyzes the conversion of succinyl-CoA to succinate. Simultaneously, the reaction generates GTP from GDP, utilizing the high-energy bond between CoA and succinate. This formation of GTP is referred to as substrate-level phosphorylation to distinguish it from ATP production during oxidative phosphorylation.

9. A 5-year-old child was rushed to emergency room after accidentally consuming fluoroacetate, a known inhibitor of TCA cycle. Which of the following enzymes is inhibited by fluoroacetate?
A. aconitase
B. citrate synthase
C. isocitrate dehydrogenase
D. malate dehydrogenase
E. succinate dehydrogenase

Answer A: Fluoroacetate is a structural analog of citrate and a strong competitive inhibitor of aconitase.

10. A 56-year-old chronic alcoholic has been brought to the emergency room in a semiconscious state. Blood biochemistry reveals hypoglycemia with a blood glucose level of 45 mg/dL. Which of the following intermediates of TCA cycle can be directly converted to phosphoenolpyruvate to trigger the pathway of gluconeogenesis?

A. α-ketoglutarate
B. malate
C. oxaloacetate
D. pyruvate
E. succinate

Answer C: The TCA cycle compound, oxaloacetate, serves as a key intermediate in gluconeogenesis. Within the mitochondria, it can be converted to phosphoenolpyruvate (PEP) via the action of PEP carboxykinase.

11. Anaplerotic reactions are those that result in replenishing intermediates in the TCA cycle. Which of the following enzymes catalyzes an anaplerotic reaction?
A. citrate synthase
B. malate dehydrogenase
C. pyruvate carboxylase
D. pyruvate kinase
E. succinyl-CoA synthetase

Answer C: Pyruvate carboxylase catalyzes the carboxylation of pyruvate-forming oxaloacetate, which can then enter the TCA cycle (anaplerotic) keeping the cycle replenished.

12. Oxaloacetate, uniformly labeled with radioactive carbon, reacts with glutamate using transaminase and pyridoxal phosphate. Which of the following percentages of the original radioactivity will be found in 2-oxoglutarate (α-ketoglutarate) formed in this reaction?
A. 0%
B. 25%
C. 50%
D. 75%
E. 100%

Answer A: In the aspartate transaminase (AST)–catalyzed reaction, the amine group from glutamate is transferred to OAA, generating aspartate from the OAA and α-ketoglutarate from the glutamate. Therefore, none of the radioactive carbon atoms from OAA will enter the TCA cycle.

13. Energy made available for useful work from metabolism can be represented as the number of moles of ATP, reduced flavoproteins, and reduced pyridine nucleotides that are formed. How many moles of NADH are formed during the conversion of 1 mole of citrate to 1 mole of oxaloacetate and 2 moles of CO_2?
A. 2
B. 3
C. 6
D. 8
E. 12

Answer B: The reduction of NAD^+ to NADH in the TCA cycle, starting with citrate, occurs at the isocitrate dehydrogenase, α-ketoglutarate dehydrogenase, and malate dehydrogenase–catalyzed reactions, thus generating 3 moles of NADH per mole of citrate.

14. There is no net synthesis of 4-carbon precursors of glucose during the metabolic breakdown of acetyl-CoA in the TCA cycle because of which of the following reason?
A. insufficient NADH for gluconeogenesis is produced in the mitochondrial matrix during oxidation-reduction reactions of the cycle
B. the mitochondrial membrane is impermeable to oxaloacetate which is trapped in the matrix
C. oxidative decarboxylation reactions prevent oxaloacetate production by producing allosteric inhibitors
D. 2 moles of CO_2 are released during each circuit of the cycle

Answer D: The 2 carbon atoms that enter the TCA cycle as acetyl-CoA are stoichiometrically released as CO_2 at the isocitrate dehydrogenase and α-ketoglutarate dehydrogenase–catalyzed reactions. Thus, there is no net carbon input into oxaloacetate, which is the major gluconeogenic precursor of the TCA cycle.

15. Regeneration of which of the following participants in the TCA cycle is dependent on the presence of oxygen?
A. ADP
B. citrate
C. α-ketoglutarate
D. NAD^+
E. succinate

Answer D: The reduced electron carriers generated via reactions of the TCA cycle (NADH and $FADH_2$) are subsequently reoxidized to NAD^+ and FAD via the oxidative phosphorylation pathway.

16. Which of the following best describes why the GTP produced in the conversion of succinyl-CoA to succinate in the TCA cycle is equivalent to ATP?
A. amino group on the C–2 position of GTP can be transferred to the C–6 position to form ATP
B. free energy of hydrolysis of the γ-phosphate of GTP is equivalent to that of ATP

C. GTP is used in biosynthetic pathways such as protein synthesis
D. salvage pathway involving phosphoribosylpyrophosphate (PRPP) can be used to regenerate GTP

Answer B: All cells contain enzymes for the interconversion of various nucleoside mono- and diphosphates into nucleoside triphosphates such as ATP. Thus, the γ-phosphate of GTP is energetically equivalent to the same phosphate in ATP. GTP can therefore, drive the synthesis of ATP from ADP via the action of nucleoside diphosphokinases.

17. The equilibrium constant for the reaction catalyzed by malate dehydrogenase (malate + $NAD^+ \leftrightarrow$ oxaloacetate + NADH + H^+) is 10^{-4}. However, in vivo, the production of oxaloacetate is favored because of which of the following?
A. the buildup of malate results in the formation of succinate
B. malate leaves the mitochondrial matrix by a symport carrier along with phosphate
C. oxaloacetate cannot cross the mitochondrial membrane and is trapped in the matrix
D. oxaloacetate is removed by citrate synthase

Answer D: Thermodynamically unfavorable reactions can be driven to proceed in the unfavorable direction if the product of the reaction is rapidly removed by a subsequent enzyme. This is the case in the TCA cycle where the OAA formed via MDH is rapidly converted to citrate via citrate synthase. As long as there is sufficient acetyl-CoA to drive the removal of OAA, the MDH reaction will proceed toward OAA synthesis.

18. Which of the following CoA derivatives serves the dual function of channeling carbon units into the TCA cycle for oxidative catabolism and acting as a precursor for lipid biosynthesis?
A. acetoacetyl-CoA
B. acetyl-CoA
C. HMG-CoA
D. malonyl-CoA
E. propionyl-CoA

Answer B: Oxidation of carbohydrates, fats, and amino acids yields acetyl-CoA. When energy demand is high, the acetyl-CoA will be completely oxidized via the TCA cycle. When energy demand is low, the excess energy can be used to drive reductive biosynthetic reactions such as fatty acid synthesis, which will utilize the acetyl-CoA as the substrate.

Checklist

✓ The entry of carbohydrate carbons into the TCA cycles occurs via the oxidative decarboxylation of pyruvate, catalyzed by the pyruvate dehydrogenase complex, PDHc.

✓ The PDHc is a large multi-subunit enzyme complex that requires 5 distinct cofactors, 4 of which are derived from vitamins.

✓ Regulation of the PDHc is complex, involving both covalent modification (phosphorylation/dephosphorylation) and numerous allosteric effectors.

✓ The TCA cycle is the terminal pathway for the complete oxidation of the by-products of carbohydrate, fatty acid, and amino acid metabolism. The common end product of catabolism of these 3 types of compound is acetyl-CoA.

✓ The acetyl-CoA, derived from carbohydrate, fatty acid, and amino acid oxidation, reacts with oxaloacetate forming citrate. Citrate then undergoes a series of oxidation and decarboxylation steps in the context of the TCA cycle to regenerate oxaloacetate while simultaneously generating reducing equivalents as NADH and $FADH_2$, as well as releasing CO_2.

CHAPTER

17 Mitochondrial Functions and Oxidative Phosphorylation

CHAPTER OUTLINE

High-Yield Terms

Mitochondrial DNA (mtDNA): the circular genome found within mitochondria, encompasses genes involved in respiratory functions of this organelle

Electrochemical half-cell: consists of an electrode and an electrolyte, 2 half-cells compose an electrochemical cell that is capable of deriving energy from chemical reactions

Ubiquinone (CoQ): a mobile component of the electron transport chain that can undergo either 1- or 2-electron reactions, transfers electrons from complexes I and II to complex III

Chemiosmotic potential: more correctly referred to as proton motive force (PMF), refers to the electrochemical gradient formed across the inner mitochondrial membrane due to the transport of protons, H^+, whose energy is used to drive ATP synthesis

Reactive oxygen species: any of a group of chemically reactive molecules containing oxygen, such as hydrogen peroxide and superoxide anion

Encephalomyopathy: a disorder most often resulting from a defect in mitochondrial function affecting both skeletal muscle and central nervous system function

Adaptive thermogenesis: the regulated production of heat in response to environmental changes in temperature and diet; for example, shivering in humans is adaptive thermogenesis

Mitochondria

Oxidative phosphorylation is a critical energy (ATP)–generating metabolic pathway that occurs within the mitochondria. Mitochondria evolved from a symbiotic relationship between aerobic bacteria and primordial eukaryotic cells. Mitochondria contain a 16-kb circular genome (mtDNA) that contains 37 genes critical for the processes oxidative phosphorylation. However, the mtDNA does not encode all of the proteins in the mitochondria. Over 900 mitochondrial proteins are actually encoded by the nuclear genome. Thirteen of the mtDNA genes encode protein subunits of respiratory complexes I, III, IV, and V. Only complex II is solely composed of proteins encoded by nuclear genes. The mtDNA genome also encodes 22 mitochondrial tRNAs and 2 rRNAs that are essential for translation of mtDNA transcripts.

Mammalian cells can have hundreds to thousands of mitochondria, and each mitochondrion contains several mtDNA genomes. This phenomenon is referred to as heteroplasmy. Also, any given mitochondrion is not a discrete, autonomous organelle because it has the capacity to fuse with a neighboring mitochondrion in the near future. Therefore, the entire mitochondrial population within any given cell is in constant flux. The concept of heteroplasmy is significant in the context of inherited disorders in mitochondrial biogenesis (discussed below). It is why the spectrum of symptoms with these types of diseases can be quite broad. In addition, because of the stochastic nature of mitochondrial inheritance during cell division, a daughter cell can occasionally inherit a population of mitochondria whose ratio of mutant to wild-type mtDNA differs significantly from that of the parental cell.

Normal biogenesis of mitochondria is triggered in response to changes in the ATP:ADP ratio and to activation of 5′ adenosine monophosphate–activated protein kinase (AMPK) (Chapter 34) which in turn results in increased expression of peroxisome proliferator–activated receptor γ coactivator-1α (PGC-1α) and nuclear respiratory factor-1 (NRF1). PGC-1α is a master transcriptional coactivator of numerous genes involved in mitochondrial biogenesis. NRF1 is a transcription factor that regulates the expression of mitochondrial transcription factor A (TFAM, for **t**ranscription **f**actor **A**, **m**itochondrial; also designated mtTFA), which is a nuclear transcription factor essential for replication, maintenance, and transcription of mitochondrial DNA.

Principles of Reduction/Oxidation (Redox) Reactions

Coupled electrochemical half-cells have the thermodynamic properties of other coupled chemical reactions. An example of a coupled redox reaction is the oxidation of NADH by the electron transport chain:

$$NADH + \tfrac{1}{2}O_2 + H^+ \rightarrow NAD^+ + H_2O$$

The thermodynamic potential of a chemical reaction is calculated from equilibrium constants and concentrations of reactants and products. Because it is not practical to measure electron concentrations directly, the electron energy potential of a redox system is determined from the electrical potential or voltage of the individual half-cells, relative to a standard half-cell. When the reactants and products of a half-cell are in their standard state and the voltage is determined relative to a standard hydrogen half-cell (whose voltage, by convention, is zero), the potential observed is defined as the standard electrode potential, E^o. If the pH of a standard cell is in the biological range, pH 7, its potential is defined as the standard biological electrode potential and designated $E^{o\prime}$. By convention, standard electrode potentials are written as potentials for reduction reactions of half-cells. The free energy of a typical reaction is calculated directly from its $E^{o\prime}$ by the Nernst equation, where n is the number of electrons involved in the reaction and F is the Faraday constant (23.06 kcal/volt/mol or 94.4 kJ/volt/mol) (Table 17-1):

$$\Delta G^{o\prime} = -nF\Delta E^{o\prime}$$

High-Yield Concept

Mitochondria are maternally inherited due to the transmission of mitochondria from the egg to the zygote. Paternal mitochondria from the sperm are selectively marked with ubiquitin and degraded.

High-Yield Concept

Redox reactions involve the transfer of electrons from one chemical species to another. The oxidized plus the reduced form of each chemical species is referred to as an electrochemical half-cell.

TABLE 17-1: Some Redox Potentials of Special Interest in Mammalian Oxidation Systems

System	E'_0 *Volts*
H^+/H_2	−0.42
NAD^+/NADH	−0.32
Lipoate; ox/red	−0.29
Acetoacetate/3-hydroxybutyrate	−0.27
Pyruvate/lactate	−0.19
Oxaloacetate/malate	−0.17
Fumarate/succinate	+0.03
Cytochrome *b*; Fe^{3+}/Fe^{2+}	+0.08
Ubiquinone; ox/red	+0.10
Cytochrome c_1; Fe^{3+}/Fe^{2+}	+0.22
Cytochrome *a*; Fe^{3+}/Fe^{2+}	+0.29
Oxygen/water	+0.82

Murray RK, Bender DA, Botham KM, Kennelly PJ, Rodwell VW, Weil PA. *Harper's Illustrated Biochemistry,* 29th ed. New York, NY: McGraw-Hill; 2012.

Energy from Cytosolic NADH

The oxidation of glucose is a major pathway for the generation of cellular energy both aerobically and anaerobically. When carried out aerobically, the NADH derived from cytosolic glycolysis is transferred into the mitochondria where it can be reoxidized and coupled to ATP synthesis. The energy yield from cytosolic NADH depends upon the transport system used to get the electrons into the mitochondria. Two shuttle mechanisms exist: the malate-aspartate shuttle (see Figure 10-2) and the glycerol phosphate shuttle (see Figure 10-3). The glycerol phosphate shuttle involves 2 different glycerol-3-phosphate dehydrogenases: one is cytosolic, acting to produce glycerol 3-phosphate, and the other is an integral protein of the inner mitochondrial membrane that acts to oxidize the glycerol 3-phosphate produced by the cytosolic enzyme. The net result of the process is that reducing equivalents from cytosolic NADH are transferred to the mitochondrial electron transport system as $FADH_2$. In some tissues, such as that of heart and muscle, mitochondrial glycerol-3-phosphate dehydrogenase is present in very low amounts, and the malate-aspartate shuttle is the dominant pathway for aerobic oxidation of cytosolic NADH.

Complexes of the Electron Transport Chain

The large quantity of NADH resulting from glycolysis (Chapter 10) and the NADH and $FADH_2$ generated from fatty acid oxidation (Chapter 25) and the TCA cycle (Chapter 16) are used to supply the energy for ATP synthesis via oxidative phosphorylation (Figure 17-1).

Oxidation of NADH and $FADH_2$, with phosphorylation of ADP to form ATP, is a process supported by the mitochondrial electron transport assembly and ATP synthase, often referred to as complex V, which are integral protein complexes of the inner mitochondrial membrane. The electron transport assembly is comprised of a series of protein complexes that catalyze sequential oxidation-reduction reactions (Figure 17-2).

The reduced electron carriers, NADH and $FADH_2$, are oxidized by a series of catalytic redox carriers that are integral proteins of the inner mitochondrial membrane. Coupled to these oxidation reduction steps is a transport process in which protons (H^+) from the mitochondrial matrix are translocated to the space between the inner and outer mitochondrial membranes (Figure 17-3). The redistribution of protons leads to formation of a proton gradient across the mitochondrial membrane. The size of the gradient is proportional to the free-energy change of the electron transfer reactions. The result of these reactions is that the redox energy of NADH is converted to the energy of the proton gradient. In the presence of ADP, protons flow down their thermodynamic gradient from outside the mitochondrion back into the mitochondrial matrix.

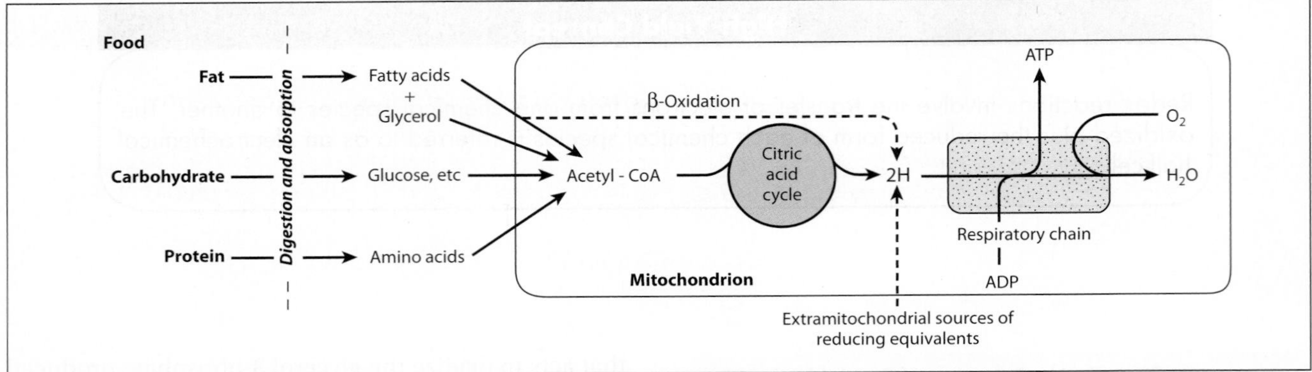

FIGURE 17-1: Role of the respiratory chain of mitochondria in the conversion of food energy to ATP. Oxidation of the major foodstuffs leads to the generation of reducing equivalents (2H) that are collected by the respiratory chain for oxidation and coupled generation of ATP. Murray RK, Bender DA, Botham KM, Kennelly PJ, Rodwell VW, Weil PA. *Harper's Illustrated Biochemistry*, 29th ed. New York, NY: McGraw-Hill; 2012.

This process is facilitated by a proton carrier in the inner mitochondrial membrane known as ATP synthase. As its name implies, this carrier is coupled to ATP synthesis (Figure 17-3).

The mitochondrial electron transport proteins are clustered into multiprotein complexes known as complexes I, II, III, and IV. Complex I, also known as NADH-CoQ oxidoreductase (also NADH-ubiquinone oxidoreductase or NADH dehydrogenase), is composed of NADH dehydrogenase with FMN as cofactor, plus non-heme iron proteins having at least 1 iron sulfur center. There are a total of 45 protein subunits in complex I. Complex I is responsible for transferring electrons from NADH to CoQ. The $\Delta E^{\circ\prime}$ for the latter transfer is 0.42 V, corresponding to a $\Delta G'$ of −19 kcal/mol of electrons transferred. With its highly exergonic free-energy change, the flow of electrons through complex I is more than adequate to drive ATP synthesis.

Complex II is also known as succinate-CoQ oxidoreductase (also succinate-ubiquinone oxidoreductase

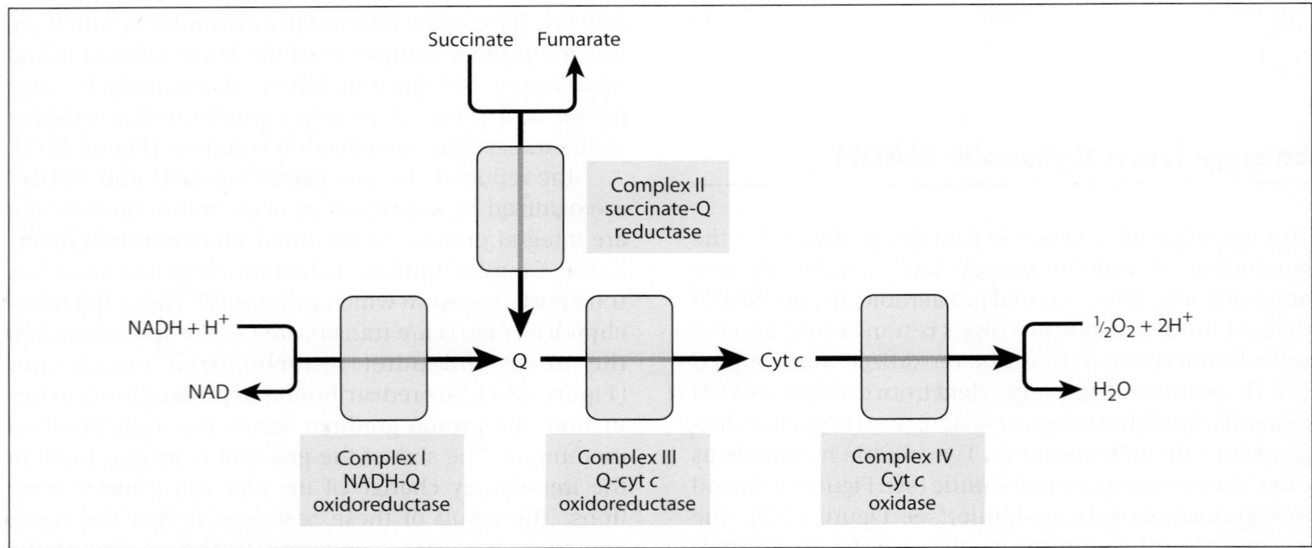

FIGURE 17-2: Overview of electron flow through the respiratory chain. (cyt, cytochrome; Q, coenzyme Q or ubiquinone.) Murray RK, Bender DA, Botham KM, Kennelly PJ, Rodwell VW, Weil PA. *Harper's Illustrated Biochemistry*, 29th ed. New York, NY: McGraw-Hill; 2012.

High-Yield Concept

Classically, the description of ATP synthesis through oxidation of reduced electron carriers indicated 3 moles of ATP could be generated for every mole of NADH and 2 moles for every mole of $FADH_2$. However, direct chemical analysis has shown that for every 2 electrons transferred from NADH to oxygen, 2.5 equivalents of ATP are synthesized and 1.5 ATP equivalents for $FADH_2$.

or succinate dehydrogenase). Complex II is composed of 4 protein subunits. The $\Delta E^{\circ\prime}$ for electron flow through complex II is about 0.05 V, corresponding to a $\Delta G'$ of –2.3 kcal/mol of electrons transferred, which is insufficient to drive ATP synthesis. The difference in free energy of electron flow through complexes I and II accounts for the fact that a pair of electrons originating from NADH and passing to oxygen supports production of 2.5 (more commonly reported as 3) equivalents of ATP, while 2 electrons from succinate (as $FADH_2$) support the production of only 1.5 (more commonly reported as 2) equivalents of ATP.

Reduced CoQ ($CoQH_2$) diffuses in the lipid phase of the membrane and donates its electrons to complex III, whose principal components are the heme proteins known as cytochromes *b* and c_1 and a non-heme iron protein, known as the Rieske iron-sulfur protein. Complex III is known as ubiquinol-cytochrome *c* oxidoreductase (also CoQ-cytochrome reductase) and is composed of 11 protein subunits. In contrast to the heme of hemoglobin and myoglobin, the heme iron of all cytochromes participates in the cyclic redox reactions of electron transport, alternating between the oxidized (Fe^{3+}) and reduced (Fe^{2+}) forms. The electron carrier from complex III to complex IV is cytochrome *c*.

Complex IV, also known as cytochrome *c* oxidase, contains the heme proteins known as cytochrome *a* and cytochrome a_3, as well as copper-containing proteins in which the copper undergoes a transition from

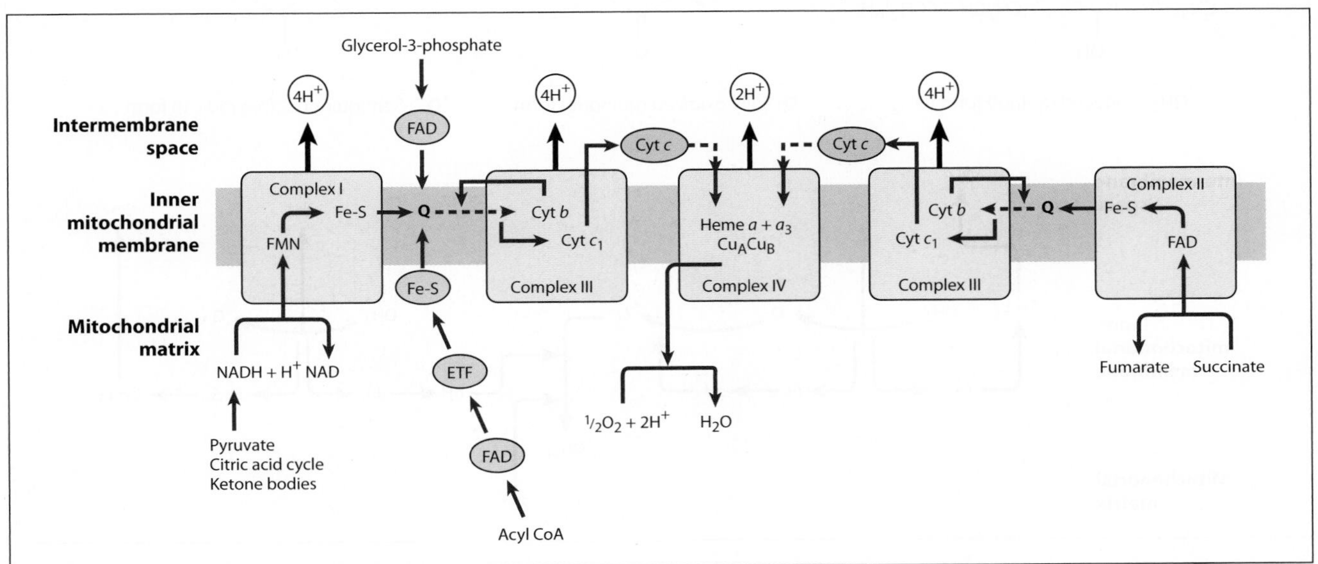

FIGURE 17-3: Flow of electrons through the respiratory chain complexes, showing the entry points for reducing equivalents from important substrates. Q and cyt c are mobile components of the system as indicated by the dotted arrows. (ETF, electron transferring flavoprotein; Fe–S, iron–sulfur protein; cyt, cytochrome; Q, coenzyme Q or ubiquinone.) Murray RK, Bender DA, Botham KM, Kennelly PJ, Rodwell VW, Weil PA. *Harper's Illustrated Biochemistry*, 29th ed. New York, NY: McGraw-Hill; 2012.

Cu^+ to Cu^{2+} during the transfer of electrons through the complex to molecular oxygen. Complex IV is composed of a total of 13 protein subunits. Oxygen is the final electron acceptor, with water being the final product of oxygen reduction.

In addition to the core protein subunits of each of the complexes of oxidative phosphorylation, there are numerous assembly factors required to ensure correct formation of each complex. The importance of the assembly factors in functional formation of these complexes can be demonstrated by the mitochondrial encephalomyopathies that result due to mutations in several of these genes. For example, GRACILE syndrome (**G**rowth **R**etardation, **A**mino aciduria, **C**holestasis, **I**ron overload, **L**actic acidosis, and **E**arly death) is caused by mutations in the *BCS1L* gene which is required for proper assembly of complex III.

Normal oxidation of NADH or $FADH_2$ is always a 2-electron reaction, with the transfer of 2 hydride ions to a flavin. A hydride ion is composed of 1 proton and 1 electron. Unlike NADH and succinate, flavins can participate in either 1-electron or 2-electron reactions; thus, flavin that is fully reduced by the dehydrogenase reactions can subsequently be oxidized by 2 sequential 1-hydride reactions. The fully reduced form of a flavin is known as the quinol form and the fully oxidized form is known as the quinone form; the intermediate containing a single electron is known as the semiquinone or semiquinol form.

Like flavins, CoQ (also known as ubiquinone) can undergo either 1- or 2-electron reactions leading to formation of the reduced quinol, the oxidized quinone, and the semiquinone intermediate (Figure 17-4). The ability of flavins and CoQ to form semiquinone intermediates is a key feature of the mitochondrial electron transport systems, since these cofactors link the obligatory 2-electron reactions of NADH and $FADH_2$ with the obligatory 1-electron reactions of the cytochromes.

The free energy available as a consequence of transferring 2 electrons from NADH or $FADH_2$ to molecular oxygen is –57 and –36 kcal/mol, respectively. Oxidative phosphorylation traps this energy as the high-energy phosphate of ATP. All of the available energy from electron flow is not captured in the synthesis of ATP and what is not is released as heat which maintains the normal human body temperature.

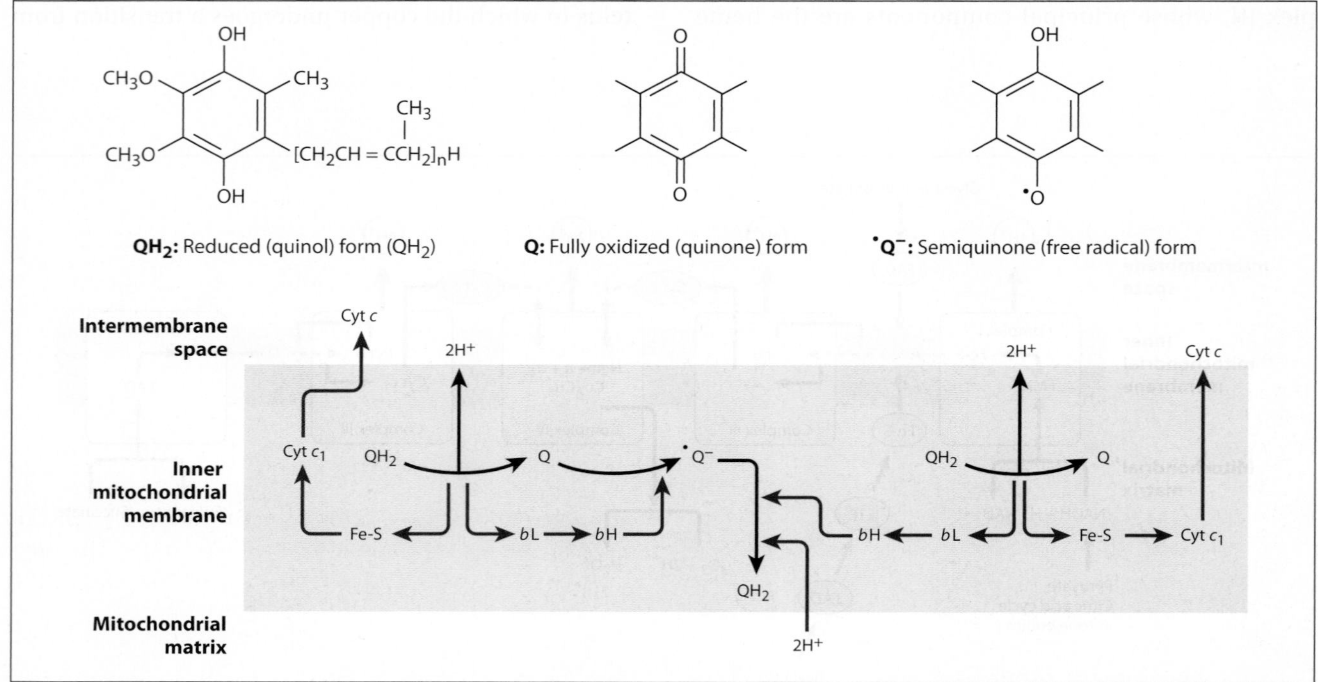

FIGURE 17-4: The Q cycle. During the oxidation of QH_2 to Q, one electron is donated to cyt *c* via a Rieske Fe–S and cyt c_1 and the second to a Q to form the semiquinone via cyt b_L and cyt b_H, with $2H^+$ being released into the intermembrane space. A similar process then occurs with a second QH_2, but in this case the second electron is donated to the semiquinone, reducing it to QH_2, and $2H^+$ are taken up from the matrix. (cyt, cytochrome; Fe–S, iron-sulfur protein; Q, coenzyme Q or ubiquinone.) Murray RK, Bender DA, Botham KM, Kennelly PJ, Rodwell VW, Weil PA. *Harper's Illustrated Biochemistry*, 29th ed. New York, NY: McGraw-Hill; 2012.

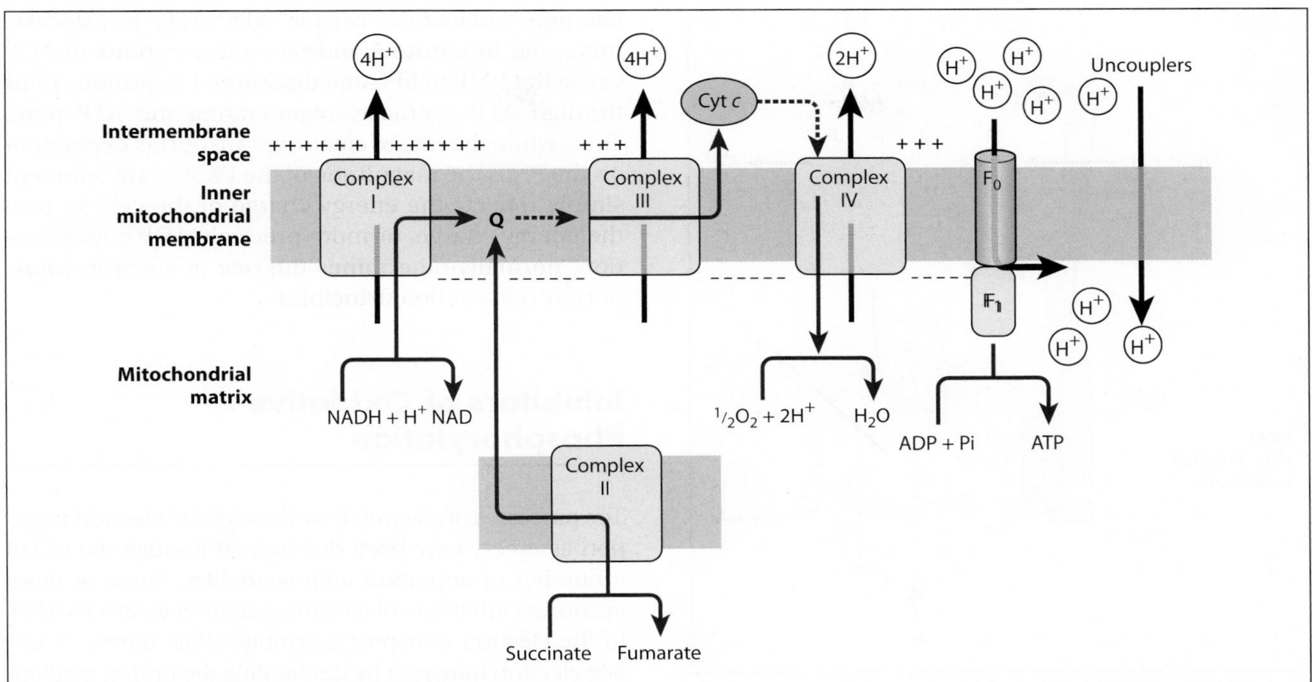

FIGURE 17-5: The chemiosmotic theory of oxidative phosphorylation. Complexes I, III, and IV act as proton pumps creating a proton gradient across the membrane, which is negative on the matrix side. The proton motive force generated drives the synthesis of ATP as the protons flow back into the matrix through the ATP synthase enzyme. Uncouplers increase the permeability of the membrane to ions, collapsing the proton gradient by allowing the H^+ to pass across without going through the ATP synthase, and thus uncouple electron flow through the respiratory complexes from ATP synthesis. (cyt, cytochrome; Q, coenzyme Q or ubiquinone.) Murray RK, Bender DA, Botham KM, Kennelly PJ, Rodwell VW, Weil PA. *Harper's Illustrated Biochemistry*, 29th ed. New York, NY: McGraw-Hill; 2012.

In order for oxidative phosphorylation to proceed, 2 principal conditions must be met. First, the inner mitochondrial membrane must be physically intact so that protons can only reenter the mitochondrion by a process coupled to ATP synthesis. Second, a high concentration of protons must be developed on the outside of the inner membrane. The energy of the proton gradient is known as the chemiosmotic potential (Figure 17-5), or PMF. The energy of this gradient is used to drive ATP synthesis as the protons are transported back down their thermodynamic gradient into the mitochondrion.

Electrons return to the mitochondrion through the integral membrane protein known as ATP synthase or complex V (Figure 17-6). ATP synthase is a multiple subunit complex that binds ADP and inorganic phosphate at its catalytic site inside the mitochondrion, and requires a proton gradient for activity in the forward direction. ATP synthase is composed of 3 fragments: F_0, which is localized in the membrane; F_1, which protrudes from the inside of the inner membrane into the matrix; and oligomycin sensitivity-conferring protein (OSCP), which connects F_0 to F_1. In damaged mitochondria, permeable to protons, the ATP synthase reaction is active in the reverse direction acting as a very efficient ATP hydrolase or ATPase (Figure 17-6).

Regulation of Oxidative Phosphorylation

Since electron transport is directly coupled to proton translocation, the flow of electrons through the electron transport system is regulated by the magnitude of the PMF. The higher the PMF, the lower the rate of electron transport, and vice versa. Under resting conditions, with a high cell energy charge, the demand for new synthesis of ATP is limited and, although the PMF is high, flow of protons back into the mitochondria through ATP synthase is minimal. When energy demands are increased, such as during vigorous muscle activity, cytosolic ADP rises and is exchanged with intramitochondrial ATP via the transmembrane

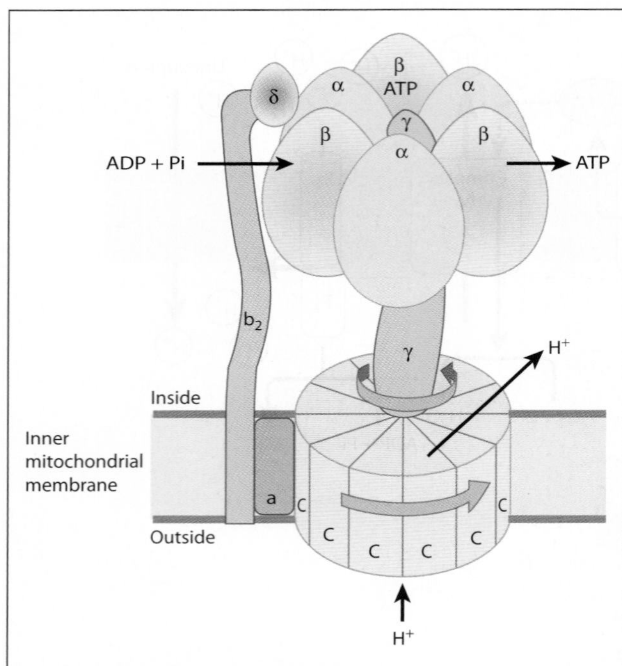

FIGURE 17-6: Mechanism of ATP production by ATP synthase. The enzyme complex consists of an F_0 subcomplex which is a disk of "C" protein subunits. Attached is a γ subunit in the form of a "bent axle." Protons passing through the disk of "C" units cause it and the attached γ subunit to rotate. The γ subunit fits inside the F_1 subcomplex of three α and three β subunits, which are fixed to the membrane and do not rotate. ADP and P_i are taken up sequentially by the β subunits to form ATP, which is expelled as the rotating γ subunit squeezes each β subunit in turn and changes its conformation. Thus, three ATP molecules are generated per revolution. For clarity, not all the subunits that have been identified are shown—eg, the "axle" also contains an ε subunit. Murray RK, Bender DA, Botham KM, Kennelly PJ, Rodwell VW, Weil PA. *Harper's Illustrated Biochemistry*, 29th ed. New York, NY: McGraw-Hill; 2012.

adenine nucleotide carrier ADP/ATP translocase. Increased intramitochondrial concentrations of ADP cause the PMF to become discharged as protons pour through ATP synthase, regenerating the ATP pool. Thus, while the rate of electron transport is dependent on the PMF, the magnitude of the PMF at any moment simply reflects the energy charge of the cell. In turn the energy charge, or more precisely ADP concentration, normally determines the rate of electron transport by mass action principles.

Inhibitors of Oxidative Phosphorylation

The processes of electron flow through the electron transport assembly have been determined through the use of a number of important antimetabolites. Some of these agents are inhibitors of electron transport at specific sites in the electron transport assembly, while others stimulate electron transport by discharging the proton gradient (Figure 17-7). For example, antimycin A is a specific inhibitor of cytochrome *b*. In the presence of antimycin A, cytochrome *b* can be reduced but not oxidized. As expected, cytochrome *c* remains oxidized in the presence of antimycin A, as do the downstream cytochromes *a* and a_3.

An important class of antimetabolites are the uncoupling agents exemplified by 2,4-dinitrophenol (DNP). Uncoupling agents act as lipophilic weak acids, associating with protons on the exterior of mitochondria, passing through the membrane with the bound proton, and dissociating the proton on the interior of the mitochondrion. These agents cause maximum respiratory rates but the transport of electrons generates no ATP, since the translocated protons do not return to the interior through ATP synthase (Table 17-2).

High-Yield Concept

The rate of electron transport is usually measured by assaying the rate of oxygen consumption and is referred to as the cellular respiratory rate. The respiratory rate is known as the state 4 rate when the energy charge is high, the concentration of ADP is low, and electron transport is limited by ADP. When ADP levels rise and inorganic phosphate is available, the flow of protons through ATP synthase is elevated and higher rates of electron transport are observed; the resultant respiratory rate is known as the state 3 rate. Thus, under physiological conditions mitochondrial respiratory activity cycles between state 3 and state 4 rates.

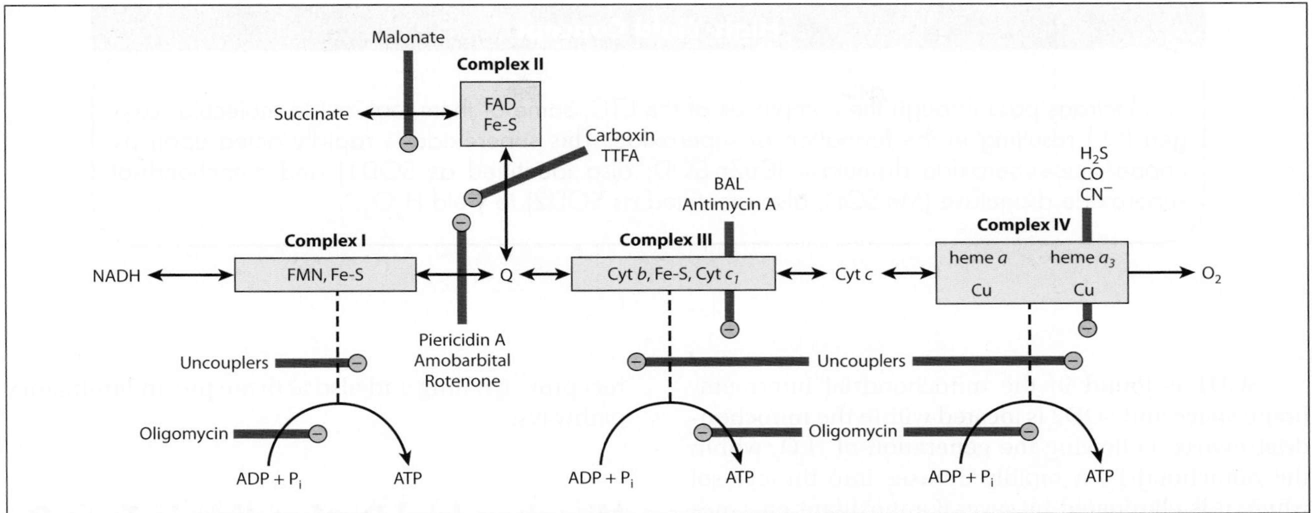

FIGURE 17-7: Sites of inhibition (⊖) of the respiratory chain by specific drugs, chemicals, and antibiotics. (BAL, dimercaprol; TTFA, an Fe-chelating agent. Murray RK, Bender DA, Botham KM, Kennelly PJ, Rodwell VW, Weil PA. *Harper's Illustrated Biochemistry*, 29th ed. New York, NY: McGraw-Hill; 2012.

Generation of Reactive Oxygen Species

The mitochondrial electron transport chain (ETC) of oxidative phosphorylation is the major site for the cellular generation of reactive oxygen species (ROS) (Figure 17-8).

TABLE 17-2: Inhibitors of Oxidative Phosphorylation

Name	*Function*	*Site of Action*
Rotenone	e^- transport inhibitor	Complex I
Amytal	e^- transport inhibitor	Complex I
Antimycin A	e^- transport inhibitor	Complex III
Cyanide	e^- transport inhibitor	Complex IV
Carbon monoxide	e^- transport inhibitor	Complex IV
Azide	e^- transport inhibitor	Complex IV
2,4, -Dinitrophenol	Uncoupling agent	Transmembrane H^+ carrier
Pentachloro-phenol	Uncoupling agent	Transmembrane H^+ carrier
Oligomycin	Inhibits ATP synthase	OSCP fraction of ATP synthase

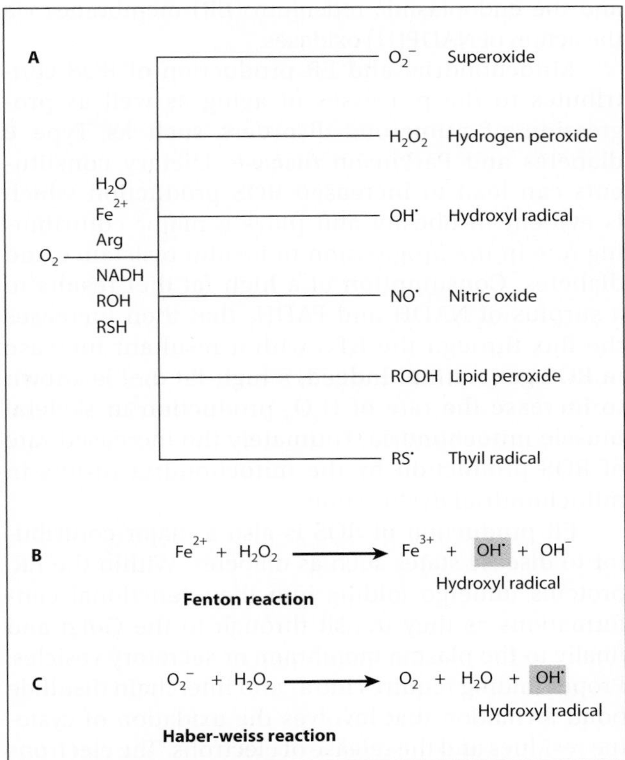

FIGURE 17-8: Reactive oxygen species (ROS) are toxic by-products of life in an aerobic environment. (A) Many types of ROS are encountered in living cells. (B) Generation of hydroxyl radical via the Fenton reaction. (C) Generation of hydroxyl radical by the Haber–Weiss reaction. Murray RK, Bender DA, Botham KM, Kennelly PJ, Rodwell VW, Weil PA. *Harper's Illustrated Biochemistry*, 29th ed. New York, NY: McGraw-Hill; 2012.

High-Yield Concept

As electrons pass through the complexes of the ETC, some of them leak out to molecular oxygen (O_2) resulting in the formation of superoxide. This superoxide is rapidly acted upon by copper-zinc-superoxide dismutase (CuZn-SOD; also identified as SOD1) and mitochondrial superoxide dismutase (Mn-SOD; also identified as SOD2) to yield H_2O_2.

SOD1 is found in the mitochondrial intermembrane space and SOD2 is located within the mitochondrial matrix. Following the generation of H_2O_2 within the mitochondria, it rapidly diffuses into the cytosol where it is eliminated by several antioxidant enzymes that include the glutathione peroxidases (GPx1-GPx4), catalase, and the peroxiredoxins (PRX1 and PRX2). Within the ETC itself the major site of ROS generation is the flavin mononucleotide (FMN) of complex I. ROS generation also occurs within the plasma membrane and the endoplasmic reticulum (ER) membranes via the action of NADP(H) oxidases.

Mitochondrial and ER production of ROS contributes to the processes of aging as well as progression of numerous disorders such as Type 2 diabetes and Parkinson disease. Dietary constituents can lead to increased ROS production which is evident in obesity and plays a major contributing role in the progression to insulin resistance and diabetes. Consumption of a high-fat diet results in a surplus of NADH and $FADH_2$ that then increases the flux through the ETC with a resultant increase in ROS generation. Indeed, a high-fat diet is known to increase the rate of H_2O_2 production in skeletal muscle mitochondria. Ultimately the increased rate of ROS production by the mitochondria results in mitochondrial dysfunction.

ER production of ROS is also a major contributor to disease states such as diabetes. Within the ER, proteins undergo folding into their functional conformations as they transit through to the Golgi and finally to the plasma membrane or secretory vesicles. Proper folding requires intra- and interchain disulfide bond formation that involves the oxidation of cysteine residues and the release of electrons. The electrons are passed to protein disulfide isomerase, then to ER oxidoreductin, and finally to the O_2-generating superoxide anion. The nutrient excess seen in obesity and diabetes may play a role in overloading the ER protein folding capacity resulting in increased ROS production. An increase in ER ROS production results in ER stress and the induction of the ER stress response pathways (see Chapter 37) that in turn impair insulin receptor signaling and also activate pro-inflammatory pathways.

Mitochondrial Dysfunction in Type 2 Diabetes and Obesity

It is well established that mitochondrial dysfunction, particularly as it relates to the processes of oxidative phosphorylation, is contributory to the development of encephalomyopathy, mitochondrial myopathy, and several age-related disorders that include neurodegenerative diseases, the metabolic syndrome, and diabetes. Indeed, with respect to diabetes, several mitochondrial biogenesis diseases (see below) manifest with diabetic complications such as mitochondrial myopathy, encephalopathy, lactic acidosis, and stroke-like episodes (MELAS) and maternally inherited diabetes and deafness (MIDD).

As pointed out earlier, normal biogenesis of mitochondria involves the transcription factors PGC-1α and NRF1. Evidence has demonstrated that both PGC-1α and NRF1 expression levels are lower in diabetic patients and in nondiabetic subjects from families with Type 2 diabetes. The expression of NRF1 is highest in skeletal muscle which is also the tissue that accounts for the largest percentage of glucose disposal in the body and, therefore, is the tissue that is most responsible for the hyperglycemia resulting from impaired insulin signaling.

Mitochondrial dysfunction results in increased production of ROS which activates stress responses leading to increased activity of MAPK and JNK. Both of these serine/threonine kinases phosphorylate IRS1 and IRS2 resulting in decreased signaling downstream of the insulin receptor. Decreased insulin receptor signaling results in decreased activation of PI3K, which is responsible for stimulating the translocation of GLUT4 to the plasma membrane allowing for increased glucose uptake. Thus, inhibition of PI3K activation results in reduced glucose uptake in skeletal muscle and adipose tissue.

High-Yield Concept

Because skeletal muscle consumes the largest amount of serum glucose, mitochondrial dysfunction in this tissue will have the greatest impact on glucose disposal. However, adipose tissue also plays an important role in glucose homeostasis and mitochondrial dysfunction in this tissue also results in impaired glucose homeostasis resulting in diabetes.

Mitochondrial dysfunction, particularly in skeletal muscle, also results in a reduction in the level of enzymes involved in fatty acid β-oxidation leading to increases in intramyocellular lipid content. Indeed, skeletal muscle metabolism of lipids is impaired in type 2 diabetics. An increased delivery of fatty acids to skeletal muscle, as well as diminished mitochondrial oxidation, results in increased intracellular content of fatty acid metabolites such as diacylglycerol (DAG), fatty acyl-CoAs, and ceramides. These metabolites of fatty acids are all known to induce the activity of protein kinase C isoforms (PKC-β and PKC-δ) that phosphorylate IRS1 and IRS2 on serine residues resulting in impaired insulin signaling downstream of the insulin receptor.

Mitochondrial Encephalomyopathies

Mitochondrial diseases are among the most common of the inherited disorders of metabolism. The mitochondrial encephalomyopathies represent a broad family of disorders resulting from defects in mitochondrial respiratory function. Due to the role of the nuclear genome in overall mitochondrial biogenesis and the process of oxidative phosphorylation, mitochondrial diseases can be inherited by maternal, autosomal, or X-chromosomal transmission. In most of these diseases the symptoms manifest due to defects in energy generation in the brain and skeletal muscle, thus they are referred to as mitochondrial encephalomyopathies.

As pointed out earlier mammalian cells can have hundreds to thousands of mitochondria, and each mitochondrion contains several mtDNA genomes. Because mitochondria are inherited from the mother, this uniparental inheritance of mtDNA means that it is possible for mtDNA mutations to accumulate slowly over successive generations until, eventually, a threshold mutant level is reached that manifests as a disease. In general, disease severity correlates with the relative proportion of mutated to intact mtDNA. A heteroplasmic person will only develop the disease if the mutant load exceeds a certain threshold. Disease severity and symptom presentation is also affected by the level of heteroplasmy since no 2 cells, even within the same individual, will harbor the same level of mutant mtDNA. This also means that the threshold level may be different for different mutations as well as for different tissues. Mitochondrial DNA mutations are also known to occur sporadically in somatic tissues. These somatic mutations may undergo clonal expansion, eventually reaching the threshold level and causing mitochondrial dysfunction at a later age. It is this latter phenomenon that suggests that accumulating mtDNA mutations, and subsequent progressive mitochondrial dysfunction, contribute to the normal processes of aging.

Due to the poor oxidative capacity in skeletal muscle, these cells are incapable of pyruvate oxidation resulting in increased reduction of the pyruvate to lactate. The lactate is released to the blood resulting in lactic acidosis which is a common symptom in many mitochondrial encephalomyopathies. Biopsy tissue from skeletal muscle of patients with these disorders is normally stained with Gomori-modified trichrome. This histological technique stains the massive subsarcolemmal proliferation in these disorders red and the muscle fibers look ragged. Indeed, the finding of ragged red fibers in skeletal muscle biopsies is a hallmark of many mitochondrial encephalomyopathies (Table 17-3).

Brown Adipose Tissue and Heat Generation

The uncoupling of proton flow releases the energy of the electrochemical proton gradient as heat (Figure 17-9). This process is a normal physiological function of brown adipose tissue (BAT). Brown adipose tissue gets its color from the high density of mitochondria in the individual adipose cells. Newborn babies contain BAT in their neck and upper

TABLE 17-3: Several Mitochondrial Encephalomyopathies

Disorder	*Genetic Defect(s)*	*Symptoms*
Kearns-Sayre syndrome, KSS	Various mitochondrial deletions are found in 78% of KSS patients	Ophthalmoplegia, weakness, ataxia, pigmentary retinopathy, loss of hearing, dementia, and seizures; nonneurological manifestations include hypertrophic and dilated cardiomyopathy, cardiac conduction abnormalities, impaired GI motility, diabetes mellitus and other endocrine abnormalities, short stature, and renal dysfunction
Alpers disease, also known as mitochondrial DNA (mtDNA) depletion syndrome-4A (MTDPS4A)	Mitochondrial DNA polymerase g	psychomotor retardation, intractable epilepsy, and liver failure in infants
MELAS: mitochondrial myopathy, encephalopathy, lactic acidosis, and stroke	Mutations in at least 10 different mitochondrial tRNA genes; commonly due to A → G mutation at nucleotide 3243 in mitochondrial $tRNA^{leu}$ (MTTL1)	Characterized by encephalopathy (seizures, dementia), recurrent stroke-like episodes at a young age, myopathy, and lactic acidosis; ataxia, deafness, pigmentary retinopathy, and short stature are seen in some patients
LHON: Leber hereditary optic neuropathy	At least 18 allelic variants due to missense mutations; 90% of patients harbor 1 of 3 mtDNA mutations at nucleotide 3460, 11778, or 14484	Begins with blurring and clouding of vision, progresses to severe loss of sharpness and color
MIDD: maternally inherited diabetes and deafness	Mutations in at least 3 different mitochondrial tRNA genes; most common mutation is A → G at nucleotide 3243 in mitochondrial $tRNA^{leu}$ (MTTL1)	Cardiomyopathy and neurological symptoms, lactic acidosis upon exercise
MERRF: myoclonic epilepsy with ragged red fibers	Mutations in at least 6 different mitochondrial tRNA genes; also caused by mutations in gene encoding complex I subunit ND5	Characterized by myoclonus, epilepsy, ataxia, and dementia; principally affected tissues are brain, heart, and skeletal muscle
Leigh syndrome	Mutations in both nuclear and mitochondrial genes; includes components of complexes I, II, III, IV, and V, and components of the pyruvate dehydrogenase complex	Infantile onset, damages primarily the brainstem and basal ganglia causing hypotonia, ophthalmoplegia, nystagmus, and psychomotor regression; mean age of death is 5 years

back that serves the function of nonshivering thermogenesis. The muscle contractions that take place in the process of shivering not only generate ATP but also produce heat. Nonshivering thermogenesis is a hormonal stimulus for heat generation without the associated muscle contractions of shivering. The process of thermogeneses in BAT is initiated by the release of free fatty acids from the triglycerides stored in the adipose cells.

The mitochondria in BAT contain a protein called uncoupling protein 1, UCP1 (also called thermogenin). There are 3 uncoupling protein genes in humans identified as UCP1, UCP2, and UCP3. UCP2 is expressed in a number of tissues, and UCP3 is expressed in skeletal and heart muscle. Only UCP1 is involved in the process of adaptive thermogenesis.

UCP1 acts as a channel in the inner mitochondrial membrane to control the permeability of the membrane to protons. When norepinephrine is released in response to cold sensation, it binds to β-adrenergic receptors on the surface of brown adipocytes triggering the activation of adenylate cyclase.

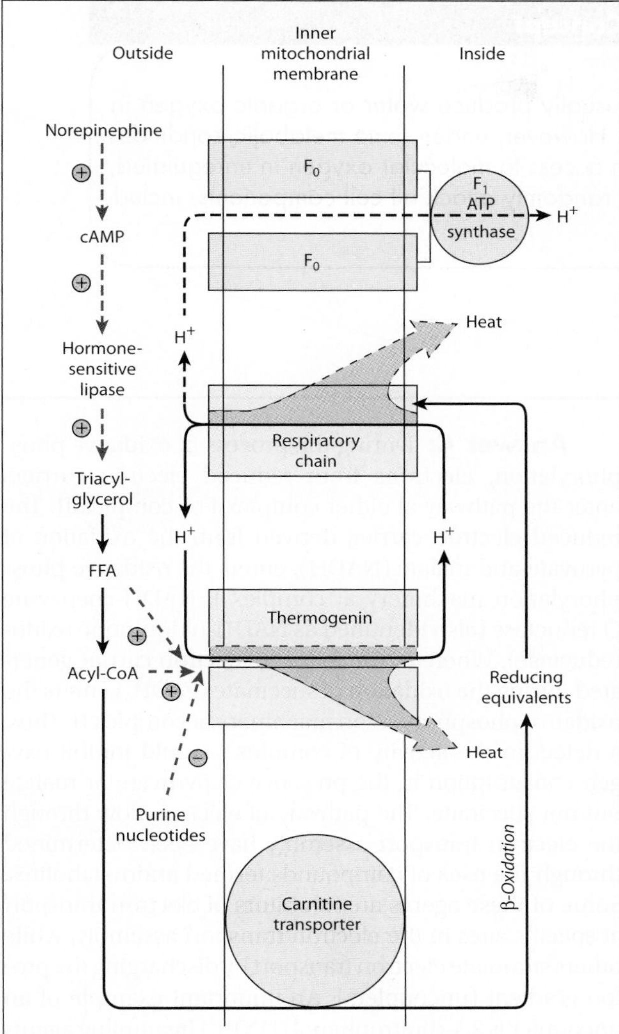

FIGURE 17-9: Thermogenesis in brown adipose tissue. Activity of the respiratory chain produces heat in addition to translocating protons. These protons dissipate more heat when returned to the inner mitochondrial compartment via thermogenin instead of via the F_1 ATP synthase, the route that generates ATP. The passage of H^+ via thermogenin is inhibited by purine nucleotides when brown adipose tissue is unstimulated. Under the influence of norepinephrine, the inhibition is removed by the production of free fatty acids (FFA) and acyl-CoA. Note the dual role of acyl-CoA in both facilitating the action of thermogenin and supplying reducing equivalents for the respiratory chain. ⊕ and ⊖ signify positive or negative regulatory effects. Murray RK, Bender DA, Botham KM, Kennelly PJ, Rodwell VW, Weil PA. *Harper's Illustrated Biochemistry*, 29th ed. New York, NY: McGraw-Hill; 2012.

Activated adenylate cyclase leads to increased production of cAMP and the concomitant activation of cAMP-dependent protein kinase (PKA) with the result being phosphorylation and activation of hormone-sensitive lipase. The released free fatty acids bind to UCP1 triggering an uncoupling of the proton gradient and the release of the energy of the gradient as heat.

Other Biological Oxidations

Oxidase complexes, like cytochrome oxidase, transfer electrons directly from NADH and other substrates to oxygen, producing water. Oxygenases, widely localized in membranes of the ER, catalyze the addition of molecular oxygen to organic molecules. There are 2 kinds of oxygenase complexes, monooxygenases and dioxygenases. Dioxygenases add the 2 atoms of molecular oxygen (O_2) to carbon and nitrogen of organic compounds. Monooxygenase complexes play a key role in detoxifying drugs and other compounds and in the normal metabolism of steroids, fatty acids, and fat-soluble vitamins. Monooxygenases act by sequentially transferring 2 electrons from NADH or NADPH to 1 of the 2 atoms of oxygen in O_2, generating H_2O from one oxygen atom and incorporating the other oxygen atom into an organic compound as a hydroxyl group (R-OH). The hydroxylated products are markedly more water soluble than their precursors and are much more readily excreted from the body. Widely used synonyms for the monooxygenases are: mixed function oxidases, hydroxylases, and mixed function hydroxylases. The chief components of monooxygenase complexes include cytochrome b_5, a cytochrome P450 (CYP), and cytochrome P450 reductase, which contains FAD plus FMN. There are at least 57 CYP genes in the human genome. Within the liver, where the bulk of drug and other xenobiotic metabolism occur, up to 50 different CYP genes are expressed.

Most tissues are replete with enzymes to protect against the random chemical reactions that ROS initiate. Free radical scavenging enzymes include the superoxide dismutases (SOD), catalase, glutathione peroxidases (GPx), and peroxiredoxins (PRX).

Superoxide dismutases convert superoxide anion to peroxide, thereby minimizing production of hydroxy radical which is the most potent of the oxygen-free radicals. Peroxides produced by SOD are also toxic. They are detoxified by conversion to water via the peroxidases such as the glutathione peroxidases. Catalase (located in peroxisomes) provides a reductant route for the degradation of H_2O_2.

High-Yield Concept

Enzymatic reactions involving molecular oxygen usually produce water or organic oxygen in well-regulated reactions having specific products. However, under some metabolic conditions (such as discussed above) unpaired electrons gain access to molecular oxygen in unregulated, nonenzymatic reactions generating ROS that can randomly attack all cell components, including proteins, lipids, and nucleic acids.

REVIEW QUESTIONS

1. You are studying the effects of a compound on the respiratory activity of isolated mitochondria. Your experiments demonstrate that oxygen consumption is normal when pyruvate and malate are used as well as when succinate is added. However, you find that the production of ATP is severely impaired with addition of the compound. These results most closely resemble the effects that would be seen by the addition of the following electron transport inhibitor to your system?

A. antimycin A
B. azide
C. dinitrophenol (DNP)
D. oligomycin
E. rotenone

Answer C: The normal flow of electrons, through the proteins of the oxidative phosphorylation machinery, is coupled with the establishment of a proton gradient across the inner mitochondrial membrane. The establishment of this pH gradient is the chemiosmotic potential that is coupled with the production of ATP. If the process of proton movement is uncoupled from the normal pathway through the ATP synthase complex, oxygen can be consumed but no ATP will be synthesized. This is the effect of uncoupling agents such as DNP, which act to discharge the proton gradient.

2. A laboratory analysis of isolated mitochondria demonstrates that oxygen consumption is normal when succinate is added but extremely low when pyruvate and malate are used. The mitchondria are subsequently shown to have normal cytochromes but a reduced iron content. The reduced pyruvate/malate oxidation is due to a defect in which of the following respiratory components?

A. cytochrome *c*
B. cytochrome oxidase
C. NADH dehydrogenase
D. succinate dehydrogenase
E. ubiquinone

Answer C: During the process of oxidative phosphorylation, electrons from reduced electron carriers enter the pathway at either complex I or complex II. The reduced electron carrier, derived from the oxidation of pyruvate and malate (NADH), enters the oxidative phosphorylation machinery at complex I, NADH-coenzyme Q reductase (also identified as NADH-ubiquinone oxidoreductase). Whereas, the reduced electron carrier generated during the oxidation of succinate ($FADH_2$) enters the oxidative phosphorylation machinery at complex II. Thus, a defect in the activity of complex I would inhibit oxygen consumption in the presence of pyruvate or malate but not succinate. The pathway of electron flow through the electron transport assembly have been determined through the uses of compounds termed antimetabolites. Some of these agents are inhibitors of electron transport at specific sites in the electron transport assembly, while others stimulate electron transport by discharging the proton gradient (uncouplers). An important example of an uncoupler is 2,4-dinitrophenol (DNP). Uncoupling agents such as DNP act as lipophilic weak acids, associating with protons on the exterior of mitochondria, passing through the membrane with the bound proton, and dissociating the proton on the interior of the mitochondrion. These agents cause maximum respiratory rates but the electron transport generates no ATP, since the translocated protons do not return to the interior through ATP synthase.

3. Which of the following statements best characterizes ATP synthase?

A. it couples ATP export from the mitochondrial matrix to ATP synthesis
B. it is soluble protein found in the mitochondrial matrix
C. its catalytic function is to synthesize ATP in a reaction driven by a chemiosmotic potential
D. oligomycin binds to ATP synthase, directly preventing ATP export
E. the low H^+ ion concentration outside mitochondria establishes an electrochemical gradient that drives ATP synthesis

Answer C: ATP synthase is the enzyme associated with oxidative phosphorylation that utilizes the energy from the chemiosmotic potential generated by electron flow coupled to the pumping of protons out of the matrix of the mitochondria across the inner mitochondrial membrane. ATP synthase uses this potential energy to synthesize ATP from ADP and P_i.

4. Which of the following enzymes catalyzes the reaction shown?

$$Fe^{2+} + O_2 + 4H^+ \rightarrow 2H_2O + Fe^{3+}$$

A. catalase
B. cytochrome *c* oxidase
C. cytochrome P450
D. peroxidase
E. superoxide dismutase

Answer B: Complex IV, also known as cytochrome *c* oxidase, contains the heme proteins known as cytochrome *a* and cytochrome a_3, as well as copper-containing proteins in which the copper undergoes a transition from Cu^+ to Cu^{2+} during the transfer of electrons from the heme iron in cytochrome *c* through the complex to molecular oxygen.

5. You are studying the effects of a compound on the respiratory activity of isolated mitochondria. Your experiments demonstrate that oxygen consumption increases as expected when pyruvate and malate are used as well as when succinate is added. Addition of the test compound results in a significant rate of oxygen consumption. These results most closely resemble the effects that would be seen by the addition of which of the following to your system?

A. antimycin A
B. carbon monoxide
C. cyanide
D. dinitrophenol
E. rotenone

Answer D: Dinitrophenol, DNP, is a chemical uncoupler of electron transport. Uncouplers cause increased oxygen consumption. DNP functions by allowing protons to flow back into the matrix of the mitochondria through the inner mitochondrial membrane which dissipates the electrochemical gradient and preventing ATP synthesis. Since the proton motive force (PMF) across the membrane is lost, there is no longer a gradient to restrict the rate of electron flow; as a result electron transport accelerates resulting in increased oxygen consumption.

6. A 9-year-old girl is brought to her physician for an assessment of potential causes for her increased vision problems. Examination demonstrates that her eye movement is impaired and she has pigmentary retinopathy. Her physician suspects the child has Kearns-Sayre syndrome which is caused by a defect in complex II of the electron transport chain. If this diagnosis is correct, oxidation of which of the following substrates would be associated with impaired electron transfer?

A. acetyl-CoA
B. α-ketoglutarate
C. malate
D. pyruvate
E. succinate

Answer E: Electrons from the oxidation of succinate, via succinate dehydrogenase, enter the electron transport chain (ETC) from $FADH_2$ at complex II. Therefore, an impairment of complex II function as in this patient would impair electron flow. Oxidation of each of the other substrates generates NADH which feeds its electrons to the ETC at complex I.

7. Reduced ubiquinone, generated during the oxidation of NADH, passes its electrons to which of the following?

A. ATP synthase
B. cytochrome *c* oxidase (complex IV)
C. cytochrome *b*
D. cytochrome *c*
E. molecular oxygen

Answer C: Reduced CoQ ($CoQH_2$) diffuses in the lipid phase of the membrane and donates its electrons to complex III, whose principal components are the heme proteins cytochromes *b* and a non-heme protein, known as the Rieske iron-sulfur protein.

8. In cases of acute cyanide poisoning, cyanide binds to the Fe^{3+} of a cytochrome. Which statement best describes this cytochrome?

A. binds carbon monoxide
B. directly oxidized by cytochrome *c*
C. directly oxidizes cytochrome *b*
D. found in the mitochondrial matrix
E. reduces cytochrome *c*

Answer A: Cyanides bind to the heme iron in cytochrome a+a_3 of complex IV. This same cytochrome is the site of carbon-monoxide binding.

9. You are the physician examining a 6-year-old boy who has been experiencing progressive muscle weakness. You perform assays on muscle biopsy tissue from this patient and find that mitochondrial oxidation of succinate is normal but that pyruvate oxidation is severely impaired. Mitochondrial extracts demonstrate that the activity of the pyruvate dehydrogenase complex (PDHc) is normal as is the activity of malate dehydrogenase. These results are consistent with the patient harboring a defect in which of the following mitochondrial components?

A. ATP synthase
B. complex I
C. complex II
D. complex III
E. complex IV

Answer B: Since the PDHc activity of the patient's mitochondria was shown to be normal but the NADH produced by this reaction could not be reoxidized via electron transport, it suggests that the defect causing the muscle weakness is in mitochondrial complex I. Succinate oxidation was normal indicating that electron flow to complex II is not impaired, further strengthening the argument that the defect lies in complex I. If ATP synthase were defective neither pyruvate nor succinate oxidation would be normal.

10. You are carrying out experiments on isolated skeletal muscle mitochondria. For these experiments you are using malate as the oxidizable substrate. Following the addition of malate you add the electron transport inhibitor cyanide. You then examine the oxidation state of various components of the electron transport chain. Which of the following would be expected to be in an oxidized state following this experiment?

A. coenzyme Q
B. complex I
C. complex II
D. complex III
E. cytochrome *c*

Answer C: Cyanide inhibits the transfer of electrons through complex IV (cytochrome oxidase). In order for any of the components of electron transport to be in an oxidized state they must have either transferred electrons to the next component downstream or never have received electrons in the first place. Oxidation of malate generates NADH which gives its electrons to complex I which then gives the electrons to coenzyme Q which then gives the electrons to complex II, then to cytochrome *c*, and finally they are passed to complex IV. Since cyanide blocks the transfer of electrons from complex IV to oxygen, all of the upstream electron acceptors will be "blocked" in the reduced state. Only complex II will have never accepted electrons and thus will be in the oxidized state under the conditions of this experiment.

11. A 6-year-old boy is brought to his pediatrician because his parents are concerned about the appearance of seizures and stroke-like episodes. Upon examination the parents reveal that their son has recently begun to exhibit a progressive incoordination in his walking and also difficulty picking up his toys. The physician notes that the patient is short for his age and an eye examination reveals pigmentary retinopathy. Analysis of blood shows elevated levels of lactic acid. These signs and symptoms are most indicative of which of the following disorders?

A. erythrocyte pyruvate kinase deficiency
B. Kearns-Sayre syndrome (KSS)
C. Leigh syndrome
D. mitochondrial myopathy, encephalopathy, lactic acidosis, and stroke-like episodes (MELAS)
E. Type 2 diabetes

Answer D: Mitochondrial biogenesis disorders are similar to lysosomal storage diseases in that there are symptom similarities between several different diseases of the class. Many of the mitochondrial encephalomyopathies are associated with hearing loss, vision problems such as pigmentary retinopathy, and neurological dysfunction. MELAS is characterized by the fact that it is also associated with the potential for severe lactic acidosis stroke-like episodes. Leigh syndrome is normally fatal before age 5 and so could be eliminated solely on the basis of the patient's age.

12. Which of the following components of mitochondrial electron transport can act as 1-electron or 2-electron carriers?

A. coenzyme Q and flavins
B. cytochrome *c*, coenzyme Q, and flavins
C. NADH, non-heme iron, cytochrome *c*, coenzyme Q, and flavins
D. non-heme iron, cytochrome *c*, coenzyme Q, and flavins

Answer A: Only coenzyme Q and the flavins are capable of both 1- and 2-electron transfer reactions. Ubiquinone can undergo either 1- or 2-electron reactions leading to formation of the reduced quinol, the oxidized quinone, and the semiquinone intermediate. NADH and $FADH_2$ can only carry out obligatory 2-electron reactions and the cytochromes can only carry out 1-electron reactions.

13. Which of the following components of the electron transport system is inhibited by oligomycin?

A. ATP synthase
B. complex I
C. complex II
D. complex III
E. complex IV

Answer A: Oligomycin is a natural antibiotic isolated from *Streptomyces diastatochromogenes* which inhibits mitochondrial ATP synthase. It inhibits the ATP-synthase by binding to the oligomycin sensitivity-conferring protein (OSCP) of the F_0 portion of the complex.

14. Biological oxidation-reduction reactions always involve which of the following?

A. direct participation of oxygen
B. formation of water
C. mitochondria
D. transfer of electron(s)
E. transfer of hydrogens

Answer D: All biological reactions which involve electron flow are considered oxidation-reduction reactions. The basic definition can be defined as one reactant becomes oxidized (loses electrons) while another becomes reduced (gains electrons).

15. The standard reduction potentials ($E^{0\prime}$) for the following half reactions are given.

$$\text{Fumarate} + 2\text{H}^+ + 2\text{e}^- \rightarrow \text{succinate} \quad E^{0\prime} = +0.031\ \text{V}$$

$$\text{FAD} + 2\text{H}^+ + 2\text{e}^- \rightarrow \text{FADH}_2 \quad E^{0\prime} = -0.219\ \text{V}$$

If you mixed succinate, fumarate, FAD, and $FADH_2$ together, all at 1-M concentrations and in the presence of succinate dehydrogenase, which of the following would happen initially?

A. fumarate and succinate would become oxidized; FAD and $FADH_2$ would become reduced
B. fumarate would become reduced, $FADH_2$ would become oxidized
C. no reaction would occur because all reactants and products are already at their standard concentrations
D. succinate would become oxidized, FAD would become reduced
E. succinate would become oxidized, $FADH_2$ would be unchanged because it is a cofactor

Answer B: The reactions as written demonstrate that the free energy available from the oxidation of $FADH_2$ is sufficient to drive the succinate dehydrogenase reaction in the direction of fumarate reduction to succinate.

16. You are examining a 1-year-old infant who is presenting with liver failure and suffers from frequent seizures. An analysis of mitochondrial function from a skeletal muscle biopsy shows a significant respiratory deficit. A molecular analysis shows that there is a deletion of the mtDNA encompassing the gene encoding DNA polymerase γ. This patient is most likely suffering from which of the following diseases?

A. Alpers disease
B. Kearns-Sayre syndrome
C. Leigh syndrome
D. MELAS
E. myoclonic epilepsy and ragged red fiber disease (MERRF)

Answer A: Alpers disease, which usually manifests in infancy, is associated with intractable seizures and a failure to meet meaningful developmental milestones. Primary symptoms of the disease are developmental delay, progressive mental retardation, hypotonia (low muscle tone), spasticity (stiffness of the limbs), and progressive dementia. The typical seizures are of a type that consists of repeated myoclonic (muscle) jerks. Experimental evidence indicates that Alpers disease is associated with deficiencies in the mtDNA-encoded DNA polymerase γ.

17. Obesity is associated with hyperlipidemia resulting in an increased delivery of fatty acid to most tissues including the pancreas. Excess fatty acid oxidation in β-cells of the pancreas results in increased reactive oxygen species (ROS) production. The increased ROS production ultimately contributes to β-cell apoptosis and the need for exogenous insulin in poorly controlled Type 2 diabetes. The deleterious effects of ROS within the pancreas are amplified due to limited expression of which of the following?

A. caspase 9
B. catalase
C. glutathione peroxidase
D. peroxiredoxin
E. superoxide dismutase

Answer B: The oxidation of fatty acids results in the generation of ROS both via mitochondrial and peroxisomal pathways. When fatty acid levels rise significantly, as in obesity, peroxisomal oxidation of fatty acids increases. The initial enzyme in peroxisomal fatty acid oxidation generates H_2O_2. The primary antioxidant enzyme tasked with removal of H_2O_2 is catalase. Pancreatic β-cells are highly susceptible to the damaging effects of H_2O_2 due to a significantly reduced level of expression of catalase compared to other tissue.

18. Which of the following best explains how the brown adipose tissue in newborns generates large amounts of heat?

A. decreased availability of carnitine
B. increased availability of carnitine
C. increased availability of fat
D. increased formation of ATP
E. mitochondrial leak of hydrogen ions

Answer E: The uncoupling of proton flow releases the energy of the electrochemical proton gradient as heat. This process is a normal physiological function of brown adipose tissue (BAT). Newborn babies contain BAT in their neck and upper back that serves the function of nonshivering thermogenesis. The mitochondria in BAT contain a protein called uncoupling protein 1, UCP1 (also called thermogenin). UCP1 acts as a channel in the inner mitochondrial membrane to control the permeability of the membrane to protons. When norepinephrine is released in response to cold sensation it binds to β-adrenergic receptors on the surface of brown adipocytes triggering the activation of adenylate cyclase. Activated adenylate cyclase leads to increased production of cAMP and the concomitant activation of PKA with the result being phosphorylation and activation of hormone-sensitive lipase. The released free fatty acids bind to UCP1 triggering an uncoupling of the proton gradient and the release of the energy of the gradient as heat.

19. A 21-year-old man is brought to the ER after being found unconscious. He is gasping, and respirations are 24/min. There is evidence that he has vomited recently. Two capsules containing potassium cyanide are found in his shirt pocket. Blood lactate concentration is 3.3 mEq/L (normal = 0.8 ± 0.4 mEq/L). Which of the following processes is most likely inhibited in this patient?

A. conversion of pyruvate to alanine
B. glycolysis
C. mitochondrial electron transport
D. mobilization of fatty acids from adipose tissue
E. release of insulin from pancreas

Answer C: Cyanide is a poison that acts by inhibiting electron flow through complex IV of the oxidative phosphorylation machinery. This prevents further mitochondrial electron transport leading to rapid decline in ATP synthesis capacity and ultimately cellular death.

20. Addition of an uncoupling agent to respiring mitochondria carrying out oxidative phosphorylation has which of the following metabolic effects?

A. activity of the TCA cycle ceases
B. ATP formation ceases, but O_2 consumption continues
C. fatty acid oxidation ceases
D. formation of ATP continues, but O_2 consumption ceases
E. NADH oxidation ceases

Answer B: The normal flow of electrons, through the proteins of the oxidative phosphorylation machinery, is coupled with the establishment of a proton gradient across the inner mitochondrial membrane. The establishment of this pH gradient is the chemiosmotic potential that is coupled with the production of ATP. If the process of proton movement is uncoupled from the normal pathway through the ATP synthase complex, oxygen can be consumed but no ATP will be synthesized. Since the PMF across the membrane is lost, there is no longer a gradient to restrict the rate of electron flow; as a result electron transport accelerates resulting in increased oxygen consumption.

21. The electron transport chain of mammalian mitochondria contains 3 multienzyme protein complexes that convert the energy of oxidation-reduction reactions into a form that can be used for the synthesis of ATP and for the uptake of solutes. This form of energy is most likely an example of which of the following?

A. high-energy phosphorylated ester
B. phosphocreatine
C. proton gradient only
D. sodium gradient only
E. sodium and potassium gradient

Answer C: The normal flow of electrons, through the proteins of the oxidative phosphorylation machinery, is coupled with the establishment of a proton gradient across the inner mitochondrial membrane. The establishment of this pH gradient is the chemiosmotic potential that is coupled with the production of ATP.

22. Which of the following is the most likely mechanism of action of a pharmacological agent that prevents ATP generation in isolated mitochondria?

A. activation of cytochrome *c*
B. decrease of NADH generation by NADH dehydrogenase
C. disruption of pH gradient across mitochondrial membrane
D. increase of transport of pyruvate through the mitochondrial membrane
E. inhibition of glyceraldehydes-3-phosphate dehydrogenase

Answer C: The normal flow of electrons, through the proteins of the oxidative phosphorylation machinery, is coupled with the establishment of a proton gradient across the inner mitochondrial membrane. The establishment of this pH gradient is the chemiosmotic potential that is coupled with the production of ATP. Any disruption in this PMF, such as with the addition of an uncoupling agent like dinitrophenol, results in a loss of the energy needed for ATP synthesis but does not prevent oxygen consumption.

23. According to the chemiosmotic theory of how oxidation and phosphorylation are coupled, which of the following processes produces the chemical gradient that drives the generation of ATP from ADP?

A. electron transport causes H^+ to penetrate the inner mitochondrial membrane
B. electron transport ejects H^+ into the intermembrane space
C. $FADH_2$ is regenerated from FAD
D. NADH is regenerated from NAD^+
E. osmotic forces cause H^+ to bind with FAD in the mitochondrial matrix

Answer B: The normal flow of electrons, through the proteins of the oxidative phosphorylation machinery, is coupled with the establishment of a proton gradient across the inner mitochondrial membrane. As electrons flow from one complex to another the energy released is used to pump protons out of the matrix into the inner membrane space. The establishment of this proton gradient is the chemiosmotic potential that is coupled with the production of ATP.

24. In a study of the regulation of body weight, the administration of exogenous leptin to mice is found to increase the activity of proton leak channels located in the inner membrane of mitochondria in adipose tissue cells. Which of the following is most likely to increase as a result of the increased transport of protons through these mitochondrial leak channels?

A. heat production
B. mitochondrial NADH concentrations
C. mitochondrial synthesis of ATP
D. NADH reduction from NAD^+
E. pH of the mitochondrial matrix

Answer A: The uncoupling of the normal process of proton flow across the inner mitochondrial membrane and coupling movement back into the matrix through ATP synthase releases the energy of the electrochemical proton gradient as heat.

25. In newborns, brown fat plays an important role in the generation of heat through which of the following actions?

A. blocking the action of hormone-sensitive lipase
B. increasing the rate of thyroxine synthesis
C. inducing of shivering by leptin
D. promoting proton leakage into mitochondria without ATP formation
E. uncoupling gluconeogenesis from triglyceride hydrolysis

Answer D: The uncoupling of proton flow releases the energy of the electrochemical proton gradient as heat. This process is a normal physiological function of brown adipose tissue (BAT). Newborn babies contain BAT in their neck and upper back that serves the function of nonshivering thermogenesis. The mitochondria in BAT contain a protein called uncoupling protein 1 (UCP1; also called thermogenin). UCP1 acts as a channel in the inner mitochondrial membrane to control the permeability of the membrane to protons. When norepinephrine is released in response to cold sensation, it binds to β-adrenergic receptors on the surface of brown adipocytes triggering the activation of adenylate cyclase. Activated adenylate cyclase leads to increased production of cAMP and the concomitant activation of PKA with the result being phosphorylation and activation of hormone-sensitive lipase. The released free fatty acids bind to UCP1 triggering an uncoupling of the proton gradient and the release of the energy of the gradient as heat.

Checklist

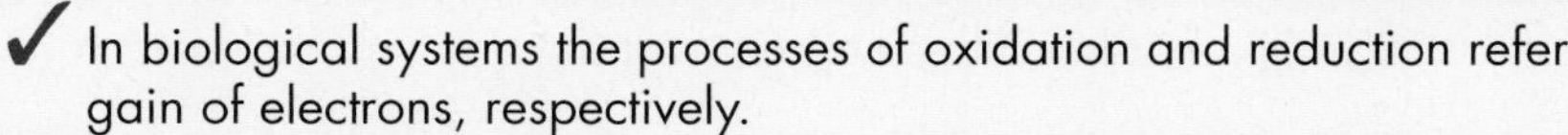

✓ In biological systems the processes of oxidation and reduction refer to the loss and gain of electrons, respectively.

✓ Mitochondria evolved from a symbiotic relationship between aerobic bacteria and primordial eukaryotic cells. The function of the mitochondria is to convert the energy from catabolic reaction into ATP via a process of electron transport.

- ✓ The energy released from the oxidation of carbohydrates, fats, and amino acids is made available to the mitochondria in the form of the educed electron carriers, NADH and $FADH_2$. The electrons from these compounds are then transferred through the electron transport chain to molecular oxygen.
- ✓ The electron transport chain is composed of 4 complexes. Three of these complexes utilize the energy of electron transport to pump protons across the inner mitochondrial membrane creating an electrochemical gradient between the inside of the mitochondria and the inner membrane space. This gradient is referred to as the proton motive force or the chemiosmotic potential and is the energy driving ATP synthesis.
- ✓ ATP synthase (sometimes referred to as complex V) is a rotary-type ATPase that spans the inner mitochondrial membrane and utilizes the energy of the proton gradient (proton motive force) to drive ATP synthesis from ADP and inorganic phosphate (P_i).
- ✓ Numerous poisons and chemicals interfere with the processes of oxidative phosphorylation, such as carbon monoxide and cyanide, both of which inhibit the activities of complex IV.
- ✓ Uncoupling agents create pores in the inner mitochondrial membrane, thereby allowing protons to flow across the membrane preventing ATP synthesis and releasing the energy as heat. This process occurs naturally in brown adipose tissue (BAT) and is catalyzed by UCP1 in a process called adaptive thermogenesis.
- ✓ The electron transport chain is the major site for the generation of cellular reactive oxygen species (ROS) occurring mainly via complex I. Excess delivery of NADH to complex I can result in some electrons passing to molecular oxygen directly generating superoxide anion. Superoxide is neutralized via the action of mitochondrial and cytosolic superoxide dismutases (SOD).
- ✓ The excess oxidation of fatty acids, as is typical in obesity, drives an increase in ROS production leading to progressive mitochondrial dysfunction. Pancreatic β-cells are especially susceptible to ROS damage and mitochondrial-triggered apoptosis contributing to the development of diabetes in overweight and obese individuals.

CHAPTER

18 Ethanol Metabolism

CHAPTER OUTLINE

High-Yield Terms

Alcohol dehydrogenase (ADH): any of a family of enzymes that catalyze the interconversion of alcohols and aldehydes or ketones; humans express multiple forms of ADH from at least 7 distinct genes

Aldehyde dehydrogenase (ALDH): any of a family of enzymes that catalyze the oxidation of aldehydes, 2 primary enzymes, ALDH1A1 and ALDH2, involved in metabolizing acetaldehyde generated during ethanol oxidation

Microsomal ethanol-oxidizing system: inducible ethanol-metabolizing system employing a cytochrome P450 enzyme (CYP2E1)

Hepatic steatosis: condition of fatty liver that can result from excess alcohol consumption

Nonalcoholic fatty liver disease (NAFLD): one cause of a fatty liver (steatosis) not due to excessive alcohol use, most common form of chronic liver disease; obesity and activation of CYP2E1 are major contributors to development of NAFLD and NASH

Nonalcoholic steatohepatitis (NASH): progression of NAFLD to state of inflammation and fibrosis, the major feature in NASH is fat in the liver, along with inflammation and cellular damage; obesity and activation of CYP2E1 are major contributors to development of NAFLD and NASH

Kupffer cell: liver resident macrophages that contribute to inflammatory responses in response to increased reactive oxygen species generation during ethanol metabolism

High-Yield Concept

It should be pointed out that humans evolved to express multiple *ADH* genes and isoforms, not for metabolism of ethanol, but to metabolize naturally occurring alcohols found in foods as well as those produced by intestinal bacteria. As an example, one form of ADH (encoded by the *ADH7* gene) is responsible for the metabolism of not only ethanol but also retinol to retinaldehyde, which is the form of vitamin A necessary for vision.

Ethanol-Metabolizing Pathways

Ethanol is a small 2-carbon alcohol that, due to its small size and alcoholic hydroxyl group, is soluble in both aqueous and lipid environments. This allows ethanol to freely pass from body fluids into cells. Since the portal circulation from the gut passes first through the liver, the bulk of ingested alcohol is metabolized in the liver. The process of ethanol oxidation involves at least 3 distinct enzymatic pathways. The most significant pathway, responsible for the bulk of ethanol metabolism, is that initiated by alcohol dehydrogenase, ADH. ADH is an NAD^+-requiring enzyme expressed at high concentrations in hepatocytes. Animal cells (primarily hepatocytes) contain cytosolic ADH, which oxidizes ethanol to acetaldehyde. Acetaldehyde then enters the mitochondria where it is oxidized to acetate by one of several aldehyde dehydrogenases (ALDHs). A cytosolic ALDH exists but is responsible for only a minor amount of acetaldehyde oxidation.

The second major pathway for ethanol metabolism is the microsomal ethanol-oxidizing system (MEOS), which involves the NADPH-dependent cytochrome P450 enzyme, CYP2E1. The MEOS pathway is induced in individuals who chronically consume alcohol.

The third pathway involves a nonoxidative pathway catalyzed by fatty acid ethyl ester (FAEE) synthase. This latter pathway results in the formation of fatty acid ethyl esters and takes place primarily in the liver and pancreas, both of which are highly susceptible to the toxic effects of alcohol.

Oxidation of ethanol can also occur in peroxisomes via the activity of catalase. However, this oxidation pathway requires the presence of a hydrogen peroxide (H_2O_2)-generating system and as such plays no major role in alcohol metabolism under normal physiological conditions (Figure 18-1).

Enzymes of Ethanol Metabolism: ADHs

In humans there are multiple isoforms of ADH encoded for by 7 different *ADH* genes. All human *ADH* genes are members of a large family of enzymes known as the medium-chain dehydrogenase/reductase (MDR) superfamily. Functional ADH exists as either a homo- or a heterodimer and the active enzymes are divided into 5 distinct classes denoted I to V.

The hepatic forms of ADH are derived from the protein subunits encoded by the class I genes: *ADH1A*, *ADH1B*, and *ADH1C*. The α-, β-, and γ-subunits encoded by these 3 genes, respectively, can form homo- and heterodimers as indicated earlier. These ADH isoforms account for the vast majority of ethanol oxidation in the liver. As a consequence of single-nucleotide polymorphisms (SNPs) in several of the *ADH* genes, there are isoforms derived from the same gene that exhibit different kinetic characteristics. For example, as shown in Table 18-1 there are 3 known polymorphisms in the *ADH1B* gene and 2 in the *ADH1C* gene. The consequences of these alleles are ADH enzymes with much higher turnover rates.

Enzymes of Ethanol Metabolism: ALDHs

There are 2 primary *ALDH* genes in humans that are responsible for the oxidation of acetaldehyde generated during the oxidation of ethanol. These genes are identified as *ALDH1A1* and *ALDH2* and encode the *ALDH1* and *ALDH2* enzymes, respectively. The ALDH1 protein is a cytosolic enzyme, while the ALDH2 protein resides in the mitochondria. The bulk of acetaldehyde oxidation occurs in the mitochondria via ALDH2. However, some oxidation will occur in the cytosol via ALDH1 as a means to help control overall levels of acetaldehyde. This latter fact is most apparent in individuals with ALDH2 alleles

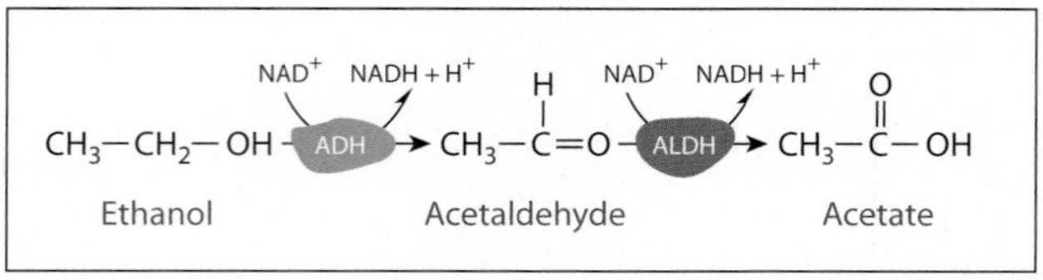

$$CH_3{-}CH_2{-}OH \xrightarrow[\text{ADH}]{NAD^+ \rightarrow NADH + H^+} CH_3{-}\overset{H}{\overset{|}{C}}{=}O \xrightarrow[\text{ALDH}]{NAD^+ \rightarrow NADH + H^+} CH_3{-}\overset{O}{\overset{\|}{C}}{-}OH$$

Ethanol — Acetaldehyde — Acetate

FIGURE 18-1: Reactions of ethanol metabolism. Reproduced with permission of themedicalbiochemistrypage, LLC.

High-Yield Concept

Due to the negative physiological effects of the ALDH2*2 allele, even heterozygous individuals are strongly protected against alcohol dependence.

TABLE 18-1: Mammalian Alcohol Dehydrogenases

Gene Name	*Gene Class*	*Protein Name*	*K_M(mM) for Ethanol*	*Primary Tissue*
ADH1A	I	α	4.0	Liver
*ADH1B*1*	I	β_1	0.05	Liver, lung
*ADH1B*2*	I	β_2	0.9	
*ADH1B*3*	I	β_3	40	
*ADH1C*1*	I	γ_1	1.0	Liver, stomach
*ADH1C*2*	I	γ_2	0.6	
ADH4	II	π	30	Liver, cornea
ADH5 (also identified as *ADHX*)	III	χ	>1000	Widely expressed
ADH6	V	ADH6	Unknown	Stomach
ADH7	IV	μ or σ	30	Liver, stomach

that exhibit low to no acetaldehyde-oxidizing capacity. Several ALDH2 polymorphisms are known to exist in various populations. Indeed, the most highly studied gene variations in alcohol-metabolizing enzymes are those in the *ALDH2* gene. The ALDH2*2 allele encodes a nearly inactive ALDH2 enzyme. This particular ALDH2 allele is responsible for the ease with which many individuals of Asian descent become intoxicated by alcohol consumption and this fact is due to the reduced rate of ethanol metabolism. In addition, because the levels of acetaldehyde in the blood of these individuals rises rapidly following alcohol consumption, it leads to the highly adverse reactions to this compound that includes severe flushing, nausea, and tachycardia.

Acetate From EtOH Metabolism and Fatty Liver

Under normal conditions, the levels of acetate in human serum is less than 0.2 mM. Therefore, the roles of acetate metabolism in mammals under normal physiological conditions remain to be established. Normal physiological sources of acetate include bacterial fermentation in the colon, which increases significantly when consuming a high-fiber diet. This intestinal acetate enters the portal circulation and is taken up by the liver where it is converted to acetyl-CoA. Intracellular generation of acetate is the consequence of the ubiquitously expressed cytosolic enzyme acetyl-CoA hydrolase.

High-Yield Concept

Humans express cytosolic and mitochondrial acetyl-CoA synthetases, AceCS1 and AceCS2, respectively. Expression of AceCS1 is under the control of SREBP-1c, which is itself transcriptionally regulated by PGC-1α.

The acetate can then be salvaged by reactivation to acetyl-CoA. In the nervous system, the neurotransmitter acetylcholine (ACh) is degraded to acetate by acetylcholinesterase. In order to replenish the pool of Ach, the acetate must be reactivated to acetyl-CoA so that it can participate in the choline acetyltransferase-catalyzed reaction. Acetate is also generated within the nucleus of all cells via the action of histone deacetylases (HDACs). As with the other sources of acetate, this nuclear acetate must be reactivated before it can be oxidized or reused. Under conditions of prolonged starvation and in Type 1 diabetes, the endogenous pathways of acetate production are the main sources for serum acetate. Following the consumption of ethanol, acetate levels can be elevated by as much as 20-fold.

Acetate, from whatever source, is converted to acetyl-CoA by ATP-dependent acetyl-CoA synthetases (AceCS) by the following reaction:

$$\text{ATP} + \text{acetate} + \text{CoA} \leftrightarrow \text{AMP} + PPi + \text{acetyl-CoA}$$

The primary causes of fatty liver syndrome (hepatic steatosis), induced by excess alcohol consumption are the altered NADH/NAD^+ levels that in turn inhibit gluconeogenesis, inhibit fatty acid oxidation, and inhibit the activity of the TCA cycle. Each of these inhibited pathways results in the diversion of acetyl-CoA into de novo fatty acid synthesis. Ethanol has also been shown to activate SREBP-1c, which results in the transcriptional activation of numerous genes involved in lipogenesis (see Chapter 19). However, given that large amounts of acetate are generated via ethanol metabolism in the liver, this can be a significant contributor to the overall pool of acetyl-CoA utilized as the precursor for fatty acid and cholesterol biosynthesis.

Microsomal Ethanol Oxidation System

Under conditions of chronic alcohol ingestion, the increased level of ethanol metabolism cannot be accounted for solely via the ADH- and ALDH-catalyzed reactions. Studies in animals demonstrated that the alcohol-induced increase in metabolism was associated with hepatic smooth endoplasmic reticulum (SER; also referred to as microsomal membranes). This ethanol-induced metabolic system is, therefore, referred to as the microsomal ethanol-oxidation system (MEOS). The MEOS contains a cytochrome-P450 activity that is distinct from ADH and is designated as CYP2E1. Induction of CYP2E1 mRNA and enzyme activity ranges from 4- to 10-fold in the liver following alcohol intake (Figure 18-2).

Given that the MEOS pathway for ethanol metabolism is induced in chronic alcoholics, the enhanced ethanol metabolism likely contributes to alcoholics' metabolic tolerance for ethanol, which in turn promotes further alcohol consumption. The activity of CYP2E1 is

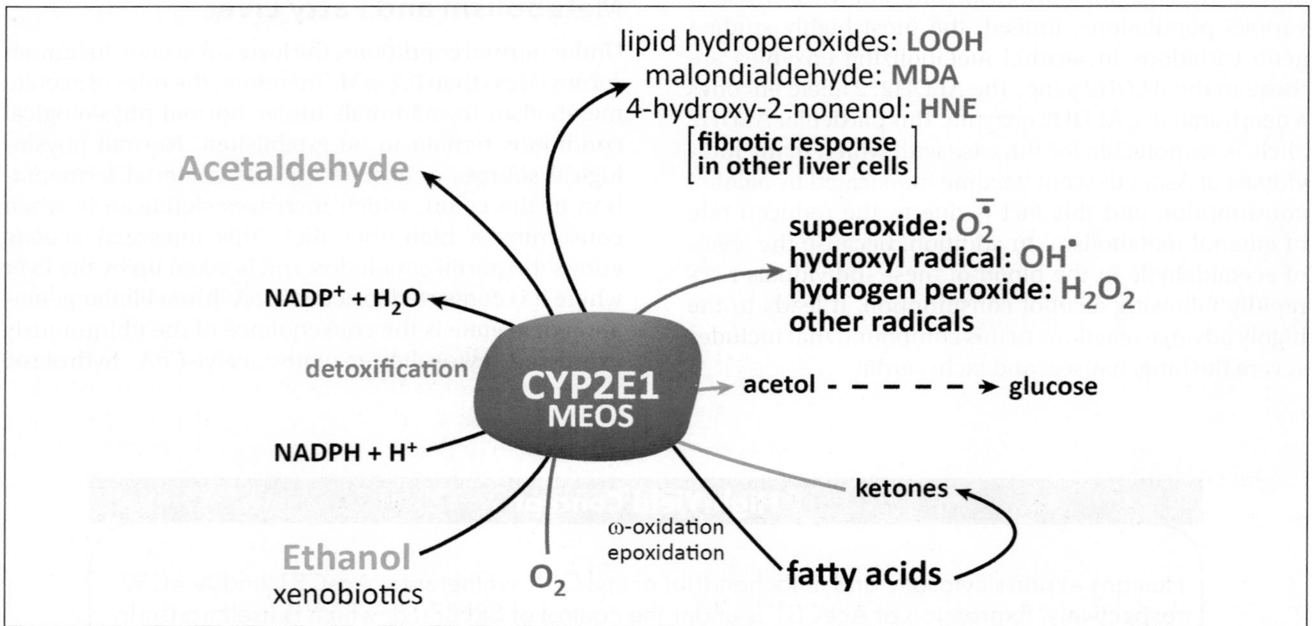

FIGURE 18-2: Physiological and toxic activities associated with hepatic CYP2E1. Reproduced with permission of themedicalbiochemistrypage, LLC.

High-Yield Concept

Increased activity of CYP2E1 results in accelerated production of lipid hydroperoxides (LOOH in the Figure 18-2) and is a significant contributor to the development of nonalcoholic fatty liver disease, NAFLD and nonalcoholic steatohepatitis, NASH. Both NAFLD and NASH are commonly associated with obesity, Type 2 diabetes, and hyperlipidemia.

also essential in the metabolism of several xenobiotics. Therefore, the increased level of expression of this enzyme in alcoholics can have a significant impact on the production of toxic metabolites and, thus, contributes to ethanol-induced liver injury. Metabolism of ethanol by CYP2E1 also results in a significant increase in free radical and acetaldehyde production, which, in turn, diminish reduced glutathione (GSH) and other defense systems against oxidative stress leading to further hepatocyte damage.

Ethanol Metabolism and Alcoholism

As indicated in Table 18-1, several alleles exist for the *ADH1B* and *ADH1C* genes. Several of these alleles have been correlated with either an increased or decreased propensity toward alcohol abuse or dependence. Of clinical significance is the fact that these associations between ADH and ALDH alleles and alcoholism are the strongest and most widely reproduced associations of any gene with this disorder.

The class I *ADH* and *ALDH2* genes play a central role in alcohol metabolism. Polymorphisms in the genes encoding ADH and ALDH produce enzymes that vary in activity. These genetic variations have been associated with an individual's susceptibility to developing alcoholism and alcohol-related tissue damage. The ADH1B alleles occur at different frequencies in different populations. For example, the ADH1B*1 form is found predominantly in Caucasian and Black populations, whereas ADH1B*2 frequency is higher in Chinese and Japanese populations and in 25% of people with Jewish ancestry. Also, African Americans and Native Americans with the ADH1B*3 allele metabolize alcohol at a faster rate than those with ADH1B*1.

Although several ALDH isozymes have been identified, only the cytosolic ALDH1 and the mitochondrial ALDH2 metabolize acetaldehyde. There is one significant genetic polymorphism of the *ALDH2* gene, resulting in allelic variants ALDH2*1 and ALDH2*2, which are virtually inactive. ALDH2*2 is present in about 50% of the Taiwanese, Chinese, and Japanese populations and shows virtually no acetaldehyde-metabolizing activity in vitro. ALDH2*2 heterozygotes, and most significantly homozygotes, show increased acetaldehyde levels after alcohol consumption and, therefore, experience significant negative physiological responses to alcohol intake.

Because polymorphisms of ADH and ALDH2 play an important role in determining peak blood acetaldehyde levels and voluntary ethanol consumption, they also influence vulnerability to alcohol dependence. A fast ADH or a slow ALDH are expected to elevate acetaldehyde levels and, thus, reduce the tolerance to alcohol consumption.

Acute and Chronic Effects of Ethanol Metabolism

The primary acute effects of ethanol consumption are the result of the altered NADH:NAD$^+$ ratio that is the consequence of both the ADH- and ALDH-catalyzed reactions. Acute effects resulting from ethanol metabolism are also due to the fact that acetaldehyde forms adducts with proteins, nucleic acids, and other compounds resulting in impaired activity of the affected compounds. Additional acute consequences of ethanol metabolism include oxygen deficits (ie, hypoxia) in the liver and the formation of highly reactive oxygen-containing molecules (ie, reactive oxygen species, ROS) that can damage other cell components.

The NADH produced in the cytosol by ADH must be reduced back to NAD$^+$ via either the malate-aspartate shuttle or the glycerol-phosphate shuttle. Thus, the ability of an individual to metabolize ethanol is dependent upon the capacity of hepatocytes to carry out either of these 2 shuttles, which in turn is affected by the rate of the TCA cycle in the mitochondria. The rate of flux through the TCA cycle is itself being negatively affected by the NADH produced by the ADH and ALDH reactions.

The reduction in NAD$^+$ impairs the flux of glucose through glycolysis at the glyceraldehyde-3-phosphate dehydrogenase reaction, thereby limiting energy production. Additionally, there is an increased rate of hepatic lactate production due to the effect of increased NADH on the direction of the hepatic lactate dehydrogenase (LDH) reaction. This reversal of the LDH reaction in hepatocytes diverts pyruvate (and also alanine) from gluconeogenesis, leading to a reduction in the capacity of the liver to deliver glucose to the blood resulting in hypoglycemia.

In addition to the negative effects of the altered NADH:NAD^+ ratio on hepatic gluconeogenesis, fatty acid oxidation is also reduced as this process requires NAD^+ as a cofactor. Concomitant with reduced fatty acid oxidation is enhanced fatty acid synthesis and increased triglyceride production by the liver. In the mitochondria, the production of acetate from acetaldehyde leads to increased levels of acetyl-CoA. Since the increased generation of NADH also reduces the activity of the TCA cycle, the acetyl-CoA is diverted to fatty acid synthesis. The reduction in cytosolic NAD^+ leads to reduced activity of glycerol-3-phosphate dehydrogenase (in the glycerol 3-phosphate to DHAP direction), resulting in increased levels of glycerol 3-phosphate which is the backbone for the synthesis of the triglycerides. Both of these 2 events lead to fatty acid deposition in the liver leading to fatty liver syndrome and excessive levels of lipids in the blood, referred to as *hyperlipidemia* (Figure 18-3).

The increased NADH must be oxidized in the mitochondria via the pathway of oxidative phosphorylation and requires an increased input of oxygen. Indeed, studies have shown that ethanol metabolism does result in increased uptake of oxygen by hepatocytes, particularly those that reside close to the artery supplying oxygen-rich blood to the liver. This results in limitations to the amount of oxygen left in the blood to adequately supply to other liver regions. This leads to significant hypoxia in perivenous hepatocytes, which are those that are located close to the vein where the cleansed blood exits the liver. The perivenous hepatocytes also are the first ones to show evidence of damage from chronic alcohol consumption, indicating the potential harmful consequences of hypoxia induced by ethanol metabolism. In addition, ethanol metabolism indirectly increases

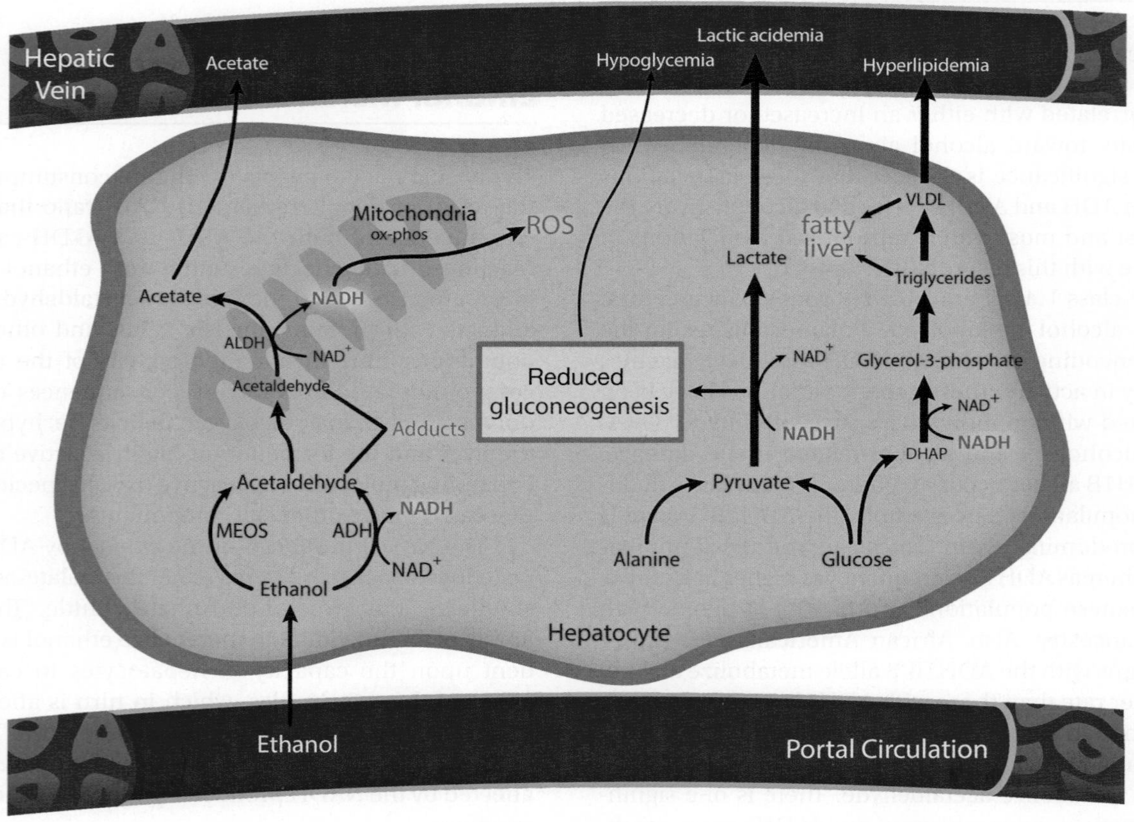

FIGURE 18-3: Acute effects of ethanol metabolism on liver functions. Reproduced with permission of themedicalbiochemistrypage, LLC.

Kupffer cell (specialized hepatic immune cells) oxygen use. When Kupffer cells become activated in response to ethanol consumption, they release various stimulatory molecules that contribute to increased metabolic activity of hepatocytes, leading to even more oxygen consumption. As a result, alcohol-induced Kupffer cell activation also contributes to the onset of hypoxia.

The acetaldehyde produced by the ADH reaction, as well as the ROS produced via CYP2E1 oxidation, both can interact with amino acids, proteins, and other biomolecules in the cell to form both stable and unstable adducts. Proteins highly susceptible to acetaldehyde-induced adduct formation include red blood cell membranes, lipoproteins, hemoglobin, albumin, collagen, tubulin, and several cytochromes including CYP2E1. Adduct formation with hemoglobin can result in reduced oxygen-binding capacity. Albumin is a major protein of the blood and among its functions is to transport fatty acids from adipose tissue. Therefore, altered albumin function could impair tissue access to energy from fatty acid oxidation. Tubulin is involved in the formation of microtubules, which are necessary for intracellular transport and cell division. Collagen is the most abundant protein in the body forming a significant portion of the connective tissue. Acetaldehyde-lysine adducts can indirectly contribute to liver damage because the body recognizes them as foreign, resulting in an immune response and antibody production. The production of these antibodies leads to immune system–mediated destruction of hepatocytes containing these adducts via a process known as immune-mediated hepatotoxicity or antibody-dependent cell-mediated cytotoxicity (ADCC).

Ethanol metabolism by CYP2E1 and NADH oxidation by the electron transport chain generate ROS that lead to lipid peroxidation. Ethanol-induced lipid peroxidation is associated with the formation of malondialdehyde (MDA) and 4-hydroxy-2-nonenal (HNE), both of which can form adducts with proteins (see Figure 18-2). Similar to the acetaldehyde-amino acid adducts, peroxy lipid-acetaldehyde adducts can induce immune responses resulting in antibody formation. Importantly, MAA adducts can induce inflammatory processes in stellate and endothelial cells of the liver. Thus, there is a close link between the production of MDA and HNE, and the formation of MAA adducts and subsequent development of liver disease.

The production of ROS is associated with cancer development, atherosclerosis, diabetes, inflammation, aging, and other harmful processes. The cell regulates ROS levels via numerous defense systems involving a variety of different antioxidant compounds (eg, glutathione). Under normal conditions, a balance between ROS production and antioxidant removal exists in cells, but this balance can be disturbed. During ethanol oxidation, ROS production increases dramatically due to induction of CYP2E1 and by activation of Kupffer cells in the liver. Both acute and chronic alcohol consumption can increase ROS production and lead to oxidative stress.

Chronic ethanol consumption and alcohol metabolism also negatively affects several other metabolic pathways, thereby contributing to the spectrum of metabolic disorders frequently found in alcoholics. These disorders include fatty liver syndromes such as NAFLD and NASH, hyperlipidemia, lactic acidosis, ketoacidosis, and hyperuricemia. The first stage of liver damage following chronic alcohol consumption is the appearance of fatty liver, which is followed by inflammation, apoptosis, fibrosis, and finally cirrhosis. Chronic alcohol consumption has also been shown to significantly enhance the risk of developing cancers of the esophagus and oral cavity as well as playing a major role in the development of liver cancer. As indicated earlier, metabolism of ethanol results in increased production of acetaldehyde and ROS. Acetaldehyde adducts are known to promote cancer development. In addition, the induction of CYP2E1 results in increased ROS production and all the associated cellular disruptions related to these reactive substances, including cancer.

REVIEW QUESTIONS

1. Induction of CYP2E1 would be expected to result in which of the following?

A. decreased rate of ethanol clearance from the blood
B. decreased rate of acetaldehyde production
C. increased level of alcohol tolerance
D. protection from alcohol-induced hepatic necrosis
E. reduced likelihood of free radical production

Answer C: The primary pathway of ethanol metabolism is that initiated by ADH. The second major pathway for ethanol metabolism is the microsomal ethanol-oxidizing system (MEOS), which involves the cytochrome P450 enzyme CYP2E1. The MEOS pathway is induced in individuals who chronically consume alcohol, resulting in higher rates of metabolism leading to increased tolerance to alcohol ingestion.

2. Which of the following chronic effects of alcohol consumption is irreversible?

A. activation of triglyceride synthesis
B. inhibition of fatty acid oxidation
C. ketoacidosis

D. lactic acidosis
E. liver cirrhosis

Answer E: Chronic ethanol consumption and alcohol metabolism contributes to the spectrum of metabolic disorders frequently found in alcoholics. These disorders include fatty liver syndromes such as NAFLD and NASH, hyperlipidemia, lactic acidosis, ketoacidosis, and hyperuricemia. The first stage of liver damage following chronic alcohol consumption is the appearance of fatty liver, which is followed by inflammation, apoptosis, fibrosis, and finally cirrhosis. These negative and toxic changes within the liver are irreversible even when alcohol consumption is terminated.

3. Acetate, derived from the oxidation of ethanol, has which of the following fate?
A. due to its toxicity it leads to necrosis of the liver
B. it directly enters the TCA cycle and is oxidized
C. it is converted into NADH via the action of ADH
D. it is excreted in the bile
E. it is taken up by nonhepatic tissues and converted to acetyl-CoA

Answer E: Acetate, from whatever source, is converted to acetyl-CoA by ATP-dependent acetyl-CoA synthetases (AceCS). Following the consumption of ethanol, acetate levels can be elevated by as much as 20-fold. The primary causes of fatty liver syndrome (hepatic steatosis), induced by excess alcohol consumption, are the altered NADH/NAD$^+$ levels that in turn inhibits gluconeogenesis, inhibits fatty acid oxidation, and inhibits the activity of the TCA cycle. Each of these inhibited pathways results in the diversion of acetyl-CoA into de novo fatty acid synthesis.

4. Which of the following events would be most likely to be observed following acute consumption of alcohol?
A. activation of fatty acid oxidation
B. increased rate of gluconeogenesis
C. increased ratio of NAD$^+$ to NADH
D. inhibition of ketogenesis
E. lactic acidosis

Answer E: The majority of the aberrant metabolic effects of ethanol intoxication stem from the actions of ADH and ALDH and the resultant cellular imbalance in the NADH:NAD$^+$ ratio. Additionally, there is an increased rate of hepatic lactate production due to the effect of increased NADH on direction of the hepatic lactate dehydrogenase (LDH) reaction. This reversal of the LDH reaction in hepatocytes results in reduced capacity of the liver to divert lactate into glucose via gluconeogenesis. resulting in elevated lactate levels in the blood, leading to lactic acidosis.

5. Alcoholism is sometimes treated with the drug disulfiram. This drug deters the consumption of alcohol by which of the following mechanisms?
A. activating the excessive metabolism of ethanol to acetate resulting in rapid inebriation with limited alcohol consumption
B. blocking the conversion of acetaldehyde to acetate resulting in rapid accumulation of toxic acetaldehyde adducts
C. inhibiting ethanol absorption so that an individual cannot become intoxicated
D. inhibiting the conversion of ethanol to acetaldehyde, thereby, causing ethanol to be excreted before it can be metabolized
E. preventing the excretion of acetate resulting in severe nausea and vomiting

Answer B: Disulfiram blocks the processing of alcohol in the body by inhibiting acetaldehyde dehydrogenase, thus causing an unpleasant reaction when alcohol is consumed due to a rapid increase in the production of toxic acetaldehyde adducts.

6. Ethanol metabolism is associated with a disruption in the NADH:NAD$^+$ ratio. Which of the following is one major consequence of this disruption?
A. altered membrane fluidity resulting in decreased hepatocyte function
B. hyperglycemia due to increased rates of hepatic gluconeogenesis
C. increased production of glycerol 3-phosphate contributing to triglyceride production
D. increased TCA cycle activity resulting in increased oxygen consumption
E potentiation of CNS activity

Answer C: The altered NADH:NAD$^+$ ratio that in turn inhibits gluconeogenesis, inhibits fatty acid oxidation and the activity of the TCA cycle. The reduction in NAD$^+$ impairs the flux of glucose through glycolysis at the glyceraldehyde-3-phosphate dehydrogenase reaction, thereby limiting energy production. The reduction in cytosolic NAD$^+$ leads to reduced activity of glycerol-3-phosphate dehydrogenase (in the glycerol 3-phosphate to DHAP direction), resulting in increased levels of glycerol 3-phosphate which is the backbone for the synthesis of the triglycerides. Both of these 2 events lead to fatty acid deposition in the liver leading to fatty liver syndrome and excessive levels of lipids in the blood, referred to as hyperlipidemia.

7. Which of the following is the primary mode of metabolism of ethanol?
   A. excretion through the kidneys
   B. exhalation from the lungs
   C. oxidation in the kidneys
   D. oxidation in the liver
   E. oxidation in the lungs

Answer D: Metabolism of ethanol occurs within the liver and involves oxidation to acetaldehyde and then to acetate catalyzed by ADH and ALDH, respectively.

8. You are examining a patient who complains of severe headaches and flushing of the face, neck, and upper chest following the consumption of a glass of white wine. After taking a history, you find that other members of his family also suffer from similar symptoms following alcohol consumption. Given this patient's symptoms and history, which of the following is most likely his associated genotype?
   A. ADH1A and ALDH2*2
   B. ADH1B*1 and ALDH2*2
   C. ADH1C*1 and ALDHA1
   D. ADH4 and ALDH1A1
   E. ADH5 and ALDH2*2

Answer B: Physiological responses to alcohol consumption are influenced by the activities of both the major ethanol-oxidizing ADH and the acetaldehyde-oxidizing ALDH isozymes. Because polymorphisms of ADH and ALDH2 play an important role in determining peak blood acetaldehyde levels and voluntary ethanol consumption, they also influence vulnerability to alcohol dependence. A fast ADH or a slow ALDH are expected to elevate acetaldehyde levels and thus result in rapid onset of undesirable side effects such as flushing, headache, and nausea. The ADH1B*1 allele has the highest rate of ethanol oxidation while the ALDH2*2 allele has little to no activity.

9. Increased activity of which of the following alleles encoding enzymes of alcohol metabolism would be expected to have the greatest effect on the susceptibility to alcoholism?
   A. ADH1A
   B. ADH1B*1
   C. ADH1C*2
   D. ALDH2*2
   E. CYP2E1

Answer B: Because polymorphisms of ADH and ALDH2 play an important role in determining peak blood acetaldehyde levels and voluntary ethanol consumption, they also influence vulnerability to alcohol dependence. A fast ADH or a slow ALDH are expected to elevate acetaldehyde levels and thus reduce alcohol drinking. The opposite would be expected such that individuals with slow ADH and normal or fast ALDH have a higher likelihood of alcoholism. Since the ADH1B*1 allele has the highest rate of ethanol oxidation, it would have the highest potential for an association with alcohol abuse. Although several CYP2E1 polymorphisms have been identified, only a few studies have been done to determine the effect on alcohol metabolism and tissue damage. In one study, the presence of the rare C–2 allele was associated with higher alcohol metabolism in Japanese alcoholics, but this effect was only seen at high blood alcohol concentrations. Individuals with the CYP2E1 RsaI polymorphism were shown to be more likely than others to abstain from alcohol consumption over their lifetimes.

10. Prolonged ethanol consumption and subsequent metabolism ultimately leads to a condition referred to as steatohepatitis or more commonly, "fatty liver syndrome." Ethanol metabolism results in alteration in the activity of which of the following enzymes, one of the consequences of which is excess lipid deposition in the liver?
   A. fatty acyl-CoA oxidase
   B. glucose-6-phosphate dehydrogenase
   C. glycerol-3-phosphate dehydrogenase
   D. lactate dehydrogenase
   E. pyruvate dehydrogenase

Answer C: The metabolism of ethanol by the liver leads to a large increase in NADH. This increase in NADH disrupts the normal processes of metabolic regulation such as hepatic gluconeogenesis, TCA cycle function, and fatty acid oxidation. Concomitant with reduced fatty acid oxidation is enhanced fatty acid synthesis and increased triglyceride production by the liver. In the mitochondria, the production of acetate from acetaldehyde leads to increased levels of acetyl-CoA. Since the increased generation of NADH also reduces the activity of the TCA cycle, the acetyl-CoA is diverted to fatty acid synthesis. The reduction in cytosolic NAD^+ leads to reduced activity of glycerol-3-phosphate dehydrogenase (in the glycerol 3-phosphate to DHAP direction) resulting in increased levels of glycerol 3-phosphate, which is the backbone for the synthesis of the triglycerides. Both of these 2 events lead to fatty acid deposition in the liver leading to fatty liver syndrome and excessive levels of lipids in the blood, referred to as hyperlipidemia.

Checklist

✓ The primary pathway for ethanol metabolism occurs within the liver and involves oxidation by ADHs and ALDHs.

✓ Alcohol dehydrogenase catalyzes a cytosolic oxidation reaction converting ethanol to acetaldehyde.

✓ The major ALDH is a mitochondrial enzyme catalyzing the oxidation of acetaldehyde to acetate; a cytosolic ALDH exists in humans but is a minor contributor to overall ethanol metabolism.

✓ Metabolism of ethanol disrupts the NADH:NAD+ ratio within the hepatocyte resulting in the inhibition of gluconeogenesis, fatty acid oxidation, and TCA cycle activity.

✓ Excess acetate from ethanol metabolism is converted to acetyl-CoA and diverted into fatty acid biosynthesis.

✓ A second major alcohol-metabolizing pathway involves the microsomal cytochrome P450 enzyme, CYP2E1, referred to as the microsomal ethanol-oxidizing system, MEOS.

✓ Chronic alcohol consumption results in induction of the CYP2E1-mediated MEOS pathway, which is a major contributor to liver cell damage due to high rates of reactive oxygen species (ROS) production.

✓ Increased ROS production during chronic ethanol metabolism is associated with cancer, atherosclerosis, diabetes, inflammation, aging, and other harmful metabolic processes.

✓ Chronic alcohol consumption leads to excess deposition of fat resulting in hepatic steatosis (fatty liver).

✓ Various alleles of ADH and ALDH are associated with variable rates of ethanol metabolism. ADH and ALDH are most frequently seen in high rates of alcoholism.

CHAPTER

19 Lipids: Fatty Acid Synthesis

CHAPTER OUTLINE

High-Yield Terms

ATP-citrate lyase (ACL): cytosolic enzyme involved in the transport of acetyl-CoA from the mitochondria to the cytosol; a nuclear ACL is involved in delivery of acetyl-CoA to histone acetyltransferases (HAT) involved in modulating gene expression at the level of epigenetic marking

Acetyl-CoA carboxylase (ACC): rate-limiting and highly regulated enzyme of de novo fatty acid synthesis

Fatty acid synthase (FAS): homodimeric enzyme that carries out all of the reactions of de novo fatty acid synthesis generating palmitic acid as the final product

Carbohydrate-response element-binding protein: major glucose-responsive transcription factor that is required for glucose-induced expression of *L-PK* and the lipogenic genes *ACC* and *FAS*

Steroyl-CoA desaturase (SCD): rate-limiting enzyme for the synthesis of mono-unsaturated fatty acids (MUFAs), primarily oleate (18:1) and palmitoleate (16:1), both of which represent the majority of MUFA present in membrane phospholipids, triglycerides, and cholesterol esters

De Novo Fatty Acid Synthesis

The pathway for fatty acid synthesis occurs in the cytoplasm, utilizes the oxidation of NADPH, and requires an activated intermediate. The activated intermediate is malonyl-CoA which is derived via carboxylation of acetyl-CoA. The synthesis of malonyl-CoA represents the first committed step as well as the rate-limiting and major regulated step of fatty acid synthesis (Figure 19-1). This reaction is catalyzed by the biotin-requiring enzyme, acetyl-CoA carboxylase (ACC). Human tissues express 2 distinct *ACC* genes identified as *ACC1* and *ACC2*. The differential regulation of these 2 genes and the encoded enzymes is discussed in the Regulation of Fatty Acid Synthesis section.

The reactions of fatty acid synthesis are catalyzed by fatty acid synthase (FAS) (Figure 19-2). All of the reactions of fatty acid synthesis take place in distinct reactive centers within the enzyme. These reactive centers are β-keto-ACP synthase, β-keto-ACP reductase, 3-OH acyl-ACP dehydratase and enoyl-CoA reductase. ACP is acyl-carrier protein but does not refer to a distinct protein but rather refers to a distinct domain of the enzyme which contains a phosphopantetheine group. The 2 reduction reactions require NADPH oxidation to $NADP^+$. The acetyl-CoA and malonyl-CoA are transferred to ACP by the action of acetyl-CoA transacylase and malonyl-CoA transacylase, respectively. The attachment of these carbon atoms to ACP allows them to enter the fatty acid synthesis cycle. The primary fatty acid synthesized by FAS is palmitate. Palmitate is then released from the enzyme and can then undergo separate elongation and/or unsaturation to yield other fatty acid molecules.

Origin of Cytoplasmic Acetyl-CoA

Acetyl-CoA is generated in the mitochondria primarily from 2 sources, the pyruvate dehydrogenase complex (PDHc) reaction and fatty acid oxidation but also can originate from the oxidation of several amino acids.

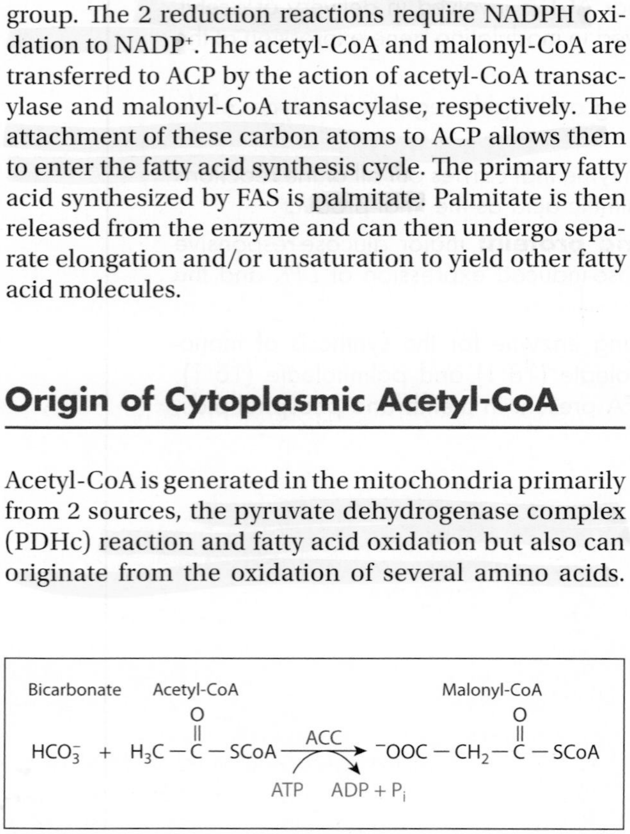

Bicarbonate + Acetyl-CoA → Malonyl-CoA

$$HCO_3^- + H_3C-\overset{O}{\overset{\|}{C}}-SCoA \xrightarrow[ATP \;\; ADP + P_i]{ACC} {}^-OOC-CH_2-\overset{O}{\overset{\|}{C}}-SCoA$$

FIGURE 19-1: Synthesis of malonyl-CoA catalyzed by acetyl-CoA carboxylase. Reproduced with permission of themedicalbiochemistrypage, LLC.

In order for these acetyl units to be utilized for fatty acid synthesis they must be transported into the cytoplasm. The shift from fatty acid oxidation and glycolytic oxidation occurs when the need for energy diminishes. This results in reduced oxidation of acetyl-CoA in the TCA cycle. Under these conditions the mitochondrial acetyl units can be stored as fat for future energy demands.

Acetyl-CoA enters the cytoplasm in the form of citrate via the tricarboxylate transport system (Figure 19-3). In the cytoplasm, citrate is converted to oxaloacetate and acetyl-CoA by the ATP-driven ATP-citrate lyase (ACL) reaction. This reaction is essentially the reverse of that catalyzed by the TCA enzyme citrate synthase except it requires the energy of ATP hydrolysis to drive it forward. The resultant oxaloacetate is converted to malate by malate dehydrogenase (MDH).

The malate produced by this pathway can undergo oxidative decarboxylation by malic enzyme. The coenzyme for this reaction is $NADP^+$-generating NADPH. The advantage of this series of reactions for converting mitochondrial acetyl-CoA into cytoplasmic acetyl-CoA is that the NADPH produced by the malic enzyme reaction can be a major source of reducing cofactor for the FAS activities.

ATP-Citrate Lyase: Role in Epigenetics

Epigenetics refers to the generation of a particular phenotype due to effects "on" a gene as opposed to effects "by" a gene. Acetylation of histones in chromatin is a major mechanism of epigenetic regulation of gene expression. Histone acetylation relies on acetyl-CoA synthetase enzymes that use acetate to produce acetyl-CoA. However, humans have only low extracellular concentrations of acetate such that there is a dependence on glucose metabolism for generation of acetyl-CoA for histone acetylation. ATP-citrate lyase (ACL) is the critical enzyme necessary to convert glucose-derived citrate into acetyl-CoA. Indeed, ACL is required for increases in histone acetylation in response to growth factor stimulation as well as during differentiation, and glucose availability can affect histone acetylation in an ACL-dependent manner. ACL activity is, therefore, required to link growth factor–induced increases in nutrient metabolism to the regulation of histone acetylation and ultimately gene expression patterns. Nutrient-responsive histone acetylation selectively alters the expression of genes required to reprogram intracellular metabolism to use glucose for ATP production and macromolecular synthesis.

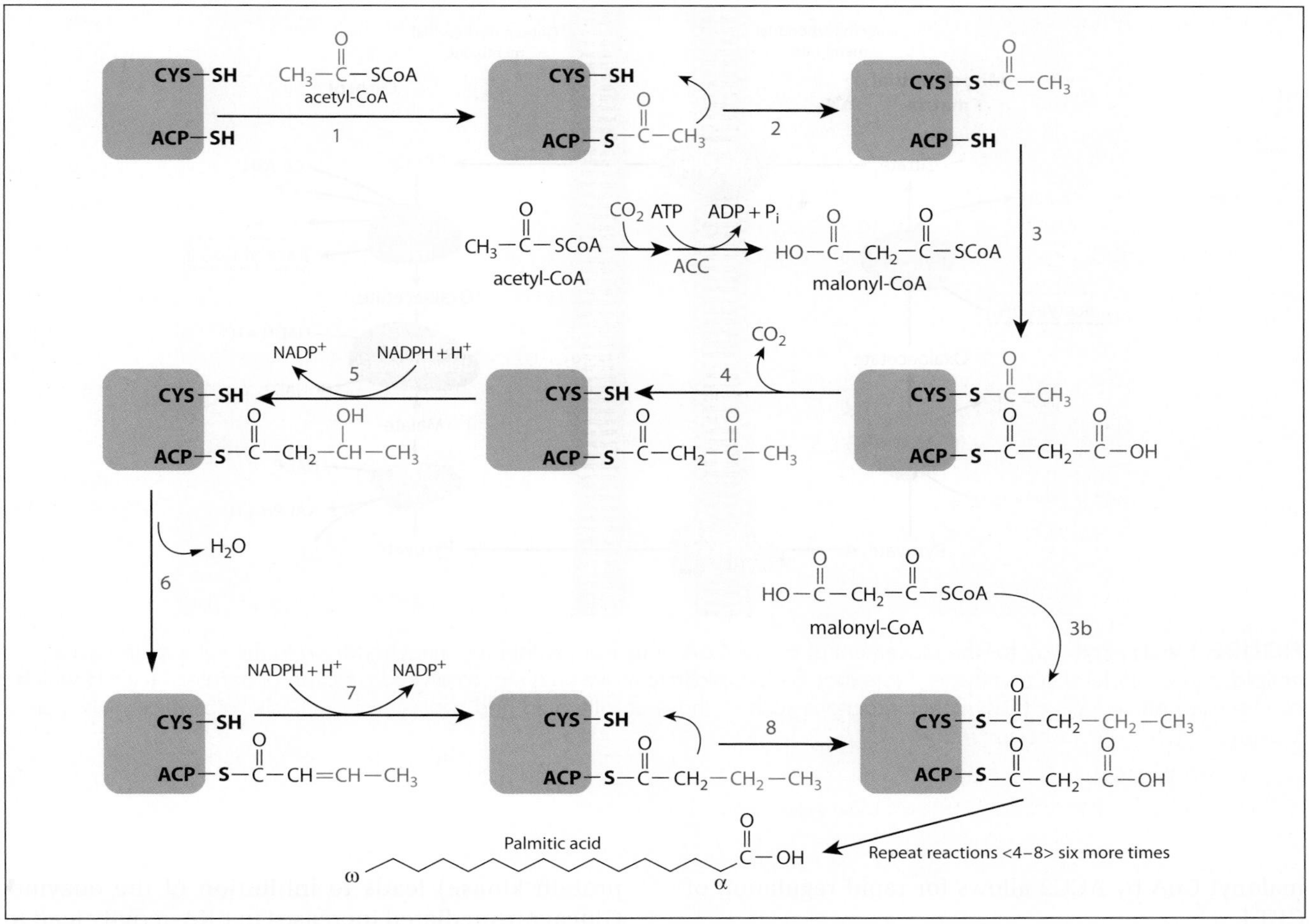

FIGURE 19-2: Reactions of fatty acid synthesis catalyzed by FAS. Only half of the normal head-to-tail (head-to-foot) dimer of functional FAS is shown. Synthesis of malonyl-CoA from CO_2 and acetyl-CoA is carried out by ACC as shown in Figure 19-1. The acetyl group is initially attached to the sulfhydryl of the 4′-phosphopantothenate of the acyl carrier protein portion of FAS (ACP-SH). This is catalyzed by malonyl/acetyl-CoA ACP transacetylase (reactions 1 and 2). This activating acetyl group represents the omega (ω) end of the newly synthesized fatty acid. Following transfer of the activating acetyl group to a cysteine sulfhydryl in the β-keto-ACP synthase portion of FAS (CYS-SH), the three carbons from a malonyl-CoA are attached to ACP-SH (reaction 3), also catalyzed by malonyl/acetyl-CoA ACP transacetylase. The acetyl group attacks the methylene group of the malonyl attached to ACP-SH catalyzed β-keto-ACP synthase (reaction 4) which also liberates the CO_2 that was added to acetyl-CoA by ACC. The resulting 3-ketoacyl group then undergoes a series of 3 reactions catalyzed by the β-keto-ACP reductase (reaction 5), 3-OH acyl-ACP dehydratase (reaction 6), and enoyl-CoA reductase (reaction 7) activities of FAS resulting in a saturated 4-carbon (butyryl) group attached to the ACP-SH. This butyryl group is then transferred to the CYS-SH (reaction 8) as for the case of the activating acetyl group. At this point another malonyl group is attached to the ACP-SH (3b) and the process begins again. Reactions 4 through 8 are repeated another 6 times, each beginning with a new malonyl group being added. At the completion of synthesis, the saturated 16-carbon fatty acid, palmitic acid, is released via the action of the thioesterase activity of FAS (palmitoyl ACP thioesterase) located in the *C*-terminal end of the enzyme. Not shown are the released CoASH groups. Reproduced with permission of themedicalbiochemistrypage, LLC.

Regulation of Fatty Acid Synthesis

There are 2 major isoforms of ACC in mammalian tissues. These are identified as ACC1 and ACC2. ACC1 is strictly cytosolic and is enriched in liver, adipose tissue, and lactating mammary tissue. ACC2 expression occurs in the heart, liver, and skeletal muscle. ACC2 has an *N*-terminal extension that contains a mitochondrial targeting motif and is found associated with carnitine palmitoyltransferase I (CPT I) involved in fatty acid oxidation (Chapter 25). The synthesis of

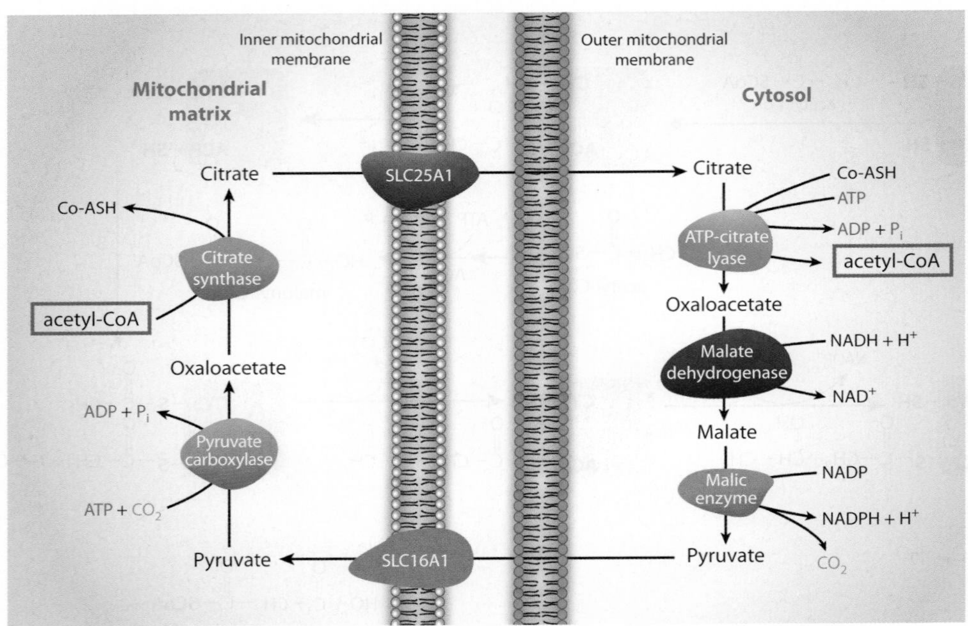

FIGURE 19-3: Pathway for the movement of acetyl-CoA units from within the mitochondrion to the cytoplasm for use in lipid and cholesterol biosynthesis. Note that the cytoplasmic malic enzyme–catalyzed reaction generates NADPH which can be used for reductive biosynthetic reactions such as those of fatty acid and cholesterol synthesis. Reproduced with permission of themedicalbiochemistrypage, LLC.

malonyl-CoA by ACC2 allows for rapid regulation of CPT I.

Both isoforms of ACC are allosterically activated by citrate and inhibited by palmitoyl-CoA and other short- and long-chain fatty acyl-CoAs. Citrate triggers the polymerization of ACC1 which leads to significant increases in its activity. Although ACC2 does not undergo significant polymerization (presumably due to its mitochondrial association), it is allosterically activated by citrate. Glutamate and other dicarboxylic acids can also allosterically activate both ACC isoforms.

ACC activity is also regulated by phosphorylation. Both ACC1 and ACC2 contain at least 8 sites that undergo phosphorylation. The sites of phosphorylation in ACC2 have not been as extensively studied as those in ACC1. Phosphorylation of ACC1 by AMPK (5′ adenosine monophosphate-activated protein kinase) leads to inhibition of the enzyme. Glucagon-mediated increases in PKA activity lead to phosphorylation of both ACC isoforms where ACC2 is a better substrate for PKA than is ACC1. The activating effects of insulin on ACC are complex and not completely resolved. It is known that insulin leads to the dephosphorylation of the AMPK-phosphorylated sites in heart ACC but not in hepatocytes or adipose tissues. At least a portion of the ACC-activating effects of insulin are related to decreases in cAMP levels (Figure 19-4).

Long-term regulation of fatty acid synthesis occurs at the level of gene expression primarily controlled by the circulating levels of insulin and glucagon. Insulin stimulates both ACC and FAS synthesis, whereas starvation leads to decreased synthesis of these enzymes.

High-Yield Concept

ACC is the rate-limiting and highly regulated step in fatty acid synthesis.

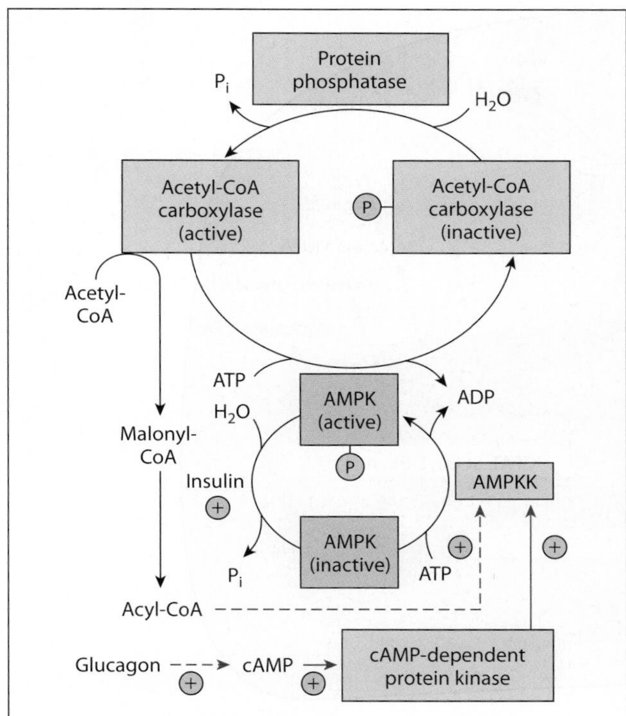

FIGURE 19-4: Regulation of acetyl-CoA carboxylase by phosphorylation/dephosphorylation. The enzyme is inactivated by phosphorylation by AMP-activated protein kinase (AMPK), which in turn is phosphorylated and activated by AMP-activated protein kinase kinase (AMPKK). Glucagon (and epinephrine) increase cAMP, and thus activate this latter enzyme via cAMP-dependent protein kinase. The kinase kinase enzyme is also believed to be activated by acyl-CoA. Insulin activates acetyl-CoA carboxylase via dephosphorylation of AMPK. Murray RK, Bender DA, Botham KM, Kennelly PJ, Rodwell VW, Weil PA. *Harper's Illustrated Biochemistry*, 29th ed. New York, NY: McGraw-Hill; 2012.

ChREBP: Master Lipid Regulator in the Liver

When glycogen stores are maximal in the liver, excess glucose is diverted into the lipid synthesis pathway. Glucose is catabolized to acetyl-CoA and the acetyl-CoA is used for de novo fatty acid synthesis. The fatty acids are then incorporated into triglycerides and exported from hepatocytes as VLDL (very-low-density lipoprotein) and ultimately stored as triglycerides in adipose tissue. A diet rich in carbohydrates leads to stimulation of both the glycolytic and lipogenic pathways. Genes encoding glucokinase (*GK*) and liver pyruvate kinase (*L-PK*) of glycolysis and ATP-citrate lyase (*ACL*), *ACC*, and *FAS* of lipogenesis are regulated by modulation of their transcription rates. These genes contain glucose- or carbohydrate-response elements (ChoREs) that are responsible for their transcriptional regulation.

One transcription factor that exerts control over glucose and lipid homeostasis is sterol-response element-binding protein (SREBP), in particular SREBP-1c (see Chapter 26). Another critical transcription factor regulating glucose and lipid homeostasis is carbohydrate-responsive element-binding protein, ChREBP.

The kinases PKA and AMPK both phosphorylate ChREBP rendering it inactive. Under conditions of low (basal) glucose concentration, ChREBP is phosphorylated and resides in the cytosol. When glucose levels rise, protein phosphatase 2A delta (PP2Aδ) removes phosphates from ChREBP allowing it to migrate to the nucleus. PP2Aδ is activated by xylulose 5-phosphate, an intermediate in the pentose phosphate pathway (PPP) (Chapter 15).

Genes whose expression is under control of ChREBP activity include *L-PK*, *ACC*, and *FAS* as well as glycerol 3-phosphate acyltransferase (GPAT) and Δ^9-stearoly-CoA desaturase 1 (SCD1). GPAT is the enzyme that esterifies glycerol 3-phospate–generating lysophosphatidic acid which is the first step in the synthesis of triglycerides (Chapter 20) and SCD1 is the rate-limiting enzyme involved in the synthesis of the major monounsaturated fatty acids, oleic acid (18:1) and palmitoleic acid (16:1), as discussed below.

The liver X receptors (LXRs) are members of the steroid/thyroid hormone superfamily of intracellular receptors that migrate to the nucleus upon ligand binding and regulate gene expression by binding to specific target sequences (Chapter 40). The LXRs are important regulators of the lipogenic gene expression profile, in part due to LXR-mediated regulation of expression of the *ChREBP* gene. In addition, glucose itself can bind

High-Yield Concept

ChREBP is a major glucose-responsive transcription factor that is required for glucose-induced expression of *L-PK* and the lipogenic genes *ACC* and *FAS*. Expression of the *ChREBP* gene is induced in the liver in response to increased glucose uptake. In addition, the activity of *ChREBP* is regulated by posttranslational modifications as well as subcellular localization.

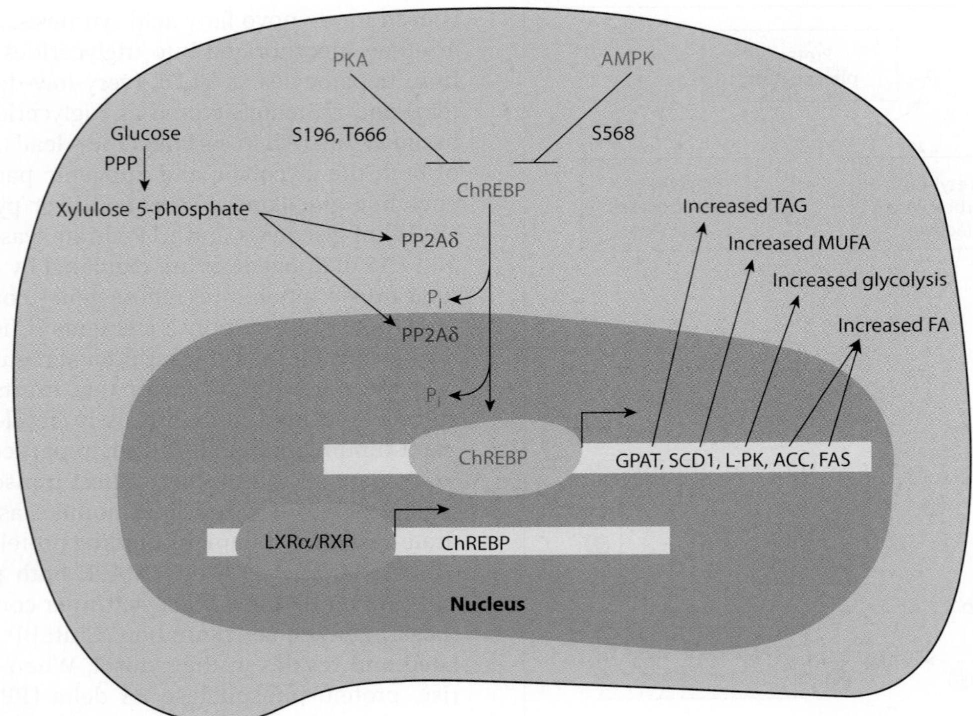

FIGURE 19-5: Role of ChREBP in the modulation of lipid and glucose homeostasis. Increased entry of glucose into the cell results in enhanced oxidation in the PPP, resulting in increased levels of xylulose-5-phosphate (X5P). X5P activates the phosphatase PP2Aδ which removes inhibitory phosphorylations on ChREBP both in the cytosol and the nucleus. Active ChREBP then can turn on the expression of numerous genes involved in the homeostasis of glucose and lipid metabolism in the liver. Activation of LXRα, by lipid ligands, results in increased expression of ChREBP in the liver, which in turn can lead to furhter modulation of lipid and glucose homeostasis. GPAT is glycerol-3-phosphate acyltransferase. SCD1 is stearoyl-CoA desaturase. L-PK is liver pyruvate kinase. ACC is acetyl-CoA carboxylase. FAS is fatty acid synthase. MUFA is monounsaturated fatty acid. The PKA and AMPK sites of phosphorylation in ChREBP are indicated where S is serine and T is threonine and the numbers refer to the specific amino acid in the ChREBP protein. PPP=pentose phosphate pathway.

and activate LXRs, thereby mediating regulation of the lipogenic pathway directly (Figure 19-5).

Elongation and Desaturation

The fatty acid product released from FAS is palmitate via the action of palmitoyl thioesterase. Elongation and unsaturation of fatty acids occurs in both the mitochondria and endoplasmic reticulum (ER) (microsomal membranes). The predominant site of these processes is in the ER membranes. Elongation involves condensation of acyl-CoA groups with malonyl-CoA. The resultant product is 2 carbons longer (CO_2 is released from malonyl-CoA as in the FAS reaction), which undergoes reduction, dehydration, and reduction yielding a saturated fatty acid. The reduction reactions of elongation require NADPH as cofactor just as for the similar reactions catalyzed by FAS. Mitochondrial elongation involves acetyl-CoA units and is a reversal of oxidation except that the final reduction utilizes NADPH instead of $FADH_2$ as cofactor (Figure 19-6).

The desaturation of fatty acids occurs in the ER membranes as well. In mammalian cells fatty acid desaturation involves 3 broad specificity fatty acyl-CoA desaturases (non-heme iron–containing enzymes). These enzymes introduce unsaturation at C5, C6, or C9. The names of these enzymes are Δ^5-eicosatrienoyl-CoA desaturase, Δ^6-oleoyl(linolenoyl)-CoA desaturase, and Δ^9-stearoyl-CoA desaturase (SCD1).

The expression of SCD1 is under the control of the transcription factor ChREBP as discussed above. The ratio of saturated to monounsaturated fatty acids in membrane phospholipids is critical to normal cellular function and alterations in this ratio have been

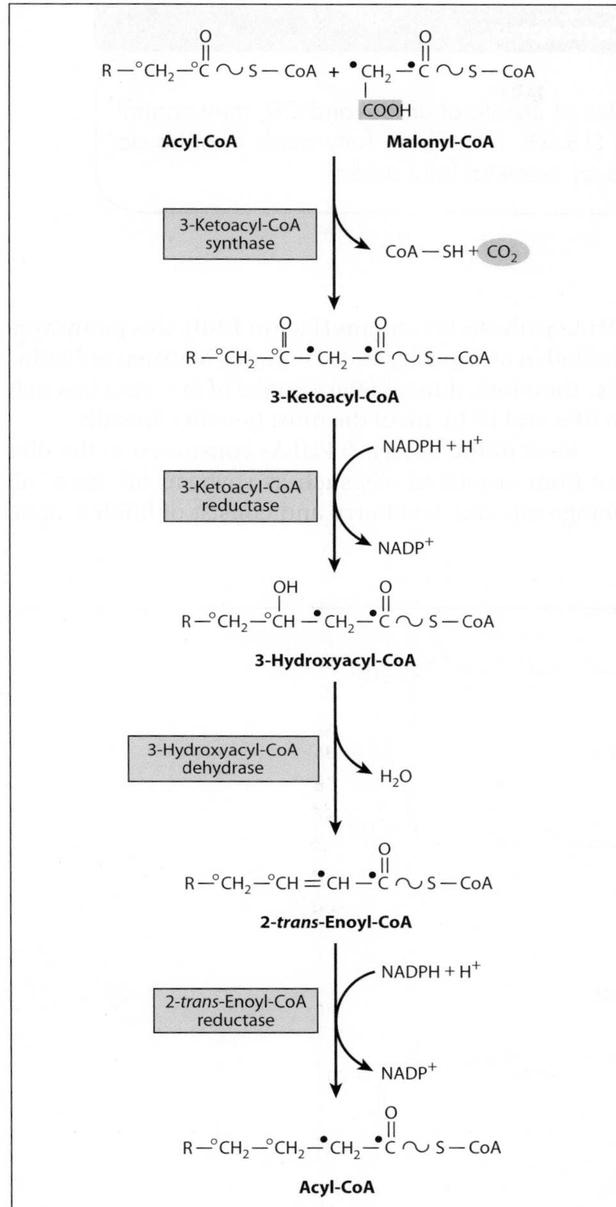

FIGURE 19-6: Microsomal elongase system for fatty acid chain elongation. NADH is also used by the reductases, but NADPH is preferred. Murray RK, Bender DA, Botham KM, Kennelly PJ, Rodwell VW, Weil PA. *Harper's Illustrated Biochemistry*, 29th ed. New York, NY: McGraw-Hill; 2012.

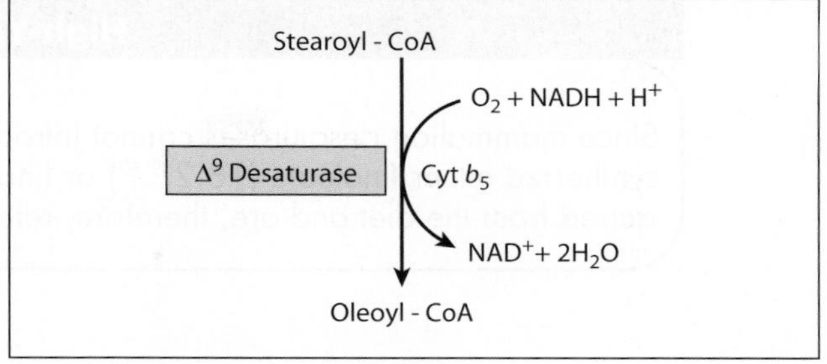

FIGURE 19-7: Microsomal Δ^9 desaturase. Murray RK, Bender DA, Botham KM, Kennelly PJ, Rodwell VW, Weil PA. *Harper's Illustrated Biochemistry*, 29th ed. New York, NY: McGraw-Hill; 2012.

correlated with diabetes, obesity, cardiovascular disease, and cancer. Thus, regulation of the expression and activity of SCD1 has important physiological significance.

The electrons transferred from the oxidized fatty acids during desaturation are transferred from the desaturases to cytochrome b_5 and then NADH-cytochrome b_5 reductase. These electrons are uncoupled from mitochondrial oxidative-phosphorylation and, therefore, do not yield ATP (Figure 19-7).

Linoleic is especially important in that it is required for the synthesis of arachidonic acid. Arachidonate is a precursor for the eicosanoids (the prostaglandins, thromboxanes, and leukotrienes). It is this role of fatty acids in eicosanoid synthesis that leads to poor growth, wound healing, and dermatitis in persons on fat-free diets. Also, linoleic acid is a constituent of epidermal cell sphingolipid that functions as the skin's water permeability barrier.

Synthesis of Biologically Active Omega-3 and omega-6 Polyunsaturated Fatty Acids

The 3 major omega-3 fatty acids utilized by human tissues are ALA, EPA, and DHA (Chapter 23). Most of the ALA consumed in the diet comes from plant sources

High-Yield Concept

SCD1 is the rate-limiting enzyme catalyzing the synthesis of monounsaturated fatty acids, primarily oleate (18:1) and palmitoleate (16:1). These 2 monounsaturated fatty acids represent the majority of monounsaturated fatty acids present in membrane phospholipids, triglycerides, and cholesterol esters.

High-Yield Concept

Since mammalian desaturases cannot introduce sites of unsaturation beyond C9, they cannot synthesize either linoleate ($18{:}2^{\Delta 9,12}$) or linolenate ($18{:}3^{\Delta 9,12,15}$). These fatty acids must be acquired from the diet and are, therefore, referred to as essential fatty acids.

such as flax seed, walnuts, pecans, hazelnuts, and kiwifruit. A small percentage of omega-3 PUFAs come from meats common to Western diets such as chicken and beef; however, this is mostly ALA. The highest concentrations of EPA and DHA are found in cold water fishes such as salmon, tuna, and herring as well as in krill. Although ALA can serve as the precursor for EPA and DHA synthesis in humans (Figure 19-8), this pathway is limited in its capacity and also varies between individuals. Therefore, direct dietary intake of omega-3 fats rich in EPA and DHA are of the most benefit clinically.

Most of the omega-6 PUFAs consumed in the diet are from vegetable oils such as soybean oil, corn oil, borage oil, and acai berry and consist of linoleic acid.

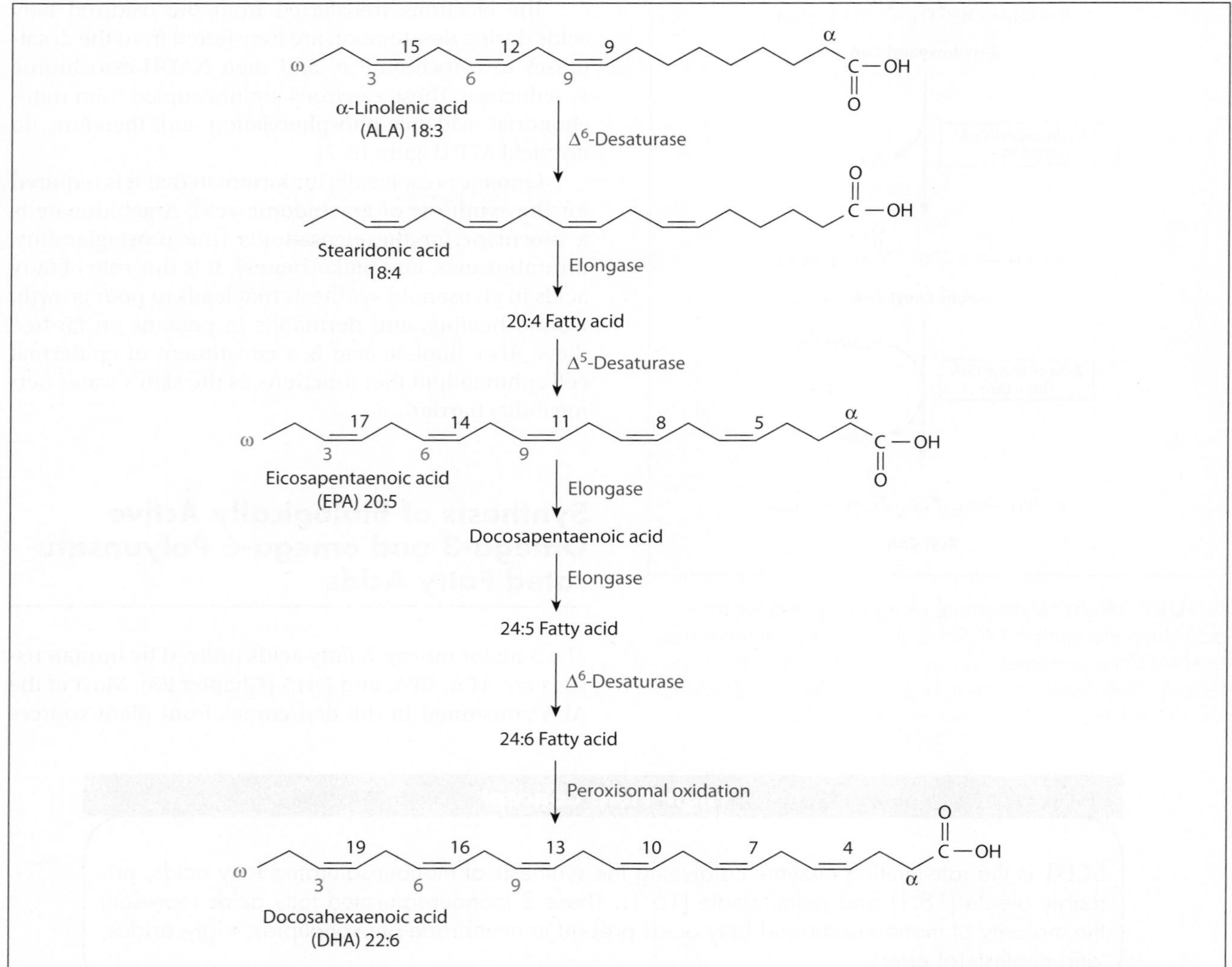

FIGURE 19-8: Pathway for ALA conversion to EPA and DHA. Reproduced with permission of themedicalbiochemistrypage, LLC.

Linoleic acid is converted to arachidonic acid through the steps outlined in Chapter 22.

Biological Activities of Omega-3 and Omega-6 PUFAs

The metabolic and clinical significances of the omega-3 PUFAs are due to the ability of these lipids to exert effects on numerous biologically important pathways as well as to serve as precursors for clinically important bioactive lipids (Chapter 23). Several G-protein–coupled receptors (GPCR, Chapter 40) can be activated by omega fatty acids and their derivatives. For example, the GPCR GPR120 is highly expressed in adipose tissue and pro-inflammatory macrophages, and this receptor is known to be activated by omega-3 PUFA. Of significance is the fact that the omega-3 fatty acids DHA and EPA exert potent anti-inflammatory effects through activation of GPR120.

The most important omega-6 PUFA is arachidonic acid which serves as the precursor for the synthesis of the biologically active eicosanoids (Chapter 22), the prostaglandins (PG), thromboxanes (TX), leukotrienes (LT), and lipoxins (LX). The arachidonate-derived eicosanoids function in diverse biological phenomena such as platelet and leukocyte activation, signaling of pain, induction of bronchoconstriction, and regulation of gastric secretions. These activities are targets of numerous pharmacological agents such as the nonsteroidal anti-inflammatory drugs (NSAIDs), COX-2 inhibitors, and leukotriene antagonists.

Dietary omega-3 PUFAs compete with the inflammatory, pyretic (fever), and pain-promoting properties imparted by omega-6 PUFAs because they displace arachidonic acid from cell membranes. In addition, omega-3 PUFAs compete with the enzymes that convert arachidonic acid into the eicosanoids. The net effect of increasing dietary consumption of omega-3 PUFAs, relative to omega-6 PUFAs, is to decrease the potential for monocytes, neutrophils, and eosinophils to synthesize potent mediators of inflammation and to reduce the ability of platelets to release TXA_2, a potent stimulator of the coagulation process. One of the most important roles of the omega-3 PUFAs, EPA and DHA, is that they serve as the precursors for potent anti-inflammatory lipids called resolvins (Rv) and protectins (PD) as outlined in Chapter 24.

REVIEW QUESTIONS

1. In studies with a particular cell line in culture you discover that the rate of mitochondrial fatty acid oxidation increases when the cells are stimulated to increase their rate of de novo fatty acid synthesis. This observation is quite unexpected since these 2 processes do not normally coincide. Which of the following enzymes involved in fatty acid synthesis is most likely to be altered thus, allowing for fat oxidation to be enhanced along with an increase in fat synthesis?

A. acetyl-CoA carboxylase 2
B. ATP-citrate lyase
C. fatty acid synthase
D. malic enzyme
E. steroyl-CoA desaturase

Answer A: During fatty acid synthesis the malonyl-CoA produced from acetyl-CoA carboxylase 2 (ACC2) directly interacts with carnitine palmitoyltransferase I (CPT I) at the outer mitochondrial membrane to prevent fatty acyl-CoA movement into the mitochondria. A defect in ACC2 activity would therefore lead to reduced inhibition of regulated mitochondrial transport of fatty acyl-CoA resulting in increased fat oxidation from the newly synthesized fatty acids.

2. You are studying fatty acid synthesis in a cell line isolated from a hepatic cancer. You discover that addition of glucose-6-phosphate does not lead to an increase in the rate of palmitic acid synthesis as is the situation in normal hepatic cells. Which of the following proteins is most likely to be altered in the hepatic cancer cells leading to the obtained results?

A. acetyl-CoA carboxylase
B. ATP-citrate lyase
C. ChREBP
D. fatty acid synthase
E. steroyl-CoA desaturase

Answer D: Regulation of de novo fatty acid synthesis takes place primarily at the level of acetyl-CoA carboxylase (ACC) but also at the level of fatty acid synthase (FAS). FAS is regulated by both short-term and long-term mechanisms. Short-term regulation is primarily the result of the allosteric activation of FAS by phosphorylated sugars, such as glucose 6-phosphate.

3. Gas chromatographic analysis of fatty acids present in cells isolated from a particular strain of mice shows little to no palmitoleic and oleic acid but expected levels of palmitic acid. A defect in which of the following proteins is most likely causing the absence of the 2 fatty acids?

A. acetyl-CoA carboxylase
B. ATP-citrate lyase

C. ChREBP
D. fatty acid synthase
E. steroyl-CoA desaturase

Answer E: The desaturation of fatty acids in mammalian cells involves 3 broad specificity fatty acyl-CoA desaturases. Steroyl-CoA desaturase (SCD1) is the rate-limiting enzyme catalyzing the synthesis of monounsaturated fatty acids, primarily oleate (18:1) and palmitoleate (16:1). These 2 monounsaturated fatty acids represent the majority of monounsaturated fatty acids present in membrane phospholipids, triglycerides, and cholesterol esters.

4. You are examining a 27-year-old female adult who presents with redness of the skin, swelling, itching, and skin lesions, several of which are oozing pus. In addition the patient complains that a bad scrape, suffered in a fall from a bike, has not properly healed even though the injury occurred several weeks ago. Patient history indicates that she started on a fat-free diet 10 months ago. Which of the following is most likely deficient in her diet leading to her current physical condition?
A. citric acid
B. linoleic acid
C. oleic acid
D. palmitic acid
E. palmitoleic acid

Answer B: Linoleic is an essential fatty acid in that it must be acquired in the diet. Linoleic acid is especially important in that it required for the synthesis of arachidonic acid. Arachidonate is a precursor for the eicosanoids (the prostaglandins, thromboxanes, and leukotrienes). It is this role of linoleic acid in eicosanoid synthesis that leads to poor growth, wound healing, and dermatitis in persons on fat-free diets.

5. You are studying the activity of acetyl-CoA carboxylase in an isolated buffered system containing the enzyme and its substrate. Addition of which of the following substances to this in vitro assay system would be expected to result in the largest decrease in malonyl-CoA production?
A. acetyl-CoA
B. citrate
C. glucose 6-phosphate
D. glutamate
E. oleic acid

Answer E: Both isoforms of ACC are allosterically activated by citrate and inhibited by palmitoyl-CoA and other short- and long-chain fatty acyl-CoAs. Citrate triggers the polymerization of ACC1 which leads to significant increases in its activity. Although ACC2 does not undergo significant polymerization (presumably due to its mitochondrial association), it is allosterically activated by citrate. Glutamate and other dicarboxylic acids can also allosterically activate both ACC isoforms.

6. Glucose is known to regulate the activity of ChREBP which in turn regulates the expression of numerous genes involved in glucose and lipid homeostasis. Which of the following proteins, whose activity rises as glucose levels rise, is involved in the signaling of glucose levels to ChREBP?
A. acetyl-CoA carboxylase
B. fatty acid synthase
C. malonyl-CoA decarboxylase
D. protein phosphatase 2Aδ
E. steroyl-CoA desaturase

Answer D: Under conditions of low (basal) glucose concentration, ChREBP is phosphorylated and resides in the cytosol. When glucose levels rise, protein phosphatase 2Aδ (PP2Aδ) is activated by xylulose 5-phosphate which is generated in the PPP. PP2Aδ dephosphorylates ChREBP allowing it to migrate into the nucleus. In the nucleus PP2Aδ carries out a second dephosphorylation which allows ChREBP to bind to specific sequence elements (ChoREs) in target genes.

7. Which of the following enzymes is most responsive to changes in the level of circulating insulin such that as insulin levels rise fatty acid synthesis is increased?
A. acetyl-CoA carboxylase
B. ATP-citrate lyase
C. fatty acid synthase
D. malonyl-CoA decarboxylase
E. steroyl-CoA desaturase

Answer A: ACC activity is inhibited by phosphorylation. Both ACC1 and ACC2 undergo phosphorylation. Glucagon-stimulated increases in cAMP and subsequently to increased PKA activity lead to phosphorylation and inhibition of ACC. The activating effects of insulin on ACC are complex but are, in part, related to reductions in cAMP levels via the insulin-mediated activation of phosphodiesterase.

8. Acetyl-CoA is transported out of the mitochondria in order to serve as a substrate for fatty acid or cholesterol synthesis. Which of the following enzymes used in this transport process provides a cofactor required for these reductive biosynthesis reactions?
A. ATP-citrate lyase
B. citrate synthase

C. malate dehydrogenase
D. malic enzyme
E. pyruvate carboxylase

Answer D: Acetyl-CoA enters the cytoplasm in the form of citrate via the tricarboxylate transport system (see Figure 19-3). In the cytoplasm, citrate is converted to oxaloacetate and acetyl-CoA by the ATP-driven ATP-citrate lyase (ACL) reaction. This reaction is essentially the reverse of that catalyzed by the TCA enzyme citrate synthase except it requires the energy of ATP hydrolysis to drive it forward. The resultant oxaloacetate is converted to malate by malate dehydrogenase (MDH). The malate produced by this pathway can undergo oxidative decarboxylation by malic enzyme. The coenzyme for this reaction is $NADP^+$-generating NADPH. The advantage of this series of reactions for converting mitochondrial acetyl-CoA into cytoplasmic acetyl-CoA is that the NADPH produced by the malic enzyme reaction can be a major source of reducing cofactor for the FAS activities.

9. Which of the following exerts a positive allosteric effect on de novo fatty acid synthesis at the level of acetyl-CoA carboxylase?
A. acetyl-CoA
B. AMPK
C. ATP
D. biotin
E. citrate

Answer E: Both isoforms of ACC are allosterically activated by citrate and inhibited by palmitoyl-CoA and other short- and long-chain fatty acyl-CoAs. Citrate triggers the polymerization of ACC1 which leads to significant increases in its activity. Although ACC2 does not undergo significant polymerization (presumably due to its mitochondrial association), it is allosterically activated by citrate. Glutamate and other dicarboxylic acids can also allosterically activate both ACC isoforms.

10. ChREBP regulates the expression of numerous genes involved in lipid and carbohydrate homeostasis. The activity of ChREBP can be modulated by AMPK-mediated phosphorylation. A defect in which of the following enzymes would most likely be apparent if ChREBP was found to be constitutively phosphorylated and inhibited?
A. AMPK
B. glucose-6-phosphate dehydrogenase
C. protein phosphatase 2Aδ
D. protein phosphatase inhibitor 1
E. SREBP

Answer C: Under conditions of low (basal) glucose concentration, ChREBP is phosphorylated and resides in the cytosol. When glucose levels rise, protein phosphatase 2Aδ (PP2Aδ) is activated by xylulose 5-phosphate which is generated in the pentose phosphate pathway. PP2Aδ dephosphorylates ChREBP allowing it to migrate into the nucleus. In the nucleus PP2Aδ carries out a second dephosphorylation which allows ChREBP to bind to specific sequence elements (ChoREs) in target genes. Therefore, a defect in the activity of PP2Ad would lead to constitutive phosphorylation and inhibition of ChREBP.

11. When cells acquire sufficient energy such that the rate of flux through the TCA cycle declines, excess acetyl-CoA that cannot be oxidized is predominantly converted into fat. In order for the carbons in mitochondrial acetyl-CoA to serve as a precursor for fat synthesis, they must be delivered to the cytosol. Which of the following represents the molecule used to transport acetyl-CoA to the cytosol?
A. acetyl-CoA
B. carnitine
C. citrate
D. β-Hydroxybutyrate
E. pyruvate

Answer C: Acetyl-CoA cannot freely diffuse across the membranes of the mitochondria, nor is there a transport mechanism to move the molecule to the cytosol. This ensures that all acetyl-CoA generated by PDH or fat oxidation will be used for energy production. However, as cellular energy demand falls, carbon atoms can be diverted into storage molecules such as glycogen and fatty acids. To move acetyl-CoA out of the mitochondria to the cytosol, it must first be converted to citrate, which can be transported by the TCA transport system.

12. The rate of transcription of the mRNA of which of the following enzymes is most likely increased in an individual on a fat-free, high-carbohydrate diet?
A. fatty acid synthase
B. fructose 1,6-bisphosphatase
C. hormone-sensitive lipase
D. phosphoenolpyruvate carboxykinase
E. pyruvate carboxylase

Answer A: Dietary composition can exert long-term effects on biochemical pathways generally exerted at the level of gene expression. A diet low in fat will trigger a need for increased de novo synthesis of fatty acids, and thus be reflected in an increased level of expression of fatty acid synthase.

Checklist

- ✓ Long-chain-fatty-acid synthesis occurs in the cytosol and requires the activities of acetyl-CoA carboxylase (ACC) and fatty acid synthase (FAS). The end product of de novo fat synthesis is palmitic acid.
- ✓ ACC represents the rate-limiting step in fatty acid synthesis. The enzyme is subject to complex short-term and long-term regulation. Two forms of ACC exist, ACC1 and ACC2 with ACC1 being primarily responsible to initiating fat synthesis and ACC2 being primarily responsible for regulating fat entry into the mitochondria
- ✓ ATP-citrate lyase (ACL) is critical for the delivery of acetyl-CoA to the cytosol from the mitochondria so that it can be used for fat synthesis. Nuclear activity of ACL is necessary for providing acetyl-CoA as a substrate for histone acetyltransferases required for regulating gene activity.
- ✓ Carbohydrate-response element-binding protein is a transcription factor critical for coordinating the expression of genes involved in lipogenesis as well as carbohydrate metabolism. The activity of ChREBP is itself regulated by the level of glucose within the cell.
- ✓ Fatty acid elongation and desaturation occurs in the membranes of the ER as well as in the mitochondria. Mammalian tissues express a limited set of desaturase enzymes and thus cannot introduce double bonds into fatty acids beyond carbon 9.
- ✓ Synthesis of omega-3 and omega-6 fatty acids and their derivatives play critical roles in the regulation of a wide range of biological activities.

CHAPTER

20 Lipids: Triglyceride and Phospholipid Synthesis

CHAPTER OUTLINE

High-Yield Terms

Triglyceride: also called *triacylglyceride* or *triacylglycerol*, major storage form of lipid in the body, composed of a glycerol backbone and 3 esterified fatty acids

Phospholipid: major lipid component of all cell membranes, composed of a glycerol backbone esterified to 2 fatty acids with phosphate esterified to the *sn*3 position, the phosphate group, with an esterified alcohol, is referred to as the polar head group of phospholipids

Lipin: a family of enzymes exhibiting both phosphatidic acid phosphatase activity involved in triglyceride synthesis and transcriptional coactivator activity regulating expression of genes involved in lipid metabolism and adipocyte differentiation

Plasmalogens: are glycerol ether phospholipids mainly of 2 types: alkyl ether (–O–CH_2–) and alkenyl ether (–O–CH=CH–); the plasmalogen platelet-activating factor (PAF) is one of the most potent biological lipids

Synthesis of Triglycerides

Triglycerides (TGs) constitute molecules of glycerol to which 3 fatty acids have been esterified. The fatty acids present in TGs are predominantly saturated. The major building block for the synthesis of TGs, in tissues other than adipose tissue, is glycerol. Adipocytes lack glycerol kinase; therefore, dihydroxyacetone phosphate (DHAP), produced during glycolysis, is the precursor for TG synthesis in adipose tissue. This means that adipocytes must have glucose to oxidize in order to store fatty acids in the form of TG. DHAP can also serve as a backbone precursor for TG synthesis in tissues other than adipose tissue, but does so to a much lesser extent than glycerol.

The glycerol backbone of TG is activated by phosphorylation at the *sn*3 position by glycerol kinase. The utilization of DHAP for the backbone is carried out through either of 2 pathways depending on whether the synthesis of TG is carried out in the mitochondria and ER or the ER and the peroxisomes. In the first situation, the action of glycerol-3-phosphate dehydrogenase (the same reaction as that used in the glycerol-phosphate shuttle) reduces DHAP to glycerol 3-phosphate. Glycerol-3-phosphate acyltransferase (GPAT) then esterifies a fatty acid to glycerol 3-phosphate, generating the monoacylglycerol phosphate structure called *lysophosphatidic acid*. The expression of the *GPAT* gene is under the influence of the transcription factor ChREBP (see Chapter 19).

The second reaction pathway utilizes the peroxisomal enzyme DHAP acyltransferase to fatty acylated DHAP to acyl-DHAP, which is then reduced by the NADPH-requiring enzyme acyl-DHAP reductase. An interesting feature of the latter pathway is that DHAP acyltransferase is one of only a few enzymes that are targeted to the peroxisomes through the recognition of a peroxisome-targeting sequence 2 (PTS2) motif in the enzyme. Most peroxisomal enzymes contain a PTS1 motif.

The fatty acids incorporated into TGs are activated to acyl-CoAs through the action of acyl-CoA synthetases. Two molecules of acyl-CoA are esterified to glycerol-3-phosphate to yield 1,2-diacylglycerol phosphate (commonly identified as phosphatidic acid). The phosphate is then removed, by phosphatidic acid phosphatase (PAP1), to yield 1,2-diacylglycerol, the substrate for addition of the third fatty acid. Intestinal monoacylglycerols, derived from the hydrolysis of dietary fats, can also serve as substrates for the synthesis of 1,2-diacylglycerols (Figure 20-1).

Lipin Genes: Triglyceride Synthesis and Transcriptional Regulation

Recent studies have identified a critical role for the enzyme PAP1 in overall TG and phospholipid homeostasis. The *lipin-1* gene (*LPIN1*) was originally identified in a mutant mouse called the fatty liver dystrophy (fld) mouse. The mutation causing this disorder was found to reside in the *LPIN1* gene. There are 3 *lipin* genes (*LPIN1, LPIN2,* and *LPIN3*) with the *LPIN1* gene encoding 3 isoforms derived through alternative splicing. These 3 lipin-1 isoforms are identified as lipin-1α, lipin-1β, and lipin-1γ. All 5 lipin proteins possess phosphatidic acid phosphatase activity that is dependent on Mg^{2+} or Mn^{2+} and phosphatidic acid as the substrate.

Lipin-1 interacts with the transcription factors PGC-1α (peroxisome proliferator-activated receptor-γ [PPARγ] coactivator 1α) and PPARα, leading to enhanced gene expression. Lipin-1 also induces the expression of the adipogenic transcription factors PPARγ and CCAAT-enhancer–binding protein α (C/EBPα). Lipin-1α induces genes that promote adipocyte differentiation while lipin-1β induces the expression of lipid-synthesizing genes such as fatty acid synthase (FAS) and diacylglycerol acyltransferase (DGAT). The interactions of lipin-1 with PPARα and PGC-1α lead to increased expression of fatty acid–oxidizing genes such as *carnitine palmitoyltransferase-1, acyl-CoA oxidase,* and *medium-chain acyl-CoA dehydrogenase (MCAD).*

Phospholipid Synthesis

Phospholipids can be synthesized by 2 mechanisms. One utilizes a CDP-activated polar head group for attachment to the phosphate of phosphatidic acid. The other utilizes CDP-activated 1,2-diacylglycerol and an inactivated polar head group (see Figure 20-1). Phospholipids are synthesized by esterification of an alcohol to the phosphate of phosphatidic acid (1,2-diacylglycerol phosphate). Most phospholipids have a saturated fatty acid on C–1 and an unsaturated fatty acid on C–2 of the glycerol backbone. The most commonly added alcohols (serine, ethanolamine, and choline) also contain nitrogen that may be positively charged, whereas glycerol and inositol do not. There are 6 major classifications of phospholipid.

1. **Phosphatidylcholine, PC:** This class of phospholipids is also called the *lecithins*. At physiological pH, phosphatidylcholines are neutral zwitterions. They contain primarily palmitic or stearic acid at carbon-1 and primarily oleic, linoleic, or linolenic acid at carbon-2. The lecithin dipalmitoyl lecithin is a component of lung or pulmonary surfactant. It contains palmitate at both carbon-1 and -2 of glycerol and is the major (80%) phospholipid found in the extracellular lipid layer lining the pulmonary alveoli. Choline is activated first by phosphorylation and then by coupling to CDP prior to attachment to phosphatidic acid. PC is also synthesized by the addition of choline to CDP-activated 1,2-diacylglycerol.

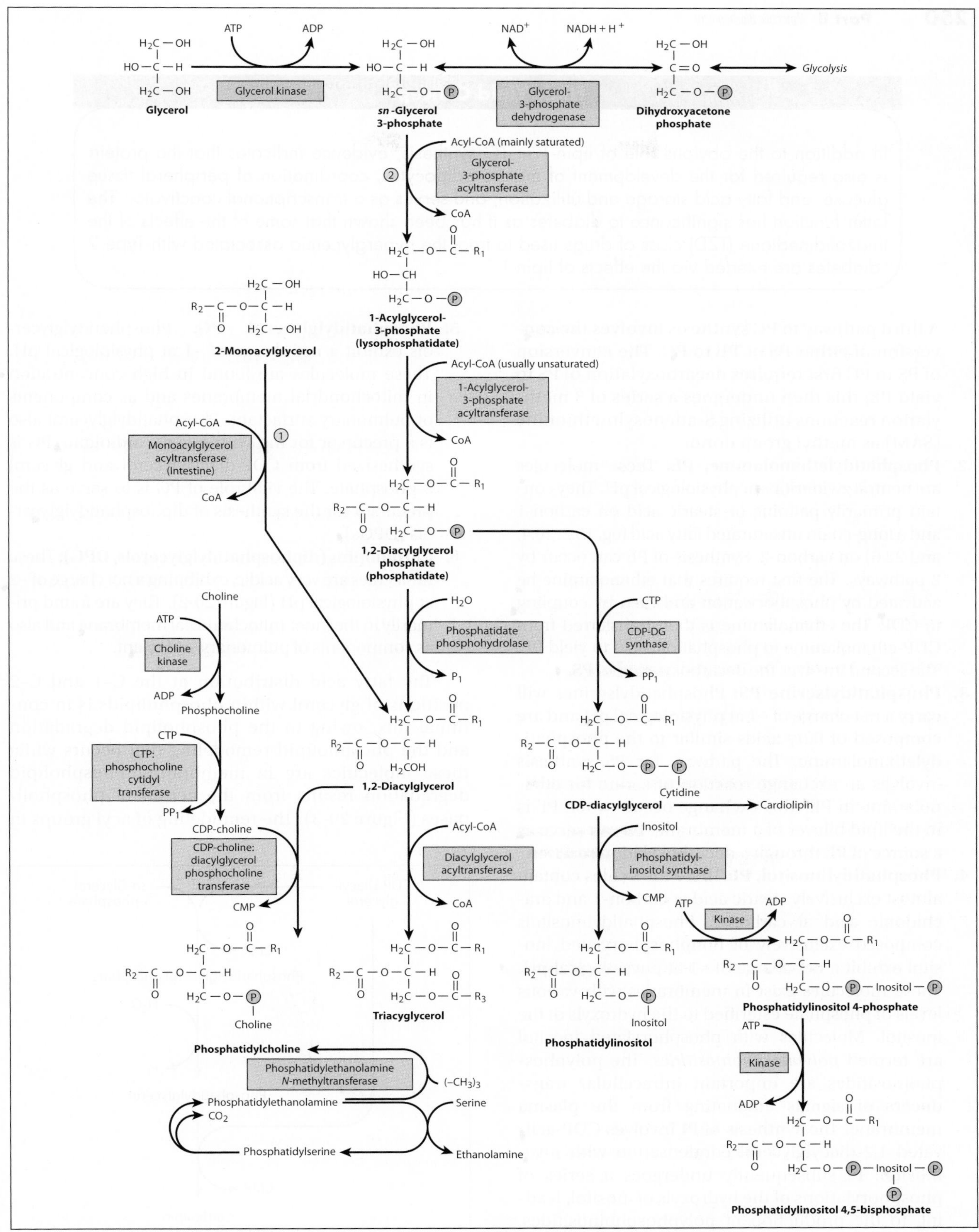

FIGURE 20-1: Biosynthesis of triacylglycerol and phospholipids. (①, Monoacylglycerol pathway; ②, glycerol phosphate pathway.) Phosphatidylethanolamine may be formed from ethanolamine by a pathway similar to that shown for the formation of phosphatidylcholine from choline. Murray RK, Bender DA, Botham KM, Kennelly PJ, Rodwell VW, Weil PA. *Harper's Illustrated Biochemistry*, 29th ed. New York, NY: McGraw-Hill; 2012.

High-Yield Concept

In addition to the obvious role of lipin-1 in TG synthesis, evidence indicates that the protein is also required for the development of mature adipocytes, coordination of peripheral tissue glucose, and fatty acid storage and utilization, and serves as a transcriptional coactivator. The latter function has significance to diabetes as it has been shown that some of the effects of the thiazolidinedione (TZD) class of drugs used to treat the hyperglycemia associated with Type 2 diabetes are exerted via the effects of lipin-1.

A third pathway to PC synthesis involves the conversion of either PS or PE to PC. The conversion of PS to PC first requires decarboxylation of PS to yield PE; this then undergoes a series of 3 methylation reactions utilizing S-adenosylmethionine (SAM) as methyl group donor.

2. **Phosphatidylethanolamine, PE:** These molecules are neutral zwitterions at physiological pH. They contain primarily palmitic or stearic acid on carbon-1 and a long-chain unsaturated fatty acid (eg, 18:2, 20:4, and 22:6) on carbon-2. Synthesis of PE can occur by 2 pathways. The first requires that ethanolamine be activated by phosphorylation and then by coupling to CDP. The ethanolamine is then transferred from CDP-ethanolamine to phosphatidic acid to yield PE. The second involves the decarboxylation of PS.
3. **Phosphatidylserine PS:** Phosphatidylserines will carry a net charge of –1 at physiological pH and are composed of fatty acids similar to the phosphatidylethanolamine. The pathway for PS synthesis involves an exchange reaction of serine for ethanolamine in PE. This exchange occurs when PE is in the lipid bilayer of a membrane. PS can serve as a source of PE through a decarboxylation reaction.
4. **Phosphatidylinositol, PI:** These molecules contain almost exclusively stearic acid at carbon-1 and arachidonic acid at carbon-2. Phosphatidylinositols composed exclusively of nonphosphorylated inositol exhibit a net charge of –1 at physiological pH. These molecules exist in membranes with various levels of phosphate esterified to the hydroxyls of the inositol. Molecules with phosphorylated inositol are termed *polyphosphoinositides*. The polyphosphoinositides are important intracellular transducers of signals emanating from the plasma membrane. The synthesis of PI involves CDP-activated 1,2-diacylglycerol condensation with *myo*-inositol. PI subsequently undergoes a series of phosphorylations of the hydroxyls of inositol, leading to the production of polyphosphoinositides. One polyphosphoinositide (phosphatidylinositol 4,5-bisphosphate, PIP_2) is a critically important membrane phospholipid involved in the transmission of signals for cell growth and differentiation from outside the cell to inside.
5. **Phosphatidylglycerol, PG:** Phosphatidylglycerols exhibit a net charge of –1 at physiological pH. These molecules are found in high concentration in mitochondrial membranes and as components of pulmonary surfactant. Phosphatidylglycerol also is a precursor for the synthesis of cardiolipin. PG is synthesized from CDP-diacylglycerol and glycerol 3-phosphate. The vital role of PG is to serve as the precursor for the synthesis of diphosphatidylglycerols (DPGs).
6. **Cardiolipins (diphosphatidylglycerols, DPG):** These molecules are very acidic, exhibiting a net charge of –2 at physiological pH (Figure 20-2). They are found primarily in the inner mitochondrial membrane and also as components of pulmonary surfactant.

The fatty acid distribution at the C-1 and C-2 positions of glycerol within phospholipids is in continual flux, owing to the phospholipid degradation and the phospholipid remodeling that occurs while these molecules are in membranes. Phospholipid degradation results from the action of phospholipases (Figure 20-3). The remodeling of acyl groups in

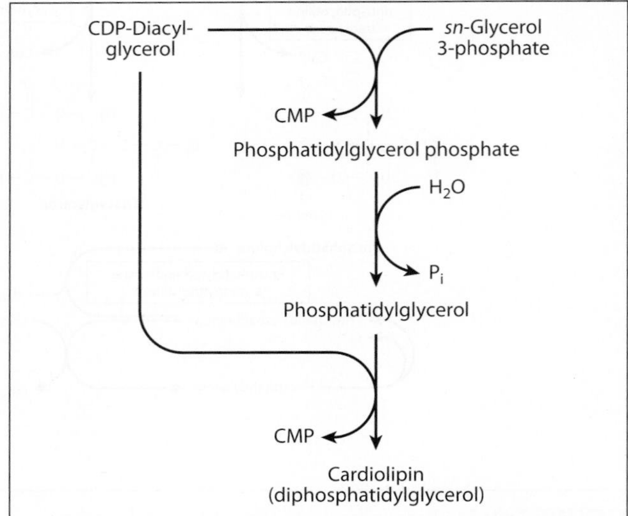

FIGURE 20-2: Biosynthesis of cardiolipin. Murray RK, Bender DA, Botham KM, Kennelly PJ, Rodwell VW, Weil PA. *Harper's Illustrated Biochemistry*, 29th ed. New York, NY: McGraw-Hill; 2012.

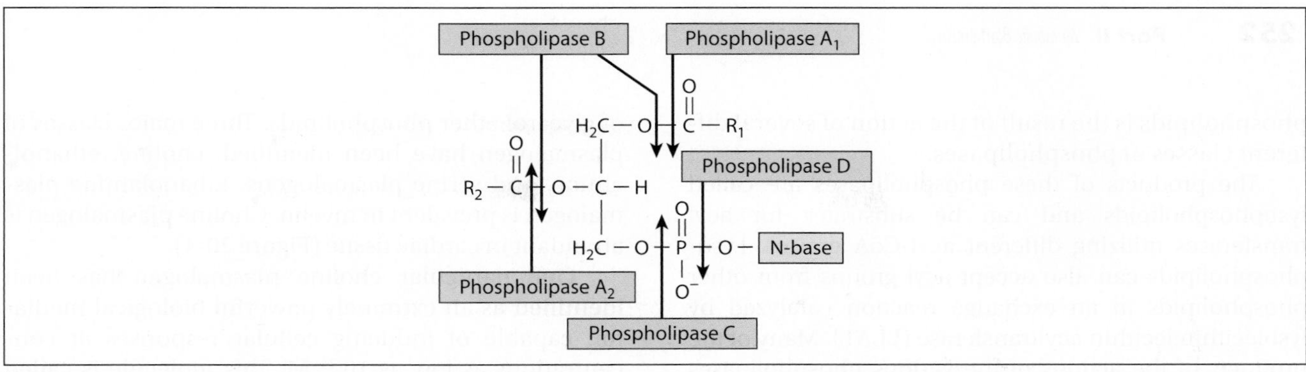

FIGURE 20-3: Sites of the hydrolytic activity of phospholipases on a phospholipid substrate. Murray RK, Bender DA, Botham KM, Kennelly PJ, Rodwell VW, Weil PA. *Harper's Illustrated Biochemistry*, 29th ed. New York, NY: McGraw-Hill; 2012.

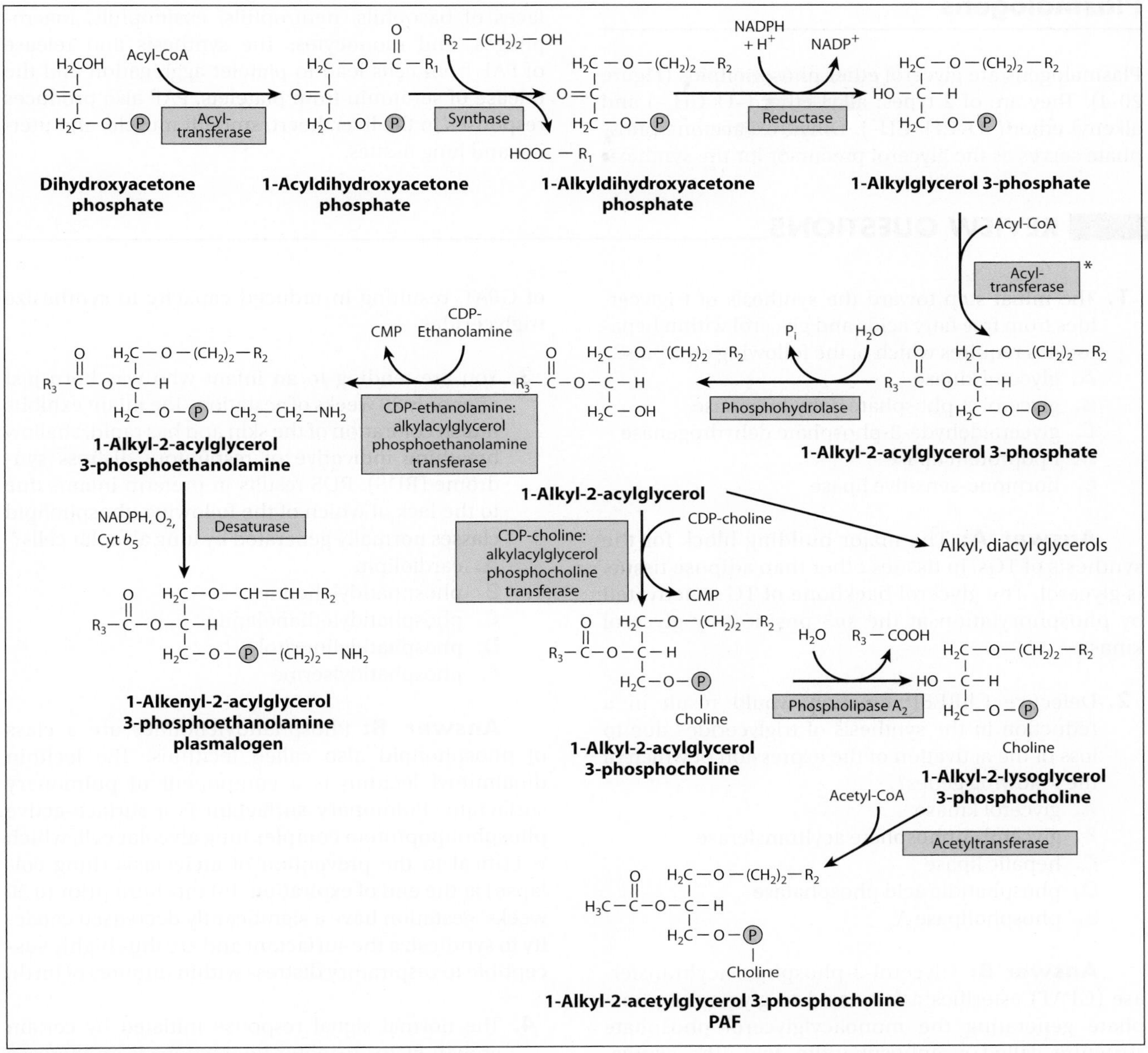

FIGURE 20-4: Biosynthesis of ether lipids, including plasmalogens, and platelet-activating factor (PAF). In the de novo pathway for PAF synthesis, acetyl-CoA is incorporated at stage*, avoiding the last 2 steps in the pathway shown here. Murray RK, Bender DA, Botham KM, Kennelly PJ, Rodwell VW, Weil PA. *Harper's Illustrated Biochemistry*, 29th ed. New York, NY: McGraw-Hill; 2012.

phospholipids is the result of the action of several different classes of phospholipases.

The products of these phospholipases are called lysophospholipids and can be substrates for acyl transferases utilizing different acyl-CoA groups. Lysophospholipids can also accept acyl groups from other phospholipids in an exchange reaction catalyzed by lysolecithin:lecithin acyltransferase (LLAT). Many of the products of the actions of the various phospholipases exert specific biological functions (see Chapter 23).

Plasmalogens

Plasmalogens are glycerol ether phospholipids (Figure 20-4). They are of 2 types: alkyl ether (–O–CH_2–) and alkenyl ether (–O–CH=CH–). Dihydroxyacetone phosphate serves as the glycerol precursor for the synthesis of glycerol ether phospholipids. Three major classes of plasmalogen have been identified: choline, ethanolamine, and serine plasmalogens. Ethanolamine plasmalogen is prevalent in myelin. Choline plasmalogen is abundant in cardiac tissue (Figure 20-4).

One particular choline plasmalogen has been identified as an extremely powerful biological mediator, capable of inducing cellular responses at concentrations as low as 10^{-11} M. This molecule is called platelet-activating factor, PAF. PAF functions as a mediator of hypersensitivity, acute inflammatory reactions, and anaphylactic shock. PAF is synthesized in response to the formation of antigen-IgE complexes on the surfaces of basophils, neutrophils, eosinophils, macrophages, and monocytes. The synthesis and release of PAF from cells lead to platelet aggregation and the release of serotonin from platelets. PAF also produces responses in the liver, heart, smooth muscle, and uterine and lung tissues.

REVIEW QUESTIONS

1. The initial step toward the synthesis of triglycerides from free fatty acids and glycerol within hepatocytes requires which of the following enzymes?
   A. glycerol kinase
   B. glycerol-3-phosphate dehydrogenase
   C. glyceraldehyde-3-phosphate dehydrogenase
   D. lipoprotein lipase
   E. hormone-sensitive lipase

Answer A: The major building block for the synthesis of TGs, in tissues other than adipose tissue, is glycerol. The glycerol backbone of TG is activated by phosphorylation at the *sn*3 position by glycerol kinase.

2. Defective ChREBP function would result in a reduction in the synthesis of triglycerides due to loss of the activation of the expression of which of the following genes?
   A. glycerol kinase
   B. glycerol-3-phosphate acyltransferase
   C. hepatic lipase
   D. phosphatidic acid phosphatase
   E. phospholipase A_2

Answer B: Glycerol-3-phosphate acyltransferase (GPAT) esterifies a fatty acid to glycerol 3-phosphate generating the monoacylglycerol phosphate structure called lysophosphatidic acid. The expression of the *GPAT* gene is under the influence of the transcription factor ChREBP. Therefore, defective ChREBP activity would result in reduced expression of GPAT, resulting in reduced capacity to synthesize triglycerides.

3. You are tending to an infant who was born just after only 28 weeks of gestation. The infant exhibits bluish coloration of the skin and has rapid, shallow breathing indicative of respiratory distress syndrome (RDS). RDS results in preterm infants due to the lack of which of the following phospholipid classes normally generated by lung alveolar cells?
   A. cardiolipin
   B. phosphatidylcholine
   C. phosphatidylethanolamine
   D. phosphatidylinositol
   E. phosphatidylserine

Answer B: Phosphatidylcholines are a class of phospholipid also called lecithins. The lecithin dipalmitoyl lecithin is a component of pulmonary surfactant. Pulmonary surfactant is a surface-active phospholipoprotein complex lung alveolar cell, which is critical to the prevention of atelectasis (lung collapse) at the end of expiration. Infants born prior to 30 weeks' gestation have a significantly decreased capacity to synthesize the surfactant and are thus highly susceptible to respiratory distress within minutes of birth.

4. The normal signal response initiated by certain growth factor-receptor interactions is an increase in the activity of protein kinase C (PKC). The activity of PKC is controlled by both calcium ion and lipid, particularly diacylglycerols. Abnormal cells that do not exhibit normal activation of PKC in response to addition of growth factor would most likely be lacking in the ability to synthesize which of the following class of phospholipid?

A. cardiolipin
B. phosphatidylcholine
C. phosphatidylethanolamine
D. phosphatidylinositol
E. phosphatidylserine

Answer D: Phosphatidylinositols with phosphorylated inositol are termed polyphosphoinositides. The polyphosphoinositides are important intracellular transducers of signals emanating from the plasma membrane. One polyphosphoinositide (phosphatidylinositol 4,5-bisphosphate, PIP_2) is a critically important membrane phospholipid involved in the transmission of signals for cell growth and differentiation from outside the cell to inside. Numerous G-protein-coupled receptors activate phospholipase A2, which releases diacylglycerol (DAG) and inositol trisphosphate (IP_3) from PIP_2. The IP_3 binds to receptors on ER membranes resulting in the release of stored calcium into the cytosol.

5. Hypersensitive individuals have IgE to specific antigens (eg, pollen, bee venom) on the surface of their leukocytes (monocytes, macrophages, basophils, eosinophils). When these individuals are challenged with antigen, the antigen-IgE complexes induce synthesis and release of which of the following physiologically potent lipids?

A. arachidonic acid
B. leukotriene B_4
C. platelet-activating factor
D. prostaglandin E_2
E. thromboxane A_2

Answer C: Platelet-activating factor (PAF) is a unique complex lipid of the plasmalogen family. PAF functions in hypersensitivity, acute inflammatory reactions, and anaphylactic shock by increased vasopermeability, vasodilation, and bronchoconstriction. Excess production of PAF production may be involved in the morbidity associated with toxic shock syndrome and strokes.

6. Activation of phospholipase D (PLD) would be expected to result in an increased level of which of the following compounds?

A. cardiolipin
B. diacylglycerol
C. dihydroxyacetone phosphate
D. platelet-activating factor
E. phosphatidic acid

Answer E: Phospholipase D hydrolyzes the alcohol esterified to the phosphate of phospholipids. The products of the action of PLD are, therefore, phosphatidic acid and the original alcohol such as inositol of ethanolamine, for example.

7. Studies on a cell line derived from a biopsy of a liver tumor demonstrate that these cells are unable to synthesize triglycerides. Which of the following enzymes is most likely defective, or missing, from these cells resulting in the loss of triglyceride synthesis?

A. glycerol kinase
B. glycerol-3-phosphate acyltransferase
C. glycerol-3-phosphate dehydrogenase
D. hepatic lipase
E. phosphatidic acid phosphatase

Answer A: Hepatocytes utilize glycerol as the building block for the synthesis of triglycerides. The glycerol backbone is activated by phosphorylation at the C-3 position by glycerol kinase. Therefore, a loss of glycerol kinase activity in these cells would most likely explain the reduced capability to synthesize triglycerides.

8. Phosphatidic acid, synthesized from glycerol 3-phosphate and 2 molecules of fatty acyl-CoA, is a key intermediate in the biosynthesis of which of the following?

A. bile salts
B. glycosphingolipids
C. phospholipids
D. prostaglandins
E. steroid hormones

Answer C: Phosphatidic acid serves as an intermediate in the synthesis of triglycerides and phospholipids. The fatty acids incorporated into triglycerides are activated to acyl-CoAs through the action of acyl-CoA synthetases. Two molecules of acyl-CoA are esterified to glycerol 3-phosphate to yield phosphatidic acid. The phosphate is then removed, by phosphatidic acid phosphatase (PAP1), to yield 1,2-diacylglycerol, the substrate for addition of the third fatty acid of a triglyceride. Phospholipids are synthesized by esterification of an alcohol to the phosphate of phosphatidic acid.

9. In adipose tissue, synthesis of triglycerides from fatty acids derived from chylomicrons requires glycolysis for the synthesis of which of the following?

A. acetyl-CoA
B. citrate
C. glycerol 3-phosphate
D. $NADP^+$
E. NADPH

Answer C: Adipocytes lack glycerol kinase; therefore, dihydroxyacetone phosphate (DHAP), produced during glycolysis, is the precursor for triglyceride synthesis in adipose tissue. The utilization of DHAP for the backbone is carried out through either of 2 pathways depending on whether the synthesis of triglycerides is carried out in the mitochondria and ER or the ER and the peroxisomes. In the former case, the action of glycerol-3-phosphate dehydrogenase converts DHAP to glycerol 3-phosphate.

10. Platelet-activating factor (PAF) causes release of arachidonic acid from membrane lipids. Which of the following enzymes is most likely responsible for this effect?

A. cyclooxygenase
B. lipoprotein lipase
C. lipoxygenase
D. phospholipase A_2
E. thromboxane synthase

Answer D: Arachidonic acid is found esterified to the *sn*2 position of the glycerol backbone of membrane phospholipids. Activation of membrane receptors, such as that which is activated by PAF, leads to activation of phospholipase A_2, which hydrolyzes the ester bond at the *sn*2 position in phospholipids.

Checklist

✓ Triglycerides represent the major storage form of lipid in the body. These molecules are synthesized from glycerol and 3 fatty acids.

✓ Adipose tissue requires glycolysis coupled to triglyceride synthesis since adipocytes do not express glycerol kinase and must acquire glycerol 3-phosphate via the reduction of the glycolytic intermediate, dihydroxyacetone phosphate catalyzed by glycerol-3-phosphate dehydrogenase.

✓ Phospholipids represent the major lipid molecules present in plasma membranes of cells. In this capacity, phospholipids serve as sources of precursor lipids for the synthesis of numerous bioactive lipid derivatives. Release of fatty acids from membrane phospholipids occurs most often in response to ligand-mediated receptor activation of PLA_2, but can also result from activation of PLD.

✓ Plasmalogens are a form of phospholipid containing an ether-linked fatty acid at the *sn*1 position of the glycerol backbone. One of the most potent plasmalogens is platelet-activating factor (PAF). PAF is a unique plasmalogen in that it contains acetate esterified to the *sn*2 position instead of a long-chain fatty acid.

CHAPTER

21 Lipids: Sphingolipids, Ceramides, and Glycosphingolipids

CHAPTER OUTLINE

High-Yield Terms

Sphingolipid: a class of lipid composed of a core of the long-chain amino alcohol, sphingosine, to which is attached a polar head group (such as a sugar) and a fatty acid via *N*-acylation

Ceramide: a class of lipid composed of a sphingosine core and a single fatty acid but no polar head group as for sphingolipids

Spingomyelins: a class of sphingolipid that contains phosphocholine as the polar head group and are, therefore, also a class of phospholipid

Saposin: a family (A, B, C, and D) of small glycoprotein activators of lysosomal hydrolases that are all derived from a single precursor, prosaposin

Hexosaminidases: dimeric enzymes composed of 2 subunits, either the α-subunit (encoded by the *HEXA* gene) and/or the β-subunit (encoded by the *HEXB* gene); various isoforms of β-hexosaminidase result from the combination of α- and β–subunits

Lysosomal storage disease: any of a large family of disorder resulting from defects in lysosomal hydrolases resulting in accumulation of incompletely degraded complex lipids, particularly of the sphingolipid family

Cherry-red spot: a finding describing the appearance of a small circular deep red choroid shape in the fovea centralis (fundus) of the eye in a variety of lipid storage diseases

Synthesis of Sphingosine and the Ceramides

The sphingolipids, like the phospholipids, are composed of a polar head group and 2 nonpolar tails. The core of a sphingolipid is the long-chain amino alcohol, sphingosine (Figure 21-1). The sphingolipids include the sphingomyelins and glycosphingolipids (the cerebrosides, sulfatides, globosides, and gangliosides). Sphingomyelins are unique in that they are also phospholipids. Sphingolipids are components of all membranes but are particularly abundant in the myelin sheath.

The initiation of the synthesis of the sphingoid bases (sphingosine, dihydrosphingosine, and ceramides) takes place via the condensation of palmitoyl-CoA and serine (Figure 21-2). This reaction occurs on the cytoplasmic face of the endoplasmic reticulum (ER) and is catalyzed by serine palmitoyltransferase (SPT). SPT is the rate-limiting enzyme of the sphingolipid biosynthesis pathway. Active SPT is a heterotrimeric enzyme composed of 2 main subunits and a third subunit that greatly enhances the activity of the enzyme complex as well as confers acyl-CoA preference to the complex.

The acylation of dihydrosphingosine (also called sphinganine) to dihydroceramide occurs through the activities of 6 different ceramide synthases (CerS) in humans. These CerS enzymes introduce fatty acids of varying lengths and degrees of unsaturation.

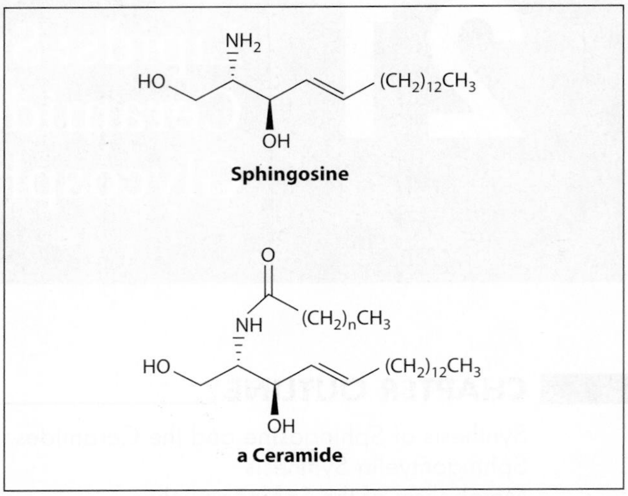

FIGURE 21-1: Structure of sphingosine and a ceramide. Reproduced with permission of themedicalbiochemistrypage, LLC.

Following conversion to ceramide, sphingosine is released via the action of ceramidase. Sphingosine can be reconverted to a ceramide by condensation with a fatty acyl-CoA catalyzed by the various CerS. There are at least 2 ceramidase genes in humans both of which are defined by their pH range of activity: acid and neutral. Acid ceramidase is encoded by the *ASAH1* gene. Defects in the human *ASAH1* gene result in Farber lipogranulomatosis (Clinical Box 21-1). Neutral ceramidase

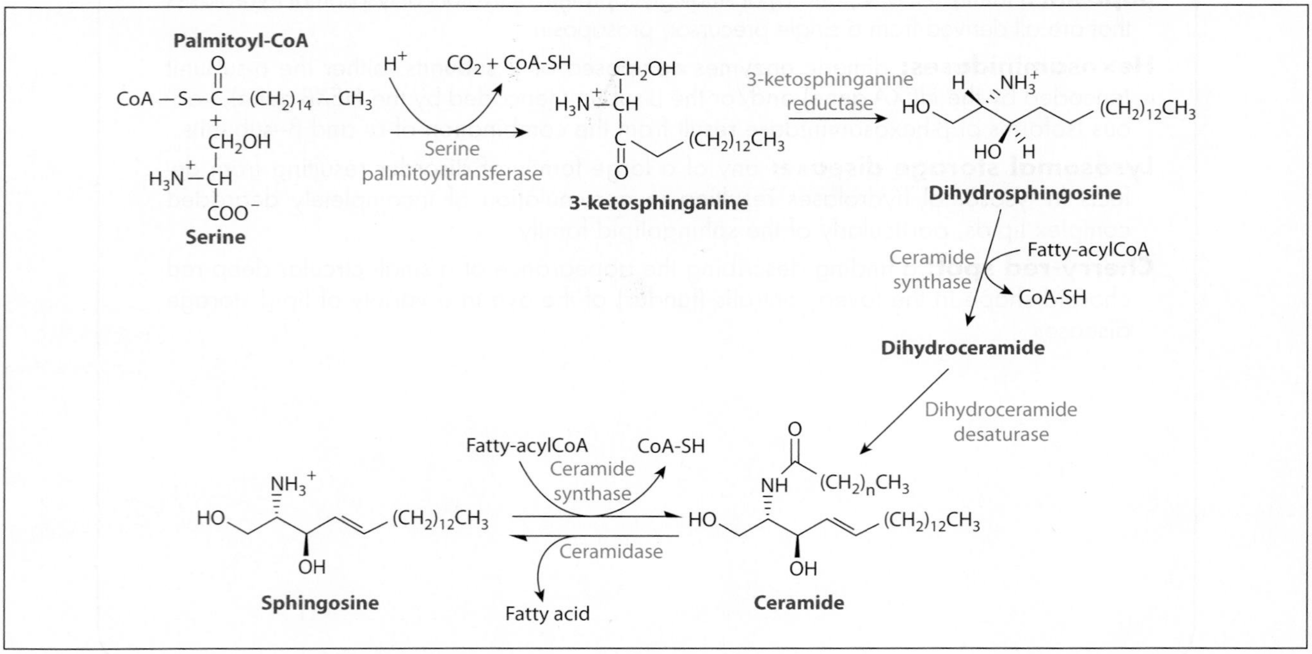

FIGURE 21-2: Pathway for sphingosine and ceramide synthesis. Reproduced with permission of themedicalbiochemistrypage, LLC.

CLINICAL BOX 21-1: FARBER LIPOGRANULOMATOSIS

Farber lipogranulomatosis belongs to a family of disorders identified as lysosomal storage diseases. This disorder is characterized by the lysosomal accumulation of ceramides. Farber lipogranulomatosis results from defects in the gene encoding the lysosomal hydrolase: acid ceramidase encoded by the *ASAH1*. Acid ceramidase catalyzes the hydrolysis of ceramides generating sphingosine and a free fatty acid. Symptoms of Farber lipogranulomatosis commonly appear during the first months after birth. The clinical manifestations are characterized by painful and progressively deformed joints, progressive hoarseness due to laryngeal involvement, and subcutaneous nodules particularly over the joints. The tissues in afflicted individuals contain granulomatous and lipid-laden macrophages. The liver, spleen, lungs, and heart are particularly affected with central nervous system involvement resulting in the progressive degeneration in psychomotor development. Farber lipogranulomatosis is a rapidly progressing disease often leading to death before 2 years of age. There are several clinical phenotypes associated with acid ceramidase deficiencies giving rise to 7 subtypes of Farber lipogranulomatosis.

Type 1 is the classic Farber disease. The characteristic clinical presentation of type 1 disease is painful swelling of the joints, especially the ankle, wrist, elbow, and knee and a hoarse cry. These symptoms are evident as early as 2 weeks of age. In many cases these patients will have an additional symptom characteristic of Tay-Sachs disease which is the "cherry-red spot" on the fundus of the eye.

Type 2 is the "intermediate" form and **type 3** is the "mild" form of the disease. These patients have longer survival period than do type 1 infants. In addition, the neurological involvement is much more mild than in type 1.

Type 4 is referred to as the "neonatal-visceral" form of the disease. Infants are extremely ill in the neonatal period. These patients will present with severe hepatosplenomegaly. In the severest cases, type 4 neonates will present as hydrops fetalis (severe fluid accumulation, usually in the brain) and die within days of birth. Unlike type 1 patients, infants with type 4 disease do not present with the characteristic features of deformed painful joints, thus, requiring biochemical assay for definitive diagnosis.

Type 5 is referred to as "neurologic progressive." As the name implies, the most striking clinical feature of type 5 disease is a progressive neurological deterioration accompanied by seizures. Joint involvement is evident but to a lesser degree than in type 1 disease. Type 5 patients also exhibit the "cherry-red spot" seen in many type 1 patients.

Type 6 is characterized by patients exhibiting both Farber lipogranulomatosis as well as Sandoff disease.

Type 7 disease results from a deficiency in prosaposin, a precursor encoding the sphingolipid activator proteins called saposins (saposin A, B, C, and D).

is encoded by the *ASAH2* gene and the enzyme is expressed in the apical membranes of the proximal and distal tubules of the kidney, endosome-like organelles in heptocytes, and in the epithelial cells of the gut. Neutral ceramidase is involved in the catabolism of dietary sphingolipids and the regulation of bioactive sphingolipid metabolites in the intestinal tract.

Sphingomyelin Synthesis

Sphingomyelins are sphingolipids that are also phospholipids (Figure 21-3). Sphingomyelins are important structural components of nerve cell membranes. The predominant sphingomyelins contain palmitic or stearic acid *N*-acylated at carbon-2 of sphingosine.

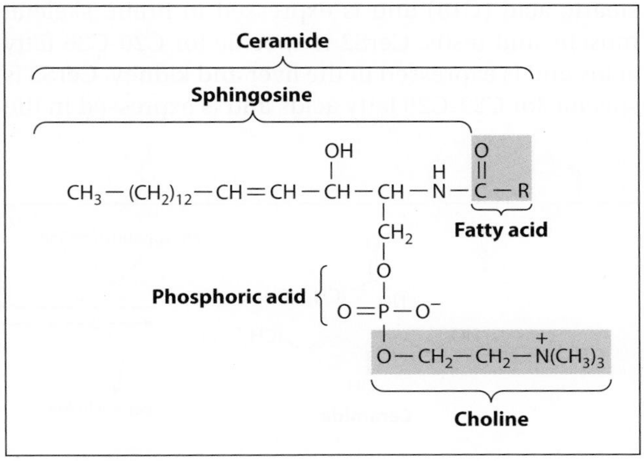

FIGURE 21-3: A sphingomyelin. Murray RK, Bender DA, Botham KM, Kennelly PJ, Rodwell VW, Weil PA. *Harper's Illustrated Biochemistry*, 29th ed. New York, NY: McGraw-Hill; 2012.

The sphingomyelins are synthesized by the transfer of phosphorylcholine from phosphatidylcholine to a ceramide in a reaction catalyzed by sphingomyelin synthases (SMS). There are 2 SMS genes in humans identified as SMS1 and SMS2. SMS1 is found in the trans-Golgi apparatus, while SMS2 is predominantly associated with the plasma membrane.

Metabolism of the Sphingomyelins

Sphingomyelins are degraded via the action of sphingomyelinases resulting in release of ceramides and phosphocholine (Figure 21-4). The sphingomyelinase in humans functions at acidic pH and is, therefore, referred to as acid sphingomyelinase (ASMase) encoded for by the sphingomyelin phosphodiesterase-1 gene (SMPD1). Defects in the *SMPD1* gene result in the lysosomal storage disease known as Niemann-Pick disease (Clinical Box 21-2).

Metabolism of the Ceramides

The overall level of ceramides in a cell is a balance between the need for sphingosine and sphingosine derivatives, such as sphingosine-1-phosphate (S1P) and the sphingomyelins. With respect to the sphingomyelins they serve a dual purpose of being important membrane phospholipids and as a reservoir for ceramides.

The conversion of both dihydrosphingosine (sphinganine) and sphingosine to ceramide is catalyzed by the ceramide synthases (CerS). Each CerS exhibits fatty acyl chain length specificity as well as differential tissue distribution. CerS1 is specific for stearic acid (C18) and is expressed in brain, skeletal muscle, and testis. CerS2 is specific for C20-C26 fatty acids and is expressed in the liver and kidney. CerS3 is specific for C22-C26 fatty acids and is expressed in the skin and testis. CerS4 is specific for C18-C20 fatty acids and is ubiquitously expressed but with highest levels in liver, heart, skin, and leukocytes. CerS5 is specific for palmitic acid (C16) and is ubiquitously expressed at low levels. CerS6 is specific for myristic (C14) and palmitic acid and is expressed at low levels in all tissues. CerS1 is structurally and functionally distinct from the other 5 CerS each of which contains a homeobox-like domain.

The clinical significance of ceramide synthesis and the activity of the CerS is evident by studies in several different types of human cancers. In this regard, CerS1 appears most significant. Head and neck squamous cell carcinomas (HNSCC) exhibit a down-regulation of C18-ceramide levels when compared to adjacent normal tissue. In addition, a balance between the levels of C16- and C18-ceramides is associated with the state of clinical progression of HNSCC. In the chemotherapy of certain cancers, CerS1 activity may also play a role. Enhanced expression of CerS1 has been shown to sensitize cells to a variety of chemotherapeutic drugs such as cisplatin, vincristine, and doxorubicin. Increased production of C18-ceramide is associated with the induction of apoptosis.

Ceramides and Insulin Resistance

Numerous lines of evidence over the past 10 years have shown that various inducers of cellular stress such as inflammatory activation, excess saturated fatty acid intake, and chemotherapeutics, result in increased rates of ceramide synthesis. In addition, there is ample evidence demonstrating that the accumulation of cellular ceramides is associated with the pathogenesis of diseases such as obesity, diabetes, atherosclerosis, and cardiomyopathy. Endogenous ceramides and glucosylceramides are known to antagonize insulin-stimulated glucose uptake and synthesis. Details of the role of ceramides in the development of insulin resistance are found in Chapter 46.

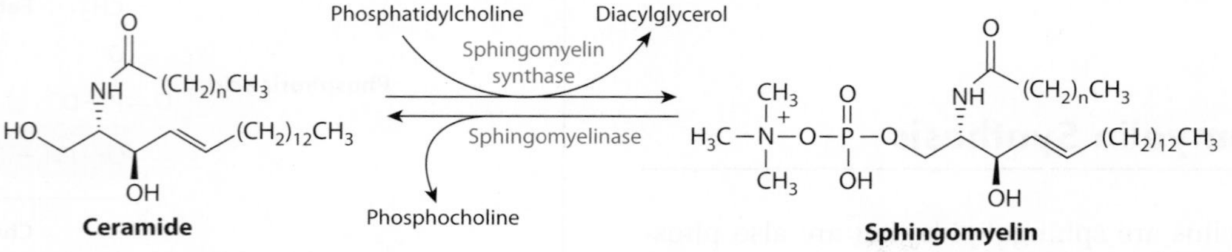

FIGURE 21-4: Interrelated metabolism of sphingomyelins and ceramides. Reproduced with permission of themedicalbiochemistrypage, LLC.

CLINICAL BOX 21-2: NIEMANN-PICK DISEASES

The Niemann-Pick (NP) diseases belong to a family of disorders identified as lysosomal storage diseases. There are 2 distinct subfamilies of NP diseases. NP type A (NPA) and type B (NPB) diseases are caused by defects in the *acid sphingomyelinase gene* (*SMPD1*). NP type C (NPC) diseases are caused by defects in a gene involved in LDL-cholesterol homeostasis identified as the *NPC1* gene. At least 95% of NPC patients contain mutations in the *NPC1* locus with the remainder harboring mutations in a second gene identified as *NPC2*. Like the protein encoded by the *NPC1* locus, the *NPC2* gene product also binds cholesterol esters.

Type A NP disease is associated with a rapidly progressing neurodegeneration leading to death by 2 to 3 years of age. In contrast, type B NP disease has a variable phenotype marked primarily by visceral involvement with little to no neurological detriment. Diagnosis of type B NP disease is usually made in early childhood by the presence of hepatosplenomegaly. The most severely affected type B patients exhibit a progressive pulmonary involvement. Both type A and type B NP diseases are characterized by the presence of the "Niemann-Pick" cell. This histologically distinct cell type is of the monocyte-macrophage lineage and is a characteristic lipid-laden foam cell. The course of type A NP disease is rapid. Infants are born following a typically normal pregnancy and delivery. Within 4 to 6 months the abdomen protrudes and hepatosplenomegaly will be diagnosed. The early neurological manifestations include hypotonia, muscular weakness, and difficulty feeding. As a consequence of the feeding difficulties and the swollen spleen, infants will exhibit a decrease in growth and body weight. By the time afflicted infants reach 6 months of age the signs of psychomotor deterioration become evident. Ophthalmic examination reveals a cherry-red spot typical of patients with Tay-Sachs disease in about 50% of type A NP infant patients. As the disease progresses, spasticity and rigidity increase and infants experience complete loss of contact with their environment.

Niemann-Pick disease type C (NPC) results from an error in the trafficking of exogenous cholesterol, thus it is more commonly referred to as a lipid trafficking disorder even though it belongs to the family of lysosomal storage diseases. The principal biochemical defect in patients with NPC is an accumulation of cholesterol, sphingolipids, and other lipids in the late endosomes/lysosomes (LE/L) of all cells. NPC is a disease characterized by fatal progressive neurodegeneration. The prevalence of NPC disease is more common than NPA and NPB disease combined. There can be significant clinical heterogeneity associated with NPC disease. Most afflicted individuals have progressive neurological disease with early lethality. The characteristic phenotypes associated with "classic" NPC disease are variable hepatosplenomegaly, progressive ataxia, dystonia, dementia, and vertical supranuclear gaze palsy (VSGP). These individuals will present in childhood and death will ensue by the second or third decade. Because of the variable clinical phenotypes of NPC disease it has been subdivided into 5 presentation classifications: perinatal, early infantile, late infantile, juvenile, and adult. VSGP is a characteristic neurological manifestation in NPC disease being found in virtually all juvenile and adult cases of the disease. Like NPA and NPB disease, NPC pathology is characterized by the presence of lipid-laden foam cells in the visceral organs and the nervous system.

A gene related to the NPC1 gene, called Niemann-Pick type C1-like 1 (NPC1L1), is expressed in the brush border cells of the small intestine and is involved in intestinal absorption of cholesterol. The cholesterol-lowering action of the drug ezemitibe (Zetia) stems from the fact that the drug binds to and interferes with the cholesterol absorption functions of NPC1L1.

Metabolism of Sphingosine-1-Phosphate

Sphingosine-1-phosphate (S1P) is a signaling sphingolipid that functions as a ligand for a family of 5 distinct G-protein–coupled receptors (GPCR). These 5 S1P receptors are differentially expressed and each is coupled to various G-proteins. The activities initiated by S1P binding to its receptors include involvement in vascular system and central nervous system development, viability and reproduction, immune cell trafficking, cell adhesion, cell survival and mitogenesis, stress responses, tissue homeostasis, angiogenesis, and metabolic regulation.

Synthesis of S1P occurs exclusively from sphingosine via the action of sphingosine kinases (Figure 21-5). Humans express 2 related sphingosine kinases encode

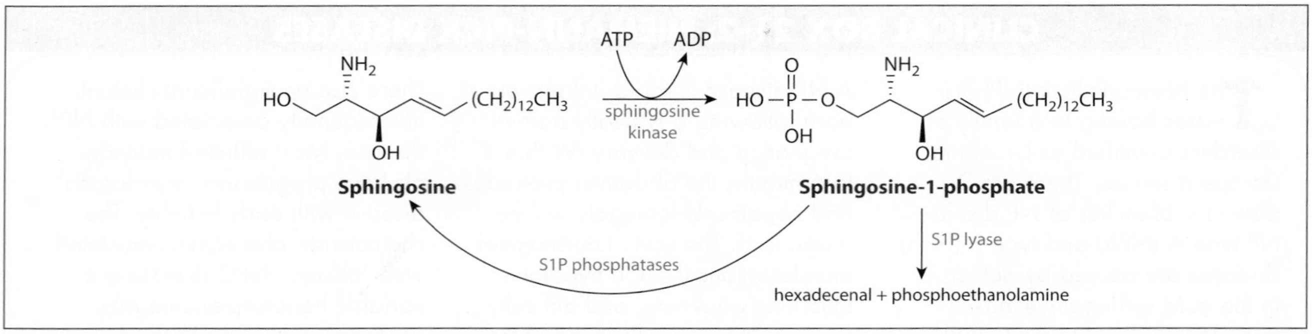

FIGURE 21-5: Synthesis and metabolism of sphingosine-1-phosphate. Reproduced with permission of themedicalbiochemistrypage, LLC.

by the *SPHK1* and *SPHK2* genes. The intermediate in sphingosine synthesis, dihydrosphingosine, is also a substrate for sphinogosine kinases. In vertebrates, S1P is secreted into the extracellular space by specific transporters, one of which is called spinster-2 homolog-2 encoded by the *SPNS2* gene. Plasma levels of S1P are high, whereas interstitial fluids contain very low levels. Hematopoietic cells and vascular endothelial cells are the major sources of the high plasma S1P concentrations. Lymphatic endothelial cells are also thought to secrete S1P into the lymphatic circulation. The majority of plasma S1P is bound to HDL (65%) with another 30% bound by albumin. Indeed, the ability of HDL to induce vasodilation and migration of endothelial cells, as well as to serve a cardioprotective role in the vasculature is dependent on S1P. Thus, the beneficial property of HDL to reduce the risk of cardiovascular disease may be due, in part, on its role as an S1P chaperone.

Degradation of S1P occurs through the action of S1P lyase or the S1P phosphatases (S1P phosphatase-1 and -2) as well as lysophospholipid phosphatase 3 (LPP3). The different S1P phosphatases remove the phosphate, thus, regenerating sphingosine which can reenter the sphingolipid metabolic pathway. When used as a substrate for phospholipid synthesis, S1P is degraded by S1P lyase to yield hexadecenal and phosphoethanolamine. Phosphoethanolamine is the direct precursor for the synthesis of the phospholipid phosphatidylethanolamine (PE). The hexadecenal is converted into hexadecenoic acid by hexadecenal dehydrogenase and then into palmitoyl-CoA. The degradation of S1P by the S1P lyase pathway serves as an important pathway for the conversion of sphingolipids into glycerolipids.

Sphingosine-1-Phosphate Activities

The first GPCR shown to bind S1P was called $S1P_1$. Because several lysophospholipid (LPL) receptors, including the S1P receptors, were independently identified in unrelated assays, there are several different names for some members of this receptor family. In particular, a group of GPCR genes that were originally identified as endothelial differentiation genes (EDGs) were later found to be the same as several of the LPL receptors. For example, $S1P_1$ is also known as EDG1 (Table 21-1).

The Glycosphingolipids

Glycosphingolipids, or glycolipids, are composed of a ceramide backbone with a wide variety of carbohydrate groups (mono- or oligosaccharides) attached to carbon-1 of sphingosine. The 4 principal classes of glycosphingolipids are the cerebrosides, sulfatides, globosides, and gangliosides (Chapter 3).

Cerebrosides have a single sugar group linked to ceramide with the most being galactose forming the galactocerebrosides. Galactocerebrosides are found predominantly in neuronal cell membranes. Galactocerebrosides are synthesized from ceramide and UDP-galactose. Excess lysosomal accumulation of glucocerebrosides is observed in Gaucher disease (Clinical Box 21-3).

Sphingolipid Metabolism Disorders

Some of the most devastating inborn errors in metabolism are those associated with defects in the enzymes responsible for the lysosomal degradation (Figure 21-6; Table 21-2) of membrane glycosphingolipids which are particularly abundant in the membranes of neural cells. Many of these disorders lead to severe psychomotor retardation and early lethality such as is the situation for Tay-Sachs disease (Clinical Box 21-4). Because the disorders are caused by defective lysosomal enzymes, with the result being lysosomal accumulation of pathway intermediates, these are often referred to as lysosomal storage diseases.

High-Yield Concept

Glucocerebrosides are only intermediates in the synthesis of complex gangliosides or are found at elevated levels only in disease states such as Gaucher disease, where there is a defect in the catabolism of the complex gangliosides. Thus, the presence of high concentrations of glucocerebrosides in cells such as monocytes and macrophages is indicative of a metabolic defect.

TABLE 21-1: Sphingosine-1-Phosphate (S1P) Receptors

S1P Receptor	*Alternative Name*	*Gene Symbol*	*G-Proteins*	*Comments*
$S1P_1$	EDG1	*S1PR1*	$G_{i/o}$	Expressed in brain, heart, spleen, liver, kidney, skeletal muscle, thymus, pancreatic β-cells, and numerous white blood cells. Within the immune system, activation of $S1P_1$ has been shown to block β-cell and T-cell chemotaxis and infiltration into tissues. In addition $S1P_1$ activation results in inhibition of late-stage maturation processes associated with T cells. Within the central nervous system $S1P_1$ is involved in astrocyte migration and increased migration of neural stem cells. Within the vasculature $S1P_1$ is involved in early vascular system development and endothelial cell functions such as adherens junction assembly and vascular smooth muscle cell development. Within the pancrease $S1P_1$ functions in islet cell survival and insulin secretion.
$S1P_2$	EDG5	*S1PR2*	$G_{i/o}$, G_q, $G_{12/13}$	Expressed in the brain, heart, spleen, liver, lung, kidney, skeletal muscle, and thymus. $S1P_2$ is involved in the development of epithelial cells, enhancing the survival of cardiac myocytes to ischemic-reperfusion injury, and hepatocyte proliferation and matrix remodeling. Within the vasculature $S1P_2$ promotes mast cell degranulation and decreases vascular smooth muscle cell responses to PDGF-induced migration. In the eye $S1P_2$ activation can result in pathologic angiogenesis and disruption in adherens junction formation.
$S1P_3$	EDG3	*S1PR3*	$G_{i/o}$, G_q, $G_{12/13}$	Expressed in the brain, heart, spleen, liver, lung, kidney, skeletal muscle, testis, and thymus. $S1P_3$ activation is associated with a worsening of sepsis, increased inflammation and coagulation. However, with respect to cardiac tissues $S1P_3$ promotes survival in response to ischemic-reperfusion injury.t
$S1P_4$	EDG6	*S1PR4*	$G_{i/o}$, $G_{12/13}$	Expressed in lymphoid tissues (leukocytes) and within a restricted subset of cells in the lung that includes airway smooth muscle cells. The primary responses to $S1P_4$ activation are increased T-cell migration and secretion of cytokines.
$S1P_5$	EDG8	*S1PR5*	G_q, $G_{12/13}$	Expressed in the brain, spleen, and the skin. Within the brain $S1P_5$ activation is associated with inhibition of migration of oligodendrocyte progenitors while increasing the survival of oligodendrocytes. $S1P_5$ also stimulates natural killer (NK) cell trafficking.

CLINICAL BOX 21-3: GAUCHER DISEASE

Gaucher disease (pronounced "go-shay") belongs to a family of disorders identified as lysosomal storage diseases. Gaucher disease is characterized by the lysosomal accumulation of glucosylceramide (glucocerebroside) which is a normal intermediate in the catabolism of globosides and gangliosides. Gaucher disease results from defects in the gene encoding the lysosomal hydrolase: acid β-glucosidase, also called glucocerebrosidase (GBA). Acid β-glucosidase exists as a homodimer and the active hydrolytic complex requires an additional activator protein. The activator of acid β-glucosidase is saposin C, a member of the saposin family of small glycoproteins. The saposins (A, B, C, and D) are all derived from a single precursor, prosaposin. The mature saposins, as well as prosaposin, activate several lysosomal hydrolases involved in the metabolism of various sphingolipids. Prosaposin is proteolytically processed to saposins A, B, C, and D, within lysosomes. The natural substrates for acid β-glucosidase are *N*-acyl-sphingosyl-1-*O*-β-D-glucosides, glucosylceramides, and various sphingosyl compounds. The physiological significance of the role of saposin C in acid β-glucosidase activity is evident in patients with a saposin C deficiency exhibiting a Gaucher-like disease phenotype.

The hallmark of Gaucher disease is the presence of lipid-engorged cells of the monocyte/macrophage lineage with a characteristic appearance in a variety of tissues. These distinctive cells contain one or more nuclei and their cytoplasm contains a striated tubular pattern described as "wrinkled tissue paper." These cells are called Gaucher cells. Clinically, Gaucher disease is classified into 3 major types. These types are determined by the absence or presence and severity of neurological involvement. Type 1 (adult, nonneuronopathic) is the most commonly occurring form of Gaucher disease and is called the nonneuronopathic type (historically called the adult form). Type 1 Gaucher disease has a broad spectrum of severity from early onset of massive hepatosplenomegaly and extensive skeletal abnormalities to patients lacking symptoms until the eighth or ninth decade of life. Type 2 (infantile, neuronopathic) Gaucher disease is characterized by onset at an early age disease. Type 2 is the acute neuronopathic form manifesting with early onset of severe central nervous system dysfunction and is usually fatal within the first 2 years of life. Abnormalities in oculomotor function are often the first manifesting symptoms in type 2 disease. Patients often thrust their heads in an attempt to compensate when following a moving object. Type 3 Gaucher disease (subacute neuronopathic) patients have later-onset neurological symptoms with a more chronic course than type 2 patients. Type 3 disease is divided into 3 subclasses. Type 3a presents with progressive neurological involvement dominated by dementia and myoclonus (involuntary muscle twitching). Type 3b presents with aggressive skeletal and visceral symptoms. The neurological symptoms are limited to horizontal supranuclear gaze palsy. Type 3c presents with neurological involvement limited to horizontal supranuclear gaze palsy, cardiac valve calcification, and corneal opacities but with little visceral involvement. Enlargement of the liver is characteristic in all Gaucher disease patients. In severe cases the liver can fill the entire abdomen. Splenomegaly is present in all but the most mildly affected individuals and even in asymptomatic individuals spleen enlargement can be found. In addition to hepatosplenomegaly, bleeding is a common presenting symptom in Gaucher disease. The most common cause of the bleeding is thrombocytopenia (deficient production of platelets).

Currently there is no effective treatment for type 2 Gaucher disease. Current treatments for type 1 and type 3 Gaucher disease include enzyme replacement therapy (ERT), bone marrow transplantation (BMT), or oral medications. ERT replaces the deficient enzyme with artificial enzymes. Currently the biotech company Genzyme, a unit of Sanofi SA, markets the drug Cerezyme for ERT treatment of Gaucher disease.

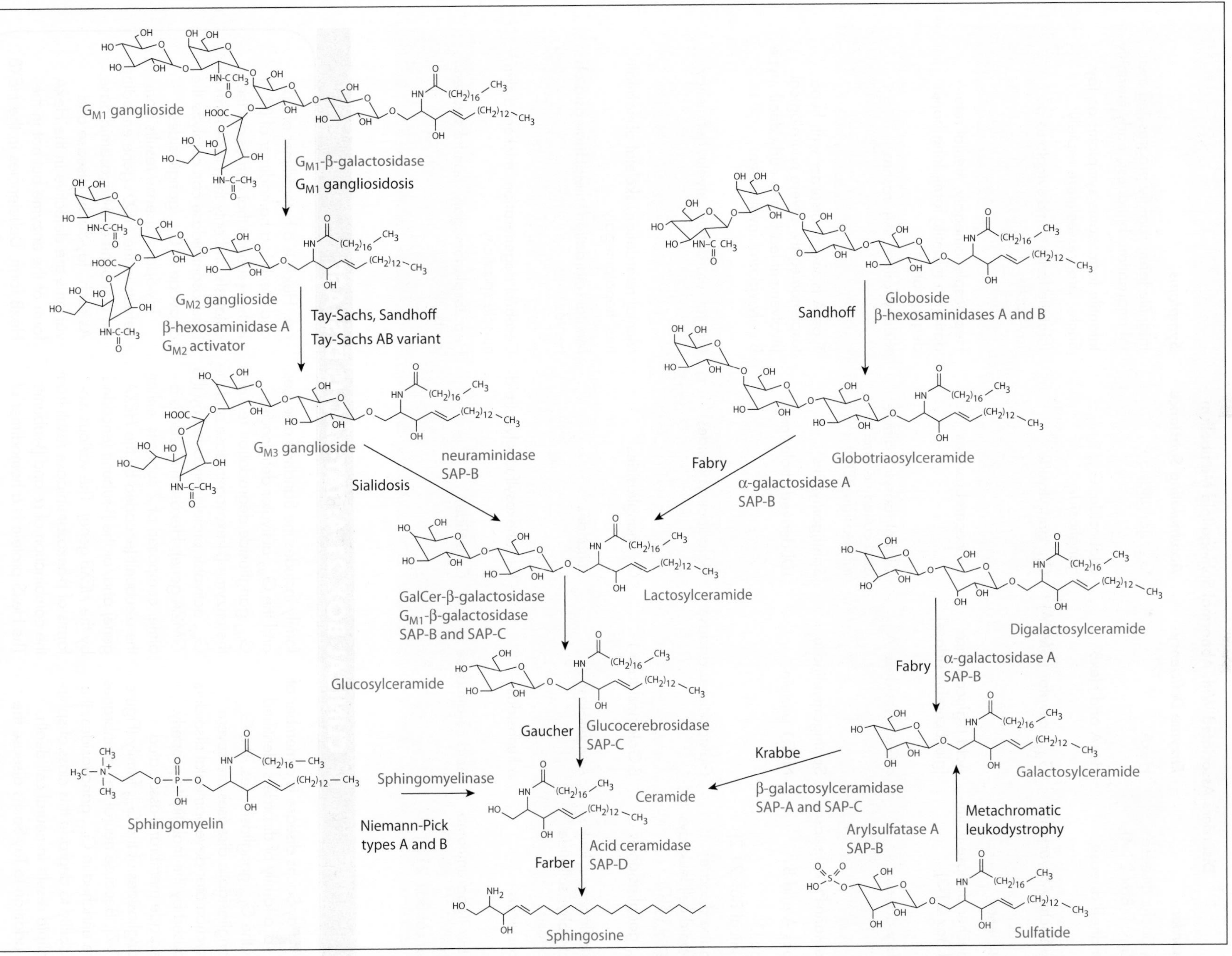

FIGURE 21-6: Pathways of glycosphingolipid metabolism. Glycosphingolipid structures are indicated in red, enzymes are indicated in green, and the disease(s) associated with defects in the indicated enzyme are shown in blue. SAP-A, SAP-B, SAP-C, and SAP-D are the saposins which are a family of small glycoproteins. The saposins (A, B, C, and D) are all derived from a single precursor, prosaposin. Reproduced with permission of themedicalbiochemistrypage, LLC.

TABLE 21-2: Disorders Associated With Abnormal Sphingolipid Metabolism

Disorder	*Enzyme Deficiency*	*Accumulating Substance*	*Symptoms*
Tay-Sachs disease (Clinical Box 21-4)	HexA	G_{M2} ganglioside	Infantile form: rapidly progressing mental retardation, blindness, early mortality
Sandhoff disease	HexA and HexB	Globoside; G_{M2} ganglioside	Infantile form: same symptoms as Tay-Sachs, progresses more rapidly
Tay-Sachs AB variant G_{M2} activator deficiency	G_{M2} activator (GM2A)	G_{M2} ganglioside	infantile form: same symptoms as Tay-Sachs
Gaucher disease (Clinical Box 21-3)	Acid β-glucosidase (glucocerebrosidase)	Glucocerebrosides	Hepatosplenomegaly, mental retardation in infantile form, long bone degeneration
Fabry disease	α-Galactosidase A	Globotriaosylceramide; also called ceramide trihexoside (CTH)	Kidney failure, skin rashes
Niemann-Pick diseases Types A and B Type C (Clinical Box 21-2)	Sphingomyelinase NPC1 protein	Sphingomyelins LDL-derived cholesterol	Type A is severe disorder with hepatosplenomegaly, severe neurological involvement leading to early death, type B only visceral involvement
Krabbe disease; globoid cell leukodystrophy (GLD)	Galactocerebrosidase	Galactocerebrosides	Mental retardation, myelin deficiency
G_{M1} gangliosidosis	β-Galactosidase-1	G_{M1} gangliosides	Mental retardation, skeletal abnormalities, hepatomegaly
Metachromatic leukodystrophy; sulfatide lipodosis	Arylsulfatase A	Sulfatides	Mental retardation, metachromasia of nerves
Fucosidosis	α-Fucosidase	Pentahexosylfucoglycolipid	Cerebral degeneration, thickened skin, muscle spasticity
Farber lipogranulomatosis (Clinical Box 21-1)	Acid ceramidase	Ceramides	Hepatosplenomegaly, painful swollen joints

CLINICAL BOX 21-4: TAY-SACHS DISEASE

Tay-Sachs disease is a member of a family of disorders identified as the G_{M2} gangliosidoses. The G_{M2} gangliosidotic diseases are severe psychomotor developmental disorders caused by the inability to properly degrade membrane-associated gangliosides of the G_{M2} family (Figure 21-7). Because neural cell membranes are enriched in G_{M2} gangliosides, the inability to degrade this class of sphingolipid results in neural cell death. In addition to Tay-Sachs disease the family includes the Sandhoff diseases and the G_{M2} activator deficiencies. G_{M2} ganglioside degradation requires the enzyme β-hexosaminidase and the G_{M2} activator protein (encoded by the *GM2A* gene). Hexosaminidase is a dimer composed of 2 subunits, either the α-subunit (encoded by the *HEXA* gene) and/or the β-subunit (encoded by the *HEXB* gene). The various isoforms of β-hexosaminidase result from the combination of α- and β-subunits. The HexS protein is a homodimer of αα, HexA is a heterodimer of αβ, and HexB is a homodimer of ββ. It is the α-subunit that carries out the catalysis and only the HexA form of β-hexosaminidase can catalyze the cleavage of G_{M2} gangliosides.

Tay-Sachs disease results from defects in the *HEXA* gene encoding the α-subunit of β-hexosaminidase. As such, Tay-Sachs disease and variants are defective in the HexA form of the enzyme but not in the HexB form. Deficiencies in the *HEXB*

CLINICAL BOX 21-4: TAY-SACHS DISEASE (*Continued*)

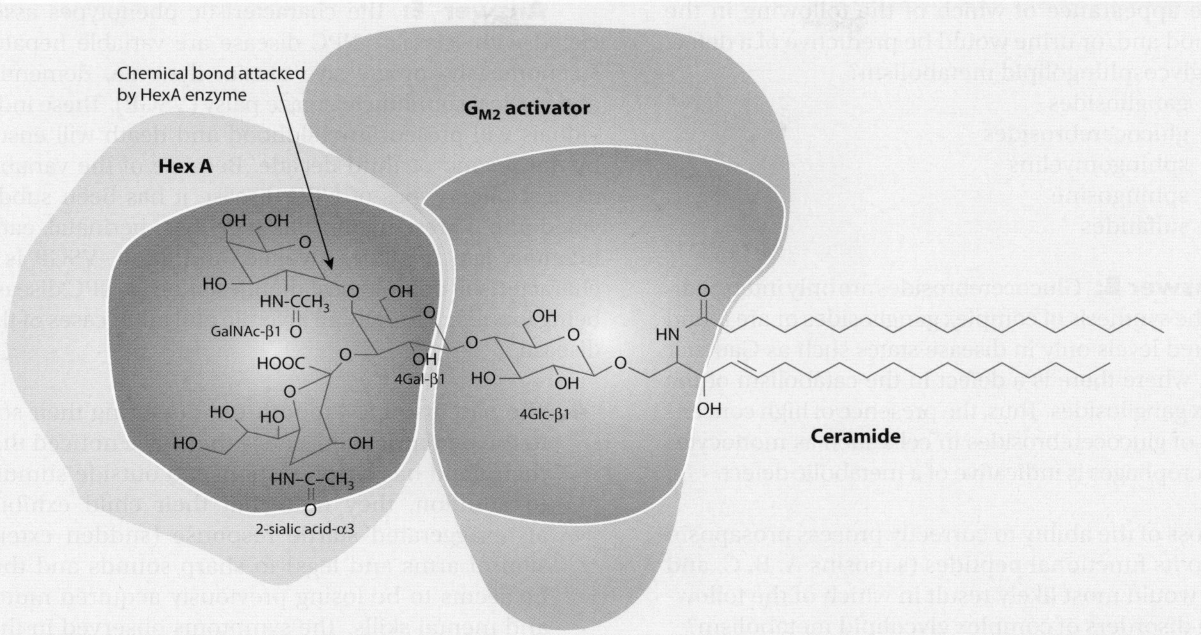

FIGURE 21-7: HexA and G_{M2} activator action on G_{M2} gangliosides. Reproduced with permission of themedicalbiochemistrypage, LLC.

gene result in Sandhoff disease and deficiencies in the *GM2A* gene result in G_{M2} activator deficiency disease, also referred to as the AB variant of Tay-Sachs disease. The eponym, Tay-Sachs disease, is reserved for the infantile forms of G_{M2} gangliosidotic diseases. The infantile forms are very severe and infants will not normally survive beyond 2 years of age. There are numerous variant mutants of the α-subunit that encompass a clinical spectrum from subacute to chronic forms of disease in which symptoms may be delayed for many years. The clinical phenotypes associated with the infantile forms of Tay-Sachs disease, Sandhoff disease, and G_{M2} activator deficiency disease are, for the most part, indistinguishable. In fact, the initial discrimination of Sandhoff disease from Tay-Sachs disease is only accomplished by enzyme assay not by clinical differential. Infants with Tay-Sachs disease appear normal at birth. Symptoms usually begin with mild motor weakness by 3 to 5 months of age. Parents will begin to notice that their afflicted child has a dull response to outside stimuli. Another early symptom is an exaggerated startle response (sudden extension of arms and legs) to sharp sounds. By 6 to 10 months of age infants will begin to show regression of prior acquired motor and mental skills. It is the loss of these activities that will normally prompt parents to seek a medical opinion. A progressive loss in visual attentiveness may lead to an ophthalmological consultation which will reveal macular pallor and the presence of the characteristic "cherry-red spot" on the fundus of the eye (Figure 21-8). At around 8 to 10 months of age the symptoms of Tay-Sachs disease begin to progress rapidly. Infants are progressively nonresponsive to parental stimulation. The exaggerated startle response becomes quite pronounced. Most frightening to parents is the onset of seizures which initially can be controlled by antiseizure medication. However, the seizures become progressively more severe and are very frequent by the end of the first year. Psychomotor deterioration increases by the second year and invariably leads to decerebrate posturing (typical of patients in persistent vegetative states), difficulty in swallowing, and increased seizure activity. Ultimately, the patient will progress to an unresponsive vegetative state with death resulting from bronchopneumonia resulting from aspiration in conjunction with a depressed cough.

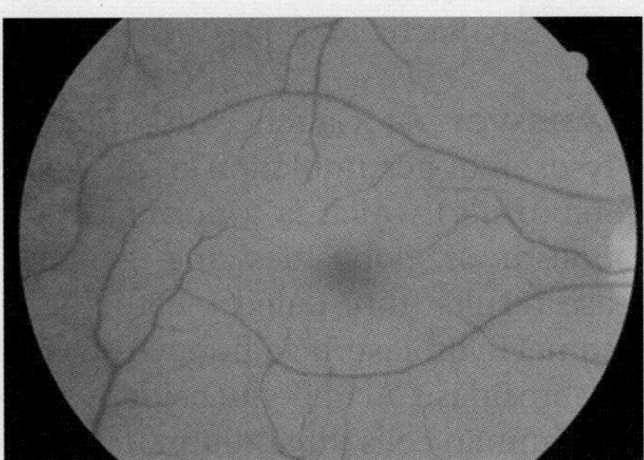

FIGURE 21-8: Typical "cherry red spot" associated with Tay-Sachs disease. Reproduced with permission of themedicalbiochemistrypage, LLC.

REVIEW QUESTIONS

1. The appearance of which of the following in the blood and/or urine would be predictive of a defect in glycosphingolipid metabolism?
A. gangliosides
B. glucocerebrosides
C. sphingomyelins
D. sphingosine
E. sulfatides

Answer B: Glucocerebrosides are only intermediates in the synthesis of complex gangliosides or are found at elevated levels only in disease states such as Gaucher disease, where there is a defect in the catabolism of the complex gangliosides. Thus, the presence of high concentrations of glucocerebrosides in cells such as monocytes and macrophages is indicative of a metabolic defect.

2. A loss of the ability to correctly process prosaposin into its functional peptides (saposins A, B, C, and D) would most likely result in which of the following disorders of complex glycolipid metabolism?
A. Gaucher disease
B. Niemann-Pick type C
C. Sandhoff disease
D. Tay-Sachs

Answer A: Gaucher disease is characterized by the lysosomal accumulation of glucosylceramide (glucocerebroside) which is a normal intermediate in the catabolism of globosides and gangliosides. Gaucher disease results from defects in the gene encoding the lysosomal hydrolase: acid β-glucosidase, also called glucocerebrosidase. Acid β-glucosidase exists as a homodimer in human cells. In addition to the enzyme itself, an active hydrolytic complex requires an additional activator protein, saposin C. The saposins (A, B, C, and D) are all derived from a single precursor, prosaposin. The mature saposins, as well as prosaposin, activate several lysosomal hydrolases involved in the metabolism of various sphingolipids. Prosaposin is proteolytically processed to saposins A, B, C, and D within lysosomes but also exists as an integral membrane protein not destined for lysosomal entry.

3. An impaired ability to look upward without raising the head is diagnostic of vertical supranuclear gaze palsy. This defect is associated with which of the following diseases?
A. Familial intrahepatic cholestasis type 1
B. Gaucher disease
C. G_{M2} activator deficiency
D. Krabbe disease
E. Niemann-Pick type C

Answer E: The characteristic phenotypes associated with "classic" NPC disease are variable hepatosplenomegaly, progressive ataxia, dystonia, dementia, and vertical supranuclear gaze palsy (VSGP). These individuals will present in childhood and death will ensue by the second or third decade. Because of the variable clinical phenotypes of NPC disease it has been subdivided into 5 presentation classifications: perinatal, early infantile, late infantile, juvenile, and adult. VSGP is a characteristic neurological manifestation in NPC disease being found in virtually all juvenile and adult cases of the disease.

4. The parents of a 7-month-old boy bring their son to the pediatrician because they have noticed that their child has a dull response to outside stimuli. In addition, they note that their child exhibits an exaggerated startle response (sudden extension of arms and legs) to sharp sounds and that he seems to be losing previously acquired motor and mental skills. The symptoms observed in this infant are most indicative of which of the following disorders?
A. Fabry disease
B. Farber lipogranulomatosis
C. Gaucher disease
D. Krabbe disease
E. Tay-Sachs disease

Answer E: Infants with Tay-Sachs disease appear normal at birth. Symptoms usually begin with mild motor weakness by 3 to 5 months of age. Parents will begin to notice that their afflicted child has a dull response to outside stimuli. Another early symptom is an exaggerated startle response. By 6 to 10 months of age infants will begin to show regression of prior acquired motor and mental skills. It is the loss of these activities that will normally prompt parents to seek a medical opinion. A progressive loss in visual attentiveness may lead to an ophthalmological consultation which will reveal macular pallor and the presence of the characteristic "cherry-red spot" on the fundus of the eye.

5. The parents of an 18-month-old girl are alarmed at the rapid deterioration in her motor skills and the appearance of an engorged belly. They note that when their daughter tries to follow the movement of an object she thrusts her head in the direction of movement as if she cannot move her eyes from side to side. Physical and laboratory examination reveals hepatosplenomegaly, skeletal lesions, dry scaly skin, and lipid-laden foam cells that have the appearance of wrinkled paper when viewed under

a microscope. What is the most likely diagnosis in this infant?
A. Fabry disease
B. Gaucher disease
C. Krabbe disease
D. Niemann-Pick disease type B1
E. Tay-Sachs disease

Answer B: The hallmark of Gaucher disease is the presence of lipid-engorged cells of the monocyte/macrophage lineage with a characteristic appearance in a variety of tissues. These distinctive cells contain one or more nuclei and their cytoplasm contains a striated tubular pattern described as "wrinkled tissue paper." These cells are called Gaucher cells.

6. An 8-month-old infant is brought to his pediatrician because he has had difficulty in feeding and frequently vomits following feedings. The parents indicate that their son had been able to sit by himself but now is incapable of doing so. Upon examination the doctor notes that the infant has obvious hepatosplenomegaly and is emaciated. Additional physical signs include thin limbs. Examination of his eyes reveals a cherry-red spot in the central part of the retina. Analysis of monocytes indicates the presence of sphingomyelin-rich lipids. The clinical findings in this infant indicate he is suffering from which of the following disorders?
A. fucosidosis
B. Gaucher disease
C. G_{M2} activator deficiency
D. Niemann-Pick disease type A1
E. Tay-Sachs disease

Answer D: Niemann-Pick disease (NPD) comprises two distinct but related types of lipid storage disorder, termed type 1 and type 2. In addition, type 1 NPD comprises two subtypes, type 1A (NPA) and type 1B (NPB), both of which result from defects in acid sphingomyelinase. The type 2 forms of NPD lead to accumulations of abnormal LDL-cholesterol. NPA is a disorder that leads to infantile mortality. NPB is variable in phenotype and is diagnosed by the presence of hepatosplenomegaly in childhood and progressive pulmonary infiltration. Pathologic characteristics of the type 1 Niemann-Pick diseases are the accumulation of histiocytic cells that result from sphingomyelin deposition in cells of the monocyte-macrophage system.

7. An adult man suffered from stable angina pectoris for 15 years, during which time there was progressive heart failure and repeated pulmonary thromboembolism. On his death at age 63, autopsy disclosed enormous cardiomyopathy (1100 g), cardiac storage of globotriaosylceramide (11 mg lipid/g wet weight), and restricted cardiocytes. Which of the following lipid storage diseases would result in these clinical findings?
A. Fabry disease
B. Gaucher disease
C. Krabbe disease
D. Niemann-Pick disease type A1
E. Tay-Sachs disease

Answer A: Fabry disease is an X-linked disorder that results from a deficiency in α-galactosidase A. This leads to the deposition of neutral glycosphingolipids with terminal α-galactosyl moieties in most tissues and fluids. Most affected tissues are heart, kidneys, and eyes. The predominant glycosphingolipid accumulated is globotriaosylceramide [galactosyl-(α1→4)-galactosyl-(β1→4)-glucosyl-(β1→1')-cer amide]. With increasing age the major symptoms of the disease are due to increasing deposition of glycosphingolipid in the cardiovascular system. Indeed, cardiac disease occurs in most hemizygous males.

8. A 4-month-old boy presents with painful progressive joint deformity (particularly the ankles, knees, elbows, and wrists), hoarse crying, and granulomatous lesions of the epiglottis and larynx leading to feeding and breathing difficulty. Biopsy of the liver indicates an accumulation of ceramides. The observed symptoms and the results of the liver biopsy are indicative of which disease?
A. Farber lipogranulomatosis
B. fucosidosis
C. Gaucher disease
D. Metachromic leukodystrophy
E. Sandhoff-Jatzkewitz disease

Answer A: Farber lipogranulomatosis is characterized by painful and progressively deformed joints and progressive hoarseness due to involvement of the larynx. Subcutaneous nodules form near the joints and over pressure points. Granulomatous lesions form in these tissues and there is an accumulation of lipid-laden macrophages. Significant accumulation of ceramide and gangliosides is observed, particularly in the liver. If these compounds accumulate in nervous tissue there may be moderate nervous dysfunction. The illness often leads to death within the first few years of life, although milder forms of the disease have been identified.

9. Clinical evidence indicates aspirin is effective in the control of numerous chronic conditions such as atherosclerosis. One of the principal cardiovascular benefits from taking aspirin is due to its ability to reduce the incidence and severity of thrombotic episodes. The anticoagulant effect of aspirin occurs through its ability to inhibit which of the following activities?

A. cyclooxygenase
B. fibrin cross-linking by factor XIIIa
C. phospholipase A_2
D. thrombin binding to activated platelets
E. von Willebrand factor

Answer A: The synthesis of the cyclic eicosanoids (the prostaglandins and the thromboxanes) begins with the cyclization of arachidonic acid. This reaction is carried out by the enzyme prostaglandin endoperoxide synthetase. This enzyme has 2 distinct activities, cyclooxygenase and a peroxidase. The activity of the cyclooxygenase domain is inhibited by a class of compounds referred to as the NSAIDs. Aspirin is of this class of drug and, therefore, inhibits the cyclooxygenase activity. The inhibition of prostaglandin synthesis has a negative effect on the process of coagulation through a reduction in the production of TXA_2, a potent activator of platelet function. Aspirin also reduces the production of prostacyclin (PGI_2) by endothelial cells. PGI_2 is a vasodilator and an inhibitor of platelet aggregation. Since endothelial cells regenerate active cyclooxygenase faster than platelets, the net effect of aspirin is more in favor of endothelial cell–mediated inhibition of the coagulation cascade.

10. Which of the following occurs in the lipidosis known as Tay-Sachs disease?

A. ganglioside G_{M2} is not catabolized by lysosomal enzymes
B. phosphoglycerides accumulate in the brain
C. synthesis of a specific ganglioside is decreased
D. synthesis of a specific ganglioside is excessive
E. xanthomas, due to cholesterol deposition, are observed

Answer A: In the genetic disorder known as Tay-Sachs disease, ganglioside G_{M2} is not catabolized. As a consequence, the ganglioside concentration is elevated many times higher than normal. The functionally absent lysosomal enzyme is β-*N*-acetylhexosaminidase (more commonly called hexosaminidase A). The elevated G_{M2} results in irreversible brain damage to infants, who usually die before the age of 3 years. Under normal conditions, this enzyme cleaves *N*-acetylgalactosamine from the oligosaccharide chain of this complex sphingolipid, allowing further catabolism to occur.

11. A 2-month-old infant suffering from increased vomiting and diarrhea is seen in the hospital and observed to have significant abdominal distention due to hepatosplenomegaly. Unfortunately, the infant does not survive. Autopsy reveals calcification of the adrenals and massive accumulation of cholesteryl esters and triglycerides in most tissues. Analysis of enzyme activity in fibroblasts and lymphocytes demonstrates a significant acid lipase (cholesteryl ester hydrolase) deficiency. These clinical findings are indicative of which of the following disorders?

A. hyperlipoproteinemia, type I (familial lipoprotein lipase deficiency)
B. I-cell disease (mucolipidosis type II)
C. Maroteaux-Lamy syndrome
D. Sanfilippo syndrome
E. Wolman disease

Answer E: Wolman disease results from a deficiency in the lysosomal acid lipase enzyme (also called cholesteryl ester hydrolase) and is very nearly always a fatal disease of infancy. Symptoms of the disorder arise from massive accumulation of cholesteryl esters and triglycerides in most tissues. Clinical manifestations include hepatosplenomegaly leading to abdominal distention, gastrointestinal abnormalities, steatorrhea, and adrenal calcification.

12. A 42-year-old man presents with hepatomegaly, jaundice, refractory ascites, and renal insufficiency. Peripheral leukocytes exhibit only 20% of normal glucocerebrosidase activity. Which of the following would explain his symptoms?

A. Fabry disease
B. Gaucher disease
C. Krabbe disease
D. Niemann-Pick disease type C2
E. Tay-Sachs disease

Answer B: Gaucher disease is characterized by the lysosomal accumulation of glucosylceramide (glucocerebroside) which is a normal intermediate in the catabolism of globosides and gangliosides. Gaucher disease results from defects in the gene encoding the lysosomal hydrolase: acid β-glucosidase, also called glucocerebrosidase The hallmark feature of Gaucher disease is the presence of lipid-engorged cells of the monocyte/macrophage lineage with a characteristic appearance in a variety of tissues. These distinctive cells contain one or more nuclei and their cytoplasm contains a striated tubular pattern described as "wrinkled tissue paper." These cells are called Gaucher cells.

13. A 30-month-old child presents with coarse facial features, corneal clouding, hepatosplenomegaly, and exhibiting disproportionate short-trunk dwarfism. Radiographic analysis indicates enlargement of the diaphyses of the long bones and irregular metaphyses, along with poorly developed epiphyseal centers. Other skeletal abnormalities typify the features comprising dystosis multiplex. The child's physical stature and the analysis of bone development indicate the child is suffering from which of the following disorders?

A. Hunter syndrome
B. Hurler syndrome
C. Maroteaux-Lamy syndrome
D. Morquio syndrome type B
E. Sanfilippo disease type A

Answer B: Although multiorgan involvement, liver and spleen enlargement, and skeletal abnormalities are common to all the mucopolysaccharidotic (MPS) diseases, each encompasses features that allow for specific diagnosis. Hurler syndrome is characterized by progressive multiorgan failure and premature death. Hallmark features include enlargement of the spleen and liver, severe skeletal deformity, and coarse facial features (which are associated with the constellation of defects referred to as dystosis multiplex). The disease results from a defect in α-L-iduronidase activity, which leads to intracellular accumulations of heparan sulfates and dermatan sulfates. The accumulation of these GAGs (glycosaminoglycans) in Hurler syndrome patients severely affect development of the skeletal system leading, primarily, to defective long bone growth plate disruption.

14. Hypersensitive individuals have IgE to specific antigens (eg, pollen, bee venom) on the surface of their leukocytes (monocytes, macrophages, basophils, eosinophils). When these individuals are challenged with antigen, the antigen-IgE complexes induce synthesis and release of which of the following physiologically potent lipids?

A. arachidonic acid
B. leukotriene B_4
C. platelet-activating factor (PAF)
D. prostaglandin E_2
E. thromboxane A_2 (TXA_2)

Answer C: Platelet-activating factor is a unique complex lipid of the plasmalogen family. PAF functions in hypersensitivity, acute inflammatory reactions, and anaphylactic shock by increased vasopermeability, vasodilation, and bronchoconstriction. Excess production of PAF production may be involved in the morbidity associated with toxic shock syndrome and strokes.

15. A 10-year-old girl exhibits the following symptoms: marked hepatomegaly, variceal bleeding, chronic bilateral pulmonary infiltrates, chronic liver disease, hepatic encephalopathy, and only 5% of normal sphingomyelinase activity in peripheral blood leukocytes. What is the most likely diagnosis?

A. Fabry disease
B. Gaucher disease
C. Krabbe disease
D. Niemann-Pick disease type B1
E. Tay-Sachs disease

Answer D: Niemann-Pick disease (NPD) comprises two distinct but related types of lipid storage disorder, termed type 1 and type 2. In addition, type 1 NPD comprises two subtypes, type 1A (NPA) and type 1B (NPB), both of which result from defects in acid sphingomyelinase. The type 2 forms of NPD lead to accumulations of abnormal LDL-cholesterol. NPA is a disorder that leads to infantile mortality. NPB is variable in phenotype and is diagnosed by the presence of hepatosplenomegaly in childhood and progressive pulmonary infiltration. Pathologic characteristics of the type 1 Niemann-Pick diseases are the accumulation of histiocytic cells that result from sphingomyelin deposition in cells of the monocyte-macrophage system.

16. A 12-month-old female infant exhibits severe developmental delay with associated macrocephaly, dysmorphic facies, hypotonia, and hepatosplenomegaly. Clouding of the corneas is not evident. A pebbly ivory-colored lesion is present over the infant's back. The activity of iduronate sulfatase in the plasma is not detectable. These symptoms are indicative of which of the following diseases?

A. Hunter syndrome
B. Hurler syndrome
C. Maroteaux-Lamy syndrome
D. Morquio B syndrome
E. Sanfilippo A syndrome

Answer A: Although multiorgan involvement, liver and spleen enlargement, and skeletal abnormalities are common to all the mucopolysaccharidotic (MPS) diseases, each encompasses specific and unique features. Each different MPS is caused by defects in different enzymes which allows for specific diagnosis. Hunter syndrome is characterized by progressive multiorgan failure and premature death. Hallmark features include enlargement of the spleen and liver, severe skeletal deformity, and coarse facial features (which are associated with the constellation of defects referred to as dystosis multiplex). Unlike Hurler syndrome, whose symptoms are similar (but more severe), Hunter syndrome does not cause corneal opacities. Hunter syndrome results from a defect in iduronidate sulfatase activity and this activity can be measured in the plasma.

17. The parents of 6-month-old are alarmed at the apparent regression of their child's pyschomotor skills. The infant has had difficulty in feeding accompanied by recurrent vomiting. Examination reveals a protuberant abdomen with clear hepatosplenomegaly. Extremities are thin and emaciation is apparent. Opthalmologic examination reveals cherry-red maculae. Histochemical examination of the monocytic fraction of the plasma demonstrates the presence of lipid-laden foam cells engorged with sphingomyelin. These findings are indicative of which of the following disorders?

A. fucosidosis
B. Gaucher disease
C. G_{M2} activator deficiency
D. Niemann-Pick disease type A1
E. Tay-Sachs disease

Answer D: For the correct answer explanation see Question 6.

18. A 71-year old man was admitted to the hospital after getting very dizzy upon rising from the toilet seat. At that time his pulse was racing and he remembers that his stool looked very different than usual. Over the last 4 or 5 weeks before the incident, the patient self-medicated with high-dose ibuprofen 3 times a day to control some pain in his hips. What is the mechanism of action for nonsteroidal anti-inflammatory drugs (NSAIDs) to cause gastrointestinal bleeding?

A. they inhibit arachidonic acid synthesis
B. they inhibit bradykinin synthesis
C. they inhibit cyclooxygenase
D. they inhibit histamine synthesis
E. they promote prostaglandin synthesis

Answer C: Nonsteroidal anti-inflammatory drugs (NSAIDs) inhibit cyclooxygenase and consequently inhibit synthesis of prostaglandins. In the stomach, prostaglandins have a cytoprotective effect through inhibition of acid secretion, enhancement of mucosal blood flow, and stimulation of bicarbonate and mucus secretion. Inhibiting these processes can cause stomach ulcers and bleeding such as described in the case.

19. Lipoxygenase converts arachidonic acid to biologically active compounds called leukotrienes. Leukotrienes have been implicated in several disease entities, including allergic asthma, where they are presumed to mediate bronchoconstriction. Introducing leukotrienes into an airway would be expected to cause which of the following responses?

A. decreased airway resistance
B. decreased dead space volume
C. increased functional residual capacity
D. increased lung compliance
E. increased total lung capacity

Answer B: Bronchiole volume contributes to dead space volume, so increasing bronchoconstriction would decrease bronchiolar volume and thus decrease dead space volume. Bronchoconstriction is a major determinant of airway resistance to air flow.

20. You are studying the effects of serum lipoproteins, of the HDL type, on the migration of endothelial cells in culture. Whereas, in one preparation of HDL from wild-type mice you observe significant increases in cell migration, a preparation from a mutant mouse line shows no increase in migration. Knowing the effects of HDL-associated lipids, which of the following lipid classes is most likely to be missing from the mutant mouse HDL preparation?

A. ceramide
B. galactocerebroside
C. G_{M2} ganglioside
D. sphingomyelin
E. sphingosine-1-phosphate

Answer E: Hematopoietic cells and vascular endothelial cells are the major sources of the high plasma S1P concentrations. Lymphatic endothelial cells are also thought to secrete S1P into the lymphatic circulation. The majority of plasma S1P is bound to HDL (65%) with another 30% bound by albumin. Recent work has demonstrated that the ability of HDL to induce vasodilation and migration of endothelial cells as well as to serve a cardioprotective role in the vasculature is dependent on S1P. These studies suggest that the beneficial property of HDL to reduce the risk of cardiovascular disease may be due, in part, on its role as an S1P chaperone.

21. You are examining cells extracted from a squamous cell tumor of the neck and find that they metabolize palmitic acid at a reduced rate compared to cells isolated from normal tissue in the same region of the neck. Which of the following lipid metabolic enzymes is most likely expressed at reduced levels in the cancer cells relative to normal cells?

A. ceramide synthase 1
B. serine palmitoyltransferase
C. sphingomyelin synthase
D. sphingomyelinase
E. sphingosine kinase

Answer B: The initiation of the synthesis of the sphingoid bases (sphingosine, dihydrosphingosine, and ceramides) takes place via the condensation of palmitoyl-CoA and serine. This reaction is catalyzed by serine palmitoyltransferase (SPT). SPT is the rate-limiting enzyme of the sphingolipid biosynthesis pathway. Reduced activity of SPT would result in reduced synthesis of ceramides. Although decreased ceramide synthase 1 activity is associated with more aggressive types of head and neck cancers, it is SPT that utilizes palmitic acid as a substrate and, thus, reduced SPT activity would be associated with reduced palmitate metabolism in these cells.

22. Which of the following lipids would most likely result in a reduced response of adipocytes to the actions of insulin?

- **A.** ceramides
- **B.** galactocerebroside
- **C.** GM_1 gangliosides
- **D.** sphingomyelins
- **E.** sphingosine-1-phosphate

Answer A: The ability of ceramides to interfere with insulin receptor signaling is the result of blocking the receptors ability to activate the downstream effector kinase, PKB/Akt. Experiments in cell culture, involving both adipocytes and skeletal muscle cells, have shown that ceramides inhibit insulin-stimulated glucose uptake by blocking translocation of GLUT4 to the plasma membrane as well as interfering with glycogen synthesis, as well as glycogen synthesis. That blockade of PKB/Akt activation is central to the effects of ceramides can be demonstrated by constitutive overexpression of PKB/Akt which negates the effects of ceramides.

23. Studies with a new cell line, derived from a cancerous tumor, reveal that normal responses to apoptotic signals to TNF-α are absent or significantly reduced when compared to normal cells from the same tissue. Further analysis reveals that the cells take up serine and palmitic acid when added to the culture media. Analysis of the levels of sphingosine show that they fluctuate with the same kinetics in both tumor-derived and normal cells. Which of the following sphingolipid metabolizing enzymes is most likely to be missing or significantly reduced in the tumor cells to explain the observations obtained?

- **A.** acid sphingomyelinase
- **B.** ceramidase
- **C.** hexosaminidase A
- **D.** serine palmitoyltransferase
- **E.** sphingosine kinase

Answer A: Ceramides play a role in apoptotic processes via the activation of the aspartate protease cathepsin D. Cathepsin D is associated with membranes and when activated by ceramides is released to the cytosol where it triggers the mitochondrial apoptosis pathway. Further evidence for the role of ceramides in negative growth responses is seen in cell cultures to which ceramide analogues are added. These types of assays demonstrate that ceramides induce oxidative stress, growth arrest, and apoptosis and/or necrosis. When derived from the sphingomyelins, ceramides are the products of the action of acid sphingomyelinase (ASMase). The importance of sphingomyelin as a source of ceramide can be evidenced by the fact that the activation of the ASAase pathway is a shared response to the effects of cytokines, stress, radiation, chemotherapeutic drugs, and pathogenic and cytotoxic agents. Several receptor- and non–receptor-mediated pathways, activated in response to stress such as those involving death ligands like TNF-α, are coupled to the activation of ASMase activity. The induction of ASMase in response to apoptotic triggers results in increased production of ceramides which then can initiate aspects of the apoptosis pathway.

24. All sphingolipid storage diseases are the result of an abnormality in which of the following processes?

- **A.** biosynthesis of cerebrosides in the Golgi complex
- **B.** biosynthesis of gangliosides in the ER
- **C.** lipid trafficking among membranes
- **D.** lysosomal catabolism of ceramide lipids
- **E.** processing of glycolipids in the Golgi complex

Answer D: The sphingolipid storage diseases are all members of the family of lysosomal storage diseases. All sphingolipids (glycosphingolipids and sphingomyelins) contain a backbone formed from polar head group attachment to ceramides. Thus, defects in lysosomal hydrolases that result in sphingolipid storage diseases are all due to the inability to fully degrade ceramide lipids.

25. A 7-month-old girl exhibits an exaggerated startle response, has decreased muscle tone, and demonstrates a loss of hearing. Previously attained developmental milestones appear to be disappearing in this infant. Physical and biochemical examinations show cherry-red spots on the retinas of both eyes and a significant reduction in hexosaminidase A activity. A diagnosis of Tay-Sachs disease is made. Which of the following properties of the lipid substrate for the deficient enzyme is the most likely cause of these symptoms?

- **A.** accumulation in cells
- **B.** failure to enter cells
- **C.** failure to form a physiologically required product
- **D.** failure to interact with a cell membrane receptor
- **E.** shunting via minor metabolic pathways

Answer A: Tay-Sachs disease is a member of a family of disorders identified as the G_{M2} gangliosidoses. The G_{M2} gangliosidotic diseases are severe psychomotor developmental disorders caused by the inability to properly degrade membrane-associated gangliosides of the G_{M2} family which then accumulate within the lysosomes of cells. Because neural cell membranes are enriched in G_{M2} gangliosides, the inability to degrade this class of sphingolipid results in neural cell death.

Checklist

✓ Sphingolipids are a class of lipid that includes the sphingomyelins and glycosphingolipids (the cerebrosides, sulfatides, globosides, and gangliosides). Sphingomyelin is the only sphingolipid class that is also phospholipid.

✓ Sphingosine is an amino alcohol that serves as the backbone of the ceramides and sphingolipids. Sphingosine is synthesized from palmitoyl-CoA and serine in a reaction initiated by serine palmitoyltransferase (SPT). SPT represents the rate-limiting step in shingolipid synthesis.

✓ Ceramides and sphingosine can be interconverted through the actions of ceramidases and ceramide synthases (CerS). Humans express 6 distinct CerS genes. Sphingomyelins and ceramides can also be interconverted via the actions of sphingomyelin synthases and sphingomyelinase.

✓ Each CerS exhibits fatty acyl chain length specificity as well as differential tissue distribution.

✓ Cellular levels of ceramides depend on a balance between the need for sphingosine and sphingosine derivatives, such as sphingosine-1-phosphate (S1P), and the sphingomyelins.

✓ Increased levels of ceramides can induce insulin resistance by blocking the ability of the insulin receptor to activate the downstream kinase, PKB/Akt. Conversely, reduced synthesis of ceramides is associated with increased growth of certain types of cancers, whereas, enhanced expression of CerS1, in particular, is associated with increased efficacy of chemotherapeutic drugs.

✓ The glycosphingolipids are major constituents of all cellular membranes and they are the major glycans of the vertebrate brain, where more than 80% of glycoconjugates are in the form of glycosphingolipids.

✓ Sphigosine-1-phosphate (S1P) is a major biologically active lysophosholipid. S1P is derived by phosphorylation of sphingosine by 2 distinct sphingosine kinases. S1P binds to, and activates, 5 functionally distinct G-protein–coupled receptors, eliciting activities that include involvement in vascular system and central nervous system development, viability and reproduction, immune cell trafficking, cell adhesion, cell survival and mitogenesis, stress responses, tissue homeostasis, angiogenesis, and metabolic regulation.

✓ Defects in lysosomal hydrolases, responsible for the degradation of membrane sphigolipids, results in potentially devastating clinical consequences. The disorders that arise due to these enzyme defects are referred to as lysosomal storage diseases.

CHAPTER 22 Lipids: The Eicosanoids: Prostaglandins, Leukotrienes, and Thromboxanes

CHAPTER OUTLINE

High-Yield Terms

Eicosanoids: a family of bioactive lipids derived via the oxidation of 20-carbon omega-3 or omega-6 polyunsaturated fatty acids, such as prostaglandins, thromboxanes, and leukotrienes

Cyclic pathway: describes the pathway, initiated by prostaglandin G/H synthase, *PGS* (also called *prostaglandin endoperoxide synthetase*), for the synthesis of arachidonic acid-derived eicosanoids containing a cyclic moiety

Linear pathway: describes the pathway, initiated through the action of lipoxygenases (LOXs), for the synthesis of arachidonic acid-derived eicosanoids with linear structure

Cyclooxygenase (COX): common name for prostaglandin G/H synthase which possesses both cyclooxygenase and peroxidase activities, 2 principal COX enzymes exist in humans, COX1 and COX2

Peptidoleukotrienes: also called the cysteinyl leukotrienes, LTC_4, LTD_4, LTE_4, and LTF_4 constitute this group of eicosanoids because of the presence of amino acids

Slow-reacting substance of anaphylaxis (SRS-A): consists of the leukotrienes LTC_4, LTD_4, and LTE_4, secreted by mast cells during anaphylactic reaction, induces slow contraction of smooth muscle resulting in bronchoconstriction

Introduction to the Eicosanoids

The principal eicosanoids consist of the prostaglandins (PG), thromboxanes (TX), leukotrienes (LT), and lipoxins (LX). The PG and TX are collectively identified as prostanoids. The nomenclature of the prostanoids includes a subscript number, which refers to the number of carbon-carbon double bonds that exist in the molecule. The majority of the biologically active prostaglandins and thromboxanes are referred to as series-2 molecules due to the presence of 2 double bonds. There are, however, important series-1 and series-3 prostaglandins and thromboxanes. The predominant leukotrienes are series-4 molecules due to the presence of 4 double bonds. Prostaglandins were originally shown to be synthesized in the prostate gland, thromboxanes from platelets (thrombocytes), and leukotrienes from leukocytes, hence the derivation of their names. The lipoxins (see Chapter 24) are anti-inflammatory lipids synthesized through *lipox*ygenase *in*teractions (hence the derivation of the name).

Overall, the various eicosanoids can be divided into 3 distinct groups dependent upon the source of origin. The series-1 and -3 prostanoids (and related leukotrienes) are derived from dietary intake of linoleic acid and α-linolenic acid (ALA), respectively, whereas the series-3 prostanoids (and series-4 leukotrienes and the lipoxins) are derived from arachidonic acid released from membrane phospholipids (Figure 22-1).

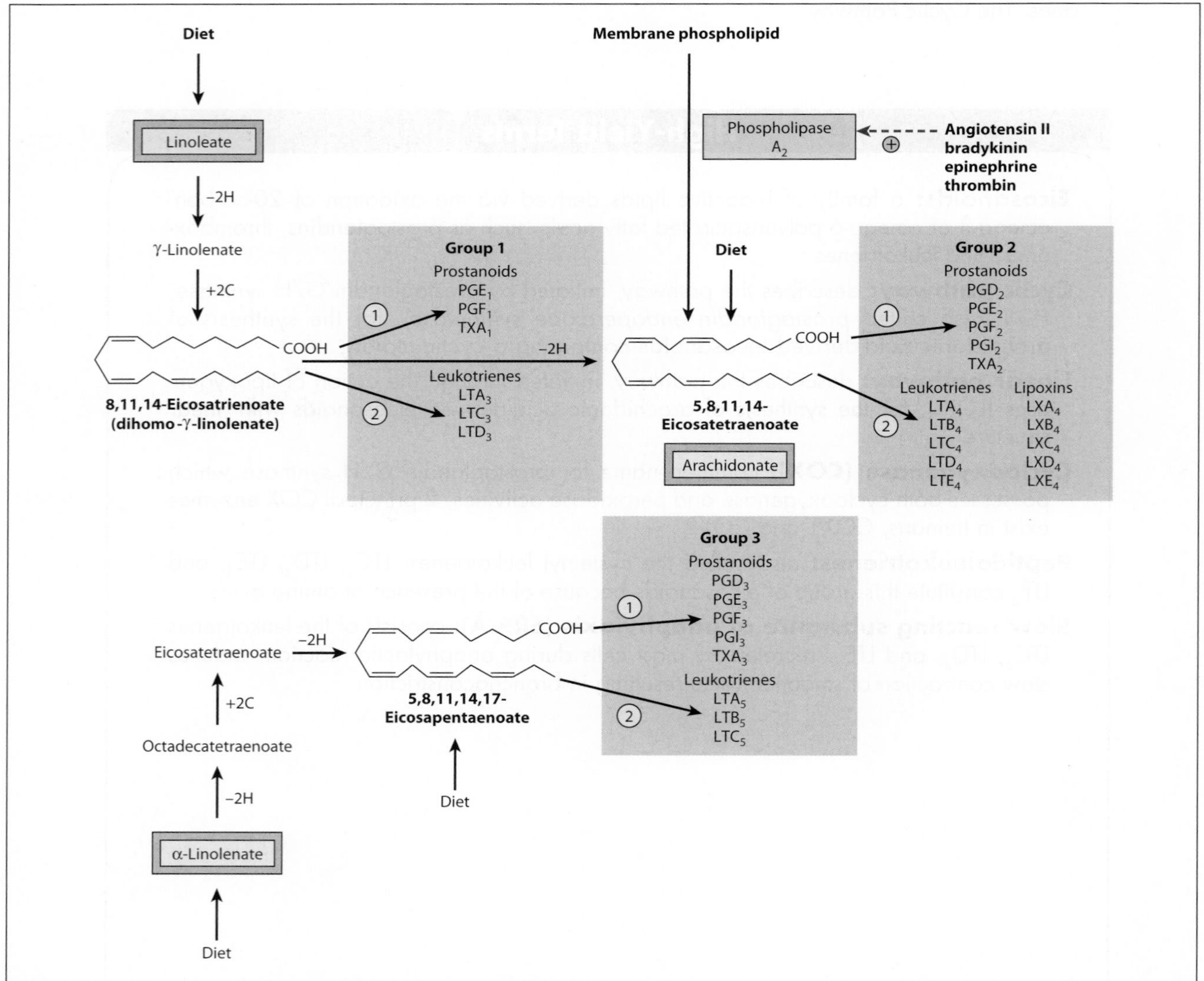

FIGURE 22-1: The 3 groups of eicosanoids and their biosynthetic origins. (①, cyclooxygenase pathway; ②, lipoxygenase pathway; LT, leukotriene; LX, lipoxin; PG, prostaglandin; PGI, prostacyclin; TX, thromboxane.) The subscript denotes the total number of double bonds in the molecule and the series to which the compound belongs. Murray RK, Bender DA, Botham KM, Kennelly PJ, Rodwell VW, Weil PA. *Harper's Illustrated Biochemistry*, 29th ed. New York, NY: McGraw-Hill; 2012.

High-Yield Concept

The eicosanoids produce a wide range of biological effects on inflammatory responses (predominantly those of the joints, skin, and eyes), on the intensity and duration of pain and fever, and on reproductive function (including the induction of labor). They also play important roles in inhibiting gastric acid secretion, regulating blood pressure through vasodilation or constriction, and inhibiting or activating platelet aggregation and thrombosis.

Arachidonic Acid Synthesis

The principal eicosanoids of biological significance to humans are a group of molecules derived from the C_{20} omega-6 polyunsaturated fatty acid (PUFA), that is, arachidonic acid. Additional biologically significant eicosanoids are derived from dihomo-γ-linolenic acid (DGLA), which is produced in the reaction pathway leading to arachidonic acid from linoleic acid. Within the cell, arachidonic acid resides predominantly at the C-2 position of membrane phospholipids and is released upon the activation of PLA_2 (see Chapter 20).

The immediate dietary precursor of arachidonate is linoleic acid, the essential fatty acid. Linoleic acid is converted to arachidonic acid through a series of 3 reactions (Figure 22-2). The activity of the Δ^6-desaturase is slow and can be further compromised due to nutritional deficiencies as well as during inflammatory conditions. Therefore, maximal capacity for synthesis of arachidonic acid occurs with ingested γ-linolenic acid (GLA), the product of the Δ^6-desaturase. GLA is converted to dihomo-γ-linolenic acid (DGLA) and then to arachidonic acid. Like the Δ^6-desaturase, the activity of the Δ^5-desaturase is limiting in arachidonic acid synthesis and its activity is also influenced by diet and environmental factors. Due to the limited activity of the Δ^5-desaturase, most of the DGLA formed from GLA is inserted into membrane phospholipids at the same C-2 position as for arachidonic acid.

Synthesis of Prostaglandins and Thromboxanes: The Cyclic Pathway

All mammalian cells except erythrocytes synthesize eicosanoids. These molecules are extremely potent; able to cause profound physiological effects at very dilute concentrations. All eicosanoids function locally at the site of synthesis, through receptor-mediated G-protein–coupled receptor (GPCR) signaling pathways. Two main pathways are involved in the biosynthesis of eicosanoids. The prostaglandins and thromboxanes are synthesized by the cyclic pathway (Figure 22-3), the leukotrienes by the linear pathway (Figure 22-4).

The cyclic pathway is initiated through the action of prostaglandin G/H synthase, *PGS* (also called *prostaglandin endoperoxide synthetase*). This enzyme possesses 2 activities, cyclooxygenase (COX) and peroxidase. There are 2 forms of the COX activity in humans. COX-1 (PGS-1) is expressed constitutively in gastric mucosa, kidney, platelets, and vascular endothelial cells. COX-2 (PGS-2) is inducible and is expressed in macrophages and monocytes in response to inflammation. The primary triggers for COX-2 induction in monocytes and macrophages are platelet-activating factor, PAF and interleukin-1, IL-1. Both COX-1 and COX-2 catalyze the 2-step conversion of arachidonic acid to PGG_2 and then to PGH_2.

The linear pathway is initiated through the action of LOXs of which there are 3 forms, 5-LOX, 12-LOX, and 15-LOX. It is 5-LOX that gives rise to the leukotrienes. The leukotrienes are synthesized by several different cell types including leukocytes, mast cells, lung, spleen, brain, and heart (Table 22-1).

Biological Activities of the Major Eicosanoids

Each of the eicosanoids function via interactions with cell-surface receptors that are members of the G-protein–coupled receptor (GPCR) family. There are at least 9 characterized prostaglandin receptors. Receptors that bind the prostaglandin D family of lipids are called the *PGD receptors* and those that bind the E-family prostaglandins are called the *PGE receptors*. The receptor for prostacyclin (PGI_2) is called the *PC receptor*. There are 2 receptors that bind LTB_4 called BLT_1 and BLT_2. The peptidoleukotrienes, LTC_4, LTD_4, and LTE_4 (also called

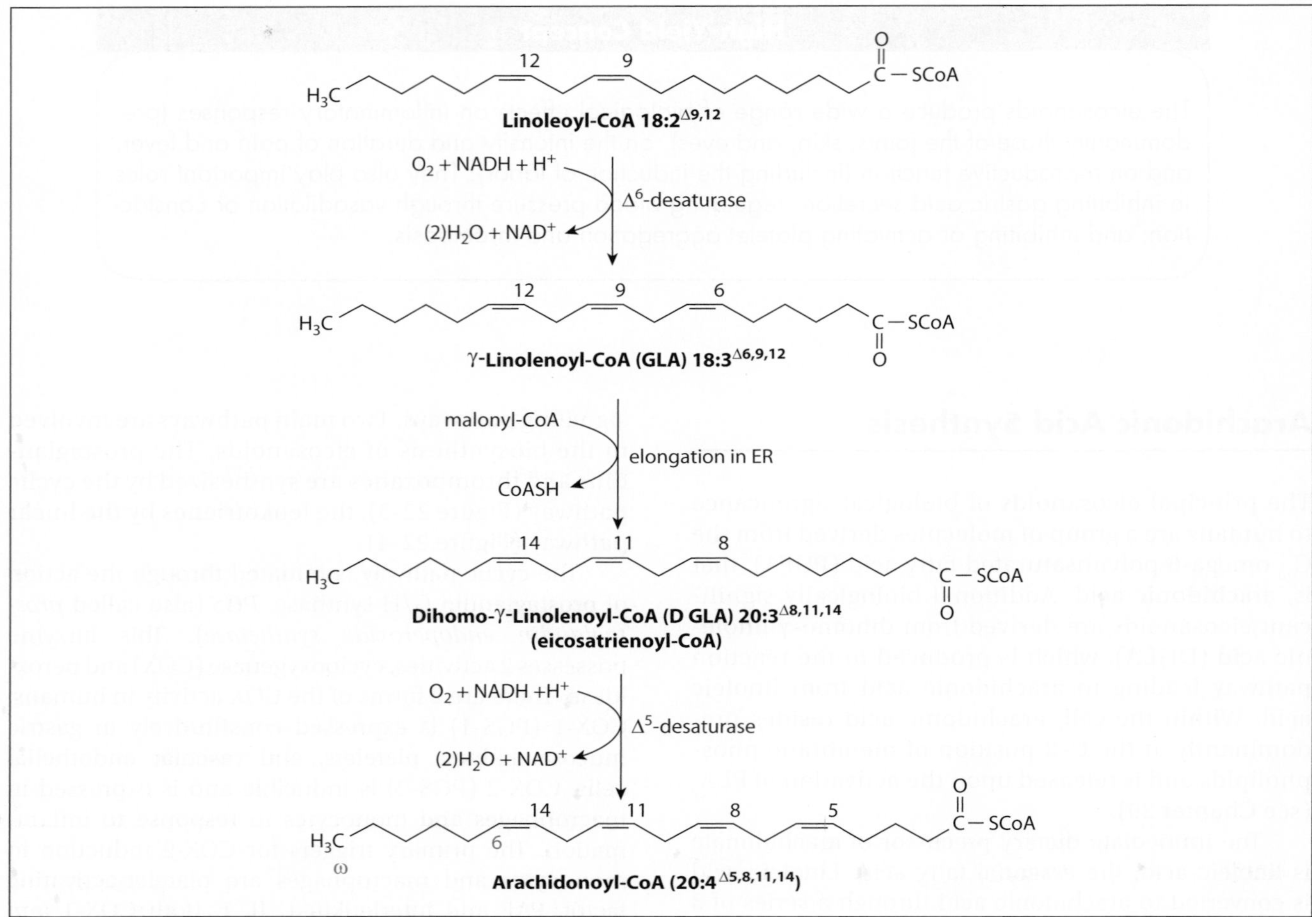

FIGURE 22-2: Synthesis of DGLA and arachidonic acid from linoleic acid. Reproduced with permission of themedicalbiochemistrypage, LLC.

the cysteinyl leukotrienes), bind to receptors called CysLT1 and CysLT2. The thromboxane receptor is called the TP receptor.

The major actions of the series-2 prostaglandins and thromboxanes (predominantly PGE_2 and TXA_2) are pro-inflammatory as are the series-4 leukotrienes (predominantly LTB_4). Thus, the use of drugs that reduce the production of these compounds would be beneficial at reducing inflammation and the associated vascular pathologies.

Aspirin is unique among the class of NSAIDs in that its actions on relief from pain (analgesia) and as an anti-inflammatory as well as a heart-protective drug are not solely due to its ability to inhibit COX activity. Because inhibition of COX-1 activity in the gut is associated with NSAID-induced ulcerations, drugs have been developed that are targeted exclusively against the inducible COX-2 activity (eg, celecoxib [Celebrex]). Another class of anti-inflammatory drug, the corticosteroidal drugs, act to inhibit PLA_2, thereby, inhibiting the release of arachidonate from membrane phospholipids and the subsequent synthesis of pro-inflammatory eicosanoids.

Research over the past 10 to 15 years has demonstrated the physiological benefits (ie, anti-inflammatory) of alternative pathways of polyunsaturated fatty acid metabolism. Much of the DGLA derived from ingested linoleic acid or GLA is diverted into membrane phospholipids due to the inefficiency of the Δ^5-desaturase catalyzing the conversion of DGLA to arachidonic acid. Incorporation of DGLA into membrane phospholipids competes with the incorporation of arachidonate so that diets enriched in GLA result in an alteration in the ratio of membrane arachidonate to DGLA. Release of membrane DGLA occurs through the action of PLA_2 just as for release of arachidonate. Once DGLA is released, it will compete with arachidonate as a substrate for the COX and LOX enzymes. The products of COX action on DGLA are series-1 prostaglandins (PGE_1) and thromboxanes (TXA_1).

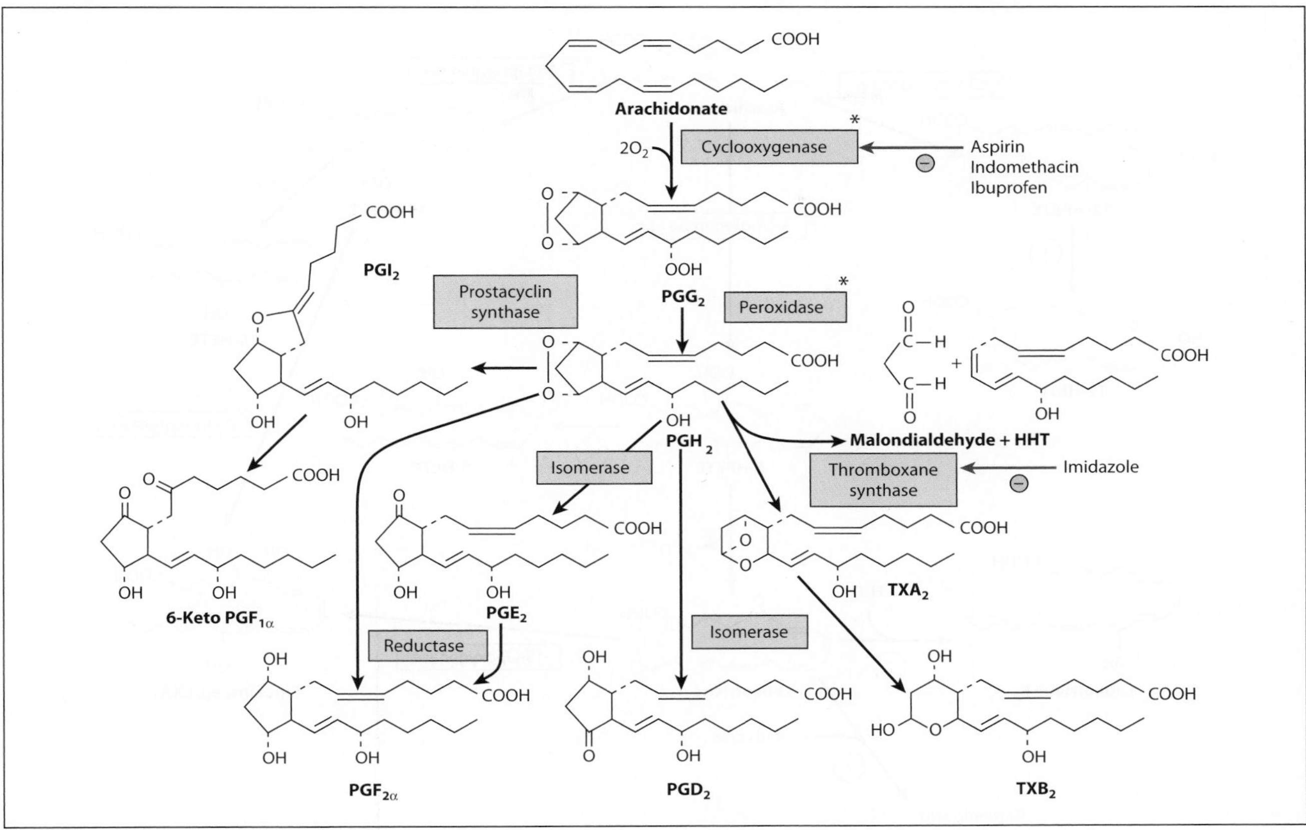

FIGURE 22-3: Conversion of arachidonic acid to prostaglandins and thromboxanes of series 2. (HHT, hydroxyheptadecatrienoate; PG, prostaglandin; PGI, prostacyclin; TX, thromboxane.) (*Both of these starred activities are attributed to the cyclooxgenase enzyme [prostaglandin H synthase]. Similar conversions occur in prostaglandins and thromboxanes of series 1 and 3.) Murray RK, Bender DA, Botham KM, Kennelly PJ, Rodwell VW, Weil PA. *Harper's Illustrated Biochemistry*, 29th ed. New York, NY: McGraw-Hill; 2012.

Although structurally similar, the series-1 eicosanoids have distinctly different biological actions. PGE_1 and TXA_1 are anti-inflammatory; they induce vasodilation and inhibit platelet aggregation. When DGLA is a substrate for 15-LOX, the product is 15-hydroxyeicosatrienoic acid (15-HETrE). 15-HETrE is a potent inhibitor of 5-LOX, which is the enzyme responsible for the conversion of arachidonic acid to LTB_4. LTB_4 is a potent inflammatory molecule through its action on neutrophils, thus, DGLA serves to inhibit inflammation via the linear eicosanoid pathway as well.

Because of the vasodilating action of PGE_1, it is used as a drug alprostadil pharmaceutically. Alprostadil is used clinically to treat newborn infants with ductal-dependent congenital heart disease. The administration of alprostadil in these infants maintains a patent ductus arteriosus until surgery can be carried out to correct the underlying

High-Yield Concept

A widely used class of drugs, the nonsteroidal anti-inflammatory drugs (NSAIDs) such as aspirin, ibuprofen, indomethacin, naproxen, and phenylbutazone all act upon the cyclooxygenase activity, inhibiting both COX-1 and COX-2.

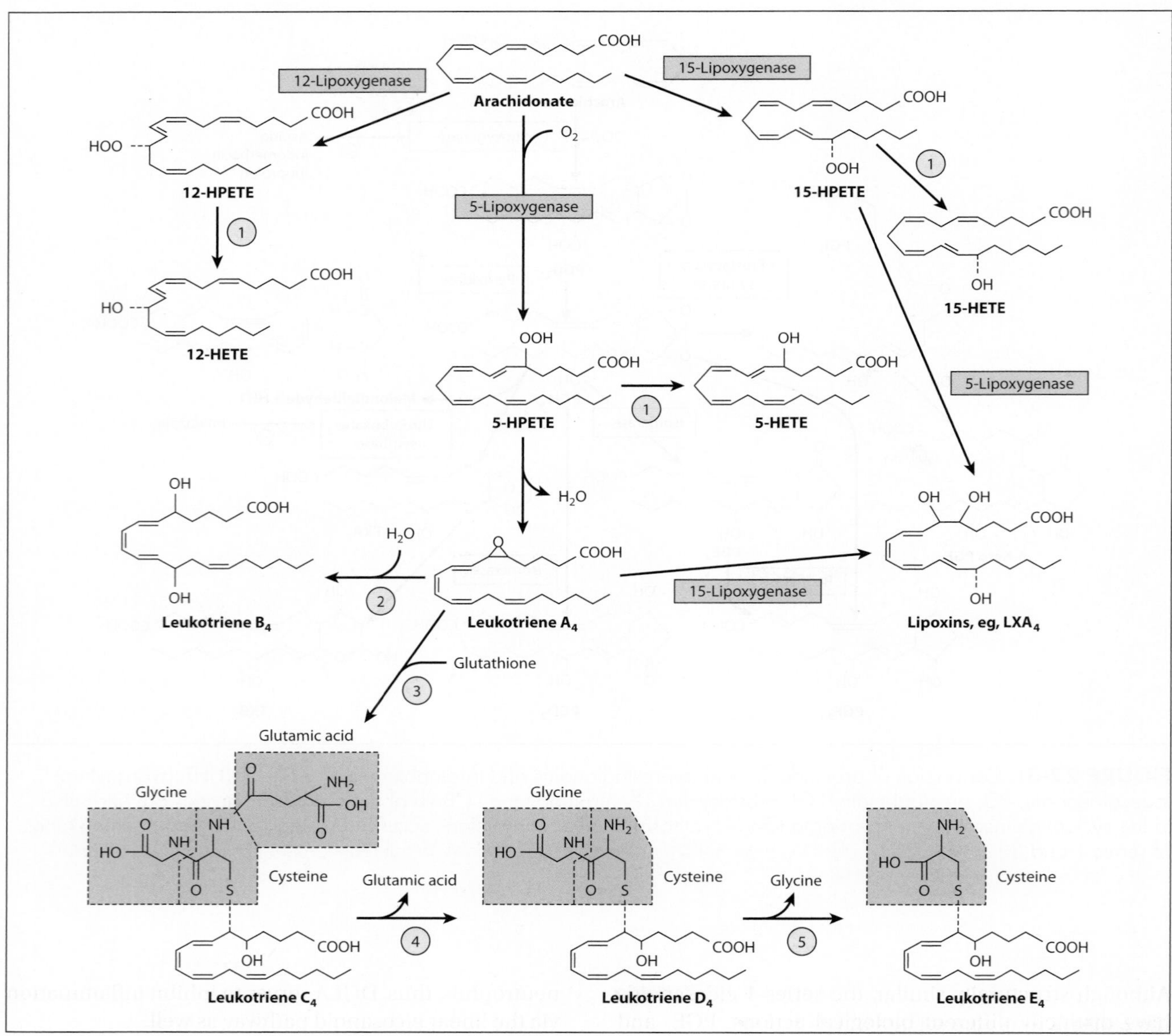

FIGURE 22-4: Conversion of arachidonic acid to leukotrienes and lipoxins of series 4 via the lipoxygenase pathway. Some similar conversions occur in series 3 and 5 leukotrienes. (①, peroxidase; ②, leukotriene A_4 epoxide hydrolase; ③, glutathione *S*-transferase; ④, γ-glutamyltranspeptidase; ⑤, cysteinyl-glycine dipeptidase; HETE, hydroxyeicosatetraenoate; HPETE, hydroperoxyeicosatetraenoate.) Murray RK, Bender DA, Botham KM, Kennelly PJ, Rodwell VW, Weil PA. *Harper's Illustrated Biochemistry*, 29th ed. New York, NY: McGraw-Hill; 2012.

heart defect. Ductus arteriosus is a normal structure of the fetal heart that allows blood to bypass circulation to the lungs since the fetus does not use his/her lungs in utero. The ductus arteriosus shunts blood flow from the left pulmonary artery to the aorta. Shortly after birth, the ductus closes due to the high levels of oxygen the newborn is exposed to at birth. However, in newborns with certain congenital heart defects, maintaining a patent ductus arteriosus is clinically significant. Alprostadil is also prescribed for the treatment of erectile dysfunction (ED) as MUSE and Caverject. MUSE is a urethral suppository and Caverject is an injectable version of the drug.

TABLE 22-1: Major Arachidonic Acid-Derived Eicosanoids

Eicosanoid	*Major Site(s) of Synthesis*	*Major Biological Activities*
PGD_2	Mast cells, eosinophils, brain	Induces inflammatory responses principally by recruiting eosinophils and basophils; induces bronchoconstriction; involved in androgenetic alopecia, inhibitors of PGD_2 being studied to treat male-pattern baldness
PGE_1		Induces vasodilation and inhibits platelet aggregation
PGE_2	Kidney, spleen, heart	Increases vasodilation and cAMP production, enhancement of the effects of bradykinin and histamine, induction of uterine contractions and platelet aggregation, maintaining the open passageway of the fetal ductus arteriosus; decreases T-cell proliferation and lymphocyte migration and secretion of IL-1α and IL-2
$PGF_2\alpha$	Kidney, spleen, heart	Increases vasoconstriction, bronchoconstriction, and smooth muscle contraction
PGH_2		Precursor to thromboxanes A_2 and B_2, induction of platelet aggregation and vasoconstriction
PGI_2	Heart, vascular endothelial cells	Inhibits platelet and leukocyte aggregation, decreases T-cell proliferation and lymphocyte migration and secretion of IL-1α and IL-2; induces vasodilation and production of cAMP
TXA_1		Induces vasodilation and inhibits platelet aggregation
TXA_2	Platelets	Induces platelet aggregation, vasoconstriction, lymphocyte proliferation, and bronchoconstriction
TXB_2	Platelets	Induces vasoconstriction
LTB_4	Monocytes, basophils, neutrophils, eosinophils, mast cells, epithelial cells	Powerful inducer of leukocyte chemotaxis and aggregation, vascular permeability, T-cell proliferation, and secretion of INF-γ, IL-1, and IL-2
LTC_4	Monocytes and alveolar macrophages, basophils, eosinophils, mast cells, epithelial cells	Component of SRS-A, microvascular vasoconstrictor, vascular permeability and bronchoconstriction, and secretion of INF-γ, recruitment of leukocytes to sites of inflammation, enhance mucus secretions in gut and airway
LTD_4	Monocytes and alveolar macrophages, eosinophils, mast cells, epithelial cells	Same as LTC_4
LTE_4	Mast cells and basophils	Same as LTC_4

SRS-A, slow-reacting substance of anaphylaxis.

REVIEW QUESTIONS

1. You are investigating a novel series 1 prostaglandin inhibitor on the activity of a section of femoral artery in culture. You have shown that the inhibitory compound directly interferes with the action of PGE_1. Which of the following activies is most likely reduced or absent in your organ culture system in the presence of this inhibitor?

- **A.** activation of 5-LOX for leukotriene synthesis
- **B.** enhancement of neutrophil adhesion
- **C.** induction of slow cardiac contraction
- **D.** platelet aggregation and activation
- **E.** relaxation of vascular smooth muscle cells

Answer E: PGE_1 is a series 1 eicosanoid derived from linoleic acid or γ-linolenic acid (GLA). This lipid induces vasodilation through relaxation of smooth muscle cells, exhibits anti-inflammatory activity, and inhibits platelet aggregation.

2. Cells isolated from the lungs of experimental mice via alveolar lavage are being studied for their responses to various lipid molecules. Results indicate that addition of arachidonic acid leads to increased production of PGE_2 but that LTA_4 is not detected. Which of the following

enzymes is most likely defective explaining the observed results?
A. COX-1
B. 5-LOX
C. LTC_4 synthase
D. prostacylin synthase
E. thromboxane synthase

Answer B: LTA_4 is an intermediate in the linear eicosanoid synthesis pathway. The linear pathway is initiated through the action of LOXs of which there are 3 forms: 5-LOX, 12-LOX, and 15-LOX. It is 5-LOX that gives rise to the leukotrienes. Therefore, loss of LTA_4 detection would most likley be due to loss of 5-LOX activity given that arachidonic acid was utilized effectively as a cyclic pathway (PGE_2) substrate.

3. You are studying the effects of a novel compound in a variety of vascular and immune system assays. Your results demonstrate that the compound exhibits actitivies very similar to a previously identified eicosanoid. These activities include inhibition of platelet and leukocyte aggregation, induction of smooth muscle relaxation, decreased proliferation of T cells, decreased lymphocyte migration, and decreased secretion of IL-1α and IL-2. Which of the following eicosanoids exhibits biological activities most closely resembling those of your test compound?
A. LTB_4
B. LTC_4
C. PGE_2
D. PGI_2
E. TXA_2

Answer D: Prostacyclin (PGI_2) is primarily synthesized by cardiac and vascular endothelial cells. Activities associated with this eicosanoid include inhibition of platelet and leukocyte aggregation, decreases in T-cell proliferation and lymphocyte migration and secretion of IL-1α and IL-2. Additional activities include smooth muscle relaxation leading to vasodilation.

4. You are examining the effects of an experimental compound on the activities of cultured sections of rat coronary artery. You determine that the compound exerts an effect identical to the natural prostaglandin, PGE_2 indicating that the compound is exerting which of the folllowing activities?
A. enhanced endothelial permeability
B. increased neutrophil adhesion
C. inhibited platelet adhesion
D. smooth muscle contraction
E. smooth muscle relaxation

Answer E: PGE_2 is one of the most potent eicosanoids and it exhibits multiple activities. These activities include the relaxation of smooth muscle cells resulting in increased vasodilation, enhancement of the effects of bradykinin and histamine, induction of uterine contractions and platelet aggregation, maintaining the open passageway of the fetal ductus arteriosus, decreasing T-cell proliferation and lymphocyte migration, and secretion of the cytokines, IL-1α and IL-2.

5. A 71-year old man was admitted to the hospital after getting very dizzy upon rising from the toilet seat. At that time, his pulse was racing and he remembers that his stool looked very different than usual. Over the last 4 or 5 weeks before the incident, the patient self-medicated with high-dose ibuprofen TID to control some pain in his hips. What is the mechanism of action for nonsteroidal anti-inflammatory drugs (NSAIDs) to cause gastrointestinal bleeding?
A. they inhibit arachidonic acid synthesis
B. they inhibit bradykinin synthesis
C. they inhibit cyclooxygenase
D. they inhibit histamine synthesis
E. they promote prostaglandin synthesis

Answer C: Nonsteroidal anti-inflammatory drugs inhibit cyclooxygenase and consequently inhibit (not promote, choice E) synthesis of prostaglandins. In the stomach, prostaglandins have a cytoprotective effect through inhibition of acid secretion, enhancement of mucosal blood flow, and stimulation of bicarbonate and mucus secretion. Inhibiting these processes can cause stomach ulcers and bleeding such as described in the case.

6. You are carrying out clinical studies aimed at determining the optimal nutritional requirements for the production of the series-2 prostaglandins. Your studies determine that this production can be met by the daily ingestion of approximately 10 g of which of the following fatty acids?
A. adipic
B. linoleic
C. palmitic
D. stearic
E. suberic

Answer B: Prostaglandins are synthesized from the 20-carbon polyunsaturated fatty acid, arachidonic acid, which itself is synthesized from the essential fatty acid, linoleic acid. Linoleic acid is termed an essential fatty acid because it contains sites of unsaturation that human tissues cannot introduce and the lipid must, therefore, be acquired in the diet.

7. In a healthy newborn soon after delivery, there is constriction of the ductus arteriosus. This process is most likely influenced by which of the following changes?

A. decreased serum calcium concentration
B. decreased serum glucose concentration
C. decreased serum prostaglandin concentration
D. increased serum calcium concentration
E. increased venous blood flow

Answer C: Due to the vasodilating action of PGE_1, it is used pharmaceutically as alprostadil to treat newborn infants with ductal-dependent congenital heart disease. The administration of alprostadil in these infants maintains a patent ductus arteriosus until surgery can be carried out to correct the underlying heart defect. Ductus arteriosus is a normal structure of the fetal heart that allows blood to bypass circulation to the lungs since the fetus does not use his/her lungs in utero. The ductus arteriosus shunts blood flow from the left pulmonary artery to the aorta. Shortly after birth, the ductus closes due to the high levels of oxygen the newborn is exposed to at birth. However, in newborns with certain congenital heart defects, maintaining a patent ductus arteriosus is clinically significant.

8. A 23-year-old woman has a severe viral respiratory infection. Her temperature is 38.9°C (102°F), but decreases after she takes aspirin. Which of the following is the most likely mechanism of action of aspirin in decreasing the fever?

A. activation of adenylate cyclase
B. blockade of the action of exogenous viral pyrogens
C. inactivation of lipoxygenase
D. inhibition of cyclooxygenase
E. prevention of mast cell degranulation

Answer D: The antipyretic (fever reducing) effects of aspirin are due to the ability of this drug to block the synthesis of pro-inflammatory and pyretic prostaglandins from arachidonic acid. The synthesis of the prostaglandins is initiated via the activity of PGS. This enzyme possesses 2 activities, COX and peroxidase. One of the actions of aspirin (acetylsalicylic acid) is the inhibition of the COX activity of PGS.

9. You are examining the effects of an experimental compound on the synthesis of series-2 prostaglandins. You find that addition of the compound to endothelial cells in culture results in the same level of inhibition as that observed for acetylsalicylate. These results indicate that the compound is inhibiting which of the following reactions of prostaglandin synthesis?

A. acetyltransferase reaction
B. desaturation reaction
C. hydrolytic reaction
D. hydroxylation reaction
E. oxygenation reaction

Answer E: The synthesis of the prostaglandins is initiated via the activity of PGS. This enzyme possesses 2 activities, COX and peroxidase. One of the actions of aspirin (acetylsalicylic acid) is the inhibition of the oxygenation activity of the COX portion of PGS and since the experimental compound exhibits the same activity, it is most likely the oxygenation reaction being inhibited.

Checklist

✓ The eicosanoids consist of the prostaglandins (PG), thromboxanes (TX), leukotrienes (LT), and lipoxins (LX) and are synthesized from 20-carbon essential omega-3 or omega-6 polyunsaturated fatty acids (PUFA).

✓ All mammalian cells, excepting erythrocytes, synthesize eicosanoids.

✓ Eicosanoids are extremely potent bioactive lipids, able to induce physiological effects at very dilute concentrations. All eicosanoids function locally at the site of synthesis, through binding to specific G-protein–coupled receptors.

✓ The omega-6 fatty acid, arachidonic acid, serves as a primary precursor lipid for the synthesis of bioactive eicosanoids. It is found esterified to the *sn*2 position of membrane phospholipids and is released upon receptor activation of PLA_2.

- ✓ Arachidonic acid synthesis is primarily initiated from the essential fatty acid, linoleic acid, but the pathway can also utilize dietary γ-linolenic acid (GLA).
- ✓ The primary prostaglandins and thromboxanes are synthesized from arachidonic acid via the cyclic pathway, which involves the enzyme PGS (more commonly called cyclooxygenase).
- ✓ The primary leukotrienes are synthesized from arachidonic acid via the linear pathway, which involves the enzyme 5-lipoxygenase (5-LOX).
- ✓ Dihomo-γ-linolenic acid (DGLA) is an intermediate in arachidonic acid synthesis that can be diverted into membrane phospholipids, where it competes with arachidonic acid. PLA_2-mediated release of DGLA results in synthesis of series-1 prostaglandins and thromboxanes, which mediate effects opposite to those of arachidonic acid-derived molecules.
- ✓ The nonsteroidal anti-inflammatory class of pharmaceutical drugs all function by blocking the cyclooxygenase activity of PGS.

CHAPTER

23 Lipids: Bioactive Lipids and Lipid-Sensing Receptors

CHAPTER OUTLINE

High-Yield Terms

Oleoylethanolamide: amide derivative of oleic acid synthesized by intestinal cells following intake in the diet, functions by binding to the fat-sensing receptor, GPR119

Lysophospholipid: represents a class of phospholipid generated via the removal of the fatty acid esterified to the *sn*1 or *sn*2 position of the glycerol backbone catalyzed by either PLA_1 or PLA_2, respectively

Bioactive Lipids and Lipid-Sensing Receptors

Until recently fats were considered mere sources of energy and as components of biological membranes. However, research over the past 10 to 15 years has demonstrated a widely diverse array of biological activities associated with fatty acids and fatty acid derivatives as well as other lipid compounds. Bioactive lipids span the gamut of structural entities from simple saturated fatty acids to complex molecules such as those derived from various omega-3 and omega-6 fatty acids and those derived from sphingosine. All bioactive lipids exert their effects through binding to specific receptors of the G-protein–coupled receptor (GPCR) family. Bioactive lipids play important roles in energy homeostasis, cell proliferation, metabolic homeostasis, and regulation of inflammatory processes.

Fatty Acids and Fatty Acid–Sensing GPCRs

Several novel GPCRs have been identified in recent years that have been shown to bind and be activated by free fatty acids and/or lipid molecules. Three tandemly encoded intronless genes on chromosome 19 were originally identified as *GPR40* (later also identified as free fatty acid receptor 1 [FFAR1]), *GPR41* (*FFAR3*), and *GPR43* (FFAR2). Subsequent to their isolation and characterization GPR40 was shown to bind and be activated by medium- and long-chain free fatty acids, whereas, GPR41 and GPR43 were shown to be activated by short-chain free fatty acids. GPR84 was identified as an orphan GPCR in a screen of differentially expressed genes in granulocytes. GPR119 and GPR120 were identified as a result of the human genome sequencing project and shown to be members of the rhodopsin-like family of GPCR (see Chapter 40).

GPR34: GPR34 belongs to the P2Y family of GPCRs to which other emerging newly identified lysophospholipid receptors, such as LPA_4/P2Y9/GPR23, LPA_5/GPR92, and LPA_6/P2Y5 belong. The natural ligand for GPR34 has recently been determined to be lysophosphatidylserine (lysoPS) which is the product of the action of phosphatidylserine (PS)-specific PLA_1 (PS-PLA_1) described below.

GPR35: GPR35 was first described to be activated by kynurenic acid (an intermediate in tryptophan catabolism that has neurotransmitter activity as an antiexcitotoxic and anticonvulsant) but is most likely the receptor for 2-arachidonyl lysophosphatidic acid (LPA). The emerging function of GPR35 demonstrates that it may be an important target involved in pain, heart disease, inflammatory bowel disease (IBD), cancer, and asthma. Expression of GPR35 is seen at highest levels in the stomach, small intestine, and colon. Expression, albeit at lower levels than in the GI, are seen in lung, uterus, spinal cord, and several types of white cells including basophils, eosinophils, mast cells peripheral monocytes, and macrophages.

GPR40: GPR40 is abundantly expressed in pancreatic β-cells and is also found in the gut in enteroendocrine cells. The preferred ligands for GPR40 are medium- to long-chain saturated fatty acids (C12-C16) as well as unsaturated fatty acids (C18-C22). GPR40 is coupled to a G_q protein that activates PLCβ upon ligand binding to the receptor. The activation of GPR40 in pancreatic β-cells results in increased cytosolic Ca^{2+} via IP_3-mediated release from the endoplasmic reticulum. The increased cytosolic Ca^{2+} can depolarize the β-cell leading to an influx of additional Ca^{2+} leading to increased secretion of insulin. This is an important mechanism by which fatty acids enhance glucose-stimulated insulin secretion (GSIS). A synthetic agonist for GPR40 is currently being tested as a potentially useful orally active antidiabetic drug.

GPR41 and GPR43: GPR41 and GPR43 are activated by short-chain fatty acids (SCFAs) such as propionic acid, butyric acid, and pentanoic acid. Both of these receptors are expressed at highest levels in adipose tissue and immune cells but are also found expressed in enteroendocrine cells of the gut. The activation of GPR41 and GPR43 is involved in adipogenesis and the production of leptin by adipose tissue. In the gut, GPR41 and GPR43 are involved in responses to SCFAs derived from gut microbiota metabolism of complex carbohydrates. Intestinal GPR41 plays a critical role in energy homeostasis and as well as control of feeding behaviors through the activated release of gut hormones such as PYY.

GPR55: GPR55 is a member of the rhodopsin-like family of GPCRs. Expression of GPR55 is highest in brain, GI system, adrenal glands, testis, endothelial cells, and numerous cancers. GPR55 was initially suggested to be a cannabinoid receptor for cannabinoid and endocannabinoid responses that are not mediated by the classical cannabinoid receptors: CB_1 and CB_2. Despite the fact that certain endocannabinoids, phytocannabinoids, and synthetic cannabinoids can act as GPR55 agonists or antagonists, the most potent GPR55 agonist characterized to date is 2-arachidonoyl lysophosphatidylinositol (LPI).

GPR84: GPR84 was originally shown to be activated by lipopolysaccharide (LPS) suggesting that medium-chain free fatty acids could be regulating inflammatory responses via interaction with GPR84. Subsequently it was demonstrated that GPR84 is a receptor for medium-chain free fatty acids such as capric acid (C10:0), undecenoic acid (C11:0), and lauric acid (C12:0). GPR84 is highly expressed in leukocytes.

GPR119: GPR119 is expressed at the highest levels in the pancreas and fetal liver with expression also seen in the GI tract, specifically the ileum and colon. GPR119 is a member of the class A family (rhodopsin-type) of GPCRs. GPR119 binds to long-chain fatty acids including oleoylethanolamide (OEA), lysophosphatidylcholine (LPC), various lipid amides, and retinoic acid. The role of GPR119 in metabolic homeostasis is described in more detail below in the section **Oleoylethanolamide**.

GPR120: Obesity and Diabetes

GPR120 is specifically activated by long-chain nonesterified fatty acids (NEFA), in particular in the intestines by α-linolenic acid (ALA). Activation of GPR120 in the intestines results in increased glucagon-like peptide 1 (GLP-1) secretion from enteroendocrine L cells (see Chapter 44). GPR120 is highly expressed in adipose tissue and pro-inflammatory macrophages. In contrast, negligible expression of GPR120 is seen in muscle, pancreatic β-cells, and hepatocytes. However, GPR120 is highly inducible in liver resident macrophage-like cells known as Kupffer cells.

Short-chain fatty acids are known to be pro-inflammatory and unsaturated fatty acids are generally neutral. In contrast the omega-3 polyunsaturated fatty acid (PUFA), DHA, and EPA exert potent anti-inflammatory effects through GPR120. The anti-inflammatory effects DHA and EPA activation of GPR120 are due to inhibition of both the Toll-like receptor (TLR) and tumor necrosis factor-α (TNF-α) inflammatory signaling pathways (Figure 23-1).

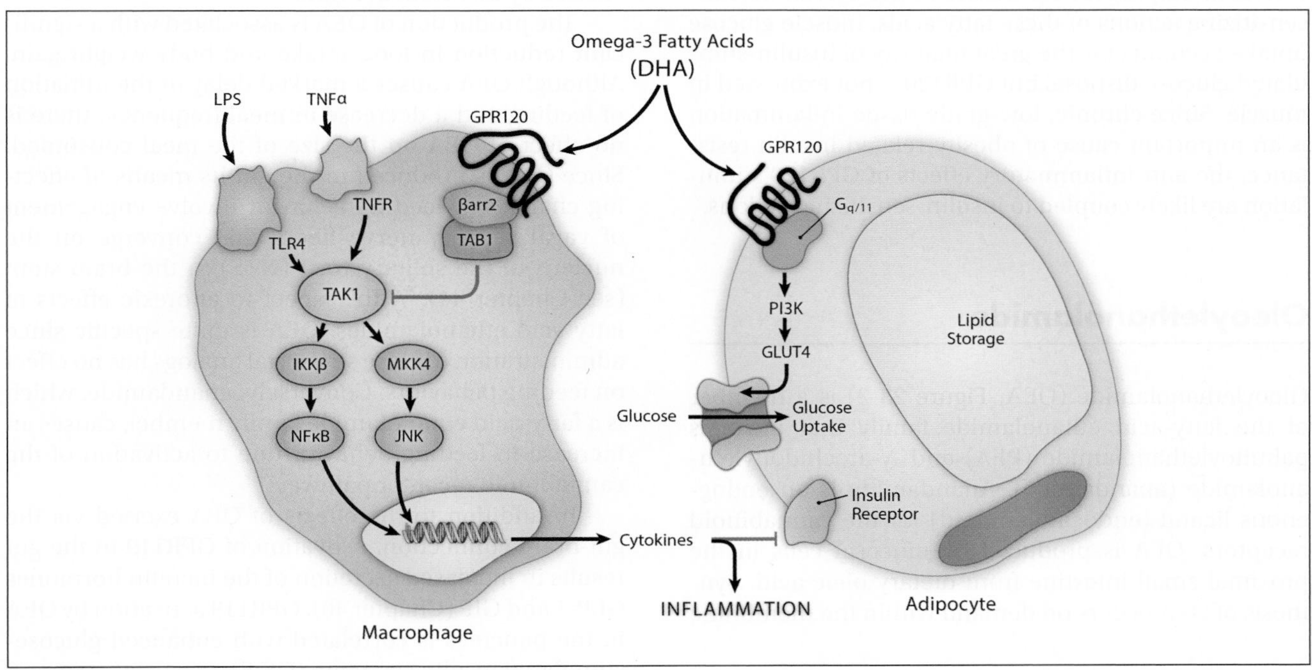

FIGURE 23-1: Diagrammatic representation of the signaling events initiated in response to DHA binding to GPR120 on macrophages and adipocytes. The mechanism of GPR120-mediated anti-inflammation involves inhibition of transforming growth factor-β–activated kinase 1 (TAK1) through a β-arrestin-2 (βarr2)–dependent effect. TAK1-binding protein (TAB1) is the activating protein for TAK1. Stimulation of GPR120 by DHA has been shown to inhibit both the Toll-like receptor 4 (TLR4) and TNF-α pro-inflammatory cascades via TAK1 inhibition. Activation of the kinases, inhibitor of nuclear factor kappa-B kinase subunit beta (IKKβ) and c-JUN *N*-terminal kinase (JNK), is common to TLR and TNF-α signaling. Nuclear factor kappa B (NFκB), one of the most important transcription factors regulating the expression of pro-inflammatory genes, is normally activated by IKKβ. JNK is normally activated by mitogen activated protein kinase kinase 4 (MKK4). The effects of GRP120 activation in macrophages are reduced secretion of pro-inflammatory cytokines which would normally interfere with insulin effects on adipose tissue. Within adipose tissue DHA-mediated activation of GRP120 results in enhanced mobilization of GLUT4 to the plasma membrane, thus, enhancing glucose uptake. Reproduced with permission of themedicalbiochemistrypage, LLC.

High-Yield Concept

Given the functions of omega-3 PUFAs in inflammation, insulin sensitization, and lipid profiles mediated through activation of GPR120 indicates that this GPCR is a critically important control point in the integration of anti-inflammatory and insulin-sensitizing responses, which may prove useful in the future development of new therapeutic approaches for the treatment of diabetes.

The TLRs are a class of noncatalytically active transmembrane receptors that are involved in mediating responses of the innate immune system.

DHA stimulation of GPR120 is also involved in glucose homeostasis in adipose tissue due to increased GLUT4 translocation to the cell surface with a subsequent increase in glucose transport into the cells. The effects of DHA on glucose uptake in adipocytes are additive to those of insulin. Although it is possible to propose that the insulin-sensitizing effects of omega-3 PUFAs in adipocytes contribute to the overall insulin-sensitizing actions of these fatty acids, muscle glucose uptake accounts for the great majority of insulin-stimulated glucose disposal but GPR120 is not expressed in muscle. Since chronic, low-grade tissue inflammation is an important cause of obesity-related insulin resistance, the anti-inflammatory effects of GPR120 stimulation are likely coupled to insulin-sensitizing actions.

Oleoylethanolamide

Oleoylethanolamide (OEA, Figure 23-2) is a member of the fatty-acid ethanolamide family that includes palmitoylethanolamide (PEA) and *N*-arachidonylethanolamide (anandamide). Anandamide is an endogenous ligand (endocannabinoid) for the cannabinoid receptors. OEA is produced by mucosal cells in the proximal small intestine from dietary oleic acid. Synthesis of OEA occurs on demand within the membrane of the intestinal mucosal cell by 2 concerted reactions. Metabolism of OEA occurs via hydrolysis to oleic acid and ethanolamine. Two enzymes are known to be responsible for OEA hydrolysis.

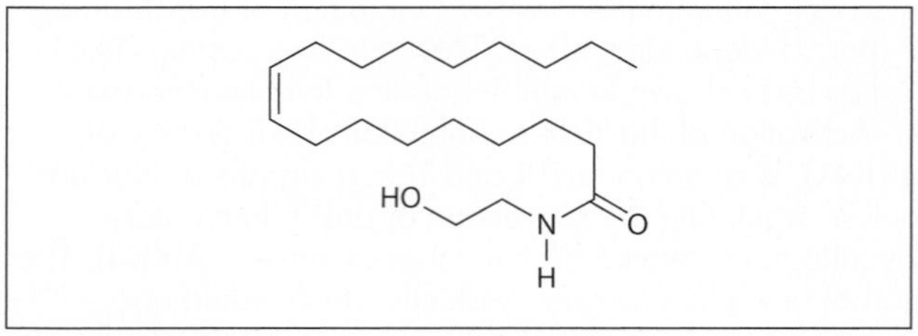

OEA has been shown to activate the fatty acid-sensing GPCR identified as GPR119 and to interact with intestinal FAT/CD36 for uptake from the gut. Indeed, OEA is the most potent ligand and likely represents the endogenous ligand for GPR119. However, its interaction with FAT/CD36 is required for the satiety response elicited by this bioactive lipid.

The production of OEA is associated with a significant reduction in food intake and body weight gain. Although OEA causes a marked delay in the initiation of feeding and a decrease in meal frequency, there is no effect of OEA on the size of the meal consumed. Since OEA is produced in the gut its means of effecting changes in feeding behavior involve engagement of vagal sensory nerve fibers that converge on the nucleus of the solitary tract (NTS) in the brain stem (see Chapter 44). With respect to anorexic effects of fatty acid ethanolamides, OEA is quite specific since administration of close structural analogs has no effect on feeding behaviors. Conversely, anandamide, which is a fatty-acid ethanolamide family member, causes an increase in feeding behavior due to activation of the cannabinoid receptor pathway.

In addition to the effects of OEA exerted via the gut-brain connection, activation of GPR119 in the gut results in increased secretion of the incretin hormones GLP-1 and GIP (Chapter 46). GPR119 activation by OEA in the pancreas is correlated with enhanced glucose-stimulated insulin secretion (GSIS).

HO N H O

FIGURE 23-2: Structure of oleoylethanolamide (OEA).

Biological Activities of Omega-3 and Omega-6 PUFAs

The metabolic and clinical significances of the omega-3 and omega-6 PUFAs are principally due to the ability of these lipids to exert effects on numerous biologically important pathways following binding to specific

High-Yield Concept

These observations indicate that GPR119 activation is associated with a dual mechanism of reducing blood glucose: acting directly through pancreatic β-cells to promote GSIS and in the gut via the stimulation of the incretins GLP-1 and GIP both of which increase insulin release from the pancreas in response to food intake. Currently there are several small molecule agonists of GPR119 in clinical trials being tested for their efficacy in treating the hyperglycemia of Type 2 diabetes as well as for their efficacy in treating obesity.

cell-surface receptors. When omega-3 and omega-6 fatty acids are consumed, they are incorporated into cell membranes in all tissues of the body. Because of this fact, dietary changes in the composition of PUFAs can have profound effects on cellular function because the membrane lipids serve as a source of precursors for the synthesis of important signaling molecules involved in cell growth and development as well as modulation of inflammation. Another important consequence of dietary alteration in fatty acid composition is the fact that omega-3 and omega-6 PUFAs compete for incorporation into cell membranes.

The most important omega-6 PUFA is arachidonic acid (Chapter 22). When cells are stimulated by a variety of external stimuli, arachidonic acid is released from cell membranes through the action of phospholipase A_2 (PLA_2). The released arachidonate then serves as the precursor for the synthesis of the biologically active eicosanoids, the prostaglandins (PG), thromboxanes (TX), leukotrienes (LT), and lipoxins (LX). The arachidonate-derived eicosanoids function in diverse biological phenomena such as platelet and leukocyte activation, signaling of pain, induction of bronchoconstriction, and regulation of gastric secretions. These activities are targets of numerous pharmacological agents such as the nonsteroidal anti-inflammatory drugs (NSAIDs), COX-2 inhibitors, and leukotriene antagonists.

Various eicosanoids are synthesized depending upon the source of the precursor PUFA. The dihomo-γ-linolenic acid (DGLA) that is synthesized from ingested linoleic acid or GLA can be diverted into membrane phospholipids due to the inefficiency of the Δ^5-desaturase catalyzing the conversion of DGLA to arachidonic acid. When DGLA is released from membrane phospholipids, it is a substrate for COX the same as arachidonic acid. However, the products of COX action on DGLA are series-1 prostaglandins which are anti-inflammatory, induce vasodilation, and inhibit platelet aggregation, effects opposite to those of series-2 prostaglandins derived from arachidonic acid.

Dietary omega-3 PUFAs compete with the inflammatory, pyretic (fever), and pain-promoting properties imparted by omega-6 PUFAs because they displace arachidonic acid from cell membranes. In addition, omega-3 PUFAs compete with the enzymes that convert arachidonic acid into the bioactive eicosanoids. The net effect of increasing dietary consumption of omega-3 PUFAs, relative to omega-6 PUFAs, is to decrease the potential for monocytes, neutrophils, and eosinophils (ie, leukocytes) to synthesize potent mediators of inflammation and to reduce the ability of platelets to release TXA_2, a potent stimulator of the coagulation process.

Probably the most important role of the omega-3 PUFAs, EPA, and DHA, is that they serve as the precursors for potent anti-inflammatory lipids called resolvins and protectins (Chapter 24). The resolvins exert their anti-inflammatory actions by promoting the resolution of inflammatory processes, hence the derivation of their name. The resolvins (Rv) are synthesized either from EPA or DHA. An additional anti-inflammatory lipid derived from DHA is protectin D1 (PD1).

The omega-3 fatty acids, DHA and EPA, have also been shown to be important for normal brain development and function. DHA is essential for proper development of the prenatal and postnatal central nervous system. The benefits of EPA appear to be in its effects on behavior and mood. In clinical studies with DHA and EPA there has been good data demonstrating benefit in treating attention-deficit hyperactivity disorder (ADHD), autism, dyspraxia (motor skills disorder), dyslexia, and aggression. In patients with affective disorders, consumption of DHA and EPA has confirmed benefits in major depressive disorder and bipolar disorder. Of significance to these effects of EPA and DHA on cognition, mood, and behavior is the fact that administration of omega-3 fatty acid–containing phospholipids (such as those present in Krill oils) are significantly better than omega-3–containing triglycerides such as those that predominate in fish oils.

Omega-3 PUFAs also regulate hepatic lipid metabolism via regulation of the expression of key enzymes involved in lipid synthesis and catabolism. Omega-3 PUFAs bind to and activate peroxisome proliferator–activated receptor-α (PPARα). Activation of PPARα results in activation of hepatic fatty acid oxidation.

Inhibition of hepatic fatty acid synthesis by omega-3 PUFAs is mediated by suppression of *SREBP-1c* gene expression, enhanced degradation of SREBP-1c mRNA, and increased proteosomal degradation of SREBP-1 proteins. The decrease in SREBP-1c expression results in a reduction in the expression levels of hepatic fatty acid synthase (FAS) and acetyl-CoA carboxylase (ACC), 2 critical enzymes of fatty acid synthesis. Because the liver plays a central role in whole-body lipid metabolism this regulatory process affects the lipid composition throughout the body, and therefore likely contributes to the onset and progression of several chronic diseases, including atherosclerosis, diabetes, and obesity.

Lysophospholipids

Lysophospholipids (LPL) are minor lipid components compared to the major membrane phospholipids such as phosphatidylcholine (PC), phosphatidylethanolamine (PE), and sphingomyelin. The LPL are generated via the actions of phospholipase A (PLA) enzymes on glycerophospholipids or sphingolipids. The LPL exert biological properties resembling those of extracellular growth factors or signaling molecules. The most biologically significant LPL are lysophosphatidic acid (LPA), lysophosphatidylinositol (LPI), lysophosphatidylcholine (LPC), sphingosine-1-phosphate (S1P; see Chapter 21), and sphingosylphosphorylcholine (SPC). Each of these LPL functions via interaction with specific GPCRs leading to autocrine or paracrine effects. The first LPL receptor identified was called LPA_1 because it bound LPA. Currently there are 15 characterized LPL receptors of which 6 are receptors for LPA.

Lysophosphatidic Acid

LPA, although being simple in structure, exerts a wide variety of cellular responses in many different cell types. LPA is produced by activated platelets, activated adipocytes, neuronal cells, as well as several other cell types. LPA is produced in the serum through the action of several different enzymes including monoacylglycerol kinase, phospholipase A_1 (PLA_1), secretory phospholipase A_2 ($sPLA_2$), and lysophospholipase D (lysoPLD). LPA is known to enhance platelet aggregation, smooth muscle contraction, cell proliferation and migration, neurite retraction, and the secretion of chemokines and cytokines. These effects of LPA are the result of binding to specific GPCRs. There are at least 6 characterized LPA receptors. LPA has also been shown to interact intracellularly with PPARγ. (Table 23-1)

Lysophosphatidylinositol

Lysophosphatidylinositol (LPI) is produced by numerous cell types and it exerts a wide range of biological effects. The receptor for LPI is the orphan GPCR identified as GPR55. However, additional studies have shown that LPI can bind and activate GPR119 which is also a receptor for OEA. Activation of GPR55 by LPI

TABLE 23-1: Lysophosphatidic Acid (LPA) Receptors

LPA Receptor	*Alternative Name*	*Gene Symbol*	*G-Proteins*	*Comments*
LPA_1	EDG2	*LPAR1*	$G_{i/o}$, G_q, $G_{12/13}$	Expressed in a wide variety of tissues; highest expression seen in brain, heart, stomach, intestines, kidney
LPA_2	EDG4	*LPAR2*	$G_{i/o}$, G_q, $G_{12/13}$	Highest levels of expression in the testes and in leukocytes; also in prostate, spleen, thymus, and pancreas
LPA_3	EDG7	LPAR3	$G_{i/o}$, G_q	Highest expression in the testes, pancreas, prostate, and heart
LPA_4	P2Y9, GPR23	*LPAR4*	G_s, $G_{i/o}$, G_q, $G_{12/13}$	Low expression in several tissues, high expression only in ovary
LPA_5	GPR92	*LPAR5*	G_q, $G_{12/13}$; possibly also G_s	More restricted pattern of expression that other LPARs, highest level seen in spleen
LPA_6	P2Y5	*LPAR6*	$G_{12/13}$	Expressed in a wide variety of tissues

binding results in increased insulin release from the pancreas, arterial contraction, and the proliferation and migration of several cell types. In addition, LPI induces calcium flux in hepatic mitochondria. In cancer cells, cytoplasmic phospholipase A_2 ($cPLA_2$) synthesizes a pool of LPI that is transported from the cell via the action of the ABCC1 transporter (see Chapter 7). Once released, LPI binds to GPR55 and activates a signaling cascade resulting in increased proliferation. Of significance is the fact that when GPR55 is downregulated in ovarian and pancreatic cancer cell lines their proliferation is inhibited.

REVIEW QUESTIONS

1. The omega-3 class of polyunsaturated fatty acids (PUFAs) exerts potent effects on neural development, cardiovascular function, and inflammation. The most active omega-3 PUFAs are DHA and EPA. These PUFA are precursors for which of the following class of biologically active lipids?

A. gangliosides
B. leukotrienes
C. prostaglandins
D. resolvins
E. thromboxanes

Answer D: The resolvins (Rv) have anti-inflammatory actions that lead to the resolution of the inflammatory processes, hence the derivation of their names as resolvins (resolution phase interaction products). The resolvins are synthesized either from eicosapentaenoic acid (EPA) or from docosahexaenoic (DHA). The D-series resolvins are derived from DHA and the E-series from EPA.

2. You are testing the activity of a fatty acid analog for efficacy in the treatment of the hyperglycemia associated with Type 2 diabetes. You find that inclusion of the compound in the diet of these test subjects results in an increased release of the gut hormone GLP-1. Which of the following fatty acid–binding receptors is most likely activated by your compound in the gut of the test subjects accounting for the observed response?

A. GPR35
B. GPR40
C. GPR41
D. GPR55
E. GPR120

Answer E: GPR120 is specifically activated by long-chain nonesterified fatty acids (NEFAs), in particular in the intestines by α-linolenic acid (ALA), an omega-3 polyunsaturated fatty acid (PUFA). Activation of GPR120 in the intestines results in increased GLP-1 secretion from enteroendocrine L cells.

3. You are testing a novel lipid molecule for its activity on vascular function in experimental animals. Your results demonstrate that the compound induces vasodilation by causing relaxation of smooth muscle. It also enhances platelet aggregation. These results indicate that your compound is most likely mimicking the effects of which of the following lipids?

A. docosahexaenoic acid, DHA
B. eicosapentaenoic acid, EPA
C. lysophosphatidic acid, LPA
D. lysophosphatidylinositol, LPI
E. oleoylethaolamide, OEA

Answer C: LPA, although being simple in structure, exerts a wide variety of cellular responses in many different cell types. LPA is known to enhance platelet aggregation, smooth muscle contraction, cell proliferation and migration, neurite retraction, and the secretion of chemokines and cytokines. The effects of LPA are the result of binding to at least 6 specific GPCRs (LPA_1-LPA_6).

4. Lysophosphatidylinositol (LPI) has been shown to induce an increase in pancreatic insulin secretion. This effect is due to increasing intracellular calcium concentration. This effect of LPI is exerted by its binding to and activating which of the following receptors?

A. GPR35
B. GPR40
C. GPR41
D. GPR55
E. GPR120

Answer D: The primary receptor for LPI is GPR55 although additional studies have shown that LPI can also bind and activate GPR119. LPI activation of GPR55 results in increased intracellular calcium concentrations. This effect of LPI is associated with increased insulin release from the pancreas, arterial contraction, and the proliferation and migration of several cell type. In addition, LPI induces calcium flux in hepatic mitochondria. The effects of LPI on intracellular calcium mobilization are blocked by GPR55 antagonists as well as in cells where GPR55 levels have been downregulated demonstrating the specificity of the role of GPR55 in LPI action.

5. You are testing a novel fatty acid–related compound for it efficacy in the treatment of obesity. When the compound is added to the chow of laboratory animals, there is a significant reduction in food intake leading to a reduction on overall body weight. You discover that the compound can bind to and activate the G-protein–coupled receptor, GPR119. Your results indicate that your test compound most likely functions similarly to which of the following lipids?

A. docosahexaenoic acid, DHA
B. eicosapentaenoic acid, EPA
C. lysophosphatidic acid, LPA
D. lysophosphatidylinositol, LPI
E. oleoylethaolamide, OEA

Answer E: Oleoylethanolamide (OEA) is produced by mucosal cells in the proximal small intestine from dietary oleic acid. OEA has been shown to activate the fatty acid–sensing GPCR identified as GPR119. When OEA is administered to laboratory animals, the result is a significant reduction in food intake and body weight gain. These effects of OEA are the result of the activation of the nuclear receptor PPARα resulting in the observed modification of feeding behavior and motor activity in laboratory animals.

6. Activation of which of the following receptors would be expected to be associated with increased glucose uptake by adipocytes?

A. GPR35
B. GPR40
C. GPR55
D. GPR119
E. GPR120

Answer D: GPR120 is highly expressed in adipose tissue and pro-inflammatory macrophages. DHA stimulation of GPR120 in adipocytes results in increased GLUT4 translocation to the cell surface with a subsequent increase in glucose transport into the cells.

7. You are testing a novel compound related to the polyunsaturated fatty acid, DHA, for its effects on the activity of macrophages in culture. Addition of this compound to your cultures results in a significant reduction in the release to the media of tumor necrosis factor-α (TNF-α). Given these observation, your test compound is most likely binding to, and activating, which of the following receptors?

A. GPR35
B. GPR40
C. GPR41
D. GPR55
E. GPR120

Answer E: The omega-3 PUFAs, DHA and EPA, exert potent anti-inflammatory effects through GPR120. It has been found that GPR120 functions as an omega-3 fatty acid receptor/sensor in pro-inflammatory macrophages and mature adipocytes. By signaling through GPR120, both DHAand EPA mediate potent anti-inflammatory effects. These effects are exerted by inhibition of the Toll-like receptor (TLR) and tumor necrosis factor-α (TNF-α) pro-inflammatory signaling pathways.

Checklist

✓ Bioactive lipids constitute a diverse array of fatty acid–derived molecules that exert their effects through binding to specific G-protein–coupled receptors (GPCRs). The most potent bioactive lipids are those derived from the essential omega-3 and omega-6 polyunsaturated fatty acids.

✓ Oleoylethanolamide (OEA) is a member of the fatty-acid ethanolamide family that includes palmitoylethanolamide (PEA) and *N*-arachidonylethanolamide (anandamide). OEA exerts its biological effects through activation of the GPR119.

✓ The phospholipases that remodel membrane phospholipids also generate a special class of bioactive lipid termed the lysophospholipids (LPLs). The LPL exerts specific biological responses via interaction with membrane receptors of the GPCR family. Lysophosphatidic acid (LPA) and lysophosphatidylinositol (LPI) are 2 of the most biologically significant LPLs.

CHAPTER

24 Lipids: Lipid Mediators of Inflammation

CHAPTER OUTLINE

High-Yield Terms

Lipoxin: anti-inflammatory and pro-resolution eicosanoids synthesized through lipoxygenase interactions

Aspirin-triggered lipoxin: epimeric lipoxins synthesized as a result of aspirin-mediated acetylation of COX-2

Eicosapentaenoic acid (EPA): an omega-3 polyunsaturated fatty acid that is a precursor for the synthesis of anti-inflammatory lipids

Docosahexaenoic acid (DHA): an omega-3 polyunsaturated fatty acid that can exert numerous activities by binding to a specific G-protein–coupled receptor (GPCR), also is a precursor for the synthesis of anti-inflammatory lipids

Polymorphonuclear leukocytes (PMN): commonly refers to neutrophils (can be any of the granulocyte family of leukocytes), characterized by the varying shapes of the nucleus which is usually lobed into 3 segments

Nonphlogistic: refers to the process of phagocytosis and clearance by macrophages within induction of inflammation

Apoptosis: the process of programmed cell death

High-Yield Concept

Once initiated, an inflammatory response must be turned off following completion of the required processes triggered by the initiating challenge. This process is referred to as *resolution of inflammation.*

As pointed out in Chapters 22 and 23, biological molecules derived from various polyunsaturated fatty acids (PUFAs) participate in the mediation of numerous physiologically relevant processes including, but not limited to, immune responses. Lipid mediators, such as the prostaglandins and leukotrienes, have been appreciated for many years for their activities that promote and enhance inflammatory responses. Through the activities of cyclooxygenase (COX-1 and COX-2) or lipoxygenase (5-LOX), leukocytes rapidly synthesize these lipid mediators from membrane-derived arachidonic acid within seconds to minutes of an acute challenge. The primary endogenous lipid mediators that are released by cells that infiltrate the site of immune challenge are prostaglandin E_2 (PGE_2) and leukotriene B_4 (LTB_4). These molecules are important for host defense, but can also inadvertently lead to tissue damage if inappropriately and/or excessively produced.

An active, coordinated program of resolution initiates in the first few hours after an inflammatory response begins. This resolution process is initiated following infiltration of granulocytes into the tissues. There are 3 types of granulocytes more commonly called neutrophils, eosinophils, and basophils. These leukocytes promote the switch of arachidonic acid–derived prostaglandin and leukotriene synthesis to that of lipoxin synthesis. The lipoxins then initiate the resolution and termination sequence. The recruitment of neutrophils to the inflammatory site ceases following the initiation of lipoxin synthesis and programmed death by apoptosis is engaged. Neutrophil apoptosis coincides with the biosynthesis of the resolvins (Rv) and protectins. These latter molecules are derived from the omega-3 PUFA, EPA and DHA.

Lipoxins

The lipoxins (LX), or the *lipox*ygenase *in*teraction products, are generated from arachidonic acid via sequential actions of lipoxygenases (including 5-LOX, 12-LOX, and 15-LOX) and subsequent reactions to give rise to specific trihydroxytetraene-containing eicosanoids (Figure 24-1). These unique lipid compounds are formed during cell–cell interactions and appear to act at both temporally and spatially distinct sites from those of the pro-inflammatory eicosanoids. The synthesis of the lipoxins triggers the natural pathways leading to termination and resolution of inflammatory responses.

Lipoxin A_4 (LXA_4) and lipoxin B_4 (LXB_4) were the first-recognized eicosanoid-related mediators that display both potent anti-inflammatory and pro-resolving actions in animal models of disease. The LX act as agonist ligands for specific GPCR resulting in the activation of cellular responses important to inflammation and inflammatory resolution. The LX and their analogs exert important activities related to airway inflammation, asthma, arthritis, cardiovascular disorders, gastrointestinal disease, periodontal disease, kidney diseases and graft-versus-host disease (GVHD), and many other diseases/disorders where uncontrolled inflammation is a key mediator of disease pathogenesis (Figure 24-1).

The synthesis of the lipoxins occurs via 3 distinct pathways, one of which is triggered via the actions of aspirin. The 2 "classical" pathways for the synthesis of the lipoxins are the result of the concerted actions of 15-LOX acting on arachidonic acid in epithelial cells

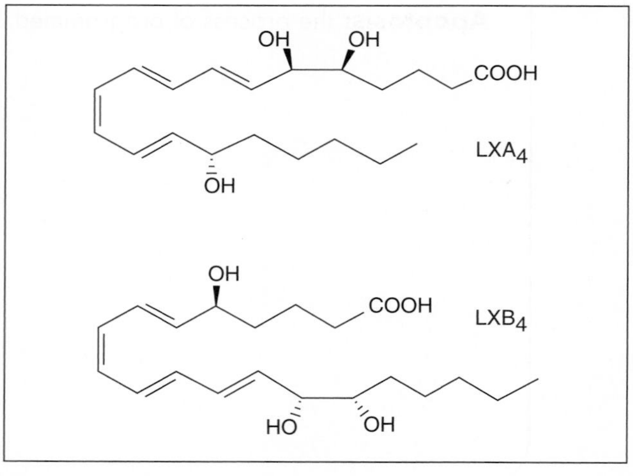

OH OH COOH LXA4 OH

OH COOH LXB4 HO OH

FIGURE 24-1: Structures of LXA_4 and LXB_4.

(eg, airway epithelia) and 5-LOX in leukocytes or through the actions of 5-LOX in leukocytes followed by 12-LOX action in platelets (Figure 24-2). This latter activity requires that platelets interact directly with adherent neutrophils as occurs only following platelet activation. Activated leukocytes that adhere to epithelial cells as a consequence inflammation (such as gastrointestinal, airway, or kidney epithelia) induce the production of lipoxins. An additional stimulus that leads to production of lipoxins is epithelial cell conversion of LTA_4 that is released from airway epithelia.

Activities of the Lipoxins

The lipoxins are potent anti-inflammatory eicosanoids and counteract the actions of the pro-inflammatory eicosanoids (primarily LTB_4 but also PGE_2 and TXA_2). The lipoxins LXA_4 and 15 epi-LXA_4 (an aspirin-triggered lipoxin) elicit their effects by binding to a specific GPCR identified as ALXR. *ALXR* is a multirecognition receptor involved in immune responses, which was originally identified as the formyl peptide receptor-like 1 (FPRL1) protein; a member of the formyl peptide receptor (FPR) family of receptors that bind *N*-formulated peptides derived by the degradation of bacteria or host cells. The FPR family of receptors is involved in mediating immune responses to infection.

Both LXA_4 and LXB_4 have been shown to promote the relaxation of the vasculature (both aortic and pulmonary relaxation). Lipoxins and the epi-lipoxins inhibit polymorphonuclear leukocyte (PMN) chemotaxis, PMN-mediated increases in vasopermeability, and PMN adhesion and migration through the endothelium. The lipoxins also stimulate phagocytosis of apoptotic PMN by monocyte-derived macrophages. PMN phagocytosis represents the resolution phase of inflammatory events.

Additional anti-inflammatory actions of the lipoxins include blocking expression of the IL-8, a pro-inflammatory chemokine produced by macrophages and endothelial cells that stimulates neutrophil migration. Actions of the lipoxins also include inhibition of the release and actions of tumor necrosis factor-α (TNF-α), and stimulation of the activity of transforming growth factor-β (TGF-β). By regulating the actions of histamine, the lipoxins also lead to a reduction in swelling due to edema. The actions of LXA_4 in some tissues lead to the production of prostacyclin (PGI_2) and nitric oxide (NO), both of which are vasodilators and may play roles in the anti-inflammatory properties of the aspirin-triggered lipoxins.

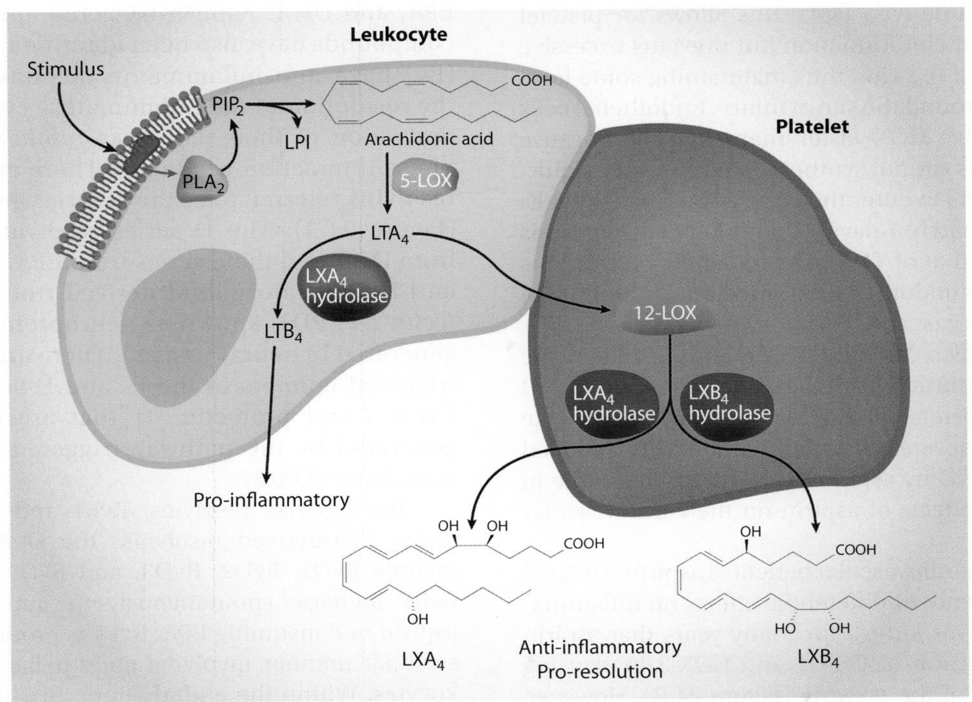

FIGURE 24-2: Pathways for the synthesis of LXA_4 and LXB_4. Reproduced with permission of themedicalbiochemistrypage, LLC.

Actions of Aspirin via Lipid Modulators of Inflammation

Aspirin is the acetylated form of salicylic acid. *Salicylate* is a common constituent of numerous medicinal plants, which have been used for thousands of years to treat pain and rheumatic fever. Salicylate has an extremely bitter taste and causes gastric irritation. This led to the development of acetylated salicylate giving rise to the advent of aspirin (acetylsalicylic acid).

In the 1970s it was determined that aspirin and other nonsteroidal anti-inflammatory drugs (NSAIDs) all exerted their effects through the inhibition of prostaglandin synthesis via the inhibition of cyclooxygenase. However, this did not explain all of the actions that were being described for aspirin, in particular the ability of aspirin to limit leukocyte migration into sites of inflammation, thereby dampening host inflammatory responses. At high doses, aspirin functions to block the prostaglandin and thromboxane-synthesizing activity of COX-1, which results in inhibition of the primary pro-inflammatory, pyretic, and pain-inducing action of these eicosanoids. In addition, aspirin is an important inhibitor of platelet activation by reducing the production of thromboxane A_2 (TXA_2). Aspirin also reduces endothelial cell production of prostacyclin (PGI_2), an inhibitor of platelet aggregation and a vasodilator. Localized to the site of coagulation is a balance between the levels of platelet-derived TXA_2 and endothelial cell-derived PGI_2. This allows for platelet aggregation and clot formation but prevents excessive accumulation of the clot, thus maintaining some level of blood flow around the site of injury. Endothelial cells regenerate active COX faster than platelets because mature platelets cannot synthesize the enzyme, requiring new platelets to enter the circulation (platelet half-life is approximately 4 days). Therefore, PGI_2 synthesis is greater than that of TXA_2. The net effect of aspirin is more in favor of endothelial cell-mediated inhibition of the coagulation cascade.

Aspirin is also the only NSAID that results in the production of nitric oxide (NO). The induction of NO by aspirin is correlated with a reduction in leukocyte accumulation at sites of inflammation. The induced production of NO by aspirin plays a significant role in the protective effects of aspirin on the cardiovascular system.

Part of the cardiovascular benefit of aspirin is related to its dose-dependent differential effects on inflammatory events. It was known for many years that aspirin inhibited the action of COX-1 and COX-2 by causing the acetylation of the enzyme (Figure 24-3). However, in endothelial and epithelial cells the aspirin-induced acetylation of COX-2 alters the enzyme activity such that it now converts arachidonic acid to 15*R* hydroxyeicosatetraenoic acid (15*R*-HETE). Only at low doses (eg, 81 mg) will aspirin elicit its most important anti-inflammatory benefits. The low-dose anti-inflammatory effects of aspirin are due to its ability to trigger the synthesis of stereoisomers (epimers) of LXA_4 and LXB_4 identified as 15 epi-LXA_4 and 15 epi-LXB_4. These compounds are referred to as aspirin-triggered lipoxins (ATL) and they exhibit biological activities similar to the lipoxins synthesized by the "classical" pathways. When produced in leukocytes, 15*R*-HETE is a substrate for 5-LOX, the product of which is then ultimately converted to the ATL (see Figure 24-3). This aspirin-triggered lipoxin synthesis pathway is initiated when activated circulating leukocytes (primarily neutrophils) adhere to the vascular endothelium.

Actions of the Resolvins and Protectins

As indicated earlier, the resolution phase of inflammation occurs following the induction of lipoxin synthesis and the initiation of neutrophil apoptosis. Neutrophil apoptosis coincides with the biosynthesis of the resolvins and protectins (Table 24-1), which are lipid mediators derived from the omega-3 PUFA, EPA, and DHA. Aspirin-triggered epimers of these compounds have also been identified. The resolvins (Rv) have anti-inflammatory actions that lead to the resolution of the inflammatory cycle, hence the derivation of their names as *resolvins* (resolution phase interaction products). There are 2 classes of resolvins referred to as the D series and the E series (Figure 24-4). The D series resolvins are derived from DHA and the E series from EPA. An additional anti-inflammatory lipid derived from DHA is *protectin D1* (PD1, known as neuroprotectin D1 when generated in neural tissues). There are also aspirin-triggered epimers of the E- and D-series resolvins (AT-Rv) and protectin D1 that are enzymatically generated by the pathway triggered when aspirin acetylates COX-2.

The E-series resolvins, RvE1 and RvE2, are the major EPA-derived resolvins. The D-series resolvins include RvD1, RvD2, RvD3, and RvD4. The levels of RvE1 increase spontaneously in individuals taking aspirin or consuming EPA. RvE1 is produced in a transcellular manner involving endothelial cells and leukocytes. Within the endothelium, EPA is converted to

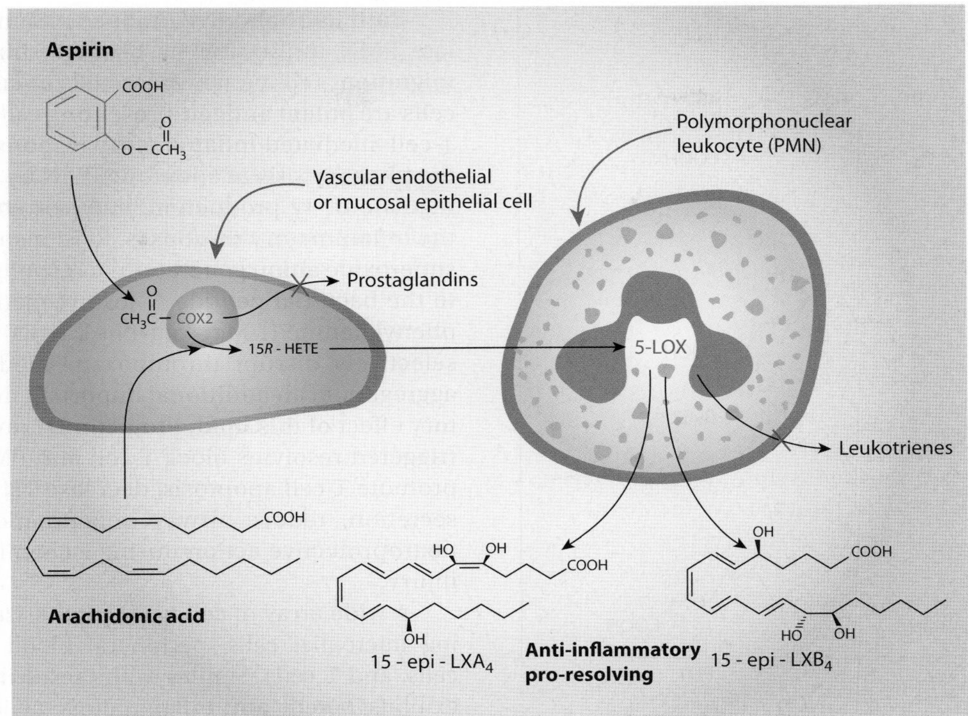

FIGURE 24-3: Synthesis of the aspirin-triggered lipoxins. Reproduced with permission of themedicalbiochemistrypage, LLC.

TABLE 24-1: Activities of the Major Lipid Mediators of Inflammation

Mediator	*Major Activities*
LXA_4 and LXB_4	Prevents vascular permeability, reduces inflammation, blocks histamine and PGE_2-mediated edema, accelerates resolution, protective in ischemia-reperfusion injury, reduces endothelial cell proliferation and migration, thus preventing atherosclerotic plaque rupture, attenuates pro-inflammatory gene expression in the gut reducing the severity of colitis, stimulates bone marrow and enhances growth of myeloid progenitors, reduces leukocyte adherence, decreases neutrophil recruitment, limits neovascularization and promotes host defense in the eye, protects against graft-versus-host disease (GVHD)
RvD1	Anti-inflammatory, limits PMN infiltration, inhibits cytokine expression in microglial cells, reduces local inflammation in the GI, and protects from GI tissue damage
RvE1 and RvE2	Reduce inflammation, limit PMN infiltration, protect the GI in colitis, reduce inflammation leading to bone loss
PD1	Reduces PMN infiltration, limits stroke damage, promotes corneal epithelial cell wound healing, protects the liver, reduces asthma and protects lung from damage, protects kidney from leukocyte-mediated tissue damage
NPD1	Downregulates pro-inflammatory cytokines and chemokines and stimulates anti-inflammatory cytokines and chemokines, reduces PMN infiltration and T-cell recruitment in peritonitis, promotes neuronal cell survival, protects from retinal injury, production reduced in Alzheimer disease

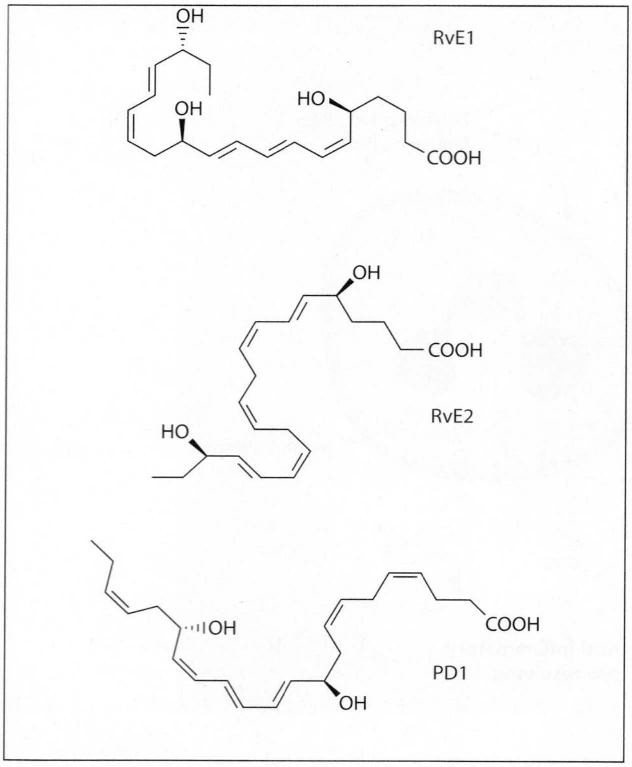

FIGURE 24-4: Structures of RvE1, RvE2, and PD1.

18*R*-HEPE (18*R*-hydroxyeicosapentaenoic acid) by COX-2 exposed to aspirin. The 18*R*-HEPE is released by the endothelial cells and taken up by adherent leukocytes, where 5-LOX activity results in its eventual conversion to RvE1.

Both RvE1 and RvE2 reduce inflammation, regulate PMN infiltration by blocking transendothelial migration, reduce dendritic cell function (dendritic cells are potent antigen-presenting cells which prime T-cell–mediated inflammatory responses), stimulate the phagocytosis of apoptotic PMN by macrophages, regulate IL-12 production, and lead to resolution of the inflammatory responses. RvE1 also inhibits PMN superoxide anion generation in response to TNF-α or to the bacterial peptide *N*-formyl-methionyl-leucyl-phenylalanine (f-Met-Leu-Phe). RvE1 is also able to selectively disrupt thromboxane-mediated platelet aggregation, an additional important anti-inflammatory effect of this lipid. Protectin D1 and the aspirin-triggered resolvins block T-cell and PMN migration, promote T-cell apoptosis, decrease TNF-α and INF-γ secretion, reduce airway inflammation, and exert neuroprotective action during ischemia-reperfusion injury.

A wide array of cell types synthesize PD1, including microglial cells, peripheral blood mononuclear cells, and T cells. Similar to the resolvins, PD1/NPD1 exhibits potent anti-inflammatory actions. PD1 is a potent regulator of allergic airway inflammation and responses to immunologic challenge by preventing the development of airway hyperreactivity and inhibiting the infiltration eosinophils and T cells into the lung tissues. Experimental data show that administration of PD1 accelerates the resolution of airway inflammation in models of allergic asthma. PD1 is also crucial to the protection of renal tissue in response to ischemic injury. Of potential clinical significance is the observation that the activity of NPD1 appears to be dysregulated in Alzheimer disease.

REVIEW QUESTIONS

1. You are studying the effects of a previously uncharacterized drug upon oral administration to experimental animals. Your tests involve examination of the effects of this compound within the gut following inducement of colitis-like symptoms. You find that administration of the drug to these animals leads to a reduction in the severity of inflammation in the gut and enhances a return to normal GI activity. Your test compound is most likely inducing the synthesis of which of the following compound?
   A. LTB_4
   B. LXA_4
   C. PCI_2
   D. PGE_2
   E. TXA_2

Answer B: The lipoxin, LXA_4, inhibits polymorphonuclear leukocyte (PMN) chemotaxis, PMN-mediated increases in vasopermeability, and PMN adhesion and migration through the endothelium resulting in an attenuation of pro-inflammatory responses in the gut. LXA_4 also stimulates phagocytosis of apoptotic PMN by monocyte-derived macrophages, which represents the resolution phase of inflammatory events.

2. A defect in which of the following enzyme activities would impair the production of the lipoxins by the classic pathway (ie, nonaspirin triggered) in neutrophils?
   A. COX-1
   B. COX-2
   C. 5-LOX

D. 12-LOX
E. 15-LOX

Answer C: In one of the classical pathways of lipoxin synthesis, the interactions between epithelial cells and neutrophils require the activities of both 15-LOX and 5-LOX. Within the epithelial cells, the PLA_2-mediated release of arachidonic acid serves as a substrate for 15-LOX and generates 15*S*-H(p)ETE. This latter compound will then diffuse out of the epithelial cells and be taken up by neutrophils where the activity of 5-LOX will then convert it into 15*S*-epoxytetraene, which is the precursor for LXA_4 synthesis.

3. The lipoxins are characterized as pro-resolving compounds because they promote the resolution of an inflammatory response. Which of the following activities is associated with this pro-resolution function?
   A. activation of TNF-α secretion
   B. inhibition of polymorphonuclear (PMN) cell apoptosis
   C. inhibition of the action of TGF-β
   D. reduction in neutrophil infiltration at the site of inflammation
   E. stimulation of IL-8 release

Answer D: Lipoxins and epi-lipoxins inhibit neutrophils (PMN) chemotaxis, PMN-mediated increases in vasopermeability, and PMN adhesion and migration through the endothelium. Additional anti-inflammatory actions of the lipoxins and aspirin-triggered lipoxins include blocking expression of the *IL-8* gene (a pro-inflammatory chemokine produced by macrophages and endothelial cells, which stimulates neutrophil migration), inhibition of the release and actions of TNF-α, and stimulation of TGF-β activity.

4. You are studying the responses of renal tissue to ischemic injury in laboratory animals. You find that in these animals there is an initial inflammatory response detectable within the renal tissue, but it does not normally abate as expected; it only worsens resulting in total renal failure. Measurements of enzyme activities in renal tubule cells indicate that PLA_2 and COX-2 are functional. The lack of synthesis of which of the following lipid mediators is the most likely cause of the failure to limit the inflammatory responses in this animal model?
   A. LTB_4
   B. PD1
   C. PGE_2
   D. RvD1
   E. TXA_2

Answer B: Although PD1 and RvD1 are both anti-inflammatory and pro-resolution lipids, the activity of PD1 is most significant in renal, airway, and neural tissues. The other 3 lipids are all pro-inflammatory molecules.

5. You are examining the lipid synthesis characteristics of mixed cell types in culture. You find that the cells normally activate PLA_2 and that you can detect the synthesis of the intermediate 15*S*-H(p)ETE. However, in this system you cannot detect the subsequent production of LXA_4. Which of the following enzymes is most likely not functional in this culture system?
   A. COX-1
   B. COX-2
   C. 5-LOX
   D. 12-LOX
   E. 15-LOX

Answer C: In one of the classical pathways of lipoxin synthesis the interactions between epithelial cells and leukocytes requires the activities of both 15-LOX and 5-LOX. Within the epithelial cells, the PLA_2-mediated release of arachidonic acid serves as a substrate for 15-LOX and generates 15*S*-H(p)ETE. This latter compound will then diffuse out of the epithelial cells and be taken up by leukocytes where the activity of 5-LOX will then convert it into 15*S*-epoxytetraene, which is the precursor for LXA_4 synthesis. Therefore, the presence of upstream activities and lipid products in the absence of LXA_4 synthesis indicates that there is a defect in the activity of 5-LOX in this system.

6. Aspirin exerts several beneficial effects within the vasculature that result in protection against intravascular inflammation and resultant atherosclerosis. These actions of aspirin involve, in part, its ability to modify the activity of lipid-synthetic enzymes. Which of the following enzymes is a target for aspirin-mediated modification resulting in an altered activity?
   A. COX-2
   B. Δ^5-desaturase
   C. 5-LOX
   D. prostacyclin synthase
   E. thromboxane synthase

Answer A: Aspirin-induced acetylation of COX-2 alters the enzyme such that it converts arachidonic acid to 15*R*-hydroxyeicosatetraenoic acid (15*R*-HETE) instead of into prostaglandin H_2 (PGH_2). 15*R*-HETE is then rapidly metabolized to the epi-lipoxins in monocytes and leukocytes through the action of 5-lipoxygenase (5-LOX).

Checklist

✓ The lipoxins are anti-inflammatory and pro-resolution eicosanoids synthesized from arachidonic acid through the concerted actions of cyclooxygenase and lipoxygenase via interactions between epithelial cells and leukocytes, or between leukocytes and platelets.

✓ The resolvins and protectins are anti-inflammatory and pro-resolution lipids derived from the omega-3 polyunsaturated fatty acids, DHA, and EPA.

✓ Aspirin modifies the activities of COX-1 and COX-2 by acting as a suicide inhibitor at high doses, at low doses aspirin-mediated acetylation of COX-2 changes its activity toward the substrate, arachidonic acid, such that instead of driving the synthesis of the prostaglandins and thromboxanes, it directs the lipid into the epimeric lipoxin synthesis pathway, deriving the aspirin-triggered lipoxins.

CHAPTER 25

Lipids: Lipolysis, Fatty Acid Oxidation, and Ketogenesis

CHAPTER OUTLINE

Dietary Origins of Lipids
Mobilization of Fat Stores
Adipose Triglyceride Lipase
Hormone-Sensitive Lipase
Monoacylglyceride Lipase
Lipid Transporters and Cellular Uptake of Fats
Mitochondrial β-Oxidation Reactions
Minor Alternative Fatty Acid Oxidation Pathway
Peroxisomal (alpha) α-Oxidation Pathway
Peroxisomal β-Oxidation Reactions
Microsomal ω-Oxidation Reactions
Regulation of Fatty Acid Metabolism
Ketogenesis
Regulation of Ketogenesis
Diabetic Ketoacidosis

High-Yield Terms

Adipose tissue triglyceride lipase (ATGL): primary rate-limiting enzyme involved in adipose tissue triglyceride metabolism

Hormone-sensitive lipase (HSL): an adipose tissue–specific hydrolase responsible for the release of fatty acids from stored triglycerides. Its activity is regulated by hormone-mediated phosphorylation

α-oxidation: peroxisomal oxidation pathway responsible for the oxidation of the methyl-substituted fatty acid, phytanic acid present at high concentration in the tissues of ruminants

β-oxidation: major pathway for oxidation of fatty acids in both the mitochondria and the peroxisomes; peroxisomal β-oxidation is also important for metabolism of dicarboxylic acids generated via the ω-oxidation pathway

ω-oxidation: a minor, but clinically significant, pathway for fatty oxidation initiated by microsomal ω-hydroxylation reactions, also involves the oxidation of dicarboxylic acids generated

Ketone body: any of the compounds, β-hydroxybutyrate, acetoacetate, and acetone, generated during hepatic ketogenesis from the substrate, acetyl-CoA

Diabetic ketoacidosis (DKA): a condition of increased plasma ketone body concentration caused by excess adipose tissue fatty acid release and hepatic fatty acid oxidation resulting from unregulated glucagon release

High-Yield Concept

Following absorption of the products of lipid digestion, the resynthesis of TGs, cholesterol esters, and phospholipids occurs. These lipid entities are then solubilized in lipoprotein complexes called chylomicrons. Chylomicrons from the intestine are then released into the blood via the lymph system for delivery to the various tissues for storage or production of energy through oxidation.

Dietary Origins of Lipids

The predominant form of dietary lipid in the human diet is triglyceride (TG or TAG). Gastrointestinal lipid digestion and absorption is discussed in Chapter 43. Briefly, the digestion of dietary triglyceride begins in the stomach with the action of gastric lipase and continues in the duodenum via the concerted actions of gastric lipase and pancreatic lipase. Digestion of dietary phospholipids takes place in the duodenum as well via the action of pancreatic phospholipase A_2 (PLA_2), yielding free fatty acids and lysophospholipids. Digestion of dietary cholesterol esters results via the action of carboxyl ester lipase (CEL). Intestinal absorption of diacyl- and monoacylglycerides, lysophospholipids, free fatty acids, and cholesterol occurs at the interface between the brush border membranes of intestinal enterocytes and the lipid micelles and involves both passive diffusion and transport protein–mediated uptake mechanisms.

Discussion of the various lipoproteins present in human circulation can be found in Chapter 28. As chylomicrons circulate in the vasculature, fatty acids are removed from the TG fraction through the action of endothelial cell–associated lipoprotein lipase (LPL). The free fatty acids are then absorbed by the cells and the glycerol is returned via the blood to the liver where it is utilized as a carbon skeleton for glucose synthesis via gluconeogenesis (Chapter 13).

Mobilization of Fat Stores

The primary sources of fatty acids for oxidation are dietary and mobilization from cellular stores. Fatty acids from the diet are absorbed from the gut, packaged into lipoprotein particles called chylomicrons within intestinal enterocytes and then delivered to cells of the body via transport in the blood. Fatty acids are stored in the form of triglycerides (TAGs or TGs) within all cells but predominantly within adipose tissue. In response to energy demands, the fatty acids of stored TGs can be mobilized for use by peripheral tissues. The release of these stored fatty acids is controlled by a complex series of interrelated cascades that result in the activation of triglyceride hydrolysis. The primary intracellular lipases involved in the mobilization of stored fatty acids are adipose triglyceride lipase (ATGL, also called desnutrin), hormone-sensitive lipase (HSL), and monoacylglyceride lipase (MGL).

Adipose Triglyceride Lipase

Adipose triglyceride lipase (ATGL)/desnutrin belongs to the family of patatin domain-containing proteins that consists of 9 human members. Because some members of the family act as phospholipases, the proteins were originally called patatin-like

High-Yield Concept

An additional lipase, lysosomal acid lipase (LAL), plays an important role in the intracellular degradation of cholesterol esters and TGs taken into cells via endocytosis and transferred to the lysosomes. The importance of LAL in overall lipid homeostasis is evidenced by the fact that LAL deficiency results in the significant accumulation of cholesterol esters in tissues such as the spleen and liver. LAL deficiency is commonly called Wolman disease.

High-Yield Concept

Of clinical significance is the recent observation that blocking perilipin-2 (Plin2) activity in mice leads to inhibition of diet-induced obesity. This response is associated with increased formation of subcutaneous beige adipocytes that express UCP1, a reduction of inflammatory foci formation in white adipose tissue (WAT) as well as reduced steatosis in the liver. Loss of Plin2 activity results in reduced energy intake and increased physical activity in response to a high-fat diet indicating that Plin2 likely contributes to diet-induced obesity, adipose tissue inflammation, and the development of hepatic steatosis.

phospholipase domain-containing proteins A1 to A9 (PNPLA1–PNPLA9). ATGL (designated PNPLA2 in the patatin domain nomenclature) preferentially hydrolyzes TGs. ATGL expression and enzyme activity are both under complex regulation. Expression of ATGL is induced by peroxisome proliferator–activated receptor (PPAR) agonists, glucocorticoids, and fasting. The level of lipase activity of ATGL (as well as HSL) does not always correlate to the level of expression of the gene. The discrepancy between ATGL and HSL mRNA level and the level of enzyme activity is the result of extensive posttranslational regulation of both of these lipases.

There are 2 known serine residues in ATGL that are subject to phosphorylation. Unlike phosphorylation of HSL (described below), ATGL phosphorylation is not PKA-dependent. Some lines of evidence suggest that AMPK phosphorylates ATGL resulting in increased lipase activity. In addition to phosphorylation regulating ATGL activity, the enzyme requires a coactivator protein for full activity. This coactivator is known as comparative gene identification-58 (CGI-58). The official nomenclature for CGI-58 is α/β-hydrolase domain-containing protein-5 (ABHD5), owing to the presence of an α/β-hydrolase domain commonly found in esterases, thioesterases, and lipases. Additional proteins that are associated with lipid droplets (LD) in adipocytes participate in the ABHD5-mediated regulation of ATGL such as perilipin-1, Plin1.

In nonadipose tissues with high rates of TG hydrolysis, such as skeletal muscle and liver, regulation of ATGL activity occurs via a mechanism distinct from that in adipose tissues. In these tissues, perilipin-1 is replaced by perilipin-5 which recruits both ATGL and ABHD5 to LD by direct binding of the enzyme and its coactivator. Other perilipins exist in cells including perilipin-2, -3, and -4 but it is unclear if these proteins are also involved in regulating the association of ATGL with LD.

Hormone-sensitive Lipase

The expression profile of hormone-sensitive lipase (HSL) essentially mirrors that of ATGL. Highest mRNA and protein concentrations are found in WAT and brown adipose tissue (BAT) with low levels of expression found in muscle, testis, steroidogenic tissues, and pancreatic islets as well as several other tissues. HSL was originally thought to be rate limiting for the catabolism of fat stores in adipose tissue and many nonadipose tissues. However, HSL actually has a higher level of activity as a diglyceride (DG) hydrolase than as a TG hydrolase. This became evident when HSL-deficient mice were produced and shown to efficiently hydrolyze TG and they do not accumulate TG in either adipose or nonadipose tissues, but they do accumulate large amounts of DGs in many tissues. It is now accepted that ATGL is responsible for the initial step of lipolysis in human adipocytes, and that HSL is rate-limiting for the catabolism of DG. HSL not only hydrolyzes DG but is also active at hydrolyzing ester bonds of many other lipids including TG, MG, cholesteryl esters, retinyl esters, and short-chain carbonic acid esters.

In adipose tissue, HSL activity is strongly induced by β-adrenergic stimulation; conversely insulin has a strong inhibitory effect. While β-adrenergic stimulation regulates ATGL primarily via recruitment of the coactivator ABHD5, HSL is a major target for PKA-mediated phosphorylation. Additional kinases, including AMPK, extracellular signal-regulated kinase (ERK), glycogen synthase kinase-4 (GSK-4), and Ca^{2+}/calmodulin-dependent kinase 1 (CAMK1), also phosphorylate HSL to modulate the activity of the enzyme. Although phosphorylation affects HSL activity, full activation requires access to LD, which in adipose tissue is mediated by Plin1 (Figure 25-1).

In nonadipose tissues, such as skeletal muscle, HSL is activated by phosphorylation in response to

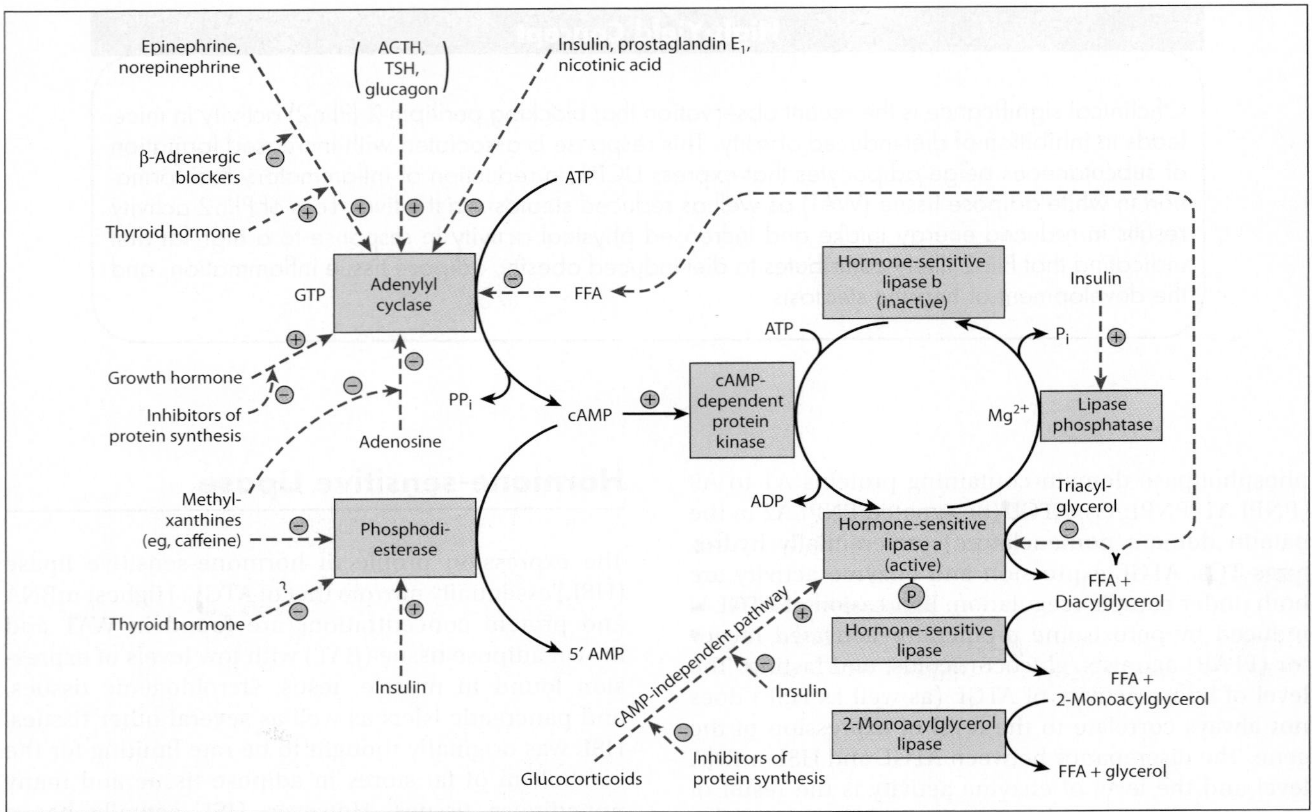

FIGURE 25-1: Control of adipose tissue lipolysis. (FFA, free fatty acids; TSH, thyroid-stimulating hormone.) Note the cascade sequence of reactions affording amplification at each step. The lipolytic stimulus is "switched off" by removal of the stimulating hormone; the action of lipase phosphatase; the inhibition of the lipase and adenylyl cyclase by high concentrations of FFA; the inhibition of adenylyl cyclase by adenosine; and the removal of cAMP by the action of phosphodiesterase. ACTH, TSH, and glucagon may not activate adenylyl cyclase in vivo since the concentration of each hormone required in vitro is much higher than is found in the circulation. Positive (⊕) and negative ⊖ regulatory effects are represented by broken lines and substrate flow by solid lines. Murray RK, Bender DA, Botham KM, Kennelly PJ, Rodwell VW, Weil PA. *Harper's Illustrated Biochemistry*, 29th ed. New York, NY McGraw-Hill; 2012.

epinephrine (β-adrenergic receptor–mediated activation of PKA) and muscle contraction (calcium release from sarcoplasmic reticulum).

Insulin-mediated deactivation of lipolysis is associated with transcriptional downregulation of ATGL and HSL expression. Insulin signaling also results in the activation of various phosphodiesterase (PDE) isoforms leading to PDE-catalyzed hydrolysis of cAMP which in turn results in reduced activation of PKA. These actions turn off lipolysis by preventing phosphorylation and activation of HSL. In addition to its peripheral action, insulin also functions within the sympathetic nervous system to inhibit lipolysis in WAT. Increased insulin levels in the brain inhibit both HSL and Plin1 phosphorylation which results in reduced HSL and ATGL activities.

Monoacylglyceride Lipase

Monoacylglyceride lipase (MGL) is considered to be the rate-limiting enzyme for the breakdown of MG that are the result of both extracellular and intracellular lipolysis pathways. The extracellular generation of MG is the result of the action of endothelial cell lipoprotein lipase (LPL) on lipoprotein particle–associated TG. Intracellular hydrolysis of TG by ATGL and HSL as well as intracellular phospholipid hydrolysis by phospholipase C (PLC) and membrane-associated DG lipase α and β results in the generation of MGL substrates.

MGL is ubiquitously expressed with highest levels of expression in adipose tissue. MGL shares homology with esterases, lysophospholipases, and haloperoxidases. MGL is critically important for efficient degradation of MG since it has been shown in mouse models that lack of MGL impairs lipolysis and is associated with increased MG levels in adipose and nonadipose tissues alike. MGL has received particular attention in recent years due to the discovery that the enzyme is responsible for the inactivation of 2-arachidonoylglycerol (2-AG) which is an endogenous cannabinoid (endocannabinoid).

Lipid Transporters and Cellular Uptake of Fats

When fatty acids are released from adipose tissue stores, they enter the circulation as free fatty acids (FFA) and are bound to albumin for transport to peripheral tissues. When the fatty acid-albumin complexes interact with cell surfaces, the dissociation of the fatty acid from albumin represents the first step of the cellular uptake process. Cellular uptake of fatty acids involves several members of the fatty acid receptor family including fatty acid translocase (FAT/CD36), plasma membrane-associated fatty acid-binding protein ($FABP_{pm}$), and at least 6 fatty acid transport proteins (FATP1-FATP6). The FATP facilitate the uptake of very-long-chain (VLCFA) and long-chain fatty acids (LCFA) (Table 25-1).

Following uptake into cells, fatty acids must be activated to acyl-CoA intermediates. Several members of the FATP family possess acyl-CoA synthetase (ACS) activity. The overall process of cellular fatty acid uptake and subsequent intracellular utilization represents a continuum of dissociation from albumin by interaction with the membrane-associated transport proteins, activation to acyl-CoA (in many cases via FATP action) followed by intracellular trafficking to sites of metabolic disposition.

Mitochondrial β-Oxidation Reactions

The primary sites of fatty acid β-oxidation are the mitochondria and the peroxisomes. Fatty acids of between 4 and 8 and between 6 and 12 carbon atoms in length, referred to as short- and medium-chain fatty acids (SCFA and MCFA), respectively, are oxidized exclusively in the mitochondria. Long-chain fatty acids (LCFA: 10-16 carbons long) are oxidized in both the mitochondria and the peroxisomes with the peroxisomes exhibiting preference for 14-carbon and longer LCFA. Very-long-chain fatty acids (VLCFA: 17-26 carbons long) are preferentially oxidized in the peroxisomes.

Fatty acids must be activated in the cytoplasm before being oxidized in the mitochondria. Activation

TABLE 25-1: Mammalian Fatty Acid Transporters

Transporter	*Comments*
FAT/CD36	Fatty acid translocase; FAT is also known as CD36 which is a member of the scavenger receptor class (class B scavenger receptors) of receptors that bind lipids and lipoproteins of the LDL family
$FABP_{pm}$	Plasma membrane–associated fatty acid–binding protein
FATP1	FATP1 is SLC27A1; FATP1 is also known as acyl-CoA synthetase very-long-chain family, member 4 (ACSVL4); highest levels of expression in adipose tissue, skeletal, and heart muscle
FATP2	FATP2 is SLC27A2; FATP2 is also known as acyl-CoA synthetase very-long-chain family, member 1 (ACSVL1) as well as very-long-chain acyl-CoA synthetase (VLCS); highest levels of expression in liver and kidney; present in peroxisome and microsomal membranes
FATP3	FATP3 is SLC27A3; FATP3 is also known as acyl-CoA synthetase very-long-chain family, member 3 (ACSVL3)
FATP4	FATP4 is SLC27A4; FATP4 is also known as acyl-CoA synthetase very-long-chain family, member 5 (ACSVL5); is the major intestinal long-chain fatty acid transporter
FATP5	FATP5 is SLC27A5; FATP5 is also known as acyl-CoA synthetase very-long-chain family, member 6 (ACSVL6), very-long-chain acyl-CoA synthetase–related protein (VLACSR), or very-long-chain acyl-CoA synthetase homolog 2 (VLCSH2); highest levels of expression in the liver; capable of activating 24- and 26-carbon VLCFAs
FATP6	FATP6 is SLC27A6; FATP6 is also known as acyl-CoA synthetase very-long-chain family, member 2 (ACSVL2), very-long-chain acyl-CoA synthetase homolog 1 (VLCSH1); expressed at highest levels in the heart; protein only detected in heart and testis; exhibits a preference for the transport of palmitic acid and linoleic acid, does not transport fatty acids less than 10-carbon long

is catalyzed by fatty acyl-CoA synthetases (also called acyl-CoA ligases or thiokinases). The net result of this activation process is the consumption of 2 molar equivalents of ATP. The process of mitochondrial fatty acid oxidation is termed β-oxidation since it occurs through the sequential removal of 2-carbon units by oxidation at the β-carbon position of the fatty acyl-CoA molecule.

$$\text{Fatty acid} + \text{ATP} + \text{CoA} \rightarrow \text{Acyl-CoA} + \text{PP}_i + \text{AMP}$$

The transport of fatty acyl-CoA into the mitochondria is accomplished via an acyl-carnitine intermediate, which itself is generated by the action of carnitine palmitoyltransferase 1 (CPT-1 or CPT-I) an enzyme that resides in the outer mitochondrial membrane (Figure 25-2 and Clinical Box 25-1). There are 3 *CPT-1* genes in humans identified as CPT-1A, CPT-1B, and CPT-1C. Expression of CPT-1A predominates in the liver and is thus, referred to as the liver isoform. CPT-1B expression predominates in skeletal muscle and is thus, referred to as the muscle isoform. CPT-1C expression is exclusive to the brain and testes. The activity of CPT-1C is distinct from those of CPT-1A and CPT-1B in that it does not act on the same types of fatty acyl-CoAs that are substrates for the latter 2 enzymes. However, CPT-1C does exhibit high-affinity malonyl-CoA binding. Following carnitine acyl-carnitine–mediated transfer of the CPT-1-generated fatty acyl-carnitines across the inner mitochondrial membrane, the fatty acyl-carnitine molecules are acted on by the inner mitochondria membrane carnitine palmitoyltransferase 2 (CPT-2 or CPT-II) regenerating the fatty acyl-CoA molecules (Figure 25-2).

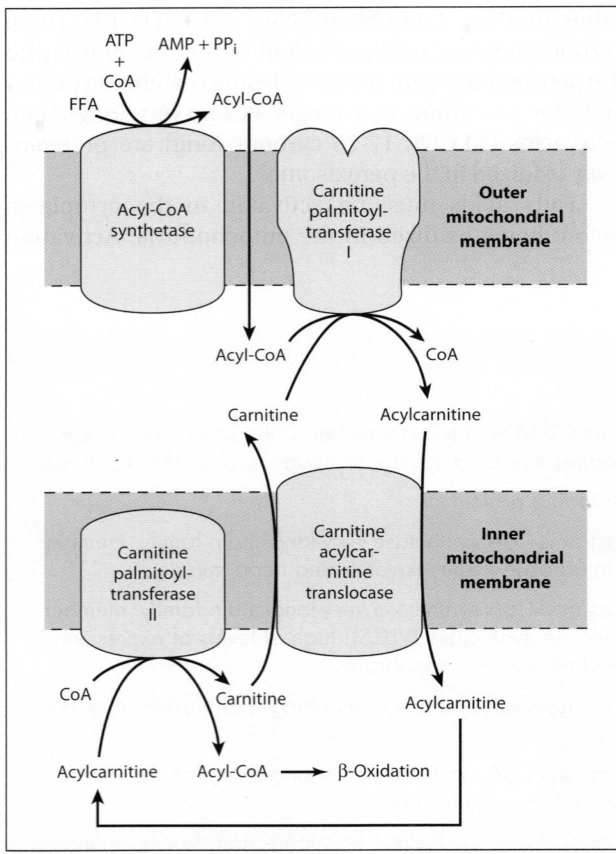

FIGURE 25-2: Role of carnitine in the transport of long-chain fatty acids through the inner mitochondrial membrane. Long-chain acyl-CoA cannot pass through the inner mitochondrial membrane, but its metabolic product, acylcarnitine, can. Murray RK, Bender DA, Botham KM, Kennelly PJ, Rodwell VW, Weil PA. *Harper's Illustrated Biochemistry*, 29th ed. New York, NY McGraw-Hill; 2012.

Each round of β-oxidation involves 4 steps that, in order, are oxidation, hydration, oxidation, and cleavage (Figure 25-3 , steps 2-5). The first oxidation step β-oxidation involves a family of FAD-dependent acyl-CoA dehydrogenases. Each of these dehydrogenases has a range of substrate specificity determined by the length of the fatty acid. Short-chain acyl-CoA dehydrogenase (SCAD, also called butyryl-CoA dehydrogenase) prefers fats of 4 to 6 carbons in length; medium-chain acyl-CoA dehydrogenase (MCAD; see Clinical Box 25-2) prefers fats of 4 to 16 carbons in length with maximal activity for C10 acyl-CoAs; long-chain acyl-CoA dehydrogenase (LCAD) prefers fats of 6 to 16 carbons in length with maximal activity for C12 acyl-CoAs. Deficiencies in several of the acyl-CoA dehydrogenases are known to result in impaired β-oxidation with MCAD deficiency being the most common form.

The next 3 steps in mitochondrial β-oxidation involve a hydration step, another oxidation step, and finally a hydrolytic reaction that requires CoA and releases acetyl-CoA and an acyl-CoA 2 carbon atoms shorter than the initial substrate. The water addition is catalyzed by an enoyl-CoA hydratase activity, the second oxidation step is catalyzed by an NAD-dependent long-chain hydroxyacyl-CoA dehydrogenase activity (3-hydroxyacyl-CoA dehydrogenase activity), and finally the cleavage into an acyl-CoA and an acetyl-CoA is catalyzed by a thiolase activity. These 3 activities are encoded in a multifunctional enzyme called the mitochondrial trifunctional protein (MTP). MTP is composed of 8 protein subunits, 4 α-subunits encoded by the *HADHA* gene, and 4 β-subunits encoded by the *HADHB* gene. The α-subunits contain the enoyl-CoA hydratase and long-chain hydroxyacyl-CoA dehydrogenase activities, while the β-subunits possess the 3-ketoacyl-CoA thiolase (β-ketothiolase or just thiolase) activity. The mammalian genome actually encodes 5 distinct enzymes with thiolase activity (Table 25-2).

Each round of β-oxidation produces 1 mole of $FADH_2$, 1 mole of NADH, and 1 mole of acetyl-CoA.

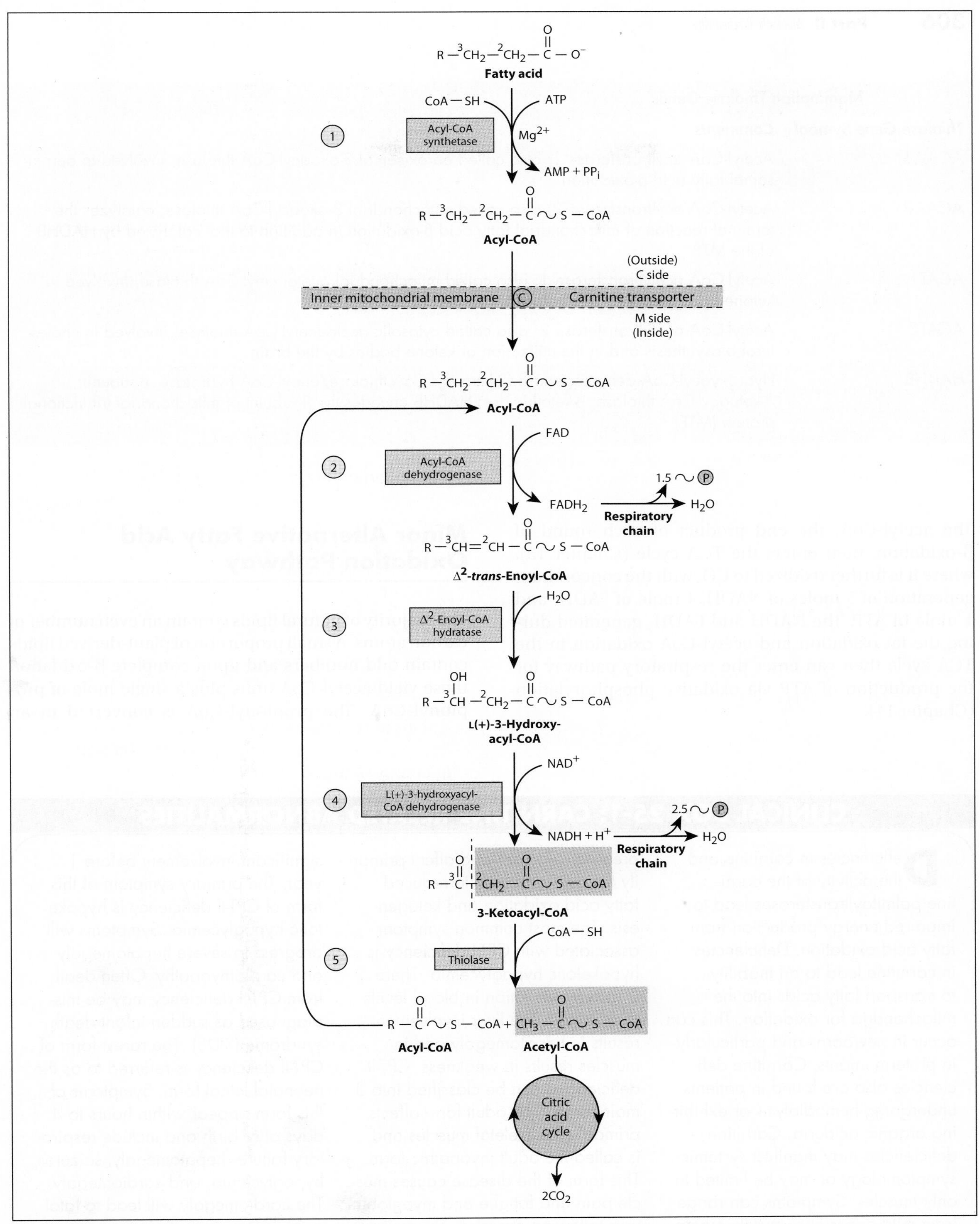

FIGURE 25-3: β-Oxidation of fatty acids. Long-chain acyl-CoA is cycled through reactions 2-5, acetyl-CoA being split off, each cycle, by thiolase (reaction 5). When the acyl radical is only 4 carbon atoms in length, 2 acetyl-CoA molecules are formed in reaction 5. Murray RK, Bender DA, Botham KM, Kennelly PJ, Rodwell VW, Weil PA. *Harper's Illustrated Biochemistry*, 29th ed. New York, NY McGraw-Hill; 2012.

TABLE 25-2: Mammalian Thiolase Genes

Thiolase Gene Symbol	*Comments*
ACAA1	Acetyl-CoA acyltransferase 1; also called peroxisomal 3-oxoacyl-CoA thiolase; involved in peroxisomal fatty acid β-oxidation
ACAA2	Acetyl-CoA acyltransferase 2; also called mitochondrial 3-oxoacyl-CoA thiolase; catalyzes the terminal reaction of mitochondrial fatty acid β-oxidation in addition to that catalyzed by HADHB of the MTP
ACAT1	Acetyl-CoA acetyltransferase 1; also called mitochondrial acetoacetyl-CoA thiolase; involved in ketone body synthesis (see below) in the liver
ACAT2	Acetyl-CoA acetyltransferase 2; also called cytosolic acetoacetyl-CoA thiolase; involved in cholesterol biosynthesis and in the utilization of ketone bodies by the brain
HADHB	Hydroxyacyl-CoA dehydrogenase/3-ketoacyl-CoA thiolase/enoyl-CoA hydratase, β-subunit; 3-ketoacyl-CoA thiolase; β-ketothiolase; HADHB encodes the β-subunit of mitochondrial trifunctional protein (MTP)

The acetyl-CoA, the end product of each round of β-oxidation, then enters the TCA cycle (Chapter 13), where it is further oxidized to CO_2 with the concomitant generation of 3 moles of NADH, 1 mole of $FADH_2$ and 1 mole of ATP. The NADH and $FADH_2$ generated during the fat oxidation and acetyl-CoA oxidation in the TCA cycle then can enter the respiratory pathway for the production of ATP via oxidative phosphorylation (Chapter 14).

Minor Alternative Fatty Acid Oxidation Pathway

The majority of natural lipids contain an even number of carbon atoms. A small proportion of plant-derived lipids contain odd numbers and upon complete β-oxidation these yield acetyl-CoA units plus a single mole of propionyl-CoA. The propionyl-CoA is converted in an

CLINICAL BOX 25-1: CARNITINE-RELATED ABNORMALITIES

Deficiencies in carnitine and the activity of the carnitine palmitoyltransferases lead to impaired energy production from fatty acid oxidation. Deficiencies in carnitine lead to an inability to transport fatty acids into the mitochondria for oxidation. This can occur in newborns and particularly in preterm infants. Carnitine deficiencies also are found in patients undergoing hemodialysis or exhibiting organic aciduria. Carnitine deficiencies may manifest systemic symptomology or may be limited to only muscles. Symptoms can range from mild occasional muscle cramping to severe weakness or even death. Treatment is by oral carnitine administration. Deficiencies in CPT-I are relatively rare and affect primarily the liver and lead to reduced fatty acid oxidation and ketogenesis. The most common symptom associated with CPT-I deficiency is hypoketotic hypoglycemia. There is also an elevation in blood levels of carnitine. The liver involvement results in hepatomegaly and in muscles results in weakness. CPT-II deficiencies can be classified into 3 main forms. The adult form affects primarily the skeletal muscles and is called the adult myopathic form. This form of the disease causes muscle pain and fatigue and myoglobinuria following exercise. The severe infantile multisystem form manifest in the first 6 to 24 months of life with most afflicted infants demonstrating significant involvement before 1 year. The primary symptom of this form of CPT-II deficiency is hypoketotic hypoglycemia. Symptoms will progress to severe hepatomegaly and cardiomyopathy. Often death from CPT-II deficiency may be misdiagnosed as sudden infant death syndrome (SIDS). The rarest form of CPT-II deficiency is referred to as the neonatal lethal form. Symptoms of this form appear within hours to 4 days after birth and include respiratory failure, hepatomegaly, seizures, hypoglycemia, and cardiomegaly. The cardiomegaly will lead to fatal arrhythmias. Carnitine acyltransferases may also be inhibited by sulfonylurea drugs such as tolbutamide and glyburide.

CLINICAL BOX 25-2: MEDIUM-CHAIN ACYL-COA DEHYDROGENASE DEFICIENCY

Medium-chain acyl-CoA dehydrogenase (MCAD), which is also called acyl-CoA dehydrogenase, medium-chain (ACADM), is so called because of the size range of its fatty acyl-CoA substrates. MCAD acts on fatty acyl-CoA molecules that range in size from 12 down to 4 carbons in length. Deficiency in MCAD is the most common defect observed in the process of mitochondrial β-oxidation of fatty acids. In fact, MCAD deficiency is one of the most common inherited disorders of metabolism occurring with a frequency of approximately 1 in 10,000 live births. The most common symptom of MCAD deficiency is episodic hypoketotic hypoglycemia brought on by fasting. Symptoms appear within the first 2 years of life. Clinical crisis is characterized by an infant presenting with episodes of vomiting and lethargy that may progress to seizures and ultimately coma. A prior upper respiratory or gastrointestinal viral infection will lead to reduced oral intake in these infants which can precipitate the acute crisis. The first episode in an infant may be fatal and the death ascribed to sudden infant death syndrome (SIDS). Autopsy results will often find marked fatty liver (hepatic steatosis) and cerebral edema. These findings are sometimes misdiagnosed as Reye syndrome especially in the circumstance where there has been a prior infection. Because the capacity of the gluconeogenesis pathway is limited in newborn infants, they are highly susceptible to the lack of brain energy from the ketones that would normally be derived from fatty acid oxidation. The defect in fatty acid oxidation leads to the presence, in the plasma and urine, of toxic metabolic intermediates such as dicarboxylic acids. Characteristic of, and diagnostic for, MCAD deficiency is the presence of octanoylcarnitine. Diagnosis can be made within 24 to 48 hours in specialized laboratories using tandem mass spectrometry (MS) of the blood for specific acylcarnitines. In MCAD deficiency the acylcarnitines that are found are highly diagnostic and specific for this disorder and include C6:0-, 4-*cis*-, and 5-*cis*-C8:1, C8:0, and 4-*cis*-C10:1 acylcarnitine species. The primary goal of treatment for MCAD deficiency patients is to provide adequate caloric intake, the avoidance of fasting and IV glucose to treat acute episodes, along with aggressive therapy during periods of infection. Anorexia can develop during infections and fever leading to mobilization of stored fatty acids. The effect of increased lipid mobilization is the production of toxic intermediates which can lead to vomiting, lethargy, coma, and even death. Treatment with oral carnitine increases the removal of these toxic intermediates.

ATP-dependent pathway to succinyl-CoA. The succinyl-CoA can then enter the TCA cycle for further oxidation (Figure 25-4).

The oxidation of unsaturated fatty acids is essentially the same process as for saturated fats, except when a double bond is encountered (Figure 25-5). In such a case, the bond is isomerized by a specific enoyl-CoA isomerase and oxidation continues. In the case of linoleate, the presence of the Δ^{12} unsaturation results in the formation of a dienoyl-CoA during oxidation. This molecule is the substrate for an additional oxidizing enzyme, the NADPH requiring 2,4-dienoyl-CoA reductase.

Peroxisomal (Alpha) α-Oxidation Pathway

Phytanic acid is a fatty acid present in the tissues of ruminants and in dairy products and is, therefore, an important dietary component of fatty acid intake.

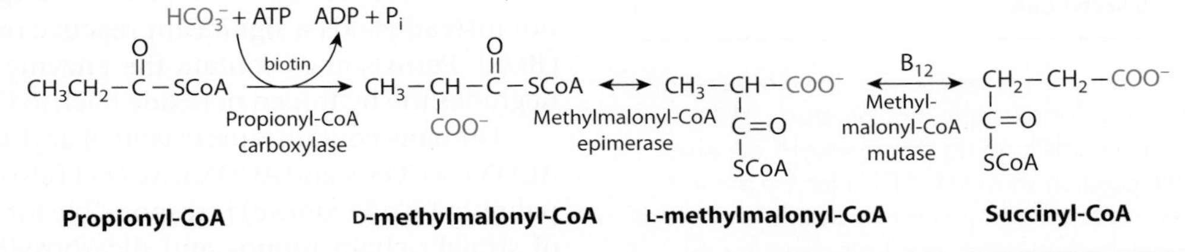

$HCO_3^- + ATP$ → $ADP + P_i$ (biotin)

$CH_3CH_2-C(=O)-SCoA$ → (Propionyl-CoA carboxylase) → $CH_3-CH(COO^-)-C(=O)-SCoA$ ⟷ (Methylmalonyl-CoA epimerase) ⟷ $CH_3-CH(COO^-)-C(=O)-SCoA$ ⟷ (B_{12}, Methyl-malonyl-CoA mutase) ⟷ $CH_2(COO^-)$... $CH_2-CH_2-COO^-$ with $C(=O)SCoA$

Propionyl-CoA | D-methylmalonyl-CoA | L-methylmalonyl-CoA | Succinyl-CoA

FIGURE 25-4: Conversion of propionyl-CoA to succinyl-CoA. Reproduced with permission of themedicalbiochemistrypage, LLC.

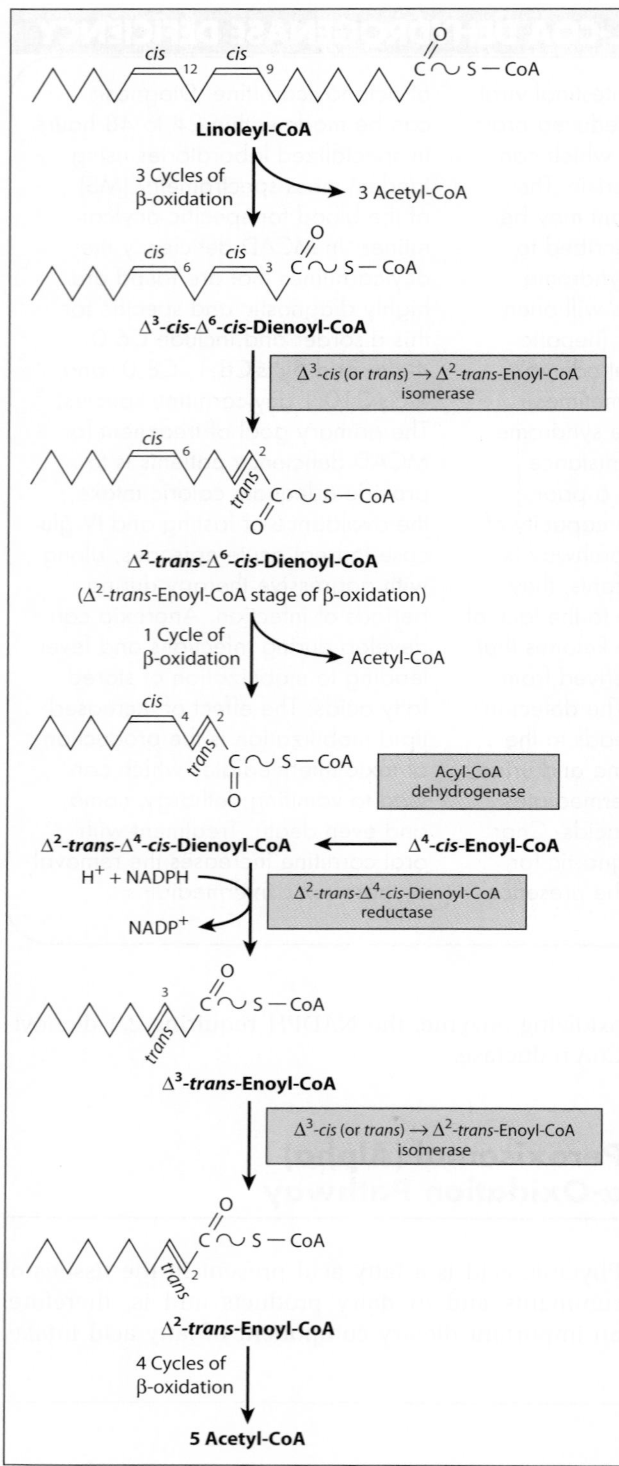

FIGURE 25-5: Sequence of reactions in the oxidation of unsaturated fatty acids, for example, linoleic acid. Δ^4-*cis*-fatty acids or fatty acids forming Δ^4-*cis*-enoyl-CoA enter the pathway at the position shown. NADPH for the dienoyl-CoA reductase step is supplied by intramitochondrial sources such as glutamate dehydrogenase, isocitrate dehydrogenase, and NAD(P)H transhydrogenase. Murray RK, Bender DA, Botham KM, Kennelly PJ, Rodwell VW, Weil PA. *Harper's Illustrated Biochemistry*, 29th ed. New York, NY McGraw-Hill; 2012.

Because phytanic acid is methylated, it cannot act as a substrate for the normal mitochondrial β-oxidation pathway. Phytanic acid is first converted to its CoA-ester and then phytanoyl-CoA serves as a substrate in an α-oxidation process, therefore, the process is referred to as α-oxidation (Figure 25-6). The α-oxidation reaction, as well as the remainder of the reactions of phytanic acid oxidation, occurs within the peroxisomes and requires a specific α-hydroxylase called phytanoyl-CoA hydroxylase (PhyH). The action of PhyH adds a hydroxyl group to the α-carbon of phytanic acid generating the 19-carbon homologue, pristanic acid. Pristanic acid then serves as a substrate for the remainder of the normal process of β-oxidation. Deficiency in PhyH activity results in the disorder known as Refsum disease. (see Clinical Box 25-3).

Peroxisomal β-Oxidation Reactions

In addition to mitochondrial oxidation of fatty acids, the peroxisomes play an important role in overall fatty acid metabolism. Very-long-chain fatty acids (VLCFAs: 17-26 carbons long) are preferentially oxidized in the peroxisomes with cerotic acid (a 26:0 fatty acid) being solely oxidized in this organelle. The peroxisomes also metabolize di- and trihydroxycholestanoic acids (bile acid intermediates); long-chain dicarboxylic acids that are produced by ω-oxidation of long-chain monocarboxylic acids (see below); pristanic acid via the α-oxidation pathway (see above); certain polyunsaturated fatty acids (PUFA) such as tetracosahexaenoic acid (24:6), which by β-oxidation yields the important PUFA docosahexaenoic acid (DHA); and certain prostaglandins and leukotrienes.

The enzymatic processes of peroxisomal β-oxidation are very similar to those of mitochondrial β-oxidation with 1 major difference (Figure 25-7). During mitochondrial oxidation the first oxidation step, catalyzed by various acyl-CoA dehydrogenases, results in the reduced electron carrier $FADH_2$ that then delivers its electrons directly to the electron transport chain for synthesis of ATP. In the peroxisome the first oxidation step is catalyzed by acyl-CoA oxidases which are coupled to the reduction of O_2 to hydrogen peroxide (H_2O_2). Thus, the reaction is not coupled to energy production but instead yields a significant reactive oxygen species (ROS). Peroxisomes contain the enzyme catalase that degrades the hydrogen peroxide back to O_2.

Humans contain 3 peroxisomal acyl-CoA oxidases, ACOX1, ACOX2, and ACOX3. ACOX1 (also referred to as palmitoyl-CoA oxidase) is responsible for the oxidation of straight-chain mono- and dicarboxylic fatty acids, VLCFAs, prostaglandins, and xenobiotics. ACOX2 (also called branched-chain acyl-CoA oxidase) is responsible for the oxidation of 2-methyl branched fatty acids

CLINICAL BOX 25-3: REFSUM DISEASE

Refsum disease (heredopathia atactica polyneuritiformis) results from a defect in fatty acid metabolism and is named after Sigvald Refsum who initially characterized the cardinal clinical features of this disease. The disorder is due to deficiencies in the peroxisomal enzyme phytanoyl-CoA hydroxylase (PhyH) which is responsible for the initial α-oxidation reaction on phytanic acid generating the 19-carbon fatty acid, pristanic acid. Pristanic acid is then oxidized by the remainder of the normal peroxisomal fatty acid β-oxidation pathway. Phytanic acid cannot be synthesized de novo in humans, so dietary sources are the exclusive origin of this fatty acid. Dairy products, meat, ruminant fats, and fish are abundant sources of phytanic acid. PhyH is localized to the peroxisomes and disorders in peroxisome biogenesis, the peroxisome biogenesis disorders, (PBDs) (eg, Zellweger syndrome) manifest with symptoms overlapping with PhyH deficiency. The cardinal clinical features of Refsum disease are retinitis pigmentosa, chronic polyneuropathy, cerebellar ataxia, and elevated protein levels in cerebrospinal fluid. Most cases have electrocardiographic changes, and some have sensorineural hearing loss and/or ichthyosis. Multiple epiphyseal dysplasia (skeletal malformations) is a conspicuous feature in some cases. Refsum disease is a slowly developing, progressive peripheral neuropathy. Progression of the disease results in severe motor weakness and muscle wasting, particularly in the lower extremities.

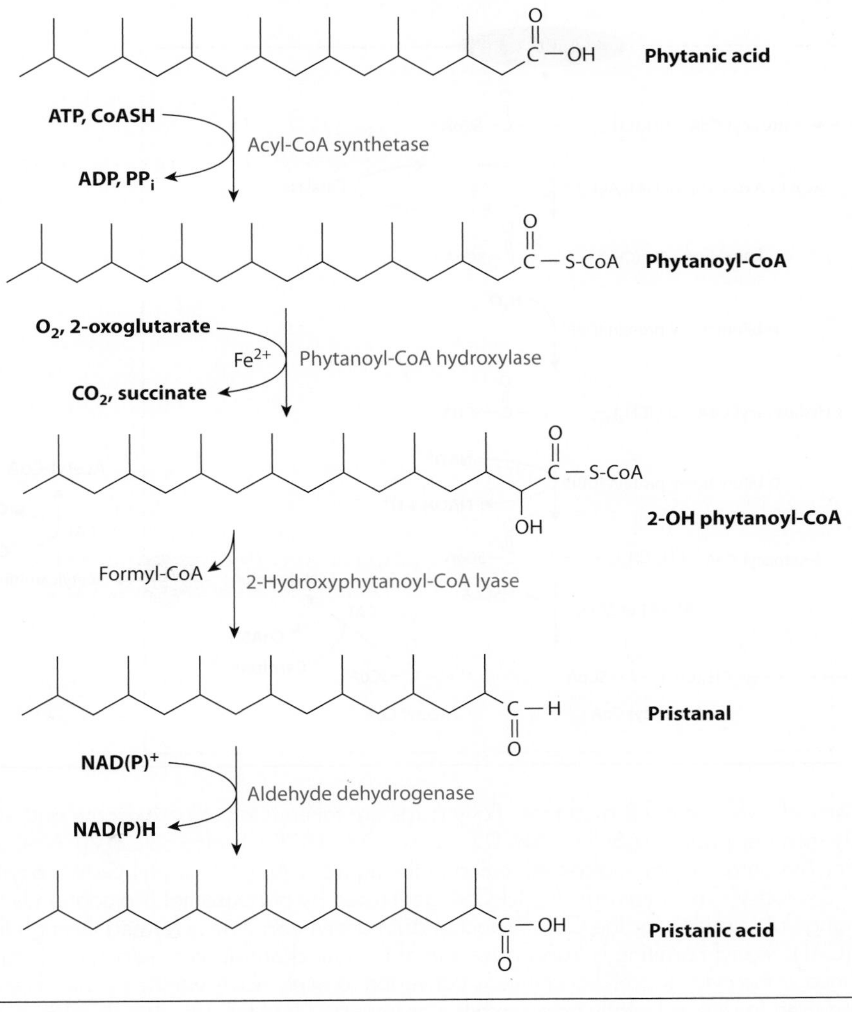

FIGURE 25-6: α-oxidation reactions involved the metabolism of phytanic acid. Reproduced with permission of themedical-biochemistrypage, LLC.

High-Yield Concept

The clinical significance of the activity of the acyl-CoA oxidases of peroxisomal β-oxidation is related to tissue specific oxidation processes. In the pancreatic β-cell there is little, if any, catalase expressed so that peroxisomal oxidation of VLCFA results in an increased release of ROS that can damage the β-cell contributing to the progressive insulin deficiency seen in obesity.

(primarily pristanic acid) and the bile acid intermediates di- and trihydroxycoprostanic acids. Expression from the human *ACOX3* gene is detected in normal tissue only at extremely low levels.

The hydration step and second oxidation step in peroxisomal β-oxidation is carried out by a single bifunctional enzyme as opposed to 2 separate enzymes as is the case for mitochondrial β-oxidation. There are 2 distinct bifunctional enzymes identified as L-bifunctional protein (LBP) and D-bifunctional protein (DBP). LBP is specific for L-3-hydroxyacyl-CoAs and DBP is specific for D-3-hydroxyacyl-CoAs. These bifunctional

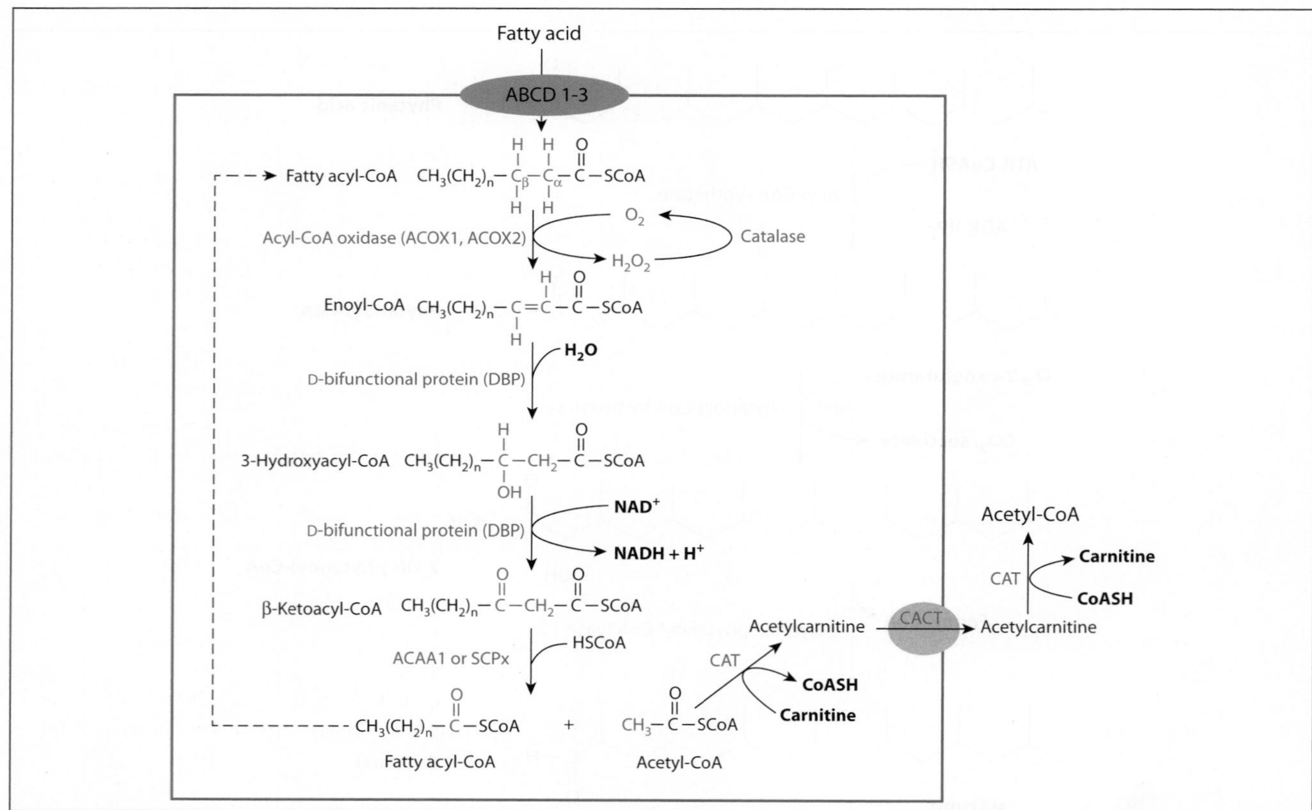

FIGURE 25-7: Pathway of peroxisomal β-oxidation. Fatty acids are taken into the peroxisome and esterified to CoA by the solute carrier family member proteins ABCD1, ABCD2, or ABCD3. ABCD1 is also called VLCFA-CoA synthetase. DBP is D-bifunctional protein. The peroxisomal thiolase indicated in the figure is ACAA1 (acetyl-CoA C-acyltransferase 1, also known as peroxisomal 3-oxoacyl-CoA thiolase). Acetyl-CoA generated by peroxisomal β-oxidation is transported out of the peroxisome after exchange of carnitine for the CoA. Mitochondrial acetyl-carnitine is formed through the action of carnitine acetyltransferase (CAT). Acetyl-carnitine is transported out of the mitochondria via the action of carnitine-acylcarnitine translocase (CACT). Once in the cytosol acetyl-carnitine is converted to acetyl-CoA via the action of cytosolic CAT. These acetyl-CoA units can be used for cytosolic fatty acid synthesis or imported into the mitochondria for oxidation in the TCA cycle. Reproduced with permission of themedicalbiochemistrypage, LLC.

High-Yield Concept

The microsomal (endoplasmic reticulum [ER]) pathway of fatty acid ω-oxidation represents a minor pathway of overall fatty acid oxidation. However, in certain pathophysiological states, such as diabetes, chronic alcohol consumption, and starvation, the ω-oxidation pathway may provide an effective means for the elimination of toxic levels of free fatty acids.

enzymes are also referred to as multifunctional proteins 1 and 2 (MFP-1 and -2) or L- and D-peroxisomal bifunctional enzymes (L-PBE and D-PBE). DBP is the primary if not exclusive enzyme involved in the oxidation of VLCFAs, pristanic acid, and di- and trihydroxycholestanoic acids. Human peroxisomes contain the thiolase (ACAA1, see Table 25-2) that catalyzes the terminal step in the peroxisomal β-oxidation pathway.

Microsomal ω-Oxidation Reactions

The pathway refers to the fact that fatty acids first undergo a hydroxylation step at the terminal (omega, ω) carbon (Figure 25-8). Human ω-hydroxylases are all members of the cytochrome P450 family (CYP) of enzymes. The CYP4A and CYP4F families that preferentially hydroxylate the terminal methyl group of 10 to 26 carbons long fatty acids are abundantly expressed in the liver and kidneys. CYP4A11 utilizes NADPH and O_2 to introduce an alcohol to the ω-CH_3– of several fatty acids including lauric (12:0), myristic (14:0), palmitic (16:0), oleic (18:1), and arachidonic acid (20:4). Following addition of the ω-hydroxyl the fatty acid is a substrate for alcohol dehydrogenase (ADH) which generates an oxo-fatty acid, followed by generation of the corresponding dicarboxylic acid via the action of aldehyde dehydrogenases (ALDH). Further metabolism then takes place via the β-oxidation pathway in peroxisomes. The CYP4F family enzyme CYP4F3A, which is expressed in leukocytes, is necessary for the ω-hydroxylation and subsequent degradation of leukotriene B_4 (Chapter 20).

Regulation of Fatty Acid Metabolism

The metabolism of fat is regulated by 2 distinct mechanisms. One is short-term regulation, which can come about through events such as substrate availability, allosteric effectors, and/or enzyme modification. The other mechanism, long-term regulation, is achieved by alteration of the rate of enzyme synthesis and turnover.

Both isoforms of ACC are allosterically activated by citrate and inhibited by palmitoyl-CoA and other short- and long-chain fatty acyl-CoAs. Citrate triggers the polymerization of ACC1 which leads to significant increases in its activity. Although ACC2 does not undergo significant polymerization, it is allosterically activated by citrate. Glutamate and other dicarboxylic acids can also allosterically activate both ACC isoforms.

ACC activity can also be affected by phosphorylation. Phosphorylation of ACC1 by AMPK leads to inhibition of the enzyme. Glucagon-stimulated increases in cAMP and subsequently to increased PKA activity also lead to phosphorylation of ACC. ACC2 is a better substrate for PKA than is ACC1. The activating effects of insulin on ACC are complex and not completely resolved but it is known that insulin leads to the dephosphorylation of ACC1 commensurate to changes in cAMP levels. Activation of α-adrenergic receptors in liver and skeletal muscle cells inhibits ACC activity as a result of phosphorylation by an as yet undetermined kinase. Fat metabolism can also be allosterically regulated by malonyl-CoA-mediated inhibition of CPT I.

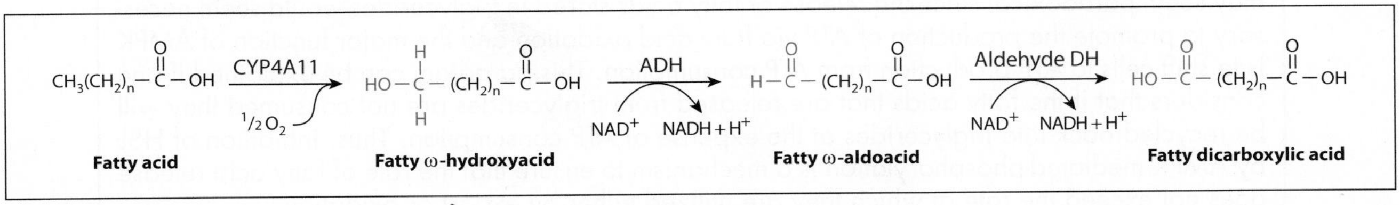

$$CH_3(CH_2)_n{-}C({=}O){-}OH \xrightarrow[\frac{1}{2}O_2]{\text{CYP4A11}} HO{-}CH_2{-}(CH_2)_n{-}C({=}O){-}OH \xrightarrow[NAD^+ \to NADH + H^+]{\text{ADH}} H{-}C({=}O){-}(CH_2)_n{-}C({=}O){-}OH \xrightarrow[NAD^+ \to NADH + H^+]{\text{Aldehyde DH}} HO{-}C({=}O){-}(CH_2)_n{-}C({=}O){-}OH$$

Fatty acid → Fatty ω-hydroxyacid → Fatty ω-aldoacid → Fatty dicarboxylic acid

FIGURE 25-8: Pathway of microsomal ω-oxidation initiated by CYP4A11. Reproduced with permission of themedicalbiochemistrypage, LLC.

High-Yield Concept

The formation of ω-hydroxylated arachidonic acid (20-hydroxyeicosatetraenoic acid, 20-HETE) by CYP4A11 plays an important role in the regulation of the cardiovascular system because 20-HETE is a known vasoconstrictor. Polymorphisms in the *CYP4A11* gene are associated with hypertension in certain populations, particularly those of Asian heritage.

Such regulation serves to prevent de novo synthesized fatty acids from entering the mitochondria and being oxidized.

Long-term regulation of fat metabolism by insulin is the result of the stimulation of ACC and FAS synthesis. Conversely, starvation leads to a decrease in the synthesis of these enzymes. Adipose tissue levels of lipoprotein lipase also are increased by insulin and decreased by starvation. However, the effects of insulin and starvation on lipoprotein lipase in the heart are just the inverse of those in adipose tissue. This sensitivity allows the heart to absorb any available fatty acids in the blood in order to oxidize them for energy production. Starvation also leads to increases in the levels of cardiac enzymes of fatty acid oxidation, and to decreases in FAS and related enzymes of synthesis.

Adipose tissue contains hormone-sensitive lipase (HSL), which is activated by PKA-dependent phosphorylation; this activation increases the release of fatty acids into the blood. This in turn leads to the increased oxidation of fatty acids in other tissues such as muscle and liver. In the liver, the net result is enhanced production of ketone bodies. This would occur under conditions in which the carbohydrate stores and gluconeogenic precursors available in the liver are not sufficient to allow increased glucose production. The increased levels of fatty acid that become available in response to glucagon or epinephrine are assured of being completely oxidized, because PKA also phosphorylates ACC leading to decreased synthesis of fatty acids.

The utilization of fatty acids, or glucose, for fuel generation exhibits reciprocal regulation via a process

High-Yield Concept

ACC is the rate-limiting step in fatty acid synthesis. There are 2 major isoforms of ACC in mammalian tissues identified as ACC1 and ACC2. ACC1 is strictly cytosolic and is enriched in liver, adipose tissue, and lactating mammary tissue. ACC2 is expressed in liver, skeletal muscle, and heart. ACC2 has an *N*-terminal extension that contains a mitochondrial targeting motif and is found associated with carnitine palmitoyltransferase I (CPT I) allowing for rapid regulation of CPT I by the malonyl-CoA produced by ACC.

High-Yield Concept

The activity of HSL is inhibited via AMPK-mediated phosphorylation. Inhibition of HSL by AMPK may seem paradoxical since the release of fatty acids stored in triglycerides would seem necessary to promote the production of ATP via fatty acid oxidation and the major function of AMPK is to shift cells to ATP production from ATP consumption. This paradigm can be explained if one considers that if the fatty acids that are released from triglycerides are not consumed they will be recycled back into triglycerides at the expense of ATP consumption. Thus, inhibition of HSL by AMPK mediated-phosphorylation is a mechanism to ensure that the rate of fatty acid release does not exceed the rate at which they are utilized either by export or oxidation.

referred to as the glucose-fatty acid cycle. Specifically, the glucose-fatty acid cycle describes the interrelationships of glucose and fatty acid oxidation as defined by fuel flux and fuel selection by various organs. The underlying theme of the glucose-fatty acid cycle is that the utilization of one nutrient (eg, glucose) directly inhibits the use of the other (in this case fatty acids) without hormonal mediation. The general interrelationships between glucose and fatty acid utilization are discussed in detail in Chapter 10.

Ketogenesis

Ketogenesis is the process of diverting the acetyl-CoA, derived primarily during high rates of fatty acid oxidation in the liver, into the synthesis of ketone bodies. The ketone bodies are acetoacetate, β-hydroxybutyrate, and acetone. The ketone bodies, principally β-hydroxybutyrate, can then be used for energy production during periods when glucose and gluconeogenesis are limiting. The synthesis of the ketone bodies occurs in the mitochondria allowing this process to be intimately coupled to rate of hepatic fatty acid oxidation. Conversely, the utilization of the ketones occurs in the cytosol.

Ketone formation begins with the condensation of 2 moles of acetyl-CoA formatting acetoacetyl-CoA (Figure 25-9). This reaction is essentially a reversal of the thiolase (HADHB or ACAA2)-catalyzed reaction of β-oxidation but is in fact catalyzed by the mitochondrial enzyme acetoacetyl-CoA thiolase encoded by the *ACAT1* gene. Acetoacetyl-CoA and an additional acetyl-CoA are converted to β-hydroxy-β-methylglutaryl-CoA (HMG-CoA) by mitochondrial HMG-CoA synthase

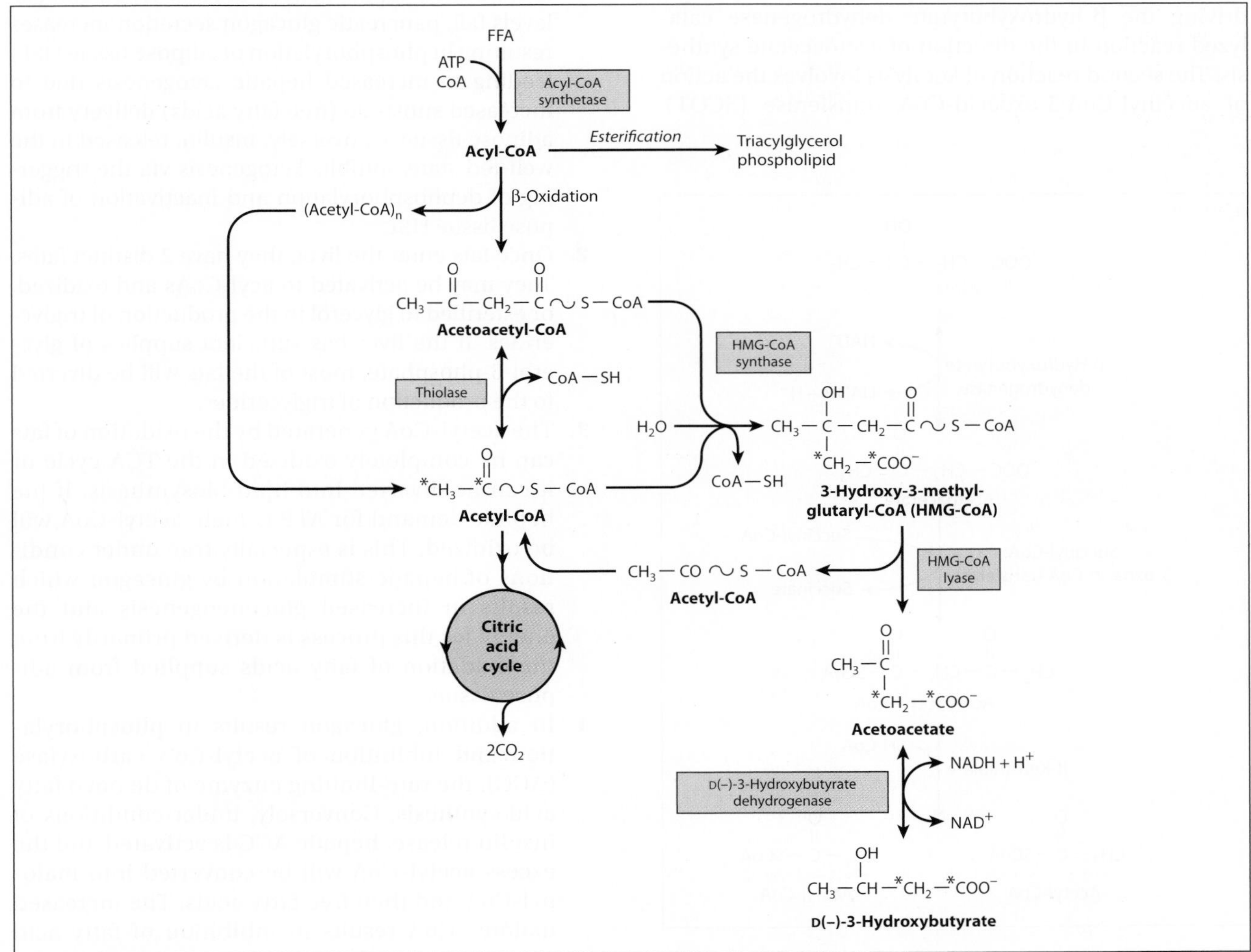

FIGURE 25-9: Pathways of ketogenesis in the liver. (FFA, free fatty acids.) Murray RK, Bender DA, Botham KM, Kennelly PJ, Rodwell VW, Weil PA. *Harper's Illustrated Biochemistry*, 29th ed. New York, NY McGraw-Hill; 2012.

(encoded by the *HMGCS2* gene), an enzyme found in large amounts only in the liver. HMG-CoA in the mitochondria is converted to acetoacetate by the action of HMG-CoA lyase. Acetoacetate can undergo spontaneous decarboxylation to acetone, or be enzymatically converted to β-hydroxybutyrate through the action of β-hydroxybutyrate dehydrogenase. The ketone bodies freely diffuse out of the mitochondria and hepatocytes and enter the circulation where they can be taken up by nonhepatic tissues such as the brain, heart, and skeletal muscle.

Ketone bodies are utilized by extrahepatic tissues via a series of cytosolic reactions that are essentially a reversal of ketone body synthesis (Figure 25-10). The initial steps involve the conversion of β-hydroxybutyrate to acetoacetate and of acetoacetate to acetoacetyl-CoA. The first step involves the reversal of the β-hydroxybutyrate dehydrogenase reaction. It is important to appreciate that under conditions where tissues are utilizing ketones for energy production their NAD^+:NADH ratios are going to be relatively high, thus driving the β-hydroxybutyrate dehydrogenase catalyzed reaction in the direction of acetoacetate synthesis. The second reaction of ketolysis involves the action of succinyl-CoA:3-oxoacid-CoA transferase (SCOT).

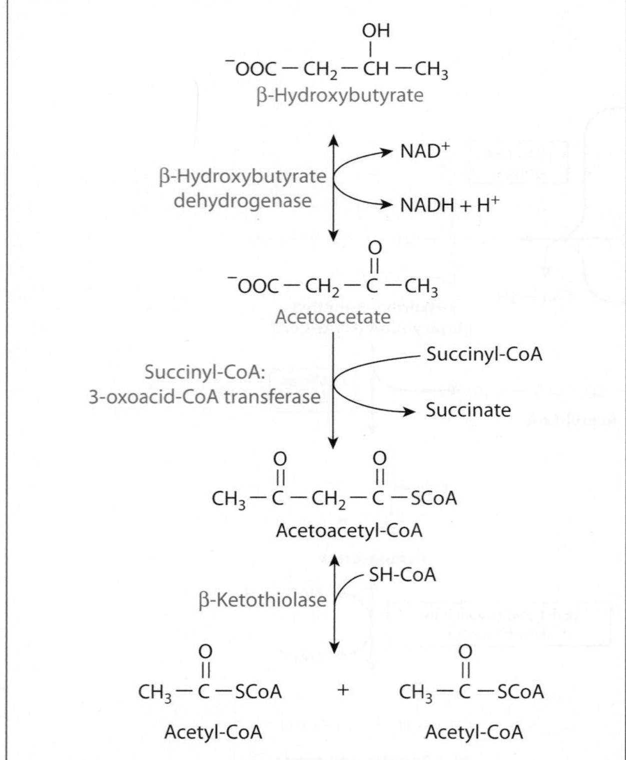

FIGURE 25-10: Reactions of ketone body utilization. Reproduced with permission of themedicalbiochemistrypage, LLC.

The latter enzyme is present at high levels in most tissues except the liver. Importantly, very low level of SCOT expression in the liver allows the liver to produce ketone bodies but not to utilize them. This ensures that extrahepatic tissues have access to ketone bodies as a fuel source during prolonged fasting and starvation.

Regulation of Ketogenesis

The level of ketone synthesis within the liver is determined by a number of factors that regulate the overall process of lipid homeostasis as well as dietary and physiological conditions.

1. Control over the release of free fatty acids from adipose tissue directly affects the level of ketogenesis in the liver. This is, of course, substrate-level regulation. Fatty acid release from adipose tissue is controlled via the activity of HSL. When glucose levels fall, pancreatic glucagon secretion increases resulting in phosphorylation of adipose tissue HSL, leading to increased hepatic ketogenesis due to increased substrate (free fatty acids) delivery from adipose tissue. Conversely, insulin, released in the well-fed state, inhibits ketogenesis via the triggering of dephosphorylation and inactivation of adipose tissue HSL.
2. Once fats enter the liver, they have 2 distinct fates. They may be activated to acyl-CoAs and oxidized, or esterified to glycerol in the production of triglycerides. If the liver has sufficient supplies of glycerol-3-phosphate, most of the fats will be diverted to the production of triglycerides.
3. The acetyl-CoA generated by the oxidation of fats can be completely oxidized in the TCA cycle or it can be diverted into lipid biosynthesis. If the hepatic demand for ATP is high, acetyl-CoA will be oxidized. This is especially true under conditions of hepatic stimulation by glucagon which results in increased gluconeogenesis and the energy for this process is derived primarily from the oxidation of fatty acids supplied from adipose tissue.
4. In addition, glucagon results in phosphorylation and inhibition of acetyl-CoA carboxylase (ACC), the rate-limiting enzyme of de novo fatty acid synthesis. Conversely, under conditions of insulin release, hepatic ACC is activated and the excess acetyl-CoA will be converted into malonyl-CoA and then free fatty acids. The increased malonyl-CoA results in inhibition of fatty acid transport into the mitochondria resulting in reduced fat oxidation and reduced production of excess acetyl-CoA.

Diabetic Ketoacidosis

The most significant disruption in the level of ketone production, leading to profound clinical manifestations, occurs in untreated Type 1 diabetes. This physiological state, diabetic ketoacidosis (DKA) results from a reduced supply of glucose (due to a significant decline in circulating insulin) and a concomitant increase in fatty acid oxidation (due to a concomitant increase in circulating glucagon). DKA is characterized by metabolic acidosis, hyperglycemia and hyperketonemia. Diagnosis of DKA is accomplished by detection of hyperketonemia and metabolic acidosis (as measured by the anion gap) in the presence of hyperglycemia. The increased production of acetyl-CoA leads to ketone body production that exceeds the ability of peripheral tissues to oxidize them. Ketone bodies are relatively strong acids (pK_a around 3.5), and their increase lowers the pH of the blood, referred to as metabolic acidosis. The resultant hyperglycemia produces an osmotic diuresis that leads to loss of water and electrolytes in the urine. The ketones are also excreted in the urine and this results in an obligatory loss of Na^+ and K^+. The loss in K^+ is large, sometimes exceeding 300 mEq/L/24 h. Initial serum K^+ is typically normal or elevated because of the extracellular migration of K^+ in response to the metabolic acidosis. The level of K^+ will fall further during treatment as insulin therapy drives K^+ into cells. If serum K^+ is not monitored and replaced as needed, life-threatening hypokalemia may develop.

REVIEW QUESTIONS

1. Parents of a 3-month-old infant arrive at the ER agitated and frightened by the extreme lethargy and near comatose state of their child. Examination shows the infant to be severely hypoglycemic accompanied by low measurable ketones in the urine and blood. Blood analysis also indicates an elevation in butyric and propionic acids and as well as C8-acylcarnitines. A deficiency in which of the following enzymes is most likely responsible for these observations?

A. CPT-I
B. hormone-sensitive lipase (HSL)
C. lipoprotein lipase (LPL)
D. long-chain acyl-CoA dehydrogenase (LCAD)
E. medium-chain acyl-CoA dehydrogenase (MCAD)

Answer E: In infants, the supply of glycogen lasts less than 6 hours and gluconeogenesis is not sufficient to maintain adequate blood glucose levels. Normally, during periods of fasting (in particular during the night) the oxidation of fatty acids provides the necessary ATP to fuel hepatic gluconeogenesis as well as ketone bodies for nonhepatic tissue energy production. In patients with MCAD deficiency there is a drastically reduced capacity to oxidize fatty acids. This leads to an increase in glucose usage with concomitant hypoglycemia. The deficit in the energy production from fatty acid oxidation, necessary for the liver to use other carbon sources, such as glycerol and amino acids, for gluconeogenesis further exacerbates the hypoglycemia. Normally, hypoglycemia is accompanied by an increase in ketone formation from the increased oxidation of fatty acids. In MCAD deficiency there is a reduced level of fatty acid oxidation, hence near-normal levels of ketones are detected in the serum.

2. Oxidation of fatty acids requires the input of energy in the form of ATP. Which of the following enzyme activities requires this energy input?

A. acyl-CoA dehydrogenases
B. acyl-CoA synthetase
C. CPT-I
D. CPT-II
E. β-ketothiolase

Answer B: Fatty acids must be activated in the cytoplasm before being oxidized in the mitochondria. Activation is catalyzed by fatty acyl-CoA synthetases (also called acyl-CoA ligases or thiokinases). The net result of this activation process is the consumption of 2 molar equivalents of ATP.

3. Very-long-chain fatty acids (VLCFA) are oxidized in the peroxisomes. The process of oxidation of these fats is referred to as which of the following?

A. α-oxidation
B. β-oxidation
C. δ-oxidation
D. γ-oxidation
E. ω-oxidation

Answer B: Oxidation of fatty acids occurs in the mitochondria and the peroxisomes via similar enzymatic pathways referred to as β-oxidation. Fatty acids of between 4 and 8 and between 6 and 12 carbon atoms in length, referred to as short- and medium-chain fatty acids (SCFAs and MCFAs), respectively, are oxidized exclusively in the mitochondria. Long-chain fatty acids

(LCFAs: 10-16 carbons long) are oxidized in both the mitochondria and the peroxisomes with the peroxisomes exhibiting preference for 14-carbon and longer LCFAs. Very-long-chain fatty acids (VLCFAs: 17-26 carbons long) are exclusively oxidized in the peroxisomes.

4. Excess delivery of free fatty acids to the pancreas results in progressive damage to the β-cells as these fats are oxidized. The primary cause of this progressive damage is due to which of the following processes?
   A. deficiency in peroxisomal oxidative capacity resulting in increased fat droplet production which results in apoptosis
   B. excess accumulation of triglycerides derived from the fatty acids
   C. increase in ER stress due to incorporation of the fats into membrane lipids triggering apoptosis
   D. increased fat oxidation in the peroxisomes results in release of cytochrome *c* triggering apoptosis
   E. limiting levels of catalase resulting in ROS excess leading to membrane lipid damage and mitochondrial dysfunction

Answer A: Peroxisomes oxidize long-chain fatty acid via a β-oxidation pathway where the first reaction generates H_2O_2 (a reactive oxygen species [ROS]) instead of $FADH_2$ as for mitochondrial β-oxidation. High-fat diet results in higher level of peroxisomal fatty acid oxidation resulting in increased levels of H_2O_2 production. Within the β-cells of the pancreas this increased ROS production cannot be tolerated due to low or no catalase production in these cells. The net result is β-cell dysfunction and triggering apoptosis.

5. Polymorphisms in the cytochrome P450 family enzyme, CYP4A11, are associated with hypertension in certain populations, particularly Asian populations. CYP4A11 belongs to a family of CYP4A enzymes responsible for the metabolism of arachidonic acid and the leukotriene, LTB_4. Which of the following represents the pathway in which the CYP4A enzymes functions?
   A. α-oxidation
   B. β-oxidation
   C. δ-oxidation
   D. γ-oxidation
   E. ω-oxidation

Answer E: The microsomal (endoplasmic reticulum [ER]) pathway of fatty acid ω-oxidation represents a minor pathway of overall fatty acid oxidation. Human ω-hydroxylases are all members of the cytochrome P450 family (CYP) of enzymes. These enzymes are abundant in the liver and kidneys. Specifically, it is members of the CYP4A and CYP4F families that preferentially hydroxylate the terminal methyl group of 10 to 26 carbons long fatty acids.

6. An individual suffers from a defect in one of the enzymes required for the synthesis of carnitine. If this individual does not have adequate intake of carnitine in the diet and is fasting, which of the following would be the most likely observation in this person compared to conditions of normal carnitine intake?
   A. elevated levels of long-chain dicarboxylic acids in the blood
   B. elevated very-long-chain fatty acid levels in the blood
   C. hyperglycemia
   D. increased levels of fatty acid oxidation
   E. increased rate of ketogenesis

Answer B: Carnitine is required for the transport of fatty acyl-CoAs from the cytosol into the mitochondria for oxidation. Limiting levels of carnitine would, therefore, result in reduced rates of mitochondrial β-oxidation of fatty acids. A reduced capacity for mitochondrial oxidation would ultimately result in a reduced capacity for cells to take fatty acids from the blood ultimately leading to hyperlipidemia. Since fatty acid oxidation would be impaired there would be reduced ketogenesis occurring and less energy production would restrict gluconeogenesis.

7. Hepatocytes deliver ketone bodies to the circulation because they lack which of the following enzymes?
   A. β-hydroxybutyrate dehydrogenase
   B. hydroxymethylglutaryl-CoA lyase
   C. hydroxymethylglutaryl-CoA synthetase
   D. succinyl-CoA: 3-oxoacid-CoA transferase
   E. the form of β-ketothiolase necessary to hydrolyze acetoacetyl-CoA

Answer D: Ketogenesis occurs in the liver from acetyl-CoA during high rates of fatty acid oxidation and during early starvation. The principal ketone bodies are acetoacetate and β-hydroxybutyrate, which are reversibly synthesized in a reaction catalyzed by β-hydroxybutyrate dehydrogenase. The liver delivers β-hydroxybutyrate to the circulation where it is taken up by nonhepatic tissue for use as an oxidizable fuel. The brain will derive much of its energy from ketone body oxidation during fasting and starvation. Within extrahepatic tissues, β-hydroxybutyrate is converted to acetoacetate by β-hydroxybutyrate dehydrogenase. Acetoacetate is reactivated to acetoacetyl-CoA in a reaction catalyzed by succinyl-CoA: 3-oxoacid-CoA-transferase (also called succinyl-CoA-acetoacetate-CoA-transferase or acetoacetate: succinyl-CoA-CoA transferase), which uses succinyl-CoA as the source of CoA. This enzyme is not present in hepatocytes. The acetoacetyl-CoA is then converted to 2 moles of acetyl-CoA by the thiolase reaction of fatty acid oxidation.

8. Which of the following symptoms can occur frequently in infants suffering from medium-chain acyl-CoA dehydrogenase (MCAD) deficiency if periods between meals are protracted?

A. bone and joint pain and thrombocytopenia
B. hyperammonemia with decreased ketones
C. hyperuricemia and darkening of the urine
D. hypoglycemia and metabolic acidosis with normal levels of ketones
E. metabolic alkalosis with decreased bicarbonate

Answer D: In infants, the supply of glycogen lasts less than 6 hours and gluconeogenesis is not sufficient to maintain adequate blood glucose levels. Normally, during periods of fasting (in particular during the night) the oxidation of fatty acids provides the necessary ATP to fuel hepatic gluconeogenesis as well as ketone bodies for nonhepatic tissue energy production. In patients with MCAD deficiency there is a drastically reduced capacity to oxidize fatty acids. This leads to an increase in glucose usage with concomitant hypoglycemia. The deficit in the energy production from fatty acid oxidation, necessary for the liver to use other carbon sources, such as glycerol and amino acids, for gluconeogenesis further exacerbates the hypoglycemia. Normally, hypoglycemia is accompanied by an increase in ketone formation from the increased oxidation of fatty acids. In MCAD deficiency there is a reduced level of fatty acid oxidation, hence near-normal levels of ketones are detected in the serum.

9. Following a minor respiratory illness, a seemingly healthy, developmentally normal 15-month-old boy exhibited repeated episodes of severe lethargy and vomiting following periods of fasting, such as during the middle of the night. The parents brought the infant to the ER following a seizure. The child was hypoglycemic and was administered 10% dextrose, but remained lethargic. Blood ammonia was high, liver function tests were slightly elevated, and his serum contained an accumulation of dicarboxylic acids. Only low levels of ketones were detectable in the urine. This infant suffers from which of the following disorders?

A. glutaric acidemia type II
B. Lesch-Nyhan syndrome
C. MCAD deficiency
D. PDH deficiency
E. type III (Cori) glycogen storage disease

Answer C: Deficiency in MCAD is the most common inherited defect in the pathways of mitochondrial fatty acid oxidation. The most common presentation of infants with this disorder is episodic hypoketotic hypoglycemia following periods of fasting. Although the first episode may be fatal, and incorrectly ascribed to sudden infant death syndrome, patients with MCAD deficiency are normal between episodes and are treated by avoidance of fasting and treatment of acute episodes with intravenous glucose. Accumulation of acylcarnitines (dicarboxylic acids) is diagnostic, in particular octanoylcarnitine.

10. A 15-year-old boy has been diagnosed with retinitis pigmentosa, peripheral polyneuropathy, and cerebellar ataxia. Analysis of his cerebrospinal fluid indicated a high protein content but no elevation of cell number. A telling clinical finding was a high level of serum phytanic acid. These findings are indicative of which of the following disorders?

A. carnitine palmitoyltransferase I deficiency
B. fragile X syndrome
C. MCAD deficiency
D. Refsum disease
E. rhizomelic chondrodysplasia punctata

Answer D: Refsum disease is the result of defects in the oxidation of phytanic acid, a lipid requiring an α-oxidation pathway. As a consequence phytanic acid accumulates in the blood and tissues. The hallmark symptoms of the disease are retinitis pigmentosa, cerebellar ataxia, chronic polyneuropathy, and an elevation in protein in the cerebrospinal fluid with no increase in cell count.

11. When fatty acids with odd numbers of carbon atoms are oxidized in the β-oxidation pathway the final product is 1 mole of acetyl-CoA and 1 mole of the 3-carbon molecule, propionyl-CoA. In order to use the propionyl carbons, the molecule is carboxylated and converted ultimately to succinyl-CoA and fed into the TCA cycle. Which of the following represents the vitamin cofactor required in one of the steps of this conversion?

A. cobalamin (B_{12})
B. pantothenic acid (B_5)
C. pyridoxine (B_6)
D. riboflavin (B_2)
E. thiamine (B_1)

Answer A: Propionyl-CoA is converted to succinyl-CoA in a series of reactions using 3 different enzymes. It is first carboxylated in an ATP-dependent reaction catalyzed by propionyl-CoA carboxylase, an enzyme that requires biotin as a cofactor. The product of the first reaction, D-methylmalonyl-CoA is then converted to L-methylmalonyl-CoA by methylmalonyl-CoA racemase. Finally, methylmalonyl-CoA is converted to succinyl-CoA by the cobalamin-requiring enzyme, methylmalonyl-CoA mutase.

12. The ability of the liver to regulate the level of blood glucose is critical for survival. A number of sources of carbon atoms of nonhepatic origin are used by the liver for gluconeogenesis. However, the net conversion of carbons from fat into carbons of glucose cannot occur in humans because of which of the following?

A. fat oxidation occurs in the mitochondria and gluconeogenesis occurs in the cytosol
B. states of catabolism and anabolism are never concurrently active
C. storage of fats occurs in adipose tissue and gluconeogenesis occurs in liver and kidney
D. the carbons of acetyl-CoA from fat oxidation are lost as CO_2 in the TCA cycle
E. the carbons of acetyl-CoA from fat oxidation inhibit conversion of pyruvate to oxaloacetate

Answer D: When the carbons of fatty acids are oxidized for energy production, the by-product of that process is the 2-carbon compound, acetyl-CoA. Acetyl-CoA can then enter the TCA cycle for complete oxidation. Although, several compounds of the TCA cycle can be directed into the gluconeogenic pathway of glucose synthesis the carbons of acetyl-CoA cannot provide a net source of carbon in that latter pathway. This is due to the fact that, following entry of the 2 carbons of acetyl-CoA into the TCA cycle, 2 carbons are lost as CO_2 during the subsequent reactions of the cycle.

13. The rate of ketone body production is determined by the relative rate of which of the following key metabolic pathways?

A. gluconeogenesis
B. glycogenolysis (muscle)
C. glycolysis
D. lipolysis
E. proteolysis

Answer D: Ketone bodies are synthesized in the liver from acetyl-CoA. Acetyl-CoA can be derived from the oxidation of pyruvate, certain amino acids, and fatty acids. By far, the largest concentration of acetyl-CoA is derived from the β-oxidation of fatty acids.

14. Serum concentrations of acetoacetate and β-hydroxybutyrate increase dramatically after a 3-day fast primarily because of the increased rate of which of the following?

A. fatty acid oxidation in the liver
B. fatty acid synthesis in the liver
C. glycogenolysis in the liver
D. glycolysis in skeletal muscle
E. protein degradation in skeletal muscle

Answer A: Fasting induces the release of fatty acids from adipose tissue triglycerides via the actions of glucagon. This signal is intended to provide the liver with the necessary energy to convert precursor carbon atoms into glucose. Prolonged fasting, such as a 3-day fast, will result in fatty acid oxidation in excess of the capacity of the liver to fully oxidize all the resulting acetyl-CoA. This will result in diversion of the acetyl-CoA into ketogenesis.

15. During a period of fasting, the principal precursor of ketone bodies in the blood is most likely to be which of the following?

A. alanine
B. glucose
C. glutamate
D. glycerol
E. palmitate

Answer E: Ketone bodies are synthesized in the liver from acetyl-CoA. Acetyl-CoA can be derived from the oxidation of pyruvate, certain amino acids, and fatty acids. By far, the largest concentration of acetyl-CoA is derived from the β-oxidation of fatty acids such as palmitic acid.

16. During prolonged starvation, the brain increases its use of which of the following substrates in blood as an energy source?

A. arachidonic acid
B. glucose
C. glycerol
D. β-hydroxybutyrate
E. palmitic acid

Answer D: During periods of fasting and starvation the liver diverts acetyl-CoA, derived from the oxidation of amino acids and fatty acids, into ketogenesis. The ketone bodies, acetoacetate and β-hydroxybutyrate, produced by the liver are then delivered to the blood and oxidized by peripheral tissues, such as the brain, for ATP production.

17. A 6-year-old boy with progressive muscle weakness is found to have a systemic defect in the production of carnitine. Therefore, this child has a limited ability to produce ATP in skeletal muscle because of a defect in the degradation of long-chain fatty acids via the β-oxidation pathway. Which of the

following is the most likely result of this defect in muscle?
A. decreased utilization of lactate
B. increased cholesterol stores
C. increased glycogen stores
D. increased triglyceride stores
E. increased utilization of acetoacetate

Answer D: When cells cannot effectively oxidize fatty acid, or are in need of storage fat, the fats are diverted into triglyceride synthesis. In an individual with a defect in carnitine synthesis, or a dietary carnitine deficiency, fatty acid oxidation will be impaired resulting in the diversion of the fats into triglycerides.

18. Synthesis and oxidation of fatty acids take place in the cytoplasm and mitochondria, respectively. Their simultaneous occurrence is prevented by malonyl-CoA, the first intermediate of fatty acid synthesis, because malonyl-CoA inhibits which of the following?
A. acetyl-CoA carboxylase
B. acyl carrier protein
C. carnitine palmitoyltransferase I
D. β-keto-acyl carrier protein reductase
E. β-keto-acyl carrier protein synthase

Answer C: Malonyl-CoA binds to the outer mitochondrial membrane carnitine palmitoyltransferase I. This action of malonyl-CoA is designed to prevent de novo synthesized palmitic acid from being diverted into the mitochondria and oxidized.

19. Which of the following compounds is required for intracellular transport of long-chain fatty acids into mitochondria for oxidation?
A. carnitine
B. ceramide
C. ceruloplasmin
D. citrate
E. cytidine

Answer A: During the pathway of fatty acid oxidation the molecules are first activated by attachment of CoA generating a fatty acyl-CoA derivative. The fatty acyl-CoA derivatives are then substrates for the enzyme carnitine palmitoyltransferase I, which substitutes carnitine for CoA generating a fatty acyl-carnitine which can then be transported across the outer mitochondrial membrane.

20. Transport of fatty acids from adipose tissue to other tissues for metabolism is primarily a function of which of the following compounds?
A. chylomicrons
B. α-lipoprotein
C. β-lipoprotein
D. plasmalogens
E. serum albumin

Answer E: When fatty acids are released from adipose tissue stores, they enter the circulation as free fatty acids (FFAs) and are bound to albumin for transport to peripheral tissues. When the fatty acid-albumin complexes interact with cell surfaces, the dissociation of the fatty acid from albumin represents the first step of the cellular uptake process.

21. During an episode of gastroenteritis that significantly compromises food intake, a 13-month-old girl develops progressive vomiting followed by coma. She is hypoglycemic and no ketone bodies are detected in the urine. A specific defect in the metabolism of which of the following is the most likely cause of these findings?
A. glycine
B. glycogen
C. insulin
D. leucine
E. long-chain fatty acids

Answer E: The symptoms observed in this patient resemble those of medium-chain acyl-CoA dehydrogenase (MCAD) deficiency. The most common presentation in MCAD deficiency is episodic hypoketotic hypoglycemia following periods of fasting.

22. A 2-year-old boy is admitted to the hospital because of generalized weakness, repeated episodes of vomiting, and coma after several days of reduced food intake because of a minor febrile illness. He is treated successfully with intravenous glucose. After 13 hours of fasting, when the child is well, his serum glucose and β-hydroxybutyrate levels are low while free carnitine concentrations are increased. Triglycerides containing only medium-chain fatty acids are fed, and the serum β-hydroxybutyrate concentration increases to the reference range. Which of the following disorders of fatty acid metabolism is the most likely diagnosis?
A. carnitine palmitoyltransferase I deficiency
B. dietary carnitine deficiency
C. fatty acyl-CoA synthetase deficiency
D. medium-chain acyl-CoA dehydrogenase deficiency
E. peroxisomal

Answer A: Deficiencies in the activity of the carnitine palmitoyltransferases lead to impaired energy production from fatty acid oxidation. Deficiencies in CPT-I are relatively rare and affect primarily the liver and lead to reduced fatty acid oxidation and ketogenesis. The most common symptom associated with CPT-I deficiency is hypoketotic hypoglycemia. There is also an elevation in blood levels of carnitine. The liver involvement results in hepatomegaly and in muscles results in weakness. A high carbohydrate, low-fat diet composed of primarily medium-chain triglycerides is required. Medium-chain fatty acids enter the mitochondria without the need for the carnitine shuttle.

23. An 8-month-old female infant is brought to the ER because her parents have been unable to fully rouse her for 3 hours. She had repeated episodes of vomiting and diarrhea the previous day, and she has not eaten for the past 12 hours. Physical examination shows lethargy and mild hepatomegaly. Serum and urine studies show no ketones. There is an abnormally increased ratio of acylcarnitine to free carnitine in urine. Which of the following is the most likely diagnosis?

A. glucose-6-phosphatase deficiency
B. maple syrup urine disease
C. medium-chain acyl-CoA dehydrogenase deficiency
D. tyrosinemia
E. Zellweger syndrome

Answer C: The most common symptom of MCAD deficiency is episodic hypoketotic hypoglycemia brought on by fasting. Symptoms appear within the first 2 years of life. Clinical crisis is characterized by an infant presenting with episodes of vomiting and lethargy that may progress to seizures and ultimately coma. Because the capacity of the gluconeogenesis pathway is limited in newborn infants, they are highly susceptible to the lack of brain energy from the ketones that would normally be derived from fatty acid oxidation.

Checklist

✓ Dietary fats are primarily in the form of triglycerides which are hydrolyzed by gastric and pancreatic lipases. The released fatty acids are then taken into intestinal enterocytes where triglycerides and phospholipids are formed and packaged into chylomicrons.

✓ Fatty acids are taken into cells via the actions of specific fatty acid transport proteins. Several transport proteins also possess acyl-CoA transferase activity, thus activating the fatty acids in conjunction with intracellular uptake

✓ Fatty acids are stored for future use as triglycerides with the major storage location being adipose tissue. Adipose tissue releases stored fats upon hormonal stimulation of the need for energy production. The fats are released through the concerted actions of ATGL, HSL, and MGL.

✓ Fatty acids are oxidized to produce large quantities of ATP. Oxidation takes place primarily within the mitochondria by a process referred to as β-oxidation that sequentially releases acetyl-CoA units that then enter the TCA cycle.

✓ Entry of fatty acyl-CoA into the mitochondria is controlled by malonyl-CoA–mediated inhibition of carnitine palmitoyltransferase I. This regulatory process connects fatty acid synthesis to fatty acid oxidation since malonyl-CoA is the product of the rate-limiting enzyme of fat synthesis.

✓ Long-chain fatty acids can undergo β-oxidation in the peroxisomes and very-long-chain fatty acids are exclusively oxidized in the peroxisome. Peroxisomal β-oxidation generates hydrogen peroxide which is metabolized primarily by catalase. Excess peroxisomal oxidation in pancreatic β-cells leads to cellular dysfunction due to limiting amounts of catalase in these cells.

✓ Ruminant fats contain significant quantities of the methyl-substituted fatty acid, phytanic acid which is oxidized in the peroxisomes via α-oxidation pathway. Defects in the α-oxidation pathway result in peroxisomal disorder called Refsum disease.

- ✓ Microsomal ω-oxidation is a minor fatty acid oxidation pathway that involves an initial hydroxylation step to the terminal ω-carbon. In certain pathophysiological states, such as diabetes, chronic alcohol consumption, and starvation, the ω-oxidation pathway provides a route for the elimination of toxic levels of free fatty acids.
- ✓ Fatty acid oxidation is regulated by the delivery of substrate to the oxidation enzymes. This reflects a balance between hormonal signals, such as insulin and glucagon, designed to control energy storage and energy production, respectively.
- ✓ Glucose and fatty acids reciprocally regulate the utilization of each other in energy generation pathways through substrate-product interactions termed the glucose-fatty acid cycle.
- ✓ Ketogenesis represents the pathway carried out in the liver to divert acetyl-CoA into carbon sources of energy, the ketone bodies, for use by the brain and other peripheral tissues primarily during periods of fasting and starvation. In Type 1 diabetes the unregulated release of glucagon leads to excess adipose tissue release of fatty acids which are converted to ketone bodies by the liver in excess of peripheral tissue utilization resulting in the condition referred to as diabetic ketoacidosis.
- ✓ Defects in enzymes of fatty acid oxidation can lead to potentially life-threatening conditions of hypoglycemia and fatty deposition in organs such as the liver resulting in cirrhosis. Additionally, peroxisomal fatty acid oxidation defects manifest with symptoms similar to the more classical peroxisomal biogenesis disorders such as Zellweger syndrome.

CHAPTER

26 Lipids: Cholesterol Metabolism

CHAPTER OUTLINE

High-Yield Terms

Cholesterol ester: product of fatty acid esterification of the 3-OH catalyzed by ACAT or LCAT

Reverse cholesterol transport: process by which cholesterol is transferred from nonhepatic cells to HDLs and then transported back to the liver via blood

LDL: low-density lipoprotein, derived from *de novo* VLDL synthesized in the liver, referred to as "bad cholesterol"

HDL: lipoprotein particle involved in reverse cholesterol transport, referred to as "good cholesterol"

SREBP2: sterol-regulated element-binding protein 2, controls the expression of genes involved in hepatic cholesterol biosynthesis

SCAP: SREBP cleavage-activating protein, cleaves the transcription factor domain from ER-embedded SREBP, allowing it to migrate to the nucleus

Insig: insulin-regulated gene, regulates the activity of SCAP

Isoprenoid: any compound containing the 5-carbon organic molecule isoprene (also called terpene) with the formula: $CH_2{=}C{-}(CH_3){-}CH{=}CH_2$

Prenylation: process of attaching isoprenoid intermediates of the cholesterol biosynthetic pathway (farnesyl pyrophosphate and geranylgeranyl pyrophosphate) to proteins

Cholesterol: Physiologically and Clinically Significant Lipid

Cholesterol is a waxy lipophilic compound of the sterol family, which contains 3 six-membered rings, a five-membered ring, and a hydroxyalcohol (Figure 26-1). That cholesterol is a critical component of normal physiological function can easily be demonstrated when its biosynthesis is disrupted or when it accumulates in excess of normal physiological requirements (see Clinical Box 26-1 and 26-2). Loss of the activity of the terminal enzyme in de novo cholesterol biosynthesis (7-dehydrocholesterol reductase [DHCR7]) results in varying degrees of developmental malformation as well as behavioral and learning disabilities encompassing the disorder known as Smith-Lemli-Opitz syndrome (see Clinical Box 26-3). At the opposite end of the spectrum, excess cholesterol, in the vasculature, is a significant contributing factor in the development of coronary artery disease, vascular dysfunction, and atherosclerosis. It is this latter consequence of abnormal cholesterol that has led to the near-universal use of cholesterol biosynthesis–inhibiting drugs in the treatment of hypercholesterolemia.

At the normal end of the spectrum, cholesterol is a critical component of biological membranes, establishing proper fluidity and permeability to the structure. The hydroxyalcohol attached to carbon-3 of the cholesterol structure plays a significant role in the mobilization and storage of cholesterol through fatty acid esterification. In addition to its role in membrane structure and function, cholesterol serves as the precursor for the synthesis of the steroid hormones (see Chapter 50), vitamin D (see Chapter 8), and the bile acids (see Chapter 27). In addition, cholesterol is metabolized by the cytochrome P450 (CYP) family of metabolic enzymes resulting in the generation of a number of oxysterols. Oxysterols serve as biologically active signaling molecules that exert their effects primarily through the activation of nuclear receptors such as the liver X receptors (LXRs, see Chapter 40) and SREBP (see later).

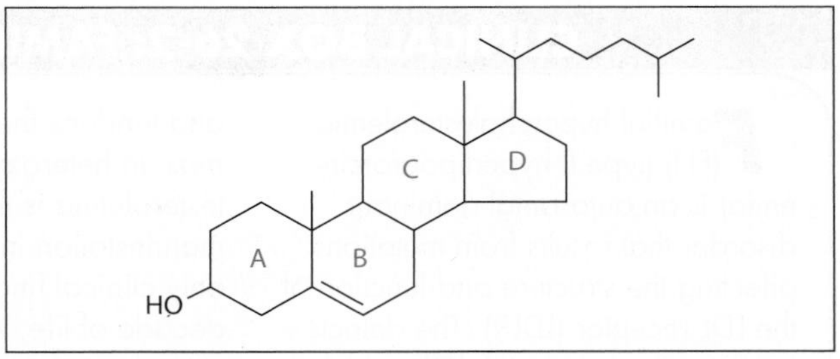

FIGURE 26-1: Structure of cholesterol.

Both dietary cholesterol and that synthesized de novo are transported through the circulation in lipoprotein particles (see Chapter 28) either as free cholesterol or as cholesterol esters with a fatty acid esterified to the carbon-3 hydroxyl group (Figure 26-2). Esterification of cholesterol is catalyzed by ratio of intracellular acyl-CoA to cholesterol acyltransferase (ACAT) or by the ratio of HDL-associated enzyme lecithin to cholesterol acyltransferase (LCAT).

CLINICAL BOX 26-1: CHOLESTEROL VALUES

Standard fasting blood tests for cholesterol will include values for total cholesterol, HDL cholesterol (so-called "good" cholesterol), and LDL cholesterol (so-called "bad" cholesterol). Family history and lifestyle, including factors such as blood pressure and whether or not one smokes, affect what would be considered ideal versus nonideal values for fasting blood lipid profiles.

Total Serum Cholesterol

<200 mg/dL = desired values

200–239 mg/dL = borderline to high risk

240 mg/dL and above = high risk

HDL Cholesterol

With HDL cholesterol the higher the better

<40 mg/dL for men and <50 mg/dL for women = higher risk

40-50 mg/dL for men and 50-60 mg/dL for women = normal values

>60 mg/dL is associated with some level of protection against heart disease

LDL Cholesterol

With LDL cholesterol the lower the better

<100 mg/dL = optimal values

100 mg/dL-129 mg/dL = optimal to near optimal

130 mg/dL-159 mg/dL = borderline high risk

160 mg/dL-189 mg/dL = high risk

190 mg/dL and higher = very high risk

CLINICAL BOX 26-2: FAMILIAL HYPERCHOLESTEROLEMIA

Familial hypercholesterolemia (FH) (type II hyperlipoproteinemia) is an autosomal dominant disorder that results from mutations affecting the structure and function of the LDL receptor (LDLR). The defects in LDLR interaction with LDL particles result in lifelong elevation of LDL cholesterol in the blood. The consequent hypercholesterolemia leads to premature coronary artery disease and atherosclerotic plaque formation. FH was the first inherited disorder that was recognized as being a cause of myocardial infarction (heart attack).

Although the disease is inherited in an autosomal dominant manner, it exhibits a gene dosage effect. Homozygous individuals are more severely affected than are heterozygotes. Heterozygotes for FH occur with a frequency of 1 in 500, which makes this disease one of the most common inherited disorders in metabolism. More than 700 different mutations in the *LDLR* gene have been identified. Of diagnostic significance is the fact that 45 different polymorphisms in the *LDLR* gene have been identified and can be detected using standard molecular biological techniques.

The clinical characteristics of FH include elevated concentrations of plasma LDL and deposition of LDL cholesterol in the arteries, tendons, and skin. Fat deposits in the arteries are called *atheromas* and in the skin and tendons they are called *xanthomas*. In heterozygotes, hypercholesterolemia is the earliest clinical manifestation in FH and remains the only clinical finding during the first decade of life. Xanthomas and the characteristic arcus cornea (whitish ring on the peripheral cornea) begin to appear in the second decade. The symptoms of coronary heart disease present in the fourth decade. At the time of death, 80% of heterozygotes will have xanthomas. The clinical picture is more uniform and severe in homozygotes. Homozygotes present with marked hypercholesterolemia at birth and it will persist throughout life. Xanthomas, arcus cornea, and atherosclerosis will develop during childhood in homozygotes. Death from myocardial infarction usually will occur before the age of 30 in homozygotes.

Five different classes of receptor mutation have been identified in FH with each class having multiple alleles. Class 1 mutations are null mutations because these result in a failure to make any detectable LDLR protein. Class 2 mutations are the most common and represent intracellular transport defects. There are 2 subclasses of class 2 mutations in FH. Class 2A mutations result in an LDLR protein that fails to be transported out of the ER. Class 2B mutations are "leaky," in that some of the newly synthesized LDLR protein is transported to the Golgi but at a reduced rate compared to wild type. The class 2B mutations are the more common type in this class of mutation. Class 3 mutations represent LDLRs that are delivered to the cell surface, but fail in their ability to bind LDL. Because there is a similarity in the class 2 and class 3 mutant alleles, it is difficult to assess which class of mutation is causing the observed FH phenotype. To accurately distinguish class 3 and class 2B alleles at the functional level, it is necessary to isolate fibroblasts from the patient and do in vitro ligand-binding assays. Class 4 mutations are the rarest and result in LDLR protein that will bind LDL, but the LDLR-LDL complexes cannot be internalized. The class 4 alleles can be divided into 2 subclasses dependent upon whether the mutations affect only the cytoplasmic domain or include mutations in the adjacent membrane-spanning domain. Class 5 mutations result in receptors that bind and internalize the LDL particle but cannot release the particles in the endosomes, so the receptors cannot recycle back to the cell surface. Class 5-type mutations may be underestimated because they can produce a phenotype that somewhat resembles that of class 3 mutations (ie, deficient LDL binding).

Cholesterol Biosynthesis

Critical Enzymes

HMG-CoA reductase (HMGR): rate-limiting enzyme of *de novo* cholesterol biosynthesis, levels of activity affected at numerous levels

7-dehydrocholesterol reductase (DHC7): terminal enzyme of de novo cholesterol biosynthesis; defects lead to defective early development, disease is called SLOS

Normal healthy adults synthesize cholesterol at a rate of approximately 1 g/d and consume approximately 0.3 g/d in the diet. Of course, this assumes a normal healthy diet that does not constitute excess cholesterol intake. A relatively constant level of cholesterol in the blood (150-200 mg/dL) is maintained primarily by controlling the level of de novo synthesis. The synthesis of cholesterol is required only to supply slightly less than

CLINICAL BOX 26-3: SMITH-LEMLI-OPITZ SYNDROME

Smith-Lemli-Opitz syndrome (SLOS) is an autosomal recessive disorder caused by defects in the terminal enzyme of cholesterol biosynthesis: 7-dehydrocholesterol reductase (DHCR7). Defects in this gene result in increased levels of 7-dehydrocholesterol and reduced levels (15%-27% of normal) of cholesterol. The highest frequency of SLOS appears in Caucasians of northern European descent with a frequency of around 1 in 20,000 to 1 in 70,000. The clinical spectrum of SLOS is very broad, ranging from the most severe form manifesting as a lethal malformation syndrome, to a relatively mild disorder that encompasses behavioral and learning disabilities. Frequent observations in SLOS infants is poor feeding and postnatal growth failure. The growth failure may necessitate the insertion of a gastronomy tube to ensure adequate nutritional support. There are distinct craniofacial anomalies associated with SLOS. These include microcephaly (head size smaller than normal), micrognathia (abnormally small lower jaw), ptosis (drooping eyelids), a small upturned nose, and cleft palate or bifid uvula. Male infants with SLOS exhibit genital abnormalities that range from a small penis to ambiguous genitalia or gender reversal. Abnormalities in limb development are common in SLOS patients and include short thumbs, postaxial polydactyly, and single palmar creases. In addition, the most common clinical finding in SLOS patients is syndactyly (fusion of digits) of the second and third toes. This latter limb deformity is found in over 95% of SLOS patients.

The developmental defects are due to defective cholesterol modification of the pattern-regulating gene *sonic hedgehog* (*Shh*). Shh is necessary for patterning events that take place in the central nervous system, during limb development, and in the formation of facial structures. Altered levels of cholesterol in SLOS also affect the normal physiochemical processes of cell membranes. One major defect that results from reduced membrane cholesterol is an inability to form ordered lipid domains that are necessary for normal signal transduction events to take place. These defects then alter normal cellular functions resulting in many of the symptoms of SLOS.

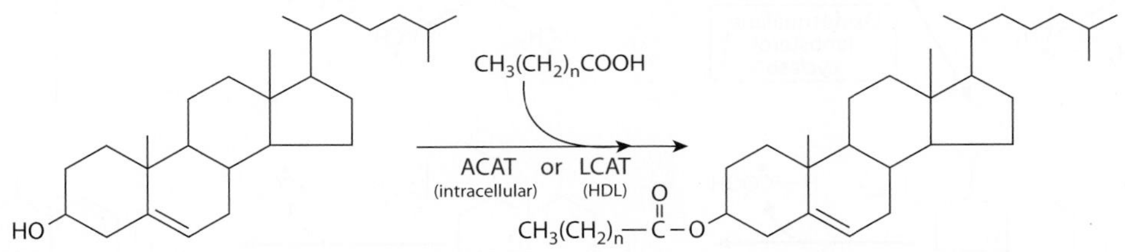

HO
$CH_3(CH_2)_nCOOH$
ACAT or LCAT
(intracellular) (HDL)
$CH_3(CH_2)_n-\overset{O}{\overset{\|}{C}}-O$

FIGURE 26-2: Fatty acid esterification of cholesterol catalyzed by ACAT (acyl-CoA cholesterol acyltransferase) or LCAT (lecithin cholesterol acyltransferase).

half of the daily bodily needs, as the rest is derived from the diet. Biosynthesis in the liver accounts for approximately 10%, and in the intestines approximately 15%, of the amount produced de novo each day.

The rate and level of cholesterol synthesis is regulated by both the dietary intake of cholesterol as well as the cholesterol contributed to the pool by de novo synthesis. Cholesterol from both diet and synthesis is utilized for the synthesis of the bile acids (see Chapter 27) and the steroid hormones (see Chapter 50) as well as being incorporated into cellular membranes. The greatest proportion of cholesterol is consumed in the synthesis of the bile acid in the liver.

Origin of Carbon Atoms in Cholesterol

The synthesis and utilization of cholesterol must be tightly regulated in order to prevent over-accumulation and abnormal deposition within the body. Of particular importance clinically is the abnormal deposition of cholesterol-rich lipoproteins in the coronary arteries. Such deposition, eventually leading to atherosclerosis (see Chapter 48), is the leading contributory factor in diseases of the coronary arteries.

Cholesterol synthesis occurs from the 2-carbon acetate group of acetyl-CoA, which can be derived from glucose oxidation (see Chapter 10), amino acid oxidation (see

Chapter 30), and lipid oxidation (see Chapter 25). Since all of these sources of acetyl-CoA originate in the mitochondria and cholesterol synthesis occurs in the cytosol, the acetyl-CoA must be transported out of the mitochondria. Acetyl-CoA transport to the cytoplasm occurs via the mechanism depicted in Figure 19-3.

Reactions of Cholesterol Synthesis

Cholesterol synthesis is a highly complex process requiring nearly 30 individual reactions that consume over 250 moles of ATP (outlined in Figure 26-3). The second reaction constitutes the rate-limiting reaction, and it is

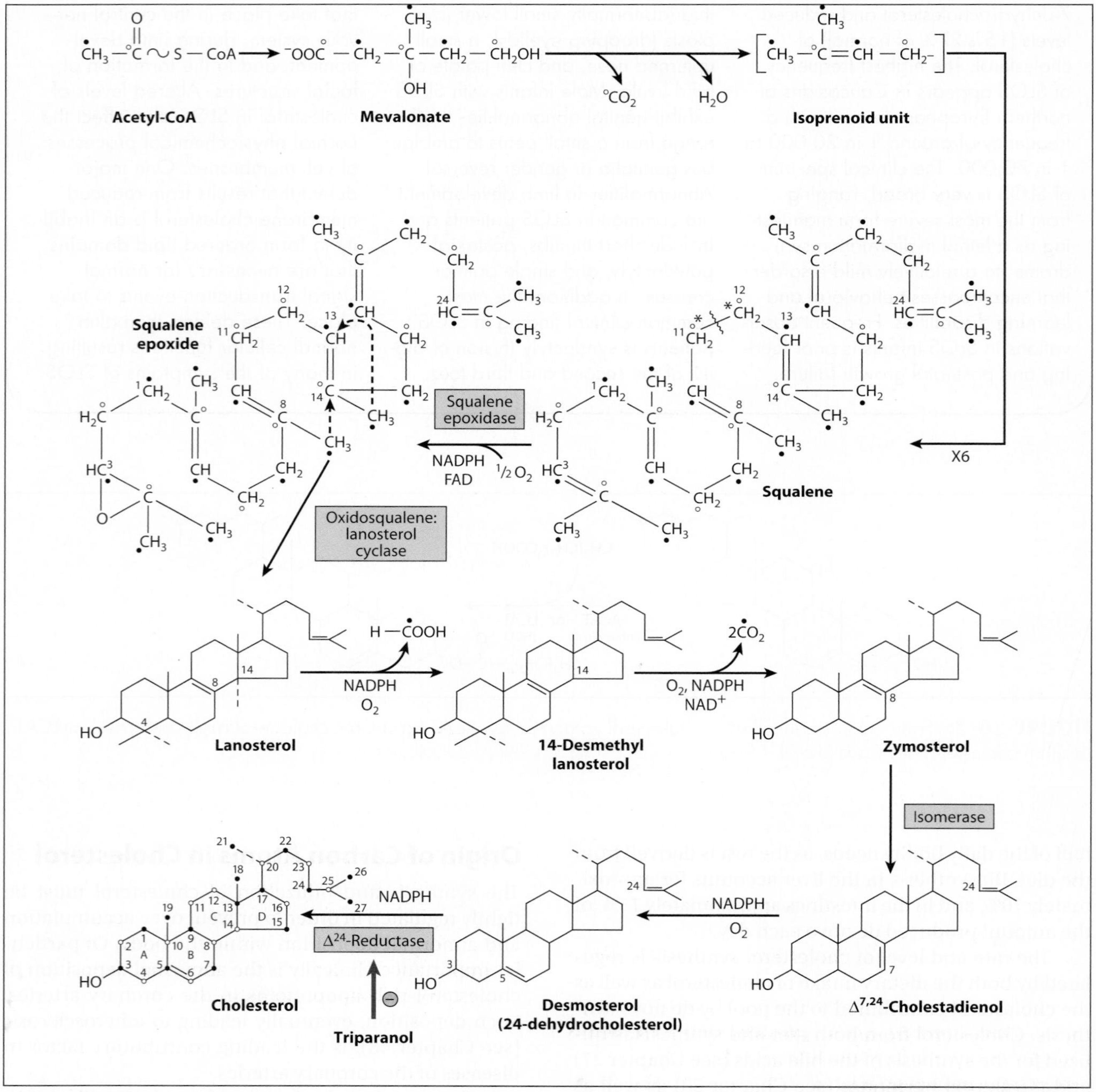

FIGURE 26-3: Biosynthesis of cholesterol. The numbered positions are those of the steroid nucleus and the open and solid circles indicate the fate of each of the carbons in the acetyl moiety of acetyl-CoA. Murray RK, Bender DA, Botham KM, Kennelly PJ, Rodwell VW, Weil PA. *Harper's Illustrated Biochemistry,* 29th ed. New York, NY: McGraw-Hill; 2012.

High-Yield Concept

Acetyl-CoA can also be synthesized from cytosolic acetate derived from cytoplasmic oxidation of ethanol, which is initiated by a cytoplasmic alcohol dehydrogenase (ADH3). The acetyl-CoA synthesis reaction is catalyzed by cytosolic acetyl-CoA synthetase (correctly named acetyl-CoA ligase). Production of acetyl-CoA from ethanol metabolism is one reason that excess alcohol consumption is a significant contributor to elevated serum cholesterol and lipid levels.

catalyzed by HMG-CoA reductase (HMGR). Cholesterol synthesis can be considered to occur in 5 major steps:

1. Acetyl-CoAs are converted to 3-hydroxy-3-methyl-glutaryl-CoA (HMG-CoA).
2. HMG-CoA is converted to mevalonate.
3. Mevalonate is converted to the isoprene-based molecule, isopentenyl pyrophosphate (IPP), with the concomitant loss of CO_2.
4. IPP is converted to squalene.
5. Squalene is converted to cholesterol.

Each mole of cholesterol begins with the condensation of 3 moles of cytoplasmic acetyl-CoA. First, 2 moles of acetyl-CoA are condensed in a reversal of the thiolase reaction, forming acetoacetyl-CoA. Acetoacetyl-CoA and a third mole of acetyl-CoA are converted to HMG-CoA by the action of cytoplasmic HMG-CoA synthase. This series of reactions is chemically identical to the reactions of ketone body synthesis (see Chapter 25) but of course occur in the cytosol, whereas, the ketone synthesis reactions occur inside the mitochondria. Although the bulk of acetoacetyl-CoA is derived via this process, it is possible for some acetoacetate, generated during ketogenesis to diffuse out of the mitochondria and be converted to acetoacetyl-CoA in the cytosol via the action of acetoacetyl-CoA synthetase.

HMG-CoA is converted to mevalonate by HMG-CoA reductase. HMGR absolutely requires NADPH as a cofactor, and 2 moles of NADPH are consumed during the conversion of HMG-CoA to mevalonate. The reaction catalyzed by HMGR is the rate-limiting step of cholesterol biosynthesis, and this enzyme is subject to complex regulatory controls (see later).

Following the synthesis of mevalonate, the compound is activated by 2 successive phosphorylations (catalyzed by mevalonate kinase and phosphomevalonate kinase), yielding 5-pyrophosphomevalonate. After phosphorylation, an ATP-dependent decarboxylation yields isopentenyl pyrophosphate (IPP), an activated isoprenoid molecule (Figure 26-4). Isopentenyl pyrophosphate is in equilibrium with its isomer, dimethylallyl pyrophosphate (DMPP). One molecule of IPP condenses with one molecule of DMPP to generate geranyl pyrophosphate (GPP). GPP further condenses with another IPP molecule to yield farnesyl pyrophosphate (FPP). Finally, the NADPH-requiring enzyme, squalene synthase, catalyzes the head-to-tail condensation of 2 molecules of FPP, yielding squalene. Like HMGR, squalene synthase is tightly associated with the endoplasmic reticulum. Squalene undergoes a 2-step cyclization to yield lanosterol. The first reaction is catalyzed by squalene monooxygenase. This enzyme uses NADPH as a cofactor to introduce molecular oxygen as an epoxide at the 2,3 position of squalene. Through a series of 19 additional reactions, lanosterol is converted to cholesterol. The terminal reaction in cholesterol biosynthesis is catalyzed by 7-dehydrocholesterol reductase. Defects in this gene results in Smith-Lemli-Opitz syndrome (SLOS, Clinical Box 26-3).

Regulation of Cholesterol Biosynthesis

The cellular supply of cholesterol is maintained at a steady level by 3 distinct mechanisms:

1. Regulation of HMGR activity and levels, which is the major site of control
2. Regulation of excess intracellular free cholesterol through the activity of ratio of acyl-CoA to cholesterol acyltransferase
3. Regulation of plasma cholesterol levels via LDL receptor-mediated uptake and HDL-mediated reverse cholesterol transport

Regulation of HMGR Activity

Regulation of HMGR activity is the primary means for controlling the level of cholesterol biosynthesis. The level of enzyme activity is regulated by 4 distinct mechanisms: (1) feedback inhibition, (2) control of gene expression, (3) rate of enzyme degradation, and (4) phosphorylation-dephosphorylation.

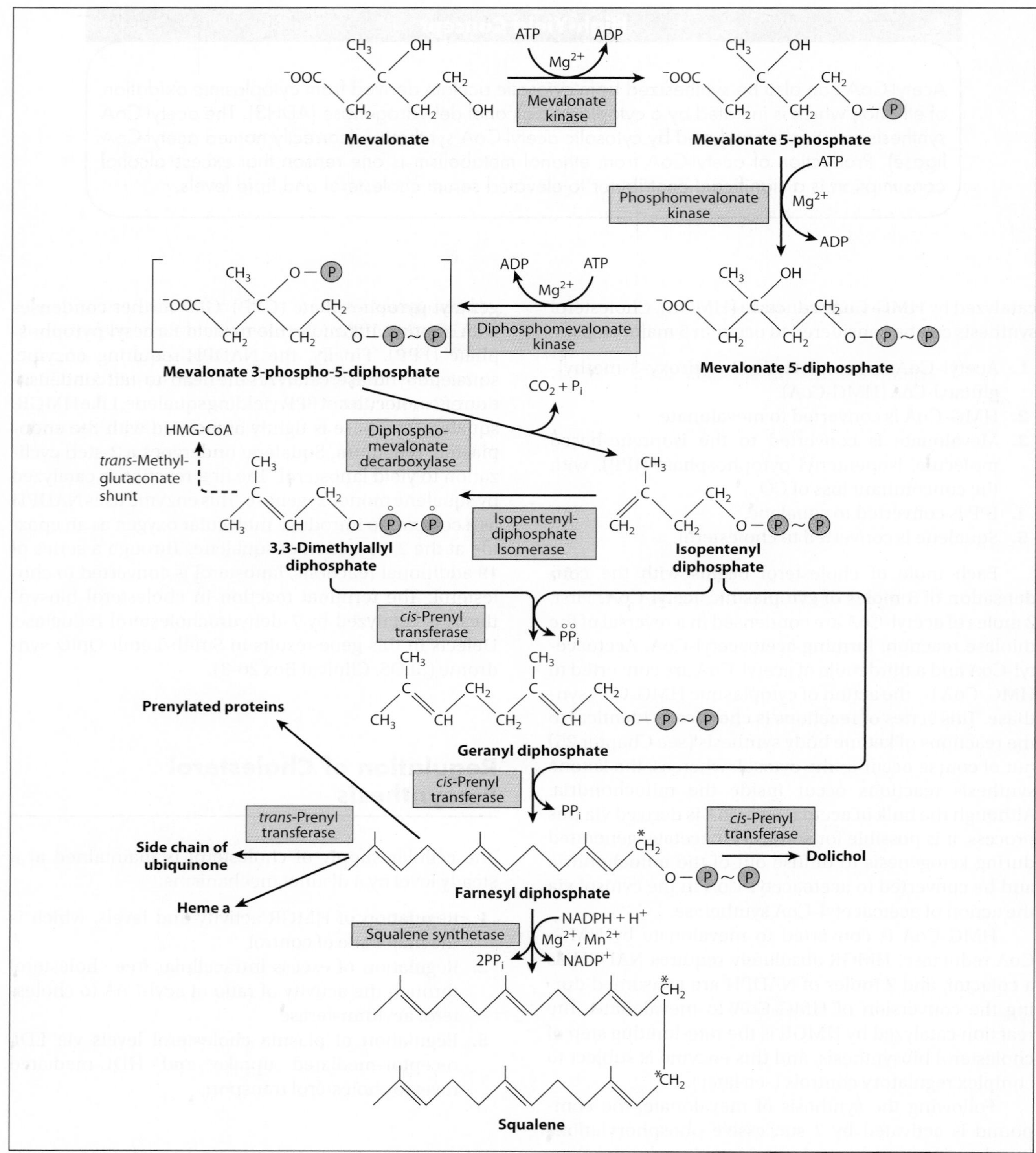

FIGURE 26-4: Biosynthesis of squalene, ubiquinone, dolichol, and other polyisoprene derivatives. (HMG-CoA, 3-hydroxy-3-methylglutaryl-CoA.) A farnesyl residue is present in heme a of cytochrome oxidase. The carbon marked with an asterisk becomes C_{11} or C_{12} in squalene. Squalene synthetase is a microsomal enzyme; all other enzymes indicated are soluble cytosolic proteins, and some are found in peroxisomes. Murray RK, Bender DA, Botham KM, Kennelly PJ, Rodwell VW, Weil PA. *Harper's Illustrated Biochemistry*, 29th edition, Copyright 2012, New York: McGraw-Hill.

The first 3 control mechanisms are exerted by cholesterol itself. Cholesterol acts as a feedback inhibitor of preexisting HMGR as well as inducing rapid degradation of the enzyme. The latter is the result of cholesterol-induced polyubiquitination of HMGR and its degradation in the proteosome (see Proteolytic Regulation of HMGR Levels section). This ability of cholesterol is a consequence of the sterol-sensing domain (SSD) of HMGR. In addition, when cholesterol is in excess the amount of mRNA for HMGR is reduced because of the decreased expression of the gene. The mechanism by which cholesterol (and other sterols) affects the transcription of the *HMGR* gene is described in the following section.

Regulation of HMGR through covalent modification occurs because of phosphorylation and dephosphorylation (Figure 26-5). The enzyme is most active in its unmodified form. Phosphorylation of the enzyme decreases its activity. HMGR is phosphorylated by AMP-activated protein kinase (AMPK).

The cAMP-signaling pathway via the regulation of PKA activity additionally controls the activity of HMGR. Since the intracellular level of cAMP is regulated by hormonal stimuli, regulation of cholesterol biosynthesis is, therefore, under hormonal control. Insulin decreases cAMP, which in turn activates cholesterol synthesis. Alternatively, glucagon and epinephrine, which increase the level of cAMP, inhibit cholesterol synthesis. In the context of HMGR regulation, PKA phosphorylates phosphoprotein phosphatase inhibitor-1 (PPI-1), leading to an increase in its activity. PPI-1 can inhibit the activity of numerous phosphatases including protein phosphatase-2C (PP-2C) and PP-2A (also known as HMGR phosphatase), which remove phosphates from AMPK and HMGR, respectively. This maintains AMPK in the phosphorylated and active state, and HMGR in the phosphorylated and inactive state. As the stimulus leading to increased cAMP production is removed, the level of phosphorylation decreases and that of

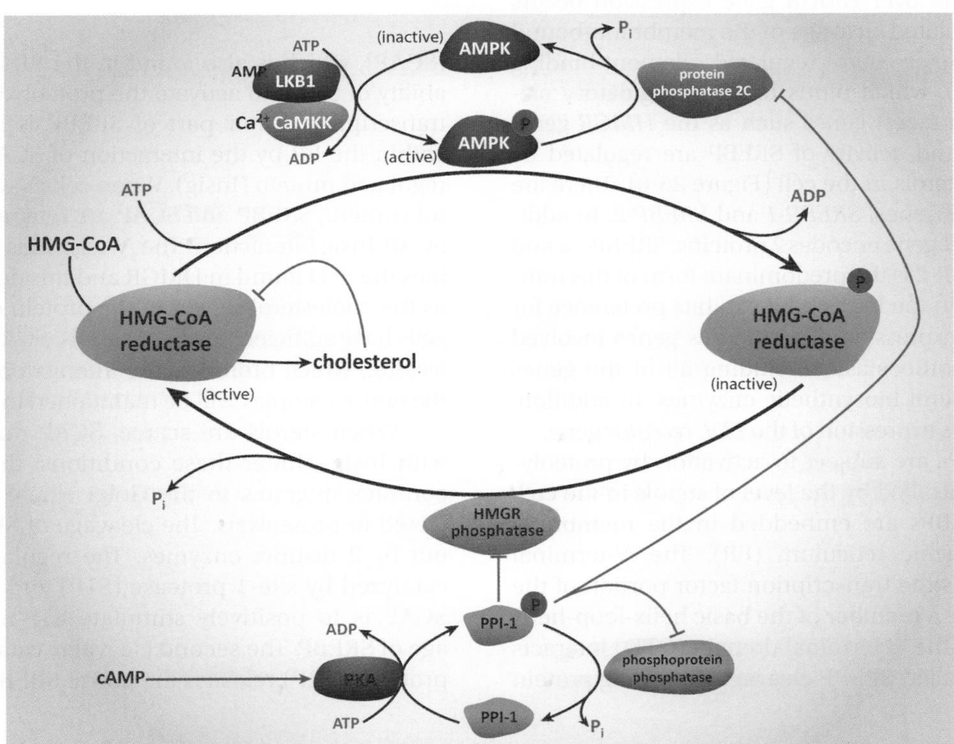

FIGURE 26-5: Regulation of HMGR by covalent modification. HMGR is most active in the dephosphorylated state. Phosphorylation is catalyzed by AMP-activated protein kinase (AMPK) an enzyme whose activity is also regulated by phosphorylation. Phosphorylation of AMPK is catalyzed by at least 2 enzymes: liver kinase B1 (LKB1) and calmodulin-dependent protein kinase kinase-beta (CaMKKβ). Hormones such as glucagon and epinephrine negatively affect cholesterol biosynthesis by increasing the activity of the inhibitor of the phosphatase inhibitor, phosphoprotein phosphatase inhibitor-1, PPI-1. Conversely, insulin stimulates the removal of phosphates and, thereby, activates HMGR activity. Additional regulation of HMGR occurs through an inhibition of its' activity as well as of its' synthesis by elevation in intracellular cholesterol levels. Reproduced with permission of themedicalbiochemistrypage, LLC.

dephosphorylation increases. The net result is a return to a higher level of HMGR activity.

SREBP and the Regulation of Cellular Sterol Levels

Long-term control of HMGR activity is exerted primarily through control of the synthesis and degradation of the enzyme. When levels of cholesterol are high, the level of expression of the *HMGR* gene is reduced. Conversely, reduced levels of cholesterol activate expression of the gene. Insulin also brings about long-term regulation of cholesterol metabolism by increasing the level of HMGR synthesis. The continual alteration of the intracellular sterol pool occurs through the regulation of key sterol-synthetic enzymes as well as by altering the levels of cell-surface LDL receptors. Regulation of the cellular pool of sterols is affected primarily by sterol-regulated transcription of key rate-limiting enzymes and by the regulated degradation of HMGR.

Sterol control over *HMGR* gene expression occurs through the regulated cleavage of the membrane-bound transcription factor sterol-regulated element-binding protein (SREBP), which binds to sterol-regulatory elements (SREs) in target genes such as the *HMGR* gene. Both the level and activity of SREBP are regulated by the amount of sterols in the cell (Figure 26-6). There are 2 distinct SREBP genes, *SREBP-1* and *SREBP-2*. In addition, the *SREBP-1* gene encodes 2 proteins, SREBP-1a and SREBP-1c. SREBP-2 is the predominant form of this transcription factor in the liver and it exhibits preference for controlling the expression of numerous genes involved in cholesterol homeostasis, including all of the genes encoding the sterol biosynthetic enzymes. In addition, SREBP-2 controls expression of the *LDL receptor* gene.

All 3 SREBPs are subject to activation by proteolysis, which is controlled by the level of sterols in the cell. Full-length SREBPs are embedded in the membrane of the endoplasmic reticulum (ER). The *N*-terminal domain contains the transcription factor portion of the protein, which is a member of the basic helix-loop-helix (bHLH) family. The *C*-terminal domain (CTD) interacts with a protein called SREBP cleavage-activating protein

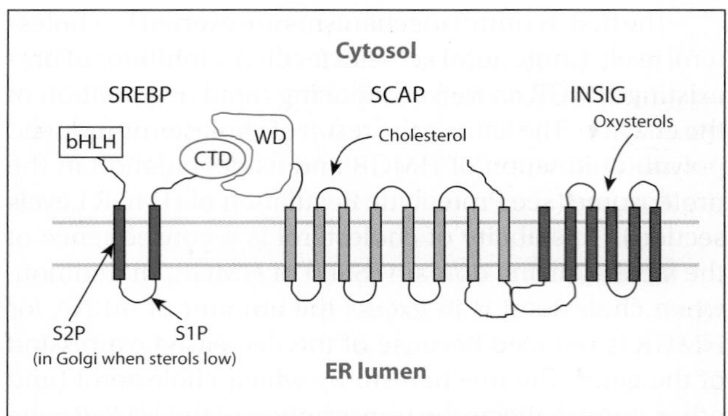

FIGURE 26-6: Regulation of SREBP by SCAP: Diagrammatic representation of the interactions between SREBP, SCAP, and *Insig* in the membrane of the ER when sterols are high. When sterols are low, SCAP does not interact with *Insig* and the SREBP-SCAP complex migrates to the Golgi where the proteases, S1P and S2P reside. bHLH, basic helix-loop-helix domain; CTD, C-terminal domain; WD, WD40 domain. Reproduced with permission of themedicalbiochemistrypage, LLC.

(SCAP), which is also found in the ER membrane. The ability of SCAP to activate the proteolytic release of the transcription factor part of SREBP is itself controlled within the ER by the interaction of SCAP with insulin-regulated protein (Insig). When cells have sufficient sterol content, SREBP and SCAP are retained in the ER via SCAP-Insig interaction. The *N*-terminus of SCAP resembles the SSD found in HMGR and this domain functions as the cholesterol sensor in the protein complex. When cells have sufficient levels of sterols, SCAP will bind cholesterol, which promotes the interaction with Insig and the entire complex will be maintained in the ER.

When sterols are scarce, SCAP does not interact with Insig. Under these conditions, the SREBP-SCAP complex migrates to the Golgi where SREBP is subjected to proteolysis. The cleavage of SREBP is carried out by 2 distinct enzymes. The regulated cleavage is catalyzed by site-1 protease (S1P) and the function of SCAP is to positively stimulate S1P-mediated cleavage of SREBP. The second cleavage, catalyzed by site- 2 protease (S2P) releases the active SREBP transcription

High-Yield Concept

AMPK is a master metabolic regulator whose activity increases the rate of ATP production and inhibits ATP consumption. AMPK activity is itself regulated via phosphorylation. In addition to regulating the activity of HMGR, AMPK activity influences the transcriptional regulation of numerous metabolic genes. Discussion of the global impact of AMPK is covered in Chapter 34.

factor to the cytosol, where it can then migrate to the nucleus. In the nucleus, the bHLH domain of SREBP will dimerize and form complexes with transcriptional coactivators leading to the activation of genes containing the SRE motif. To control the level of SREBP-mediated transcription, the soluble bHLH domain is itself subject to rapid proteolysis.

Proteolytic Regulation of HMGR Levels

The stability of HMGR is regulated as the rate of flux through the mevalonate synthesis pathway changes. When the flux is high, the rate of HMGR degradation is also high. When the flux is low, degradation of HMGR decreases. This phenomenon can easily be observed in the presence of the statin drugs as discussed in the section Treatment of Hypercholesterolemia. When sterol levels increase in cells, there is a concomitant increase in the rate of HMGR degradation. The degradation of HMGR occurs within the proteosome, a multiprotein complex dedicated to protein degradation (see Chapter 37). The primary signal-directing proteins to the proteosome is *ubiquitination*. HMGR has been shown to be ubiquitinated prior to its degradation. The primary sterol-regulating HMGR degradation is cholesterol itself. As the levels of free cholesterol increase in cells, the rate of HMGR degradation increases.

The Utilization of Cholesterol

Cholesterol is transported in the plasma predominantly as cholesteryl esters associated with lipoproteins (see Chapter 28). Dietary cholesterol is transported from the small intestine to the liver within chylomicrons. Cholesterol synthesized by the liver, as well as any dietary cholesterol in the liver that exceeds hepatic needs, is transported in the serum within LDLs. The liver synthesizes VLDLs and these are converted to LDLs through the action of endothelial cell–associated lipoprotein lipase. Cholesterol found in plasma membranes can be extracted by HDLs and esterified by the HDL-associated enzyme LCAT. The cholesterol acquired from peripheral tissues by HDLs can then be transferred to VLDLs and LDLs via the action of cholesteryl ester transfer protein (CETP), which is associated with HDLs. Reverse cholesterol transport allows peripheral cholesterol to be returned to the liver in LDLs. Ultimately, cholesterol is excreted in the bile as free cholesterol or as bile salts following conversion to bile acids in the liver.

Treatment of Hypercholesterolemia

Drug treatment to lower plasma lipoproteins and/or cholesterol is primarily aimed at reducing the risk of atherosclerosis and subsequent coronary artery disease that exists in patients with elevated circulating lipids (see Clinical Box 26-1). Drug therapy usually is considered as an option only if nonpharmacologic interventions (altered diet and exercise) have failed to lower plasma lipids.

Atorvastatin (Lipitor), simvastatin (Zocor), lovastatin (Mevacor)

These drugs are fungal HMGR inhibitors and are members of the family of drugs referred to as the statins. The net result of treatment is an increased cellular uptake of LDLs, since the intracellular synthesis of cholesterol is inhibited and cells are therefore dependent on extracellular sources of cholesterol. However, since mevalonate (the product of the HMGR reaction) is required for the synthesis of other important isoprenoid compounds besides cholesterol, long-term treatments carry some risk of toxicity. The most common untoward side effect of the statin drugs is muscle weakness and pain. A component of the natural cholesterol-lowering supplement, red yeast rice, is in fact a statin-like compound.

The statins have become recognized as a class of drugs capable of more pharmacologic benefits than just lowering blood cholesterol levels via their actions on HMGR. Part of the cardiac benefit of the statins relates to their ability to regulate the production of S-nitrosylated cycloxoxygenase-2 (COX-2). COX-2 is an inducible enzyme involved in the synthesis of the prostaglandins and thromboxanes as well as the lipoxins and resolvins (see Chapter 24). Evidence has shown that statins activate inducible nitric oxide synthase (iNOS), leading to nitrosylation of COX-2. The S-nitrosylated COX-2 enzyme produces the lipid compound 15*R*-hydroxyeicosatetraenoic acid (15*R*-HETE) which is then converted via the action of 5-lipoxygenase (5-LOX) to the epimeric lipoxin, 15-epi-LXA_4. This latter compound is the same as the aspirin-triggered lipoxin (ATL) that results from the aspirin-induced acetylation of COX-2 (see Chapter 24). Therefore, part of the beneficial effects of the statins is exerted via the actions of the lipoxin family of anti-inflammatory lipids.

Additional anti-inflammatory actions of the statins result from a reduction in the prenylation of numerous pro-inflammatory modulators. Prenylation refers to the addition of the 15-carbon farnesyl group or the 20-carbon geranylgeranyl group to acceptor proteins. These isoprenoid groups are derived from the cholesterol biosynthetic pathway as outlined earlier. The prenylation of proteins allows them to be anchored to cell membranes. In addition to cell membrane attachment, prenylation is known to be important for protein–protein interactions. Thus, inhibition of this posttranslational modification by the statins interferes with the important functions of many signaling proteins.

Nicotinic acid

Nicotinic acid reduces the plasma levels of both VLDLs and LDLs by inhibiting hepatic VLDL secretion, as well as suppressing the flux of free fatty acid (FFA) release from adipose tissue by inhibiting lipolysis. In addition, nicotinic acid administration increases the circulating levels of HDLs. Patient compliance with nicotinic acid administration is sometimes compromised because of the unpleasant side effect of flushing. Recent evidence has shown that nicotinic acid binds to and activates the G-protein–coupled receptor identified as GPR109A (also called HM74A or PUMA-G). The identity of a receptor to which nicotinic acid binds allows for the development of new drug therapies that activate the same receptor but that may lack the negative side effect of flushing associated with nicotinic acid.

Gemfibrozil (Lopid), Fenofibrate (TriCor)

These compounds (called fibrates) are derivatives of fibric acid and although used clinically since the 1930s were only recently discovered to exert some of their lipid-lowering effects via the activation of peroxisome proliferation. Specifically, the fibrates were found to be activators of the peroxisome proliferator–activated receptor-α (PPAR-α) class of proteins (see Chapter 40). The naturally occurring ligands for PPAR-α are leukotriene B_4 (LTB_4), unsaturated fatty acids, and oxidized components of VLDLs and LDLs. Fibrates result in the activation of PPAR-α in liver and muscle. In the liver this leads to increased β-oxidation of fatty acids, thereby decreasing the liver's secretion of triacylglycerol- and cholesterol-rich VLDLs, as well as increased clearance of chylomicron remnants, increased levels of HDLs, and increased lipoprotein lipase activity, which in turn promotes rapid VLDL turnover.

Cholestyramine or colestipol (resins)

These compounds are nonabsorbable resins that bind bile acids in the gut, which are then not reabsorbed but excreted. The drop in bile acid reabsorption releases a hepatic feedback-inhibitory mechanism that limits bile acid synthesis. As a result, a greater amount of cholesterol is converted to bile acids to maintain a steady level in the circulation. Additionally, the synthesis of LDL receptors increases to allow increased cholesterol uptake for bile acid synthesis, and the overall effect is a reduction in plasma cholesterol. This treatment is ineffective in patients who are homozygous for familial hypercholesterolemia (FH), since they are completely deficient in LDL receptors (FH, see Clinical Box 26-2).

Ezetimibe

This drug is sold under the trade names Zetia or Ezetrol and is also combined with the statin drug simvastatin and sold as Vytorin or Inegy. Ezetimibe reduces cholesterol uptake from the gut by inhibiting the intestinal brush border transporter involved in absorption of cholesterol. This transporter is known as Niemann-Pick type C1-like 1 (NPC1L1). Ezetimibe is usually prescribed for patients who cannot tolerate a statin drug or a high-dose statin regimen. The combination drug of ezetimibe and simvastatin has shown efficacy equal to or slightly greater than atorvastatin (Lipitor) alone at reducing circulating cholesterol levels.

REVIEW QUESTIONS

1. You have been studying the pathway of cholesterol biosynthesis using a cell line derived from a human hepatoma. You discover that, unlike in nontransformed liver cells, the addition of oxysterols, such as 25-hydroxycholesterol, does not lead to reduced measurements of newly synthesized cholesterol. These observations indicate that normal regulation of an enzyme in cholesterol biosynthesis is defective in these cancer cells. Which of the following enzymes is the most likely candidate for this loss of regulation?

A. acetoacetyl-CoA thiolase (ACAT2)
B. 7-dehydrocholesterol reductase (DHCR7)
C. HMG-CoA reductase (HMGR)
D. HMG-CoA synthase
E. mevalonate kinase

Answer C: Oxysterols regulate the activity of the transcription factor SREBP-1c. When oxysterol or cholesterol levels are elevated, there is an inhibition of the release of SREBP-1c from the Golgi membrane, thereby, reducing the SREBP-1c-mediated transcriptional activation of numerous target genes including *HMGR*. Normal oxysterol regulation of SREBP-1c would lead to reduced cholesterol synthesis due, in part, to reduced expression of HMGR. Thus, continued transcriptional activation of target genes by SREBP-1c, even in the presence of oxysterols, would be measurable with continued cholesterol synthesis due to unregulated transcription of HMGR.

2. Activation of which of the following enzymes, involved in the regulation of cholesterol biogenesis, occurs in response to an altered ATP:ADP ratio?

A. AMP-activated kinase (AMPK)
B. HMG-CoA reductase phosphatase
C. protein phosphatase 2C
D. protein phosphatase inhibitor-1
E. protein kinase A (PKA)

Answer A: Regulation of HMG-CoA reductase (HMGR) is controlled primarily by a short-term regulatory cascade that results in phosphorylation of the enzyme. Once phosphorylated, HMGR is much less active and thus, cholesterol biosynthesis will be reduced. In order to return to a more active state, the phosphorylated sites on HMGR must be dephosphorylated. All of the enzyme choices listed are involved in regulation of HMGR activity, however, only AMP-activated kinase (AMPK) activity is affected by alteration in the ATP:ADP ratio in cells. When ATP levels fall, AMP levels will rise and AMPK becomes fully activated. Phosphorylation of HMGR by AMPK results in reduced cholesterol synthesis, which results in reduced ATP consumption.

3. The statin class of drugs that are currently used to control hypercholesterolemia function to lower circulating levels of cholesterol by which of the following mechanisms?

A. increasing the elimination of bile acids leading to increased diversion of cholesterol into bile acid production
B. increasing the synthesis of apoB-100 resulting in increased elimination of cholesterol through the action of low-density lipoprotein (LDL) uptake by the liver
C. decreasing the absorption of dietary cholesterol from the intestines
D. inhibiting the interaction of LDLs with the hepatic LDL receptor
E. inhibiting the rate-limiting step in cholesterol biosynthesis

Answer E: The statins are a class of drugs derived from a compound originally isolated from red yeast (*Monascus purpurus*) used to ferment white rice (commonly called red yeast rice). The original compound isolated from red yeast is called lovastatin and marketed in the United States as the drug Mevacor. These drugs all inhibit the activity of the rate-limiting enzyme in cholesterol biosynthesis, HMG-CoA reductase.

4. Glucagon binding to liver cells induces an increase in intracellular cAMP concentration. The rate-limiting step in cholesterol biosynthesis is regulated as a consequence of this glucagon-mediated rise in cAMP. The effect of increased cAMP on the rate of cholesterol biosynthesis occurs because of which of the following?

A. AMP-regulated kinase (AMPK) is activated and directly phosphorylates human HMG-CoA reductase (HMGR), leading to an increase in the activity of the latter enzyme
B. cAMP-dependent protein kinase (PKA) is activated and directly phosphorylates HMGR, reducing the activity of the latter enzyme
C. PKA is activated and phosphorylates AMPK, which then phosphorylates and activates HMGR
D. PKA activation results in a reduced level of phosphate removal from HMG-CoA reductase so that the latter enzyme is kept less active.
E. the increased cAMP directly inhibits HMGR via allosteric interaction

Answer D: Activation of PKA in hepatocytes will lead to increased phosphorylation of protein phosphatase inhibitor-1 (PPI-1) which will, in turn, lead to decreased activity of HMGR phosphatase. The reduced level of phosphate removal from HMGR will keep this enzyme in a less active state. The net effect will be a reduction in cholesterol biosynthesis, which will preserve ATP for use in gluconeogenesis, a primary response of liver to glucagon stimulation.

5. You are studying cell line in which you discover that SREBP-2 is less tightly bound to the membranes of the ER. Examination of these cells shows no increase in cholesterol biosynthetic gene expression and no observable binding of SREBP-2 to the SREBP-response element (SRE) of a known target gene. These observations can best be explained by a mutation in which of the following proteins?

A. Insig
B. SCAP
C. site 1 protease (S1P)
D. site 2 protease (S2P)
E. SREBP-1c

Answer D: The most likely mutated protein in this case would be S2P. The reduced binding of SREBP-2 to ER membranes could most easily be explained by the normal activity of S1P. However, inability to fully release SREBP-2 would be due to ineffective S2P activity. Since S1P activity is likely normal, the mutation is not likely to be in Insig or SCAP either. The activity of SREBP-1c would have no bearing on the release of SREBP-2 from membranes.

6. Which of the following proteins/enzymes is directly responsive to elevation in sterols, leading to a reduction in the transcriptional activation of the gene encoding HMG-CoA reductase?

A. AMPK
B. HMG-CoA reductase phosphatase
C. SCAP
D. site-1 protease (S1P)
E. SREBP-1c

Answer C: Sterols, particularly cholesterol, interact with SCAP and regulate the interaction of SCAP with the various SREBP proteins in the ER membrane.

When sterols interact with SCAP, it results in SCAP retaining SREBP in the ER membrane such that it cannot migrate to the Golgi apparatus, where is would be acted upon by S1P. When sterol levels drop, the interaction between SCAP and SREBP is reduced and SREBP can migrate to the Golgi and be released from the membrane via the concerted actions of S1P and S2P.

7. The major source of acetyl-CoA for the synthesis of cholesterol is derived from cytosolic citrate. Examination of a hepatic cell line shows that despite a loss of expression of ATP-citrate lyase (ACL), these cells continue to have the capacity to synthesize cholesterol. The most likely explanation for this observation is related to the fact that an additional pathway is active. Which of the following enzymes is involved in this pathway?

A. acetyl-CoA synthetase
B. acetyl-CoA acyltransferase 1 (ACAT1)
C. acetoacetyl-CoA synthetase
D. HMG-CoA reductase
E. HMG-CoA synthase

Answer C: During ketogenesis, mitochondrial acetoacetate can diffuse to the cytosol where it is converted to acetoacetyl-CoA via the cytosolic enzyme, acetoacetyl-CoA synthetase. The resulting acetoacetyl-CoA could then serve as a direct substrate for incorporation into cholesterol. It is important to understand, however, that although this reaction process can occur, under conditions where ketogenesis is occurring in the liver the level of active HMGR would be significantly reduced.

8. A 35-year-old man who has suffered a heart attack has a serum total cholesterol concentration of 500 mg/dL. His father died at 30 years of age from a massive heart attack, and one of his 2 younger siblings also has an increased serum concentration of total cholesterol. This patient most likely has a disorder caused by an autosomal dominant allele affecting which of the following components of cholesterol metabolism?

A. acyl-CoA acyltransferase (ACAT)
B. HMG-CoA reductase (HMGR)
C. low-density lipoprotein (LDL) receptor
D. lysosomal cholesterol esterase
E. plasma lipoprotein lipase

Answer C: The patient is most likely exhibiting symptoms related to familial hypercholesterolemia (FH). FH is an autosomal dominant inherited disease affecting the *LDL receptor* gene leading to significant elevation in plasma LDL levels and total cholesterol. Patients who are heterozygous for an FH allele will manifest with total serum cholesterol levels between 300 and 600 mg/dL.

9. A 22-year-old man is being examined by his physician because he is concerned about growths on his eyelids. He is 180 cm (5 ft 11 in) tall and weighs 85 kg (188 lb); BMI is 26 kg/m^2. Physical examination shows no other abnormalities except for xanthelasmas. Serum studies show a total cholesterol concentration of 300 mg/dL, HDL-cholesterol concentration of 37 mg/dL, and triglyceride concentration of 3500 mg/dL. Which of the following is the most likely cause of these findings?

A. essential fatty acid deficiency
B. hepatic lipase deficiency
C. HMG-CoA reductase deficiency
D. leptin deficiency
E. lipoprotein lipase deficiency

Answer E: The most telling finding in this patient is the massively elevated levels of triglycerides. Loss of, or reduced, activity of lipoprotein lipase would lead to a decreased capacity to remove fatty acids from the triglycerides in circulating lipoprotein particles, thus causing the significant increase in serum triglycerides.

10. A 65-year-old man, who has been taking lovastatin to control his hypercholesterolemia, is found to have significantly reduced levels of glycoproteins in the plasma membranes of several cell types including red blood cells. The most likely cause of these changes in glycoprotein levels is a decrease in which of the following?

A. bile acids
B. cholesterol
C. coenzyme Q
D. dolichol phosphate
E. insulin

Answer D: Inhibition of de novo cholesterol biosynthesis with the use of statin drugs, such as lovastatin, leads to reduction in the synthesis of several isoprenoid compounds such as dolichol phosphate. The reduction in dolichol production leads to inhibition of the ability to effectively carry off *N*-linked glycosylation of many cellular proteins (see Chapter 34).

11. Which of the following enzymes would be expected to exert the greatest negative effect on the rate of cholesterol biosynthesis?

A. acetyl-CoA carboxylase (ACC)
B. AMP-regulated kinase (AMPK)
C. cGMP-dependent protein kinase (PKG)
D. HMG-CoA reductase (HMGR)
E. malonyl-CoA decarboxylase (MCD)

Answer B: HMG-CoA reductase is the rate-limiting enzyme of cholesterol biosynthesis and the major site for regulation of this metabolic pathway. Regulation of HMGR through covalent modification occurs as a result of phosphorylation and dephosphorylation. The enzyme is most active in its unmodified form. Phosphorylation of the enzyme decreases its activity. HMGR is phosphorylated by AMPK, which itself is activated via phosphorylation. Increased AMPK activity would, therefore, have a significant negative impact on the rate of HMGR activity.

12. Cholestyramine is a drug used to reduce serum cholesterol. It functions through binding bile salts and thereby, interferes with normal enterohepatic circulation of bile salts in the feces. Use of this drug would be associated with increased fecal amounts of which of the following compounds?

A. bilirubin
B. cholesterol
C. deoxycholate
D. glucuronate
E. palmitate

Answer C: Cholestyramine is a drug belonging to the bile-binding resin class of cholesterol-lowering drugs. These drugs function by binding bile acids in the gut, thereby, preventing their reuptake. Inhibition of bile acid uptake into the enterohepatic circulation will result in increased bile salt concentrations in the feces, including deoxycholate, a primary bile salt.

13. Like all biosynthetic reactions, synthesis of cholesterol requires the input of energy in the form of ATP. In addition, cholesterol biosynthesis is dependent upon input of cytoplasmic precursor carbon atoms in the form of acetyl-CoA. Which of the following enzymes, each of which plays a role in cholesterol synthesis, is most dependent upon ATP for maximal activity?

A. citrate synthase
B. 7-dehydrocholesterol reductase (DHCR7)
C. HMG-CoA reductase (HMGR)
D. malate dehydrogenase
E. pyruvate carboxylase

Answer E: The cytoplasmic acetyl-CoA required for de novo cholesterol biosynthesis is primarily derived from mitochondrial acetyl-CoA. The movement of acetyl-CoA from the mitochondria to the cytosol requires several enzymes including pyruvate carboxylase and citrate synthase. Pyruvate is the only one that is dependent upon ATP for activity.

14. You are examining a 6-month-old infant who presents with a series of distinctive craniofacial and limb abnormalities. These abnormalities include microcephaly, micrognathia, ptosis, cleft palate, short thumbs, and syndactyly of the second and third toes. You suspect the infant is suffering from Smith-Lemli-Opitz syndrome and order a confirmatory test that includes analysis of the activity of which of the following enzymes?

A. ATP-citrate lyase
B. 7-dehydrocholesterol reductase
C. HMG-CoA reductase
D. mevalonate kinase
E. pyruvate carboxylase

Answer B: Smith-Lemli-Opitz syndrome (SLOS) is caused by mutations in the gene encoding the terminal enzyme in cholesterol biosynthesis, that is, 7-dehydrocholesterol reductase.

15. Which of the following best explains the mechanism by which insulin action can result in increased hepatic cholesterol biosynthesis?

A. insulin action results in phosphorylation of SCAP leading to increased release of SREBP-1c
B. insulin action results in reduced levels of cAMP with consequent reduction in active PKA-mediated phosphorylation of SCAP
C. insulin action results in reduced levels of cAMP with consequent reduction in active PKA-mediated phosphorylation of HMG-CoA reductase
D. insulin action causes reduced levels of cAMP, which lead to reduced PKA-mediated phosphorylation of protein phosphatase inhibitor 1 (PPI-1)
E. insulin action leads to tyrosine phosphorylation of AMPK, causing loss of the AMPK-mediated inhibition of HMG-CoA reductase

Answer D: One of the effects, within cells such as hepatocytes, of insulin activation of its receptor is activation of phosphodiesterase. Phosphodiesterase catalyzes the hydrolysis of cAMP to AMP. Reduced levels of cAMP lead to decreased activation of PKA. With respect to cholesterol biosynthesis, PKA normally phosphorylates PPI-1, which when phosphorylated prevents phosphate removal from HMG-CoA reductase (HMGR) by HMGR phosphatase. The reduction in the activity of PPI-1 results in increased HMGR phosphatase activity. Removal of phosphates from HMGR returns it to its more active state. Thus, the net effect of insulin is an increase in the synthesis of cholesterol via its effects on HMGR activity.

16. You are examining a patient you suspect is afflicted with Smith-Lemli-Opitz syndrome (SLOS), which is associated with mild to severe developmental abnormalities. Knowing that this disorder is the consequence of a defect in cholesterol biosynthesis,

measurement of the blood levels of which of the following compounds would be most diagnostic of SLOS?
A. acetyl-CoA
B. 7-dehydrocholesterol
C. HMG-CoA
D. lanosterol
E. mevalonate

Answer B: Smith-Lemli-Opitz syndrome is caused by mutations in the gene encoding the terminal enzyme in cholesterol biosynthesis, that is, 7-dehydrocholesterol reductase. The enzyme converts 7-dehydrocholesterol to cholesterol. Therefore, defects in this gene result in increased serum levels of 7-dehydrocholesterol and reduced levels (15%-27% of normal) of cholesterol.

17. In familial hypercholesterolemia, cholesterol is deposited in various tissues because of the high concentration of LDL cholesterol in the plasma. Of particular concern is the oxidation of the excess LDL to form oxidized LDL (oxLDL). The oxLDL is taken up by macrophages, which become engorged to form foam cells. Which statement best describes the formation of foam cells?
A. cholesterol cannot be extracted from macrophages by HDL
B. expression of the receptors for oxLDL is increased in the macrophages
C. LDL enters by pinocytosis to form foam cells
D. LDL receptors on peripheral cells are upregulated
E. there is increased synthesis of cholesterol in macrophages as a result

Answer B: There are a number of cell surface receptors that bind lipoproteins of the LDL family, such as the classic LDL receptor and the LDL receptor–related proteins. Modified LDL, such as oxLDL, does not bind to the LDL receptor. Instead, these lipoprotein particles are taken up into macrophages via the scavenger receptor, FAT/CD36. Presentation of this receptor on macrophage plasma membranes is not downregulated in response to oxLDL uptake as is the case for the LDL receptor. Conversely, uptake of oxLDL by macrophages leads to increased density of FAT/CD36 on these cells.

18. A patient presents with very high levels of serum cholesterol. After a series of tests, it is concluded that the patient has high circulating levels of LDL cholesterol, but has normal levels of the hepatic LDL receptor. Which of the following could best explain the observations in this patient?
A. hepatocytes from the patient are defective in the selective removal of cholesterol from the LDL complex
B. hepatocytes from the patient have decreased levels of acyl-CoA:cholesterol acyltransferase ratio
C. the absence of the enzyme lipoprotein lipase in the endothelial cells of the liver
D. the patient has a mutated form of apoB-100
E. there is an altered level of phosphorylation of the LDL receptor

Answer D: LDL is taken up by cells via LDL receptor-mediated endocytosis. In order for LDL receptors to recognize and bind LDL, they require the presence of both apoB-100 and apoE (the LDL receptor is also called the apoB-100/apoE receptor). Therefore, in this patient with elevated serum LDL in the presence of normal levels of hepatic LDL receptors, the most likely possible cause is a defective apoB-100 protein associated with the circulating LDL.

19. A patient presents in your office with very high levels of serum cholesterol. He states that he has tried to follow the diet and exercise regimen you gave him last year. You decide that this patient would benefit by taking a drug of the statin class. This class of drug is effective in treating hypercholesterolemia because it has which of the following effects?
A. binds cholesterol, preventing it from being absorbed by the intestine
B. decreases the stability of HMG-CoA reductase
C. directly prevents the deposition of cholesterol on artery walls
D. inhibits the enzyme HMG-CoA reductase
E. stimulates phosphorylation of HMG-CoA reductase

Answer D: The statin drugs are fungal-derived HMG-CoA reductase (HMGR) inhibitors.

20. Free cholesterol can affect cholesterol metabolism in the body by inhibiting cholesterol biosynthesis. Which of the following most closely reflects the mechanism by which cholesterol suppresses its own synthesis?
A. condensation of acetyl-CoA and acetoacetyl-CoA to form hydroxymethyl glutaryl-CoA
B. cyclizing of squalene to form lanosterol
C. formation of mevalonate from hydroxymethyl glutaryl-CoA
D. kinase that phosphorylates hydroxymethyl glutaryl-CoA reductase
E. reduction of 7-dehydrocholesterol to form cholesterol

Answer C: Regulation of HMG-CoA reductase (HMGR) activity is the primary means for controlling the level of cholesterol biosynthesis. This enzyme catalyzes the conversion of mevalonate to hydroxymethyl glutaryl-CoA. HMGR activity is controlled by 4 distinct mechanisms: feedback inhibition, control of gene expression, rate of enzyme degradation, and phosphorylation-dephosphorylation. The first 3 control mechanisms are exerted by cholesterol itself. Cholesterol acts as a feedback inhibitor of preexisting HMGR as well as inducing rapid degradation of the enzyme. In addition, when cholesterol is in excess, the amount of mRNA for HMGR is reduced because of decreased expression of the gene.

21. Which of the following vitamins can be used in high doses to treat hypercholesterolemia?

A. folic acid
B. niacin
C. pyridoxine
D. riboflavin
E. thiamine

Answer B: Nicotinic acid, derived from niacin, reduces the plasma levels of both VLDLs and LDLs by inhibiting hepatic VLDL secretion, as well as suppressing the flux of FFA release from adipose tissue by inhibiting lipolysis. In addition, nicotinic administration strongly increases the circulating levels of HDLs. Patient compliance with nicotinic acid administration is sometimes compromised because of the unpleasant side effect of flushing (strong cutaneous vasodilation).

22. A 65-year-old woman is brought to the emergency room by her husband because she is experiencing chest pain radiating to her left arm. The attending physician diagnoses her as suffering from a mild myocardial infarction and prescribes appropriate intervention. Blood work reveals her total cholesterol to be 280 mg/dL, so a statin is prescribed. Statin drugs inhibit the activity of HMG-CoA reductase. Which of the following best describes how taking statin drugs leads to reduced serum cholesterol and LDL levels?

A. it decreases the serum level of LDL by promoting catabolism
B. it increases the serum level of HDL, thereby promoting increased reverse cholesterol transport
C. it inhibits synthesis of LDL receptors
D. it inhibits the formation of LDL from IDL
E. it inhibits the rate-limiting step in cholesterol biosynthesis

Answer E: The statin drugs inhibit HMG-CoA, which is the rate-limiting enzyme in de novo cholesterol biosynthesis. Thus, inhibition of cholesterol synthesis reduces the amount of free and LDL-associated cholesterol in the serum.

23. A 35-year-old woman presents with crushing substernal chest pain and shortness of breath. A coronary artery is occluded due to an atherosclerotic plaque, and she is diagnosed with having a myocardial infarction. Her serum cholesterol level is 700 mg/dL. She has a family history of hypercholesterolemia. Which of the following is the inherited defect in individuals with familial hypercholesterolemia?

A. abnormal LDL receptors
B. high activity of HMG-CoA reductase
C. increased conversion of VLDL to LDL
D. low activity of 7-α hydroxylase
E. reduced plasma concentration of HDL

Answer A: Familial hypercholesterolemia, FH (type II hyperlipoproteinemia), is an autosomal dominant disorder that results from mutations affecting the structure and function of the cell-surface receptor that binds plasma LDLs, removing them from the circulation. The defects in LDL-receptor (LDLR) interaction result in lifelong elevation of LDL-cholesterol in the blood. The resultant hypercholesterolemia leads to premature coronary artery disease and atherosclerotic plaque formation.

24. Which of the following compounds directly inhibits the expression of the *HMG-CoA reductase* gene?

A. cholesterol
B. HMG-CoA
C. isopentenyl pyrophosphate
D. lanosterol
E. squalene

Answer A: Regulation of HMG-CoA reductase (HMGR) activity is the primary means for controlling the level of cholesterol biosynthesis. This enzyme catalyzes the conversion of mevalonate to hydroxymethyl glutaryl-CoA. HMGR activity is controlled by 4 distinct mechanisms: feedback inhibition, control of gene expression, rate of enzyme degradation, and phosphorylation-dephosphorylation. The first 3 control mechanisms are exerted by cholesterol itself. Cholesterol acts as a feedback inhibitor of preexisting HMGR as well as inducing rapid degradation of the enzyme. In addition, when cholesterol is in excess, the amount of mRNA for HMGR is reduced because of decreased expression of the gene.

25. A 23-year-old woman presents with low red blood cell count, corneal opacities, and renal insufficiency.

She is diagnosed with lecithin:cholesterol acyltransferase (LCAT) ratio deficiency. In which of the following reactions LCAT is involved?

A. converting cholesterol to cholesterol esters
B. hydrolysis of HDL
C. promoting uptake of HDL into liver cells
D. transfer of cholesterol esters from HDL to VLDL
E. uptake of cholesterol from liver cells

Answer A: The primary mechanism by which HDL acquires peripheral tissue cholesterol is via an interaction with macrophages in the subendothelial spaces of the tissues. The free cholesterol transferred from macrophages to HDL is esterified by HDL-associated LCAT. LCAT is synthesized in the liver and so named because it transfers a fatty acid from the C-2 position of lecithin to the C-3-OH of cholesterol, generating a cholesteryl ester and lysolecithin.

26. An autopsy is conducted on a stillborn female fetus exhibiting multiple lethal congenital malformations and osteosclerosis. Analysis of lipids accumulated in tissues showed high levels of desmosterol and extremely low levels of cholesterol. Given the skeletal malformations and the lipid profiles obtained from this fetus, the pathologist makes a diagnosis of desmosterolosis. Which of the following enzymes was most likely defective in this fetus resulting in the lethality?

A. 7-dehydrocholesterol reductase
B. 24-dehydrocholesterol reductase
C. HMG-CoA reductase
D. mevalonate kinase
E. squalene monooxygenase

Answer B: Desmosterolosis is an extremely rare disorder, but the presentations are useful for an understanding of the role of cholesterol in early neonatal developments. Skeletal abnormalities found in desmosterolosis are similar to, but more severe than, those presenting in SLOS. Desmosterolosis results from a defect in the gene encoding 3-β-hydroxysterol δ-24-reductase (DHCR24), which catalyzes the reduction of the δ-24 double bond of sterol intermediates during cholesterol biosynthesis. Loss of DHCR4, therefore, causes a loss of cholesterol production with accumulation of the intermediate, desmosterol.

Checklist

- ✓ Cholesterol is required for synthesis of the bile acids required for lipid digestion and absorption, synthesis of the steroid hormones, and incorporation into membranes and lipoprotein particles.
- ✓ Cholesterol synthesis occurs in the cytosol, and mitochondrially derived acetyl-CoA must first be transported to the cytosol as citrate.
- ✓ Cholesterol synthesis requires many reactions, some of which generate byproducts that are utilized in other important biological processes.
- ✓ Cholesterol synthesis is tightly regulated at the level of HMGR activity and level.
- ✓ The master metabolic regulator, AMPK, is a critical enzyme in the control of HMGR activity.
- ✓ Transcriptional regulation of genes involved in cholesterol biosynthesis (eg, HMGR) occurs via regulated activity of SREBP.
- ✓ Defects in the terminal enzyme of cholesterol biosynthesis, 7-dehydrocholesterol reductase (DHCR7), result in SLOS.
- ✓ FH is one of the most common genetic causes of hypercholesterolemia.
- ✓ Hypercholesterolemia can be treated by several approaches, with the statin drugs being the most prescribed class.

CHAPTER 27 Lipids: Bile Acid Metabolism

CHAPTER OUTLINE

High-Yield Terms

Classic (neutral) pathway: major pathway for bile acid synthesis, initiated from cholesterol via the action of CYP7A1, both cholic and chenodeoxycholic acid synthesized via the classic pathway

Acidic pathway: alternative, minor pathway for bile acid synthesis initiated via the action of sterol 27-hydroxylase (CYP27A1), only chenodeoxycholic acid synthesized via the acidic pathway

CYP7A1: 7α-hydroxylase, rate-limiting enzyme in the classic pathway of bile acid synthesis

Primary bile acids: the end products of hepatic bile acid synthesis and includes cholic acid and chenodeoxycholic acid

Secondary bile acids: products of the actions of intestinal bacteria on the primary bile acids generating deoxycholate (from cholate) and lithocholate (from chenodeoxycholate)

Enterohepatic circulation: the circulation of bile acids, or other substances, from the liver to the gallbladder, followed by secretion into the small intestine, absorption by intestinal enterocytes, and transport back to the liver

Farnesoid X receptors (FXR): nuclear receptors for bile acids and bile acid metabolites; regulate the expression of genes involved in bile acid synthesis

Guggulsterone: the term for any resin collected by tapping the trunk of a tree is called guggul (or guggal) and the lipid component of this extract is called guggulsterone (also called guggul lipid)

High-Yield Concept

Although the acidic pathway is not a major route for human bile acid synthesis, it is an important one as demonstrated by the phenotype presenting in a newborn harboring a mutation in the CYP7B1 gene. This infant presented with severe cholestasis (blockage in bile flow from liver) with cirrhosis and liver dysfunction.

Bile Acid Synthesis Pathways

The end products of cholesterol utilization are the bile acids. Indeed, synthesis of bile acids is one of the predominant mechanisms for the excretion of excess cholesterol. However, the excretion of cholesterol in the form of bile acids is insufficient to compensate for an excess dietary intake of cholesterol.

Although several of the enzymes involved in bile acid synthesis are active in many cell types, the liver is the only organ where their complete biosynthesis can occur. Although bile acid synthesis constitutes the route of catabolism of cholesterol, these compounds are also important in the solubilization of dietary cholesterol, lipids, and essential nutrients, thus promoting their delivery to the liver. Synthesis of a full complement of bile acids requires 17 individual enzymes and occurs in multiple intracellular compartments that include the cytosol, endoplasmic reticulum (ER), mitochondria, and peroxisomes. The genes encoding several of the enzymes of bile acid synthesis are under tight regulatory control to ensure that the necessary level of bile acid production is coordinated to changing metabolic conditions. Given the fact that many bile acid metabolites are cytotoxic, it is understandable why their synthesis needs to be tightly controlled.

The major pathway for the synthesis of the bile acids is initiated via hydroxylation of cholesterol at the 7 position via the action of cholesterol 7α-hydroxylase (CYP7A1) which is an ER-localized enzyme. CYP7A1 is a member of the cytochrome P450 family of metabolic enzymes. This pathway is depicted in highly abbreviated fashion in Figure 27-1. The pathway initiated by

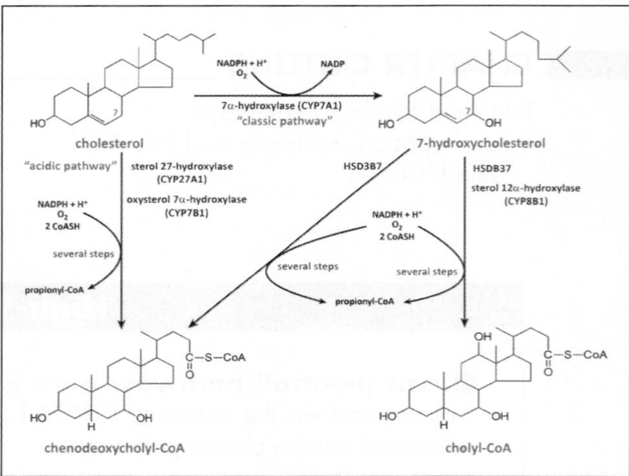

FIGURE 27-1: Synthesis of the 2 primary bile acids, cholic acid (CA) and chenodeoxycholic acid (CDCA). The reaction catalyzed by the 7α-hydroxylase (CYP7A1) is the rate-limiting step in bile acid synthesis. Expression of CYP7A1 occurs only in the liver. Conversion of 7α-hydroxycholesterol to the bile acids requires several steps not shown in detail in this image. Only the relevant cofactors needed for the synthesis steps are shown. Sterol 12α-hydroxylase (CYB8B1) controls the synthesis of cholic acid and as such is under tight transcriptional control (see text). Reproduced with permission of themedicalbiochemistrypage, LLC.

CYP7A1 is referred to as the "classic" or "neutral" pathway of bile acid synthesis.

There is an alternative pathway that involves hydroxylation of cholesterol at the 27 position by the mitochondrial enzyme sterol 27-hydroxylase (CYP27A1). This alternative pathway is referred to as the "acidic"

High-Yield Concept

The hydroxyl group on cholesterol at the 3 position is in the β-orientation and must be epimerized to the α-orientation during the synthesis of the bile acids. This epimerization is initiated by conversion of the 3β-hydroxyl to a 3-oxo group catalyzed by 3β-hydroxy-Δ^5-C_{27}-steroid oxidoreductase (HSD3B7). Evidence that this reaction is critical for bile acid synthesis and function is demonstrated in children harboring mutations in the HSD3B7 gene. These children develop progressive liver disease that is characterized by cholestatic jaundice.

CLINICAL BOX 27-1: INBORN ERRORS IN BILE ACID SYNTHESIS

Several inborn errors in metabolism are due to defects in genes of bile acid synthesis and are associated with liver failure in early childhood to progressive neuropathies in adults. Metabolic disorders associated with bile acid synthesis and metabolism are broadly classified as primary or secondary disorders. Primary disorders involve inherited deficiencies in enzymes responsible for catalyzing key reactions in the synthesis of cholic and chenodeoxycholic acids. Bile acid disorders classified as secondary refer to metabolic defects that impact primary bile acid synthesis but that are not due to defects in the enzymes responsible for synthesis. Secondary disorders of bile acid metabolism include peroxisomal disorders such as Zellweger syndrome and related peroxisomal biogenesis disorders and Smith-Lemli-Opitz syndrome which results from a deficiency of 7-dehydrocholesterol reductase (DHCR7) (Table 27-1).

pathway of bile acid synthesis. In humans this alternative bile acid synthesis pathway accounts for no more than 6% of total bile acid production. The bile acid intermediates generated via the action of CYP27A1 are subsequently hydroxylated on the 7 position by oxysterol 7α-hydroxylase (CYP7B1). Numerous disorders have been identified that result from mutations in the genes of bile synthesis (Clinical Box 27-1 and Table 27-1)

Following the action of HSD3B7 the bile acid intermediates can proceed via two pathways whose end products are chenodeoxycholic acid (CDCA) and cholic acid (CA). The distribution of these 2 bile acids is determined by the activity of sterol 12α-hydroxylase (CYP8B1). The intermediates of the HSD3B7 reaction that are acted on by CYP8B1 become CA and those that escape the action of the enzyme will become CDCA. Therefore, the activity of the CYP8B1 gene will determine the ratio of CA to CDCA. The CYP8B1 gene is subject to regulation by bile acids themselves via their ability to regulate the action of the nuclear receptor FXR.

The most abundant bile acids in human bile are chenodeoxycholic acid (45%) and cholic acid (31%). These are referred to as the primary bile acids. Before the primary bile acids are secreted into the canalicular lumen they are conjugated via an amide bond at the terminal carboxyl group with either of the amino acids glycine or taurine. These conjugation reactions yield glycoconjugates and tauroconjugates, respectively (Figure 27-2). This conjugation process increases the amphipathic nature of the bile acids making them more easily secretable as well as less cytotoxic. The conjugated bile acids are the major solutes in human bile.

Enterohepatic Circulation and Bile Acid Modification

Following secretion by the liver, the bile acids enter the bile canaliculi which join with the bile ductules which then form the bile ducts (Figure 27-3). Bile acids are carried from the liver through these ducts to the gallbladder, where they are stored for future use. In the gallbladder bile acids are concentrated up to 1000 fold. Excess bile accumulation in the bile canaliculi and the gallbladder is a primary cause of gallstones (Clinical Box 27-2). Following stimulation by food intake the gallbladder releases the bile into the duodenum, via the action of the gut hormone cholecystokinin, CCK (Chapter 44), where they aid in the emulsification of dietary lipids.

Within the intestines the primary bile acids are acted upon by bacteria and undergo a deconjugation process that removes the glycine and taurine residues. The deconjugated bile acids are either excreted (only a small percentage) or reabsorbed by the gut and returned to the liver. Anaerobic bacteria present in the colon modify the primary bile acids converting them to the secondary bile acids, identified as deoxycholate (from cholate) and lithocholate (from chenodeoxycholate). Both primary and secondary bile acids are reabsorbed by the intestines and delivered back to the liver via the portal circulation. Indeed, as much as 95% of total bile acid synthesized by the liver is absorbed by the distal ileum and returned to the liver. This process of secretion from the liver to the gallbladder and then to the intestines and finally reabsorption is termed the enterohepatic circulation.

Regulation of Bile Acid Homeostasis

Bile acids, in particular chenodeoxycholic acid (CDCA) and cholic acid (CA), can regulate the expression of genes involved in their synthesis, thereby creating a feedback loop. This regulatory pathway involves a class of nuclear receptors called the farnesoid X receptors, FXR. The FXR genes are expressed at highest levels in the intestine and liver. Bile acids and bile acid metabolites bind to and activate the transcriptional activity of FXR.

One major target of FXR is the small heterodimer partner (SHP) gene. Activation of SHP expression by FXR represses the expression of the cholesterol

TABLE 27-1: Primary Disorders in Bile Acid Synthesis

Affected Enzyme	*Gene Symbol*	*Phenotype/Comments*
Cholesterol 7α-hydroxylase	*CYP7A1*	No liver dysfunction, clinical phenotype manifests with markedly elevated total cholesterol as well as LDL, premature gallstones, premature coronary and peripheral vascular disease, elevated serum cholesterol is not responsive to statin drug therapy
Sterol 27-hydroxylase	*CYP27A1*	Progressive neurological dysfunction, neonatal cholestasis, bilateral cataracts, chronic diarrhea
Oxysterol 7α-hydroxylase	*CYP7B1*	A single case has been reported, a 10-week-old boy presented with severe progressive cholestasis, hepatosplenomegaly, cirrhosis, and liver failure, serum ALT and AST were markedly elevated
3β-hydroxy-Δ^5-C_{27}-steroid oxidoreductase	*HSD3B7*	Most commonly reported defect in bile acid synthesis, heterogeneous clinical presentation that includes progressive jaundice, hepatomegaly, pruritus, malabsorption with resultant steatorrhea (fatty diarrhea), fat-soluble vitamin deficiency, rickets
Δ^4-3-oxosteroid 5β-reductase	*AKR1C4*	Similar clinical manifestation to HSD3B7 deficiency, although with earlier presentation afflicted infants will have a more severe liver disease with rapid progression to cirrhosis and death if no clinical intervention is undertaken, liver function tests will show marked elevation in AST and ALT, serum tests show elevated conjugated bilirubin, coagulopathy will also be evident
2-methylacyl-CoA racemase	*AMACR*	First reported in 3 adults who presented with a sensory motor neuropathy, also found in a 10-week-old infant who had severe fat-soluble vitamin deficiencies, hematochezia (passage of bright red stool), and mild cholestatic liver disease

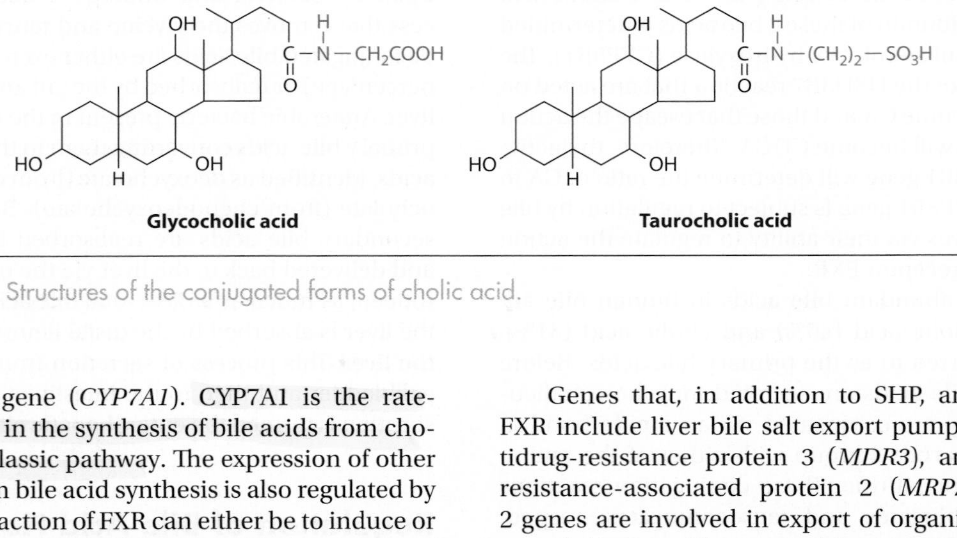

FIGURE 27-2: Structures of the conjugated forms of cholic acid.

7α-hydroxylase gene (*CYP7A1*). CYP7A1 is the rate-limiting enzyme in the synthesis of bile acids from cholesterol via the classic pathway. The expression of other genes involved in bile acid synthesis is also regulated by FXR action. The action of FXR can either be to induce or to repress the expression of these genes. The activity of FXR has been shown to be affected by guggal lipids (see Clinical Box 27-3). Genes that are repressed, in addition to *CYP7A1*, include *SREBP-1c*, sterol 12α-hydroxylase (*CYP8B1*), and the Na^+-taurocholate cotransporting polypeptide (*NTCP*). *NTCP* is involved in hepatic uptake of bile acids through the sinusoidal/basolateral membrane. Bile acid–mediated repression of *NTCP* gene expression results in reduced uptake of bile acids, which in turn protects the liver from the toxic effects of excess bile acid accumulation. Bile acids also repress the transcription of the Na^+-independent organic anion transporting polypeptide 1B1 (OATP1B1).

Genes that, in addition to SHP, are induced by FXR include liver bile salt export pump (*BSEP*), multidrug-resistance protein 3 (*MDR3*), and multidrug-resistance-associated protein 2 (*MRP2*). The latter 2 genes are involved in export of organic compounds out of the liver. The normal function of *MDR3* is the translocation of phospholipids through the canalicular membrane of hepatocytes. Thus, it is inferred that the bile acid–mediated increase in *MDR3* expression is necessary to allow hepatocytes to respond to bile acid toxicity via the formation of cholesterol, phospholipid, and bile acid–containing micelles. *BSEP* is involved in the process of exporting bile acids out of hepatocytes, thus reducing their toxicity to these cells. Mutations in *BSEP* and *MDR3* are associated with familial intrahepatic cholestasis type 2 and 3, respectively. Mutations in *MRP2* are associated with Dubin-Johnson syndrome, a form of inherited hyperbilirubinemia (see Chapter 33).

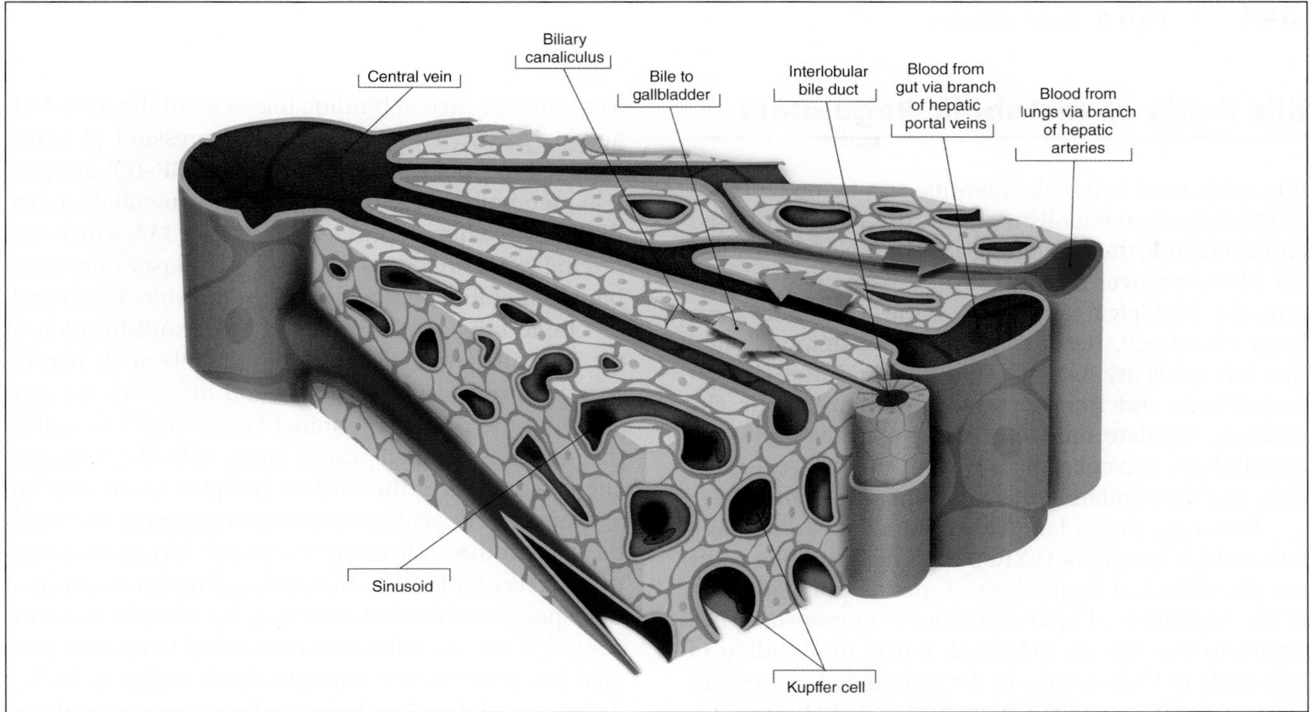

FIGURE 27-3: Structure of a liver portal lobule. Liver lobules represent small subdivisions of the liver defined at the histological level as opposed to the four major anatomic lobes. Kuppffer cells are specialized liver-resident macrophages. Reproduced with permission of themedicalbiochemistrypage, LLC.

CLINICAL BOX 27-2: GALLSTONES

Gallstones are hard, pebble-like deposits that form inside the gallbladder. The clinical term for this condition is cholelithiasis. Gallstones may be as small as a grain of sand or as large as a golf ball. Gallstones are more common in women, Native Americans, and other ethnic groups, and people older than 40 years. Gallstones may also run in families. There are a variety of causes for the formation of gallstones. There are 2 main types of gallstones, those composed primarily of cholesterol and those composed of bilirubin. Gallstones formed from cholesterol are the most common type. Gallstones formed from too much bilirubin in the bile are called pigment stones. Gallstones can remain asymptomatic for many years. Migration of the stones into the ductal system of the gallbladder can result in obstruction of bile flow resulting in inflammation. If a large stone blocks either the cystic duct or the common bile duct (called choledocholithiasis), symptoms will include a cramping pain in the middle to right upper abdomen. This is known as biliary colic. The pain goes away if the stone passes into the duodenum via the common bile duct. Once gallstones become symptomatic, definitive surgical intervention with excision of the gallbladder (cholecystectomy) is usually indicated. Cholecystectomy is among the most frequently performed abdominal surgical procedures.

CLINICAL BOX 27-3: AYURVEDIC MEDICINE

In the Ayurvedic tradition of medicine, any resin that is collected by tapping the trunk of a tree is called guggul (or guggal). The cholesterol-lowering action of the guggul from the Mukul myrrh tree (*Commiphora mukul*) of India is a function of the lipid component of this extract, called guggulsterone (also called guggul lipid). Guggulsterone is an antagonist of FXR. However, in addition to its effects on FXR function, guggulsterone has been shown to activate the pregnane X receptor (PXR), which is another member of the nuclear receptor superfamily. PXR is a recognized receptor for lithocholic acid and other bile acid precursors. PXR activation leads to repression of bile acid synthesis due to its physical association with hepatocyte nuclear factor 4α (HNF4α) causing this transcription factor to no longer be able to associate with the transcriptional coactivator PGC1α (PPARγ coactivator 1α) which ultimately leads to loss of transcription factor activation of CYP7A1.

Bile Acids as Metabolic Regulators

Bile acids were originally identified as being involved in cholesterol metabolism and in the process of lipid emulsification, thereby aiding absorption of dietary lipids. However, over the past several years new insights into the biological activities of the bile acids have been elucidated. Recent findings have demonstrated that bile acids are involved in the control of their own metabolism and transport via the enterohepatic circulation, regulate lipid metabolism, regulate glucose metabolism, control signaling events in liver regeneration, and the regulation of overall energy expenditure.

Following the isolation and characterization of the farnesoid X receptors (FXRs), for which the bile acids are physiological ligands, the functions of bile acids in the regulation of lipid and glucose homeostasis has begun to emerge. As indicated above, the binding of bile acids to FXRs results in the attenuated expression of several genes involved in overall bile acid homeostasis. However, genes involved in bile acid metabolism are not the only ones that are regulated by FXR action as a consequence of binding bile acid. In the liver, FXR action is known to regulate the expression of genes involved in lipid metabolism (eg, SREBP-1c), lipoprotein metabolism (eg, apoC-II), glucose metabolism (eg, PEPCK), and hepatoprotection (eg, CYP3A4, which was originally identified as nifedipine oxidase; nifedipine being a member of the calcium channel blocker drugs).

In addition to their roles in lipid emulsification in the intestine and activating FXR, the bile acids participate in various signal transduction processes via activation of the c-JUN *N*-terminal kinase (JNK) as well as the mitogen-activated protein kinase (MAPK) pathways. Other members of the nuclear receptor family that are activated by bile acids are the pregnane X receptor (PXR), the constitutive androstane receptor (CAR), and the vitamin D receptor (VDR). An additional receptor activated in response to bile acids that may have implications for control of obesity is the transmembrane G-protein–coupled bile acid receptor 1 (originally identified as TGR5). Activation of TGR5 in brown adipose tissue results in activation of uncoupling protein 1, UCP1 (also called thermogenin) leading to enhanced energy expenditure.

REVIEW QUESTIONS

1. The Ayurvedic practice of medicine, native to India, has demonstrated a cholesterol-lowering benefit to the guggul lipid extract from the myrrh tree, guggulsterone. This lipid extract has been shown in laboratory studies to activate the expression of a gene involved in the regulation of bile acid metabolism. Which of the following genes is activated by guggul lipids?

A. 7α-hydroxylase (CYP7A1)
B. farnesoid X receptor (FXR)
C. pregnane X receptor (PXR)
D. multidrug-resistance protein 3 (MDR3)
E. small heterodimer partner (SHP)

Answer C: In the Ayurvedic tradition of medicine, any resin that is collected by tapping the trunk of a tree is called guggul (or guggal). The cholesterol-lowering action of the guggul from the Mukul myrrh tree (*Commiphora mukul*) of India is that a lipid component of this extract called guggulsterone (also called guggul lipid) is an antagonist to FXR. However, in addition to its effects on FXR function, guggulsterone has been shown to activate the pregnane X receptor (PXR) which is another member of the nuclear receptor superfamily. PXR is a recognized receptor for lithocholic acid and other bile acid precursors. PXR activation leads to repression of bile acid synthesis due to its physical association with hepatocyte nuclear factor 4α (HNF4α) causing this transcription factor to no longer be able to associate with the transcriptional coactivator PGC1α (PPARγ coactivator 1α) which ultimately leads to loss of transcription factor activation of CYP7A1.

2. A 2-year-old girl who is exhibiting a failure to thrive is diagnosed with hepatic failure and cholestasis. Her pediatrician suspects the girl is suffering from familial intrahepatic cholestasis. Which of the following genes is likely harboring a mutation resulting in the observed symptoms?

A. 7α-hydroxylase (*CYP7A1*)
B. bile salt export pump (*BSEP*)
C. farnesoid X receptor (*FXR*)
D. pregnane X receptor (PXR)
E. sodium (Na^+)-taurocholate cotransporting polypeptide (*NTCP*)

Answer B: *BSEP* is a member of the ABC family of transporters (*BSEP* is also identified as *ABCB11*) and it is involved in the process of exporting bile acids out of hepatocytes thus reducing their toxicity to these cells. Mutation in *BSEP* is associated with familial intrahepatic cholestasis type 2.

3. You are measuring bile acid metabolites produced by a cell line isolated from a hepatoma. Mass spec and gas chromatographic studies indicate that the cell line produces chenodeoxycholic acid and related metabolites but does not produce cholic acid nor any metabolites of this compound. Which of the following is the most likely enzyme missing or defective in these cells?

A. 7-dehydrocholesterol reductase (DHC7R)
B. 3β-hydroxy Δ^5 C_{27}-steroid oxidoreductase (HSD3B7)
C. 7α-hydroxylase (CYP7A1)
D. oxysterol 7α-hydroxylase (CYP7B1)
E. sterol 27-hydroxylase (CYP27A1)

Answer C: The major pathway for the synthesis of the bile acids is initiated via hydroxylation of cholesterol at the 7 position via the action of cholesterol 7α-hydroxylase (CYP7A1). The pathway initiated by CYP7A1 is referred to as the "classic" or "neutral" pathway of bile acid synthesis. The hydroxyl group on cholesterol at the 3 position is in the β-orientation and must be epimerized to the α-orientation during the synthesis of the bile acids. This epimerization is initiated by conversion of the 3β-hydroxyl to a 3-oxo group catalyzed by 3β-hydroxy-Δ^5-C_{27}-steroid oxidoreductase (HSD3B7). Following the action of HSD3B7 the bile acid intermediates can proceed via 2 pathways whose end products are chenodeoxycholic acid (CDCA) and cholic acid (CA). The alternative bile acid synthesis pathway initiated by sterol 27-hydroxylase (CYP27A1) yields chenodeoxycholic acid, the same as for the classic pathway initiated by CYP7A1. However, the acidic pathway does not lead to the synthesis of cholic acid.

4. A 5-month-old infant is brought to her pediatrician because her parents are concerned about her general failure to thrive and a progressive yellowing of her eyes and skin. Upon examination it is noted the infant has slightly bowing legs indicative of rickets, hepatomegaly, poorly clotting blood, and fatty diarrhea. The rickets-like symptoms and the fatty stool are indicative of lipid maladsorption. The pediatrician makes a diagnosis of a bile acid metabolism disorder. Which of the following enzymes is likely to be defective in this infant?

A. bile salt export protein (BSEP)
B. 3β-hydroxy Δ^5 C_{27}-steroid oxidoreductase (HSD3B7)
C. 7α-hydroxylase (CYP7A1)
D. multidrug-resistance-associated protein 2 (MRP2)
E. sterol 27-hydroxylase (CYP27A1)

Answer B: Defects in 3β-hydroxy Δ^5 C_{27}-steroid oxidoreductase (HSD3B7) are the most commonly reported inborn errors in bile acid synthesis. The disorder is characterized by neonatal onset of progressive liver disease with cholestatic jaundice and malabsorption of lipids and lipid-soluble vitamins from the gastrointestinal tract resulting from a primary failure to synthesize bile acids. Affected infants also show failure to thrive, secondary coagulopathy, progressive jaundice, hepatomegaly, and malabsorption with resultant steatorrhea (fatty diarrhea).

5. You have generated a line of transgenic mice in which the gene encoding the transcription factor, small heterodimer partner (SHP) has been disabled specifically in hepatocytes. Which of the following genes, involved in bile acid metabolism, would most likely exhibit unregulated expression in the livers of these mice?

A. bile salt export protein (BSEP)
B. farnesoid X receptor (FXR)
C. 3β-hydroxy-Δ^5-C_{27}-steroid oxidoreductase (HSD3B7)
D. 7α-hydroxylase (CYP7A1)
E. multidrug-resistance-associated protein 2 (MRP2)

Answer D: Expression of SHP is normally controlled through the action of the FXR family of transcription factors. Activation of SHP expression by FXR results in inhibition of transcription of SHP target genes. Of significance to bile acid synthesis, SHP represses the expression of the cholesterol 7α-hydroxylase gene (CYP7A1). CYP7A1 is the rate-limiting enzyme in the synthesis of bile acids from cholesterol via the classic pathway. Loss of SHP expression would, therefore, result in unregulated CYP7A1 expression.

6. Bile acids have been shown to control their own metabolism and transport via the enterohepatic circulation, regulate lipid metabolism, regulate glucose metabolism, and regulate overall energy expenditure. These effects of the bile acids are exerted via the binding to and activation of which of the following?

A. ChREBP
B. farnesoid X receptor (FXR)
C. 7α-hydroxylase (CYP7A1)
D. SREBP-1c
E. sterol 27-hydroxylase (CYP27A1)

Answer B: Bile acids, in particular chenodeoxycholic acid (CDCA) and cholic acid (CA), can regulate the expression of genes involved in their synthesis, thereby creating a feedback loop. The elucidation of this regulatory pathway came about as a consequence of the isolation of a class of receptors called the farnesoid X receptors (FXRs), which were shown to bind to bile acids.

7. A 6-month-old infant presents with progressive neurological dysfunction, cholestasis, bilateral cataracts, and chronic diarrhea. A diagnosis is made of a bile acid metabolism defect due to deficiency in the sterol 27-hydroxylase gene. Which of the following would be expected to be an additional finding in this infant?

A. decreased overall levels of chenodeoxycholic acid
B. decreased overall levels of cholic acid
C. elevated cholesterol in the gallbladder
D. elevated taurocholic acid in the biliary canaliculi
E. increased deoxycholic acid in the gallbladder

Answer B: The alternative bile acid synthesis pathway involves hydroxylation of cholesterol at the 27 position by the mitochondrial enzyme sterol 27-hydroxylase (CYP27A1). This alternative pathway is referred to as the "acidic" pathway of bile acid synthesis. The product of this pathway is chenodeoxycholic acid, the same as for the classic pathway initiated by CYP7A1. However, the acidic pathway does not lead to the synthesis of cholic acid; so this bile acid and its metabolites would be reduced in individuals with a deficiency in CYP27A1. Although the acidic pathway accounts for no more than 6% of total bile acid production, it is an important as evidenced by the symptoms seen in infants harboring the defective gene.

8. Which of the following modifications increases the working pH range and amphipathic nature of bile acids?

A. conjugation to taurine or glycine
B. dehydroxylation by intestinal bacteria
C. esterification
D. formation of sodium or potassium salts
E. 7α-hydroxylation

Answer A: Bile acids are modified, prior to secretion from the liver into the bile canaliculi, by addition of the amino acid glycine or taurine. The addition of these amino groups increases amphipathic nature of bile acids making them more easily secretable as well as less cytotoxic.

Checklist

✓ Bile acids represent the major pathway for the metabolism of cholesterol.

✓ Bile acids are synthesized in the liver, stored within the gallbladder, and secreted into the intestines, via the actions of cholecystokinin (CCK), in response to food intake in order to aid in the solubilization of lipids and lipid-soluble vitamins.

✓ The most abundant bile acids in human bile are chenodeoxycholic acid (45%) and cholic acid (31%) which are referred to as the primary bile acids.

✓ Bile acids are modified, prior to secretion into the bile canaliculi, by amino acid addition which increases their amphipathic nature making them more easily secretable as well as less cytotoxic.

✓ Within the intestines the primary bile acids are acted upon by bacteria and undergo a deconjugation process that removes the glycine and taurine residues. Anaerobic bacteria present in the colon modify the primary bile acids converting them to the secondary bile acids, identified as deoxycholate (from cholate) and lithocholate (from chenodeoxycholate).

✓ Both primary and secondary bile acids are reabsorbed by the intestines and delivered back to the liver via the portal circulation which results in as much as 95% of total bile acid synthesized by the liver being returned to the liver. This process of secretion from the liver to the gallbladder and then to the intestines and finally reabsorption is termed the enterohepatic circulation.

✓ Bile acids and bile acid metabolites are bioactive lipids that bind to transcription factors of the nuclear receptor family leading to a wide range of biological effects.

✓ Defects in enzymes of bile acid metabolism and membrane transport of bile acids can result in liver dysfunction, cholestatic liver disease, cirrhosis, progressive jaundice, and fatty diarrhea (steatorrhea).

CHAPTER

28 Lipids: Lipoproteins

CHAPTER OUTLINE

High-Yield Terms

Lipoprotein: complex of variable protein and lipid composition responsible for transport of fats throughout the body

Apolipoprotein: lipid-binding proteins of lipoprotein complexes

Apolipoprotein A-IV (apoA-IV): synthesized in intestines and hypothalamus, synthesis increased upon fat consumption, inhibits desire for food intake

Chylomicron: lipoprotein complex generated from dietary lipids within the enterocytes of the intestines

VLDL: lipoprotein complex generated from endogenous (or dietary) lipids within the liver, circulation in the vasculature leads to progressive loss of fatty acids converting these lipoproteins to IDL and finally LDL

HDL: high-density lipoprotein involved in the removal of cholesterol from peripheral tissue for return to the liver; the process is referred to as reverse cholesterol transport (RCT)

Space of Disse: the space between hepatic sinusoidal endothelium and hepatocytes, LDL and chylomicron remnants can be modified here prior to binding receptors on hepatocytes

Acyl-CoA-cholesterol acyltransferase (ACAT): key intracellular enzyme for esterifying cholesterol

Lecithin:cholesterol acyltransferase (LCAT) ratio: key HDL-associated enzyme involved in the esterification of cholesterol, removed from peripheral tissue, prior to exchange for triglyceride with VLDL and LDL

Cholesterol ester transfer protein (CETP): HDL-associated protein that transfers cholesterol esters from HDLs to VLDL and LDL in exchange of triglycerides from the VLDL/LDL to HDL

Paraoxonases (PON): HDL-associated enzymes that impart antioxidant activity of HDL toward LDL

Lipoprotein-associated phospholipase A_2 (Lp-PLA$_2$): is one of 2 forms of platelet-activating factor acetylhydrolase (PAF-AH), major HDL-associated hydrolase that is responsible for the hydrolysis of oxidized phospholipids

Lipoprotein(a) (Lp[a]): clinically significant apolipoprotein disulfide bonded to apoB-100 in LDL, easily oxidized and phagocytosed by macrophages-enhancing pro-inflammatory responses, inhibits the process of fibrin clot dissolution

Biochemically, a lipoprotein represents a complex assembly of both proteins and lipids. The major lipoproteins are those found in the plasma and are responsible for the mobilization of lipids, primarily fats, throughout the body. The lipid portion of lipoproteins consists of cholesterol, cholesterol esters, triglycerides, and/or phospholipids. Lipoproteins can be derived from dietary lipids via synthesis in enterocytes of the intestine or from endogenous lipids via synthesis in the liver. The generalization of lipoprotein types is defined by the amount of protein and lipid as depicted in Table 28-1.

The proteins associated with lipoproteins are referred to as apolipoproteins or often just apoproteins. Different apolipoproteins are found in functionally distinct lipoproteins types. There are 2 major types of apolipoproteins distinguished by the secondary structural motifs present in the proteins. The apolipoprotein A (apoA) proteins are composed primarily of alpha helices. These apoproteins form reversible complexes with the lipids of lipoproteins. The apolipoprotein B (apoB) proteins are composed primarily of β-sheet structures and form irreversible complexes with the lipids of lipoproteins. In addition to the apoA and apoB family of proteins, there are apoC, apoD, and apoE proteins. Several functionally significant apolipoproteins are described in Table 28-2.

TABLE 28-1: Composition of the Lipoproteins in Plasma of Humans

				Composition			
Lipoprotein	***Source***	***Diameter (nm)***	***Density (g/mL)***	***Protein (%)***	***Lipid (%)***	***Main Lipid Components***	***Apolipoproteins***
Chylomicrons	Intestine	90-1000	< 0.95	1-2	98-99	Triacylglycerol	A-I, A-II, A-IV,[1] B-48, C-I, C-II, C-III, E
Chylomicron remnants	Chylomicrons	45-150	< 1.006	6-8	92-94	Triacylglycerol, phospholipids, cholesterol	B-48, E
VLDL	Liver (intestine)	30-90	0.95-1.006	7-10	90-93	Triacylglycerol	B-100, C-I, C-II, C-III
IDL	VLDL	25-35	1.006-1.019	11	89	Triacylglycerol, cholesterol	B-100, E
LDL	VLDL	20-25	1.019-1.063	21	79	Cholesterol	B-100
HDL	Liver, intestine, VLDL, chylomicrons					Phospholipids, cholesterol	A-I, A-II, A-IV, C-I, C-II, C-III, D,[2] E
HDL_1		20-25	1.019-1.063	32	68		
HDL_2		10-20	1.063-1.125	33	67		
HDL_3		5-10	1.125-1.210	57	43		
Preβ-HDL[3]		< 5	> 1.210				A-I
Albumin/free fatty acids	Adipose tissue		> 1.281	99	1	Free fatty acids	

[1]Secreted with chylomicrons but transfers to HDL.
[2]Associated with HDL_2 and HDL_3 subfractions.
[3]Part of a minor fraction known as very high density lipoproteins (VHDL).
Abbreviations: HDL, high-density lipoproteins; IDL, intermediate-density lipoproteins; LDL, low-density lipoproteins; VLDL, very low density lipoproteins.
Murray RK, Bender DA, Botham KM, Kennelly PJ, Rodwell VW, Weil PA. *Harper's Illustrated Biochemistry*, 29th ed. New York, NY: McGraw-Hill; 2012.

TABLE 28-2: Major Apolipoprotein Classifications

Apolipoprotein—MW (Da)	*Lipoprotein Association*	*Function and Comments*
apoA-I—29,016	Chylomicrons, HDL	Major protein of HDL, binds ABCA1 on macrophages, critical antioxidant protein of HDL, activates lecithin:cholesterol acyltransferase (LCAT)
apoA-II—17,400	Chylomicrons, HDL	Primarily in HDL, enhances hepatic lipase activity
apoA-IV—46,000	Chylomicrons and HDL	Present in triacylglycerol-rich lipoproteins; synthesized in small intestine, synthesis activated by PYY, acts in central nervous system to inhibit food intake
apoB-48—241,000	Chylomicrons	Exclusively found in chylomicrons, derived from *apoB-100* gene by RNA editing in intestinal epithelium; lacks the LDL receptor-binding domain of apoB-100
apoB-100—513,000	VLDL, IDL, and LDL	Major protein of LDL, binds to LDL receptor; one of the longest-known proteins in humans
apoC-I—7,600	Chylomicrons, VLDL, IDL, and HDL	May also activate LCAT
apoC-II—8, 916	Chylomicrons, VLDL, IDL, and HDL	Activates lipoprotein lipase
apoC-III—8,750	Chylomicrons, VLDL, IDL, and HDL	Inhibits lipoprotein lipase, interferes with hepatic uptake and catabolism of apoB–containing lipoproteins, appears to enhance the catabolism of HDL particles, enhances monocyte adhesion to vascular endothelial cells, activates inflammatory signaling pathways
apoD—33,000	HDL	Closely associated with LCAT
Cholesterol ester transfer protein (CETP)	HDL	Plasma glycoprotein secreted primarily from the liver and is associated with cholesteryl ester transfer from HDL to LDL and VLDL in exchange for triglycerides
apoE—34,000 (at least 3 alleles [E_2, E_3, E_4] each of which have multiple isoforms)	Chylomicron remnants, VLDL, IDL, and HDL	Binds to LDL receptor, apo$E_{\varepsilon\text{-}4}$ allele amplification associated with late-onset Alzheimer disease
apoH—50,000 (also known as β_2-glycoprotein I)	Negatively charged surfaces	Inhibit serotonin release from platelets, alters ADP-mediated platelet aggregation
apo(a)—at least 19 different alleles; protein ranges in size from 300,000-800,000	LDL	Disulfide bonded to apoB-100, forms a complex with LDL identified as lipoprotein(a) (Lp[a]); strongly resembles plasminogen; may deliver cholesterol to sites of vascular injury, high-risk association with premature coronary artery disease and stroke

Apolipoprotein A-IV and the Control of Feeding Behaviors

Apolipoprotein A-IV (apoA-IV) is synthesized exclusively in the small intestine and the hypothalamus. Intestinal synthesis of apoA-IV increases in response to ingestion and absorption of fat, and it is subsequently incorporated into chylomicrons and delivered to the circulation via the lymphatic system. Systemic apoA-IV has been shown to have effects in the CNS involving the sensation of satiety.

Intestinal apoA-IV

Following the consumption of fat, the absorption of the lipid content stimulates the synthesis and secretion of apoA-IV by the intestines. Chylomicrons serve as the inducing signal for apoA-IV transcription and secretion; however, the precise mechanism by which the transcriptional enhancement is affected is currently undetermined. A signal is released by the distal gut during active lipid absorption, which is capable of stimulating apoA-IV synthesis in the proximal gut and this signal is the ileal peptide protein tyrosine tyrosine (PYY).

High-Yield Concept

Chronic consumption of a high-fat diet leads to significant reduction in apoA-IV mRNA levels and the response of hypothalamic *apoA-IV* gene expression to dietary lipids. Therefore, it is highly likely that dysregulation of hypothalamic apoA-IV could contribute to diet-induced obesity.

Although transcription of apoA-IV increases rapidly following fat ingestion, within 90 minutes the level of apoA-IV transcription is once again reduced. This reduction is a result of increased leptin secretion. Although numerous studies have demonstrated a negative correlation between leptin levels and apoA-IV expression, the mechanism by which this effect is exerted is not fully understood. There are leptin receptors in the gut and, therefore, leptin binding to these receptors could lead to direct effects on intestinal enterocytes.

Hypothalamic apoA-IV and Satiety

Expression of apoA-IV in the hypothalamus, a site intimately involved in regulating energy homeostasis, indicates that the effects exerted, on appetite, by apoA-IV are due to direct hypothalamic synthesis and secretion. This can be demonstrated by blocking apoA-IV actions by central injection of antibodies to the protein. Experiments of this type result in increased food consumption in experimental animals. Additional studies have shown that apoA-IV is involved in inhibiting food intake following the ingestion of fat. When apoA-IV containing chylomicrons are infused, there is marked suppression of food intake during the first 30 minutes following administration. If apoA-IV is removed from the chylomicrons prior to infusion, there is no observed effect on food intake. Alternatively, if apoA-IV itself is infused, suppression of food intake is the same as that seen with infusion of chylomicrons.

Chylomicrons

Chylomicrons are assembled in intestinal enterocytes as a means to transport dietary cholesterol and triglycerides to the rest of the body. Chylomicrons are, therefore, the molecules formed to mobilize dietary (exogenous) lipids (see Figure 28-1). The predominant lipids of chylomicrons are triglycerides (see Table 28-1). The apolipoproteins that predominate before chylomicrons enter the circulation include apoB-48, apoA-I, apoA-II, and apoA-IV, where apoB-48 is found exclusively in chylomicrons.

Chylomicrons leave the intestine via the lymphatic system and enter the circulation at the left subclavian vein. In the bloodstream, chylomicrons acquire apoC-II and apoE from plasma HDL. In the capillaries of adipose tissue and muscle, the fatty acids of chylomicrons are removed from the triglycerides by the action of lipoprotein lipase (LPL), which is found on the surface of the endothelial cells of the capillaries (Figure 28-2). The apoC-II in the chylomicrons activates LPL in the presence of phospholipid. During the removal of fatty acids, a substantial portion of phospholipid apoA and apoC is transferred to HDL. The loss of apoC-II prevents LPL from further degrading the chylomicron remnants.

Chylomicron remnants, containing primarily cholesterol esters, apoE and apoB-48, are then delivered to, and taken up by, the liver. The remnant particle must be of a sufficiently small size such that can pass through the fenestrated endothelial cells lining the hepatic sinusoids and enter into the space of Disse. Chylomicron remnants can then be taken up by hepatocytes via interaction with the LDL receptor, which requires apoE (Figure 28-3). In addition, in the space of Disse chylomicron remnants can accumulate additional apoE that is secreted free into the space. This latter process allows the remnant to be taken up via the chylomicron remnant receptor, which is a member of the LDL receptor-related protein (LRP) family. The recognition of chylomicron remnants by the hepatic remnant receptor also requires apoE. Chylomicron remnants can also remain sequestered in the space of Disse by binding of apoE to heparan sulfate proteoglycans and/or binding of apoB-48 to hepatic lipase. While sequestered, chylomicron remnants may be further metabolized, which increases apoE and lysophospholipid content allowing for transfer to LDL receptors or LRP for hepatic uptake.

VLDL, IDL, and LDL

Whereas chylomicrons represent the form of lipoprotein complex responsible for dietary lipid transport, very low density lipoproteins (VLDL) are the complexes involved in the transport of lipid (primarily triglyceride) from the liver to the extrahepatic tissues. In addition to triglycerides, VLDL contain some cholesterol and cholesterol esters, phospholipids, and the

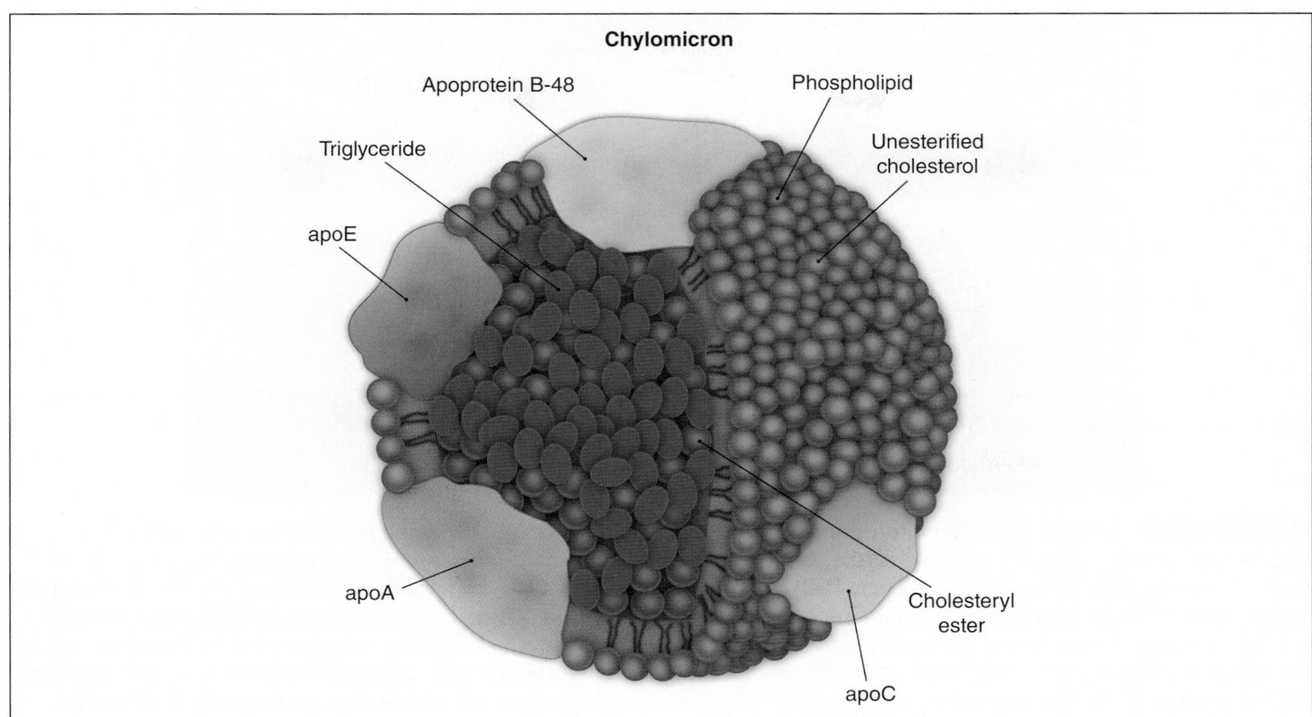

FIGURE 28-1: Structure of a chylomicron as a representative structure of a typical lipoprotein particle. Image demonstrates the outer layer of phospholipid and free cholesterol with primarily triglycerides and cholesteryl esters internally. Included in chylomicrons and other lipoprotein cores but not shown are triglycerides (TG). Each lipoprotein type, chylomicron, LDL, and HDL, contains apolipoproteins. Apolipoprotein B-48 (apoB-48) is specific for chylomicrons just as apoB-100 is specific for LDL. Reproduced with permission of themedicalbiochemistrypage, LLC.

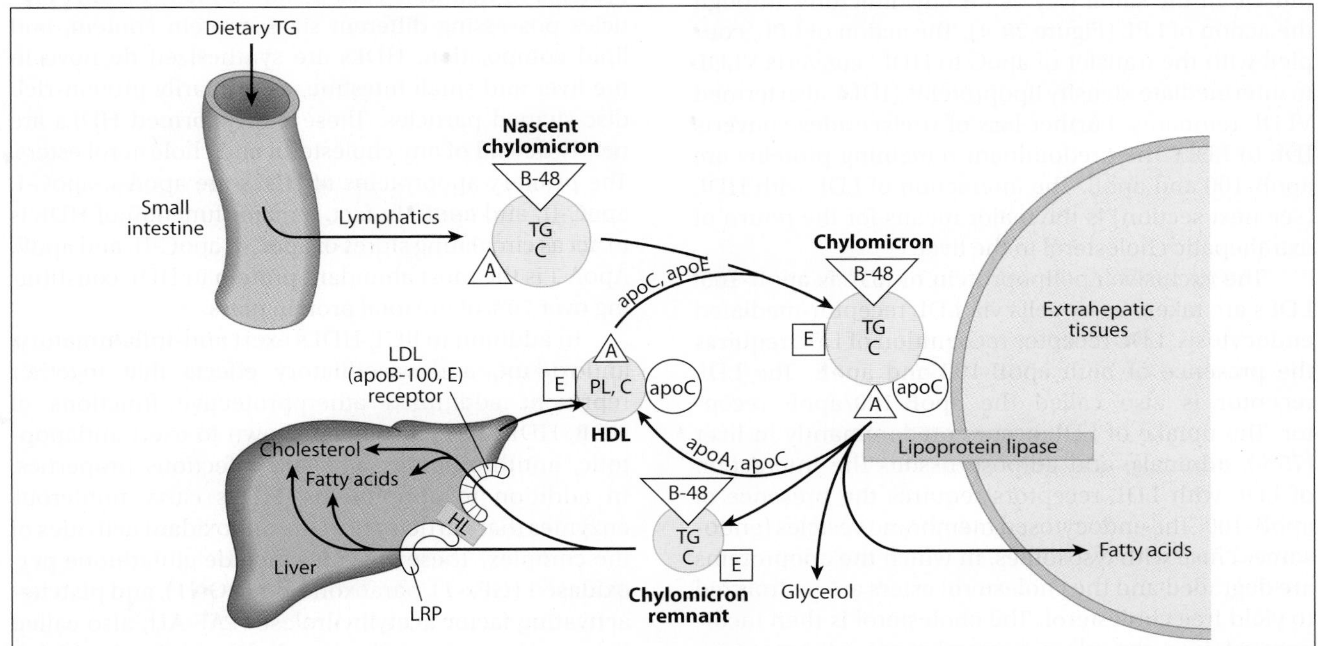

FIGURE 28-2: Metabolic fate of chylomicrons. (A, apolipoprotein A; B-48, apolipoprotein B-48; C, cholesterol and cholesteryl ester; E, apolipoprotein E; HDL, high-density lipoprotein; HL, hepatic lipase; LRP, LDL-receptor-related protein; PL, phospholipid; TG, triacylglycerol.) Only the predominant lipids are shown. Murray RK, Bender DA, Botham KM, Kennelly PJ, Rodwell VW, Weil PA. *Harper's Illustrated Biochemistry,* 29th ed. New York, NY: McGraw-Hill; 2012.

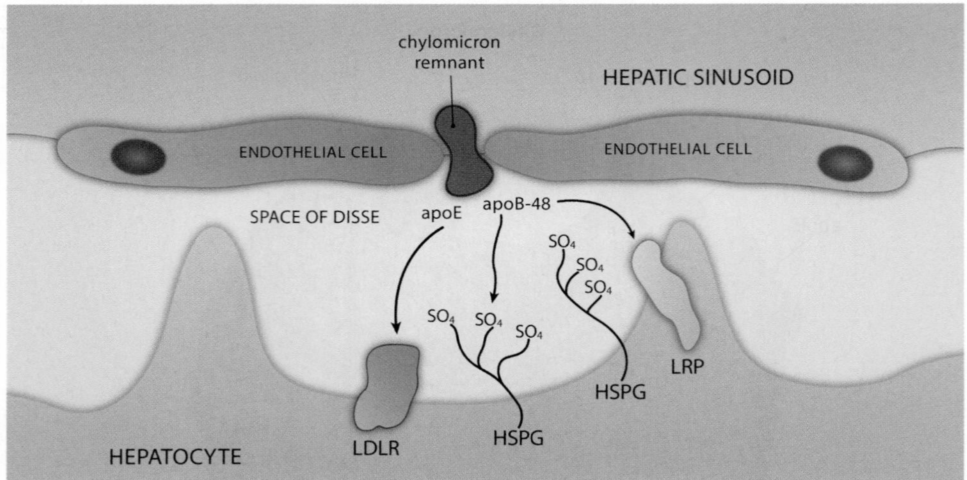

FIGURE 28-3: Uptake of chylomicron remnants by the liver. The space between hepatic sinusoidal endothelium and hepatocytes is called the space of Disse. Chylomicron remnants containing primarily cholesterol esters apoE, and apoB-48 are rapidly taken up by the liver. The remnants that pass through the endothelial lining of the hepatic sinusoid in the space of Disse interact with specific receptors as well as heparin-sulfated proteoglycans (HSPG). Hepatocyte uptake of remnants is initiated by sequestration of the particles on HSPG followed by receptor-mediated endocytosis of the remnants. The receptor-mediated endocytic process may be mediated by LDL receptors (LDLR) and/or LDL receptor-related protein (LRP). The interaction of remnants with HSPG involves apoB-48 and the interaction with LDLR or LRP involves apoE.

apoproteins, apoB-100, apoC-I, apoC-II, apoC-III, and apoE. Like nascent chylomicrons, newly released VLDL obtain apoC and apoE from circulating HDL. The fatty acid portion of VLDL is released into adipose tissue and muscle in the same way as for chylomicrons, through the action of LPL (Figure 28-4). The action of LPL, coupled with the transfer of apoC to HDL, converts VLDL to intermediate-density lipoproteins (IDL), also termed VLDL remnants. Further loss of triglycerides converts IDL to LDL. The predominant remaining proteins are apoB-100 and apoE. The interaction of LDL with HDL (see next section) is the major means for the return of extrahepatic cholesterol to the liver.

The exclusive apolipoprotein of LDL is apoB-100. LDLs are taken up by cells via LDL receptor-mediated endocytosis. LDL receptor recognition of LDL requires the presence of both apoB-100 and apoE. The LDL receptor is also called the apoB-100/apoE receptor. The uptake of LDL occurs predominantly in liver (75%), adrenals, and adipose tissue. The interaction of LDL with LDL receptors requires the presence of apoB-100. The endocytosed membrane vesicles (endosomes) fuse with lysosomes, in which the apoproteins are degraded and the cholesterol esters are hydrolyzed to yield free cholesterol. The cholesterol is then incorporated into the plasma membranes as necessary. Excess intracellular cholesterol is re-esterified by acyl-CoA-cholesterol acyltransferase (ACAT) for intracellular storage.

High-Density Lipoproteins

HDLs represent a heterogeneous population of lipoproteins in that they exist as functionally distinct particles possessing different sizes, protein content, and lipid composition. HDLs are synthesized de novo in the liver and small intestine, as primarily protein-rich disc-shaped particles. These newly formed HDLs are nearly devoid of any cholesterol and cholesterol esters. The primary apoproteins of HDLs are apoA-I, apoC-I, apoC-II, and apoE. In fact, a major function of HDL is to act as circulating stores of apoC-I, apoC-II, and apoE. ApoA-I is the most abundant protein in HDL constituting over 70% of the total protein mass.

In addition to RCT, HDLs exert anti-inflammatory, antioxidant, and vasodilatory effects that together represent additional atheroprotective functions of HDL. HDLs have also been shown to exert antiapoptotic, antithrombotic, and anti-infectious properties. In addition to apoproteins, HDLs carry numerous enzymes that participate in the antioxidant activities of the complex. These enzymes include glutathione peroxidase 1 (GPx-1), paraoxonase 1 (PON1), and platelet-activating factor acetylhydrolase (PAF-AH, also called lipoprotein-associated phospholipase A_2, Lp-PLA_2). With respect to the various atheroprotective functions of HDL, it is the small dense particles (referred to as HDL_3) that are the most beneficial.

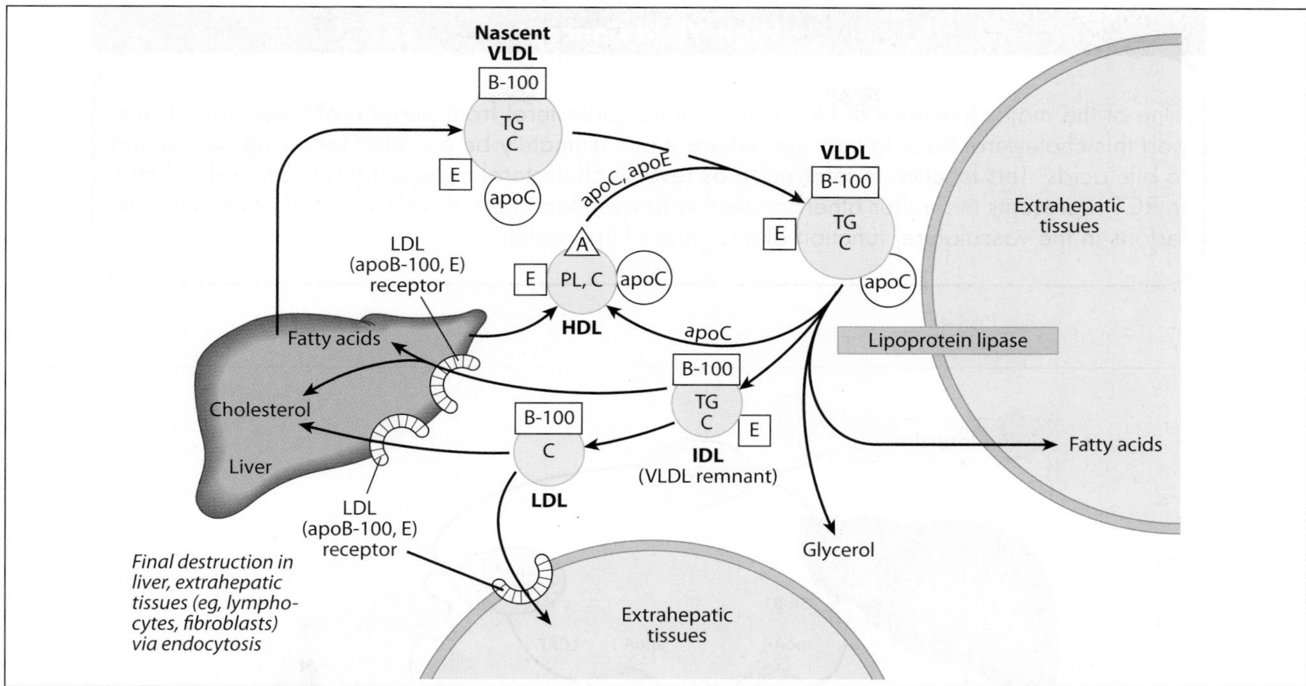

FIGURE 28-4: Metabolic fate of very low density lipoproteins (VLDL) and production of low-density lipoproteins (LDL). (A, apolipoprotein A; B-100, apolipoprotein B-100; C, cholesterol and cholesteryl ester; E, apolipoprotein E; HDL, high-density lipoprotein; IDL, intermediate-density lipoprotein; PL, phospholipid; TG, triacylglycerol.) Only the predominant lipids are shown. It is possible that some IDL is also metabolized via the low-density lipoprotein receptor–related protein (LRP). Murray RK, Bender DA, Botham KM, Kennelly PJ, Rodwell VW, Weil PA. *Harper's Illustrated Biochemistry,* 29th ed. New York, NY: McGraw-Hill; 2012.

The primary mechanism by which HDLs acquire peripheral tissue cholesterol is via an interaction with monocyte-derived macrophages in the subendothelial spaces of the tissues (Figure 28-5). Macrophages bind nascent HDL, that contains primarily apoA-I, through interaction with the ATP-binding cassette transport protein A1 (ABCA1). The transfer of cholesterol from macrophages via the action of ABCA1 results in the formation of nascent discoidal lipoprotein particles termed pre-β HDL. The free cholesterol transferred in this way is esterified by HDL-associated lecithin:cholesterol-acyltransferase (LCAT) ratio. LCAT is synthesized in the liver and so named because it transfers a fatty acid from the C-2 position of lecithin to the C-3-OH of cholesterol, generating a cholesterol ester and lysolecithin. The activity of LCAT requires interaction with apoA-I. The cholesterol esters formed via LCAT activity are internalized into the hydrophobic core of the pre-β HDL particle. As pre-β HDL particles enlarge with progressive uptake of cholesterol, they become larger and spherical

High-Yield Concept

The consumption of alcohol is associated with either a protective or a negative effect on the level of circulating LDL. Low-level alcohol consumption, particularly red wines, which contain the antioxidant resveratrol, appear to be beneficial with respect to cardiovascular health. Resveratrol consumption is associated with a reduced risk of cardiovascular, cerebrovascular, and peripheral vascular disease. One major effect of resveratrol in the blood is the prevention of oxidation of LDL, forming oxidized LDL (oxLDL). OxLDL contribute significantly to the development of atherosclerosis. Conversely excess alcohol consumption is associated with the development of fatty liver, which in turn impairs the ability of the liver to take up LDL via the LDL receptor resulting in increased LDL in the circulation.

High-Yield Concept

One of the major functions of HDL is to acquire cholesterol from peripheral tissues and transport this cholesterol back to the liver, where it can ultimately be excreted following conversion to bile acids. This function is referred to as reverse cholesterol transport (RCT). The role of HDL in RCT represents the major atheroprotective (prevention of the development of atherosclerotic lesions in the vasculature) function of this class of lipoprotein.

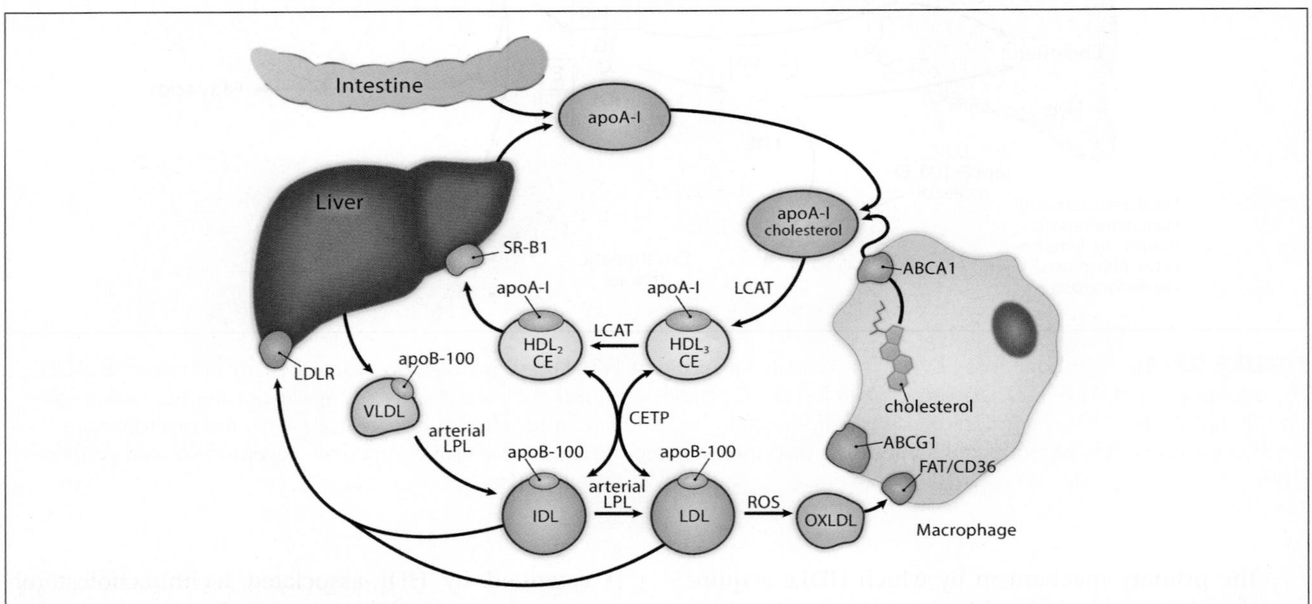

FIGURE 28-5: Details of the interactions between HDL and LDL within the vasculature. As indicated in the text, HDL begins as protein-rich discoidal structures, composed primarily of apoA-I, produced by the liver and intestines. Within the vasculature, apoA-I interacts with the ATP-binding cassette transporter, ABCA1 (such as is diagrammed for interaction with macrophages) and extracts cholesterol from cells. Through the action of LCAT, the apoA-I–associated cholesterol is esterified forming cholesterol esters. This process results in the generation of HDL_3 particles. As the HDL_3 particles continue through the circulation, they pick up more cholesterol and through the action of LCAT, generate more cholesterol esters. As HDL migrates through the vasculature, there is an interaction between them and IDL and LDL. This interaction occurs through the action of CETP, which exchanges the cholesterol esters in the HDL for triglycerides from LDL. This interaction results in the conversion of HDL_3 particles to HDL_2. The differences between these 2 types of HDL particle are detailed in Table 28-1. HDL can also remove cholesterol from cells via interaction with the ATP-binding cassette transporter ABCG1. Approximately 20% of HDL uptake of cellular cholesterol occurs via ABCG1. HDL is then removed from the circulation by the liver through binding of the HDL to hepatic scavenger receptor SR-B1. Cholesterol ester–rich IDL and LDL can return to the liver and be taken up through interaction with the LDL receptor (LDLR). Within the vasculature, the generation of ROS results in oxidation of lipid components of LDL, generating oxidized LDL (oxLDL) that is taken up by the macrophages via the scavenger receptor, FAT/CD36.

generating the HDL_3 and then HDL_2 particles. HDLs also extract cholesterol from cell surface membranes, which involves the action of the ATP-binding cassette protein G1 (ABCG1). Approximately 20% of HDL uptake of peripheral tissue cholesterol occurs via the ABCG1-mediated pathway. The importance of ABCA1 in RCT is evident in individuals harboring defects in *ABCA1* gene. These individuals suffer from a disorder called Tangier disease, which is characterized by 2 clinical hallmarks; enlarged lipid-laden tonsils and low-serum HDL (see Clinical Box 28-1). Cholesterol-rich HDLs return to the liver, where they bind to a receptor that is a member of the scavenger receptor family, specifically the scavenger receptor B1 (SR-B1). HDL binding to SR-B1 does not result in internalization as in the case of LDL receptor-mediated endocytosis. The cholesterol esters of HDLs are taken up by the hepatocytes through caveolae while the HDLs and SR-B1 remain on the plasma membrane.

CLINICAL BOX 28-1: TANGIER DISEASE

Tangier disease (TD) is an autosomal recessive disorder resulting from defects in the ATP-binding cassette (*ABC*) transporter family gene encoding ABCA1. The disease is so named because it was originally identified in 2 individuals living on Tangier Island, Virginia. Tangier disease is a rare disease with only around 50 cases identified worldwide. Although a rare disease, the identification of the gene defective in the disease and an analysis of the function of the encoded transporter protein have provided insight into overall cellular cholesterol homeostasis. Expression of the *ABCA1* gene is highest in placenta, liver, lung, and adrenal glands. Numerous pathways of transcriptional regulation of ABCA1 have been identified including cAMP, nuclear receptors (such as LXRs, RXRs, and PPARs), hormones, and cytokines. The involvement of cytokines in the regulation of ABCA1 expression demonstrates the crosstalk between cellular cholesterol management and inflammatory responses. Pro-inflammatory cytokines such as tumor necrosis factor-α (TNF-α) and interleukin-1β (IL-1β) interfere with the transcriptional enhancement of ABCA1 exerted by LXRs. The predominant site of ABCA1 protein localization is the plasma membrane. In nonhepatic tissue, the role of ABCA1 is to promote the efflux of cholesterol principally to the HDL class of lipoprotein particles, which in turn transport the cholesterol back to the liver for catabolism. The clinical hallmarks of Tangier disease are a lack of HDL and apoA-I. The clinical manifestations of Tangier disease are related to an accumulation of cholesterol esters in reticuloendothelial tissues (eg, tonsils, lymph nodes, spleen, thymus, and bone marrow). The first symptom seen in almost all Tangier disease patients is enlarged tonsils that appear orange in color. Additional typical clinical findings include splenomegaly, a variable incidence of cardiovascular disease, and peripheral neuropathy.

Reverse cholesterol transport also involves the transfer of cholesterol esters from HDL to VLDL and LDL. This transfer requires the activity of the plasma glycoprotein cholesterol ester transfer protein (CETP). The transfer of cholesterol esters from HDL to VLDL involves a reciprocal exchange of triglycerides from the VLDL to the HDL. This action allows excess cellular cholesterol to be returned to the liver through the LDL receptor. Additionally, when HDL particles become enriched with triglycerides they are better substrates for the action of hepatic lipase (see Figure 28-5).

In the absence of systemic inflammation, many of the enzymes and apolipoproteins associated with HDL play important roles in reducing the amount of oxidized lipid to which peripheral tissues are exposed. Some of these important proteins are apoA-I, PON1, GPx, and PAF-AH. However, when an individual has an ongoing systemic inflammatory state, these antioxidant proteins can be dissociated from the HDL or become inactivated resulting in the increased generation of oxidized and peroxidized lipids, which are proatherogenic.

Antioxidant and Anti-inflammatory Activities of HDL

In addition to their role in RCT, HDLs exert important anti-inflammatory and antioxidant properties within the vasculature. Various apolipoproteins associated with HDLs have been shown to be critical for these beneficial effects of HDL.

Apolipoprotein A-I: In addition to reverse cholesterol transport, apoA-I can remove oxidized phospholipids from oxidized LDL (oxLDL) and from cells. Specific methionine residues of apoA-I have been shown to directly reduce cholesterol ester hydroperoxides and phosphatidylcholine hydroperoxides.

Apolipoprotein A-II: ApoA-II–enriched HDLs support highly effective RCT from macrophages and also protect VLDL from oxidation more efficiently than apoA-II–deficient HDL. Recent clinical studies in human patients show that the higher the plasma apoA-II concentration, the lower is the risk of developing coronary heart disease (CHD).

Apolipoprotein A-IV: ApoA-IV has multiple activities related to lipid and lipoprotein metabolism as well as the control of feeding behaviors. ApoA-IV participates in RCT by promoting cholesterol efflux as well as by activation of LCAT. ApoA-IV has also been shown to have antioxidant, anti-inflammatory, and antiatherosclerotic actions.

Paraoxonases 1 and 3: Paraoxonases are a family of enzymes that hydrolyze organophosphates. Paraoxonase 1 (PON1) is synthesized in the liver and is carried in the serum by HDL. PON1 possesses antioxidant properties, in particular it prevents the oxidation of LDL. PON1 has been shown to enhance cholesterol efflux from macrophages by promoting

HDL binding mediated by ABCA1, which in turn results in a reduction of pro-inflammatory signaling by these cells. In human clinical studies, a higher level of PON1 activity is associated with a lower incidence of major cardiovascular events. Other pathological conditions in humans that are associated with oxidative stress, such as rheumatoid arthritis and Alzheimer disease, are frequently associated with reduced activity of PON1. PON3, which is another HDL-associated paraoxonase, has also been shown to prevent the oxidation of LDL.

Platelet-activating factor acetylhydrolase (PAF-AH): There are 2 major forms of PAF-AH, cytosolic and plasma lipoprotein associated. The plasma form of PAF-AH (lipoprotein-associated PLA_2, Lp-PLA_2) circulates bound to HDL. Lp-PLA_2 is a major HDL-associated hydrolase responsible for the hydrolysis of oxidized phospholipids. In humans, Lp-PLA_2 deficiency is associated with increases in cardiovascular disease, while conversely circulating levels of Lp-PLA_2 serve as an independent marker of the risk for developing CHD.

Glutathione peroxidase 1: Glutathione peroxidase 1 (GPx-1) has been shown to reduce lipid hydroperoxides to corresponding hydroxides, effectively detoxifying these types of abnormally modified lipids. Numerous human clinical studies indicated that GPx-1 provides a protective role against the development of atherosclerosis.

Sphingosine-1-phosphate (S1P): S1P is a bioactive lysophospholipid involved in a number of physiologically important pathways (see Chapter 21). HDLs are the most prominent carriers of S1P. Indeed, many of the biological effects of HDLs are mediated, in part, via S1P binding to its cell surface receptors. Effects of HDL on endothelial cells, such as migration, proliferation, and angiogenesis, are mediated, in part, by S1P associated with HDL. HDL-associated S1P inhibits pro-inflammatory responses, such as the generation of reactive oxygen species, activation of NAD(P)H oxidase, and the production of monocyte chemoattractant protein-1. While the HDL-associated forms of S1P exhibit these anti-inflammatory effects, free plasma S1P can activate inflammatory events dependent upon the receptor subtype to which it binds.

Therapeutic Benefits of Elevating HDL

Numerous epidemiological and clinical studies have demonstrated a direct correlation between the circulating levels of HDL cholesterol (most often abbreviated HDL-c) and a reduction in the potential for atherosclerosis and CHD. Individuals with levels of HDL above 50 mg/dL are several time less likely to experience CHD than individuals with levels below 40 mg/dL. In addition, clinical studies involving increases in circulating HDL levels correlate with a reduced incidence of CHD. Thus, there is precedence for therapies aimed at raising HDL levels in the treatment and prevention of atherosclerosis and CHD.

Cholesterol ester transfer protein (CETP) plays a critical role in HDL metabolism by facilitating the exchange of cholesterol esters from HDL for triglycerides in apoB-containing lipoproteins, such as LDL and VLDL (see Figure 28-5). The activity of CETP directly lowers the cholesterol levels of HDL and enhances HDL catabolism by providing HDL with the triglyceride substrate of hepatic lipase. Thus, CETP plays a critical role in the regulation of circulating levels of HDL, LDL, and apoA-I. The potential for the therapeutic use of CETP inhibitors in humans was first suggested when it was discovered in 1985 that a small Japanese population had an inborn error in the *CETP* gene leading to hyperalphalipoproteinemia and very high HDL levels. CETP inhibitors currently being tested in clinical trials are anacetrapib and dalcetrapib.

Lipoprotein Receptors

LDL Receptors

LDL returns cholesterol to the liver via the interaction of LDL with the LDL receptor (also called the apoB-100/apoE receptor). The sole apoprotein present in LDL is apoB-100, which is required for interaction with the LDL receptor. The LDL receptor is a polypeptide of 839 amino acids that spans the plasma membrane. An extracellular domain is responsible for apoB-100/apoE binding. The intracellular domain is responsible for the clustering of LDL receptors into regions of the plasma membrane termed *coated pits*. Once LDL binds the receptor, the complexes are rapidly internalized (endocytosed). ATP-dependent proton pumps lower the pH in the endosomes, which results in dissociation of LDL from the receptor. The LDL receptors are then recycled to the plasma membrane and the LDL-containing endosomes fuse with lysosomes. Acid hydrolases of the lysosomes degrade the apoproteins and release free fatty acids and cholesterol. The free cholesterol is either incorporated into plasma membranes or esterified (by ACAT) and stored within the cell.

LDL Receptor-Related Proteins

The LDL receptor-related protein (LRP) family represents a group of structurally-related transmembrane proteins involved in a diverse range of biological activities including lipid metabolism, nutrient transport, protection against atherosclerosis, as well as numerous developmental processes. The LDL receptor (LDLR) represents the founding member of this family of proteins. The LRP include LRP1, LRP1b, LRP2 (also called megalin), LRP4 (also called MEGF7 for multiple epidermal growth factor-like domains protein 7), LRP5/6, LRP8 (also called apolipoprotein E receptor 2), the VLDL receptor (VLDLR), and LR11/SorLA1 (LDL receptor relative with 11 ligand-binding repeats/sorting protein-related receptor containing LDLR class A repeats). LRP1 (also known as CD91 or α_2-macroglobulin receptor) is expressed in numerous tissues and is known to be involved in diverse activities that include lipoprotein transport, modulation of platelet-derived growth factor receptor-β (PDGFRβ) signaling, regulation of cell-surface protease activity, and the control of cellular entry of bacteria and viruses. LRP1 has been shown to bind more than 40 different ligands that include lipoproteins, extracellular matrix proteins, cytokines and growth factors, protease and protease inhibitor complexes, and viruses. This diverse array of ligands clearly demonstrates that LRP1 is involved in numerous biological and physiological processes.

Scavenger Receptors

The founding member of the scavenger receptor family was identified in studies that were attempting to determine the mechanism by which LDL accumulated in macrophages in atherosclerotic plaques. Macrophages ingest a variety of negatively charged macromolecules that includes modified LDL, such as oxidized LDL (oxLDL). Subsequent research determined that the scavenger receptor family consists of several families that are identified as class A receptors, class B receptors, mucin-like receptors, and endothelial receptors. After binding ligand, the scavenger receptors can either be internalized, similar to the process of internalization of LDL receptors, or they can remain on the cell surface and transfer lipid into the cell through caveolae. The class A receptors include the type 1 and 2 macrophage scavenger receptors. The class B receptors include CD36 and scavenger receptor class B type 1 (SR-B1). The CD36 receptor is also known as fatty acid translocase (FAT) and it is one of the receptors responsible for the cellular uptake of fatty acids (see Chapter 23). CD36 and SR-B1 are closely related multi-ligand receptors and are recognized mostly for their roles in lipid and lipoprotein metabolism. The SR-B1 protein has been shown to be the endogenous receptor for HDL in the liver.

Abnormal Lipoproteins and the Lipoproteinemias

Lipoprotein (a) (Lp[a]) is composed of a common LDL nucleus linked to a molecule of apolipoprotein(a) (apo[a]) by disulfide bonds to apoB-100. When attached to apoB-100, the apo(a) protein surrounds the LDL molecule. Numerous epidemiological studies have demonstrated that elevated plasma levels of Lp(a) are a significant risk factor for the development of atherosclerotic disease (see Chapter 48). Apo(a) contains numerous secondary structures called Kringle domains and the protein exhibits a variability in size in different individuals due to a polymorphism caused by a variable number of the Kringle domains. The Kringle domains of apo(a) exhibit 75%-85% similarity to the Kringle domains of plasminogen, which is involved in the process of hemostasis (see Chapter 51).

When in the circulation, Lp(a) particles can be affected by oxidative modification similar to that of the other plasma lipoprotein particles. Lp(a) and oxidized Lp(a) (oxLp[a]) particles interact with macrophages via scavenger receptor uptake leading to cholesterol accumulation and foam cell formation. Indeed, oxLp(a) are phagocytosed more rapidly than other lipoprotein particles and, therefore, accumulate in the subendothelial space at high levels. This process can lead to progression of atherogenesis, thus accounting for the direct correlation between the plasma level of Lp(a) and coronary artery disease. In addition to oxidation of Lp(a) leading to increased foam cell production, glycation of the particle also may contribute to atherogenesis. In fact, there is a strong correlation in the level of glycated Lp(a) and the severity of hyperglycemia observed in poorly controlled type 2 diabetes.

Lp(a) has been shown to competitively inhibit the binding of plasminogen to its receptor on endothelial cells as well as to its binding sites on fibrinogen and fibrin. The normal function of plasminogen is to degrade the fibrin mesh in blood clots. This interference of plasminogen binding leads to reduced surface-dependent activation of plasminogen to plasmin (Figure 28-6). Therefore, high plasma concentrations of Lp(a) may represent a source of antifibrinolytic activity. In addition to the role of Lp(a) in inhibiting plasminogen binding, Lp(a) has been shown to inhibit the release of tissue plasminogen activator (t-PA) from endothelial cells. With reduced release of t-PA, there is decreased conversion of plasminogen to plasmin. This, along with the Lp(a)-mediated interference in plasminogen binding to fibrin clots results in a significant negative effect on the ability to dissolve blood clots. Lp(a) also stimulates the production of plasminogen activator inhibitor-1 (PAI-1), leading to a reduced ability of tissue t-PA to activate the process of clot dissolution.

Fortunately, few individuals carry the inherited defects in lipoprotein metabolism that lead to hyper- or hypolipoproteinemias (Table 28-3 and Table 28-4, respectively). Of the many disorders of lipoprotein metabolism, familial hypercholesterolemia (FH) may be the most prevalent in the general population (see Clinical Box 26-2).

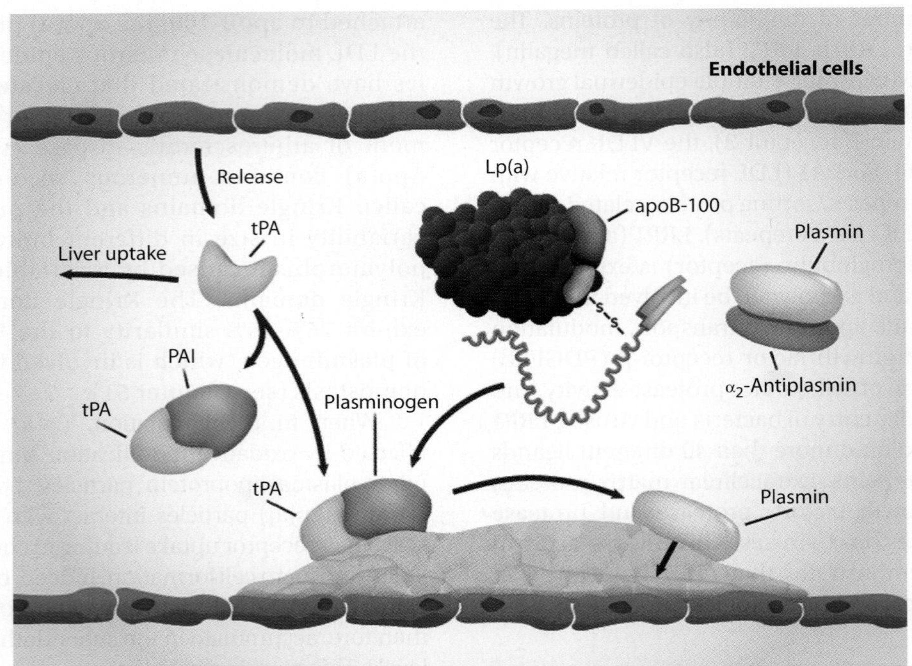

FIGURE 28-6: Mechanism of Lp(a) interference with normal fibrinolysis. The apo(a) protein disulfide bonded to apoB-100 in LDL contains Kringle domains that interfere with plasminogen binding to fibrin clots and also interfere with the ability of tPA to hydrolyze plasminogen to active plasmin, thereby, interfering with the normal course of fibrin clot dissolution. Reproduced with permission of themedicalbiochemistrypage, LLC.

TABLE 28-3: The Hyperlipoproteinemias

Disorder	*Defect*	*Comments*
Type I (familial LPL deficiency, familial hyperchylomicronemia)	(**a**) Deficiency of LPL (**b**) Production of abnormal LPL (**c**) apoC-II deficiency	Slow chylomicron clearance, reduced LDL and HDL levels; treated by low fat/complex carbohydrate diet; no increased risk of coronary artery disease
Familial hypercholesterolemia (FH) Type IIA hyperlipoproteinemia	Four classes of LDL receptor defect	Reduced LDL clearance leads to hypercholesterolemia, resulting in atherosclerosis and coronary artery disease
Type III (familial dysbetalipoproteinemia, remnant removal disease, broad β-disease, apoE deficiency)	Hepatic remnant clearance impaired due to apoE abnormality; patients only express the apoE_2 isoform that interacts poorly with the apoE receptor	Causes xanthomas, hypercholesterolemia, and atherosclerosis in peripheral and coronary arteries due to elevated levels of chylomicrons and VLDL
Type IV (familial hypertriacylglyceridemia)	Elevated production of VLDL associated with glucose intolerance and hyperinsulinemia	Frequently associated with Type-II non–insulin-dependent diabetes mellitus, obesity, alcoholism, or administration of progestational hormones; elevated cholesterol as a result of increased VLDL
Type V, familial	Elevated chylomicrons and VLDL due to unknown cause	Hypertriacylglyceridemia and hypercholesterolemia with decreased LDL and HDL
Type II hyperlipoproteinemia (familial hyperalphalipoproteinemia)	Increased level of HDL	A rare condition that is beneficial for health and longevity
Type II (familial hyperbetalipoproteinemia)	Increased LDL production and delayed clearance of triglycerides and fatty acids	Strongly associated with increased risk of coronary artery disease

TABLE 28-3: **The Hyperlipoproteinemias (*Continued*)**

Disorder	*Defect*	*Comments*
Familial ligand-defective apoB	Two different mutations: Gln for Arg (amino acid 3500) or Cys for Arg (amino acid 3531); both lead to reduced affinity of LDL for LDL receptor	Dramatic increase in LDL levels; no effect on HDL, VLDL, or plasma triglyceride levels; significant cause of hypercholesterolemia and premature coronary artery disease
Familial LCAT deficiency (Norum disease, fish eye disease)	Absence of LCAT leads to inability of HDL to take up cholesterol (reverse cholesterol transport)	Decreased levels of plasma cholesterol esters and lysolecithin; abnormal LDL (Lp-X) and VLDL; diffuse corneal opacities, target cell hemolytic anemia, and proteinuria with renal failure
Wolman disease (cholesteryl ester storage disease)	Defect in lysosomal cholesterol ester hydrolase; affects metabolism of LDL	Reduced LDL clearance leads to hypercholesterolemia, resulting in atherosclerosis and coronary artery disease
Heparin-releasable hepatic triglyceride lipase deficiency	Deficiency of the lipase leads to accumulation of triacylglycerol-rich HDL and VLDL remnants (IDL)	Causes xanthomas and coronary artery disease

TABLE 28-4: **The Hypolipoproteinemias**

Disorder	*Defect*	*Comments*
Abetalipoproteinemia (acanthocytosis, Bassen-Kornzweig syndrome)	No chylomicrons, VLDL or LDL, due to defect in apoB expression	Rare defect; intestine and liver accumulate, malabsorption of fat, retinitis pigmentosa, ataxic neuropathic disease, erythrocytes have thorny appearance
Familial hypobetalipoproteinemia	At least 20 different *apoB* gene mutations identified, LDL concentrations 10%-20% of normal, VLDL slightly lower, HDL normal	Mild or no pathological changes
Tangier disease (see Clinical Box 25-1)	Reduced HDL concentrations, no effect on chylomicron or VLDL production	Tendency to hypertriglyceridemia; some elevation in VLDL; hypertrophic tonsils with orange appearance

REVIEW QUESTIONS

1. An increase in which of the following apolipoproteins would most likely be associated with a reduced risk for the development of atherosclerosis?

A. apo(a)
B. apoA-I
C. apoC-I
D. apoC-II
E. apoE

Answer E: The cellular uptake of cholesterol from LDL occurs following the interaction of LDL with the LDL receptor (also called the apoB-100/apoE receptor). Both apoB-100, which is exclusively associated with LDL, and apoE are required for LDL receptor-mediated endocytosis of LDL. The importance of apoE in cholesterol uptake by LDL receptors has been demonstrated in transgenic mice lacking functional *apoE* genes. These mice develop severe atherosclerotic lesions at 10 weeks of age. Therefore, increased levels of apoE would be associated with a higher hepatic uptake of LDL, leading to reduced levels in the blood.

2. The hypercholesterolemia that is associated with familial hypercholesterolemia is due to which of the following?

A. abnormally elevated production of LDL
B. abnormally elevated production of VLDL by the liver

C. abnormally reduced production of HDL, resulting in a diminished capacity of reverse cholesterol transport
D. defective LDL receptors leading to reduced uptake of plasma LDL and IDL
E. defective remnant receptors on hepatic cells, leading to reduced uptake of chylomicron remnants

Answer D: Familial hypercholesterolemia, FH (type II hyperlipoproteinemia), is an autosomal dominant disorder that results from mutations affecting the structure and function of the cell-surface receptor that binds plasma LDL, removing them from the circulation. The defects in LDL-receptor (LDLR) interaction result in lifelong elevation of LDL-cholesterol in the blood. The resultant hypercholesterolemia leads to premature coronary artery disease and atherosclerotic plaque formation.

3. A 13-year-old girl presents with extensive eruptive xanthomas and hepatosplenomegaly. She does not have type 1 or type 2 diabetes as an analysis of circulating insulin and glucose levels indicates they are normal. Examination of plasma indicates that it quite milky, indicating a lipemia. Analysis of the lipid content of the plasma shows a massive accumulation of chylomicrons and triglycerides. The teenager is placed on a fat-free diet, which reduces the lipemia and all of the other clinical manifestations. A deficiency in which of the following apolipoproteins would account for the observed symptoms of this particular hyperlipoproteinemia?
A. apoA-I
B. apoA-IV
C. apoB-100
D. apoC-II
E. apoE

Answer D: ApoC-II is present in chylomicrons, LDL, and HDL and is required for the activation of the endothelial cell–associated triglyceride lipase called lipoprotein lipase (LPL). Loss, or defective activity, of apoC-II would result in circulating lipoproteins of all types enriched in triglyceride, leading to hypertriglyceridemia.

4. A deficiency in which of the following proteins would have the most significant effect on the ability of HDL to deliver nonhepatic cholesterol to LDL?
A. apoB-48
B. apoB-100
C. apoE
D. cholesteryl ester transfer protein (CETP)
E. lecithin:cholesterol acyltransferase (LCAT) ratio

Answer D: Cholesterol ester transfer protein (CETP) is a plasma glycoprotein secreted primarily from the liver and plays a critical role in HDL metabolism by facilitating the exchange of cholesterol esters (CE) from HDL for triglycerides (TG) in apoB–containing lipoproteins, such as LDL and VLDL. The activity of CETP directly lowers the cholesterol levels of HDLs and enhances HDL catabolism by providing HDLs with the TG substrate of hepatic lipase. Thus, CETP plays a critical role in the regulation of circulating levels of HDL, LDL, and apoA-I. It has also been shown that most of the cholesterol in mice, who naturally lack CETP, is found in HDL and these mice are relatively resistant to atherosclerosis.

5. Overexpression of Lp-PLA$_2$ is associated with an increased risk of cardiovascular disease. Which of the following represents a primary mechanism for this effect of the enzyme?
A. binding to the LDL receptor on hepatocytes
B. disulfide bonding to apoB-100 in LDL
C. hydrolysis of oxidized phospholipids
D. inactivation of platelet-activating factor
E. interaction with tissue plasminogen activator

Answer C: The enzymatic activity of Lp-PLA$_2$ is specific for short chain acyl groups (up to 9 methylene groups) at the *sn*2 position of phospholipids. When PAF is the substrate for Lp-PLA$_2$, the products are lyso-PAF and acetate. When phospholipids of the phosphatidylcholine (PC) family are oxidized by free radical activity (referred to as oxPL), they can be a substrate for Lp-PLA$_2$ even if the unsaturated fatty acid at the *sn*2 position is longer than 9 carbon atoms. The ability of Lp-PLA$_2$ to recognize oxPL as substrates is due to the presence of aldehydic or carboxylic moieties at the omega (w) end of the *sn*2-peroxidized fatty acyl residues. The products of Lp-PLA$_2$ activity on oxPL are oxidized free fatty acids (oxFFAs) and lyso-PC. Numerous types of oxPL have been identified in oxidized LDL (oxLDL) particles and many of them exhibit biological activity and exert key effects in atherogenesis.

6. A 2-month-old male child is presented with microcephaly (head size smaller than normal), micrognathia (abnormally small lower jaw), ptosis (drooping eyelids), a small upturned nose, cleft palate, and ambiguous genitalia. Following biochemical analysis it is determined that the infant has highly elevated levels of 7-dehydrocholesterol in his tissues. These findings are indicative of which of the following disorders?
A. Dubin-Johnson syndrome
B. familial intrahepatic cholestasis type 2
C. Rotor syndrome
D. Smith-Lemli-Opitz syndrome
E. Tangier disease

Answer D: Smith-Lemli-Opitz syndrome (SLOS) is an autosomal recessive disorder resulting from a defect in cholesterol synthesis. The defect resides in the terminal enzyme of the cholesterol biosynthesis pathway, namely 7-dehydrocholesterol reductase. Defects in this gene result in increased levels of 7-dehydrocholesterol and reduced levels (15%-27% of normal) of cholesterol in SLOS patients. The clinical spectrum of SLOS is very broad, ranging from the most severe form manifesting as a lethal malformation syndrome, to a relatively mild disorder that encompasses behavioral and learning disabilities. A frequent observation in SLOS infants is poor feeding and postnatal growth failure. There are distinct craniofacial anomalies associated with SLOS, which include microcephaly (head size smaller than normal), micrognathia (abnormally small lower jaw), ptosis (drooping eyelids), a small upturned nose, and cleft palate or bifid uvula. Male infants with SLOS exhibit genital abnormalities that range from a small penis to ambiguous genitalia or gender reversal. Abnormalities in limb development are common in SLOS patients and include short thumbs, postaxial polydactyly, and single palmar creases. In addition, the most common clinical finding in SLOS patients is syndactyly (fusion of digits) of the second and third toes. This latter limb deformity is found in over 95% of SLOS patients.

7. Lipoprotein lipase (LPL) is the endothelial cell–associated enzyme necessary for release of fatty acids from circulating lipoproteins. Which of the following apolipoproteins is required to activate LPL-mediated release of fatty acids from chylomicrons?
A. apoA
B. apoB-48
C. apoB-100
D. apoC-II
E. apoE

Answer D: ApoC-II is present in chylomicrons, LDL, and HDL and is required for the activation of the endothelial cell–associated triglyceride lipase called lipoprotein lipase (LPL).

8. A 28-year-old man has the following symptoms: diffuse grayish corneal opacities, anemia, proteinuria, and hyperlipemia. His renal function is compromised and serum albumin level is elevated. Plasma triglycerides and unesterified cholesterol levels are elevated, as are levels of phosphatidylcholine. These symptoms are indicative of which of the following lipoprotein-associated disorder?
A. Bassen-Kornzweig syndrome
B. familial hypercholesterolemia (FH)
C. familial hypertriacylglycerolemia
D. familial lecithin-cholesterol acyltransferase (LCAT) deficiency
E. Wolman disease

Answer D: Familial LCAT deficiency is also called fish eye disease or Norum disease. This hyperlipoproteinemia is associated with diffuse corneal opacities, renal failure with proteinuria, and decreased levels of plasma cholesterol esters with associated accumulation of unesterified cholesterol in many tissues. In addition, the serum contains abnormal LDL (Lp-X) and VLDL.

9. Which of the following apoproteins is found exclusively associated with chylomicrons?
A. apoA
B. apoB-48
C. apoC-II
D. apoD
E. apoE

Answer B: Chylomicrons are assembled in the intestinal mucosa as a means to transport dietary cholesterol and triglycerides to the rest of the body. The apolipoproteins that predominate before the chylomicrons enter the circulation include apoB-48, apoA-I, apoA-II, and apoA-IV, where apoB-48 is exclusively associated with chylomicrons.

10. High plasma levels of the lipoprotein particle identified as lipoprotein(a) (Lp[a]) have been shown to be a primary risk factor for coronary heart disease and stroke. Lp(a) is a unique lipoprotein assembled from low-density lipoprotein (LDL) and a single glycoprotein called apolipoprotein(a) (apo[a]). Apo(a) is associated with LDL via a disulfide linkage to which other apolipoprotein?
A. apoA-I
B. apoB-48
C. apoB-100
D. apoC-II
E. apoE

Answer C: Lp(a) is composed of a common LDL nucleus linked to a molecule of apolipoprotein(a) (apo[a]) by disulfide bonds between a cysteine residue in a Kringle-IV (KIV) type 9 domain in apo(a) and a cysteine residue in apolipoprotein B-100 (apoB-100).

11. A 16-year-old teenager boy presents with moderate to severe epigastric pain. Physical examination reveals extensive eruptive xanthomas and hepatosplenomegaly. A blood sample reveals milky plasma. Which of the following is the most likely lipoprotein to be elevated in the plasma of this patient accounting for the milky appearance?
A. apo(a)
B. chylomicrons
C. HDL
D. IDL
E. LDL

Answer B: Chylomicrons are assembled in the intestinal mucosa as a means to transport dietary cholesterol and triglycerides to the rest of the body. Chylomicrons leave the intestine via the lymphatic system and enter the circulation at the left subclavian vein. High levels of chylomicrons in the blood can give it a milky appearance. The term *chyle* refers to the milky fluid consisting of lymph and emulsified fats or free fatty acids, which is how the term chylomicron was derived.

12. Laboratory results for a patient with uncontrolled type 1 diabetes reveal hyperglycemia (634 mg/dL) and hypertriglyceridemia (498 mg/dL). Which of the following represents the most likely cause of the hypertriglyceridemia in this patient?

A. absence of hormone-sensitive lipase
B. decreased lipoprotein lipase activity
C. deficiency in apoprotein C-II
D. deficiency in LDL receptors
E. increased hepatic triglyceride synthesis

Answer B: The triglyceride components of VLDL and chylomicron are hydrolyzed to free fatty acids and glycerol in the capillaries of tissues such as liver, adipose tissue, and skeletal muscle by the actions of lipoprotein lipase (LPL) and hepatic triglyceride lipase (HTGL, also called hepatic lipase, HL). Insulin exerts numerous effects on overall metabolic homeostasis. One of the effects of insulin, which relates to the symptoms in this patient, is the regulation of the expression of LPL on the surface of endothelial cells. Since type 1 diabetics do not synthesize insulin, they do not properly regulate the level of LPL, which contributes to hypertriglyceridemia in these individuals.

13. A 23-year-old female presents with low red blood cell count, corneal opacities, and renal insufficiency. She is diagnosed with a deficiency in ratio of lecithin to cholesterol acyltransferase (LCAT). In which of the following reactions is LCAT involved?

A. converting cholesterol to cholesterol esters
B. hydrolysis of HDL
C. promoting uptake of HDL into liver cells
D. transfer of cholesterol esters from HDL to VLDL
E. uptake of cholesterol from liver cells

Answer A: The primary mechanism by which HDL acquires peripheral tissue cholesterol is via an interaction with macrophages in the subendothelial spaces of the tissues. The free cholesterol transferred from macrophages to HDL is esterified by HDL-associated LCAT. LCAT is synthesized in the liver and so named because it transfers a fatty acid from the C–2 position of lecithin to the C–3–OH of cholesterol, generating a cholesterol ester and lysolecithin.

14. You have referred a 27-year-old woman to a lipid research center for investigation of moderate hypertriglyceridemia. Analysis of her serum revealed the presence of abnormal lipid and lipoprotein profiles. Both HDL and LDL were less dense than normal and showed significant elevations in triglyceride content with the mass of triglycerides approximately the same as that of cholesterol. A deficiency in which of the following is the most likely cause of the observed lipid abnormalities?

A. apoB-100
B. cholesterol ester transfer protein (CETP)
C. hepatic triglyceride lipase
D. lecithin-cholesterol acyltransferase (LCAT)
E. lipoprotein lipase

Answer C: Hepatic triglyceride lipase (HTGL, also called hepatic lipase, HL) is an enzyme that is made primarily by hepatocytes that hydrolyzes phospholipids and triglycerides of plasma lipoproteins. The potential significance of the HTGL pathway is that it provides the hepatocyte with a mechanism for the uptake of a subset of phospholipids enriched in unsaturated fatty acids and may allow the uptake of cholesteryl ester, free cholesterol, and phospholipid without catabolism of HDL apolipoproteins. HTGL can hydrolyze triglyceride and phospholipid in all lipoproteins, but is predominant in the conversion of intermediate-density lipoproteins to LDL and the conversion of postprandial triglyceride-rich HDL into the postabsorptive triglyceride-poor HDL. HTGL plays a secondary role in the clearance of chylomicron remnants by the liver. A prominent feature of HTGL deficiency is the increase in HDL cholesterol and an approximately 10-fold increase in HDL triglyceride.

15. You are carrying out a clinical trial of a new investigational drug for the treatment of hypercholesterolemia. Results of your studies indicate that consumption of the drug results in clear elevation in the level of circulating HDL in most of the test subjects. Given these results, which of the following proteins is most likely the target of the investigational drug?

A. apoB-100
B. apoC-II
C. cholesterol ester transfer protein (CETP)
D. hepatic triglyceride lipase (HTGL)
E. lecithin-cholesterol acyltransferase (LCAT)

Answer C: Cholesterol ester transfer protein (CETP) is plasma glycoprotein secreted primarily from the liver and plays a critical role in HDL metabolism by facilitating the exchange of cholesteryl esters (CE) from HDL for triglycerides (TG) in apoB–containing lipoproteins, such as LDL and VLDL. The activity of CETP directly lowers the cholesterol levels of HDL and enhances HDL catabolism by providing HDL with the TG substrate of hepatic lipase. Thus, CETP plays a critical role in the regulation of circulating levels of HDL, LDL, and apoA-I. It has also been shown that most of the cholesterol in mice, who naturally lack CETP, is found in HDL and these mice are relatively resistant to atherosclerosis. The potential for the therapeutic use of CETP inhibitors in humans was first suggested when it was discovered that a small Japanese population had an inborn error in the *CETP* gene, leading to hyperalphalipoproteinemia and very high HDL levels.

16. Obesity is an epidemic in the United States and other industrialized countries, resulting in significant health consequences and expense. Therefore, discovering novel therapies for modifying food intake would have particular benefits to the treatment of obesity. Recent work has demonstrated that feeding behaviors are reduced following the consumption of fat through the actions of which of the following apolipoproteins?

A. apoA-IV
B. apoB-100
C. apoB-48
D. apoC-II
E. apoE

Answer A: Apolipoprotein A-IV (apoA-IV) is synthesized exclusively in the small intestine and the hypothalamus. Intestinal synthesis of apoA-IV increases in response to ingestion and absorption of fat, and it is subsequently incorporated into chylomicrons and delivered to the circulation via the lymphatic system. Systemic apoA-IV has been shown to have effects in the CNS involving the sensation of satiety. Studies in laboratory animals have indicated that the effects exerted on appetite by apoA-IV may be due to direct hypothalamic synthesis and secretion. This is demonstrated by blocking apoA-IV actions via central injection of antibodies to the protein, which results in increased food consumption. Additional studies have shown that apoA-IV is involved in inhibiting food intake following the ingestion of fat.

17. You are studying the activities of a compound that is purported to be an inhibitor of the antioxidant functions of HDL. Administration of this compound to experimental animals does indeed result in elevated levels of oxidized LDL (oxLDL) in the plasma. Which of the following proteins is the most likely target of this compound accounting for the reduced antioxidant function of HDL?

A. apoA-I
B. apoC-II
C. apoE
D. cholesterol ester transfer protein (CETP)
E. lecithin-cholesterol acyltransferase (LCAT)

Answer A: Numerous lines of evidence demonstrate that apoA-I is a major antiatherogenic and antioxidant factor in HDL due to its critical role in the HDL-mediated process of reverse cholesterol transport. In addition to reverse cholesterol transport, apoA-I can remove oxidized phospholipids from oxidized LDLs (oxLDLs) and from cells. Specific methionine residues (Met112 and Met148) of apoA-I have been shown to directly reduce cholesterol ester hydroperoxides and phosphatidylcholine hydroperoxides.

18. Which of the following statements best distinguishes VLDL from chylomicrons?

A. only chylomicrons are involved in the delivery of triglyceride to the adipocyte
B. only chylomicrons are produced by the liver
C. only chylomicrons contain phospholipids and cholesteryl esters
D. only VLDL are produced during periods of starvation
E. VLDL have a higher percentage of triglyceride than chylomicrons

Answer D: Chylomicrons are assembled in the intestinal mucosa as a means to transport dietary cholesterol and triglycerides to the rest of the body. Chylomicrons are, therefore, the molecules formed to mobilize dietary (exogenous) lipids and would, therefore, not be produced during periods of starvation or fasting.

19. Plasma triglyceride derived from dietary fats is transported in the plasma as which of the following?

A. albumin complexes
B. chylomicrons
C. HDL
D. LDL
E. VLDL

Answer B: See the answer to Question 18 for explanation.

20. An increased plasma concentration of cholesterol is most likely to be caused by a deficiency of which of the following?

A. bile acid synthetic enzymes
B. HDL receptors
C. 3-hydroxy-3-methylglutaryl-CoA (HMG-CoA) reductase
D. insulin receptors
E. LDL receptors

Answer E: The liver takes up LDL (and IDL) after they have interacted with the LDL receptor to form a complex, which is endocytosed by the cell. For LDL receptors in the liver to recognize LDL, they require the presence of both apoB-100 and apoE (the LDL receptor is also called the apoB-100/apoE receptor). Lack of functional LDL receptors is associated with hypercholesterolemia and the increased development of atherosclerotic plaques, leading to coronary heart disease.

21. A 23-year-old man is found to be incapable of producing chylomicrons. Which of the following is the most likely consequence of this disorder?
A. fasting hyperglycemia
B. impaired absorption of dietary lipids
C. increased risk of hypertriglyceridemia
D. increased risk of lactic acidosis
E. increased serum urea nitrogen concentration

Answer B: Chylomicrons are assembled in the intestinal mucosa as a means to transport dietary cholesterol and triglycerides to the rest of the body. Chylomicrons are, therefore, the molecules formed to mobilize dietary (exogenous) lipids. Failure to produce chylomicrons would, therefore, lead to impaired absorption of dietary lipids.

22. A 30-year-old woman is brought to the physician because of a rash on her arms for 2 months and severe abdominal pain for the past 24 hours. She indicates that she has had intermittent upper abdominal pain during the past 1 to 2 years. Physical examination shows yellow papules on the extensor surfaces of the upper extremities. Palpation of the epigastric region of her abdomen causes pain. Her blood work shows serum amylase activity is increased and fasting serum concentrations of chylomicrons and triglycerides are markedly increased. Which of the following changes in apolipoprotein concentrations is most likely in this patient?
A. decreased apoA-I
B. decreased apoB-III
C. decreased apoC-II
D increased apoB-100
E. increased apoE

Answer C: ApoC-II is present in chylomicrons, LDL, and HDL and is required for the activation of the endothelial cell–associated triglyceride lipase called lipoprotein lipase (LPL). Loss, or defective activity, of apoC-II would result in circulating lipoproteins of all types enriched in triglyceride, leading to hypertriglyceridemia. Additional symptoms associated with apoC-II deficiency include eruptive xanthomas, pancreatitis, and hepatosplenomegaly. The hepatosplenomegaly is the cause of the episodic epigastric pain.

23. A genetically based deficiency of which of the following will most likely result in decreased lipoprotein lipase activity?
A. apoC-II
B. bile salt deconjugase
C. ceruloplasmin
D. hormone-sensitive lipase
E. pancreatic lipase

Answer A: ApoC-II is present in chylomicrons, LDL, and HDL and is required for the activation of the endothelial cell–associated triglyceride lipase called lipoprotein lipase (LPL). Loss, or defective activity, of apoC-II would result in circulating lipoproteins of all types enriched in triglyceride leading to hypertriglyceridemia.

24. The primary function of LDL is to transport which of the following?
A. cholesterol to peripheral tissues
B. cholesterol from tissues to the liver
C. dietary-derived lipid to the liver
D. free fatty acids from adipocytes
E. triglycerides to adipocytes

Answer A: The dietary intake of both fat and carbohydrate, in excess of the needs of the body, leads to their conversion into triglycerides in the liver. These triglycerides are packaged into VLDL and released into the circulation for delivery to the various tissues (primarily muscle and adipose tissue) for storage or production of energy through oxidation. VLDL are, therefore, the molecules formed to transport endogenously derived triglycerides to extrahepatic tissues. The fatty acid portion of VLDL is released to the tissues through the action of lipoprotein lipase, which leads to increasing density of VLDL to IDL and LDL.

25. A 40-year-old man with a 10-year history of type 1 diabetes mellitus comes to the physician for a routine examination. He was diagnosed with pancreatitis 25 years ago after a 2-year history of recurrent abdominal pain. Physical examination shows a thin habitus and abdominal tenderness. After a 12-hour fast, his serum triglyceride concentration is 4000 mg/dL (normal = 60-134). Intravenous heparin is administered in order to examine the patient's lipoprotein lipase activity. Plasma lipoprotein lipase activity is assayed and is extremely deficient in this man's blood. Which of the following proteins is most likely deficient in this patient?
A. apoA-I
B. apoB-48
C. apoB-100
D. apoC-II
E. apoE

Answer D: ApoC-II is present in chylomicrons, LDL, and HDL and is required for the activation of the endothelial cell–associated triglyceride lipase called lipoprotein lipase (LPL). Loss, or defective activity, of apoC-II would result in circulating lipoproteins of all types enriched in triglyceride, leading to hypertriglyceridemia. Additional symptoms associated with apoC-II deficiency include eruptive xanthomas, pancreatitis, and hepatosplenomegaly. The hepatosplenomegaly is the cause of the abdominal tenderness.

26. A 20-year-old man comes to the physician because of recurrent episodes of acute abdominal pain since childhood. The pain usually occurs after eating a meal with a rich dessert. Physical examination shows a small number of xanthomas on the buttocks and knees. A fasting lipid analysis shows milky plasma; there is markedly increased serum concentration of triglycerides and chylomicrons. His serum LDL-cholesterol concentration is within the reference range, and serum HDL-cholesterol concentration is decreased. This patient most likely has a defect of which of the following proteins?

A. apoA-I
B. apoC-II
C. apoE
D. HDL receptor
E. LDL receptor

Answer B: ApoC-II is present in chylomicrons, LDL, and HDL and is required for the activation of the endothelial cell–associated triglyceride lipase called lipoprotein lipase (LPL). Loss, or defective activity, of apoC-II would result in circulating lipoproteins of all types enriched in triglyceride leading to hypertriglyceridemia. Additional symptoms associated with apoC-II deficiency include eruptive xanthomas, pancreatitis, and hepatosplenomegaly. The hepatosplenomegaly is the cause of the acute abdominal pain.

27. Cholesterol is transported in the bloodstream in LDL, which bind to specific membrane receptors on the peripheral tissue cell membranes. The cholesterol then enters these cells by which of the following mechanisms?

A. carrier-mediated diffusion on the cholesterol-specific carrier in the cell membrane
B. cholesterol-specific gated channel
C. endocytosis, where it is released from the LDL in the lysosomes
D. by first being converted to cholesterol esters by plasma enzyme lecithin-cholesterol acyltransferase (LCAT)

Answer C: The LDLs, formed as triglycerides, are removed from circulating VLDL. The liver takes up LDL after they have interacted with the LDL receptor to form a complex, which is endocytosed by the cell. For LDL receptors in the liver to recognize IDLs, they require the presence of both apoB-100 and apoE (the LDL receptor is also called the apoB-100/apoE receptor).

28. Which of the following is involved in the transport of newly synthesized triglycerides from the liver to adipose tissue?

A. chylomicrons
B. HDL
C. IDL
D. LDL
E. VLDL

Answer E: Hepatic triglycerides are packaged into VLDL and released into the circulation for delivery to the various tissues (primarily muscle and adipose tissue) for storage or production of energy through oxidation. VLDL are, therefore, the molecules formed to transport endogenously derived triglycerides to extra-hepatic tissues.

29. A defect in which of the following proteins or complexes would result in the inability of HDL to transfer peripheral tissue cholesterol to circulating LDL?

A. acyl-CoA:cholesterol acyltransferase (ACAT) ratio
B. clathrin
C. lecithin-cholesterol acyltransferase (LCAT)
D lipoprotein lipase
E. phosphorylated mannose residue

Answer C: HDLs acquire peripheral tissue-free cholesterol, which is then esterified by HDL-associated LCAT. LCAT is synthesized in the liver and so named because it transfers a fatty acid from the C–2 position of lecithin to the C–3–OH of cholesterol, generating a cholesterol ester and lysolecithin. The activity of LCAT requires interaction with apoA-I, which is found on the surface of HDL. As HDLs migrate through the vasculature, there is an interaction between them and IDL and LDL. This interaction occurs through the action of CETP, which exchanges the cholesterol esters in the HDL for triglycerides from LDL. A loss of LCAT activity would result in the inability of HDL to esterify cholesterol, which would, therefore, result in the inability of HDL to transfer the cholesterol esters to LDL.

30. Which of the following is most likely to occur to the LDL receptor after it has been dissociated from LDL in the acidic early endosome?

A. digested by proteasomes in the cytosol after release from the endosome
B. recycled back to the cell membrane from the endosome in transport vesicle
C. recycled into a vesicle in the *trans*-Golgi complex and transported to the cell membrane

D. transcytosis
E. transferred to lysosomes where it is degraded by lysosomal enzymes

Answer B: The LDL receptor is a polypeptide of 839 amino acids that spans the plasma membrane. An extracellular domain is responsible for apoB-100/apoE binding. The intracellular domain is responsible for the clustering of LDL receptors into regions of the plasma membrane termed *coated pits.* Once LDL binds the receptor, the complexes are rapidly internalized (endocytosed). ATP-dependent proton pumps lower the pH in the endosomes, which results in dissociation of the LDL from the receptor. The portion of the endosomal membranes harboring the receptor are then recycled to the plasma membrane.

Checklist

- ✓ 3 Lipid transport, both dietary lipids and endogenous lipids, takes place in the blood associated with proteins in complexes referred to as lipoproteins.
- ✓ Dietary lipoproteins are called chylomicrons and endogenous lipoproteins are either very low-density lipoproteins (VLDLs) or high-density lipoproteins (HDLs).
- ✓ Chylomicrons are synthesized in the intestinal enterocytes and are composed primarily of triglyceride and apolipoproteins. These lipoproteins are delivered to the circulation through the subclavian vein via the lymphatic system.
- ✓ VLDLs are synthesized in the liver to deliver fatty acid (triglyceride) and cholesterol to peripheral tissues. As they circulate and lose lipid, they become progressively more dense, becoming low-density lipoproteins (LDLs). HDLs begin as apolipoprotein A-I and acquire cholesterol via interactions with peripheral tissues and macrophages; they acquire triglycerides from VLDL and LDL.
- ✓ LDLs are highly susceptible to oxidation (oxLDL) and are then preferentially phagocytosed by macrophages inducing pro-inflammatory responses from these cells. This phenomenon is a major reason for LDLs being referred to as "bad cholesterol."
- ✓ HDLs play a critical role in the removal of cholesterol from macrophages and other peripheral tissues and return the cholesterol to the liver either directly or through exchange to VLDL and LDL. This process is referred to as reverse cholesterol transport (RCT) and is the reason why HDLs are often referred to as "good cholesterol."
- ✓ Numerous HDL-associated proteins are critical for the antioxidant and anti-inflammatory properties of these lipoproteins. Pharmacological elevation in plasma levels of HDL is beneficial in the prevention of atherosclerosis and coronary heart disease (CHD); inhibition of CETP has demonstrated efficacy in increasing circulating HDL levels.
- ✓ Lipoproteins such as, chylomicrons, LDL, and HDL, bind to specific cell-surface receptors and are either internalized or deliver constituents such as cholesterol to cell to which they bind. LDL receptors require the presence of both apoB-100 and apoE for maximal binding. Chylomicron remnants can bind to the LDL receptor, LDL receptor–related protein (LRP), or to heparin sulfate proteoglycans (HSPG) in the space of Disse in the liver. HDLs bind to the scavenger receptor, SR-B1, on hepatocytes to deliver cholesterol to this tissue.
- ✓ Defects in overall lipoprotein synthesis and metabolism can lead to severe clinical outcomes associated with hypercholesterolemia and result in atherosclerosis and CHD. Familial hypercholesterolemia (FH) results from defects in LDL receptor–mediated hepatic LDL uptake and is the most common inherited disorder of lipoprotein metabolism.

CHAPTER

29 Nitrogen: Nitrogen Homeostasis and Disposal via Urea

CHAPTER OUTLINE

High-Yield Terms

Aminotransferase: any of a family of enzymes that catalyze the transfer of an amino group between a α-amino acid and an α-keto acid

AST and ALT: aspartate aminotransferase (AST; also called serum glutamate-oxaloacetate aminotransferase, [SGOT]) and alanine transaminase (ALT; also called serum glutamate-pyruvate aminotransferase [SGPT]), the two prevalent liver enzymes whose elevations in the blood have been used as clinical markers of tissue damage

Glucose-alanine cycle: mechanism for skeletal muscle to eliminate nitrogen while replenishing its glucose supply. Glucose oxidation produces pyruvate which can undergo transamination to alanine; the alanine then enters the blood stream and is transported to the liver where it is converted back to pyruvate, which is then a source of carbon atoms for gluconeogenesis

Urea: nitrogen compound composed of 2 amino groups ($-NH_2$) joined by a carbonyl ($-C=O$) functional group; is the main nitrogen-containing substance in human urine

Kwashiorkor: an acute form of childhood protein-energy malnutrition with adequate caloric intake; characterized by edema, irritability, anorexia, ulcerating dermatoses, and an enlarged liver with fatty infiltrates

Nitrogen Distribution From Biosphere

Humans are totally dependent on other organisms for converting atmospheric nitrogen into forms available to the body. Nitrogen fixation is carried out by bacterial nitrogenases forming reduced nitrogen, NH_4^+, which can then be used by all organisms to form amino acids (Figure 29-1).

Reduced nitrogen enters the human body as dietary free amino acids, protein, and the ammonia produced by intestinal tract bacteria. A pair of principal enzymes, glutamate dehydrogenase and glutamine synthetase, incorporates this ammonia into carbon skeletons generating the amino acids glutamate and glutamine, respectively. Amino and amide groups from these 2 amino acids are then freely transferred to other carbon skeletons by transamination (Figure 29-2) and transamidation reactions.

Aminotransferases exist for all amino acids except threonine and lysine. The most common compounds involved as a donor/acceptor pair in transamination reactions are glutamate and α-ketoglutarate (2-oxoglutarate), which participate in reactions with many different aminotransferases. Serum aminotransferases AST and ALT have been used as clinical markers of tissue damage, with increasing serum levels indicating an increased extent of damage. Alanine transaminase has an important function in the delivery of skeletal muscle carbon and nitrogen (in the form of alanine) to the liver. In skeletal muscle, pyruvate is transaminated to alanine, thus affording an additional route of nitrogen transport from muscle to liver. In the liver, alanine transaminase transfers the ammonia to α-ketoglutarate and regenerates pyruvate. The pyruvate can then be diverted into gluconeogenesis. This process is referred to as the glucose-alanine cycle (Chapter 13).

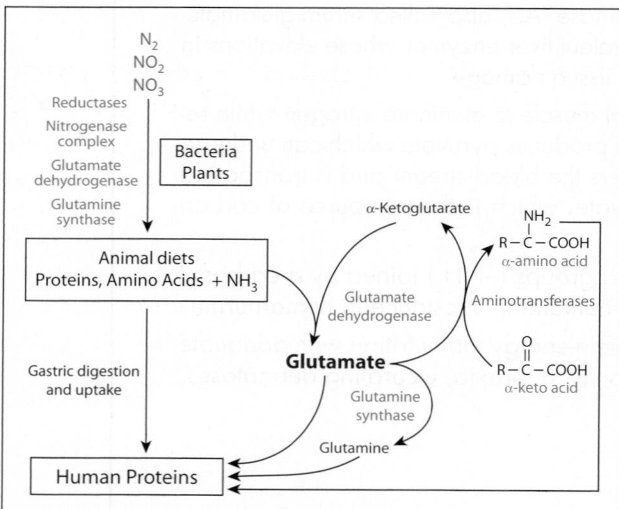

FIGURE 29-1: Overview of the flow of nitrogen in the biosphere. Nitrogen, nitrites, and nitrates are acted upon by bacteria (nitrogen fixation) and plants and we assimilate these compounds as protein in our diets. Ammonia incorporation in animals occurs through the actions of glutamate dehydrogenase and glutamine synthase. Glutamate plays the central role in mammalian nitrogen flow, serving as both a nitrogen donor and nitrogen acceptor. Reproduced with permission of themedicalbiochemistrypage, LLC.

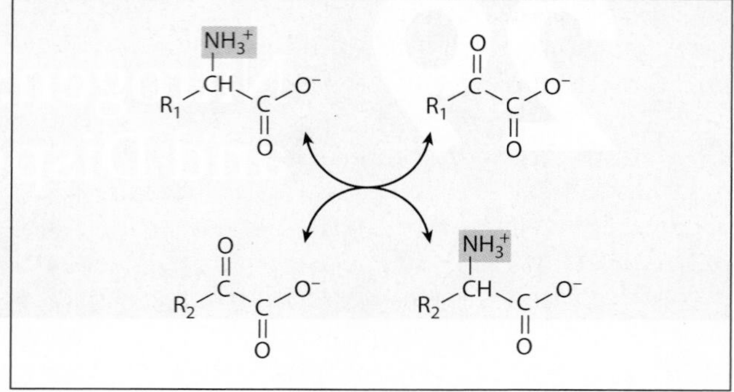

FIGURE 29-2: Transamination. The reaction is freely reversible with an equilibrium constant close to unity. Murray RK, Bender DA, Botham KM, Kennelly PJ, Rodwell VW, Weil PA. *Harper's Illustrated Biochemistry*, 29th ed. New York: McGraw-Hill; 2012.

The Glutamate Dehydrogenase Reaction

Glutamate dehydrogenase is considered a gateway enzyme of energy and nitrogen homeostasis (Figure 29-3). The enzyme utilizes NAD⁺ in the direction of nitrogen liberation and NADP⁺ for nitrogen incorporation. In the forward reaction glutamate dehydrogenase is important in converting free ammonia and α-ketoglutarate to glutamate, forming one of the 20 amino acids required for protein synthesis. On the other hand, the reverse reaction is a key anapleurotic process linking amino

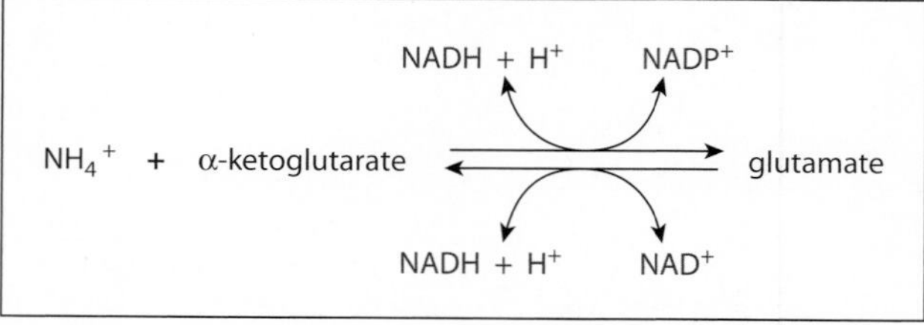

FIGURE 29-3: Glutamate dehydrogenase reaction. Reproduced with permission of themedicalbiochemistrypage, LLC.

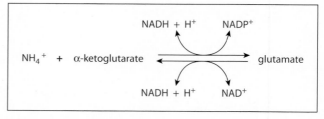

acid metabolism with TCA cycle activity. In the reverse reaction, glutamate dehydrogenase provides an oxidizable carbon source used for the production of energy as well as a reduced electron carrier, NADH.

As expected for a branch point enzyme with an important link to energy metabolism, glutamate dehydrogenase is regulated by the cell energy charge. ATP and GTP are positive allosteric effectors of the formation of glutamate, whereas ADP and GDP are positive allosteric effectors of the reverse reaction. Thus, when the level of ATP is high, conversion of glutamate to α-ketoglutarate is limited; when the cellular energy charge is low, glutamate is converted to ammonia and α-ketoglutarate which can then be oxidized in the TCA cycle. Glutamate is also a principal amino donor to other amino acids in subsequent transamination reactions.

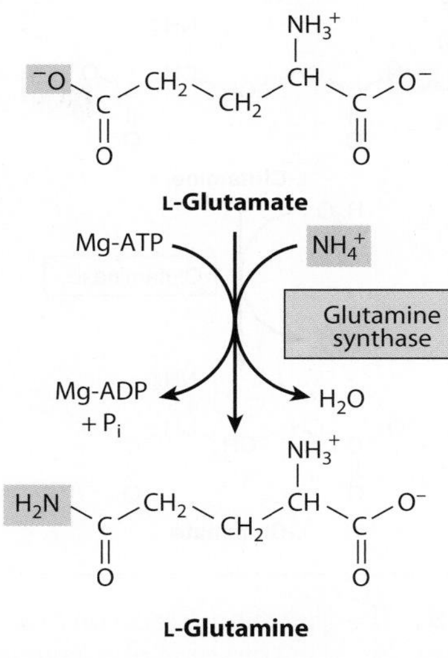

FIGURE 29-4: The glutamine synthase reaction strongly favors glutamine synthesis. Murray RK, Bender DA, Botham KM, Kennelly PJ, Rodwell VW, Weil PA. *Harper's Illustrated Biochemistry,* 29th ed. New York: McGraw-Hill; 2012.

The Glutamine Synthetase Reaction

The glutamine synthetase reaction (Figure 29-4) is also important to nitrogen homeostasis in several respects. First it produces glutamine, one of the 20 major amino acids. Second, in animals, glutamine is the major amino acid found in the circulatory system. Its role there is to carry ammonia to and from various tissues but principally from peripheral tissues to the kidney, where the amide nitrogen is hydrolyzed by the enzyme glutaminase (Figure 29-5); this process regenerates glutamate and free ammonium ion, which is excreted in the urine. Note that, in this function, ammonia arising in peripheral tissues is transported in the blood in a nonionizable form which has none of the neurotoxic or alkalosis-generating properties of free ammonia.

Liver contains both glutamine synthetase and glutaminase but the enzymes are localized in different

High-Yield Concept

The multiple roles of glutamate in nitrogen homeostasis make it a gateway between free ammonia and the amino groups of most amino acids.

High-Yield Concept

When acidosis occurs the body will divert more glutamine from the liver to the kidney. This allows for the conservation of bicarbonate ion since the incorporation of ammonia into urea requires bicarbonate. When glutamine enters the kidney, glutaminase releases 1 mole of ammonia generating glutamate and then glutamate dehydrogenase releases another mole of ammonia generating α-ketoglutarate. The ammonia will ionize to ammonium ion (NH_4^+), which is excreted. The net effect is a reduction in the concentration of hydrogen ion [H^+], and thus an increase in the pH of the blood.

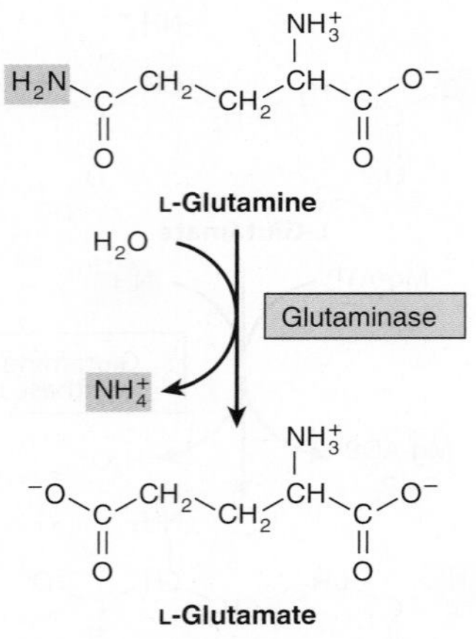

FIGURE 29-5: The glutaminase reaction proceeds essentially irreversibly in the direction of glutamate and NH_4^+ formation. Note that the *amide* nitrogen, not the α-amino nitrogen, is removed. Murray RK, Bender DA, Botham KM, Kennelly PJ, Rodwell VW, Weil PA. *Harper's Illustrated Biochemistry*, 29th ed. New York: McGraw-Hill; 2012.

cellular segments. This ensures that the liver is neither a net producer nor consumer of glutamine. The differences in cellular locations of these 2 enzymes allow the liver to scavenge ammonia that has not been incorporated into urea. The enzymes of the urea cycle are located in the same cells as those that contain glutaminase. The result of the differential distribution of these 2 hepatic enzymes makes it possible to control ammonia incorporation into urea or glutamine.

Digestive Tract Nitrogen

While glutamate, glutamine, and the remaining nonessential amino acids can be made by animals, the majority of the amino acids found in human tissues come from dietary sources. The details of protein digestion and amino acid uptake by the intestines are covered in Chapter 43. Since humans can neither synthesize the branched carbon chains found in branched chain amino acids or the ring systems found in phenylalanine and the aromatic amino acids nor incorporate sulfur into covalently bonded structures, there are 10 so-called essential amino acids (see Table 30-1) that must be supplied from the diet. However, depending on the composition of the diet and physiological state of an individual, one or another of the nonessential amino acids may also become a required dietary component. For example, arginine is only normally considered to be an essential amino acid during early childhood development because enough for adult needs is made by the urea cycle.

In addition to the amino acids obtained from the diet, many other nitrogenous compounds are found in the intestine. Most of these compounds are bacterial products of protein degradation with some exhibiting powerful pharmacological (vasopressor) effects (Table 29-1).

TABLE 29-1: Nitrogenous Products of Intestinal Bacterial Activity

	Products	
Substrates	***Vasopressor Amines***	***Other***
Lysine	Cadaverine	
Arginine	Agmatine	
Tyrosine	Tyramine	
Ornithine	Putrescine	
Histidine	Histamine	
Tryptophan		Indole and skatole
All amino acids		NH_4^+

High-Yield Concept

Normal, healthy adults are generally in nitrogen balance, with intake and excretion being very well matched. Young growing children, adults recovering from major illness, and pregnant women are often in positive nitrogen balance. Their intake of nitrogen exceeds their loss as net protein synthesis proceeds. When more nitrogen is excreted than is incorporated into the body, an individual is in negative nitrogen balance. Insufficient quantities of even one essential amino acid are adequate to turn an otherwise normal individual into one with a negative nitrogen balance.

Nitrogen Balance

Unlike fats and carbohydrates, nitrogen has no designated storage depots in the body. Since the half-life of many proteins is short (on the order of hours), insufficient dietary quantities of even 1 amino acid can quickly limit the synthesis and lower the body levels of many essential proteins. The result of limited synthesis and normal rates of protein degradation is that the balance of nitrogen intake and nitrogen excretion is rapidly and significantly altered.

The biological value of dietary proteins is related to the extent to which they provide all the necessary amino acids. Proteins of animal origin generally have a high biological value; plant proteins have a wide range of values from almost none to quite high. In general, plant proteins are deficient in lysine, methionine, and tryptophan and are much less concentrated and less digestible than animal proteins. The absence of lysine in low-grade cereal proteins, used as a dietary mainstay in many underdeveloped countries, leads to an inability to synthesize protein (because of missing essential amino acids) and ultimately to a syndrome known as kwashiorkor, common among children in these countries.

Removal of Nitrogen from Amino Acids

The dominant reactions involved in removing amino acid nitrogen from the body are known as transaminations (see Figure 29-2). This class of reactions funnels nitrogen from all free amino acids into a small number of compounds; then, either they are oxidatively deaminated, producing ammonia, or their amine groups are converted to urea by the urea cycle. Transaminations involve moving a α-amino group from a donor α-amino acid to the keto carbon of an acceptor α-keto acid. These reversible reactions are catalyzed by a group of intracellular enzymes known as aminotransferases, which generally employ covalently bound pyridoxal phosphate as a cofactor. However, some aminotransferases employ pyruvate as a cofactor.

Aminotransferases exist for all amino acids except threonine and lysine. The most common compounds involved as a donor/acceptor pair in transamination reactions are glutamate and α-ketoglutarate, which participate in reactions with many different aminotransferases.

Alanine transaminase has an important function in the delivery of skeletal muscle carbon and nitrogen to the liver. In skeletal muscle, pyruvate is transaminated to alanine allowing for waste nitrogen from amino acid oxidation to be transported from muscle to liver. In the liver, alanine transaminase transfers the ammonia to α-ketoglutarate and regenerates pyruvate. The pyruvate can then be diverted into gluconeogenesis. This process is referred to as the glucose-alanine cycle (see Figure 13-2).

Because of the participation of α-ketoglutarate in numerous transaminations, glutamate is a prominent intermediate in nitrogen elimination as well as in anabolic pathways. Glutamate, formed in the course of nitrogen elimination, is either oxidatively deaminated by liver glutamate dehydrogenase forming ammonia, or converted to glutamine by glutamine synthetase and transported to kidney tubule cells. There the glutamine is sequentially deamidated by glutaminase and deaminated by kidney glutamate dehydrogenase. The ammonia produced in the latter two reactions is excreted as NH_4^+ in the urine, where it helps maintain urine pH in the normal range of pH4 to pH8. The extensive production of ammonia by peripheral tissue or hepatic glutamate dehydrogenase is not feasible because of the highly toxic effects of circulating ammonia. Normal serum ammonium concentrations are in the range of 20 to 40 μM, and an increase in circulating ammonia to about 400 μM causes alkalosis and neurotoxicity.

In the peroxisomes of mammalian tissues, especially liver, there exists a minor enzymatic pathway for the removal of amino groups from amino acids.

High-Yield Concept

Serum aminotransferases such as aspartate aminotransferase (AST; also called serum glutamate-oxaloacetate aminotransferase [SGOT]) and alanine transaminase (ALT; also called serum glutamate-pyruvate aminotransferase [SGPT]) have been used as clinical markers of tissue damage, with increasing serum levels indicating an increased extent of damage.

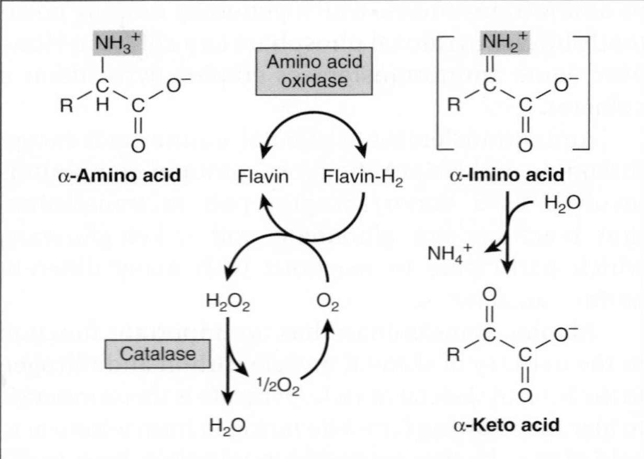

FIGURE 29-6: Oxidative deamination catalyzed by L-amino acid oxidase (L-α-amino acid: O_2 oxidoreductase). The α-imino acid, shown in brackets, is not a stable intermediate. Murray RK, Bender DA, Botham KM, Kennelly PJ, Rodwell VW, Weil PA. *Harper's Illustrated Biochemistry,* 29th ed. New York: McGraw-Hill; 2012.

L-amino acid oxidase is FMN-linked and has broad specificity for the L-amino acids (Figure 29-6). A number of substances, including oxygen, can act as electron acceptors from the flavoproteins. If oxygen is the acceptor the product is hydrogen peroxide, which is then rapidly degraded by the catalases found in liver and other tissues. Missing or defective biogenesis of peroxisomes or L-amino acid oxidase is commonly associated with oculogyric crisis (OGC; spasmodic movements of the eyeballs that last several minutes to hours) and causes generalized hyperaminoacidemia and hyperaminoaciduria, generally leading to neurotoxicity and early death.

The Urea Cycle

Although glutamine transport to the kidneys and the concerted actions of glutaminase and glutamate dehydrogenase can support a pathway for the elimination of waste nitrogen, about 80% of the excreted nitrogen is in the form of urea. The formation of urea takes place in the liver, in a series of reactions that are distributed between the mitochondrial matrix and the cytosol. The series of reactions that form urea is known as the *urea cycle* or the *Krebs-Henseleit cycle* (Figure 29-7).

The essential features of the urea cycle reactions are as follows: Arginine from the diet or from protein breakdown is cleaved by the cytosolic enzyme arginase, generating urea and ornithine. In subsequent reactions of the urea cycle a new urea residue is built on the ornithine, regenerating arginine and perpetuating the cycle.

Ornithine, arising in the cytosol, is transported to the mitochondrial matrix via the action of ornithine translocase encoded by the *ORNT1* gene. The *ORNT1* transporter is a member of the solute carrier family of transporters and as such is also identified as SLC25A15. In the mitochondria ornithine transcabamoylase (OTC) catalyzes the condensation of ornithine with carbamoyl phosphate, producing citrulline. The energy for the reaction is provided by the high-energy anhydride of carbamoyl phosphate.

The carbamoyl phosphate is synthesized from bicarbonate (HCO_3^-) and ammonium (NH_4^+) ions via the action of carbamoyl phosphate synthetase I (CPS-I). This reaction is energetically expensive consuming 2 molar equivalents of ATP. Humans express 2 carbamoyl phosphate synthetases: a mitochondrial enzyme, CPS-I, which forms carbamoyl phosphate destined for inclusion in the urea cycle, and a cytosolic synthetase (CPS-II), which is involved in pyrimidine nucleotide biosynthesis.

Concomitant with ornithine transport into the mitochondria is the export of citrulline by SLC25A15 to the cytosol, where the remaining reactions of the cycle take place. Also important in the function of the urea cycle is the mitochondrial transporter called citrin (see Clinical Box 29-1). Citrin is involved in the mitochondrial uptake of glutamate and export of aspartate and as such functions in the malate-aspartate shuttle. Citrin is a Ca^{2+}-dependent mitochondrial solute transporter that is also a member of the solute carrier family of transporters identified as SLC25A13.

In a 2-step reaction, catalyzed by cytosolic argininosuccinate synthetase, citrulline and aspartate are condensed to form argininosuccinate. The reaction involves the addition of AMP (from ATP) to the amido carbonyl of citrulline, forming an activated intermediate and the subsequent addition of aspartate to form argininosuccinate. Arginine and fumarate are produced from argininosuccinate by the cytosolic enzyme argininosuccinate lyase (also called argininosuccinase). In the final step of the cycle arginase cleaves urea from arginine, regenerating cytosolic ornithine, which can be transported to the mitochondrial matrix for another round of urea synthesis. The fumarate, generated via the action of arginiosuccinate lyase, is reconverted to aspartate for use in the argininosuccinate synthetase reaction. This occurs through the actions of cytosolic versions of the TCA cycle enzymes, fumarase (which yields malate) and malate dehydrogenase (which yields oxaloacetate).

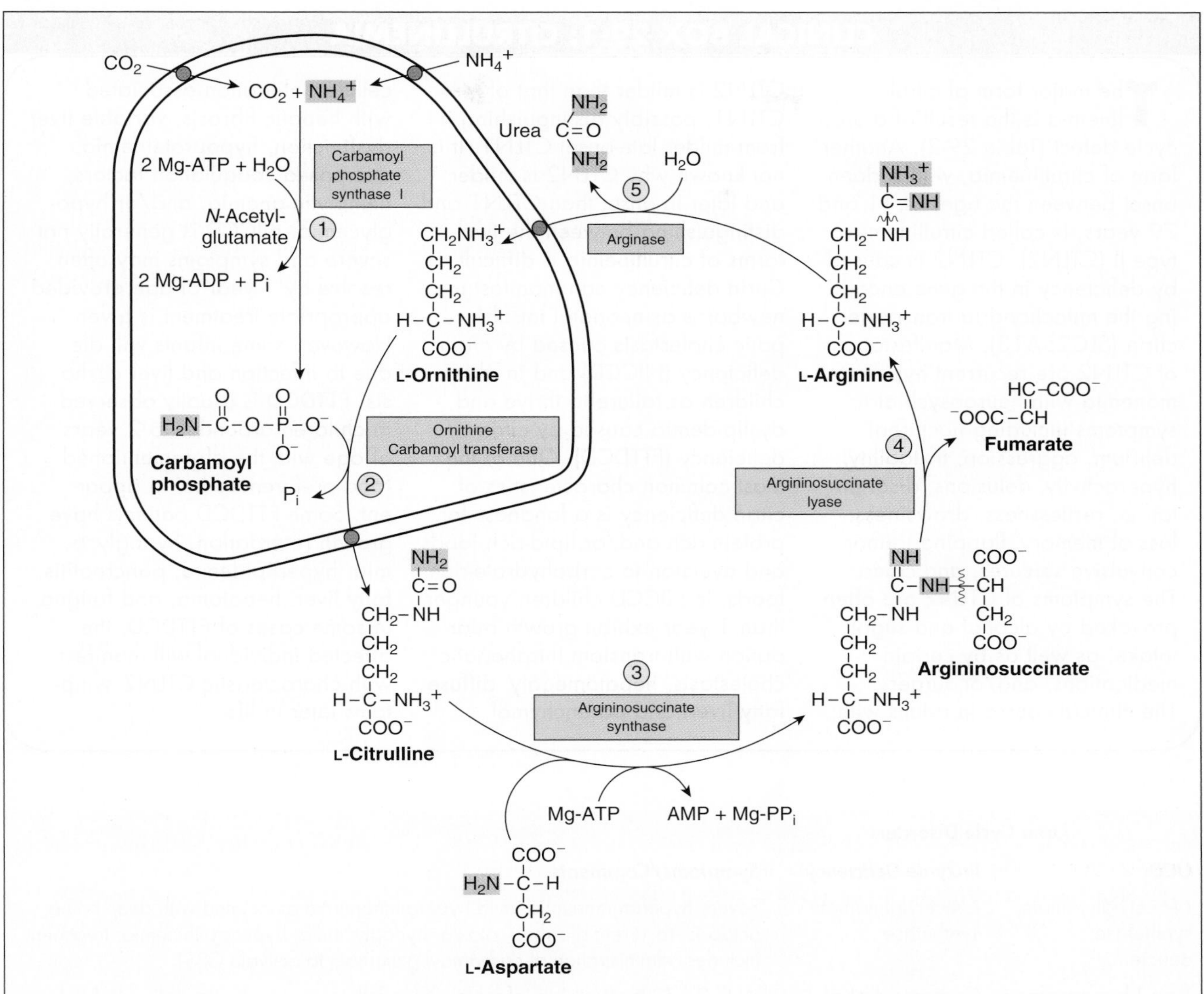

FIGURE 29-7: Reactions and intermediates of urea biosynthesis. The nitrogen-containing groups that contribute to the formation of urea are shaded. Reactions ① and ② occur in the matrix of liver mitochondria and reactions ③, ④, and ⑤ in liver cytosol. CO_2 (as bicarbonate), ammonium ion, ornithine, and citrulline enter the mitochondrial matrix via specific carriers (see red dots) present in the inner membrane of liver mitochondria. Murray RK, Bender DA, Botham KM, Kennelly PJ, Rodwell VW, Weil PA. *Harper's Illustrated Biochemistry*, 29th ed. New York: McGraw-Hill; 2012.

The oxaloacetate is then transaminated to aspartate by AST, which can then be used in another round of the urea cycle.

Beginning and ending with ornithine, the reactions of the cycle consume 3 equivalents of ATP and a total of 4 high-energy nucleotide phosphates. Urea is the only new compound generated by the cycle; all other intermediates and reactants are recycled. The energy consumed in the production of urea is more than recovered by the release of energy formed during the synthesis of the urea cycle intermediates. Ammonia released during the glutamate dehydrogenase reaction is coupled to the formation of NADH. In addition, when fumarate is converted back to aspartate, the malate dehydrogenase reaction used to convert malate to oxaloacetate generates a mole of NADH. These two moles of NADH are oxidized in the mitochondria yielding 4 to 6 moles of ATP depending upon the shuttle mechanism employed for NADH transport.

CLINICAL BOX 29-1: CITRULLINEMIA

The major form of citrullinemia is the result of a urea cycle defect (Table 29-2). Another form of citrullinemia, with sudden onset between the ages of 11 and 79 years, is called citrullinemia type II (CTLN2). CTLN2 is caused by deficiency in the gene encoding the mitochondria transporter citrin (SLC25A13). Manifestations of CTLN2 are recurrent hyperammonemia with neuropsychiatric symptoms including nocturnal delirium, aggression, irritability, hyperactivity, delusions, disorientation, restlessness, drowsiness, loss of memory, flapping tremor, convulsive seizures, and coma. The symptoms of CTLN2 are often provoked by alcohol and sugar intake, as well as by certain medications, and/or surgery. The clinical course in adults with CTLN2 is milder than that of CTLN1, possibly distinguishing it from milder late-onset CTLN1. It is not known why CTLN2 is milder and later in onset than CTLN1 and distinguishing between the two forms of citrullinemia is difficult. Citrin deficiency can manifest in newborns as neonatal intrahepatic cholestasis caused by citrin deficiency (NICCD) and in older children as failure to thrive and dyslipidemia caused by citrin deficiency (FTTDCD). One of the most common characteristics of citrin deficiency is a fondness for protein-rich and/or lipid-rich foods and aversion to carbohydrate-rich foods. In NICCD children younger than 1 year exhibit growth retardation with transient intrahepatic cholestasis, hepatomegaly, diffuse fatty liver, and parenchymal cellular infiltration associated with hepatic fibrosis, variable liver dysfunction, hypoproteinemia, decreased coagulation factors, hemolytic anemia, and/or hypoglycemia. NICCD is generally not severe and symptoms may often resolve by 1 year of age provided appropriate treatment is given. However, some infants will die due to infection and liver cirrhosis. FTTDCD is usually observed in children around 1 to 2 years of age with the aforementioned food preferences being apparent. Some FTTDCD patients have growth retardation, hypoglycemia, hyperlipidemia, pancreatitis, fatty liver, hepatoma, and fatigue. In some cases of FTTDCD, the affected individual will manifest with characteristic CTLN2 symptoms later in life.

TABLE 29-2: Urea Cycle Disorders

UCD	*Enzyme Deficiency*	*Symptoms/Comments*
N-acetylglutamate synthetase deficiency	*N*-acetylglutamate synthetase	Severe hyperammonemia, mild hyperammonemia associated with deep coma, acidosis, recurrent diarrhea, ataxia, hypoglycemia, hyperornithinemia: treatment includes administration of carbamoyl glutamate to activate CPS-I
Type I hyperammonemia, CPSD	Carbamoyl phosphate synthetase I	With 24-72 h after birth infant becomes lethargic, needs stimulation to feed, vomiting, increasing lethargy, hypothermia, and hyperventilation; without measurement of serum ammonia levels and appropriate intervention infant will die: treatment with arginine, which activates *N*-acetylglutamate synthetase
Type 2 hyperammonemia, OTCD	Ornithine transcarbamoylase	Most commonly occurring UCD, only X-linked UCD, ammonia and amino acids elevated in serum, increased serum orotic acid due to mitochondrial carbamoylphosphate entering cytosol and being incorporated into pyrimidine nucleotides which leads to excess production and consequently excess catabolic products: treat with high-carbohydrate, low-protein diet, ammonia detoxification with sodium phenylacetate or sodium benzoate
Citrullinemia type I (CTLN1), ASD	Argininosuccinate synthetase	Episodic hyperammonemia, vomiting, lethargy, ataxia, seizures, eventual coma: treat with arginine administration to enhance citrulline excretion, also with sodium benzoate for ammonia detoxification
Argininosuccinic aciduria, ALD	Argininosuccinate lyase (argininosuccinase)	Episodic symptoms similar to classic citrullinemia, elevated plasma and cerebral spinal fluid argininosuccinate; usually a fatal disorder: treat with arginine and sodium benzoate
Hyperargininemia, AD	Arginase	Rare UCD, progressive spastic quadriplegia and mental retardation; ammonia and arginine high in cerebral spinal fluid and serum; arginine, lysine, and ornithine high in urine: treatment includes diet of essential amino acids excluding arginine, low-protein diet

Regulation of the Urea Cycle

The urea cycle operates only to eliminate excess nitrogen. On high-protein diets the carbon skeletons of the amino acids are oxidized for energy or stored as fat and glycogen, but the amino nitrogen must be excreted. To facilitate this process, enzymes of the urea cycle are controlled at the gene level. With long-term changes in the quantity of dietary protein, changes of 20 fold or greater in the concentration of cycle enzymes are observed. When dietary proteins increase significantly, enzyme concentrations rise. On return to a balanced diet, enzyme levels decline. Under conditions of starvation, enzyme levels rise as proteins are degraded and amino acid carbon skeletons are used to provide energy, thus increasing the quantity of nitrogen that must be excreted.

Short-term regulation of the cycle occurs principally at CPS-I, which is relatively inactive in the absence of its allosteric activator *N*-acetylglutamate. The steady-state concentration of *N*-acetylglutamate is set by the concentration of its components acetyl-CoA and glutamate and by arginine, which is a positive allosteric effector of *N*-acetylglutamate synthase (Figure 29-8).

Urea Cycle Disorders

A complete lack of any one of the enzymes of the urea cycle will result in death shortly after birth. However, deficiencies in each of the enzymes of the urea cycle, including *N*-acetylglutamate synthase, have been identified. These disorders are referred to as urea cycle disorders (UCDs). A common thread to most UCD is hyperammonemia leading to ammonia intoxication. Blood chemistry will also show elevations in glutamine. In addition to hyperammonemia, UCD all present with encephalopathy and respiratory alkalosis. The most dramatic presentation of UCD symptoms occurs in neonates between 24 and 48 hours after birth. Afflicted infants exhibit progressively deteriorating symptoms due to the elevated ammonium levels. Deficiencies in arginase do not lead to symptomatic hyperammonemia as severe or as commonly as in the other UCD. Deficiencies in CPS-I (CPSD), OTC (OTCD), argininosuccinate synthetase (ASD), and argininosuccinate lyase (ALD) comprise the common neonatal UCD.

Clinical symptoms are most severe when the UCD is at the level of CPS-I. Symptoms of the UCD usually arise at birth and encompass ataxia, convulsions, lethargy, poor feeding, and, eventually, coma and death if not recognized and treated properly. In fact, the mortality rate is 100% for UCD that are left undiagnosed. Several UCD manifest with late-onset and in these cases the symptoms are hyperactivity, hepatomegaly, and an avoidance of high-protein foods (Table 29-2).

When making a diagnosis of neonatal UCD based upon presenting symptoms and observed hyperammonemia, it is possible to make a differential diagnosis as to which of the 4 enzyme deficiencies is the cause through a series of tests (Figure 29-9).

In general, the treatment of UCD involves the reduction of protein in the diet, removal of excess ammonia, and replacement of intermediates missing from the urea cycle. Administration of levulose reduces ammonia through its action of acidifying the colon. Antibiotics can be administered to kill intestinal ammonia producing bacteria. Sodium benzoate and sodium phenylacetate can be administered to covalently bind glycine (forming hippurate) and glutamine (forming phenylacetylglutamine), respectively. These latter compounds, which contain the ammonia nitrogen, are excreted in the feces. Ammunol is an FDA-approved intravenous solution of 10% sodium benzoate and 10% sodium phenylacetate used in the treatment

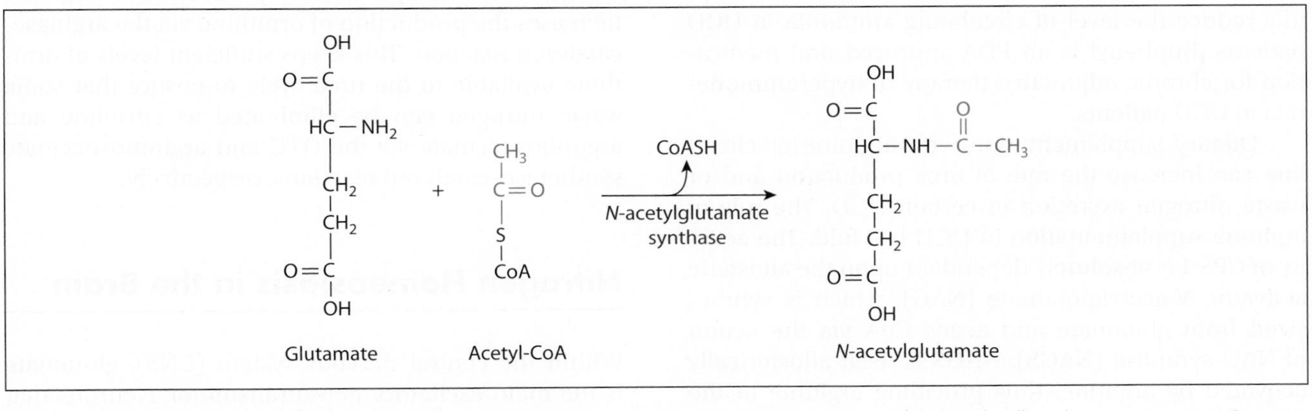

FIGURE 29-8: *N*-acetylglutamate synthetase reaction. Reproduced with permission of themedicalbiochemistrypage, LLC.

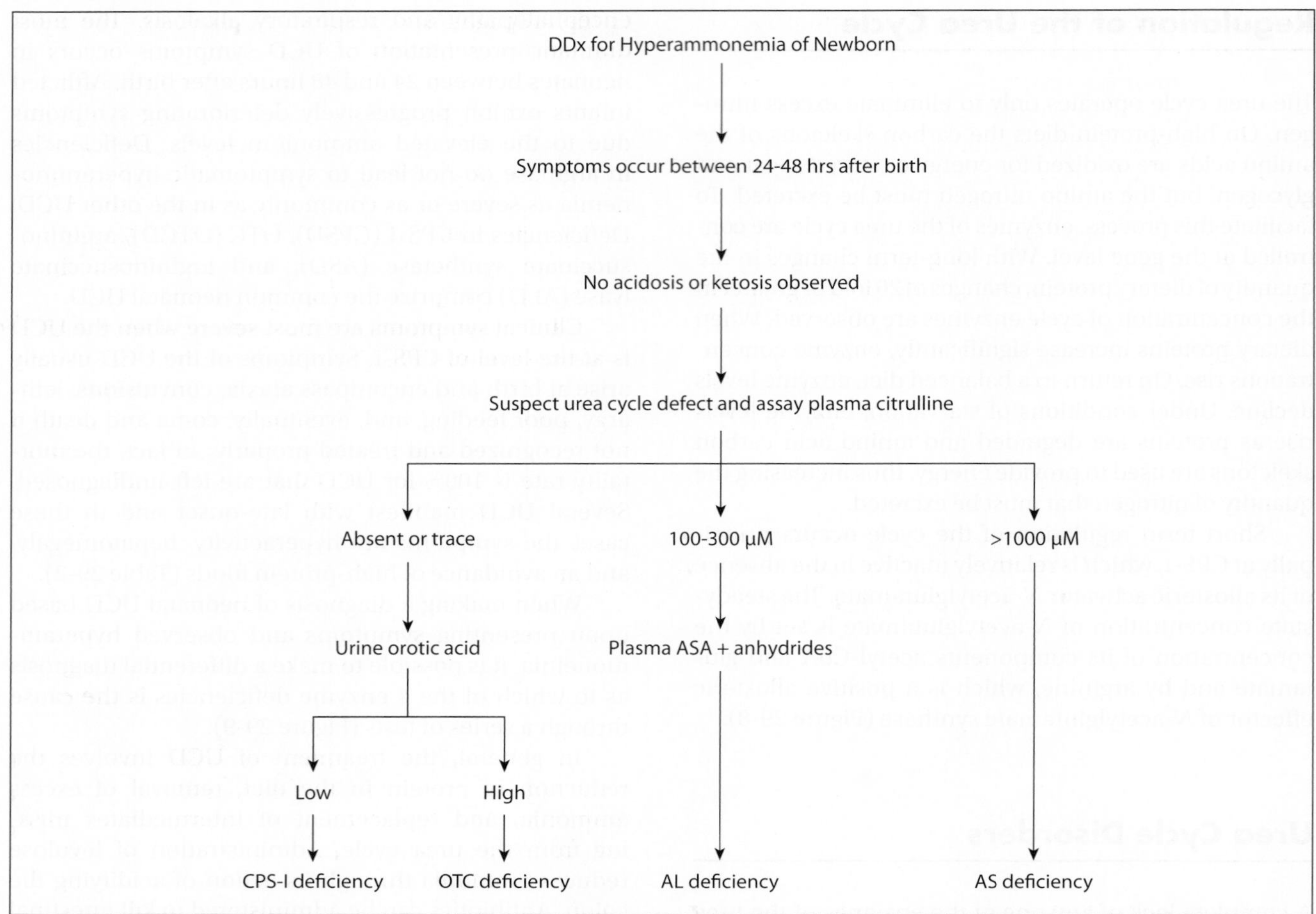

FIGURE 29-9: Schema for the differential diagnosis (DDx) of neonatal UCDs. The presentation of hyperammonemia between 24 and 48 hours after birth (but not before 24 hours after birth) would likely indicate an UCD. This diagnosis can be confirmed by the absence of acidosis or ketosis. The first diagnostic test is to assay for plasma levels of citrulline. Moderately high levels are indicative of argininosuccinate lyase deficiency (ALD) and extremely high levels indicative of argininosuccinate synthetase deficiency (ASD). If no, or trace, citrulline is detected then analysis of urine orotic acid can be used to distinguish between CPS-I deficiency (CPSD) and OTC deficiency (OTCD). Reproduced with permission of themedicalbiochemistrypage, LLC.

of the acute hyperammonemia in UCD patients. However, hemodialysis is the only effective means to rapidly reduce the level of circulating ammonia in UCD patients. Buphenyl is an FDA-approved oral medication for chronic adjunctive therapy of hyperammonemia in UCD patients.

Dietary supplementation with arginine or citrulline can increase the rate of urea production and/or waste nitrogen excretion in certain UCD. The role of arginine supplementation in UCD is 2 fold. The activity of CPS-I is absolutely dependent upon the allosteric activator *N*-acetylglutamate (NAG), which is synthesized from glutamate and acetyl-CoA via the action of NAG synthase (NAGS). NAGS is itself allosterically activated by arginine, thus providing arginine in the diet which in turn can increase the level of active CPS-I driving more ammonia into carbamoyl phosphate. Secondly, the consumption of large amounts of arginine increases the production of ornithine via the arginase-catalyzed reaction. This keeps sufficient levels of ornithine available to the urea cycle to ensure that some waste nitrogen can be eliminated as citrulline and argininosuccinate via the OTC and argininosuccinate synthetase–catalyzed reactions, respectively.

Nitrogen Homeostasis in the Brain

Within the central nervous system (CNS), glutamate is the main excitatory neurotransmitter. Neurons that respond to glutamate are referred to as glutaminergic neurons. Glutaminergic neurons are responsible for the mediation of many vital processes such as the encoding of information, the formation and retrieval of memories, spatial recognition, and the maintenance of consciousness. Excessive excitation of glutamate receptors has been associated with the pathophysiology of hypoxic injury, hypoglycemia, stroke, and epilepsy.

Within the CNS there is an interaction between the cerebral blood flow, neurons, and the protective astrocytes that regulates the metabolism of glutamate, glutamine, and ammonia. This process is referred to as the glutamate-glutamine cycle (Figure 29-10) and it is a critical metabolic process central to overall brain glutamate metabolism. Using presynaptic neurons as the starting point the cycle begins with the release of glutamate from presynaptic secretory vesicles in response to the propagation of a nerve impulse along the axon. The release of glutamate is a Ca^{2+}-dependent process that involves fusion of glutamate-containing presynaptic vesicles with the neuronal membrane. Following release of the glutamate into the synapse it must be rapidly removed to prevent overexcitation of the postsynaptic neurons. Synaptic glutamate is removed by 3 distinct processes. It can be taken up into the postsynaptic cell; it can undergo reuptake into the presynaptic cell from which it was released; or it can be taken up by a third nonneuronal cell, the astrocyte. Postsynaptic neurons remove little glutamate from the synapse and although there is active reuptake into presynaptic neurons the latter process is less important than transport into astrocytes. Glutamate uptake by astrocytes is mediated by Na^+-independent and Na^+-dependent systems.

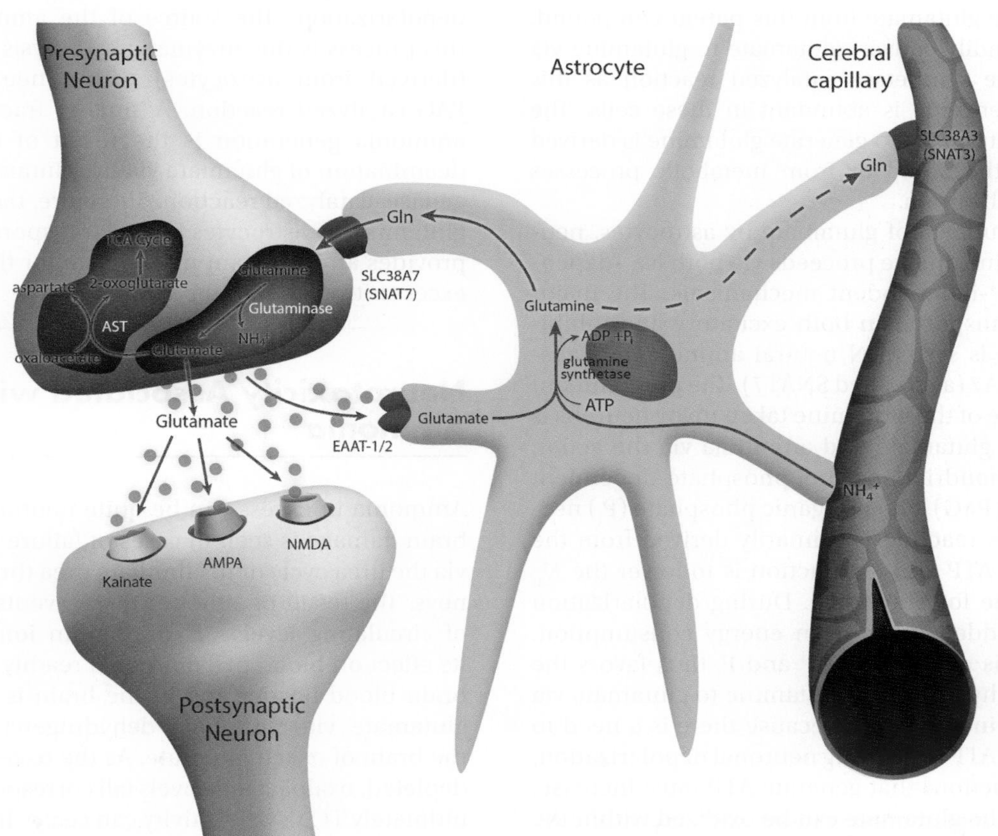

FIGURE 29-10: Brain glutamate-glutamine cycle. Ammonium ion (NH_4^+) in the blood is taken up by astrocytes and incorporated into glutamate via glutamine synthetase. The glutamine then is transported to presynaptic neurons via SLC38A7 (also called sodium-coupled neutral amino acid transporter 7, SNAT7). Within the presynaptic neuron glutamate is formed from the glutamine via the action of glutaminase. The glutamate is packaged in secretory vesicles for release following activation of an action potential. Glutamate in the synaptic cleft can be taken up by astrocytes via the EAAT1 and EAAT2 transporters (excitatory amino acid transporters 1 and 2; also known as glial high-affinity glutamate transporters). Within the astrocyte, the glutamate is converted back to glutamine. Some of the astrocyte glutamine can be transported into the blood via the action of the transporter SLC38A3 (also called sodium-coupled neutral amino acid transporter 3, SNAT3). Reproduced with permission of themedicalbiochemistrypage, LLC.

The Na^+-dependent systems have high affinity for glutamate and are the predominant glutamate-uptake mechanism in the CNS. There are 2 distinct astrocytic Na^+-dependent glutamate transporters identified as EAAT1 (excitatory amino acid transporter 1; also called GLAST) and EAAT2 (also called GLT1).

Following uptake of glutamate, astrocytes have the ability to dispose of the amino acid via export into the blood through capillaries that abut the foot processes of the astrocytes. The problem with glutamate disposal via this mechanism is that it would eventually result in a net loss of carbon and nitrogen from the CNS. In fact, the outcome of astrocyte glutamate uptake is its conversion to glutamine. Glutamine thus serves as a "reservoir" for glutamate but in the form of a nonneuroactive compound. In addition, the incorporation of ammonia into glutamate in the astrocyte serves as a mechanism to buffer brain ammonia.

Release of glutamine from astrocytes allows neurons to derive glutamate from this parent compound. Astrocytes readily convert glutamate to glutamine via the glutamine synthetase–catalyzed reaction as this microsomal enzyme is abundant in these cells. The ammonia that is used to generate glutamine is derived from either the blood or from metabolic processes occurring in the brain.

Like the uptake of glutamate by astrocytes, neuronal glutamine uptake proceeds via both Na^+-dependent and Na^+-independent mechanisms. The major glutamine transporter in both excitatory and inhibitory neurons is system N neutral amino acid transporter SLC38A7 (also called SNAT7). The predominant metabolic fate of the glutamine taken up by neurons is hydrolysis to glutamate and ammonia via the action of the mitochondrial enzyme, phosphate-dependent glutaminase (PAG). The inorganic phosphate (P_i) necessary for this reaction is primarily derived from the hydrolysis of ATP and its function is to lower the K_M of the enzyme for glutamine. During depolarization there is a sudden increase in energy consumption. The hydrolysis of ATP to ADP and P_i thus favors the concomitant hydrolysis of glutamine to glutamate via the resulting increased P_i. Because there is a need to replenish the ATP lost during neuronal depolarization, metabolic reactions that generate ATP must increase. A portion of the glutamate can be oxidized within the nerve cells following transamination. The principal transamination reaction involves aspartate aminotransferase (AST) and yields α-ketoglutarate which is a substrate in the TCA cycle. Glutamine, therefore, is not simply a precursor to neuronal glutamate but a potential fuel, which, like glucose, supports neuronal energy requirements.

During periods of basal metabolism glucose serves as the major metabolic fuel of the brain. During starvation, ketone body synthesis by the liver provides the brain with major fuels during periods when glucose is scarce. Although, as indicated, the brain oxidizes glutamate, there is little passage of either glutamate or glutamine across the blood-brain barrier. Therefore, neither amino acid can serve as a conventional metabolic substrate. Nevertheless, both amino acids are important to overall brain energy production. During periods of hypoglycemia, the consumption of glutamate and glutamine increases. Similarly, during periods of acidosis, when glycolytic flux is restricted, astrocytes increase consumption of both glutamate and glutamine. Although the glutamate-glutamine cycle implies a net release of glutamine by astrocytes, these cells also can oxidize glutamine.

A final consideration in the context of CNS nitrogen homeostasis is the means by which the brain disposes of waste nitrogen since the brain cannot synthesize urea. The brain generates ammonia and its level of generation rises sharply during neuronal depolarization. The source of the ammonia during this process is the enzymatic hydrolysis of glutamine (derived from astrocytes) within neurons via the PAG-catalyzed reaction. A smaller fraction of brain ammonia generation is the result of the oxidative deamination of glutamate via the glutamate dehydrogenase–catalyzed reaction. Therefore, the synthesis of glutamine by astrocytes and its transport to the blood provides an important mechanism for the removal of excess nitrogen from the brain.

Neurotoxicity Associated with Ammonia

Ammonia in excess can be quite neurotoxic. Marked brain damage is seen in cases of failure to make urea via the urea cycle or to eliminate urea through the kidneys. The result of either of these events is a buildup of circulating levels of ammonium ion. Aside from its effect on blood pH, ammonia readily traverses the brain-blood barrier and in the brain is converted to glutamate via glutamate dehydrogenase, depleting the brain of α-ketoglutarate. As the α-ketoglutarate is depleted, oxaloacetate levels fall correspondingly, and ultimately TCA cycle activity can cease. In the absence of aerobic oxidative phosphorylation and TCA cycle activity, irreparable cell damage and neural cell death ensue.

In addition, the increased glutamate leads to increased glutamine formation via simple mass action principles, driving the glutamine synthetase reaction. This depletes glutamate stores which are needed in neural tissue since glutamate is both a neurotransmitter and a precursor for the synthesis of γ-aminobutyrate: GABA, another neurotransmitter. Therefore, reductions in brain glutamate affect energy production as well as neurotransmission.

Additional untoward consequences of hyperammonemia have been attributed to an increase in neural glutamine concentration. Astrocyte cell volume is controlled by intracellular organic osmolyte metabolism. One important organic osmolyte in these cells is glutamine. As glutamine levels rise in the brain, concomitant with increased ammonia uptake, the volume of fluid within astrocytes can also increase resulting in the cerebral edema seen in infants with hyperammonemia caused by UCD. However, the current model of the role of brain glutamine concentration in the neurotoxicity associated with hyperammonemia relates to its adverse effects on mitochondrial function. Under conditions of hyperammonemia, the accumulation of ammonia in brain cells (in particular astrocytes) potentiates glutamine toxicity by facilitating its uptake into mitochondria. The increased mitochondrial uptake of glutamine leads to increased mitochondrial ammonia production triggering mitochondrial impairment, and an ensuing chain of deleterious events leading to astrocyte dysfunction, swelling, and brain edema.

REVIEW QUESTIONS

1. The waste nitrogen from skeletal amino acid catabolism is diverted to the liver for incorporation into urea in which of the following compounds?

A. alanine
B. asparagine
C. aspartate
D. glutamate
E. phenylalanine

Answer A: Alanine transaminase has an important function in the delivery of skeletal muscle carbon and nitrogen (in the form of alanine) to the liver. In skeletal muscle, pyruvate is transaminated to alanine, thus affording an additional route of nitrogen transport from muscle to liver. In the liver, alanine transaminase transfers the ammonia to α-ketoglutarate and regenerates pyruvate. The pyruvate can then be diverted into gluconeogenesis. This process is referred to as the glucose-alanine cycle.

2. When the body becomes acidotic the liver and the kidneys play central roles in reactions designed to reduce the pH of the blood. Which of the following constitutes the primary critical hepatic reaction occurring during periods of acidosis?

A. ammonia incorporation into glutamate forming glutamine
B. ammonia incorporation into α-ketoglutarate forming glutamate
C. glutamine conversion to glutamate releasing ammonia
D. glutamine conversion to α-ketoglutarate releasing ammonia
E. increased production of urea to dispose of ammonia

Answer A: Major reactions that involve the regulation of plasma pH as well as the level of circulating ammonia involve the hepatic and renal enzymes glutamate dehydrogenase (GDH), glutamine synthase (GS), and glutaminase. The liver compartmentalizes GS and glutaminase in order to control the flow of ammonia into glutamine or urea. Under acidotic conditions the liver diverts ammonia to glutamine via the GS reaction. The glutamine then enters the circulation. In fact, glutamine is the major amino acid of the circulation and its role is to ferry ammonia to and from various tissues. In the kidneys, glutamine is hydrolyzed by glutaminase (yielding glutamate) releasing the ammonia to the urine. There the ammonia ionizes to ammonium ion, NH_4^+, which reduces the circulating concentration of hydrogen ion resulting in an increase in the pH. Additionally, the glutamate can be converted to α-ketoglutarate yielding another mole of ammonia, which is ionized by hydrogen ions further increasing the pH.

3. Glutamate dehydrogenase is an extremely important enzyme involved in nitrogen homeostasis. This enzyme catalyzes a reversible reaction that either incorporates or liberates ammonium ion. When catalyzing the reaction in the direction of ammonium ion liberation, the enzyme is allosterically activated by which of the following?

A. adenosine diphosphate (ADP)
B. adenosine triphosphate (ATP)
C. citrate
D. glutamine
E. guanosine triphosphate (GTP)

Answer A: Glutamate dehydrogenase uses both nicotinamide nucleotide cofactors; NAD^+ in the direction of nitrogen liberation and NADPH for nitrogen incorporation. The reaction catalyzing the liberation of ammonia and α-ketoglutarate from glutamate is a key anaplerotic process linking amino acid metabolism with TCA cycle activity. This reaction allows glutamate to play an important role in energy metabolism. Glutamate dehydrogenase provides an oxidizable carbon source used for the production of energy as well as a reduced electron carrier, NADH. In the forward reaction, as shown in Figure 29-3, glutamate dehydrogenase is important in converting free ammonia and α-ketoglutarate to glutamate, forming one of the 20 amino acids required for protein synthesis. As expected for a branch point enzyme with an important link to energy metabolism, glutamate dehydrogenase is regulated by the cell energy charge.

4. Which of the following represents the major compound of the circulation responsible for transport of nitrogen?
A. alanine
B. asparagine
C. glutamate
D. glutamine
E. uric acid

Answer D: Glutamine is the major amino acid found in the circulatory system. Its role there is to carry ammonia to and from various tissues but principally from peripheral tissues to the kidney, where the amide nitrogen is hydrolyzed by the enzyme glutaminase; this process regenerates glutamate and free ammonium ion, which is excreted in the urine.

5. Under acidotic conditions the liver will divert which of the following compounds to the kidneys as a means to increase the pH?
A. ammonia
B. asparagine
C. glutamate
D. glutamine
E. urea

Answer D: Major reactions that involve the regulation of plasma pH as well as the level of circulating ammonia involve the hepatic and renal enzymes glutamate dehydrogenase (GDH), glutamine synthase (GS), and glutaminase. The liver compartmentalizes GS and glutaminase in order to control the flow of ammonia into glutamine or urea. Under acidotic conditions the liver diverts ammonia to glutamine via the GS reaction. The glutamine then enters the circulation. In fact, glutamine is the major amino acid of the circulation and its role is to ferry ammonia to and from various tissues. In the kidneys, glutamine is hydrolyzed by glutaminase (yielding glutamate) releasing the ammonia to the urine. There the ammonia ionizes to ammonium ion, NH_4^+, which reduces the circulating concentration of hydrogen ion resulting in an increase in the pH. Additionally, the glutamate can be converted to α-ketoglutarate yielding another mole of ammonia, which is ionized by hydrogen ions further increasing the pH.

6. You are examining a 6-month-old infant who is experiencing feeding difficulty and generalized hypotonia of the limbs. Additional symptoms reported to you by the infant's parents are strange eye movements tending to cause the eyeballs to rotate up that occur several times a day. Laboratory results indicate significant aminoaciduria and aminoacidemia. Which of the following enzymes is most likely defective in the infant?
A. L-amino acid oxidase
B. asparaginase
C. carbamoyl phosphate synthetase I
D. glutamate dehydrogenase
E. glutaminase

Answer A: In the peroxisomes of mammalian tissues, especially liver, there exists a minor enzymatic pathway for the removal of amino groups from amino acids. L-amino acid oxidase is FMN-linked and has broad specificity for the L-amino acids. A number of substances, including oxygen, can act as electron acceptors from the flavoproteins. If oxygen is the acceptor the product is hydrogen peroxide, which is then rapidly degraded by the catalases found in liver and other tissues. Missing or defective L-amino acid oxidase is commonly associated with oculogyric crisis (OGC; spasmodic movements of the eyeballs that lasts several minute to hours) and causes generalized hyperaminoacidemia and hyperaminoaciduria, generally leading to neurotoxicity and early death.

7. A deficiency of argininosuccinate synthetase (ASD) can be suspected in a neonate with elevated serum ammonia. To discriminate the fact that the hyperammonemia is indeed due to ASD and not due to a deficiency in other urea cycle enzymes, one can assay for the serum concentration of citrulline and orotic acid. Which of the following would best describe the expected findings?
A. both citrulline and orotate levels will be low
B. citrulline levels will be absent but orotate will be elevated
C. citrulline levels will be low but orotate levels will be elevated
D. citrulline levels will be 300 times normal, orotate will be near normal

Answer D: A urea cycle disorder (UCD) is likely in a neonate that has elevated serum ammonia appearing, not before, but between 24 and 48 hours after a normal term delivery. There are 3 hallmark symptoms associated with UCD. These are hyperammonemia, encephalopathy, and respiratory alkalosis. Thus, elevated serum ammonia is not, in and of itself, indicative of a specific defect in the urea cycle. An analysis of the levels of various amino and organic acids in the plasma and urine is the primary key to determining which defect led to the elevation in serum ammonia. Differential diagnosis of neonatal hyperammonemia as a consequence of a UCD can be accomplished by measurement of plasma citrulline and urinary orotic acid levels. Shown in Figure 29-9 is the standard differential diagnosis chart for determining which of the 4 possible neonatal UCDs are the causes of the hyperammonemia. First, the hyperammonemia appears in the absence of any significant acidosis or ketosis. If analysis of serum citrulline demonstrates that it is >1000 μM, it is confirmed that the clinical symptoms are due to a deficiency in argininosuccinate synthetase. In this circumstance, it is not necessary to assay for levels of urinary orotic acid, but they would be expected to be normal.

8. A newborn that developed seizures 2 days after birth was diagnosed with elevated serum NH_4^+, glutamate, and alanine. A neonatal urea cycle defect was suspected so a urinalysis was performed to assay for orotic acid and serum assayed for citrulline. The levels of both were found not to be elevated. A defect in which enzyme of the urea cycle would most likely account for the symptoms observed in this infant?

A. arginase
B. argininosuccinate lyase
C. argininosuccinate synthetase
D. carbamoyl phosphate synthetase I (CPS-I)
E. ornithine transcarbamoylase (OTC)

Answer D: Differential diagnosis of neonatal hyperammonemia, as a consequence of a UCD can be accomplished by measurement of plasma citrulline and urinary orotic acid levels. Refer to Figure 29-9 which shows the standard differential diagnosis chart for determining which of the 4 possible neonatal UCDs are the causes of the hyperammonemia. First, the hyperammonemia appears in the absence of any significant acidosis or ketosis. If analysis of serum cuitrulline demonstrates undetectable levels, then deficiencies in argininosuccinate lyase and argininosuccinate synthetase can be eliminated as causes of the symptoms. Assay for levels of urinary orotic acid will allow a discrimination between carbamoyl phosphate synthetase I and ornithine transcarbamoylase deficiencies. Since the levels of orotic acid were found to be insignificant, the symptoms must be due to deficiency in carbamoyl phosphate synthetase I.

9. A 2-day-old infant is brought to the ER suffering a seizure. Analysis of serum NH_4^+ reveals it to be quite high. Suspecting a urea cycle impairment the ER physician initiates hemodialysis which reduces the NH_4^+ levels. Subsequent to the hemodialysis the infant is treated with supplemental arginine which maintains the reduction in serum NH_4^+. The ability of arginine to render this effect stems from it's role in activating the synthesis of an activator of one of the enzymes of the urea cycle. Which of the following represents this potent activator whose synthesis is induced by arginine?

A. argininosuccinate
B. bicarbonate ion
C. fumarate
D. *N*-acetylcysteine
E. *N*-acetylglutamate

Answer E: Short-term regulation of the urea cycle occurs principally at carbamoyl phosphate synthetase I (CPS-I)–catalyzed step. CPS-I is relatively inactive in the absence of its obligate activator *N*-acetylglutamate. The steady-state concentration of *N*-acetylglutamate is set by the concentration of its components acetyl-CoA and glutamate and by arginine, which is a positive allosteric effector of *N*-acetylglutamate synthase.

10. A child was born at home and developed seizures 2 days after birth. Upon examination in the ER it was found that the infant had elevated serum NH_4^+, glutamate, and alanine. The ER physician suspected that the child was suffering from a defect in the urea cycle and ordered a urinalysis to assess the level of orotic acid and the serum was assayed for the level of citrulline. Orotic acid levels were above normal and citrulline was barely detectable. A defect in which enzyme of the urea cycle would most likely account for the symptoms observed in this infant?

A. arginase
B. argininosuccinate lyase
C. argininosuccinate synthetase
D. carbamoyl phosphate synthetase I (CPS-I)
E. ornithine transcarbamoylase (OTC)

Answer E: Differential diagnosis of neonatal hyperammonemia as a consequence of a UCD can be accomplished by measurement of plasma citrulline and urinary orotic acid levels. Refer to Figure 29-9 which shows the standard differential diagnosis chart for determining which of the 4 possible neonatal UCDs are the causes of the hyperammonemia. First, the hyperammonemia appears in the absence of any significant acidosis or ketosis. If analysis of serum cuitrulline demonstrates undetectable levels, then deficiencies in argininosuccinate lyase and argininosuccinate synthetase can be eliminated as causes of the symptoms.

Assay for levels of urinary orotic acid will allow a discrimination between carbamoyl phosphate synthetase I and ornithine transcarbamoylase deficiencies. Since the levels of orotic acid were found to be elevated, the symptoms must be due to deficiency in ornithine transcarbamoylase (OTC).

11. An individual harboring a mutation in OTC would be expected to exhibit which of the following measurable abnormalities?
A. citrullinemia
B. elevated urinary excretion of argininosuccinic acid
C. elevation in blood orotic acid
D. excess production of foam cells
E. uric acid deposition in the joints

Answer C: A deficiency in OTC results in one of the urea cycle defect diseases, which are the major causes of hyperammonemia in the newborn. Differentiation of which urea cycle enzyme is defective and causing the hyperammonemia can be accomplished by analysis of the levels of the various intermediates in the cycle (see Figure 29-9). Since a defect in OTC prevents incorporation of carbamoyl phosphate into ornithine, the carbamoylphosphate will leave the mitochondria and serve as a precursor for the synthesis of the pyrimidine nucleotides in excess of the need, leading to an elevation of orotic acid (pyrimidine intermediate) in the blood.

12. A 2-day-old infant boy delivered by normal labor (with no known prenatal risk factors) has become lethargic and requires stimulation for feeding. When vomiting and hyperventilation ensued, routine laboratory results showed blood urea nitrogen (BUN) less than 1 mg/dL. The infant quickly lapses into a coma and was placed on a ventilator. Bulging of the fontanel suggested an intracranial hemorrhage, but a CT scan revealed only cerebral edema. Within several hours, the infant dies. Death is ascribed to sepsis; however, a postmortem analysis of the plasma samples taken at admission showed dramatically elevated serum ammonia and citrulline levels 100 times normal. Which of the following represents the enzyme deficiency associated with these severe neonatal symptoms?
A. argininosuccinate synthetase
B. carbamoylphosphate synthetase I
C. 3-Hydroxy-3-methylglutaryl-CoA (HMG-CoA) lyase
D. medium-chain acyl-CoA dehydrogenase
E. pyruvate carboxylase

Answer A: The clinical presentation of patients with defects in several enzymes of urea synthesis is virtually identical. These enzymes are CPS-I, ornithine transcarbamoylase (OTC), argininosuccinate synthetase (AS), and argininosuccinase. The hallmark of these urea cycle enzyme defects is a normal birth with no known prenatal risk factors. Within 24–72 hours after birth the infant becomes lethargic and requires stimulation for feeding. Additional symptoms develop within hours, including vomiting, increased lethargy, hypothermia, and hyperventilation. The hyperventilation is often misdiagnosed as pulmonary disease. Sepsis is often suspected. Routine blood work indicates a reduced BUN. Lack of proper intervention will lead to coma and death. Correct analysis of hyperammonemia is paramount to proper treatment as this is indicative of a urea cycle defect when presenting in the newborn. Analysis of plasma amino acids can aid in the differentiation of which enzyme is defective. Elevated citrulline (to 100 times normal levels) results from a deficiency in AS.

13. Neonatal urea cycle defects are usually misdiagnosed because of a failure to assess which of the following?
A. level of ammonia in the blood
B. level of argininosuccinate in the blood
C. level of citrulline in the blood
D. level of orotic acid in the urine
E. odor of acetone on the breath

Answer A: Seemingly normal full-term infants suffering from urea cycle defects will usually become lethargic and need stimulation to feed within 24–72 hours after birth. When presented in the emergency many will be comatose. One obvious outward clinical sign will be a bulging fontanel due to the ammonia-induced encephalopathy. If a correct diagnosis of hyperammonemia is not made in a timely manner these infants will die.

14. Which of the following would most likely be associated with a negative nitrogen balance?
A. consuming a high-protein diet
B. neonatal development
C. post-starvation feeding
D. pregnancy
E. surgical recovery

Answer A: Unlike fats and carbohydrates, nitrogen has no designated storage depots in the body. Since the half-life of many proteins is short (on the order of hours), increased dietary intake of protein will result in an concomitant increase in amino acid degradation resulting in increased nitrogen excretion. When more nitrogen is excreted than is incorporated into the body, an individual is in negative nitrogen balance. Normal, healthy adults are generally in nitrogen balance, with intake and excretion being very well matched. Young growing children, adults recovering from major illness, and pregnant women are often in positive nitrogen balance. Their intake of nitrogen exceeds their loss as net protein synthesis proceeds.

15. An unconscious 37-year-old man is brought to the ER. His wife reports that they were at home having dinner celebrating his birthday. She indicates that normally he does not drink but they were having champagne for the celebration. She indicates that shortly after they finished the bottle he became disorientated and irritable and then he began experiencing delusions. When he began to have a seizure she called 911. By the time the ambulance arrived he was unconscious. Blood tests taken when he was admitted show significantly elevated serum ammonia. A deficiency in which of the following enzymes is most likely the cause of this patients symptoms?

A. alanine transaminase
B. asparaginase
C. citrin
D. glutamate dehydrogenase
E. glutaminase

Answer C: Citrullinemia type II (CTLN2) is caused by deficiency in the gene encoding the mitochondria transporter citrin (SLC25A13). Manifestations of CTLN2 are recurrent hyperammonemia with neuropsychiatric symptoms including nocturnal delirium, aggression, irritability, hyperactivity, delusions, disorientation, restlessness, drowsiness, loss of memory, flapping tremor, convulsive seizures, and coma. The symptoms of CTLN2 are often provoked by alcohol and sugar intake, as well as by certain medications, and/or surgery.

16. A child was born at home and developed seizures 2 days after birth. Upon examination in the ER it was found that the infant had elevated serum NH_4^+, glutamate, and alanine. The ER physician suspected that the child was suffering from a defect in the urea cycle. Which of the following is the most appropriate course of action to take with this patient?

A. administer arginine via IV
B. administer glucose via IV
C. change the infants formula to one with no protein
D. give the infant fluids and continue to monitor symptoms
E. immediate hemodialysis

Answer E: In general, the treatment of UCD involves the reduction of protein in the diet, removal of excess ammonia, and replacement of intermediates missing from the urea cycle. Administration of levulose reduces ammonia through its action of acidifying the colon. Antibiotics can be administered to kill intestinal ammonia producing bacteria. Sodium benzoate and sodium phenylacetate can be administered to covalently bind glycine (forming hippurate) and glutamine (forming phenylacetylglutamine), respectively. However, hemodialysis is the only effective means to rapidly reduce the level of circulating ammonia in UCD patients.

17. Which of the following vitamins is critically important in the overall process of nitrogen transfer from α-amino acids to α-keto acids?

A. riboflavin
B. thiamine
C. vitamin B_6
D. vitamin B_{12}
E. vitamin C

Answer C: The dominant reactions involved in removing amino acid nitrogen from the body are known as transaminations. Transaminations involve moving an α-amino group from a donor α-amino acid to the keto carbon of an acceptor α-keto acid. These reversible reactions are catalyzed by a group of intracellular enzymes known as aminotransferases, which generally employ covalently bound pyridoxal phosphate as a cofactor.

18. Under which of the following conditions would you most likely expect the glutamate dehydrogenase reaction to proceed in the direction of glutamate synthesis?

A. high ATP:ADP ratio
B. high NADH levels
C. high NADPH levels
D. low NADH levels
E. low NADPH levels

Answer C: Glutamate dehydrogenase utilizes both nicotinamide nucleotide cofactors; NAD^+ in the direction of nitrogen liberation and $NADP^+$ for nitrogen incorporation. In the forward reaction (as shown in Figure 29-3) glutamate dehydrogenase is important in converting free ammonia and α-ketoglutarate to glutamate. The reverse reaction is a key anapleurotic process linking amino acid metabolism with TCA cycle activity. In the reverse reaction, glutamate dehydrogenase provides an oxidizable carbon source used for the production of energy as well as a reduced electron carrier, NADH. As expected for a branch point enzyme with an important link to energy metabolism, glutamate dehydrogenase is regulated by the cell energy charge. ATP and GTP are positive allosteric effectors of the formation of glutamate, whereas ADP and GDP are positive allosteric effectors of the reverse reaction. Thus, when the level of ATP is high, conversion of glutamate to α-ketoglutarate and other TCA cycle intermediates is limited; when the cellular energy charge is low, glutamate is converted to ammonia and oxidizable TCA cycle intermediates.

19. The most abundant end product of nitrogen metabolism in humans is which of the following?

A. allantoin
B. ammonium ion
C. glutamine
D. urea
E. uric acid

Answer C: Glutamate plays the central role in mammalian nitrogen flow, serving as both a nitrogen donor and nitrogen acceptor. Glutamine is the nitrogen repository found in the circulatory system. Its role there is to carry ammonia to and from various tissues but principally from peripheral tissues to the kidney. In the kidneys, glutamine is hydrolyzed by glutaminase (yielding glutamate) releasing the ammonia to the urine. Additionally, the glutamate can be converted to α-ketoglutarate yielding another mole of ammonia which is excreted.

20. Which of the following ketoacids provides the carbon skeleton for an amino acid capable of carrying 2 atoms of nitrogen per molecule from other tissues to the liver and kidney via the blood?

A. acetoacetate
B. α-ketoglutarate
C. α-ketoisocaproic acid
D. oxaloacetate
E. pyruvate

Answer B: α-Ketoglutarate is capable of accepting 2 moles of ammonia, first via the action of glutamate dehydrogenase yielding glutamate and then via glutamine synthetase yielding glutamaine. Glutamate plays the central role in mammalian nitrogen flow, serving as both a nitrogen donor and nitrogen acceptor. Glutamine is the nitrogen repository found in the circulatory system. Its role there is to carry ammonia to and from various tissues but principally from peripheral tissues to the kidney.

21. A 3-day-old newborn female with a deficiency of mitochondrial carbamoyl phosphate synthetase I develops seizures and lapses into a coma. Which of the following changes in blood concentration is the most likely cause?

A. decreased glucose
B. increased ammonia
C. increased ketone bodies
D. increased lactate
E. increased urea

Answer B: A deficiency in carbamoyl phosphate synthetase I is reflective of a urea cycle disorder. A common thread to most UCDs is hyperammonemia leading to ammonia intoxication.

22. A 2-day-old male newborn develops lethargy, poor feeding, vomiting, and rapid respirations. He was delivered at term after an uncomplicated pregnancy. His brother died in infancy. He has been breast-fed since birth. Serum studies indicate an increased ammonia concentration and a nondetectable citrulline concentration. Urine orotic acid concentration is markedly increased. A deficiency in which of the following enzyme activities is the most likely cause of these findings?

A. branched-chain α-keto acid dehydrogenase
B. glucose 6-phosphatase
C. hypoxanthine-guaninephosphoribosyltransferase
D. medium-chain acyl-CoA dehydrogenase
E. ornithine transcarbmoylase

Answer E: Differential diagnosis of neonatal hyperammonemia, as a consequence of a UCD can be accomplished by measurement of plasma citrulline and urinary orotic acid levels. Refer to Figure 29-9 which shows the standard differential diagnosis chart for determining which of the 4 possible neonatal UCDs are the causes of the hyperammonemia. First, the hyperammonemia appears in the absence of any significant acidosis or ketosis. If analysis of serum cuitrulline demonstrates undetectable levels, then deficiencies in argininosuccinate lyase and argininosuccinate synthetase can be eliminated as causes of the symptoms. Assay for levels of urinary orotic acid will allow a discrimination between carbamoyl phosphate synthetase I and ornithine transcarbamoylase deficiencies. Since the levels of orotic acid were found to be elevated, the symptoms must be due to deficiency in ornithine transcarbamoylase (OTC).

23. Which of the following enzymes plays a key role in the formation of ammonium ions in the proximal renal tubule?

A. carbonic anhydrase
B. glucokinae
C. glutaminase
D. Na^+/K^+-ATPase
E. PKA

Answer C: Major reactions that involve the regulation of plasma pH as well as the level of circulating ammonia involve the hepatic and renal enzymes glutamate dehydrogenase (GDH), glutamine synthase (GS), and glutaminase. Under acidotic conditions the liver diverts ammonia to glutamine via the GS reaction. The glutamine then enters the circulation. In the kidneys, glutamine is hydrolyzed by glutaminase (yielding glutamate) releasing the ammonia to the urine. There the ammonia ionizes to ammonium ion, NH_4^+, which reduces the circulating concentration of hydrogen ion resulting in an increase in the pH.

Checklist

- ✓ Nitrogen from the biosphere enters the human body as dietary free amino acids, protein, and the ammonia produced by intestinal tract bacteria. Glutamate dehydrogenase and glutamine synthetase effect the conversion of ammonia into the amino acids glutamate and glutamine, respectively. Amino and amide groups from these 2 substances are freely transferred to other carbon skeletons by transamination and transamidation reactions.
- ✓ Glutamate dehydrogenase and glutamine synthetase represent the major nitrogen-mobilizing enzymes in the body. Glutamate dehydrogenase is considered a gateway enzyme serving to regulate energy production and waste removal during amino acid metabolism.
- ✓ Glutamine is the major form of nontoxic nitrogen in the circulation. In this capacity, it plays a major role in delivery waste nitrogen to the kidneys for excretion and also the release of the nitrogen allows the kidneys to balance fluid pH.
- ✓ Nitrogen homeostasis in the brain is critical for maintaining adequate levels of the neurotransmitter glutamate and to prevent nitrogen toxicity. Within the CNS there is an interaction between the cerebral blood flow, neurons, and the protective astrocytes that regulates the metabolism of glutamate, glutamine, and ammonia. This process is referred to as the glutamate-glutamine cycle and it is a critical metabolic process central to overall brain glutamate metabolism.
- ✓ The urea cycle represent the primary pathway for converting waste nitrogen from amino acid catabolism into a soluble nontoxic substance that is easily excreted. The cycle takes place both in the cytosol and the mitochondria of hepatocytes.
- ✓ Defects in enzymes of the urea cycle are the primary cause of potentially severe and fatal hyperammonemia. The earlier in the cycle a defect is encountered, the higher the potential for more severe hyperammonemia.
- ✓ Treatment of urea cycle disorders is principally aimed at controlling the level of free ammonia. This includes the reduction of protein in the diet, removal of excess ammonia, and replacement of intermediates missing from the urea cycle.

CHAPTER

30 Nitrogen: Amino Acid Metabolism

CHAPTER OUTLINE

High-Yield Terms

Glucogenic: relating to amino acids whose catabolic products can be used for net glucose synthesis during gluconeogenesis

Ketogenic: relating to amino acids whose catabolic products enter the tricarboxylic acid (TCA) cycle but cannot be used for net glucose synthesis during gluconeogenesis

Essential amino acid: any amino acid that cannot be formed de novo or from other precursor compounds within mammalian cells

Glutamate dehydrogenase: critical enzyme catalyzing the interconversion of glutamate and α-ketoglutarate, serves as a gateway reaction between cellular energy demands and nitrogen homeostasis

Asparaginase: enzyme catalyzing the deamination of asparagine to aspartate, enzyme is used clinically as a chemotherapeutic treatment for certain leukemias

Cystathionine β-synthase: enzyme involved in cysteine biosynthesis, deficiencies are most common cause of homocystinurias

Glycine cleavage complex: also called glycine decarboxylase, enzyme-catabolizing glycine, defects in activity cause glycine encephalopathy

Phenylketonuria (PKU): a particular form of hyperphenylalaninemia resulting from defects in the phenylalanine hydroxylase gene

Branched-chain amino acid: consists of leucine, isoleucine, and lysine; defects in the catabolic enzyme branched-chain keto acid dehydrogenase (BCKD) result in Maple syrup urine disease (MSUD)

Alkaptonuria: first inherited error in metabolism to be characterized, benign disease caused by defects in the tyrosine-catabolizing enzyme homogentisate oxidase, urine of afflicted patients turns brown on exposure to air

Amino Acid Uptake

All tissues have some capability for synthesis of the nonessential amino acids, amino acid remodeling, and conversion of nonamino acid carbon skeletons into amino acids and other derivatives that contain nitrogen. However, many amino acids cannot be synthesized by mammalian cells nor derived from other precursors and so must be acquired from the diet. The process of protein digestion followed by peptide and amino acid uptake by the gut is described in detail in Chapter 43. Briefly, proteins are degraded to free amino acids, di- and tripeptides by gut and pancreatic peptidases. Intestinal uptake of amino acids involves several different Na^+-dependent amino acid transporters present in the apical membrane of intestinal luminal brush border cells. These include acidic, basic, and neutral amino acid transporters, as well as a proline and glycine transporter. The inability to effectively absorb amino acids from the gut can lead to serious developmental and physiologic consequences, such as in the case of Hartnup disorder (Clinical Box 30-1).

Metabolic Classifications of Amino Acids

In times of both dietary surplus and fasting/starvation, the potentially toxic nitrogen of amino acids is eliminated via transaminations, deamination, and urea formation; the carbon skeletons are generally conserved as carbohydrate, via gluconeogenesis, or as fatty acid via fatty acid synthesis pathways. In this respect, amino acids fall into 3 categories: glucogenic, ketogenic, or glucogenic and ketogenic. Glucogenic amino acids are those that give rise to a net production of pyruvate or TCA cycle intermediates, such as α-ketoglutarate or oxaloacetate, all of which are precursors to glucose via gluconeogenesis. All amino acids except lysine and leucine are at least partly glucogenic. Lysine and leucine are the only amino acids that are solely ketogenic, giving rise only to acetyl-CoA or acetoacetyl-CoA, neither of which can bring about net glucose production.

A small group of amino acids comprised of isoleucine, phenylalanine, threonine, tryptophan, and tyrosine give rise to both glucose and fatty acid precursors and are thus characterized as being glucogenic and ketogenic. Finally, it should be recognized that amino acids have a third possible fate. During times of starvation, the reduced carbon skeleton is used for energy production, with the result that it is oxidized to CO_2 and H_2O (Table 30-1).

The amino acids arginine, methionine, and phenylalanine are considered essential for reasons not directly related to lack of synthesis. Arginine is synthesized by mammalian cells but at a rate that is insufficient to meet the growth needs of the body and the majority that is synthesized is cleaved to form urea. Methionine is required in large amounts to produce cysteine if the latter amino acid is not adequately supplied in the diet. Similarly, phenylalanine is needed in large amounts to form tyrosine if the latter is not adequately supplied in the diet.

CLINICAL BOX 30-1: HARTNUP DISORDER

Hartnup disorder was first described in 1956 in the Hartnup family in London as a renal aminoaciduria of neutral amino acids associated with a pellagra-like skin rash and episodes of cerebellar ataxia. The disorder is caused by a defect in neutral amino acid transport in the apical brush border membranes of the small intestine and in kidney proximal tubules. The transporter is a member of the solute carrier family, specifically the SLC6A19 transporter. SLC6A19 is also known as the system B(0)–neutral amino acid transporter 1 (B[0]AT1). SLC6A19 is responsible for the transport of neutral amino acids in a Na^+-dependent transport reaction. The lack of intestinal tryptophan transport is responsible for most if not all clinical phenotypes of Hartnup disorder. The pellagra-like skin rash seen on sun-exposed areas of skin in Hartnup disorder patients is most likely the result of nicotinamide deficiency due to a lack of tryptophan, which is a precursor for its synthesis. Symptoms of Hartnup disorder may begin in infancy or early childhood, but sometimes they begin as late as early adulthood. Symptoms may be triggered by sunlight, fever, drugs, or emotional or physical stress. Most symptoms occur sporadically and are caused by a deficiency of niacin. When Hartnup disorder manifests during infancy, the symptoms can be variable in clinical presentation. These symptoms include failure to thrive, photosensitivity, intermittent ataxia, nystagmus, and tremor.

TABLE 30-1: Essential vs Nonessential Amino Acids

Nonessential	*Essential*
Alanine	Arginine
Asparagine	Histidine
Aspartate	Isoleucine
Cysteine	Leucine
Glutamate	Lysine
Glutamine	Methionine
Glycine	Phenylalanine
Proline	Threonine
Serine	Tryptophan
Tyrosine	Valine

Glutamate and Glutamine Metabolism

Glutamate is synthesized by the reductive amination of α-ketoglutarate catalyzed by glutamate dehydrogenase (see Figure 29-3). As discussed in the Chapter 29, the glutamate dehydrogenase reaction plays a central role in overall nitrogen homeostasis. In addition, glutamate is synthesized from α-ketoglutarate via the action of several different aminotransferases, with the amino nitrogen being donated by a number of different amino acids. In this capacity, glutamate serves as the major "transporter" of waste nitrogen during amino acid catabolism.

Glutamine is produced from glutamate by a transamidation reaction catalyzed by the ATP-dependent enzyme glutamine synthetase (see Figure 29-4).

Aminotransferase reactions are readily reversible. The direction of any individual transamination depends principally on the concentration of reactants and products. By contrast, transamidation reactions, which are dependent on ATP, are considered irreversible. As a consequence, the degradation of glutamine takes place by a hydrolytic pathway rather than by a reversal of the pathway by which it was formed.

Glutaminase (see Figure 29-5) is an important kidney tubule enzyme involved in converting glutamine (primarily from liver) to glutamate and NH_4^+, with the NH_4^+ being excreted in the urine. Glutaminase activity is present in many other tissues as well, although its activity is not nearly as prominent as in the kidney. Of particular significance to renal control of blood pH, the glutamate produced from glutamine can be catabolized to α-ketoglutarate and another mole of NH_4^+ via the action of glutamate dehydrogenase. The α-ketoglutarate can serve as precursor for renal gluconeogenesis (see Chapter 13), making glutamine a glucogenic amino acid.

Aspartate and Asparagine Metabolism

Like glutamate, aspartate is synthesized by a simple 1-step transamination reaction catalyzed by aspartate aminotransferase (AST) (Figure 30-1). This reaction uses the aspartate α-keto acid analog, oxaloacetate (OAA), and glutamate as the amino donor. AST is also historically referred to as serum glutamate-oxalate transaminase (SGOT). The transfer of nitrogen to OAA is an important component of substrate generation (aspartate) for the production of ornithine in the urea cycle (see Chapter 29).

Asparagine is synthesized from aspartate via the action of asparagine synthetase (Figure 30-2) which, like glutamine synthetase, is an ATP-dependent aminotransferase reaction. Aspartate can also be formed by deamination of asparagine catalyzed by asparaginase (Figure 30-3). Asparaginase has utility as an anti-cancer drug due to the role of asparagine in hematopoietic cancers (Clinical Box 30-2).

Alanine and the Glucose-Alanine Cycle

Aside from its role in protein synthesis, alanine is second only to glutamine in prominence as a circulating amino acid. In this capacity, it serves a unique role in the transfer of nitrogen from peripheral tissues to the liver. Alanine is transferred to the circulation by many tissues, but mainly by muscle, in which alanine is formed from pyruvate at a rate proportional to intracellular pyruvate levels. Liver accumulates plasma alanine, reverses the transamination that occurs in muscle, and

High-Yield Concept

Glutamine represents the major nitrogen-carrying compound in the blood and as such plays a critical role in overall nitrogen homeostasis (see Chapter 29).

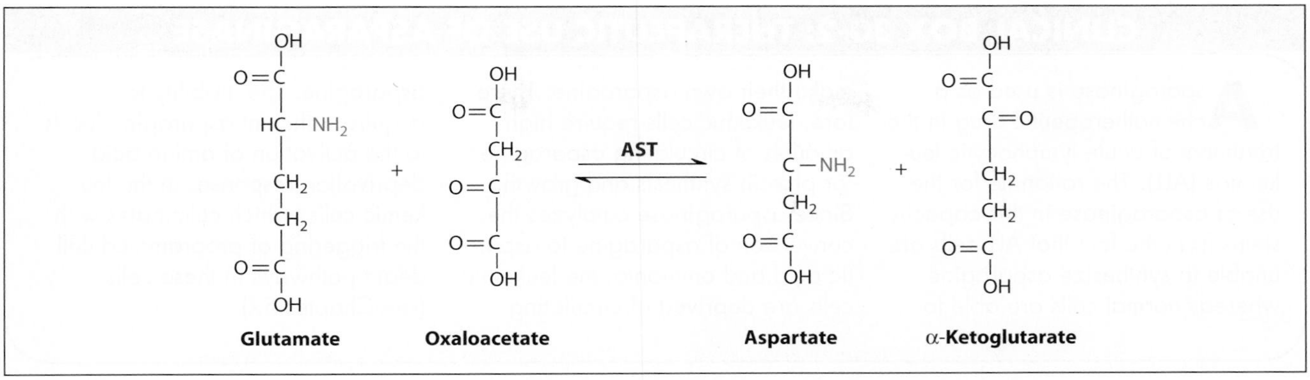

Glutamate + Oxaloacetate ⇌ (AST) Aspartate + α-Ketoglutarate

FIGURE 30-1: Aspartate aminotransferase (AST) reaction. Reproduced with permission of themedicalbiochemistrypage, LLC.

Aspartate + Glutamine → (ATP → AMP + PP_i; Asparagine synthetase) Asparagine + Glutamate

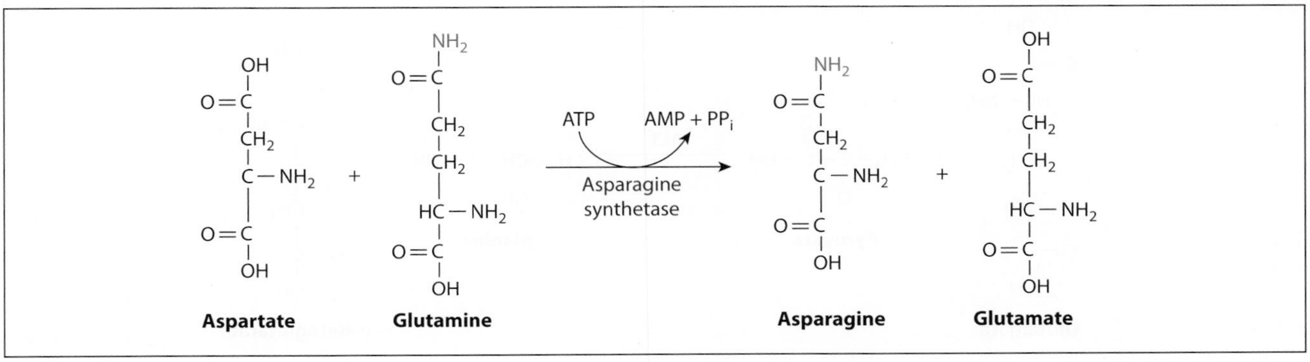

FIGURE 30-2: Asparagine synthetase reaction. Reproduced with permission of themedicalbiochemistrypage, LLC.

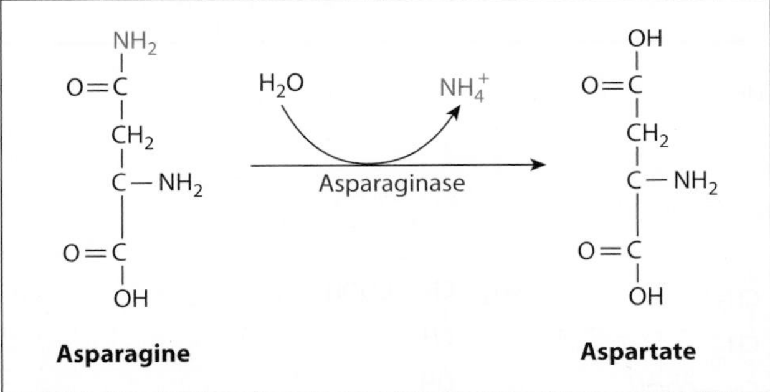

FIGURE 30-3: Asparaginase reaction. Reproduced with permission of themedicalbiochemistrypage, LLC.

proportionately increases urea production. The pyruvate is either oxidized (see Chapter 16) or converted to glucose via gluconeogenesis (see Chapter 13). When alanine transfer from muscle to liver is coupled with glucose transport from liver back to muscle, the process is known as the *glucose-alanine cycle* (see Figure 13-2).

There are 2 main pathways to production of alanine: directly from protein degradation, and via the transamination of pyruvate by alanine transaminase (ALT) (Figure 30-4). ALT is also historically referred to as serum glutamate-pyruvate transaminase (SGPT).

Cysteine and Methionine Metabolism

Cysteine and methionine metabolism are interrelated as the sulfur for cysteine synthesis comes from methionine (Figure 30-5). In cysteine synthesis, homocysteine condenses with serine to produce cystathionine, which is subsequently cleaved by cystathionase to produce cysteine and α-ketobutyrate. The sum of the latter 2 reactions is known as *trans-sulfuration*. The α-ketobutyrate from this reaction is first converted to propionyl-CoA and then via a 3-step process (see Figure 25-4) to the TCA cycle intermediate, succinyl-CoA. Other than protein, the most important product of cysteine metabolism is the bile salt precursor taurine, which is used to form the bile acid conjugates, taurocholate and taurochenodeoxycholate (see Chapter 27).

The 2 key enzymes of this pathway, cystathionine β–synthase (CBS) and cystathionase (cystathionine lyase), use pyridoxal phosphate as a cofactor. In addition, both enzymes are under regulatory control. Cystathionase is negatively regulated by the allosteric effector, cysteine. Cysteine also inhibits the expression of the *CBS* gene.

Genetic defects have been identified in both the *CBS* and the cystathionase genes. Missing or impaired *CBS* leads to homocystinuria (Clinical Box 30-3).

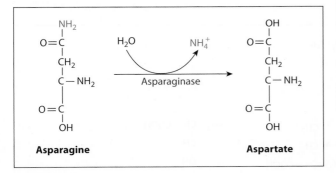

CLINICAL BOX 30-2: THERAPEUTIC USE OF ASPARAGINASE

Asparaginase is used as a chemotherapeutic drug in the treatment of acute lymphocytic leukemias (ALL). The rationale for the use of asparaginase in this capacity stems from the fact that ALL cells are unable to synthesize asparagine, whereas normal cells are able to make their own asparagine. Therefore, leukemic cells require high amounts of circulating asparagine for protein synthesis and growth. Since asparaginase catalyzes the conversion of asparagine to aspartic acid and ammonia, the leukemic cells are deprived of circulating asparagine. The inability to acquire sufficient asparagine leads to the activation of amino acid deprivation responses in the leukemic cells, which culminates with the triggering of programmed cell death pathways in these cells (see Chapter 52).

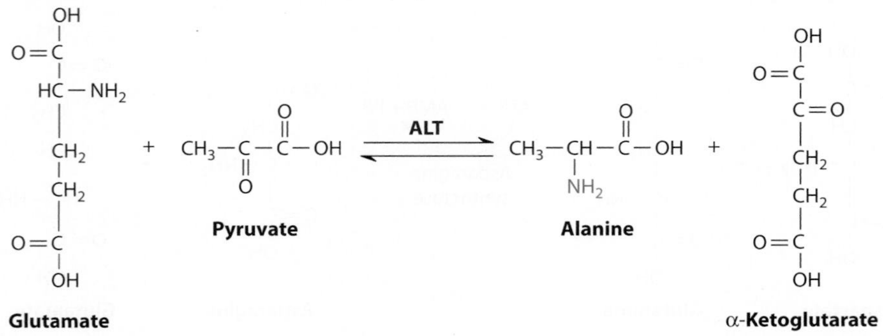

$$\text{Glutamate} + \underset{\text{Pyruvate}}{CH_3-CO-COOH} \underset{}{\overset{\text{ALT}}{\rightleftharpoons}} \underset{\text{Alanine}}{CH_3-CH(NH_2)-COOH} + \alpha\text{-Ketoglutarate}$$

FIGURE 30-4: Alanine transaminase (ALT) reaction. Reproduced with permission of themedicalbiochemistrypage, LLC.

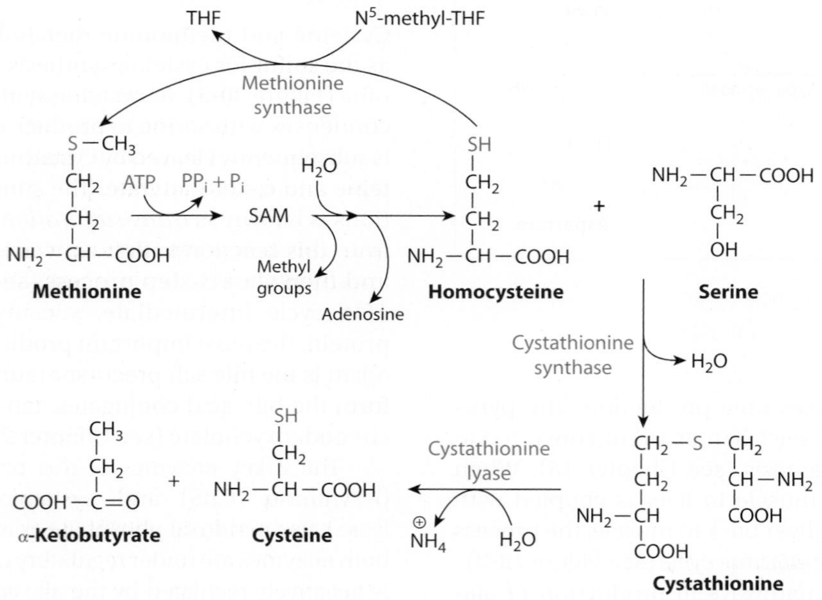

FIGURE 30-5: Utilization of methionine in the synthesis of cysteine. Reproduced with permission of themedicalbiochemistrypage, LLC.

High-Yield Concept

Cystathionase can also transfer sulfur from one cysteine to another, generating thiocysteine and pyruvate. Transamination of cysteine yields β-mercaptopyruvate, which then reacts with sulfite (SO_3^{2-}), to produce thiosulfate ($S_2O_3^{2-}$) and pyruvate. Both thiocysteine and thiosulfate can be used by the enzyme rhodanese to incorporate sulfur into cyanide (CN^-), thereby detoxifying the cyanide to thiocyanate.

CLINICAL BOX 30-3: HOMOCYSTINURIA

Homocystinurias represent a family of inherited disorders resulting from defects in several of the genes involved in the conversion of methionine to cysteine. As the name implies, these disorders result in elevated levels of homocysteine in the urine. In addition, patients excrete elevated levels of methionine and metabolites of homocysteine. The most common causes of homocystinuria are defects in the cystathionine β-synthase (*CBS*) gene. Homocystinuria is often associated with mental retardation, although the complete syndrome is multifaceted and many individuals with this disease are mentally normal, while others experience variable levels of developmental delay along with learning problems. Common symptoms of homocystinuria are dislocated optic lenses, osteoporosis, lengthening and thinning of the long bones, and an increased risk of abnormal blood clotting (thromboembolism). Some instances of genetic homocystinuria respond favorably to pyridoxine therapy, suggesting that in these cases the defect in *CBS* is a decreased affinity for the cofactor, pyridoxal phosphate.

Homocystinuria can also result from vitamin deficiencies due to the role of the co-factor forms of B_6, B_{12}, and folate in the overall metabolism of methionine. Vitamin B_6 (as pyridoxal phosphate) is required for the activity of CBS and the homocystinuria that results with B_6 deficiency is also associated with elevated methionine levels in the blood. Vitamin B_{12} and folate (as N^5-methyl-THF) are required for the methionine synthase reaction so a deficiency of either vitamin can result in homocystinuria presenting with reduced levels of plasma methionine. The enzyme methylmalonyl-CoA mutase (see Chapter 25) also requires B_{12} and so a homocystinuria resulting from a deficiency in this vitamin is also associated with methylmalonic academia. Indeed, the measurement of serum methionine and methylmalonic acid in cases of homocystinuria allows for a differential diagnosis of the nutritional (non-genetic) cause.

Missing or impaired cystathionase leads to excretion of cystathionine in the urine but does not have any other untoward effects. Rare cases have been found in which cystathionase is defective and operates at a low level, resulting in methioninuria with no other consequences.

While cysteine readily oxidizes to form the disulfide cystine, cells contain little if any free cystine. The cystine is rapidly converted to cysteine in a reaction catalyzed by cystine reductase (Figure 30-6). An additionally important enzyme activity utilizes glutathione

High-Yield Concept

Elevated levels of homocysteine in the blood have been shown to correlate with cardiovascular dysfunction. The role of homocysteine in cardiovascular disease is related to its ability to induce a state of inflammation. Homocysteine serves as a negatively charged surface that attracts the contact phase of the intrinsic pathway of blood coagulation (see Chapter 51). Activation of the intrinsic coagulation cascade leads to inappropriate thrombolytic events as well as resulting in increases in inflammatory cytokine release from leukocytes that are activated as a result of the procoagulant state.

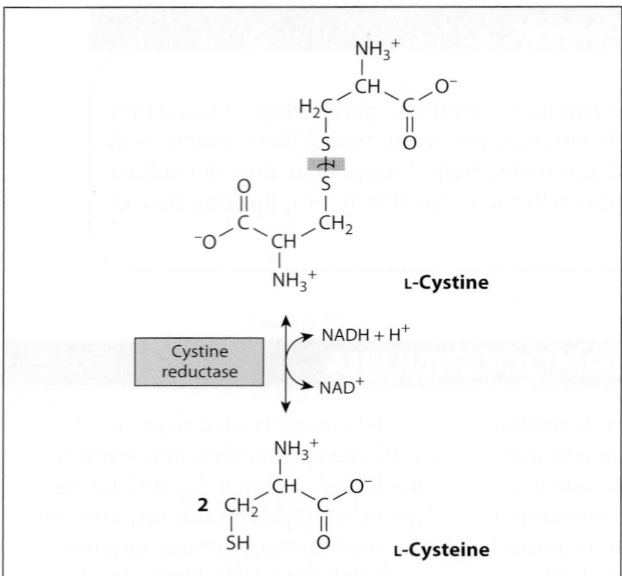

FIGURE 30-6: Reduction of cystine to cysteine in the cystine reductase reaction. Murray RK, Bender DA, Botham KM, Kennelly PJ, Rodwell VW, Weil PA. *Harper's Illustrated Biochemistry,* 29th ed. New York, NY: McGraw-Hill; 2012.

in the reduction of cystine to cysteine. In this reaction, catalyzed by glutathione-cystine transhydrogenase, glutathione (GSH) is oxidized to glutathione disulfide (GSSG) while cystine is reduced to cysteine.

There are several pathways for cysteine catabolism. The major catabolic pathway in animals is via cysteine dioxygenase that oxidizes the cysteine sulfhydryl to sulfonate, producing the intermediate cysteine sulfonate (Figure 30-7). Cysteine sulfonate can serve as a biosynthetic intermediate undergoing decarboxylation and oxidation to produce taurine used in bile acid metabolism. Catabolism of cysteine sulfonate yields bisulfite (HSO_3^-) and pyruvate. Sulfite oxidase converts HSO_3^- to sulfate, SO_4^- and H_2O_2 with the sulfate serving as a substrate for the formation of 3′-phosphoadenosine-5′-phosphosulfate (PAPS). PAPS is used for the transfer of sulfate to biological molecules such as the sugars of the glycosphingolipids (see Chapter 21).

In additional to its role as a precursor for cysteine synthesis and as an amino acid for protein synthesis, methionine serves an important role in numerous methylation reactions in the form of *S*-adenosylmethionine, SAM (also abbreviated AdoMet). The synthesis of SAM is catalyzed by methionine adenosyltransferase (Figure 30-8). The most important reactions involving SAM as methyl donor are those of catecholamine synthesis (see Chapter 31). The result of methyl transfer is the conversion of SAM to *S*-adenosylhomocysteine. *S*-adenosylhomocysteine is then cleaved by adenosylhomocysteinase to yield homocysteine and adenosine.

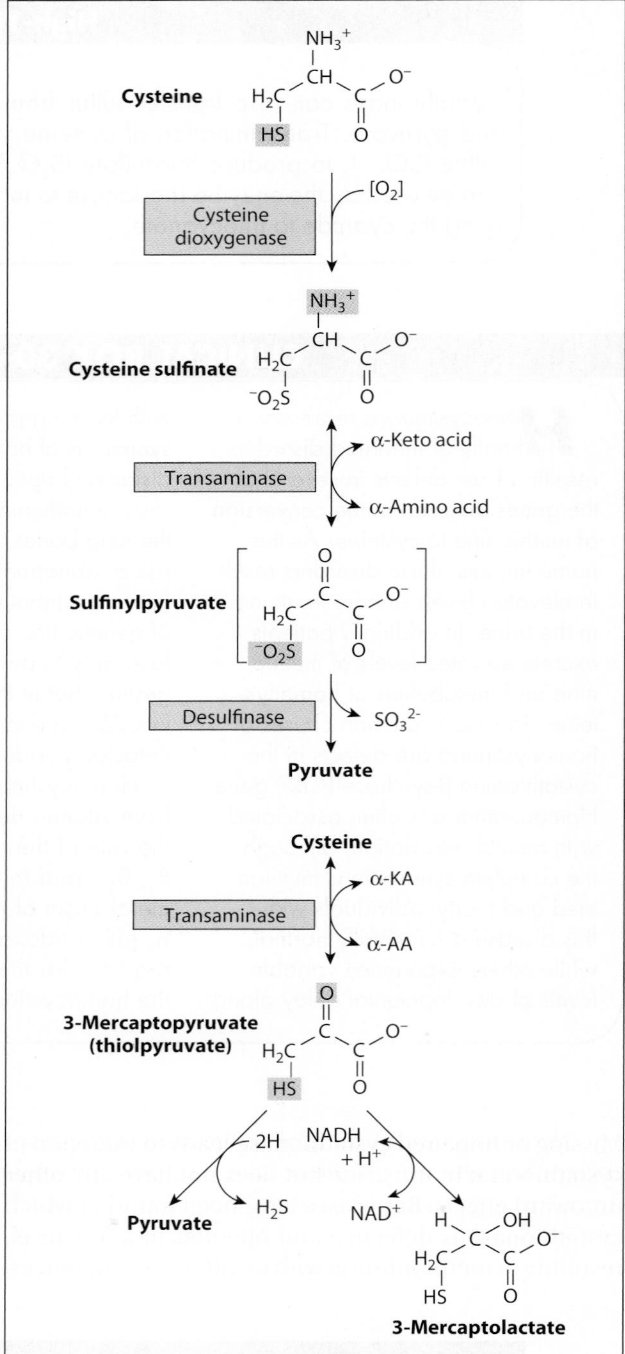

FIGURE 30-7: Two pathways catabolize L-cysteine: the cysteine sulfinate pathway (*top*) and the 3-mercaptopyruvate pathway (*bottom*). Murray RK, Bender DA, Botham KM, Kennelly PJ, Rodwell VW, Weil PA. *Harper's Illustrated Biochemistry,* 29th ed. New York, NY: McGraw-Hill; 2012.

Homocysteine can be converted back to methionine by methionine synthase (see Figure 30-5). The principal catabolic fate of methionine is the conversion to cysteine.

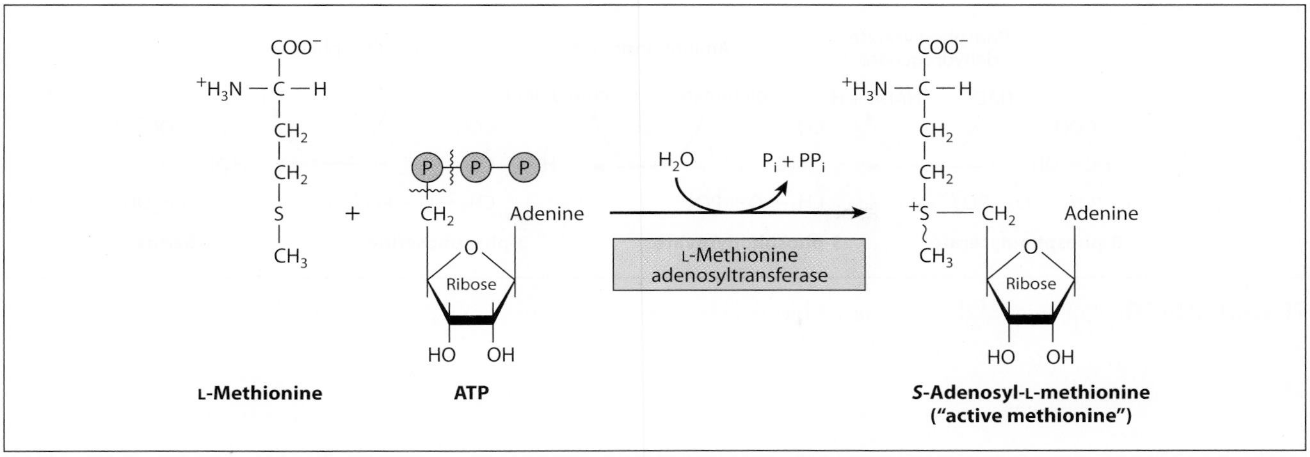

COO^- | $^+H_3N-C-H$ | CH_2 | CH_2 | S | CH_3 + ATP (P~P~P, CH_2, Adenine, Ribose, HO OH) → (H_2O in, $P_i + PP_i$ out; L-Methionine adenosyltransferase) → COO^- | $^+H_3N-C-H$ | CH_2 | CH_2 | ^+S — CH_2 Adenine, ~CH_3, Ribose, HO OH

L-Methionine **ATP** ***S*-Adenosyl-L-methionine ("active methionine")**

FIGURE 30-8: Formation of *S*-adenosylmethionine. ~CH_3 represents the high group transfer potential of "active methionine." Murray RK, Bender DA, Botham KM, Kennelly PJ, Rodwell VW, Weil PA. *Harper's Illustrated Biochemistry*, 29th ed. New York, NY: McGraw-Hill; 2012.

Glycine and Serine Metabolism

Glycine is involved in many anabolic reactions other than protein synthesis, including the synthesis of purine nucleotides, heme, glutathione, creatine, and serine. The main pathway to glycine synthesis is a 1-step reversible reaction catalyzed by serine hydroxymethyltransferase (SHMT). This enzyme is a member of the family of 1-carbon transferases and is also known as glycine hydroxymethyltransferase (Figure 30-9). This reaction involves the transfer of the hydroxymethyl group from serine to tetrahydrofolate (THF), producing glycine and N^5,N^{10}-methylene-THF. There are mitochondrial and cytosolic versions of serine hydroxymethyltransferase. The cytosolic enzyme is referred to as SHMT1 and the mitochondrial enzyme is SHMT2.

The main pathway to de novo biosynthesis of serine utilizes the glycolytic intermediate 3-phosphoglycerate (Figure 30-10). An NADH-linked dehydrogenase converts 3-phosphoglycerate into a keto acid, 3-phosphopyruvate, suitable for subsequent transamination. Aminotransferase activity with glutamate as a donor produces 3-phosphoserine, which is converted to serine by phosphoserine phosphatase. Serine can also be derived from glycine (and *vice versa*) via the SHMT-catalyzed reaction (Figure 30-11).

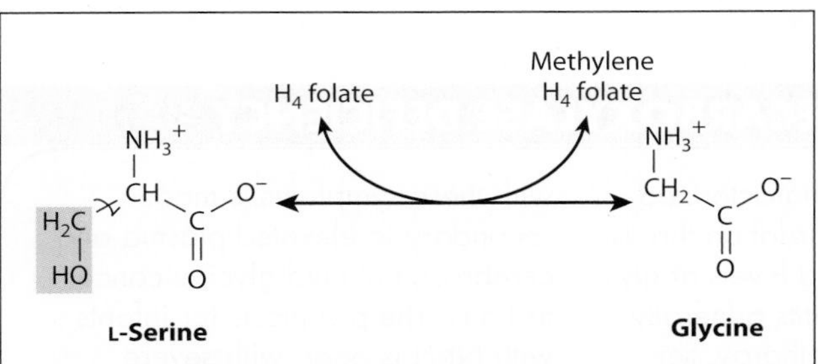

FIGURE 30-9: Interconversion of serine and glycine by serine hydroxymethyltransferase. (H_4 folate, tetrahydrofolate). Murray RK, Bender DA, Botham KM, Kennelly PJ, Rodwell VW, Weil PA. *Harper's Illustrated Biochemistry*, 29th ed. New York, NY: McGraw-Hill; 2012.

The catabolism of serine occurs via its conversion first to glycine. Glycine can then be oxidized by glycine decarboxylase (also referred to as the glycine cleavage complex, GCC) to yield ammonia, CO_2, and a second equivalent of N^5,N^{10}-methylene-THF. Glycine decarboxylase is a mitochondrial enzyme complex composed of 4 distinct proteins identified as H, L, P, and T. The H protein is a lipoic acid–containing protein. The L protein is a dihydrolipoamide dehydrogenase (DLD) similar to the DLD subunit of the pyruvate dehydrogenase and α-ketoglutarate (2-oxoglutarate) dehydrogenase complexes. The P protein is a pyridoxal phosphate-dependent glycine decarboxylase. The T protein is a tetrahydrofolate-requiring aminotransferase. Loss of activity of glycine decarboxylase (GCC) is associated with severe mental retardation (Clinical Box 30-4).

Glycine is coreleased with γ-aminobutyric acid (GABA) (see Chapter 31), which is the primary inhibitory neurotransmitter. Glycine action as a neurotransmitter is a function of the amino acid binding to a specific receptor, GlyR. GlyR is a member of the nicotinic acid receptor superfamily that includes the $GABA_A$ receptor ($GABA_AR$), the excitatory nicotinic acetylcholine receptors (nAChR), and the serotonin type 3 receptor ($5HT_3$). GlyR is a ligand-gated inotropic receptor that is a chloride channel. In addition to glycine, GlyR can be activated by several other small amino acids such as alanine and taurine. Glycine is also involved in the modulation of excitatory

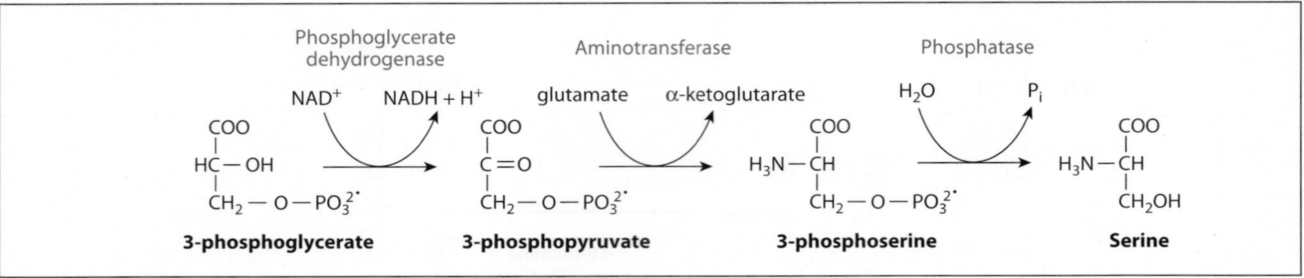

FIGURE 30-10: Pathway of de novo serine biosynthesis. Reproduced with permission of themedicalbiochemistrypage, LLC.

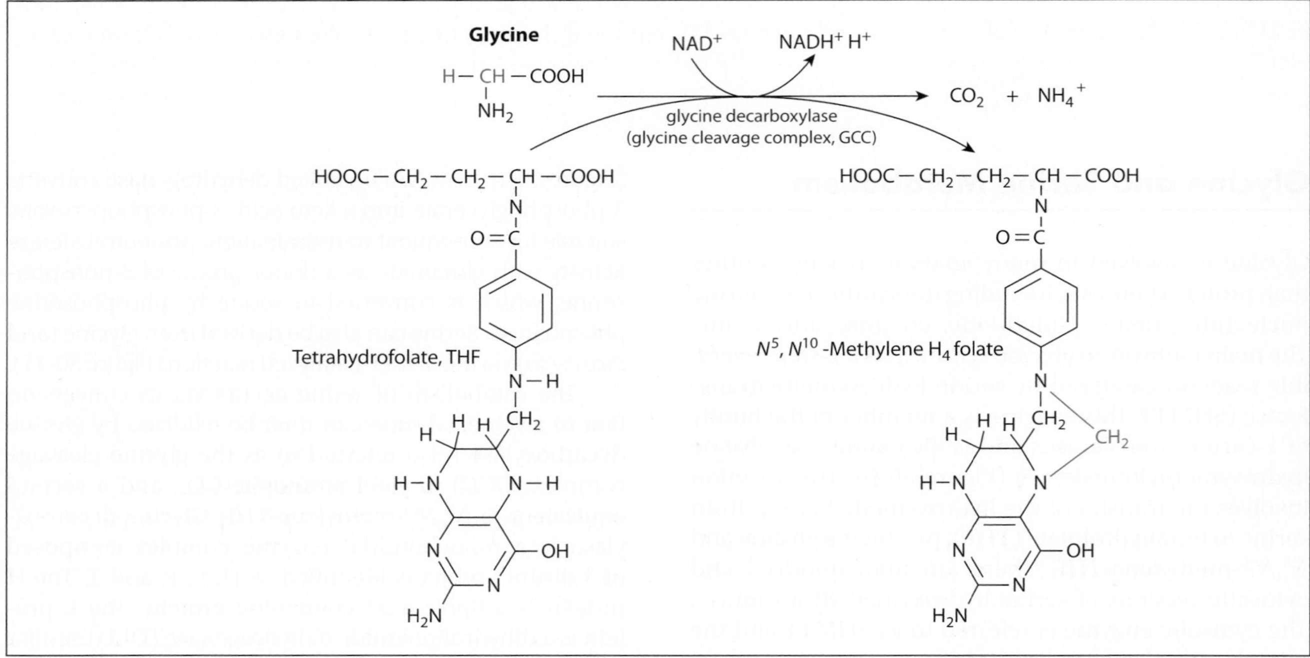

FIGURE 30-11: Reaction catalyzed by glycine decarboxylase. Reproduced with permission of themedicalbiochemistrypage, LLC.

CLINICAL BOX 30-4: GLYCINE DECARBOXYLASE DEFICIENCY

Nonketotic hyperglycinemia (NKH) is an autosomal recessive inborn error of glycine metabolism due to deficiencies in the H, P, or T proteins of the glycine decarboxylase complex. Mutations in the P protein are the most common. NKH, also known as glycine encephalopathy, is characterized by severe mental retardation that is due to highly elevated levels of glycine in the CNS. Infants generally present with severe lethargy, seizures, and respiratory depression requiring mechanical ventilation. A diagnosis of NKH associated with these symptoms is made secondary to elevated plasma and cerebrospinal fluid glycine concentrations. The prognosis for infants with NKH is poor, with severe neurologic impairment, intractable seizures, and death common before 5 years of age.

High-Yield Concept

In addition to its role in proteins synthesis and the formation of serine, glycine functions in the central nervous system as a major inhibitory neurotransmitter. In this capacity, glycine participates in regulating signals that process motor and sensory information that permits movement, vision, and audition.

neurotransmission exerted via glutamate binding to *N*-methyl-d-aspartate (NMDA) receptors.

Arginine, Ornithine, and Proline Metabolism

The synthesis and catabolism of arginine in mammals takes place within the context of the urea cycle (see Chapter 29). Synthesis occurs from citrulline and aspartate via the actions of argininosuccinate synthetase and argininosuccinate lyase. If arginine is needed for protein synthesis, it can be diverted away from the urea cycle, otherwise it is subsequently catabolized to urea and ornithine via the action of arginase.

Glutamate is the precursor of both proline and ornithine (Figure 30-12), with glutamate semialdehyde being a branch point intermediate leading to one or the other of these 2 products. While ornithine is not one of the 20 amino acids used in protein synthesis, it plays a significant role as the acceptor of carbamoyl phosphate in the urea cycle. Ornithine serves an additional important role as the precursor for the synthesis of the polyamines. The production

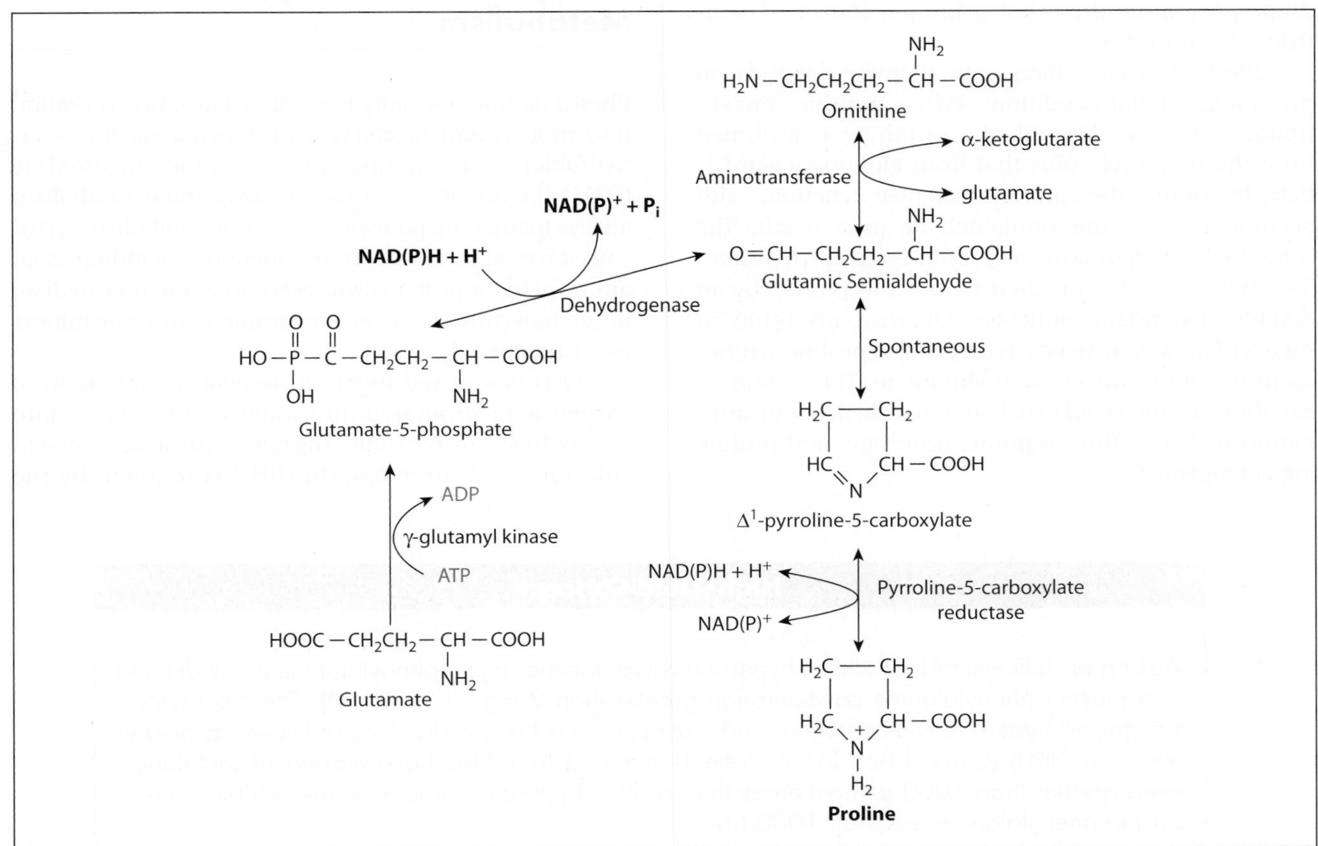

FIGURE 30-12: Synthesis of ornithine and proline. Reproduced with permission of themedicalbiochemistrypage, LLC.

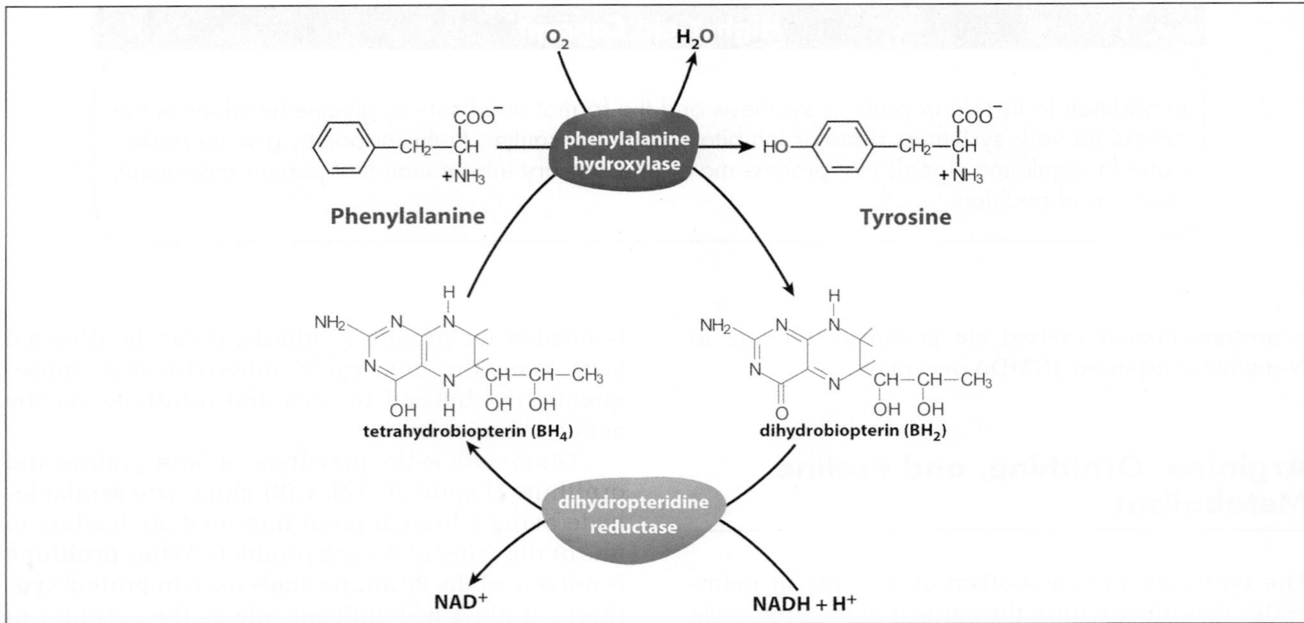

FIGURE 30-13: Biosynthesis of tyrosine from phenylalanine. Reproduced with permission of themedicalbiochemistrypage, LLC.

of ornithine from glutamate is important when dietary arginine, the other principal source of ornithine, is limited.

The fate of glutamate semialdehyde depends on prevailing cellular conditions. When arginine concentrations become elevated, the ornithine contributed from the urea cycle plus that from glutamate semialdehyde inhibit the aminotransferase reaction, with accumulation of the semialdehyde as a result. The semialdehyde spontaneously cyclizes to Δ^1-pyrroline-5-carboxylate, which is then reduced to proline by an NADPH-dependent reductase. Likewise, ornithine, in excess of urea cycle needs, is diverted to proline synthesis or it can be converted to glutamate. The glutamate can then be converted to α-ketoglutarate in a transamination reaction. Thus arginine, ornithine, and proline are glucogenic.

Phenylalanine and Tyrosine Metabolism

Phenylalanine normally has only 2 fates: incorporation into protein and production of tyrosine via the tetrahydrobiopterin-requiring phenylalanine hydroxylase (PAH) (Figure 30-13). Thus, phenylalanine catabolism always follows the pathway of tyrosine catabolism. Tyrosine serves several important functions, including as an amino acid for protein synthesis and as an intermediate in the biosynthesis of catecholamine neurotransmitters (see Chapter 31).

PAH is a mixed-function oxygenase: one atom of oxygen is incorporated into water and the other into the hydroxyl of tyrosine. The tetrahydrofolate-related cofactor tetrahydrobiopterin (BH_4) is required by the

High-Yield Concept

Missing or deficient PAH results in hyperphenylalaninemia. Hyperphenylalaninemia is defined as a plasma phenylalanine concentration greater than 2 mg/dL (120 μM). The most widely recognized hyperphenylalaninemia (and most severe) is the genetic disease known as phenylketonuria (PKU) (Clinical Box 30-5). Patients suffering from PKU have plasma phenylalanine levels greater than 1000 μM, whereas the non-PKU hyperphenylalaninemias exhibit levels of plasma phenylalanine less than 1000 μM.

CLINICAL BOX 30-5: HYPERPHENYLALANINEMIAS: PKU

Phenylketonuria (PKU) is an autosomal recessive disorder resulting from defects in the metabolism of phenylalanine. PKU is a hyperphenylalaninemia with multifactorial causes. There are several hyperphenylalaninemias that are not PKU and are called non-PKU hyperphenylalaninemias (HPA). Hyperphenylalaninemia is defined as a plasma phenylalanine concentration greater than 120 μM. PKU is characterized by plasma phenylalanine greater than 1000 μM and HPA have plasma phenylalanine amounts that are less than 1000 μM. PKU is caused by mutations in the phenylalanine hydroxylase (*PAH*) gene. Because the reaction catalyzed by PAH involves tetrahydrobiopterin (BH_4) as a cofactor, the HPA can result from defects in any of the several genes required for synthesis and recycling of BH_4. Removal of excess phenylalanine normally proceeds via the tyrosine biosynthesis reaction and then via tyrosine catabolism. Because BH_4 is involved in additional hydroxylation reactions, notably tryptophan and tyrosine in the brain in the formation of serotonin and the catecholamines, respectively, it is important to correctly diagnose any HPA as being the result of abnormal BH_4 homeostasis or defects in PAH. The major clinical manifestation associated with PKU and many HPA is impaired cognitive development and function. The mental retardation is caused by the accumulation of phenylalanine, which becomes a major donor of amino groups in aminotransferase activity and depletes neural tissue of α-ketoglutarate. This absence of α-ketoglutarate in the brain shuts down the TCA cycle and the associated production of aerobic energy, which is essential to normal brain development. The product of phenylalanine transamination, phenylpyruvic acid, is reduced to phenylacetate (Figure 30-14) and all 3 compounds appear in the urine.

The presence of phenylacetate in the urine imparts a "mousy" odor. Currently in this country (and many others as well), newborns are routinely screened for PKU by measurement of serum phenylalanine levels. In order to classify the phenotype of PKU into severe and less severe forms, as well as to exclude BH_4-deficient HPA, it is necessary to measure the plasma, urine, and cerebrospinal fluid levels of phenylalanine, pterins, and the derivatives of the neurotransmitters derived from tryptophan and tyrosine. The mainstay in treatment of PKU is the low-phenylalanine diet. Optimal treatment requires both early onset (hence the utility of the postnatal assessments in this country) and continuous treatment throughout the adolescence and possibly for life. Because of the necessity for phenylalanine in protein synthesis and neurotransmitter synthesis, it is important to carefully control the intake of the amino acid.

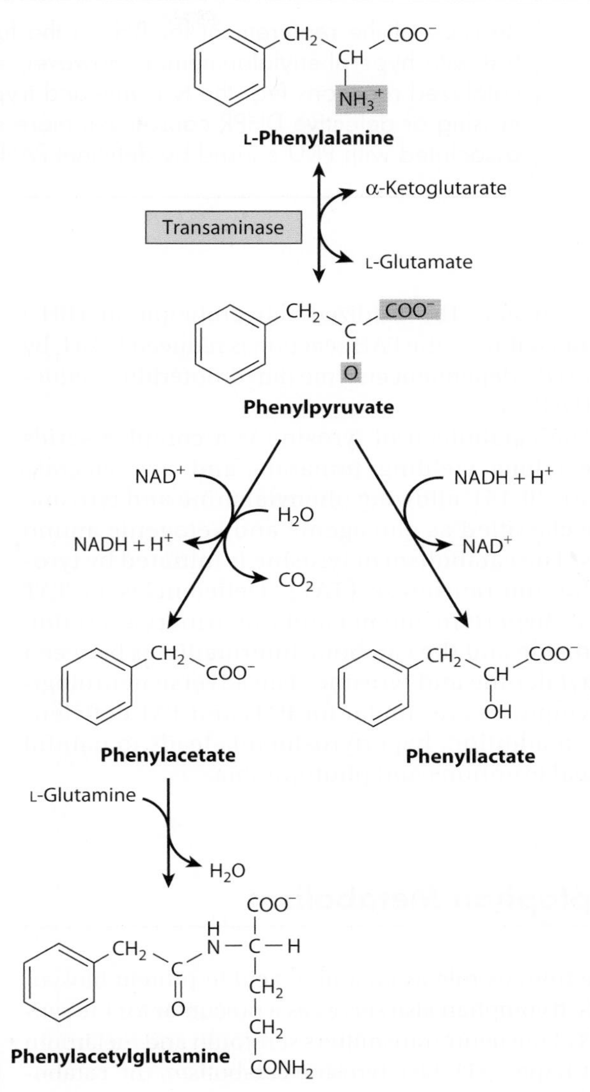

FIGURE 30-14: Alternative pathways of phenylalanine catabolism in phenylketonuria. The reactions also occur in normal liver tissue but are of minor significance. Murray RK, Bender DA, Botham KM, Kennelly PJ, Rodwell VW, Weil PA. *Harper's Illustrated Biochemistry*, 29th ed. New York, NY: McGraw-Hill; 2012.

High-Yield Concept

Because of the requirement for BH_4 in the function of PAH, deficiencies in DHPR can manifest with hyperphenylalaninemia. However, since BH_4 is a cofactor in several other enzyme-catalyzed reactions (eg, the tyrosine- and tryptophan-derived neurotransmitters), the effects of missing or defective DHPR cause even more severe neurological difficulties than those usually associated with PKU caused by deficient PAH activity.

PAH reaction. The oxidized dihydrobiopterin (BH_2) generated during the PAH reaction is reduced to BH_4 by the NADH-dependent enzyme dihydropteridine reductase (DHPR).

The catabolism of tyrosine is a complex series of reactions yielding fumarate and acetoacetate (Figure 30-15), allowing phenylalanine and tyrosine to be classified as glucogenic and ketogenic amino acids. The catabolism of tyrosine is initiated by tyrosine aminotransferase (TAT). Deficiencies in TAT lead to hypertyrosinemia and the urinary excretion of tyrosine and the catabolic intermediates between phenylalanine and tyrosine. The adverse neurological symptoms are similar for PAH and TAT deficiencies. In addition, hypertyrosinemia leads to painful corneal eruptions and photophobia.

Tryptophan Metabolism

Aside from its role as an amino acid in protein biosynthesis, tryptophan also serves as a precursor for the synthesis of the neurotransmitters serotonin and melatonin (see Chapter 31). Like tyrosine catabolism, the catabolism of tryptophan occurs via a complex series of reactions (Figure 30-16). There are a number of important side reactions that can occur during the catabolism of tryptophan.

Kynurenine is the first key branch point intermediate in tryptophan catabolism. It can undergo deamination in a standard transamination reaction yielding kynurenic acid. Kynurenic acid and its metabolites act as antiexcitotoxics and anticonvulsives. High levels of kynurenic acid are found in the urine of individuals suffering from schizophrenia. Kynurenic acid can also act as a noncompetitive antagonist at the glycine-binding site of the NMDA receptor. The NMDA receptor is a key component of the glutaminergic neurotransmission system involved in the pathophysiology of schizophrenia, thus explaining the potential role of kynurenic acid in schizophrenia.

An important kynurenine catabolic reaction occurs in the liver. In this catabolic pathway, the kynurenine is nonenzymatically cyclized to quinolate and then via a transamination and several rearrangements yields limited amounts of nicotinic acid, which leads to production of a small amount of NAD^+ and $NADP^+$.

Threonine Catabolism

There are at least 3 pathways for threonine catabolism that have been identified in mammals. These pathways utilize the enzymes serine/threonine dehydratase, threonine aldolase (more commonly called serine hydroxymethyltransferase, SHMT), and threonine dehydrogenase. The threonine dehydrogenase gene in humans appears to be

High-Yield Concept

The first inborn error in metabolism ever recognized, alkaptonuria, was demonstrated to be the result of a defect in phenylalanine and tyrosine catabolism. Alkaptonuria is caused by defective homogentisic acid oxidase. Homogentisic acid accumulation is relatively innocuous, causing urine to darken on exposure to air, but no life-threatening effects accompany the disease. The only untoward consequence of alkaptonuria is ochronosis (bluish-black discoloration of the tissues) and arthritis.

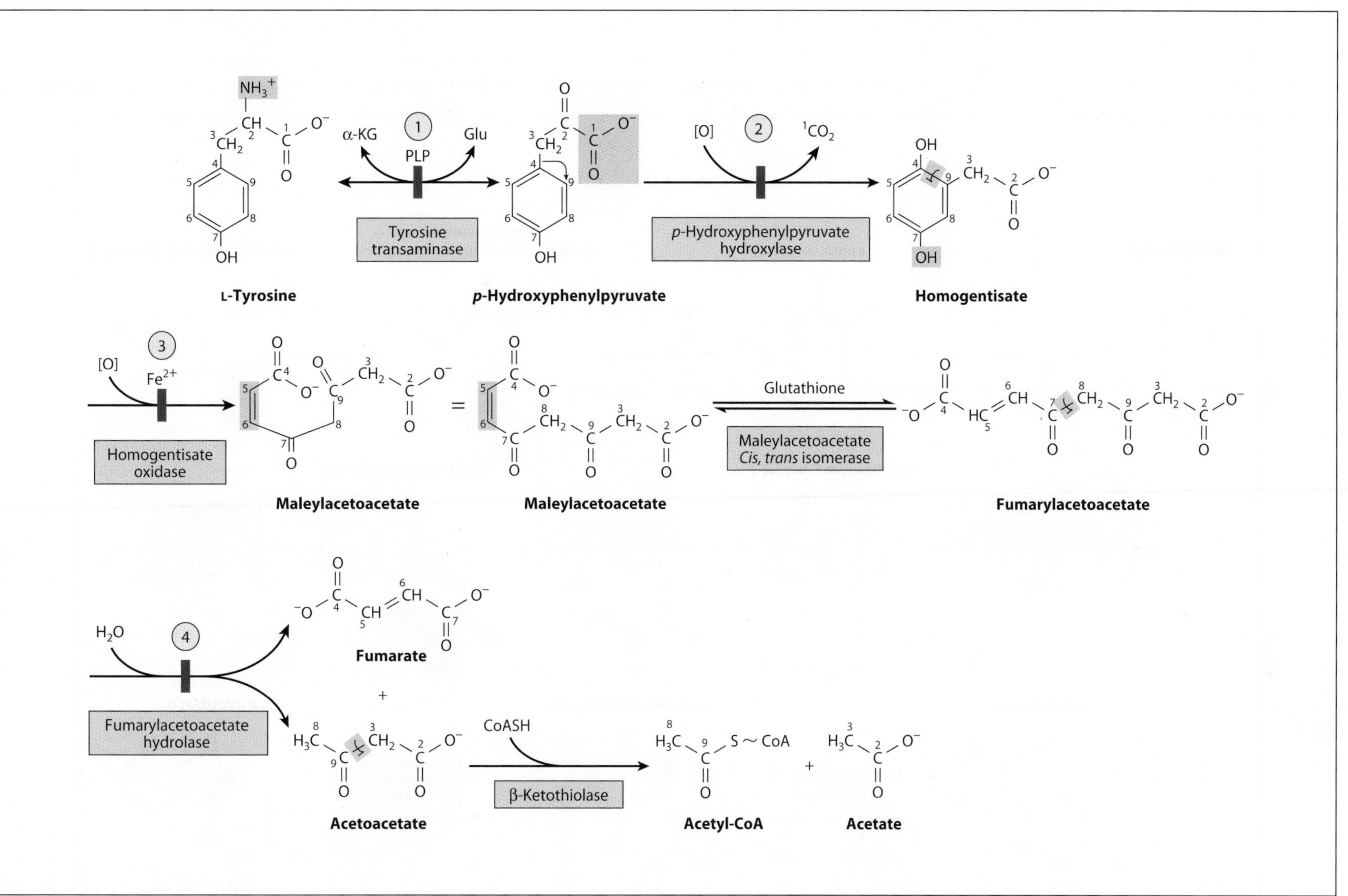

FIGURE 30-15: Intermediates in tyrosine catabolism. Carbons are numbered to emphasize their ultimate fate. (α-KG, α-ketoglutarate; Glu, glutamate; PLP, pyridoxal phosphate.) Red bars indicate the probable sites of the inherited metabolic defects in 1 type II tyrosinemia; 2 neonatal tyrosinemia; 3 alkaptonuria; and 4 type I tyrosinemia, or tyrosinosis. Murray RK, Bender DA, Botham KM, Kennelly PJ, Rodwell VW, Weil PA. *Harper's Illustrated Biochemistry*, 29th ed. New York, NY: McGraw-Hill; 2012.

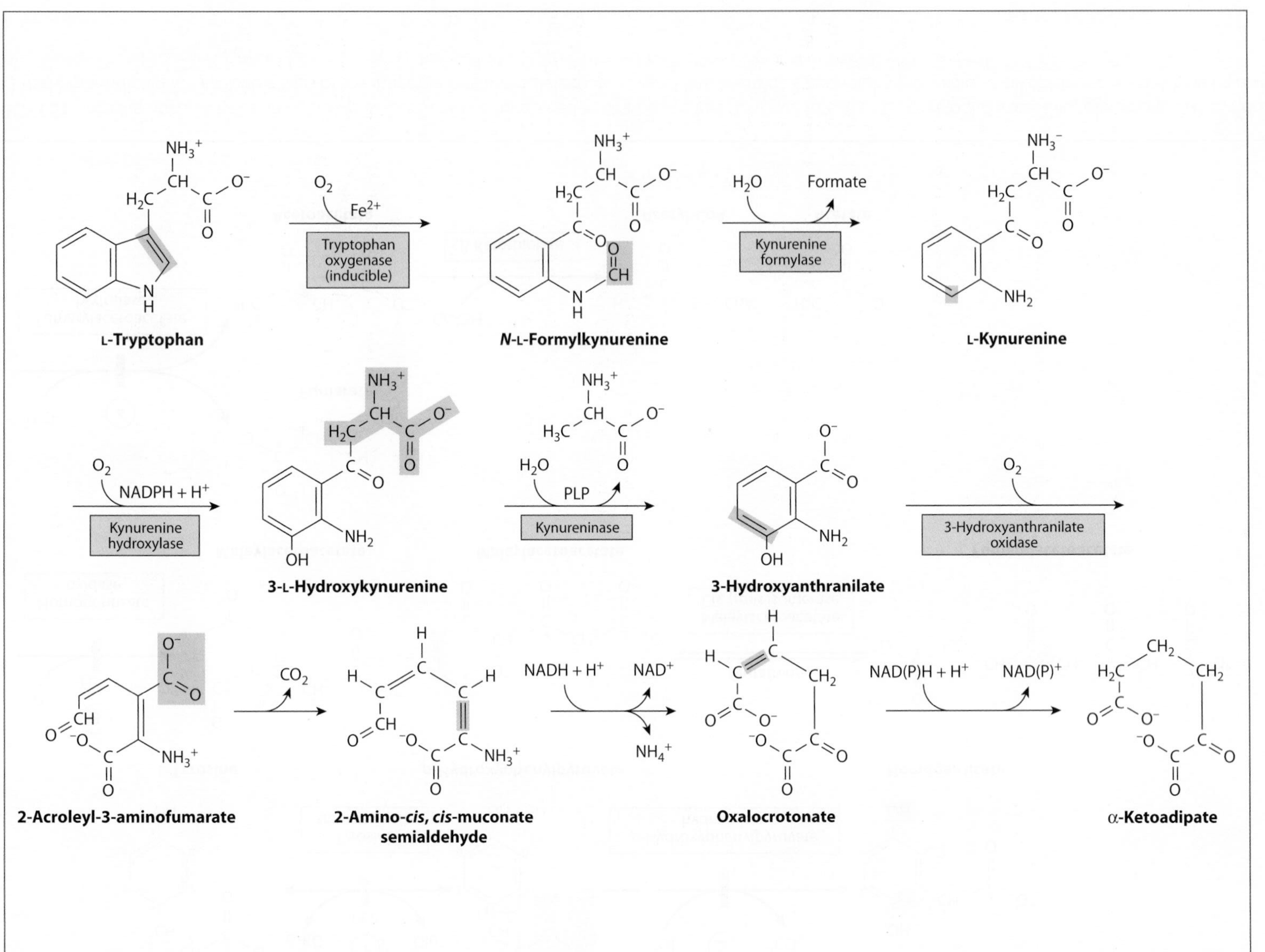

FIGURE 30-16: Reactions and intermediates in the catabolism of L-tryptophan. (PLP, pyridoxal phosphate.) Murray RK, Bender DA, Botham KM, Kennelly PJ, Rodwell VW, Weil PA. *Harper's Illustrated Biochemistry,* 29th ed. New York, NY: McGraw-Hill; 2012.

nonfunctional due to the incorporation of 3 inactivating mutations.

The principal threonine-catabolizing pathway in humans is initiated via the cytosolic serine/threonine dehydratase pathway, which yields α-ketobutyrate. The α-ketobutyrate is converted to propionyl-CoA and finally to the TCA cycle intermediate, succinyl-CoA. Serine/threonine dehydratase is expressed at high levels only in the liver. In newborn infants, catabolism of threonine occurs exclusively via the action of the serine/threonine dehydratase. Therefore, it is presumed that this is the predominant threonine-catabolizing pathway in humans.

A second cytosolic pathway for threonine catabolism utilizes SHMT, which was described earlier for serine and glycine metabolism (Figure 30-17). This

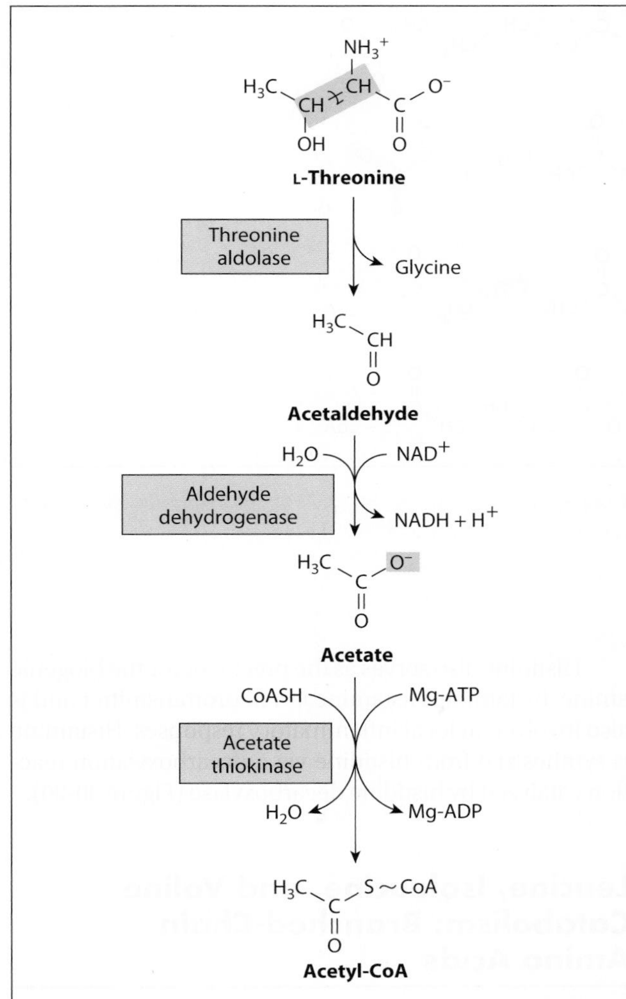

FIGURE 30-17: Intermediates in the conversion of threonine to glycine and acetyl-CoA. Murray RK, Bender DA, Botham KM, Kennelly PJ, Rodwell VW, Weil PA. *Harper's Illustrated Biochemistry*, 29th ed. New York, NY: McGraw-Hill; 2012.

1-carbon transferase is alternatively named glycine hydroxymethyltransferase or threonine aldolase. The products of this threonine-catabolic pathway are acetyl-CoA and glycine. Glycine can be converted to serine via SHMT and the serine is then catabolized as described, yielding pyruvate and NH_4^+.

Lysine Catabolism

Like all amino acids, catabolism of lysine can initiate from uptake of dietary lysine or from the breakdown of intracellular protein. There are several, at least 3, pathways for lysine catabolism but the primary pathway utilized within the liver is one that begins with the formation of an adduct between lysine and α-ketoglutarate called saccharopine (Figure 30-18). This catabolic pathway is, therefore, referred to as the saccharopine pathway. Lysine catabolism via this pathway is unusual in that the ε-amino group is transferred to α-ketoglutarate and into the general nitrogen pool. The first 2 reactions of the saccharopine pathway are catalyzed by the bifunctional enzyme α-aminoadipic semialdehyde synthase (AASS). The *N*-terminal half of the enzyme harbors the lysine-to-2-oxoglutarate reductase activity and the *C*-terminal half harbors the saccharopine dehydrogenase activity. The ultimate end product of lysine catabolism, via this pathway, is acetoacetyl-CoA.

Genetic deficiencies in either of the first 2 reactions of the saccharopine pathway of lysine catabolism result in familial hyperlysinemia. Since these 2 reactions are catalyzed by the bifunctional enzyme AASS, defects can be found in either activity. These deficiencies are observed in individuals who excrete large quantities of urinary lysine and some saccharopine. The lysinemia and associated lysinuria are benign.

Lysine is also important as a precursor for the synthesis of carnitine, required for the transport of fatty acids into the mitochondria for oxidation. Free lysine does not serve as the precursor for this reaction, however, the modified lysine found in certain proteins does so. Some proteins modify lysine to trimethyllysine, using SAM as the methyl donor to transfer methyl groups to the ε-amino of the lysine side chain. Hydrolysis of proteins containing trimethyllysine provides the substrate for the subsequent conversion to carnitine.

Histidine Catabolism

Histidine catabolism begins with release of the α-amino group catalyzed by histidase, introducing a double bond into the molecule (Figure 30-19). As a result, the

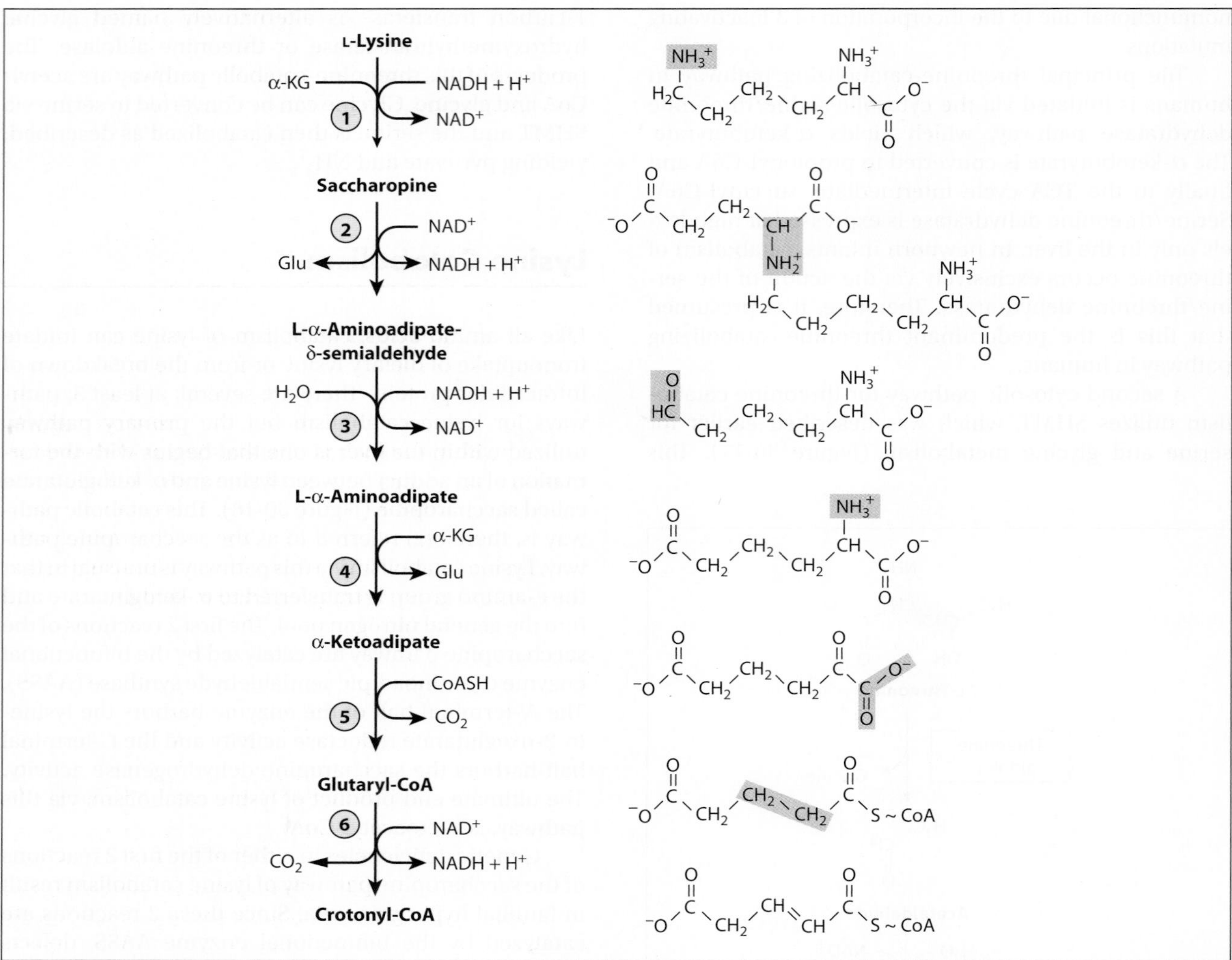

FIGURE 30-18: Reactions and intermediates in the catabolism of L-lysine. Murray RK, Bender DA, Botham KM, Kennelly PJ, Rodwell VW, Weil PA. *Harper's Illustrated Biochemistry*, 29th ed. New York, NY: McGraw-Hill; 2012.

deaminated product, urocanate, is not the usual α-keto acid associated with loss of α-amino nitrogens. Another key feature of histidine catabolism is that it serves as a source of ring nitrogen to combine with tetrahydrofolate (THF), producing the 1-carbon THF intermediate known as N^5-formimino THF. The end product of histidine catabolism is glutamate, making histidine one of the glucogenic amino acids.

The principal genetic deficiency associated with histidine metabolism is absence or deficiency of the first enzyme of the pathway, histidase. The resultant histidinemia is relatively benign. The disease, which is of relatively high incidence (1 in 10,000), is most easily detected by the absence of urocanate from skin and sweat, where it is normally found in relative abundance.

Histidine also serves as the precursor for the biogenic amine, histamine. Histamine is a neurotransmitter and is also involved in local inflammatory responses. Histamine is synthesized from histidine via a decarboxylation reaction catalyzed by histidine decarboxylase (Figure 30-20).

Leucine, Isoleucine, and Valine Catabolism: Branched-Chain Amino Acids

Leucine, isoleucine, and valine are the branched-chain amino acids (BCAAs). The catabolism of all 3 of these amino acids uses the same enzymes in the first 2 steps. The first step in each case is a transamination using a

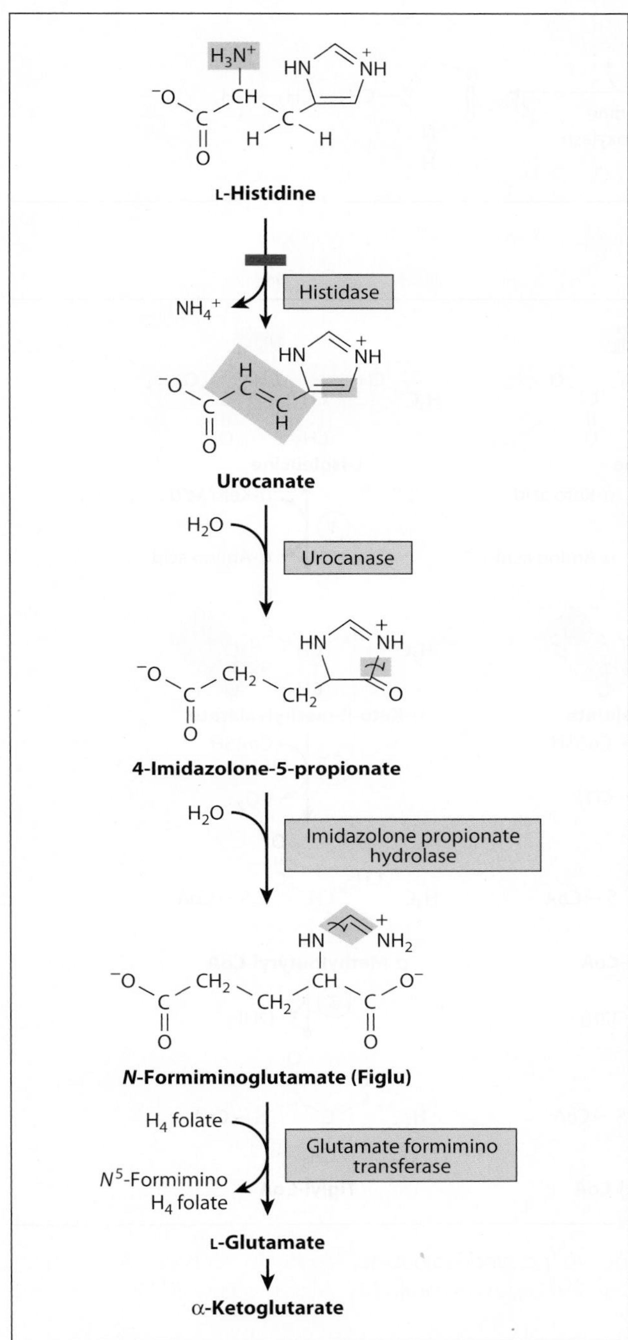

FIGURE 30-19: Catabolism of L-histidine to α-ketoglutarate. (H_4 folate, tetrahydrofolate.) The red bar indicates the site of an inherited metabolic defect. Murray RK, Bender DA, Botham KM, Kennelly PJ, Rodwell VW, Weil PA. *Harper's Illustrated Biochemistry,* 29th ed. New York, NY: McGraw-Hill; 2012.

BCAA aminotransferase (termed a *branched-chain aminotransferase, BCAT*), with α-ketoglutarate as amine acceptor. There are 2 genes encoding BCAT identified as BCAT1 and BCAT2. BCAT1 encodes a cytosolic version of the enzyme identified as BCATc, and BCAT2 encodes a mitochondrial version designated BCATm. The 3 different α-keto acids that result from the BCAT reaction are oxidized using a common branched-chain α-keto acid dehydrogenase (BCKD), yielding the 3 different CoA derivatives (Figure 30-21). Subsequently, the metabolic pathways diverge, producing many intermediates.

The principal product from valine is propionyl CoA, the glucogenic precursor of succinyl-CoA. Isoleucine catabolism terminates with production of acetyl-CoA and propionyl CoA; thus isoleucine is both glucogenic and ketogenic. Leucine gives rise to acetyl-CoA and acetoacetyl-CoA, and is thus classified as strictly ketogenic.

There are a number of genetic diseases associated with faulty catabolism of the BCAAs. The most common defect is in the branched-chain α-keto acid dehydrogenase (BCKD). Since there is only 1 dehydrogenase enzyme for all 3 amino acids, all 3 α-keto acids accumulate and are excreted in the urine. The disease is known as Maple syrup urine disease (Clinical Box 30-6) because of the characteristic odor of the urine in afflicted individuals.

Leucine Signaling and Metabolic Regulation

Numerous studies have shown that diets high in protein increase fatty acid oxidation and overall energy expenditure and thus, promote weight loss. In addition, high-protein diets are known to improve glucose homeostasis and, therefore, can have a positive impact on insulin sensitivity and diabetes. In studies on obese humans, subjects that consumed a milk whey protein–enriched diet exhibited demonstrable improvement in fatty liver symptoms (hepatic steatosis) and reduced plasma lipid profiles. In studies examining the effects of dietary protein on energy expenditure, appetite suppression, and weight loss, whey protein is the more beneficial source when comparing the effects of consumption of whey proteins, soy proteins, or casein.

Whey proteins are enriched in the branched-chain amino acids (BCAAs) leucine, isoleucine, and valine and are thus, excellent sources of energy production in skeletal muscle as well as serving as building blocks for muscle protein synthesis. Leucine has been proposed to be the primary mediator of the metabolic changes that occur when consuming a high protein diet. At the molecular level, leucine has been shown to activate the metabolic regulatory kinase known as mammalian target of rapamycin (mTOR) (see Chapters 37 and 46). Activation of skeletal muscle mTOR results in increased protein synthesis and thus, increased energy expenditure. Hypothalamic mTOR activation is also involved in the regulation of feeding behaviors. Of note

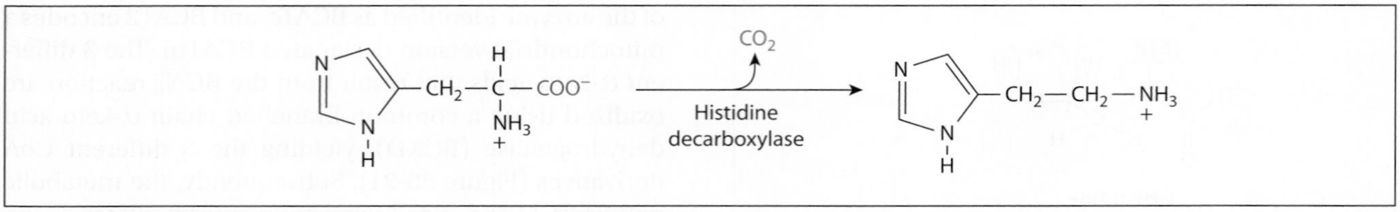

CO_2

Histidine decarboxylase

FIGURE 30-20: Synthesis of histamine. Reproduced with permission of themedicalbiochemistrypage, LLC.

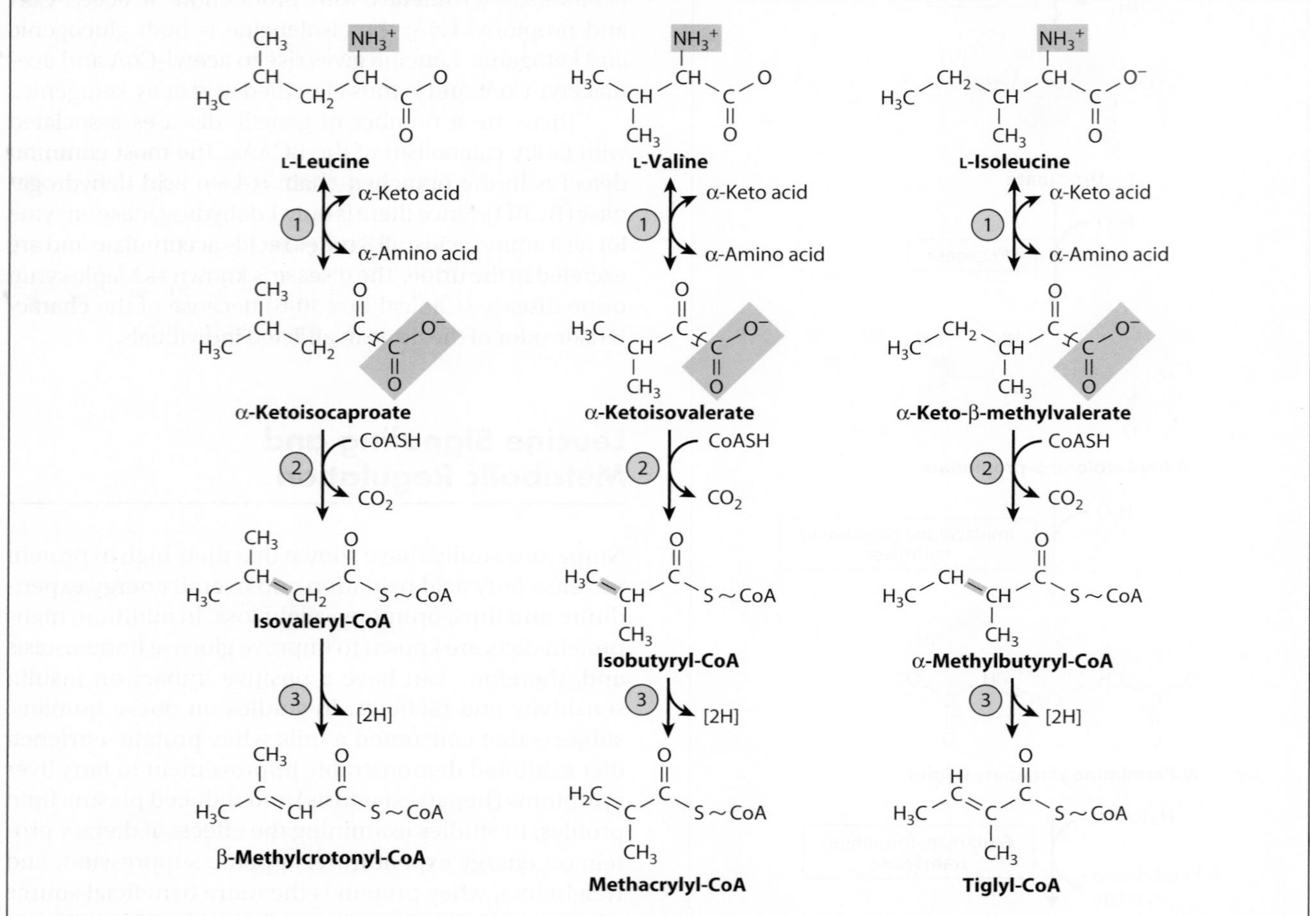

FIGURE 30-21: The first 3 reactions in the catabolism of leucine, valine, and isoleucine. Murray RK, Bender DA, Botham KM, Kennelly PJ, Rodwell VW, Weil PA. *Harper's Illustrated Biochemistry*, 29th ed. New York, NY: McGraw-Hill; 2012.

is the fact that direct injection of leucine into the hypothalamus results in increased mTOR signaling, leading to decreased feeding behavior and body weight. This effect is unique to leucine, as direct injection of valine, another BCAA, does not result in hypothalamic mTOR activation nor reductions in food intake or body weight.

Most of the work in laboratory animals demonstrates that the positive effects of increased leucine intake or high-protein diets are most pronounced when the animals are also consuming a high-fat diet. Therefore, it is suggested that there are definite benefits for overweight and obese individuals to increase their intake of leucine and/or total protein as a means for appetite and weight control. However, although high-protein diets or leucine supplementation are important considerations in a healthy diet, the total amount consumed must be taken into account so as not to lead to excess mTOR activation, which can exacerbate insulin resistance particularly in overweight individuals.

CLINICAL BOX 30-6: MAPLE SYRUP URINE DISEASE

Maple syrup urine disease (*MSUD*), also called branched-chain aminoaciduria, is so called because the urine of affected individuals smells like maple syrup or burnt sugar. MSUD results from deficiencies in BCKD, leading to an accumulation of leucine, isoleucine, and lysine and their corresponding branched-chain α-keto acids (BCKA). MSUD is an autosomal recessive disorder with a worldwide distribution of approximately 1 in 185,000 persons. The BCAAs represent approximately 35% to 40% of the essential amino acids in skeletal muscle. Following the ingestion of protein, the BCAAs represent about 60% of the increase in amino acids in the blood. In skeletal muscle, the BCAAs represent a significant source of carbon atom as an alternate to lipid and carbohydrate as a source of energy. The BCAAs are also actively metabolized for energy in the heart, kidneys, brain, and adipose tissue. In the liver, oxidation of the BCAAs provides significant carbon for the production of the ketone bodies used by the brain during periods of fasting. The BCKD complex is a multimeric enzyme composed of 3 catalytic subunits. The E1 portion of the complex is a thiamine pyrophosphate (TPP)-dependent decarboxylase with a subunit structure of $\alpha_2\beta_2$. The E2 portion is a transacylase composed of 24 lipoic acid–containing polypeptides. The E3 portion is a homodimeric flavoprotein. The activity of BCKD is regulated by 2 additional subunits, a kinase and a phosphatase that, respectively, reversibly phosphorylate and dephosphorylate the complex. The phosphorylated enzyme is inactive. The genetic heterogeneity in MSUD patients can be explained by the complexity in the structure of BCKD. There are 4 molecular phenotypes of MSUD based upon the affected locus. Type IA is due to mutations in the *E1α* gene. Type IB is due to mutations in the *E1β* gene. Type II is due to mutations in the *E2* gene. Type III is due to mutations in the *E3* gene. Based upon the overall clinical presentation as well as a particular patient's response to thiamine administration, MSUD patients can be divided into 5 phenotypic classifications.

Classic: Classic MSUD is defined by neonatal onset of encephalopathy and is the most severe form of the disorder. The levels of the BCAA, especially leucine, are dramatically elevated in the blood, urine, and cerebrospinal fluid of afflicted infants. The presence of alloisoleucine in the fluids is diagnostic of MSUD. The level of BCKD activity in classic MSUD patients is less than 2% of the normal. Affected infants appear normal at birth, but symptoms develop rapidly, appearing by 4 to 7 days after birth. The first distinctive signs are lethargy and little interest in feeding. As the disease progresses, infants will exhibit weight loss and progressive neurological deterioration. Neurological signs will alternate from hypo- to hypertonia and extension of the arms resembling decerebrate posturing. At this time, the characteristic burnt sugar or maple syrup odor to the urine is apparent. If left untreated infants will develop seizures, lapse into a coma, and die. The prognosis for untreated infants is poor, with death occurring within several months of birth due to complications of metabolic crisis and neurological deterioration.

Intermediate: Intermediate MSUD is distinguished from classic in that patients do not experience the severity of classic MSUD in the neonatal period. Infants will have persistent elevation in BCAAs in body fluids as well as neurological impairment. The level of BCKD in intermediate MSUD individuals ranges from 3% to 30% of normal. Many intermediate MSUD patients do not experience the acute metabolic decompensation present in classic MSUD.

Intermittent: In patients with the intermittent form of MSUD, the activity of BCKD ranges from 5% to 50% of normal. These individuals will show normal early development with normal intelligence. During periods when patients are asymptomatic, their fluid levels of BCAA will be normal. These patients are, however, at risk for acute metabolic decompensation during periods of stress. Initial symptoms of the intermittent form of MSUD usually appear between 5 months and 2 years of age in association with an infection.

Thiamine responsive: There is a similar course of progress in the symptoms of thiamine-responsive MSUD patients to that seen in intermediate MSUD patients. Plasma BCAA levels are around 5 times normal and alloisoleucine is characteristically detectable in these patients. Administration of thiamine and consumption of a low-protein diet results in a reduction of BCAA levels to normal. Withdrawal of thiamine treatment results in a rapid rebound in the elevation of plasma BCAA concentration. These responses to thiamine are the reason for this classification of MSUD. There is a wide range of heterogeneity in thiamine-responsive MSUD patients and thiamine treatment alone is insufficient to result in lower levels of BCAA.

Dihydrolipoyl dehydrogenase (E3) deficient: As the name of this classification implies, this form of MSUD is due to a deficiency in the E3 component of the BCKD complex. This form of MSUD is very rare with only 20 reported cases. The symptoms of the E3-deficient form are similar to those of intermediate MSUD, but there is an accompanying severe lactic acidosis. Infants with the E3-deficient form of MSUD are relatively normal for the first few months of life. Persistent lactic acidosis will be seen to develop between 2 and 6 months of age.

REVIEW QUESTIONS

1. You are examining a pediatric patient brought to you by his parents because they are disturbed by his progressive mood changes and apparent hightened anxiety. Physical examination shows pellegra-like skin eruptions and signs of cerebellar ataxia that include unsteady gait and uncoordinated eye movements. Serum and urinalysis show significant aminoacidemia and aciduria. These signs and symptoms are most likely due to which of the following disorders?

A. alkaptonuria
B. glycine decarboxylase deficiency (GCC deficiency)
C. Hartnup disorder
D. maple syrup urine disease
E. PKU

Answer C: Hartnup disorder is caused by a defect in neutral amino acid transport in the apical brush border membranes of the small intestine and in kidney proximal tubules. The lack of intestinal tryptophan transport is responsible for most if not all clinical phenotypes of Hartnup disorder. The pellagra-like skin rash seen on sun-exposed areas of skin in Hartnup disorder patients is most likely the result of nicotinamide deficiency due to a lack of tryptophan, which is a precursor for its synthesis. Symptoms of Hartnup disorder may begin in infancy or early childhood, but sometimes they begin as late as early adulthood. Symptoms may be triggered by sunlight, fever, drugs, or emotional or physical stress. Most symptoms occur sporadically and are caused by a deficiency of niacin. When Hartnup disorder manifests during infancy, the symptoms can be variable in clinical presentation. These symptoms include failure to thrive, photosensitivity, intermittent ataxia, nystagmus, and tremor.

2. You are examining an infant brought to your office due to the onset of seizures. The parents report that their baby has also exhibited a progressive lack of energy, feeding difficulties, hypotonia, abnormal jerking movements, and difficulty breathing. These symptoms are suggestive of a defect in the processes of neurotransmission and thus, are most likely due to which of the following disorders?

A. alkaptonuria
B. glycine decarboxylase deficiency (GCC deficiency)
C. Hartnup disorder
D. maple syrup urine disease
E. PKU

Answer B: Nonketotic hyperglycinemia (NKH) is an autosomal recessive inborn error of glycine metabolism due to deficiencies in the H, P, or T proteins of the glycine decarboxylase complex. NKH, also known as glycine encephalopathy, is characterized by severe mental retardation that is due to highly elevated levels of glycine in the CNS. Infants generally present with severe lethargy, seizures, and respiratory depression requiring mechanical ventilation. A diagnosis of NKH associated with these symptoms is made secondary to elevated plasma and cerebrospinal fluid glycine concentrations. The prognosis for infants with NKH is poor, with severe neurologic impairment, intractable seizures, and death common before 5 years of age.

3. A deficiency in one of the critical enzymes involved in the catabolism of the branched-chain amino acids results in neonatal vomiting, lethargy, and poor suckling behavior. Progressive neurological signs include decerebrate posturing. Which one of the following disorders corresponds to this defect?

A. alkaptonuria
B. homocystinuria
C. isovaleric acidemia
D. maple syrup urine disease
E. phenylketonuria (PKU)

Answer D: Maple syrup urine disease (MSUD), also called branched-chain aminoaciduria, is so called because the urine of affected individuals smells like maple syrup or burnt sugar. MSUD results from deficiencies in BCKD, leading to an accumulation of leucine, isoleucine, and lysine and their corresponding branched-chain α-keto acids (BCKA). Classic MSUD is defined by neonatal onset of encephalopathy and is the most severe form of the disorder. The levels of the BCAA, especially leucine, are dramatically elevated in the blood, urine, and cerebrospinal fluid of afflicted infants. Affected infants appear normal at birth but symptoms develop rapidly appearing by 4 to 7 days after birth. The first distinctive signs are lethargy and little interest in feeding. As the disease progresses, infants will exhibit weight loss and progressive neurological deterioration. Neurological signs will alternate from hypo- to hypertonia and extension of the arms resembling decerebrate posturing. At this time, the characteristic burnt sugar or maple syrup odor to the urine is apparent.

4. The parents of a 3-month-old infant rush their child to the ER following a seizure. Blood work indicates the child is hyperphenylalaninemic with serum phenylalanine measured at 650 μM. The attending physician suspects the infant has PKU and places the infant on a low-phenylalanine diet. Upon follow-up 3-days later, the level of serum phenylalanine is found to be reduced to 250 μM. However, while at home, the infant developed progressive movement disorders, difficulty swallowing, seizures, and elevated body temperature. A defect in which of the following enzymes would best explain the hyperphenylalaninemia and the lack of positive outcome on the low phenylalanine treatment?

A. dihydropteridine reductase
B. nitric oxide synthase
C. phenylalanine hydroxylase
D. tryptophan hydroxylase
E. tyrosine hydroxylase

Answer A: Several hyperphenylalaninemias are not PKU and are called non-PKU hyperphenylalaninemias (HPA). Hyperphenylalaninemia is defined as a plasma phenylalanine concentration greater than 120 μM. PKU is characterized by plasma phenylalanine greater than 1000 μM and HPA have plasma phenylalanine amounts that are less than 1000 μM. Dihydropteridine reductase (DHPR) deficiency leads to neurological signs at age 4 or 5 months, although clinical signs are often obvious from birth. The principal symptoms include psychomotor retardation, tonicity disorders, drowsiness, irritability, abnormal movements, hyperthermia, hypersalivation, and difficult swallowing.

5. A 10-year-old girl is brought to her pediatrician for a routine examination. The child is thin and has long fingers and toes, dislocated lenses, and mental retardation. Enzyme studies show an inability to convert homocysteine to cystathionine by cystathionine β-synthase. Newborn screening would have been able to identify the metabolic disorder present in this girl through the measurement of an increased serum concentration of which of the following amino acids?

A. leucine
B. methionine
C. phenylalanine
D. serine
E. tyrosine

Answer B: The most common causes of homocystinuria are defects in the cystathionine β-synthase (*CBS*) gene. *CBS* is involved in the conversion of methionine to cysteine and so a deficiency in the enzyme can be suspected in cases where there are elevated levels of methionine in the blood. Homocystinuria is often associated with mental retardation, although the complete syndrome is multifaceted and many individuals with this disease are mentally normal, while others experience variable levels of developmental delay along with learning problems. Common symptoms of homocystinuria are dislocated optic lenses, osteoporosis, lengthening and thinning of the long bones, and an increased risk of abnormal blood clotting (thromboembolism).

6. A 2-year-old boy is hospitalized with chronic diarrhea. He exhibits considerable weight loss such that he is only about 70% of expected weight for age. His muscles show significant atrophy, but he still has normal subcutaneous adipose tissue. His abdomen is distended, and he has some areas of scaly peeling skin. These findings are most consistent with which of the following conditions?

A. hepatic cirrhosis
B. infectious hepatitis
C. kwashiorkor
D. marasmus
E. nephrosis

Answer C: Kwashiorkor is a condition resulting from inadequate protein intake. Early symptoms include fatigue, irritability, and lethargy. As protein deprivation continues, one sees growth failure, loss of muscle mass, generalized swelling (edema), and decreased immunity. A large, protuberant belly is common in children suffering from this disorder.

7. A mother has brought her 3-month-old baby to the pediatrician and indicates that the infant is lethargic and has poor suckling and seems uninterested in eating. In addition, the mother notes that the baby's diapers often smell like burnt sugar. This infant likely has a defect in which of the following enzymes?

A. branched-chain α-keto acid dehydrogenase
B. cystathionine synthase
C. glycine cleavage complex (GCC)
D. homogentisate oxidase
E. phenylalanine hydroxylase

Answer A: The symptoms exhibited by the infant are reflective of maple syrup urine disease (MSUD). This disease is caused by defects in branched-chain α-keto acid dehydrogenase, one of the enzymes used in the catabolism of the branched-chain amino acids (BCAAs) and the associated branched-chain α-keto acids (BCKAs). The classical symptom of this disease is the odor of burnt sugar in the diapers of afflicted infants. Left untreated, infants will die in the first few months of life from recurrent metabolic crisis and neurologic deterioration.

8. Infants exhibiting profound metabolic ketoacidosis, muscular hypotonia, developmental retardation, and who have very large accumulations of methylmalonic acid in their blood and urine suffer from a disorder known as methylmalonic acidemia.

This disorder results from a defect in which of the following enzymes?

A. homogentisic acid oxidase
B. α-keto acid dehydrogenase
C. methylmalonyl-CoA mutase
D. phenylalanine hydroxylase
E. tyrosine aminotransferase

Answer C: Defects in methylmalonyl-CoA mutase activity comprise 4 distinct genotypes whose clinical symptoms are remarkably similar. Characteristic findings in methylmalonyl-CoA mutase deficiency include failure to thrive leading to developmental abnormalities, recurrent vomiting, respiratory distress, hepatomegaly, and muscular hypotonia. In addition, patients have severely elevated levels of methylmalonic acid in the blood and urine. Unaffected individuals have near-undetectable levels of methylmalonate in their plasma, whereas, affected individuals have been found to have levels ranging from 3 to 40 mg/dL in their blood.

9. A 5-month-old infant who has been experiencing lethargy, recurrent vomiting, respiratory distress, and muscular hypotonia is brought to the emergency room near-comatose. Lab results indicate severe metabolic ketoacidosis associated with an extreme accumulation of methylmalonic acid in the blood and urine. Negative findings for pernicious anemia or other hematologic or neurologic symptoms of cobalamin deficiency indicate that the infant is suffering a defect in which of the following enzymes?

A. malonyl-CoA decarboxylase
B. methionine synthase
C. methylmalonyl-CoA mutase
D. methylmalonyl-CoA racemase
E. propionyl-CoA carboxylase

Answer C: TCA cycle–mediated oxidation of propionyl-CoA, derived from the β-oxidation of fatty acids with an odd number of carbon atoms or from catabolism of several amino acids (eg, valine and isoleucine), requires that it first be converted to succinyl-CoA. Methylmalonyl-CoA mutase is the terminal enzyme in this conversion process. The most common physical symptoms seen in patients with defective methylmalonyl-CoA mutase activity are failure to thrive, lethargy, vomiting, muscular hypotonia, and respiratory distress. Characteristic laboratory findings will be methylmalonic acidemia.

10. A 3-month-old infant experienced several severe seizures and was brought to the doctor for testing. The test results showed hyperphenylalaninemia and the doctor diagnosed PKU as the likely disease causing the seizures. The infant was placed on a low-phenylalanine diet but developed progressive neurological symptoms and died 6 months later. A defect in which of the following enzymes would best explain the observations and outcomes in this case

A. dihydropteridine reductase
B. nitric oxide synthase
C. phenylalanine hydroxylase
D. tryptophan hydroxylase
E. tyrosine hydroxylase

Answer A: The pathway for conversion of phenylalanine (F) to tyrosine (Y), catalyzed by phenylalanine hydroxylase (PAH), is shown in Figure 30-13. The conversion of F to Y is not only necessary for Y biogenesis but is also the first step in the catabolism of F. Classic PKU manifests with hyperphenylalaninemia, excretion of metabolites of transaminated pheylalanine (phenylpyruvate, phenylacetate, and phenyllactate), and severe mental retardation. PKU is the result of defects in PAH. However, as shown in Figure 30-13, PAH requires tetrahydrobiopterin (BH_4) as a cofactor, which is converted to dihydrobiopterin (BH_2) during the PAH reaction. Conversion of BH_2 back to BH_4 requires an additional enzyme, dihydropteridine reductase (DHPR). Defects in DHPR will result in reduced activity of any enzyme requiring BH_4 as a cofactor. Thus, defective DHPR will result in defective phenylalanine metabolism and lead to hyperphenylalaninemia with similar but distinct consequences to PKU. One distinction is that patients with DHPR defects do not respond to dietary restrictions in phenylalanine as effectively as do classic PKU patients.

11. The action of many vasodilators within the vasculature involves the influx of calcium ions. A defect in which of the following proteins would most likely result in reduced effectiveness of these types of drugs?

A. adenylate cyclase
B. calmodulin
C. eNOS (NOS-3)
D. cGMP phosphodiesterase
E. guanylate cyclase

Answer B: Increases in intracellular calcium levels effects changes in various metabolic processes in part by binding to the calmodulin subunits of numerous proteins. The principal clinical actions of vasodilators that involve calcium mobilization due to their interactions with calmodulin or calmodulin-related proteins leads to reduced activation of Ca^{2+}-regulated enzymes in certain tissues, such as myosin light chain kinase in vascular smooth muscle.

12. A 9-year-old boy is stung on the arm by a wasp and very rapidly develops redness and swelling at the site of the sting. Which of the following substances is most responsible for these early changes?

A. bradykinin
B. complement 3a
C. histamine
D. leukotriene B_4
E. thromboxane A_2

Answer C: Histamine is a preformed inflammatory mediator found principally in mast cells and basophils that has a major role in the early vascular changes of inflammation, that is, dilation of precapillary arterioles, which produces the local redness (rubor) and warmth (calor), and the increased permeability of postcapillary venules, which produces the swelling (tumor).

13. A male infant is diagnosed with phenylketonuria (PKU) on newborn screening. Which of the following amino acids must be present in his diet to prevent a negative nitrogen balance?

A. alanine
B. cysteine
C. glutamine
D. serine
E. tyrosine

Answer E: A deficiency in phenylalanine hydroxylase (PAH) is the cause of PKU. Tyrosine is produced in cells by hydroxylating the essential amino acid phenylalanine and this reaction is catalyzed by PAH. Half of the phenylalanine required goes into the production of tyrosine; if the diet is rich in tyrosine itself, the requirements for phenylalanine are reduced by about 50%.

14. A 5-year-old boy with severe mental retardation is brought to the physician because of a 4-week history of progressively frequent generalized tonic-clonic seizures. There is no available record of newborn screening. He has blond hair and blue eyes. Physical examination shows patches of itchy, dry, thickened skin on the face, neck, and inner creases of the elbows and knees. Serum studies for amino acid concentrations are pending. Urine studies show increased concentrations of phenylpyruvic and phenyllactic acids. The activity of which of the following enzymes is most likely defective in this patient?

A. fumarylacetoacetate hydrolase
B. *p*-hydroxyphenylpyruvate dehydrogenase
C. phenylalanine hydroxylase
D. phenylalanine transaminase
E. tyrosine transaminase

Answer C: Missing or deficient phenylalanine hydroxylase results in *hyperphenylalaninemia*. The most widely recognized hyperphenylalaninemia (and most severe) is phenylketonuria (PKU). Untreated PKU leads to severe mental retardation. The mental retardation is caused by the accumulation of phenylalanine, which becomes a major donor of amino groups in aminotransferase activity and depletes neural tissue of α-ketoglutarate. The product of phenylalanine transamination, phenylpyruvic acid, is reduced to phenylacetate and phenyllactate, and all 3 compounds appear in the urine.

15. A 5-year-old girl with moderate mental retardation is brought to the physician by her mother who is concerned that her daughter has been having difficulty with her vision for weeks. Physical examination shows a fair complexion and malar erythema. Ophthalmologic examination shows dislocated lenses bilaterally. She has long, slender hands and fingers. Blood tests reveal her cystathionine concentration is below normal. This patient is most likely to have an increased urine concentration of which of the following amino acids?

A. alanine
B. arginine
C. cysteine
D. leucine
E. methionine

Answer E: The most common causes of homocystinuria are defects in the cystathionine β-synthase (*CBS*) gene. CBS is involved in the conversion of methionine to cysteine and so a deficiency in the enzyme can be suspected in cases where there are elevated levels of methionine in the blood.

16. A 22-year-old man comes to the physician 1 week after an episode of severe right flank pain that resolved with the passing of a renal calculus. His 25-year-old brother had similar symptoms 1 year ago. This patient most likely has an increased urine concentration of which of the following amino acids?

A. argininosuccinate and citrulline
B. glycine and alanine
C. lysine and cystine
D. methionine and homocystine
E. phenylalanine and tyrosine

Answer C: Cystinuria is a cause of persistent kidney stones (renal calculi). It is a disease involving the defective transepithelial transport of cystine and dibasic amino acids, such as lysine, in the kidney and intestine, and is one of many causes of kidney stones.

17. In using dietary restriction of phenylalanine to manage a 2-month-old girl who has phenylketonuria, which of the following should be added to the diet?
A. aspartate
B. cytosine
C. serine
D. tryptophan
E. tyrosine

Answer E: A deficiency in phenylalanine hydroxylase (PAH) is the cause of PKU. Tyrosine is produced in cells by hydroxylating the essential amino acid phenylalanine and this reaction is catalyzed by PAH. Half of the phenylalanine required goes into the production of tyrosine; if the diet is rich in tyrosine itself, the requirements for phenylalanine are reduced by about 50%.

18. The primary source of urinary ammonia (NH_3 or NH_4^+) is which of the following?
A. catabolism of glutamine within renal cells
B. catabolism of polyamines within renal cells
C. filtered ammonia
D. filtered glutamine
E. synthesis of alanine within renal cells

Answer A: Glutamine is the major amino acid of the circulation and its role is to ferry ammonia to and from various tissues. In the kidneys, glutamine is hydrolyzed by glutaminase (yielding glutamate), releasing the ammonia into the urine. There, the ammonia ionizes to ammonium ion, NH_4^+, which reduces the circulating concentration of hydrogen ion resulting in an increase in the pH. Additionally, the glutamate can be converted to α-ketoglutarate yielding another mole of ammonia, which is ionized by hydrogen ions further increasing the pH.

19. Which of the following is the amino acid in proteins that is most sensitive to air oxidation?
A. arginine
B. cysteine
C. histidine
D. methionine
E. serine

Answer B: The side chain of cysteine contains a reactive sulfur that can become oxidized, forming intermolecular disulfide bonds. Exposure of cysteine to air, such as could be the case in highly oxygen-rich tissue like erythrocytes, can result in oxidation of the sulfur.

20. The γ-amide of which of the following amino acids is a source of nitrogen in many biosynthetic reaction?
A. aspartate
B. γ-aminobutyric acid (GABA)
C. glutamine
D. histidine
E. lysine

Answer C: Glutamine is a major reservoir of nitrogen ($-NH_2$) in the body. The enzyme glutaminase releases one mole of ammonia from glutamine forming glutamate. Glutamate can be acted on by glutamate dehydrogenase to yield another mole of ammonia and α-ketoglutarate. The nitrogen, thus released, is available for use in other biosynthetic reaction.

21. A 6-day-old newborn, who is being breast-fed, is brought to the ER because he is unresponsive. He has been vomiting and is lethargic for the past 2 days. Examination shows an obtunded infant with hypertonia and muscle rigidity. A peculiar odor of burnt sugar is noted in his diaper. The plasma concentration of which of the following amino acids is most likely to be increased in this patient?
A. cysteine
B. homocysteine
C. leucine
D. phenylalanine
E. tyrosine

Answer C: Maple syrup urine disease (MSUD), also called branched-chain aminoaciduria, is so called because the urine of affected individuals smells like maple syrup or burnt sugar. MSUD results from a deficiency in an enzyme, branched-chain α-keto acid dehydrogenase (BCKD), that is involved in the catabolism of the branched-chain amino acids (BCAAs), leucine, isoleucine, and valine.

22. An 11-month-old boy is brought to the physician because of lethargy and irritability for the past 3 days, since a diagnosis of a middle ear infection. The physician prescribed an antibiotic to treat the ear infection. Laboratory studies show metabolic acidosis and an increased plasma valine concentration. Which of the following amino acid concentrations are most likely to be increased in this patient's blood if he has maple syrup urine disease?
A. arginine and lysine
B. asparagine and glutamine
C. homocysteine and cysteine
D. leucine and isoleucine
E. phenylalanine and tyrosine

Answer D: Maple syrup urine disease (MSUD), also called branched-chain aminoaciduria, is so called because the urine of affected individuals smells like maple syrup or burnt sugar. MSUD results from a deficiency in an enzyme, branched-chain α-keto acid dehydrogenase (BCKD), that is involved in the catabolism of the branched-chain amino acids (BCAAs) leucine, isoleucine, and valine.

23. A 1-month-old male newborn is brought to the physician for a routine examination. His parents both have olive-colored skin, dark hair, and dark eyes. Physical examination shows hypopigmentation of the skin, light blonde hair, and translucent irises. The inherited disorder that causes this phenotypic expression is most likely due to a defect in the metabolism of which of the following?

A. epinephrine
B. phenylalanine
C. serotonin
D. tryptophan
E. tyrosine

Answer E: Albinism is a congenital disorder characterized by the complete or partial absence of pigment in the skin, hair, and eyes due to absence or defect of tyrosinase. Tyrosinase is responsible for the conversion of tyrosine to the skin pigment melanin.

24. A 55-year-old man who has been suffering from chronic liver disease is diagnosed with elevated serum ammonia concentration. Failure of the liver to synthesize which of the following compounds most likely contributes to the increased serum ammonia concentration in this patient?

A. bilirubin
B. glutamine
C. heme
D. inosine
E. tyrosine

Answer B: Major hepatic reactions that involve the regulation of the level of circulating ammonia, include the enzymes glutamate dehydrogenase (GDH), glutamine synthase (GS), and glutaminase. The liver compartmentalizes GS and glutaminase in order to control the flow of ammonia into glutamine or urea. Under acidotic conditions, the liver diverts ammonia to glutamine via the GS reaction. The glutamine then enters the circulation. In fact, glutamine is the major amino acid of the circulation and its role is to ferry ammonia to and from various tissues.

25. A 5-day-old female newborn, who is breast-fed, is brought to the ER because of a 2-day history of poor feeding and vomiting. Physical examination shows lethargy, dehydration, hypertonicity, and rigidity of the extremities. There is a sweet odor of maple syrup in the newborn's diaper. Laboratory studies show metabolic acidosis, ketosis, and hypoglycemia. Following treatment of this patient's acute condition, long-term therapy is begun. This therapy is most likely to restrict which of the following substances?

A. galactose, fructose, and lactose
B. leucine, isoleucine, and valine
C. methionine, homocysteine, and cystathionine
D. ornithine, citrulline, and arginine
E. phenylalanine and tyrosine

Answer B: Maple syrup urine disease (MSUD), also called branched-chain aminoaciduria, is so called because the urine of affected individuals smells like maple syrup or burnt sugar. MSUD results from a deficiency in an enzyme, branched-chain α-keto acid dehydrogenase (BCKD), that is involved in the catabolism of the branched-chain amino acids (BCAAs) leucine, isoleucine, and valine.

26. A 23-year-old woman is brought to the ER because of a 1-hour history of severe pain and coldness of her left leg. History taking indicates that she dropped out of high school in the 10th grade due to difficulty with comprehension. Intelligence testing demonstrated her IQ to be 80 at that time. Her parents and 2 older siblings have normal intelligence and have no history of these symptoms. Ophthalmologic examination shows a partially dislocated lens in the right eye. Physical examination shows mottling and loss of pulses in the left lower extremity and foot. Arteriography of the left lower extremity shows thrombosis of the femoral artery. This patient most likely has a metabolic disorder involving which of the following amino acid?

A. glycine
B. homocysteine
C. leucine
D. phenylalanine
E. tyrosine

Answer B: Homocystinurias represent a family of inherited disorders resulting from defects in several of the genes involved in the conversion of methionine to cysteine. These disorders result in elevated levels of homocysteine, metabolites of homocysteine, and methionine in the urine. Homocystinuria is often associated with mental retardation, although the complete syndrome is multifaceted and many individuals with this disease are mentally normal, while others experience variable levels of developmental delay along with learning problems. Common symptoms of homocystinuria are dislocated optic lenses, osteoporosis, lengthening and thinning of the long bones, and an increased risk of abnormal blood clotting (thromboembolism).

27. A 2-year-old girl is brought to the physician because of failure to thrive. She was diagnosed with phenylketonuria on a routine neonatal screening. Her weight and height are currently well below normal for her age. She is following a low-phenylalanine diet. Her plasma phenylalanine concentration is within the reference range. The most appropriate next step is measurement of the concentration of which of the following in the plasma?

A. arginine
B. histidine
C. lysine
D. tryptophan
E. tyrosine

Answer E: A deficiency in phenylalanine hydroxylase (PAH) is the cause of PKU. Tyrosine is produced in cells by hydroxylating the essential amino acid phenylalanine and this reaction is catalyzed by PAH. Half of the phenylalanine required goes into the production of tyrosine; if the diet is rich in tyrosine itself, the requirements for phenylalanine are reduced by about 50%. Since this patient is on a diet restricting phenylalanine, it is necessary to periodically assay for serum tyrosine levels to ensure there is adequate amounts in the diet.

28. A 2-week-old girl of north European descent is found to have a blood methionine concentration of 1500 μM (normal <50) on newborn screening. Physical examination shows no abnormalities. Which of the following enzymes is most likely to be deficient in this patient's liver?

A. branched-chain α-keto acid dehydrogenase
B. cystathionine β-synthase
C. methionine synthase
D. phenylalanine hydroxylase
E. tyrosine aminotransferase

Answer B: The most common causes of homocystinuria are defects in the cystathionine β-synthase (*CBS*) gene. CBS is involved in the conversion of methionine to cysteine and so a deficiency in the enzyme can be suspected in cases where there are elevated levels of methionine in the blood.

29. During periods of drought, the leaves of desert trees often become a dietary staple for certain populations. Which of the following amino acids, present in sufficient quantity in the leaves, satisfies an essential nutrient requirement?

A. alanine
B. aspartate
C. glutamate
D. methionine
E. tyrosine

Answer D: Essential amino acids are so-called because they cannot be synthesized at all or in adequate amounts to serve the needs of the body. Of the amino acids listed, only methionine is an essential amino acid and is thus likely to be present in the leaves of the desert trees.

30. A 7-month-old boy has failed to gain weight normally. His diet consists of a diluted milk formula. His weight and length are below normal for his age, and he appears emaciated. His temperature is below normal, and his pulse is slow. Which of the following is the most likely cause of his condition?

A. chronic renal failure
B. deficiency of growth hormone
C. hypothyroidism
D. kwashiorkor
E. marasmus

Answer E: Marasmus is generally known as the gradual wasting away of the body due to severe malnutrition or inadequate absorption of food. It is a severe form of malnutrition caused by inadequate intake of proteins and calories. A child with marasmus looks emaciated and body weight is reduced to less than 60% of the normal body weight for the age. Marasmus can be distinguished from kwashiorkor in that kwashiorkor is protein deficiency with adequate energy intake whereas marasmus is inadequate energy intake in all forms, including protein.

Checklist

✓ Amino acids serve at least 2 critically important functions in cells. They are precursors for protein synthesis and conversely they can be oxidized to yield energy for ATP synthesis. Many amino acids serve additional functions in the body such as the neurotransmitter amino acids and amino acid derivatives.

✓ Dietary amino acids are absorbed via the action of specific intestinal enterocyte transporter proteins. Deficiency in the neutral amino acid transporter, found in the intestines and the kidneys, is the cause of Hartnup disorder.

✓ Amino acids are classified as essential if they cannot be synthesized by cells of the body or derived from precursor compounds.

✓ Oxidation of amino acids yields carbon compounds that can serve as precursors for glucose synthesis via gluconeogenesis or compounds that can only be delivered to the TCA cycle for further oxidation. The former are referred to as glucogenic amino acids, the latter as ketogenic.

✓ Glutamate and glutamine are 2 of the most important metabolic amino acids in the body; they serve as reservoirs of nitrogen and as the carbon skeletons for the TCA cycle intermediate, α-ketoglutarate. Glutamine is the major nitrogen-containing compound in the blood.

✓ Glutamate serves as the precursor for the synthesis of the neurotransmitter, GABA.

✓ Alanine plays a critical role in the delivery of waste nitrogen, primarily from skeletal muscle, to the liver. The carbon skeleton of alanine is pyruvate that can be used for glucose synthesis. This process is termed the glucose-alanine cycle.

✓ Methionine serves as the precursor for the synthesis of cysteine; deficiency in cystathione b-synthase is the major cause of homocysteinurias. Methionine is also the precursor for *S*-adenosylmethione, which is the principal methyl donor for the synthesis of the catecholamines and polyamines.

✓ Glycine and serine are interconverted via the action of serine-hydroxymethyltransferase. Serine can be synthesized from a glycolytic intermediate. Glycine is a neurotransmitter and also serves as a precursor in the synthesis of heme, creatine, and purine neuclotides.

✓ Tyrosine is derived from the hydroxylation of phenylalanine. Deficiency in the enzyme catalyzing this reaction results in the hyperphenyalaninemia called PKU. Tyrosine also serves as the precursor for the synthesis of the catecholamines.

✓ Tryptophan serves an important role as the precursor for the synthesis of serotonin and melatonin.

✓ Lysine serves as the precursor for the synthesis of carnitine that is required for mitochondrial uptake of fatty acids.

✓ Histodine serves as the precursor for the neurotransmitter histamine.

✓ Leucine, isoleucine, and valine are the branched-chain amino acids. Catabolism of these amino acids initially involves the same 2 enzymes. Deficiency in one of these enzymes, branched-chain a-keto-acid decarboxylase (BCKD), is the cause of maple syrup urine disease.

✓ Leucine is the primary mediator of the satiety effects associated with the consumption of a high-protein diet. At the molecular level, leucine has been shown to activate the metabolic regulatory kinase known as mammalian target of rapamycin, mTOR, Activation of skeletal muscle mTOR results in increased energy expenditure, whereas, hypothalamic mTOR activation reduces the desire for food intake.

CHAPTER

31 Nitrogen: Amino Acid–Derived Biomolecules

CHAPTER OUTLINE

High-Yield Terms

Endothelium-derived relaxing factor (EDRF): produced and released by vascular endothelium to promote smooth muscle relaxation; was found to be nitric oxide, NO

Catecholamines: neurotransmitter family derived from tyrosine, a catechol is an organic compound composed of a benzene ring and at least 2 hydroxyl groups attached, hence the derivation of the name of these compounds

Norepinephrine (noradrenaline): principal catecholamine neurotransmitter of sympathetic postganglionic nerves, its actions are exerted by binding to receptors of the adrenergic family

Epinephrine (adrenaline): a catecholamine neurotransmitter and hormone that modulates numerous function in the body by binding to receptors of the adrenergic family

Dopamine: a catecholamine neurotransmitter that plays a major role in the reward-driven learning processes in the CNS, functions by binding dopaminergic receptors

Glutathione: a tripeptide composed of glutamate, cysteine, and glycine that serves as a critical biological reductant; it is also conjugated to drugs to make them more water soluble and is involved in amino acid transport across cell membranes

Polyamine: any of a family of organic compounds having 2 or more primary amino groups ($-NH_2$), biologically important polyamines are involved in DNA replication, ion channel modulation, and blood-brain barrier permeability

Several amino acids possess distinct biochemical functions unrelated to their roles in protein synthesis and as sources of oxidizable carbon. Numerous biologically active compounds are derived from the amino acids such as signaling molecules and neurotransmitters.

Nitric Oxide Synthesis and Function

Vasodilators, such bradykinin, do not exert their effects upon the vascular smooth muscle cell in the absence of the overlying endothelium. For example, when bradykinin binds to bradykinin B_2 receptors on the surface of endothelial cells, a signal cascade, coupled to the activation phospholipase Cβ (PLCβ), is initiated. The PLCβ-mediated release of inositol trisphosphate, IP_3 (from membrane-associated phosphatidylinositol-4,5-bisphosphate, PIP_2), leads to the release of intracellular stores of Ca^{2+}. In turn, the elevation in Ca^{2+} leads to the liberation of endothelium-derived relaxing factor (EDRF) which then diffuses into the adjacent smooth muscle. EDRF was found to be the free radical diatomic gas, NO. NO is formed by the action of NO synthase (NOS) on the amino acid arginine (Figure 31-1).

NO can also be formed from nitrite, derived from vasodilator drugs such as glycerin trinitrate (nitroglycerin) during their metabolism. The half-life of NO is extremely short, lasting only 2-4 seconds. This is because it is a highly reactive free radical and interacts with oxygen and superoxide. NO is inhibited by hemoglobin and other heme proteins which bind it tightly.

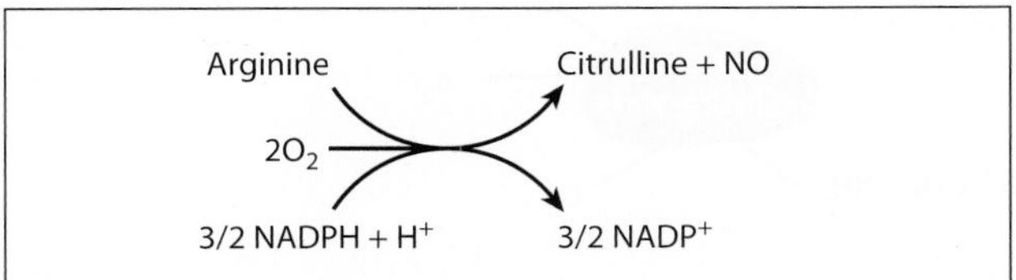

FIGURE 31-1: The reaction catalyzed by nitric oxide synthase. Murray RK, Bender DA, Botham KM, Kennelly PJ, Rodwell VW, Weil PA. *Harper's Illustrated Biochemistry*, 29th ed. New York: McGraw-Hill; 2012.

Within smooth muscle cells, NO reacts with the heme moiety of a soluble guanylyl cyclase, resulting in activation of the latter and a consequent elevation of intracellular levels of cGMP. The net effect is the activation of cGMP-dependent protein kinase (PKG) and the phosphorylation of substrates leading to smooth muscle cell relaxation.

Both eNOS and nNOS are constitutively expressed and regulated by Ca^{2+}. The calcium regulation is imparted by the associated calmodulin subunits, thus explaining how vasodilators such as acetylcholine effect smooth muscle relaxation as a consequence of increasing intracellular endothelial cell calcium levels. Although iNOS contains calmodulin subunits, its activity is unaffected by changes in Ca^{2+} concentration. iNOS is transcriptionally activated in macrophages, neutrophils, and smooth muscle cells.

The major functions of NO production through activation of iNOS are associated with the bactericidal and tumoricidal actions of macrophages. Overproduction of NO via iNOS is associated with cytokine-induced septic shock such as occurs postoperatively in patients with bacterial infections. Bacteria produce endotoxins such as lipopolysaccharide (LPS) that activate iNOS in macrophages.

NO is also generated by cells of the immune system and as such is involved in nonspecific host defense mechanisms and macrophage-mediated killing. NO also inhibits the proliferation of tumor cells and microorganisms. Additional cellular responses to NO include induction of apoptosis (programmed cell death), DNA breakage, and mutation.

Chemical inhibitors of NOS are available and can markedly decrease production of NO. The effect is a dramatic increase in blood pressure due to vasoconstriction. Another important cardiovascular effect of NO is exerted through the production of cGMP, which acts to inhibit platelet aggregation.

Tyrosine-Derived Neurotransmitters

The majority of tyrosine that does not get incorporated into proteins is catabolized for energy production. One other significant fate of tyrosine is conversion to the

High-Yield Concept

There are 3 isozymes of NOS in mammalian cells: neuronal NOS (nNOS), also called NOS-1; inducible or macrophage NOS (iNOS), also called NOS-2; endothelial NOS (eNOS), also called NOS-3. Nitric oxide synthases are very complex enzymes, employing 5 redox cofactors: NADPH, FAD, FMN, heme, and tetrahydrobiopterin (BH_4 is also sometimes written as H_4B).

High-Yield Concept

Nitric oxide is involved in a number of other important cellular processes in addition to its impact on vascular smooth muscle cells. Events initiated by NO that are important for blood coagulation include inhibition of platelet aggregation and adhesion and inhibition of neutrophil adhesion to platelets and to the vascular endothelium.

catecholamines. The catecholamine neurotransmitters are dopamine, norepinephrine, and epinephrine (Figure 31-2).

Norepinephrine is the principal neurotransmitter of sympathetic postganglionic nerves. Norepinephrine functions as a stress hormone and also regulates vascular tone resulting in increases in blood pressure. Epinephrine exerts numerous functions in the body that include regulation of heart rate, vascular tone, and alterations in metabolic processes.

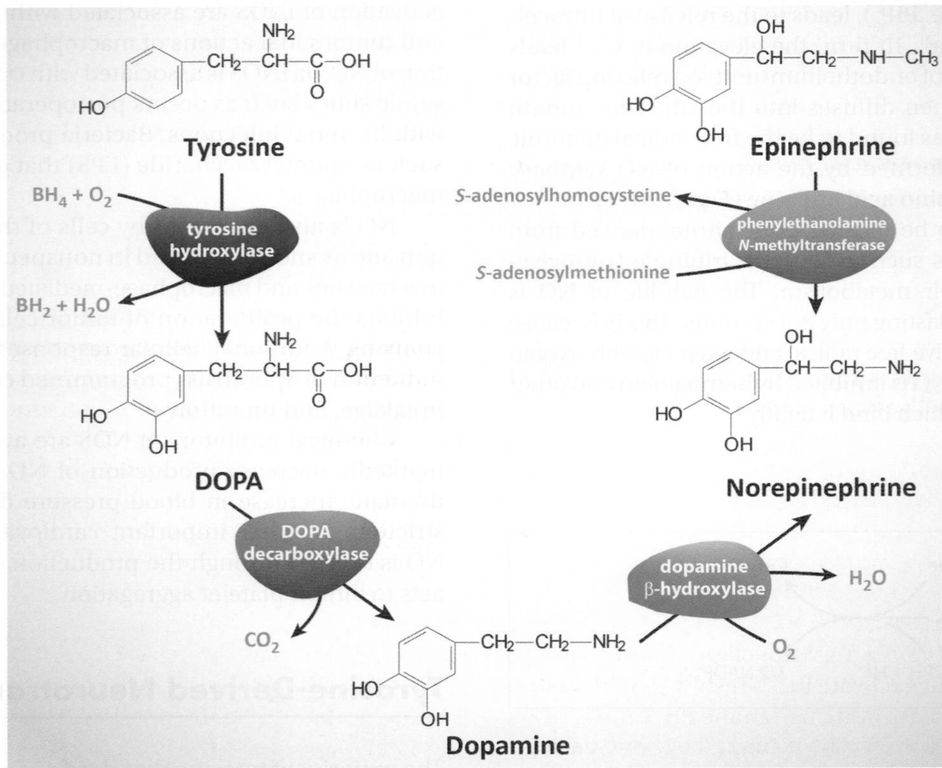

FIGURE 31-2: Synthesis of the catecholamines from tyrosine. Reproduced with permission of themedicalbiochemistrypage, LLC.

High-Yield Concept

Both epinephrine and norepinephrine actions underlie the fight-or-flight response which encompasses increased heart rate, increased blood flow to skeletal muscle, and increased glucose mobilization from glycogen.

High-Yield Concept

Tyrosine is transported into catecholamine-secreting neurons and adrenal medullary cells where catecholamine synthesis takes place. The site of synthesis is why these neurotransmitters are also referred to as adrenergic neurotransmitters and their receptors are called adrenergic receptors.

The first step in the process requires tyrosine hydroxylase, which like phenylalanine hydroxylase requires tetrahydrobiopterin (BH_4) as cofactor. The dependence of tyrosine hydroxylase on BH_4 necessitates the coupling to the action of dihydropteridine reductase (DHPR) as is the situation for phenylalanine hydroxylase (Chapter 30) and tryptophan hydroxylase (see below).

The hydroxylation reaction generates DOPA (3,4-dihydrophenylalanine, also called L-DOPA). DOPA decarboxylase converts DOPA to dopamine, dopamine β-hydroxylase converts dopamine to norepinephrine, and phenylethanolamine *N*-methyltransferase converts norepinephrine to epinephrine. This latter reaction is one of several in the body that uses *S*-adenosylmethionine (SAM) as a methyl donor generating *S*-adenosylhomocysteine. Within the substantia nigra and some other regions of the brain, synthesis proceeds only to dopamine. Within the adrenal medulla dopamine is converted to norepinephrine and epinephrine. Once synthesized, dopamine, norepinephrine, and epinephrine are packaged in granulated vesicles. Within these vesicles, norepinephrine and epinephrine are bound to ATP and a protein called chromogranin A.

The actions of norepinephrine and epinephrine are exerted via receptor-mediated signal transduction events. There are 3 distinct types of adrenergic receptors: α_1, α_2, β. Within each class of adrenergic receptor there are several subclasses. The α_1 class contains the α_{1A}, α_{1B}, and α_{1D} receptors. The α_1 receptor class is coupled to G_q-type G-proteins that activate PLCβ resulting in increases in IP_3 and DAG release from membrane PIP_2. The α_2 class contains the α_{2A}, α_{2B}, and α_{2C} receptors. The α_2 class of adrenergic receptor is coupled to G_i-type G-proteins that inhibit the activation of adenylate cyclase, and therefore activation results in reductions in cAMP levels. The β class of receptors is composed of three subtypes: β_1, β_2, and β_3 each of which couple to G_s-type G-proteins resulting in activation of adenylate cyclase and increases in cAMP with concomitant activation of PKA.

Dopamine binds to dopaminergic receptors identified as D-type receptors and there are 4 subclasses identified as D_1, D_2, D_4, and D_5. Activation of the dopaminergic receptors results in activation of adenylate cyclase (D_1 and D_5) or inhibition of adenylate cyclase (D_2 and D_4).

Epinephrine and norepinephrine are catabolized (Figure 31-3) to inactive compounds through the sequential actions of catecholamine-*O*-methyltransferase (COMT) and monoamine oxidase (MAO). Compounds that inhibit the action of MAO have been shown to have beneficial effects in the treatment of clinical depression, even when tricyclic antidepressants are ineffective. The utility of MAO inhibitors was discovered serendipitously when patients treated for tuberculosis with isoniazid showed signs of an improvement in mood; isoniazid was subsequently found to work by inhibiting MAO.

Tryptophan-Derived Neurotransmitters

Tryptophan serves as the precursor for the synthesis of serotonin (5-hydroxytryptamine, 5-HT), and melatonin (*N*-acetyl-5-methoxytryptamine). Serotonin is synthesized through 2-step process involving a tetrahydrobiopterin-dependent hydroxylation reaction (catalyzed by tryptophan 5-monooxygenase, also called tryptophan hydroxylase) and then a decarboxylation catalyzed by aromatic L-amino acid decarboxylase (Figure 31-4). The hydroxylase is normally not saturated and as a result an increased uptake of tryptophan in the diet will lead to increased brain serotonin content.

Serotonin is present at highest concentrations in platelets and in the gastrointestinal tract. Lesser amounts are found in the brain and the retina. Serotonin containing neurons have their cell bodies in the midline raphe nuclei of the brain stem and project to portions of the hypothalamus, the limbic system, the neocortex, and the spinal cord. After release from serotonergic neurons, most of the released serotonin is recaptured by an active reuptake mechanism. The function of the antidepressant, fluoxetine, and related drugs called selective serotonin reuptake inhibitors (SSRI) is to inhibit this reuptake process, thereby resulting in prolonged serotonin presence in the synaptic cleft.

The function of serotonin is exerted upon its interaction with specific receptors. Several serotonin receptors

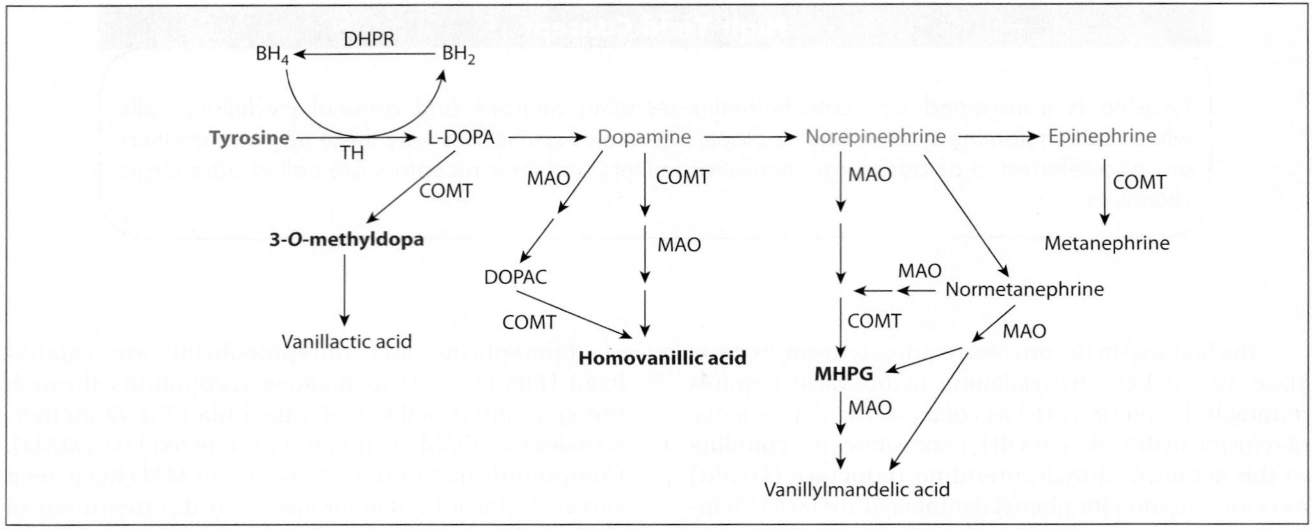

FIGURE 31-3: Metabolism of the catecholamine neurotransmitters. Only clinically important enzymes are included in this diagram. The catabolic by-products of the catecholamines, whose levels in the cerebrospinal fluid are indicative of defects in catabolism, are in blue underlined text. TH, tyrosine hydroxylase; DHPR, dihydropteridine reductase; BH_2, dihydrobiopterin; BH_4, tetrahydrobiopterin; MAO, monoamine oxidase; COMT, catecholamine-*O*-methyltransferase; MHPG, 3-methoxy-4-hydroxyphenylglycol; DOPAC, dihydroxyphenylacetic acid. Reproduced with permission of themedicalbiochemistrypage, LLC.

have been cloned and are identified as $5HT_1$, $5HT_2$, $5HT_3$, $5HT_4$, $5HT_5$, $5HT_6$, and $5HT_7$. Within the $5HT_1$ group there are subtypes $5HT_{1A}$, $5HT_{1B}$, $5HT_{1D}$, $5HT_{1E}$, and $5HT_{1F}$. There are 3 $5HT_2$ subtypes, $5HT_{2A}$, $5HT_{2B}$, and $5HT_{2C}$ as well as 2 $5HT_5$ subtypes, $5HT_{5A}$ and $5HT_{5B}$. Most of these receptors are coupled to G-proteins that affect the activities of either adenylate cyclase or phospholipase Cβ (PLCβ). The $5HT_3$ receptors are ion channels.

Some serotonin receptors are presynaptic and others postsynaptic. The $5HT_{2A}$ receptors mediate platelet aggregation and smooth muscle contraction. The $5HT_{2C}$ receptors are suspected in control of food intake as mice lacking this gene become obese from increased food intake and are also subject to fatal seizures. The $5HT_3$ receptors are present in the gastrointestinal tract and are related to vomiting. Also present in the gastrointestinal tract are $5HT_4$receptors where they function in secretion and peristalsis. The $5HT_6$ and $5HT_7$ receptors are distributed throughout the limbic system of the brain and the $5HT_6$ receptors have high affinity for antidepressant drugs.

Melatonin is derived from serotonin within the pineal gland and the retina, where the necessary *N*-acetyltransferase enzyme is expressed. The pineal parenchymal cells secrete melatonin into the blood and cerebrospinal fluid. Synthesis and secretion of melatonin increases during the dark period of the day and is maintained at a low level during daylight hours. This diurnal variation in melatonin synthesis is brought about by norepinephrine secreted by the postganglionic sympathetic nerves that innervate the pineal gland. The effects of norepinephrine are exerted through interaction with β-adrenergic receptors. This leads to increased levels of cAMP, which in turn activate the *N*-acetyltransferase required for melatonin synthesis. Melatonin functions by inhibiting the synthesis and secretion of other neurotransmitters such as dopamine and GABA.

GABA: Inhibitory Neurotransmitter

Several amino acids and amino acid derivatives have distinct excitatory or inhibitory effects upon the nervous system. The glutamate derivative, γ-aminobutyrate (GABA; also called 4-aminobutyrate) is a major inhibitor of presynaptic transmission in the CNS, and also in the retina. Neurons that secrete GABA are termed GABAergic neurons.

The formation of GABA occurs via a metabolic pathway referred to as the GABA shunt (Figure 31-5). Glucose is the principal precursor for GABA production via its conversion to α-ketoglutarate in the TCA cycle. Within the context of the GABA shunt the α-ketoglutarate is transaminated to glutamate by GABA α-oxoglutarate transaminase (GABA-T). Glutamic acid decarboxylase (GAD) catalyzes the decarboxylation of glutamic acid to form GABA. There are 2 GAD genes in humans identified as GAD1 and GAD2. The GAD isoforms produced by these 2 genes are identified as GAD67 (GAD1 gene:

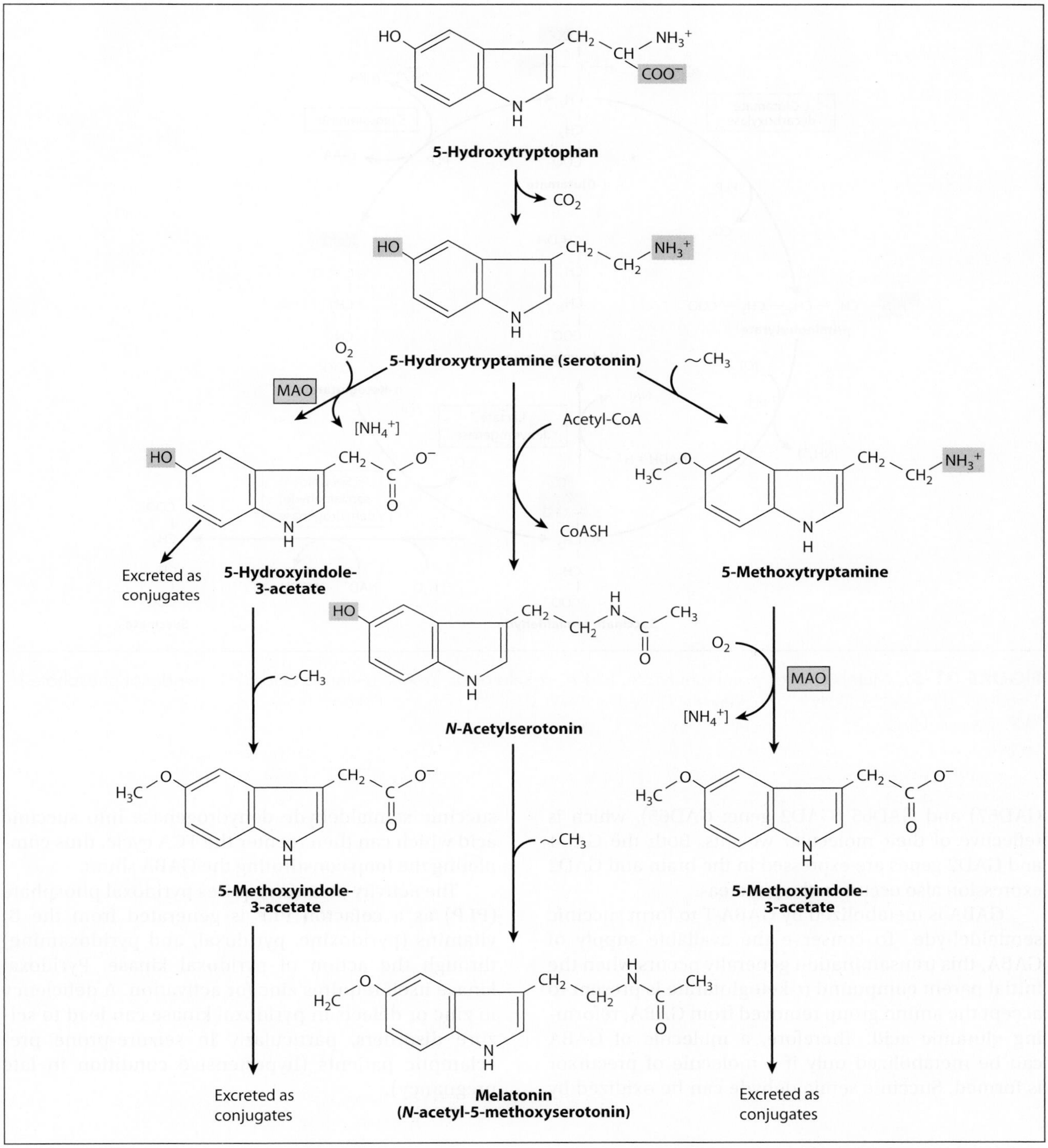

HO
CH_2
CH
NH_3^+
COO^-
N
H
5-Hydroxytryptophan
CO_2
HO
CH_2
CH_2
NH_3^+
N
H
O_2
5-Hydroxytryptamine (serotonin)
~CH_3
MAO
$[NH_4^+]$
Acetyl-CoA
HO
CH_2
C
O^-
O
N
H
H_3C
O
CH_2
CH_2
NH_3^+
N
H
CoASH
Excreted as conjugates
5-Hydroxyindole-3-acetate
5-Methoxytryptamine
HO
CH_2
CH_2
H
N
C
CH_3
O
N
H
O_2
MAO
~CH_3
$[NH_4^+]$
***N*-Acetylserotonin**
H_3C
O
CH_2
C
O^-
O
N
H
H_3C
O
CH_2
C
O^-
O
N
H
~CH_3
5-Methoxyindole-3-acetate
5-Methoxyindole-3-acetate
H_3C
O
CH_2
CH_2
H
N
C
CH_3
O
N
H
Excreted as conjugates
Melatonin (*N*-acetyl-5-methoxyserotonin)
Excreted as conjugates

FIGURE 31-4: Biosynthesis and metabolism of serotonin and melatonin. ($[NH_4^+]$, by transamination; MAO, monoamine oxidase; ~CH_3, from *S*-adenosylmethionine.) Murray RK, Bender DA, Botham KM, Kennelly PJ, Rodwell VW, Weil PA. *Harper's Illustrated Biochemistry*, 29th ed. New York: McGraw-Hill; 2012.

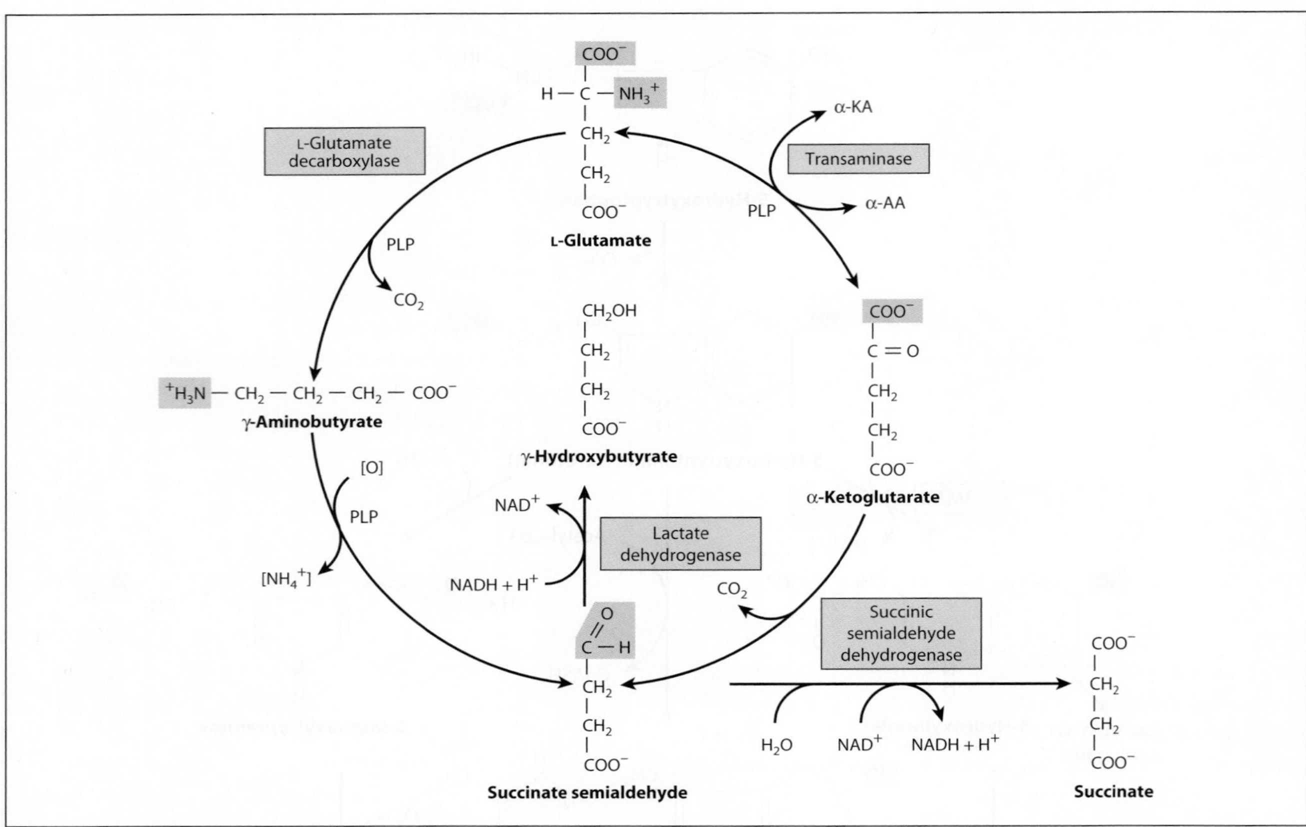

FIGURE 31-5: Metabolism of γ-aminobutyrate. (α-KA, α-keto acids; α-AA, α-amino acids; PLP, pyridoxal phosphate.) Murray RK, Bender DA, Botham KM, Kennelly PJ, Rodwell VW, Weil PA. *Harper's Illustrated Biochemistry,* 29th ed. New York: McGraw-Hill; 2012.

GAD67) and GAD65 (GAD2 gene: GAD65), which is reflective of their molecular weights. Both the GAD1 and GAD2 genes are expressed in the brain and GAD2 expression also occurs in the pancreas.

GABA is metabolized by GABA-T to form succinic semialdehyde. To conserve the available supply of GABA, this transamination generally occurs when the initial parent compound α-ketoglutarate is present to accept the amino group removed from GABA, reforming glutamic acid. Therefore, a molecule of GABA can be metabolized only if a molecule of precursor is formed. Succinic semialdehyde can be oxidized by succinic semialdehyde dehydrogenase into succinic acid which can then reenter the TCA cycle, thus completing the loop constituting the GABA shunt.

The activity of GAD requires pyridoxal phosphate (PLP) as a cofactor. PLP is generated from the B_6 vitamins (pyridoxine, pyridoxal, and pyridoxamine) through the action of pyridoxal kinase. Pyridoxal kinase itself requires zinc for activation. A deficiency in zinc or defects in pyridoxal kinase can lead to seizure disorders, particularly in seizure-prone preeclamptic patients (hypertensive condition in late pregnancy).

High-Yield Concept

The presence of anti-GAD antibodies (both anti-GAD65 and anti-GAD67) is a strong predictor of the future development of Type 1 diabetes in high-risk populations.

GABA exerts its effects by binding to 2 distinct receptors, GABA-A and GABA-B. The GABA-A receptors form a Cl^- channel. The binding of GABA to GABA-A receptors increases the Cl^- conductance of presynaptic neurons. The anxiolytic drugs of the benzodiazepine family exert their soothing effects by potentiating the responses of GABA-A receptors to GABA binding. The GABA-B receptors are coupled to an intracellular G-protein and act by increasing conductance of an associated K^+ channel.

Creatine and Creatinine Biosynthesis

Creatine is synthesized in the liver by methylation of guanidinoacetate using SAM as the methyl donor (Figure 31-6). Guanidinoacetate itself is formed in the kidney from the amino acids arginine and glycine.

Creatine is used as a storage form of high energy phosphate. The phosphate of ATP is transferred to creatine, generating creatine phosphate, through the action of creatine phosphokinase. The reaction is reversible such that when energy demand is high (eg, during muscle exertion), creatine phosphate donates its phosphate to ADP to yield ATP.

Glutathione Functions

Glutathione (abbreviated GSH) is a tripeptide composed of glutamate, cysteine, and glycine that has numerous important functions within cells. Glutathione serves as a reductant; is conjugated to drugs to make them more water soluble; is involved in amino acid transport across cell membranes (the γ-glutamyl cycle); is a substrate for the peptidoleukotrienes; serves as a cofactor for some enzymatic reactions; and plays a role as an aid in the rearrangement of protein disulfide bonds. GSH is synthesized in the cytosol of all mammalian cells (Figure 31-7). The rate of GSH synthesis is dependent upon the availability of cysteine and the activity of the rate-limiting enzyme, γ-glutamylcysteine synthetase (GCS). Numerous conditions can alter the level of GSH synthesis via changes in GCS activity and GCS gene expression such as oxidative stress, antioxidant levels, hormones, cell proliferation, and diabetes mellitus.

Endogenously produced hydrogen peroxide (H_2O_2) is reduced by GSH in the presence of selenium-dependent glutathione peroxidase. Hydrogen peroxide can also be reduced by catalase, which is present only in the peroxisomes. In the mitochondria, GSH is particularly important because mitochondria lack catalase.

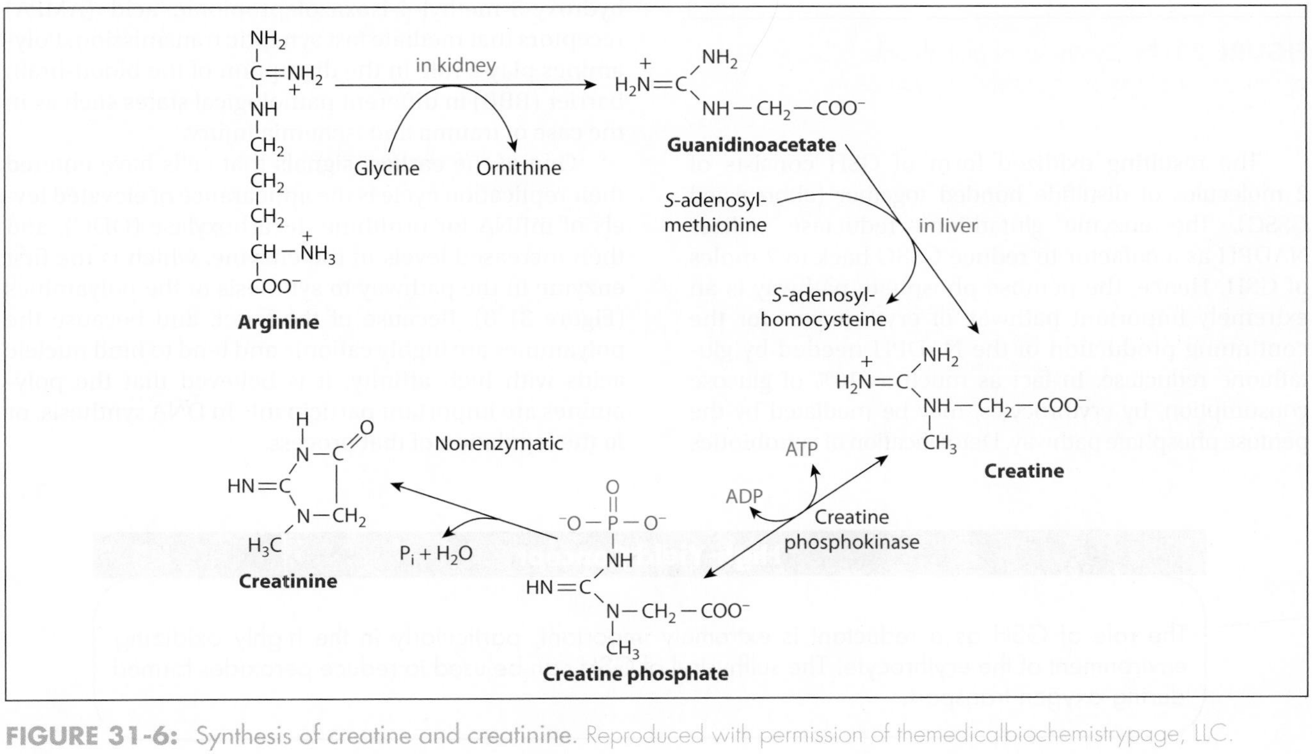

FIGURE 31-6: Synthesis of creatine and creatinine. Reproduced with permission of themedicalbiochemistrypage, LLC.

High-Yield Concept

Both creatine and creatine phosphate are found in muscle, brain, and blood. Creatinine is formed in muscle from creatine phosphate by a nonenzymatic dehydration and loss of phosphate. The amount of creatinine produced is related to muscle mass and remains remarkably constant from day to day. Creatinine is excreted by the kidneys and the level of excretion (creatinine clearance rate) is a measure of renal function.

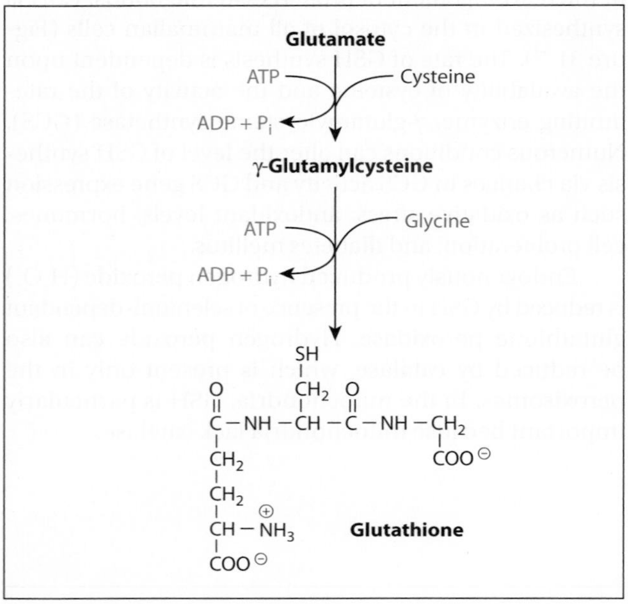

Glutamate
ATP → ADP + P_i ; Cysteine
γ-Glutamylcysteine
ATP → ADP + P_i ; Glycine
Glutathione

FIGURE 31-7: Synthesis of glutathione. Reproduced with permission of themedicalbiochemistrypage, LLC.

The resulting oxidized form of GSH consists of 2 molecules of disulfide bonded together (abbreviated GSSG). The enzyme glutathione reductase utilizes NADPH as a cofactor to reduce GSSG back to 2 moles of GSH. Hence, the pentose phosphate pathway is an extremely important pathway of erythrocytes for the continuing production of the NADPH needed by glutathione reductase. In fact as much as 10% of glucose consumption, by erythrocytes, may be mediated by the pentose phosphate pathway. Detoxification of xenobiotics or their metabolites is another major function of GSH. These compounds form conjugates with GSH either spontaneously or enzymatically in reactions catalyzed by GSH *S*-transferase. The conjugates formed are usually excreted from the cell, and in the case of the liver they are excreted in the bile.

Polyamine Biosynthesis

Polyamines are organic compounds that contain 2 or more primary amine groups ($-NH_2$). The biologically significant polyamines include putrescine, spermine, and spermidine that are involved in stabilizing DNA during the replication process. Polyamines also are important modulators of the activities of several types of ion channels such as the glutamate receptors called the *N*-methyl-D-aspartate (NMDA) and α-amino-3-hydroxy-5-methyl-4-isoxazolepropionic acid (AMPA) receptors that mediate fast synaptic transmission. Polyamines play a role in the disruption of the blood-brain barrier (BBB) in different pathological states such as in the case of trauma and ischemia injury.

One of the earliest signals that cells have entered their replication cycle is the appearance of elevated levels of mRNA for ornithine decarboxylase (ODC), and then increased levels of the enzyme, which is the first enzyme in the pathway to synthesis of the polyamines (Figure 31-8). Because of the latter, and because the polyamines are highly cationic and tend to bind nucleic acids with high affinity, it is believed that the polyamines are important participants in DNA synthesis, or in the regulation of that process.

High-Yield Concept

The role of GSH as a reductant is extremely important, particularly in the highly oxidizing environment of the erythrocyte. The sulfhydryl of GSH can be used to reduce peroxides formed during oxygen transport.

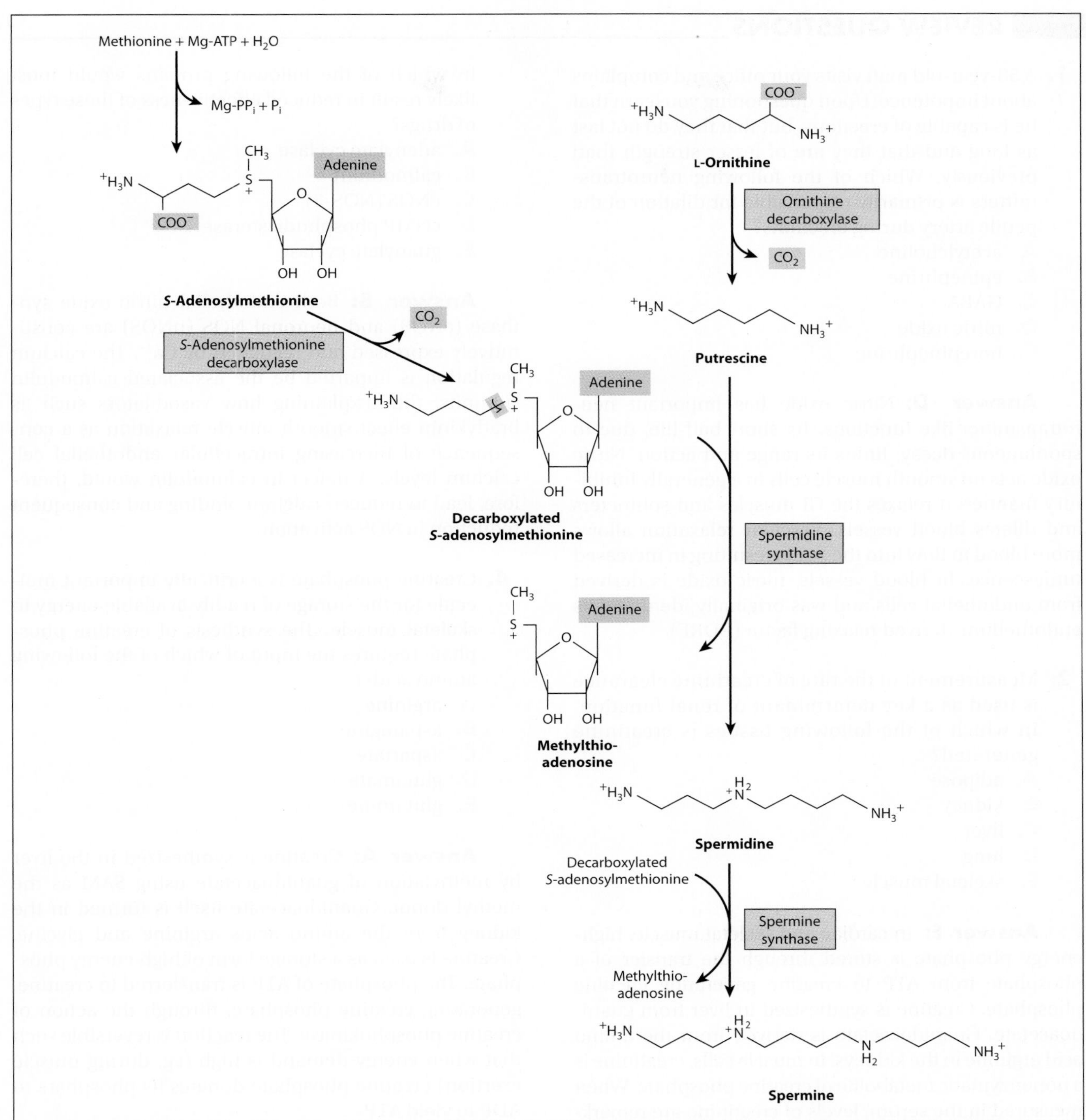

FIGURE 31-8: Intermediates and enzymes that participate in the biosynthesis of spermidine and spermine. Murray RK, Bender DA, Botham KM, Kennelly PJ, Rodwell VW, Weil PA. *Harper's Illustrated Biochemistry*, 29th ed. New York: McGraw-Hill; 2012.

The key features of the pathway are that it involves putrescine, an ornithine catabolite, and *S*-adenosylmethionine (SAM) as a donor of 2 propylamine residues. The first propylamine conjugation yields spermidine and addition of another to spermidine yields spermine.

The butylamino group of spermidine is used in a posttranslational modification reaction important to the process of translation. A specific lysine residue in the translational initiation factor eIF-4D is modified. Following the modification the residue is hydroxylated yielding a residue in the protein termed hypusine.

REVIEW QUESTIONS

1. A 58-year-old man visits your office and complains about impotence. Upon questioning you learn that he is capable of erections, but that they do not last as long and that they are of lesser strength than previously. Which of the following neurotransmitters is primarily responsible for dilation of the penile artery during erections?
   A. acetylcholine
   B. epinephrine
   C. GABA
   D. nitric oxide
   E. norepinephrine

Answer D: Nitric oxide has important neurotransmitter-like functions. Its short half-life, due to spontaneous decay, limits its range and action. Nitric oxide acts on smooth muscle cells in a generally inhibitory manner; it relaxes the GI muscles and sphincters and dilates blood vessels. Vascular relaxation allows more blood to flow into the penis resulting in increased tumescence. In blood vessels, nitric oxide is derived from endothelial cells and was originally identified as endothelium-derived relaxing factor (EDRF).

2. Measurement of the rate of creatinine clearance is used as a key determinant of renal function. In which of the following tissues is creatinine generated?
   A. adipose
   B. kidney
   C. liver
   D. lung
   E. skeletal muscle

Answer E: In cardiac and skeletal muscle, high-energy phosphate is stored through the transfer of a phosphate from ATP to creatine generating creatine phosphate. Creatine is synthesized in liver from guanidoacetate. Guanidoacetate is derived from the amino acid arginine in the kidneys. In muscle cells, creatinine is a nonenzymatic metabolite of creatine phosphate. When measured in the serum, levels of creatinine are remarkably constant from day to day and are proportional to muscle mass. In renal dysfunction, the clearance of creatinine will be impaired and its levels will therefore rise in the serum. Although creatine is synthesized in the liver from guanidoacetate, which is produced in the kidney, it is not used by these 2 tissues. Once synthesized, creatine is transported to cardiac and skeletal muscle where it is phosphorylated and stored for future energy needs.

3. The action of many vasodilators within the vasculature involves the influx of calcium ions. A defect in which of the following proteins would most likely result in reduced effectiveness of these types of drugs?
   A. adenylate cyclase
   B. calmodulin
   C. eNOS (NOS-3)
   D. cGMP phosphodiesterase
   E. guanylate cyclase

Answer B: Both endothelial nitric oxide synthase (eNOS) and neuronal NOS (nNOS) are constitutively expressed and regulated by Ca^{2+}. The calcium regulation is imparted be the associated calmodulin subunits, thus explaining how vasodilators such as bradykinin effect smooth muscle relaxation as a consequence of increasing intracellular endothelial cell calcium levels. A defect in calmodulin would, therefore, lead to reduced calcium binding and consequent reduction in NOS activation.

4. Creatine phosphate is a critically important molecule for the storage of readily available energy in skeletal muscle. The synthesis of creatine phosphate requires the input of which of the following amino acids?
   A. arginine
   B. asparagine
   C. aspartate
   D. glutamate
   E. glutamine

Answer A: Creatine is synthesized in the liver by methylation of guanidoacetate using SAM as the methyl donor. Guanidoacetate itself is formed in the kidney from the amino acids arginine and glycine. Creatine is used as a storage form of high energy phosphate. The phosphate of ATP is transferred to creatine, generating creatine phosphate, through the action of creatine phosphokinase. The reaction is reversible such that when energy demand is high (eg, during muscle exertion) creatine phosphate donates its phosphate to ADP to yield ATP.

5. A 50-year-old man comes to the physician because of difficulty sleeping. History taking indicates insomnia is most likely caused by work-related stress. Before recommending pharmacological intervention, the physician suggests drinking a glass of warm milk and eating a turkey sandwich before bedtime. Which of the following precursors of serotonin is found in these foods?
   A. γ-aminobutyric acid (GABA)
   B. arginine

C. dopamine
D. tryptophan
E. tyrosine

Answer D: Serotonin is derived from the amino acid tryptophan. Low serotonin levels result in sleep disruption and sleep disorders, including insomnia. Stress is a common cause of low serotonin levels, resulting in a snowballing feedback cycle of disrupted sleep, depression, anxiety, and fatigue during the day.

6. You are studying the effects of mineral depletion in laboratory mice. These mice are fed a chow lacking in the trace metal zinc for a period of 2 weeks. Analysis of neurotransmitter levels and function at this time indicates that GABA production is significantly reduced. Which of the following symptoms is most likely to be observed in these mice as a result of the effects of the zinc restricted diet?
A. activation of the process of emesis (vomiting)
B. enhancement in reward-driven learning processes
C. enhancement in the activity of excitatory nerve fibers
D. stimulation of appetite
E. stimulation of hormone release from the pituitary

Answer C: The amino acid derivative, γ-aminobutyrate (GABA) is a major inhibitor of presynaptic transmission in the CNS, and also in the retina. Neurons that secrete GABA are termed GABAergic. The activity of GAD requires pyridoxal phosphate (PLP) as a cofactor. PLP is generated from the B_6 vitamins through the action of pyridoxal kinase. Pyridoxal kinase itself requires zinc for activation. A deficiency in zinc or defects in pyridoxal kinase can lead to seizure disorders, particularly in seizure-prone preeclamptic patients (hypertensive condition in late pregnancy).

7. A 37-year-old 32-week pregnant woman is brought to the emergency room after suffering several seizures. Additional symptoms found in this patient are swollen hands and feet, blood pressure 165/125, right quadrant belly pain, and significant proteinuria. The ER physician suspects the woman is suffering from preeclampsia. Additional blood work indicates a deficiency in zinc. Which of the following amino acids serves as substrate for an important enzyme whose activity is impaired by a deficiency in zinc and could therefore explain the signs and symptoms in this patient?
A. glycine
B. glutamate
C. arginine
D. tyrosine
E. tryptophan

Answer: The glutamate derivative, γ-aminobutyrate (GABA; also called 4-aminobutyrate) is a major inhibitor of presynaptic transmission in the CNS. Glutamic acid decarboxylase (GAD) catalyzes the decarboxylation of glutamic acid to form GABA. The activity of GAD requires pyridoxal phosphate (PLP) as a cofactor. PLP is generated through the action of pyridoxal kinase. Pyridoxal kinase itself requires zinc for activation. A deficiency in zinc or defects in pyridoxal kinase can lead to seizure disorders, particularly as seen in this preeclamptic patient.

8. You are studying the replication characteristics of a cell line in culture. You find that the DNA in these cells fragments easily and does not replicate well. Analysis of components of the replication machinery and associated compounds shows that the levels of spermidine and spermine are significantly reduced compared to normal cells. A deficiency in which of the following enzymes could best explain the observations made with these cells?
A. cystathionine β-synthase
B. glutamate dehydrogenase
D. methionine synthase
C. γ-glutamylcysteine synthetase
E. ornithine decarboxylase

Answer E: Spermine and spermidine are polyamines whose functions include stabilization of DNA during the processes of replication. The initial step in polyamine synthesis is catalyzed by ornithine decarboxylase (ODC), which decarboxylates the amino acid ornithine producing putrescine.

9. You are examining the characteristics of erythrocytes from a patient who suffers from recurrent episodes of mild hemolytic anemia. Your analysis of these cells shows that they are highly sensitive to oxidative stress likely due to the fact that they contain significantly less glutathione than normal erythrocytes. A deficiency in which of the following enzymes is likely in these erythrocytes?
A. cystathionine β-synthase
B. glutamate dehydrogenase
C. γ-glutamylcysteine synthetase
D. methionine synthase
E. ornithine decarboxylase

Answer C: Glutathione (GSH) is synthesized in the cytosol of all mammalian cells. The rate of GSH synthesis is dependent upon the availability of cysteine and the activity of the rate-limiting enzyme, γ-glutamylcysteine synthetase (GCS).

10. During a clinical study, an investigator examines the effects of monoamine oxidase inhibitors to treat certain types of major depressive and phobic anxiety disorders. The concentration of which of the following compounds is most likely to be increased as a result of this treatment?

A. γ-aminobutyric acid, GABA
B. dihydroxyphenylalanine
C. epinephrine
D. tryptophan
E. tyrosine

Answer C: Epinephrine and norepinephrine are catabolized to inactive compounds through the sequential actions of catecholamine-*O*-methyltransferase (COMT) and monoamine oxidase (MAO). Compounds that inhibit the action of MAO have been shown to have beneficial effects in the treatment of clinical depression and anxiety disorders.

11. Genetic engineering has been used to create a strain of mice that are unable to synthesize dopamine. These mice can survive embryonic development only if they are rescued by the provision of an external source of dopamine. Which of the following genes would be the most likely target for inactivation to produce such dopamine-deficient mice?

A. glutamate decarboxylase
B. histidine decarboxylase
C. phenylethanolamine *N*-methyltransferase
D. tryptophan hydroxylase
E. tyrosine hydroxylase

Answer E: Tyrosine is the amino acid precursor for the synthesis of the catecholamines. The catecholamine neurotransmitters are dopamine, norepinephrine, and epinephrine. Tyrosine is transported into catecholamine-secreting neurons and adrenal medullary cells where catecholamine synthesis takes place. The first step in the process requires tyrosine hydroxylase. The hydroxylation reaction generates DOPA (3,4-dihydrophenylalanine); then DOPA decarboxylase converts DOPA to dopamine.

12. Overproduction of which of the following hormones by a neoplasm is best diagnosed by an increase in urinary excretion of vanillylmandelic acid?

A. ACTH
B. aldosterone
C. calcitonin
D. epinephrine
E. glucocorticoids

Answer D: Epinephrine and norepinephrine are catabolized to inactive compounds through the sequential actions of catecholamine-*O*-methyltransferase (COMT) and monoamine oxidase (MAO). The terminal catabolic product of the actions of these 2 enzymes is vanillylmandelic acid.

Checklist

✓ Nitric oxide is a major regulator of blood pressure, vascular homeostasis, coagulation, and immune functions. It is synthesized from the amino acid arginine via the action of 3 different nitric oxide synthases, NOS.

✓ The catecholamines are a family of neurotransmitters and hormones derived from the amino acid tyrosine. This family includes norepinephrine, epinephrine, and dopamine. Norepinephrine and epinephrine regulate cardiac, vascular, and metabolic processes of the periphery, whereas, dopamine functions primarily within the CNS regulating reward circuitry.

✓ Serotonin and melatonin are neurotransmitters derived from the amino acid tryptophan. Serotonin (5-hydroxytryptamine, 5-HT) functions within the periphery, primarily the GI tract, and in the CNS. Within the CNS serotonin is a crucial regulator of affect, and drugs that increase its life time at nerve endings promote increases in mood and behavior. Melatonin is diurnally synthesized and primarily regulates sleep-wake cycles.

✓ GABA is the major inhibitory neurotransmitter in the CNS. It is synthesized from the amino acid glutamate.

✓ Creatine phosphate is a major intramyocellular energy storage molecule, readily capable of donating its high-energy phosphate to ADP generating ATP via the action of creatine kinase (creatine phosphokinase). Creatine phosphate spontaneously dephosphorylates to creatinine which is excreted in the urine at a constant rate. The creatinine clearance rate is a measure of renal function.

✓ Glutathione is a major biological reductant important for detoxification of reactive oxygen species and oxidized macromolecules particularly membrane lipids. Glutathione is a tripeptide composed of glutamate, cysteine, and glycine.

✓ Biological polyamines are synthesized from the amino acid ornithine and comprise putrescine, spermine, and spermidine. The polyamines are involved in numerous functions in the body such as the stabilization of DNA during replication.

CHAPTER 32 Nitrogen: Nucleotide Metabolism

CHAPTER OUTLINE

Nucleotide Metabolism
Purine Nucleotide Biosynthesis
Regulation of Purine Nucleotide Synthesis
Catabolism and Salvage of Purine Nucleotides
Disorders of Purine Metabolism
Pyrimidine Nucleotide Biosynthesis
- Regulation of Pyrimidine Biosynthesis
- Catabolism of Pyrimidine Nucleotides
- Formation of Deoxyribonucleotides
- Regulation of dNTP Formation

Nucleotide Interconversions

High-Yield Terms

5-phosphoribosyl-1-pyrophosphate (PRPP): activated form of ribose used in de novo synthesis of purine and pyrimidine nucleotides

Gout: a disorder that is related to excess production and deposition of uric acid crystals; does not occur in the absence of hyperuricemia

Severe-combined immunodeficiency (SCID): a disorder related to defects in the activity of the purine nucleotide catabolism enzyme, adenosine deaminase (ADA)

Tumor lysis syndrome (TLS): potentially fatal condition characterized by acute urate nephropathy, resulting from significant increases in purine nucleotide degradation from dying cancer cells

Nucleotide Metabolism

The metabolic requirements for the nucleotides and their cognate bases can be met by either dietary intake or synthesis de novo from low-molecular weight precursors. Indeed, the ability to salvage nucleotides from sources within the body essentially alleviates any nutritional requirement for nucleotides. Thus the purine and pyrimidine bases are not required in the diet. The hydrolysis and uptake of dietary nucleic acids is covered in Chapter 43. The salvage pathways are a major source of nucleotides for synthesis of DNA, RNA, and enzyme cofactors.

Both the de novo synthesis and salvage pathways of purine and pyrimidine nucleotide biosynthesis utilize an activated sugar intermediate: 5-phosphoribosyl-1-pyrophosphate (PRPP), which is generated by the action of PRPP synthetase (Figure 32-1).

Purine Nucleotide Biosynthesis

The major site of purine synthesis is in the liver. Synthesis of the purine nucleotides begins with PRPP and leads to the first fully formed nucleotide, inosine 5′-monophosphate (IMP) (Figure 32-2). In purine nucleotide biosynthesis, the base is constructed upon the ribose by several amidotransferase and transformylation reactions. The synthesis of IMP requires 5 moles of ATP, 2 moles of glutamine, 1 mole of glycine, 1 mole of CO_2, 1 mole of aspartate, and 2 moles of formate. The formyl moieties are carried on tetrahydrofolate (THF) in the form of N^5,N^{10}-methenyl-THF and N^{10}-formyl-THF.

IMP represents a branch point for purine biosynthesis because it can be converted into either AMP or GMP through 2 distinct reaction pathways (Figure 32-3). The pathway leading to AMP requires energy in the form of GTP; that leading to GMP requires energy in the form of ATP. The utilization of GTP in the pathway to AMP synthesis allows the cell to control the proportions of AMP and GMP to near equivalence. The accumulation of excess GTP will lead to accelerated AMP synthesis from IMP instead at the expense of GMP synthesis. Conversely, since the conversion of IMP to GMP requires ATP, the accumulation of excess ATP leads to accelerated synthesis of GMP over that of AMP.

Regulation of Purine Nucleotide Synthesis

The essential rate-limiting steps in purine biosynthesis occur at the first 2 reactions of the pathway (Figure 32-4). The synthesis of PRPP by PRPP synthetase is feedback inhibited by purine-5′-nucleotides (predominantly AMP and GMP). Combinatorial effects of those 3 nucleotides are greatest, for example, inhibition is maximal when the correct concentration of both adenine and guanine nucleotides is achieved. The amidotransferase reaction catalyzed by PRPP amidotransferase is also feedback inhibited by binding ATP, ADP, and AMP at 1 inhibitory site and GTP, GDP, and GMP at another. Conversely, the activity of the enzyme is stimulated by PRPP. Additionally, purine biosynthesis is regulated in the branch pathways from IMP to AMP and GMP (Figure 32-5). The accumulation of excess ATP leads to accelerated synthesis of GMP and excess GTP leads to accelerated synthesis of AMP.

Catabolism and Salvage of Purine Nucleotides

Catabolism of the purine nucleotides leads ultimately to the production of uric acid (Figure 32-6), which is insoluble and is excreted in the urine as sodium urate crystals.

The synthesis of nucleotides from the purine bases and purine nucleosides takes place in a series of steps known as the *salvage pathways* (Figure 32-7). The free purine bases, adenine, guanine, and hypoxanthine, can

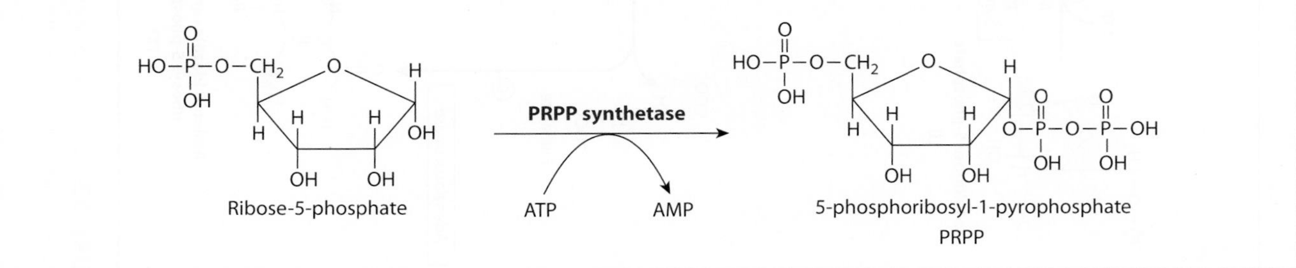

HO–P(=O)(OH)–O–CH₂ … Ribose-5-phosphate —PRPP synthetase (ATP → AMP)→ 5-phosphoribosyl-1-pyrophosphate PRPP

FIGURE 32-1: PRPP synthetase reaction. Reproduced with permission of themedicalbiochemistrypage, LLC.

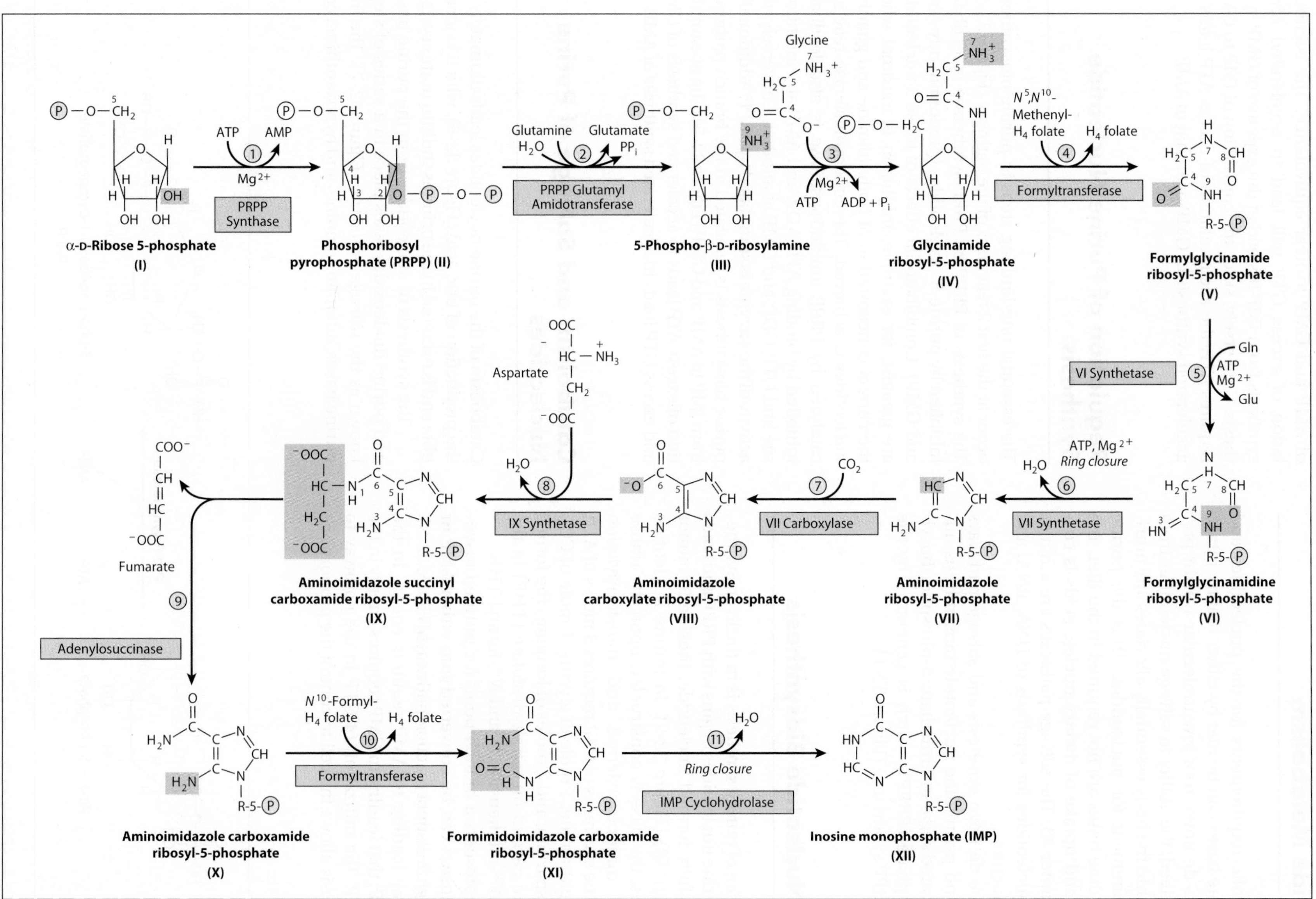

FIGURE 32-2: Purine biosynthesis from ribose 5-phosphate and ATP. (P, PO_3^{2-} or PO_2^{-}.) Murray RK, Bender DA, Botham KM, Kennelly PJ, Rodwell VW, Weil PA. *Harper's Illustrated Biochemistry,* 29th ed. New York, NY: McGraw-Hill; 2012.

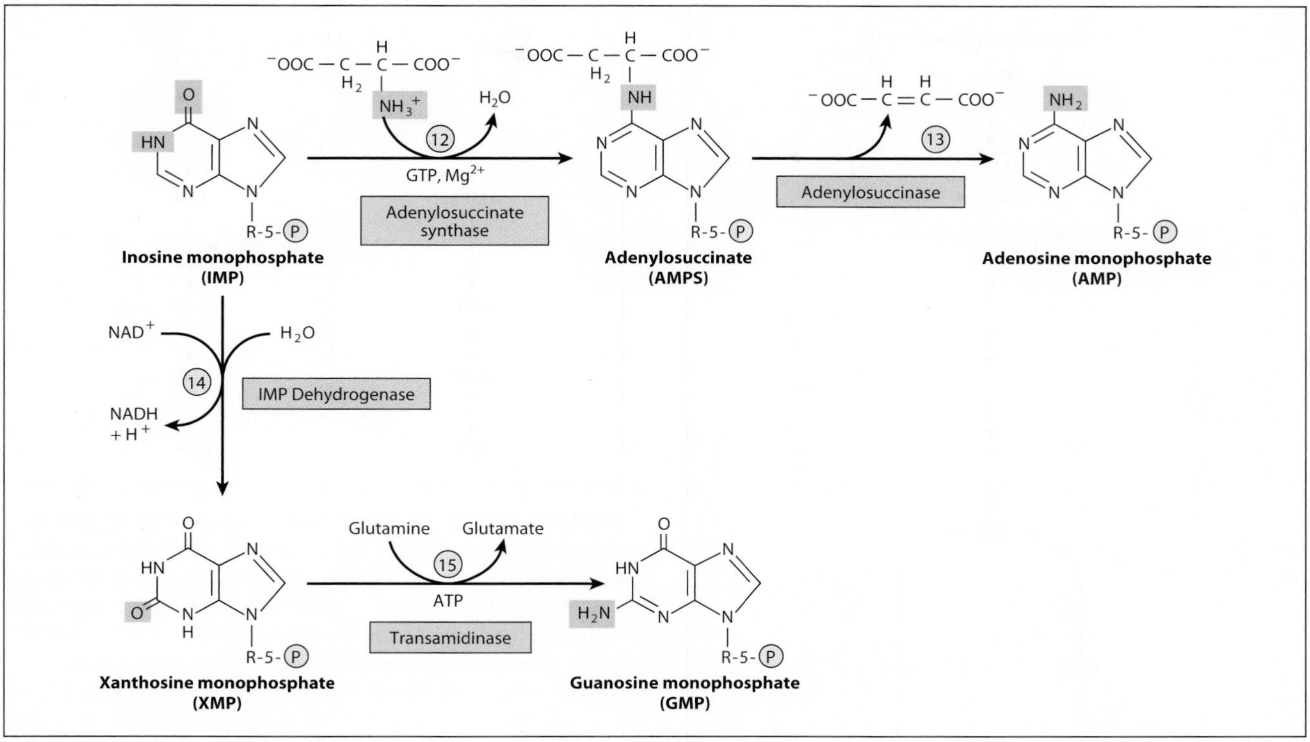

FIGURE 32-3: Conversion of IMP to AMP and GMP. Murray RK, Bender DA, Botham KM, Kennelly PJ, Rodwell VW, Weil PA. *Harper's Illustrated Biochemistry*, 29th ed. New York, NY: McGraw-Hill; 2012.

be reconverted to their corresponding nucleotides by phosphoribosylation. The 2 key transferase enzymes that are involved in the salvage of purines are adenosine phosphoribosyltransferase (APRT) and hypoxanthine-guanine phosphoribosyltransferase (HGPRT). A critically important enzyme of purine salvage in rapidly dividing cells is adenosine deaminase (ADA), which catalyzes the deamination of adenosine to inosine.

Disorders of Purine Metabolism

The clinical problems associated with nucleotide metabolism in humans are predominantly the result of abnormal catabolism of the purines. The clinical consequences of abnormal purine metabolism range from mild to severe and even fatal disorders. Clinical manifestations of abnormal purine catabolism arise from the insolubility of the degradation byproduct, uric acid. *Gout* (Clinical Box 32-1) is a condition that results from the precipitation of urate as monosodium urate (MSU) or calcium pyrophosphate dihydrate (CPPD) crystals in the synovial fluid of the joints, leading to severe inflammation and arthritis.

Two severe disorders are associated with defects in purine metabolism: Lesch-Nyhan syndrome (Clinical Box 32-2) and severe combined immunodeficiency disease (SCID) (Clinical Box 32-3). Lesch-Nyhan syndrome results from the loss of a functional *HGPRT* gene and SCID is most often (90%) caused by a deficiency in the enzyme adenosine deaminase (ADA). The glycogen storage disease, von Gierke disease, (see Clinical Box 14-1) also leads to excessive uric acid production and gouty symptoms.

Pyrimidine Nucleotide Biosynthesis

The synthesis of pyrimidine nucleotides is less complex than that of the purines since the base is chemically much simpler (Figure 32-8). The first completed pyrimidine base (orotate monophosphate, OMP) is derived from 1 mole of glutamine, 1 mole of ATP, 1 mole of CO_2, and 1 mole of aspartate. An additional mole of glutamine and ATP are required in the conversion of UTP to CTP. The synthesis of pyrimidines differs in 2 significant ways from that of purines. First, the ring structure is assembled as a free base, not built upon PRPP. PRPP is

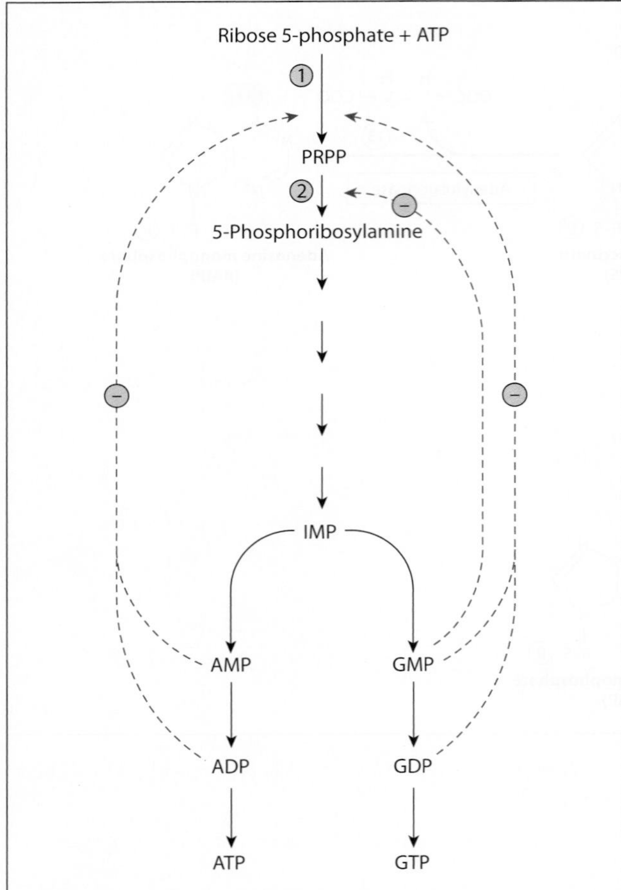

FIGURE 32-4: Control of the rate of de novo purine nucleotide biosynthesis. Reactions 1 and 2 are catalyzed by PRPP synthase and by PRPP glutamyl amidotransferase, respectively. Solid lines represent chemical flow. Broken red lines represent feedback inhibition by intermediates of the pathway. Murray RK, Bender DA, Botham KM, Kennelly PJ, Rodwell VW, Weil PA. *Harper's Illustrated Biochemistry*, 29th ed. New York, NY: McGraw-Hill; 2012.

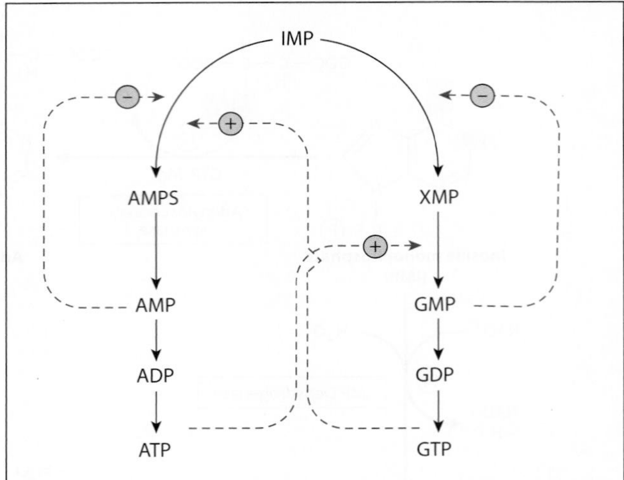

FIGURE 32-5: Regulation of the conversion of IMP to adenosine nucleotides and guanosine nucleotides. Solid lines represent chemical flow. Broken green lines represent positive feedback loops +, and broken red lines represent negative feedback loops ⊖. Abbreviations include AMPS (adenylosuccinate) and XMP (xanthosine monophosphate), whose structures are given in Figure 32–3 . Murray RK, Bender DA, Botham KM, Kennelly PJ, Rodwell VW, Weil PA. *Harper's Illustrated Biochemistry*, 29th ed. New York, NY: McGraw-Hill; 2012.

added to the first fully formed pyrimidine base (orotic acid), forming orotate monophosphate (OMP), which is subsequently decarboxylated to UMP. Second, there is no branch in the pyrimidine synthesis pathway. UMP is phosphorylated twice to yield UTP (ATP is the phosphate donor). The first phosphorylation is catalyzed by uridylate kinase and the second by ubiquitous nucleoside diphosphate kinase. Finally UTP is aminated by the action of CTP synthase, generating CTP.

The de novo pathway to deoxythymidine triphosphate (dTTP) synthesis first requires the use of dUMP from the metabolism of either UDP or CDP. The dUMP is converted to dTMP by the action of thymidylate synthase. The unique property of the action of thymidylate synthase is that the tetrahydrofolate (THF) cofactor (N^5, N^{10}-methylene-THF) is converted to dihydrofolate (DHF), the only such reaction yielding DHF from THF. In order for the thymidylate synthase reaction to continue, THF must be regenerated from DHF. This is accomplished through the action of dihydrofolate reductase (DHFR). The crucial role of DHFR in thymidine nucleotide biosynthesis makes it an ideal target for chemotherapeutic agents (see later). The salvage pathway to dTTP synthesis involves the enzyme thymidine kinase, which can use either thymidine or deoxyuridine as substrate. The activity of thymidine kinase is unique in that it fluctuates with the cell cycle, rising to peak activity during the phase of DNA synthesis.

Regulation of Pyrimidine Biosynthesis

The regulation of pyrimidine synthesis occurs mainly at the first step catalyzed by aspartate transcarbamoylase (ATCase). ATCase is a multifunctional enzyme in mammalian cells, capable of catalyzing the formation of carbamoyl phosphate, carbamoyl aspartate, and dihydroorotate. The carbamoyl synthetase activity of this complex is termed *carbamoyl phosphate synthetase II (CPS-II)* as opposed to CPS-I, which is involved in the urea cycle (Chapter 29). The CPS-II domain of ATCase is activated by ATP and inhibited

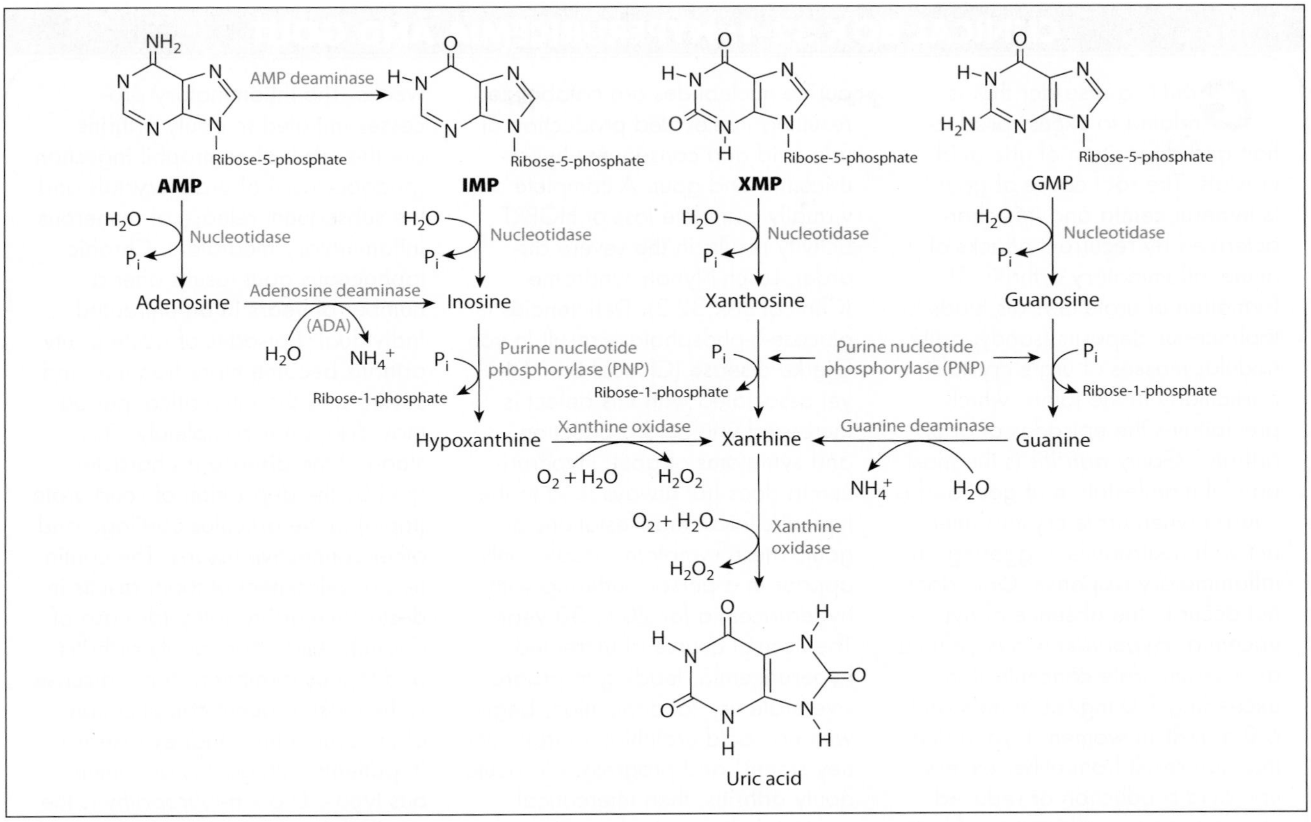

FIGURE 32-6: Pathways of purine nucleotide catabolism. Reproduced with permission of themedicalbiochemistrypage, LLC.

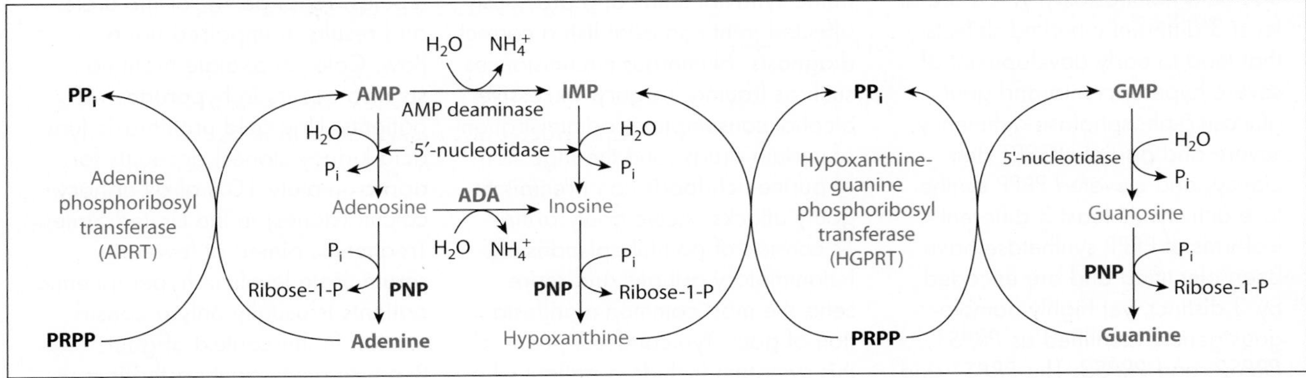

FIGURE 32-7: Pathways of purine nucleotide salvage. ADA, adenosine deaminase; PNP, purine nucleotide phosphorylase. Reproduced with permission of themedicalbiochemistrypage, LLC.

by UDP, UTP, dUTP, and CTP. As in the regulation of purine synthesis, ATP levels also regulate pyrimidine biosynthesis at the level of PRPP formation. An increase in the level of PRPP results in an activation of pyrimidine synthesis. There is also regulation of OMP decarboxylase: this enzyme is competitively inhibited by UMP and, to a lesser degree, by CMP. Finally, CTP synthase is feedback inhibited by CTP and activated by GTP.

Catabolism of Pyrimidine Nucleotides

Catabolism of the pyrimidine nucleotides leads ultimately to β-alanine (when CMP and UMP are degraded)

CLINICAL BOX 32-1: HYPERURICEMIA AND GOUT

Gout is a disorder that is related to excess production and deposition of uric acid crystals. The root cause of gout is hyperuricemia and it is characterized by recurrent attacks of acute inflammatory arthritis. The formation of urate crystals leads to tophaceous deposits (sandy, gritty, nodular masses of urate crystals), particularly in the joints, which precipitates the episodes of gouty arthritis. *Gouty arthritis* is the most painful manifestation of gout and is caused when urate crystals interact with neutrophils, triggering an inflammatory response. Gout does not occur in the absence of hyperuricemia. *Hyperuricemia* is defined as a serum urate concentration exceeding 7.0 mg/dL in men and 6.0 mg/dL in women. Hyperuricemia can result from either excess uric acid production or reduced excretion or a combination of both mechanisms. Primary gout is a biochemically and genetically heterogeneous disorder resulting from inborn metabolic errors that alter uric acid homeostasis. There are at least 3 different inherited defects that lead to early development of severe hyperuricemia and gout: glucose-6-phosphatase deficiency; severe and partial HGPRT deficiency; and elevated PRPP synthetase activity. At least 3 different isoforms of PRPP synthetase have been identified and are encoded by 3 distinct, yet highly homologous genes, identified as *PRPS1*, *PRPS2*, and *PRPS3*. The *PRPS1* and *PRPS2* genes are found on the X chromosome and the *PRPS3* gene is found on chromosome 7. Mutations in the *PRPS* genes that result in superactivity lead to enhanced production of PRPP. Increased levels of PRPP, in turn, drive enhanced purine nucleotide synthesis in excess of the needs of the body. Thus, the excess purine nucleotides are catabolized, resulting in elevated production of uric acid and consequent hyperuricemia and gout. A complete or virtually complete loss of HGPRT activity results in the severe disorder, Lesch-Nyhan syndrome (Clinical Box 32-2). Deficiencies in glucose-6-phosphatase result in von Gierke disease (Clinical Box 14-1), yet associated with this defect is increased uric acid production and symptoms of gout. Hyperuricemia does not always lead to the typical clinical manifestations of gout. These symptoms usually only appear in a person suffering with hyperuricemia for 20 to 30 years. The normal course of untreated hyperuricemia, leading to progressive urate crystal deposition, begins with uric acid urolithiasis (urate kidney stones) and progresses to acute gouty arthritis, then intercritical gout and chronic tophaceous gout. *Intercritical gout* refers to the period between gouty attacks. Diagnosis of gout during these periods is difficult, but analysis for urate crystals in the synovial fluids of a previously affected joint can establish a correct diagnosis. Numerous circumstances such as trauma, surgery, excessive alcohol consumption, administration of certain drugs, and the ingestion of purine-rich foods can precipitate gouty attacks. *Acute gouty arthritis* consists of painful episodes of inflammatory arthritis and represents the most common manifestation of gout. Typical descriptions of this symptom include a patient who goes to bed and is awakened by severe pain in the large toe, which may also be experienced in the heel, instep, or ankle. The pain can become so severe that a simple act of cloth touching the area becomes unbearable. Gouty arthritis attacks usually dissipate within several hours, but can also last for several weeks. The inflammatory processes initiated in gouty arthritis are the result of neutrophil ingestion (phagocytosis) of urate crystals and the subsequent release of numerous inflammatory mediators. Chronic tophaceous gout results after a number of years in an untreated individual. Episodes of acute gouty arthritis become more frequent and severe and the intercritical period may disappear completely. This stage of the disease is characterized by the deposition of solid urate (tophi) in the articular cartilage and other connective tissues. The continued development of tophi results in destructive arthropathy (disease of a joint). Aside from gouty arthritis and tophus formation, renal disease is the most frequent complication of hyperuricemia. Kidney disease in patients with gout is of numerous types. *Urate nephropathy* is the result of the deposition of monosodium urate crystals in the renal interstitial tissue. *Uric acid nephropathy* is caused by the deposition of uric acid crystals in the collecting tubules, renal pelvis, or the ureter and results in impaired urine flow. Calcium oxalate urolithiasis also occurs in hyperuricemic patients. Uric acid urolithiasis (uric acid kidney stones) accounts for approximately 10% of all urinary calculi (stones) in the United States. Treatments aimed at lowering serum urate levels in hyperuricemic patients is usually only a consideration in the context of gout. Because acute gouty arthritis is an inflammatory event, treatment with anti-inflammatory drugs is often successful in reducing the symptoms. The most commonly prescribed drug for reducing the production of uric acid is the xanthine oxidase inhibitor, allopurinol.

CLINICAL BOX 32-2: LESCH-NYHAN SYNDROME

Lesch-Nyhan syndrome (LNS) is a disorder related to defects in the activity of HGPRT. HGPRT catalyzes the interconversions of hypoxanthine and IMP and guanine and GMP. There are 3 overlapping clinical syndromes associated with deficiencies in HGPRT activity. Individuals that have less than 1.5% residual enzyme activity exhibit debilitating neurologic disability, behavioral abnormalities that include impulsive and self-mutilating behaviors, and varying degrees of cognitive disability in addition to overproduction of uric acid. This most severe of the 3 clinical syndromes is LNS. Patients with 1.5% to 8% of residual enzyme activity exhibit neurologic disability that ranges from clumsiness to debilitating pyramidal (CNS neurons involved in voluntary motor movement) and extrapyramidal motor dysfunction in addition to overproduction of uric acid. In cases where at least 8% of normal HGPRT activity is present, patients exhibit overproduction of uric acid and associated hyperuricemia, renal lithiasis, and gout. The latter circumstance (partial deficiency with at least 8% enzyme activity) is commonly referred to as *Kelley-Seegmiller syndrome*. Lesch-Nyhan syndrome is inherited as an X-linked recessive disorder with an incidence of approximately 1:380,000. Since it is an X-linked disease, it is found almost exclusively in males although affected females have been identified, albeit very rarely. The characteristic clinical features of the LNS are mental retardation, spastic cerebral palsy, choreoathetosis, uric acid urinary stones, and self-destructive biting of fingers and lips. The overall clinical features of LNS can be divided into 3 broad categories. These include uric acid overproduction and its associated consequences (eg, gouty arthritis and renal lithiasis), neurobehavioral dysfunction indicative of central nervous system involvement, and growth retardation. All patients with LNS manifest with profound motor dysfunction that is recognizable within the first 3 to 9 months of life. Infants fail to develop the ability to hold up their heads or to sit unaided. Further motor development will be delayed and the onset of pyramidal and extrapyramidal signs becomes evident by 1 to 2 years of age. In LNS patients there are 3 major signs of pyramidal dysfunction: spasticity, hyperreflexia, and the extensor plantar reflex (also known as the Babinski reflex). Extrapyramidal dysfunction in LNS patients is primarily evident as dystonia (sustained muscle contractions causing twisting and repetitive movements or abnormal postures), although many patients also exhibit choreoathetosis (involuntary movement disorder in association with slow continuous writhing particularly of the hands and feet). Most commonly associated with LNS is the behavioral dysfunction manifest with impulsivity and self-mutilation, particularly of the lips, fingers, and tongue. LNS patients will often strike out at people around them, spit on people, and use foul language. These symptoms are analogous to the uncontrollable compulsions associated with Tourette syndrome. The self-injury behavior is clearly an involuntary action as most LNS patients will learn to call out for help when they feel the compulsive behavior overtaking them, or they will sit on their hands or wear socks or gloves to limit the self-injurious behavior.

or β-aminoisobutyrate (when dTMP is degraded) and NH_3 and CO_2 (Figure 32-9). The β-alanine and β-aminoisobutyrate serve as $-NH_2$ donors in transamination of α-ketoglutarate to glutamate. Subsequent reactions convert the resultant α-ketoacid products to malonyl-CoA, which can be diverted to fatty acid synthesis, or methylmalonyl-CoA, which is converted to succinyl-CoA and can be shunted to the TCA cycle.

Because the products of pyrimidine catabolism are water soluble, there are few clinical signs or symptoms. However, in cases of hyperuricemia caused by overproduction of PRPP, there will be excess production of pyrimidine nucleotides evidenced by increased excretion of β-alanine. Two inherited disorders affecting pyrimidine biosynthesis are the result of deficiencies in the bifunctional enzyme catalyzing the last two steps of UMP synthesis, orotate phosphoribosyltransferase and OMP decarboxylase. These deficiencies result in orotic aciduria that causes retarded growth and severe anemia due to development of hypochromic erythrocytes and megaloblastic bone marrow. Leukopenia is also common in orotic acidurias. These disorders can be treated with uridine and/or cytidine, which increase UMP production via the action of ubiquitous nucleoside kinases. The UMP then inhibits CPS-II, thus attenuating orotic acid production.

Formation of Deoxyribonucleotides

A typical cell contains 5 to 10 times as much RNA (mRNAs, rRNAs, and tRNAs) as DNA. Therefore, the majority of de novo nucleotide biosynthesis and

CLINICAL BOX 32-3: SEVERE COMBINED IMMUNODEFICIENCY SYNDROME, SCID

Severe combined immunodeficiency disease (SCID) is a disorder related to defects in the activity of adenosine deaminase (ADA). SCID is inherited as an autosomal recessive disorder with an incidence as high as 1:200,000. ADA catalyzes the irreversible deamination of adenosine and deoxyadenosine to inosine and 2′-deoxyinosine, respectively. Although ADA activity is found in all tissues of the body, the highest concentrations are found in the thymus and other lymphoid tissues. In addition to the differences in levels of ADA in various tissues, the enzyme is also developmentally regulated such that immature thymocytes express higher levels than do mature thymocytes. The level of expression of ADA also decreases as B cells mature. In ADA deficiency, there is an elevation in the level of adenosine and 2′-deoxyadenosine levels in the blood and urine are also elevated. The consequences of the elevations in these 2 ADA substrates are impaired lymphocyte differentiation, function, and viability, which results in lymphopenia and severe immunodeficiency. Increases in 2′-deoxyadenosine results in dramatic increases in cellular dATP pools. The consequence of increased dATP is an inhibition of ribonucleotide reductase (RR), the enzyme responsible for generating deoxyribonucleotides necessary for DNA replication. The inhibition of RR leads to a block in DNA replication that is critical for the expansion of lymphocytes in response to an antigenic challenge. Deoxy-ATP also induces DNA strand breakage in nondividing lymphocytes via a direct activation of caspase 9 involved in apoptosis. In addition, *S*-adenosylhomocysteine hydrolase activity is markedly inhibited by 2′-deoxyadenosine, resulting in accumulation of *S*-adenosylhomocysteine that in turn results in reduced synthesis of *S*-adenosylmethionine, a critical substrate in transmethylation reactions. Although not all forms of SCID are caused by defects in ADA, greater than 85% of all ADA-deficient patients are infants with SCID. Infants with SCID usually present within the first month of life with failure to thrive and life-threatening interstitial pneumonitis (inflammation of the walls of the airs sacs of the lungs). Pneumonia is often caused by *Pneumocystis carinii* or a viral infection. The gastrointestinal tract, as well as the skin, is also frequently involved in initial infections. Candidiasis is first observed as "diaper rash" but then progresses to an extensive infection involving the skin, oral, and esophageal mucosa and the vagina in female patients. Persistent infections prompt most parents to have their baby examined, and SCID is thus often diagnosed by 1 to 2 months of age from a determination of immune function. Most SCID patients lack both cell-mediated (T cell) and humoral (B cell) immunity, thus the derivation of the disease name: severe combined immunodeficiency. Because this disease is severely life-threatening, most patients do not survive for more than a few months. If immunological function is not restored, SCID is always fatal by 1 to 2 years of age. The most effective treatment for SCID is bone marrow transplantation. Enzyme replacement therapy (ERT) has proved effective in treating some (but not all) ADA-deficient SCID patients. The most common treatment is to use intramuscular injection of highly purified bovine ADA coupled to the inert polymer, monomethoxy polyethylene glycol (PEG-ADA). The use of PEG-ADA therapy is sometimes warranted in SCID patients who are too ill to undergo bone marrow transplantation.

CLINICAL BOX 32-4: TUMOR LYSIS SYNDROME

Chemotherapeutic treatment of leukemias, non-Hodgkin lymphomas, and Burkitt lymphomas often results in tumor lysis syndrome (TLS). TLS is caused by massive tumor cell lysis, with the release of large amounts of potassium, phosphate, and nucleic acids into the systemic circulation. Catabolism of the purine nucleic acids to uric acid leads to hyperuricemia. The dramatic increase in uric acid excretion can result in the precipitation of uric acid in the renal tubules and can also induce renal vasoconstriction, impaired autoregulation, decreased renal blood flow, and inflammation, referred to as acute urate nephropathy. Hyperphosphatemia with calcium phosphate deposition in the renal tubules can also cause acute kidney injury. Treatment of TLS includes aggressive hydration and diuresis, monitoring of electrolyte abnormalities, and control of hyperuricemia with allopurinol and rasburicase.

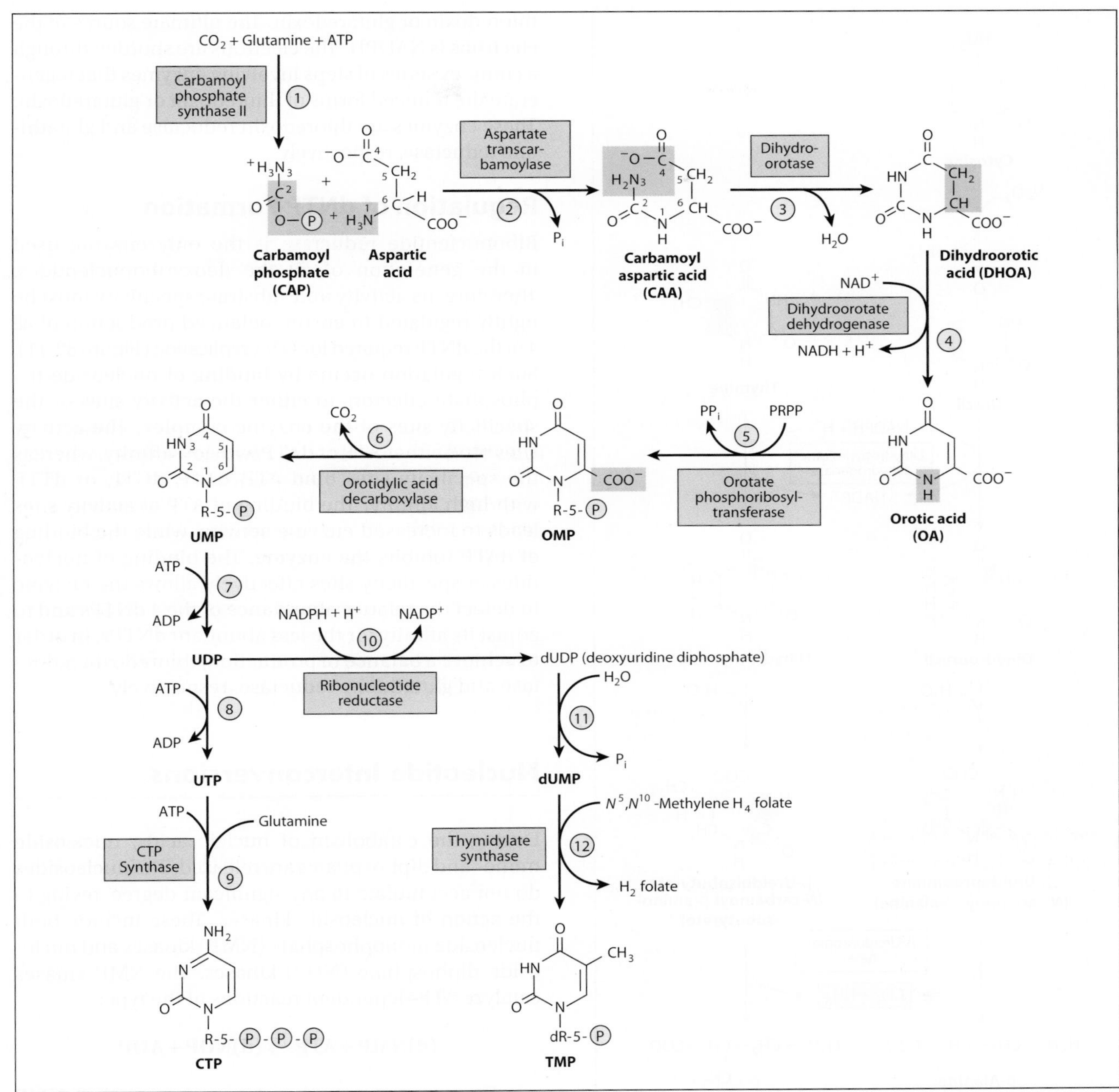

FIGURE 32-8: The biosynthetic pathway for pyrimidine nucleotides. Murray RK, Bender DA, Botham KM, Kennelly PJ, Rodwell VW, Weil PA. *Harper's Illustrated Biochemistry*, 29th ed. New York, NY: McGraw-Hill; 2012.

nucleotide salvage is the production of rNTP. However, because proliferating cells need to replicate their genomes, the production of dNTP is also necessary. This process begins with the reduction of rNDP, catalyzed by ribonucleotide reductase (RR), and followed by phosphorylation to yield the dNTP (Figure 32-10). The phosphorylation of dNDP to dNTP is catalyzed by nucleoside diphosphate kinases that also phosphorylate rNDP to rNTP, using ATP as the phosphate donor.

Ribonucleotide reductase is a multifunctional enzyme that contains redox-active thiol groups for the transfer of electrons during the reduction reactions. In the process of reducing the rNDP to a dNDP, RR becomes oxidized. RR is reduced in turn by either

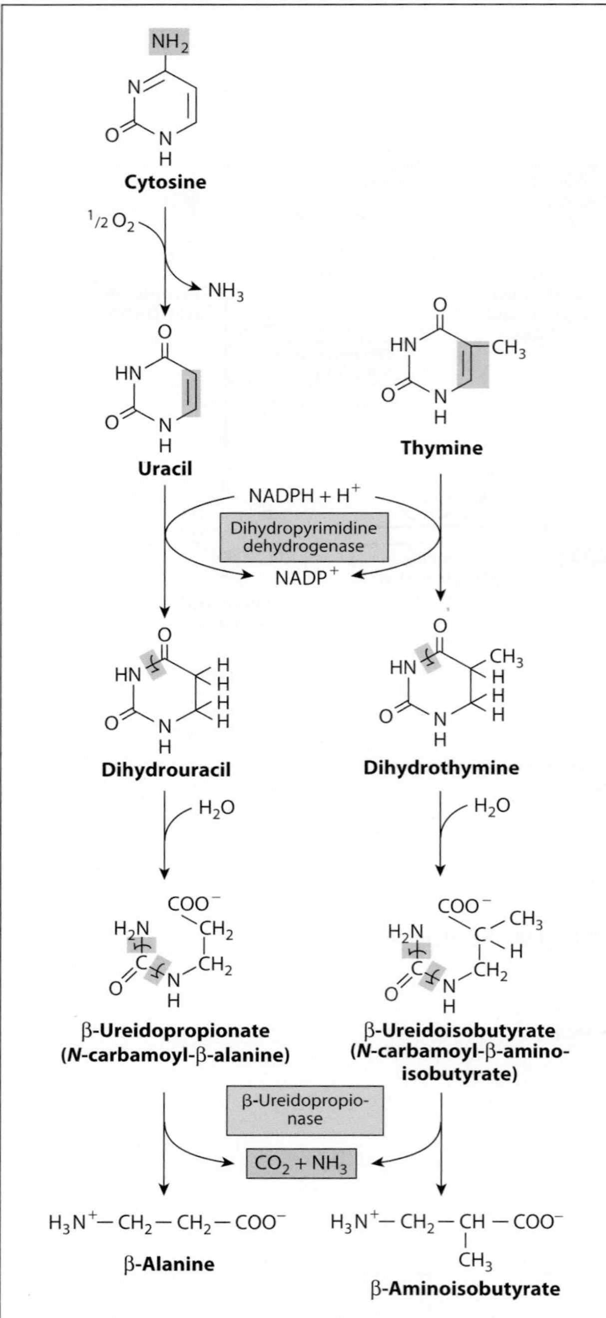

FIGURE 32-9: Catabolism of pyrimidines. Hepatic β-ureidopropionase catalyzes the formation of both β-alanine and β-aminoisobutryrate from their pyrimidine precursors. Murray RK, Bender DA, Botham KM, Kennelly PJ, Rodwell VW, Weil PA. *Harper's Illustrated Biochemistry*, 29th ed. New York, NY: McGraw-Hill; 2012.

thioredoxin or glutaredoxin. The ultimate source of the electrons is NADPH. The electrons are shuttled through a complex series of steps involving enzymes that regenerate the reduced forms of thioredoxin or glutaredoxin. These enzymes are thioredoxin reductase and glutathione reductase, respectively.

Regulation of dNTP Formation

Ribonucleotide reductase is the only enzyme used in the generation of all the deoxyribonucleotides. Therefore, its activity and substrate specificity must be tightly regulated to ensure balanced production of all 4 of the dNTP required for DNA replication (Figure 32-11). Such regulation occurs by binding of nucleoside triphosphate effectors to either the activity sites or the specificity sites of the enzyme complex. The activity sites bind either ATP or dATP with low affinity, whereas the specificity sites bind ATP, dATP, dGTP, or dTTP with high affinity. The binding of ATP at activity sites leads to increased enzyme activity, while the binding of dATP inhibits the enzyme. The binding of nucleotides at specificity sites effectively allows the enzyme to detect the relative abundance of the 4 dNTPs and to adjust its affinity for the less abundant dNTPs, in order to achieve a balance of production, thioredoxin reductase and glutathione reductase, respectively.

Nucleotide Interconversions

During the catabolism of nucleic acids, nucleoside mono- and diphosphates are released. The nucleosides do not accumulate to any significant degree, owing to the action of nucleoside kinases. These include both nucleoside monophosphate (NMP) kinases and nucleoside diphosphate (NDP) kinases. The NMP kinases catalyze ATP-dependent reactions of the type:

$$\text{(d)NMP} + \text{ATP} \leftrightarrow \text{(d)NDP} + \text{ADP}$$

The enzyme adenylate kinase is a critical NMP kinase whose activity is important for ensuring adequate levels of energy in cells, particularly liver and muscle. The reaction catalyzed by adenylate kinase is:

$$\text{2ADP} \leftrightarrow \text{AMP} + \text{ATP}$$

The NDP kinases catalyze reactions of the type:

$$N_1TP + N_2DP \leftrightarrow N_1DP + N_2TP$$

Nucleobase
HO–P–O–P–O–CH2
OH OH
H H H
OH OH OH
NDP

H_2O

Nucleobase
HO–P–O–P–O–CH2
OH OH
H H H
OH OH H
dNDP

Ribonucleotide reductase SH SH
Ribonucleotide reductase S–S

Thioredoxin S–S
Thioredoxin SH SH
Glutaredoxin S–S
Glutaredoxin SH SH

Thioredoxin reductase
FADH2 **FAD**
NADP+ **NADPH + H+**

2 GSH **GSSG**
Glutathione reductase
NADP+ **NADPH + H+**

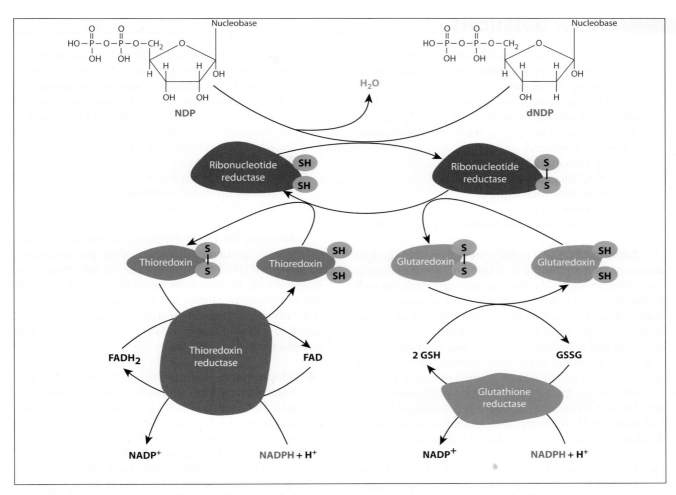

FIGURE 32-10: Reactions of ribonucleotide reductase. Reproduced with permission of themedicalbiochemistrypage, LLC.

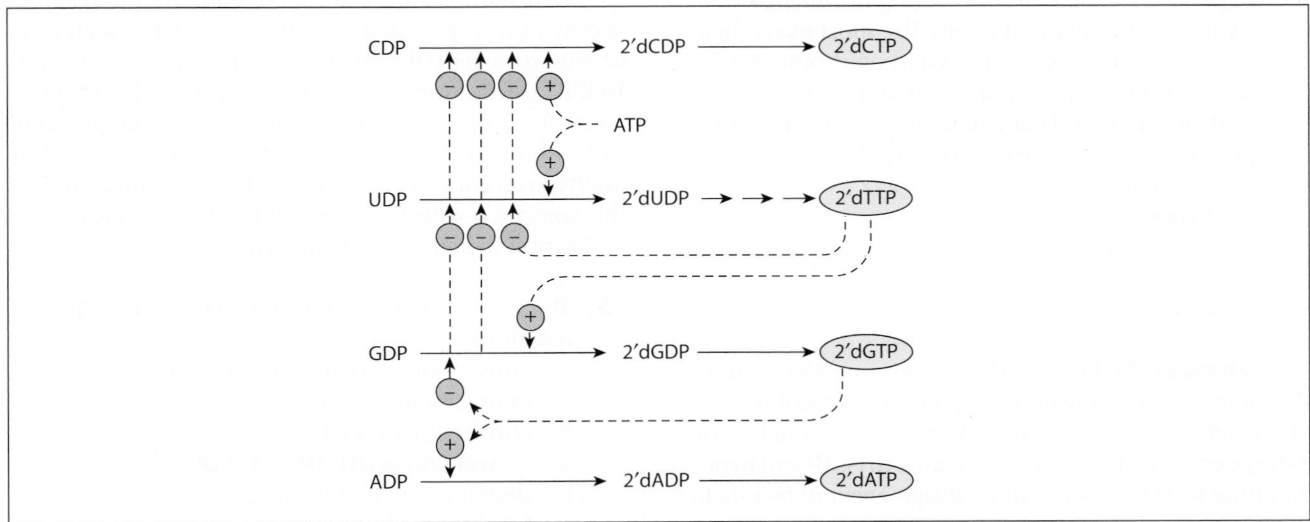

FIGURE 32-11: **Regulation of ribonucleotide reductase.** Solid lines represent direction of deoxynucleotide formation. Dashed lines represent either positive (⊕) or negative (⊖) feedback regulation. Murray RK, Bender DA, Botham KM, Kennelly PJ, Rodwell VW, Weil PA. Harper's Illustrated Biochemistry, 29th ed. New York, NY: McGraw-Hill; 2012.

REVIEW QUESTIONS

1. You are treating a 4-year-old child who has been afflicted with recurrent infections. The child exhibits retarded development, weakness, and weight loss. Physical examination also shows absent tonsils and blood work reveals a lack of lymphocytes. These signs and symptoms are due to which of the following disorders?
   A. hyperuricemia
   B. Kelley-Seegmiller syndrome
   C. Lesch-Nyhan syndrome
   D. orotic aciduria
   E. severe-combined immunodeficiency (SCID)

Answer E: SCID usually presents within the first month of life with failure to thrive and life-threatening interstitial pneumonitis. The gastrointestinal tract as well as the skin is also frequently involved in initial infections. Candidiasis is first observed as "diaper rash" but then progresses to an extensive infection involving the skin, oral and esophageal mucosa, and the vagina. Persistent infections prompt most parents to have their baby examined and SCID is thus often diagnosed by 1 to 2 months of age from a determination of immune function. Most SCID patients lack both cell-mediated (T cell) and humoral (B cell) immunity, thus the derivation of the disease name: severe combined immunodeficiency.

2. You are examining a 7-year-old male child who exhibits delayed motor development, overexaggerated reflexes, and spasticity. In addition, the boy has a tendency to chew his lips and fingers often causing tissue damage and bleeding and has painful, swollen, and inflamed joints. The most likely diagnosis in this case is Lesch-Nyhan syndrome. Analysis of blood from this patient would be expected to find elevated levels of which of the following compounds related to the observed findings?
   A. citrulline
   B. hypoxanthine
   C. lactic acid
   D. orotic acid
   E. uric acid

Answer E: Lesch-Nyhan syndrome results from deficiencies in hypoxanthine-guanine phosphoribosyltransferase (HGPRT). HGPRT is a purine nucleotide salvage enzyme that converts guanine to GMP and hypoxanthine to IMP. Loss of this salvage enzyme results in increased rates of purine nucleotide catabolism whose end product is uric acid.

3. You are examining a 5-year-old male child who has been exhibiting a tendency to bite his lower lip to the point of bleeding as well as chewing on his fingertips. Physical examination demonstrates swollen tender joints, and blood workup indicates elevated uric acid levels. These symptoms and lab results are indicative of a deficiency in which of the following enzymes?
   A. adenosine deaminase
   B. adenosine phosphoribosyltransferase
   C. AMP deaminase
   D. hypoxanthine-guanine phosphoribosyltransferase
   E. thymidylate synthase

Answer D: Lesch-Nyhan syndrome results from deficiencies in hypoxanthine-guanine phosphoribosyltransferase (HGPRT). The disorder is inherited as an X-linked trait. Patients with this defect exhibit not only severe symptoms of gout but also a severe malfunction of the nervous system. In the most serious cases, patients resort to self-mutilation. Death usually occurs before patients reach their 20th year.

4. Allopurinol is an inhibitor of xanthine oxidase. Administration of allopurinol to a patient with gout and normal HGPRT levels would be expected to lead to which of the following?
   A. decreased levels of PRPP
   B. decreased xanthine in the blood
   C. increased *de novo* synthesis of IMP
   D. increased hypoxanthine in the urine
   E. increased urate in the urine

Answer D: Most forms of gout are the result of excess purine production and consequent catabolism or due to a partial deficiency in the salvage enzyme, HGPRT. Most forms of gout can be treated by administering the antimetabolite allopurinol that strongly inhibits xanthine oxidase. The substrates for xanthine oxidase are hypoxanthine and xanthine; therefore, inhibition of the enzyme results in increased levels of hypoxanthine and xanthine in the blood and urine.

5. Thioredoxin is involved in which of the following reactions?
   A. conversion of a ribonucleotide to a deoxyribonucleotide
   B. conversion of AMP to ATP
   C. conversion of dUMP to dTMP
   D. degradation of nucleoproteins
   E. inhibition of xanthine oxidase as a treatment for gout

Answer A: Ribonucleotide reductase (RR) is a multifunctional enzyme that contains redox-active thiol groups for the transfer of electrons during the reduction reactions. In the process of reducing the rNDP to a dNDP, RR becomes oxidized. RR is reduced in turn, by either thioredoxin or glutaredoxin. The ultimate source of the electrons is NADPH. The electrons are shuttled through a complex series of steps involving enzymes that regenerate the reduced forms of thioredoxin or glutaredoxin. These enzymes are thioredoxin reductase and glutathione reductase, respectively.

6. An enzyme system, isolated from the liver, converts deoxyuridine-5′-phosphate (dUMP) to thymidine-5′-phosphate (dTMP). Which of the following participates in this reaction?
A. ATP
B. N^5,N^{10}-methylene tetrahydrofolic acid
C. *S*-adenosylmethionine
D. thioredoxin
E. vitamin B_{12}

Answer B: The de novo pathway to dTTP synthesis first requires the use of dUMP from the metabolism of either UDP or CDP. The dUMP is converted to dTMP by the action of thymidylate synthase. The methyl group is donated by N^5,N^{10}-methylene tetrahydrofolate.

7. 5-Fluorouracil is utilized as a chemotherapeutic agent because of its ability to interfere with the function of which of the following enzymes?
A. dihydrobiopterin reductase
B. dihydrofolate reductase
C. dihydropyrimidine dehydrogenase
D. glycine synthase
E. thymidylate synthase

Answer E: Tetrahydrofolate (THF) is regenerated from the dihydrofolate (DHF) product of the thymidylate synthase reaction by the action of dihydrofolate reductase (DHFR). Cells that are unable to regenerate THF suffer defective DNA synthesis and eventual death. For this reason, it is therapeutically possible to target rapidly proliferating cells over nonproliferating cells through the inhibition of thymidylate synthase. A class of molecule used to inhibit thymidylate synthase is called the *suicide substrates* because they irreversibly inhibit the enzyme. Molecules of this class include 5-fluorouracil and 5-fluorodeoxyuridine. Both are converted within cells to 5-fluorodeoxyuridylate (FdUMP). It is this drug metabolite that inhibits thymidylate synthase.

8. Methotrexate is an inhibitor of which of the following enzymes?
A. dihydrofolate reductase
B. 5-methyl-tetrahydrofolate transferase
C. ribonucleotide reductase
D. thymidylate synthase
E. xanthine oxidase

Answer A: Tetrahydrofolate (THF) is regenerated from the dihydrofolate (DHF) product of the thymidylate synthase reaction by the action of dihydrofolate reductase (DHFR). Cells that are unable to regenerate THF suffer defective DNA synthesis and eventual death. Many anticancer drugs act directly to inhibit thymidylate synthase, or indirectly, by inhibiting DHFR. Many DHFR inhibitors have been synthesized, including methotrexate, aminopterin, and trimethoprim. Each of these is an analog of folic acid.

9. The parents of a 1-year-old boy are alarmed at the increasing frequency of their child biting his lips and finger tips. In addition, on several occasions they have noticed what appears to be "orange sand" in their son's diapers. They report to their pediatrician that they believe their child is delayed in acquiring motor skills such as holding up his head and sitting unaided. Clinical tests performed on serum and urine indicate a 3-fold increase in serum uric acid and a 10-fold elevation in the urinary ratio of uric acid to creatinine. These findings are suggestive of which of the following disorders?
A. adenosine deaminase deficiency
B. adenylosuccinate lyase deficiency
C. Lesch-Nyhan disease
D. purine nucleotide phosphorylase deficiency
E. orotic aciduria

Answer C: Deficiencies in the purine nucleotide salvage enzyme, HGPRT, cause 3 overlapping clinical syndromes. The most severe deficiency (patients having <1.5% residual enzyme activity) results in debilitating neurologic disability, overproduction of uric acid, and behavioral abnormalities that include impulsive and self-injurious activities such as biting finger tips and lips. This severe form of HGPRT deficiency is referred to as Lesch-Nyhan disease. The overproduction of uric acid leads to symptoms of gout and the appearance of "orange sand" in the urine.

10. A 37-year-old man presents with tophaceous deposits within the articular cartilage, synovium, tendons, tendon sheaths, pinnae, and the soft tissue on the extensor surface of the forearms. These clinical observations suggest the patient is suffering from which of the following disorders?
A. ADA deficiency
B. gout
C. Lesch-Nyhan syndrome

D. purine nucleoside phosphorylase (PNP) deficiency
E. von Gierke disease

Answer B: Gout is characterized by elevated levels of uric acid in the blood and urine. Uric acid is the end product of purine catabolism and excess production results from a variety of metabolic abnormalities that lead to overproduction of purines via the de novo pathway. Uric acid is very insoluble and when generated in large amounts will precipitate as uric acid crystals in the joints of the extremities and in renal interstitial tissue. These deposits are gritty or sandy in nature and thus are termed tophaceous deposits.

11. The initial reaction of the de novo synthesis pathway for pyrimidine nucleotides begins with glutamine and CO_2 and is complete with the formation of uridine monophosphate. Which of the following represents the rate-limiting enzyme in this pathway?
A. aspartate transcarbamoylase
B. orotate monophosphate decarboxylase
C. phosphoribosylpyrophosphate amido transferase
D. PRPP synthetase
E. ribonucleotide reductase

Answer A: The regulation of pyrimidine synthesis occurs primarily at the first step catalyzed by the rate-limiting enzyme of the pathway, aspartate transcarbamoylase (ATCase). ATCase is a multifunctional enzyme in mammalian cells, capable of catalyzing the formation of carbamoyl phosphate, carbamoyl aspartate, and dihydroorotate.

12. Severe combined immunodeficiency disease (SCID) is characterized by a complete lack of cell-mediated and humoral immunity. This disorder results from a deficiency in which of the following enzymes?
A. adenosine deaminase
B. asparatate transcarbamoylase
C. hypoxanthine-guanine phosphoribosyltransferase
D. orotic acid decarboxylase
E. purine nucleotide phosphorylase

Answer A: Severe combined immunodeficiency disease (SCID) is a disorder related to defects in the activity of the purine nucleotide catabolism enzyme, adenosine deaminase (ADA).

13. Following a relatively normal early developmental period, a 6-month-old boy becomes pale and lethargic and begins to show signs of deteriorating motor skill. The infant has severe megaloblastic anemia; however, serum measurements of iron, folate, vitamins B_{12}, and B_6 demonstrate they are within normal range. Urine samples were clear when fresh, but when left to stand for several hours showed an abundant white precipitate that was composed of fine needle-shaped crystals. Analysis of the crystals identified them as orotic acid. Significant clinical improvement would be expected to be observed in this infant following oral administration of which of the following compounds?
A. adenosine
B. cytidine
C. guanosine
D. thymidine
E. uridine

Answer E: Hereditary orotic aciduria results from a defect in the de novo synthesis of pyrimidines. The defect is in the bifunctional enzyme that catalyzes the last 2 steps in the de novo pathway, conversion of orotic acid to OMP and OMP to UMP. Administration of uridine allows afflicted individuals to produce sufficient levels of cytidine nucleotides via the salvage pathways. Treatment with uridine leads to a return of normal blood hemoglobin levels, and bone marrow will become normoblastic.

14. You are attending to a patient who manifests with orotic aciduria. You suspect a defect in pyrimidine nucleotide biosynthesis, but aside from the orotic aciduria there are no other classical symptoms apparent in this patient, such as megaloblastic anemia, and the activity of UMP synthetase is normal. Which of the following enzymes is most likely deficient in this patient leading to the orotic aciduria?
A. aspartate transcarbamoylase
B. ornithine transcarbamoylase
C. thymidine synthase
D. orotate phosphoribosyltransferase
E. orotidine-5′-phosphate carboxylase

Answer E: Orotic aciduria can be the result of a deficiency in the urea cycle enzyme ornithine transcarbamoylase (OTC). A deficiency in OTC results in the urea cycle carbamoyl phosphate being transported from the mitochondria to the cytosol. Within the cytosol, the carbamoyl phosphate can serve as an intermediate in pyrimidine nucleotide synthesis, bypassing the regulated rate-limiting step catalyzed by ATCase. This will lead to synthesis in excess of the demands of the cells, resulting in increased orotic acid production.

15. A nucleoside analogue that is being screened as a potential anticancer agent causes gout in clinical trials. Which of the following actions of this drug may cause gout?
   A. inhibits carbamoyl phosphate synthetase
   B. inhibits the conversion of dihydrofolate to tetrahydrofolate
   C. inhibits xanthine oxidase
   D. interferes with feedback control of phosphoribosylpyrophosphate (PRPP) synthesis
   E. interferes with feedback control of thymidylate synthase

Answer D: Both the salvage and de novo synthesis pathways of purine metabolism utilize an activated sugar intermediate, 5-phosphoribosyl-1-pyrophosphate (PRPP). PRPP is generated by the action of PRPP synthetase. The synthesis of PRPP by PRPP synthetase is feedback inhibited by purine-5′-nucleotides (predominantly AMP and GMP) and activated by ribose-5-phosphate. Inhibition of purine salvage pathways leads to a reduction in the production of purine-5′-nucleotides, resulting in reduced inhibition of PRPP synthetase. Higher activity of PRPP synthetase results in excess purine nucleotide synthesis and as a consequence, increased catabolism of the excess purines to uric acid, resulting in hyperuricemia (gout).

16. Which of the following groups of amino acids are nitrogen donors in purine ring biosynthesis?
   A. arginine, lysine, histidine
   B. asparagine, lysine, histidine
   C. glutamate, histidine, aspartate
   D. glutamine, glycine, aspartate
   E. glycine, proline, lysine

Answer D: Synthesis of the purine nucleotides requires 5 moles of ATP, 2 moles of glutamine, 1 mole of glycine, 1 mole of CO_2, 1 mole of aspartate, and 2 moles of formate.

17. Ribose-5-phosphate is activated for participation in nucleotide biosynthesis by conversion to which of the following derivatives?
   A. ADP ribose
   B. CDP ribose
   C. GDP ribose
   D. UDP ribose
   E. 5-phosphoribosyl-1-pyrophosphate

Answer E: Both the salvage and de novo synthesis pathways of purine and pyrimidine biosynthesis lead to production of nucleoside-5′-phosphates through the utilization of an activated sugar intermediate. The activated sugar used is 5-phosphoribosyl-1-pyrophosphate (PRPP). PRPP is generated by the action of PRPP synthetase.

18. In the synthesis of pyrimidines, which of the following molecules is a direct precursor of the pyrimidine ring?
   A. aspartate
   B. fumarate
   C. glutamate
   D. glycine
   E. 5-phosphoribosyl-1-pyrophosphate

Answer A: Synthesis of the pyrimidines requires 1 mole of glutamine, 1 mole of ATP, and 1 mole of CO_2 (which form carbamoyl phosphate) and 1 mole of aspartate. An additional mole of glutamine and ATP are required in the conversion of UTP to CTP.

19. A 30-year-old man comes to the ER because he has had constant severe pain in his right ankle over the past 24 hours. His uncle also had episodes of pain in single joints. The ankle is swollen and warm. Serum uric acid concentration is increased. Which of the following enzyme activities is most likely to be decreased in this patient?
   A. adenosine deaminase
   B. carbamoyl phosphate synthetase
   C. hypoxanthine guanine phosphoribosyltransferase
   D. ribonucleotide reductase
   E. thymidylate synthase

Answer C: Gout is characterized by elevated levels of uric acid in the blood and urine. Uric acid is the end product of purine catabolism and excess production results from a variety of metabolic abnormalities that lead to overproduction of purines via the de novo pathway. Uric acid is very insoluble and when generated in large amounts will precipitate as uric acid crystals in the joints of the extremities. There are at least 3 different inherited defects that lead to early development of severe hyperuricemia and gout. One of these is deficiency in the purine salvage enzyme, hypoxanthine-guanine phosphoribosyltransferase (HGPRT).

20. A 10-year-old boy who has begun chemotherapy for acute myelogenous leukemia awakens at night with fever and severe pain in the ankles. Treatment with over-the-counter analgesics does not resolve the pain. The next morning, he has pain with urination and blood in the urine. Increased degradation of which of the following compounds most likely caused this patient's symptoms?
   A. amino acids
   B. fatty acids
   C. purines
   D. pyrimidines
   E. vitamin C

Answer C: Chemotherapeutic treatment of leukemias often results in tumor lysis syndrome (TLS). TLS is a severe and potentially life-threatening complication in patients with cancer occurring most frequently as a consequence of chemotherapy, radiotherapy, or immunotherapy. The hyperuricemia associated with TLS is the result of significantly increased catabolism of purine nucleotides in the dying cancer cells. The hyperuricemia can lead to acute uric acid nephropathy and kidney failure.

21. A 6-year-old boy with moderate mental retardation is brought to the physician for a follow-up examination. He has had choreoathetoid movements since the age of 16 months. He has been biting his lips and fingers for the past 2 months. His older brother has a similar condition. Physical examination shows spasticity of the lower limbs. Laboratory studies show an increased serum uric acid concentration and an increased urinary excretion of uric acid. His increased serum uric acid concentration is most likely due to which of the following?

A. deficient amidophosphoribosyltransferase activity
B. deficient hypoxanthine guanine phosphoribosyltransferase activity
C. deficient xanthine oxidase activity
D. increased adenosine phosphoribosyltransferase activity
E. increased adenosine deaminase activity

Answer B: This patient is exhibiting symptoms of Lesch-Nyhan syndrome (LNS). Lesch-Nyhan syndrome is a disorder related to defects in the activity of the purine nucleotide salvage enzyme, hypoxanthine-guanine phosphoribosyltransferase (HGPRT). The characteristic clinical features of the LNS are mental retardation, spastic cerebral palsy, choreoathetosis, uric acid urinary stones, and self-destructive biting of fingers and lips. The overall clinical features of LNS can be divided into 3 broad categories: uric acid overproduction and its associated consequences (eg, gouty arthritis and renal lithiasis) neurobehavioral dysfunction indicative of central nervous system involvement, and growth retardation.

22. The gouty arthritis in patients with Lesch-Nyhan syndrome results from a genetic defect in which of the following enzymes?

A. adenosine phosphoribosyltransferase
B. glutathione reductase
C. hypoxanthine guanine phosphoribosyltransferase
D. phosphoribosylpyrophosphate amidotransferase
E. xanthine oxidase

Answer C: Lesch-Nyhan syndrome is a disorder related to defects in the activity of the purine nucleotide salvage enzyme, hypoxanthine-guanine phosphoribosyltransferase (HGPRT). The characteristic clinical features of the LNS are mental retardation, spastic cerebral palsy, choreoathetosis, uric acid urinary stones, and self-destructive biting of fingers and lips. The uric acid overproduction and its associated consequences (eg, gouty arthritis) are the result of a block in purine nucleotide salvage, leading to increased catabolism to uric acid.

23. A 7-year-old boy is brought to the physician by his mother for a follow-up examination. He has had choreoathetosis, spasticity, and mental retardation since infancy and self-mutilation for 3 years. Laboratory studies show an increased serum uric acid concentration. The enzyme deficiency causing this disorder increases serum uric acid concentration by which of the following changes in purine metabolism?

A. decreased activity of xanthine oxidase
B. decreased formation of adenosine monophosphate
C. decreased utilization of phosphoribosylpyrophosphate (PRPP) in salvage
D. increased activity of adenosine deaminase
E. increased activity of PRPP synthetase

Answer C: This patient is exhibiting symptoms of Lesch-Nyhan syndrome (LNS). Lesch-Nyhan syndrome is a disorder related to defects in the activity of the purine nucleotide salvage enzyme, hypoxanthine-guanine phosphoribosyltransferase (HGPRT). The characteristic clinical features of the LNS are mental retardation, spastic cerebral palsy, choreoathetosis, uric acid urinary stones, and self-destructive biting of fingers and lips. The uric acid overproduction and its associated consequences (eg, gouty arthritis) are the result of a block in purine nucleotide salvage, leading to increased catabolism to uric acid resulting in hyperuricemia.

24. A 63-year-old woman comes to the physician for a follow-up examination. She has metastatic breast cancer treated with cyclophosphamide and fluorouracil. Thymidylate synthase, which is required for deoxynucleotide synthesis, is one target of fluorouracil. Which of the following is a substrate for thymidylate synthase?

A. dCMP
B. dCTP
C. dUDP
D. dUMP
E. dUTP

Answer D: The de novo pathway to dTTP synthesis first requires the use of dUMP from the metabolism of either UDP or CDP. The dUMP is converted to dTMP by the action of thymidylate synthase.

25. A 4-month-old boy is brought to the physician because of failure to thrive since birth. He is below the 5th percentile for length and at the 100th percentile for weight. Physical examination shows a doll-like face and marked hepatomegaly. After a 4-hour fast, serum studies show a decreased glucose concentration and increased concentrations of lactate, triglycerides, and uric acid. Which of the following is the most likely mechanism for the increased serum uric acid concentration in this patient?

A. decreased hepatic amidophosphoribosyltransferase activity
B. decreased hepatic hypoxanthine-guanine phosphoribosyltransferase activity
C. decreased hepatic phosphoribosylpyrophosphate activity
D. increased degradation of hepatic purine nucleotides
E. increased degradation of hepatic pyrimidine nucleotides

Answer D: This patient most likely has a deficiency in the purine nucleotide salvage enzyme, hypoxanthine-guanine phosphoribosyltransferase (HGPRT). The uric acid overproduction, and its associated consequences (eg, gouty arthritis), are likely the result of a block in purine nucleotide salvage, leading to increased catabolism to uric acid resulting in hyperuricemia.

26. A 3-year-old boy develops renal failure from hyperuricemia on the second day of cytosine arabinoside therapy for acute myelogenous leukemia. Which of the following is the most likely cause of his hyperuricemia?

A. increased catabolism of purines that are released from lysed leukemic cells
B. inhibition of orotic acid production via the urea cycle
C. inhibition of renal tubular transport by cytosine arabinoside
D. inhibition of uric acid for renal excretion by ketone bodies
E. overproduction of hypoxanthine-guanine phosphoribosyltransferase (HGPRT) by the leukemic cells

Answer A: Chemotherapeutic treatment of leukemias often results in tumor lysis syndrome, TLS. TLS is a severe and potentially life-threatening complication in patients with cancer occurring most frequently as a consequence of chemotherapy, radiotherapy, or immunotherapy. The hyperuricemia associated with TLS is the result of significantly increased catabolism of purine nucleotides in the dying cancer cells. The hyperuricemia can lead to acute uric acid nephropathy and kidney failure.

Checklist

✓ The nucleotides found in cells are derivatives of the heterocyclic highly basic, compounds, purine and pyrimidine.

✓ Nucleosides are composed of a nucleobase (purine or pyrimidine) attached to ribose but containing no phosphate. Nucleotides are the result of phosphate addition to nucleosides and they can be either mono-, di-, or triphosphate modified.

✓ The triphosphate and diphosphate groups of nucleotides are phosphoanhydride bonds imparting high transfer energy for participation in covalent bond synthesis, such as in the case of ATP.

✓ The nomenclature for the atoms in nucleosides and nucleotides includes a prime (′) designation to distinguish the atoms in the sugar from those in the base.

✓ Polynucleotides are composed of 2 or more nucleotides linked together via a phosphodiester bond between the 5′ phosphate of the sugar in one nucleotide and the 3′ hydroxyl of the sugar in another nucleotide. The common left-to-right nomenclature for polynucleotides is 5′→ 3′: for example, 5′-pApGpCpT-3′ or just 5′-AGCT-3′.

- ✓ Cyclic adenosine and guanine nucleotides act as second messengers in signal transduction events.
- ✓ Nucleotide analogs are used as antimicrobial and anticancer agents via their ability to interfere with nucleotide biosynthesis or DNA replication.
- ✓ Both purine and pyrimidine nucleotide biosynthesis involves the use of the activated form of ribose-5-phosphate, 5-phosphoribosyl-1-pyrophosphate (PRPP)
- ✓ Efficient dietary uptake, de novo synthesis, and intracellular salvage of nucleotides ensures that they are dietarily nonessential.
- ✓ Purine nucleotide synthesis proceeds with the initial construction of the nucleobase, which is then added to PRPP. The first fully formed purine nucleotide is IMP that serves as a branch point for synthesis of AMP and GMP. ATP levels regulate GMP synthesis and GTP levels regulate AMP synthesis.
- ✓ The catabolism of purine nucleotides produces the insoluble product, uric acid. Excess purine degradation can lead to hyperuricemia and ultimately to gout.
- ✓ Purine nucleotides are efficiently savaged, rendering de novo synthesis unnecessary except in conditions of rapid cell proliferation. Deficiencies in several salvage enzymes lead to a range of disorders from those with mild symptoms of hyperuricemia to potentially life-threatening immunodeficiency.
- ✓ Pyrimidine nucleotide synthesis proceeds via the construction of the nucleobase on PRPP. The first fully formed pyrimidine nucleotide is UMP. Following phosphorylation to UTP, some is converted to CTP via the action of CTP synthetase.
- ✓ Catabolism of pyrimidine nucleotides results in water-soluble products, so there are no clinical manifestations of increased catabolism.
- ✓ Thymidine nucleotides are synthesized from dUMP. Since thymidine nucleotide is almost exclusively associated with DNA, the enzymes that are involved in its synthesis are targets of chemotherapeutic agents.
- ✓ Synthesis of the deoxynucleotide is catalyzed by ribonucleotide reductase (RR). Following the reaction, the oxidized form of RR must be reduced and this is catalyzed by thioredoxin or glutaredoxin and involves the enzymes thioredoxin reductase and glutathione reductase.
- ✓ Ribonucleotide reductase activity is strongly inhibited by ATP and dATP.

CHAPTER

33 Nitrogen: Heme Metabolism

CHAPTER OUTLINE

Porphyrins and Heme
Synthesis of Porphyrins and Heme
Regulation of Heme Biosynthesis
Heme Catabolism
Abnormalities in Heme Metabolism

High-Yield Terms

Porphyrin: a group of aromatic organic compounds composed of 4 modified pyrrole subunits interconnected at their α-carbon atoms via methine bridges

Porphyria: any of a group of rare inherited or acquired disorders of enzymes involved in the production of the porphyrins and heme

Hemin: protoporphyrin IX containing a ferric (Fe^{3+}) iron, as opposed to heme which contains ferrous (Fe^{2+}) iron

Reticuloendothelial cells: a collective term for cells of the immune system that primarily comprises macrophages and monocytes but may include all phagocytic cells

Bilirubin: open chain yellowish breakdown product of heme catabolism

Kernicterus: bilirubin-induced brain dysfunction, also called bilirubin encephalopathy

Sideroblastic anemia: a disease in which the bone marrow produces ringed sideroblasts rather than healthy erythrocytes, sideroblasts are abnormal nucleated erythroblasts with granules of iron in perinuclear mitochondria

Porphyrins and Heme

The porphyrins (Figure 33-1) are a group of aromatic organic compounds composed of 4 modified pyrrole subunits interconnected at their α-carbon atoms via methine bridges (=CH–). These compounds are highly conjugated systems and as such they typically have very intense absorption bands in the visible region and may be deeply colored. Indeed, the name porphyrin comes from a Greek word for purple. In humans, the most clinically significant porphyrins are the hemes; heme *a*, heme *b*, and heme *c*. Heme *b* is called protoporphyrin IX and it contains 4 methyl, 2 vinyl, and 2 propionic acid substituents. Heme *b* is the prosthetic group that binds oxygen in erythrocytes and is the pigment that induces the reddish color of blood. Heme *a* and heme *c* are prosthetic groups of several cytochromes, particularly of the electron transport chain (Chapter 17). Many additional proteins contain a heme prosthetic group with the largest family of such proteins being the cytochrome P450 (CYP) enzymes, many of which are involved in xenobiotic metabolism in the liver.

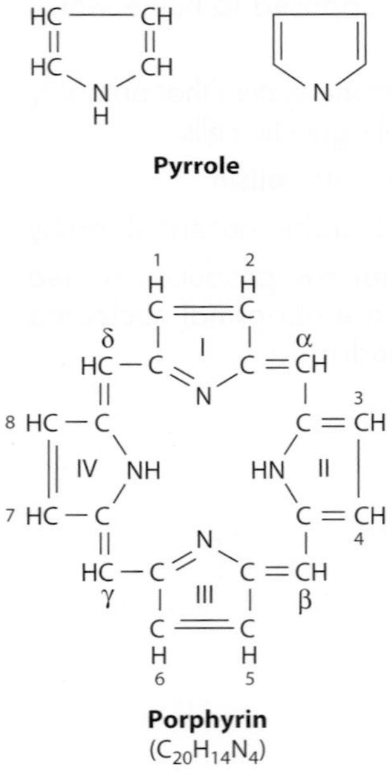

Pyrrole

Porphyrin
($C_{20}H_{14}N_4$)

FIGURE 33-1: The porphyrin molecule. Rings are labeled I, II, III, and IV. Substituent positions on the rings are labeled 1, 2, 3, 4, 5, 6, 7, and 8. The methyne bridges (=HC—) are labeled α, β, γ, and δ. The numbering system used is that of Hans Fischer. Murray RK, Bender DA, Botham KM, Kennelly PJ, Rodwell VW, Weil PA. *Harper's Illustrated Biochemistry*, 29th ed. New York: McGraw-Hill; 2012.

Synthesis of Porphyrins and Heme

The first reaction in heme biosynthesis takes place in the mitochondrion and involves the condensation of 1 glycine and 1 succinyl-CoA by the pyridoxal phosphate-containing enzyme, δ-aminolevulinic acid synthase (ALAS) (Figure 33-2). Delta-aminolevulinic acid (ALA) is also called 5-aminolevulinic acid. This reaction is both the rate-limiting reaction of heme biosynthesis and the most highly regulated reaction. There are 2 forms of ALAS. ALAS1 is considered a house-keeping gene and is expressed in all cells. ALAS2 is an erythroid-specific form of the enzyme and is expressed only in fetal liver and adult bone marrow.

Mitochondrial ALA is transported to the cytosol, where ALA dehydratase (also called porphobilinogen synthase) dimerizes 2 molecules of ALA to produce the pyrrole-ring compound porphobilinogen (see Figure 33-2). The next step in the pathway involves the head-to-tail condensation of 4 molecules of porphobilinogen to produce the linear tetrapyrrole intermediate, hydroxymethylbilane catalyzed by porphobilinogen deaminase, PBG deaminase (Figure 33-3). PBG deaminase is also called hydroxymethylbilane synthase or uroporphyrinogen I synthase. Hydroxymethylbilane has 2 main fates. The most important is regulated, enzymatic conversion to uroporphyrinogen III, the next intermediate on the path to heme. This step is mediated by a holoenzyme comprised of uroporphyrinogen synthase plus a protein known as uroporphyrinogen III cosynthase. Hydroxymethylbilane can also non-enzymatically cyclize forming uroporphyrinogen I (see Figure 33-3).

In the cytosol, the acetate substituents of uroporphyrinogen (normal uroporphyrinogen III or abnormal uroporphyrinogen I) are all decarboxylated by the enzyme uroporphyrinogen decarboxylase (Figure 33-4). The resultant products have methyl groups in place of acetate and are known as coproporphyrinogens, with coproporphyrinogen III being the important normal intermediate in heme synthesis. Coproporphyrinogen III is transported back into the mitochondria, where 2 propionate residues are decarboxylated, yielding vinyl substituents on the 2 pyrrole rings. The colorless product is protoporphyrinogen IX. In the mitochondrion, protoporphyrinogen IX is converted to protoporphyrin IX by protoporphyrinogen IX oxidase. The oxidase reaction requires molecular oxygen and results in the loss of 6 protons and 6 electrons, yielding a completely conjugated ring system, which is responsible for the characteristic red color to hemes. The final reaction in heme synthesis also takes place in the mitochondrion and involves the insertion of the iron atom into the ring system generating heme *b*. The enzyme catalyzing this reaction is known as ferrochelatase.

High-Yield Concept

Clinical problems associated with heme metabolism are of 2 types. Disorders that arise from defects in the enzymes of heme biosynthesis are termed the **porphyrias** and cause elevations in the levels of intermediates in heme synthesis in the serum and urine. Inherited disorders in bilirubin metabolism lead to **hyperbilirubinemia** which is the root cause of **jaundice**.

High-Yield Concept

Deficiencies of ALAS2 result in a disorder called X-linked sideroblastic anemia, XLSA. Sideroblasts are erythroblasts with non-heme iron–containing organelles, called siderosomes. XLSA has also been called congenital sideroblastic anemia, hereditary sideroblastic anemia, hereditary iron-loading anemia, X-linked hypochromic anemia, hereditary hypochromic anemia, and hereditary anemia.

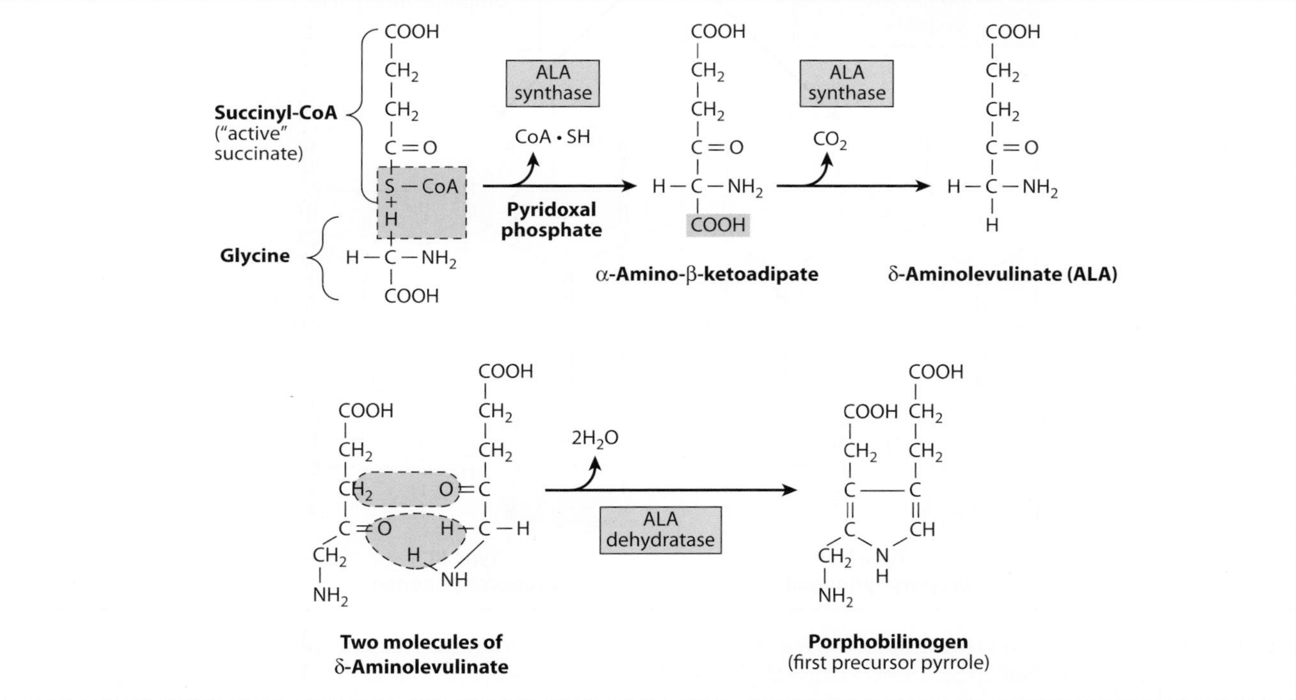

FIGURE 33-2: Biosynthesis of porphobilinogen. ALA synthase occurs in the mitochondria, whereas ALA dehydratase is present in the cytosol. Murray RK, Bender DA, Botham KM, Kennelly PJ, Rodwell VW, Weil PA. *Harper's Illustrated Biochemistry*, 29th ed. New York: McGraw-Hill; 2012.

High-Yield Concept

The enzymes ferrochelatase, ALA synthase, and ALA dehydratase are highly sensitive to inhibition by heavy metal poisoning. Indeed, a characteristic of lead poisoning is an increase in ALA in the circulation in the absence of an increase in porphobilinogen.

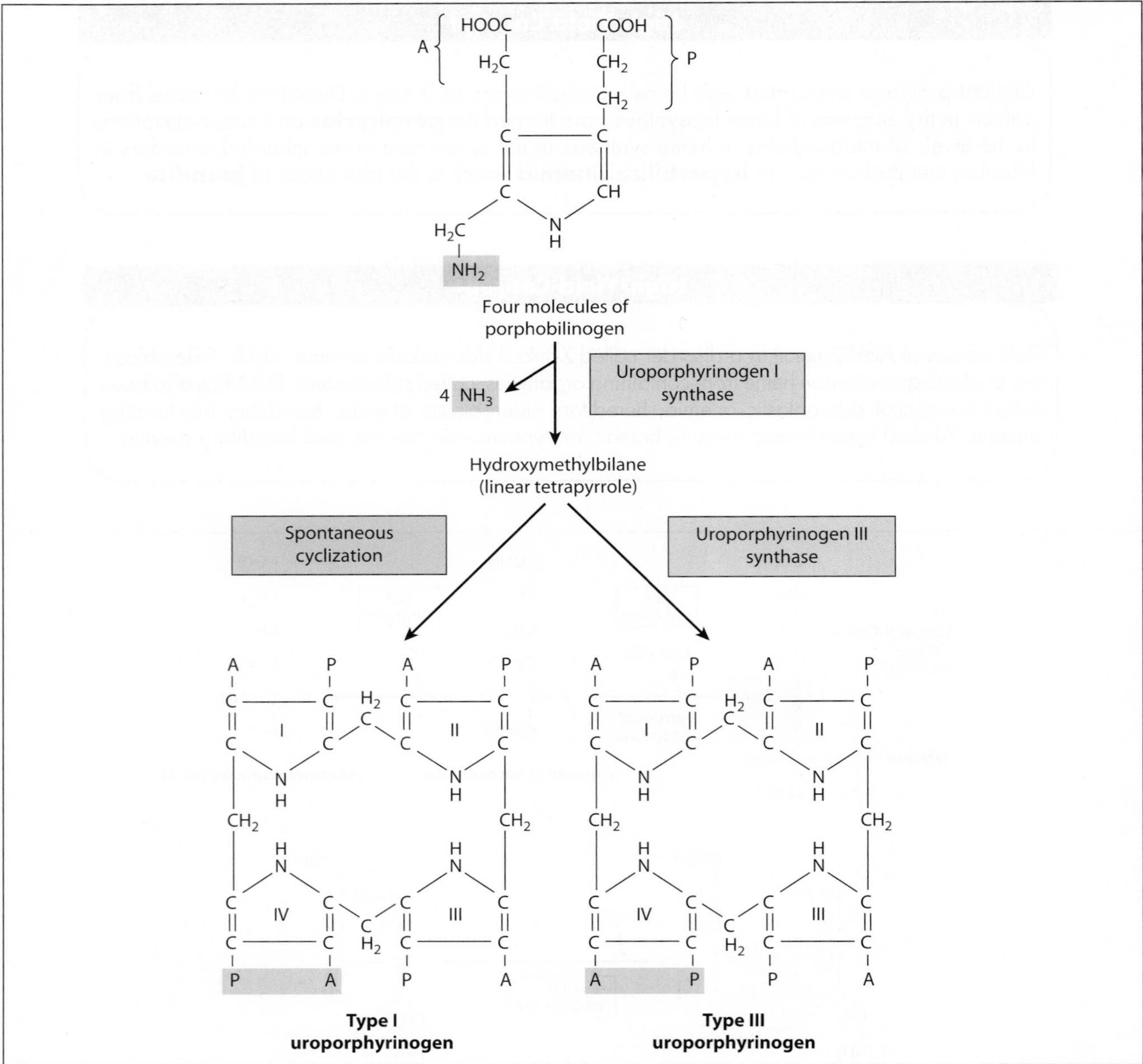

FIGURE 33-3: Conversion of porphobilinogen to uroporphyrinogens. Uroporphyrinogen synthase I is also called porphobilinogen (PBG) deaminase or hydroxymethylbilane (HMB) synthase. Murray RK, Bender DA, Botham KM, Kennelly PJ, Rodwell VW, Weil PA. *Harper's Illustrated Biochemistry*, 29th ed. New York: McGraw-Hill; 2012.

Regulation of Heme Biosynthesis

Although heme is synthesized in virtually all tissues, the principal sites of synthesis are erythroid cells (≈85%) and hepatocytes. The differences in these 2 tissues and their needs for heme result in quite different mechanisms for regulation of heme biosynthesis.

In hepatocytes, heme is required for incorporation into the cytochromes, in particular, the P450 class of cytochromes that are important for detoxification. In addition numerous cytochromes of the oxidative-phosphorylation pathway contain heme. The rate-limiting step in hepatic heme biosynthesis occurs at the ALAS catalyzed step, which represents the committed step in heme synthesis. The Fe^{3+} oxidation product of heme is termed hemin. Hemin acts as a feedback inhibitor of ALAS. Hemin also inhibits the synthesis of ALAS and inhibits its transport from the cytosol into the mitochondria.

In erythroid cells all of the heme is synthesized for incorporation into hemoglobin and occurs only upon differentiation when synthesis of hemoglobin proceeds.

High-Yield Concept

The heme oxygenase reaction is the only one that is known to produce CO. Most of the CO is excreted through the lungs, with the result that the CO content of expired air is a direct measure of the activity of heme oxygenase in an individual.

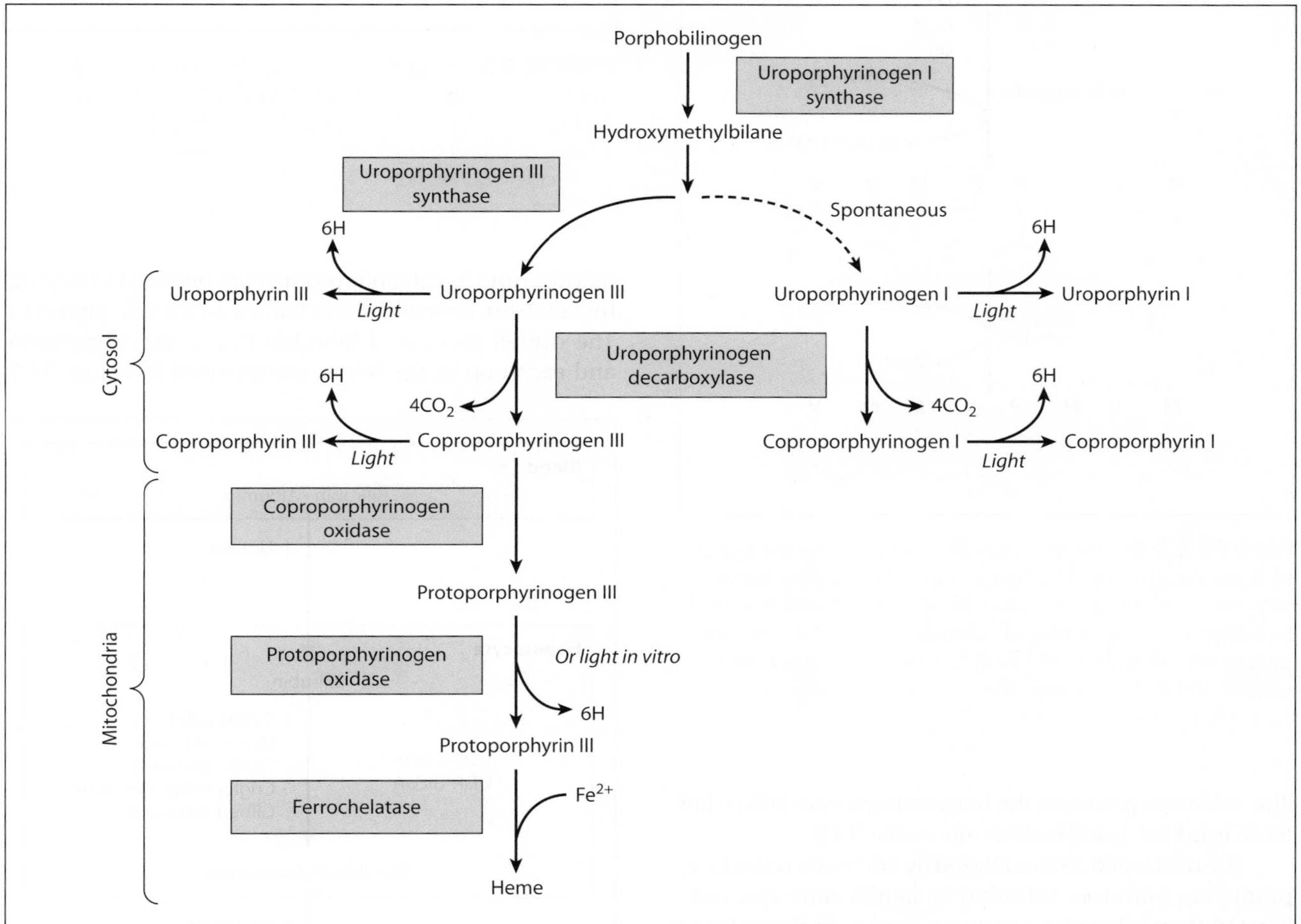

FIGURE 33-4: Steps in the biosynthesis of the porphyrin derivatives from porphobilinogen. Uroporphyrinogen I synthase is also called porphobilinogen deaminase or hydroxymethylbilane synthase. Murray RK, Bender DA, Botham KM, Kennelly PJ, Rodwell VW, Weil PA. *Harper's Illustrated Biochemistry*, 29th ed. New York: McGraw-Hill; 2012.

In mature erythrocytes both heme and hemoglobin syntheses cease. The heme and hemoglobin must, therefore, survive for the life of the erythrocyte (normally this is around 120 days). In reticulocytes, heme stimulates protein synthesis (see Chapter 37).

Heme Catabolism

The largest repository of heme in the human body is in erythrocytes. The daily turnover of these cells results in the release of about 6 g/d of hemoglobin. In the catabolism of the heme from hemoglobin the porphyrin ring is hydrophobic and must be solubilized for it to be excreted. In addition, the iron must be conserved for new heme synthesis. Senescent erythrocytes, and heme from other sources, are engulfed by cells of the reticuloendothelial system. The globin proteins are recycled or degraded into amino acids which are, in turn, recycled or catabolized as needed.

Heme is oxidized, with the heme ring being opened by the endoplasmic reticulum enzyme, heme oxygenase (Figure 33-5). This oxidation step requires heme as a substrate, and any hemin (Fe^{3+}) is reduced to heme (Fe^{2+}) first.

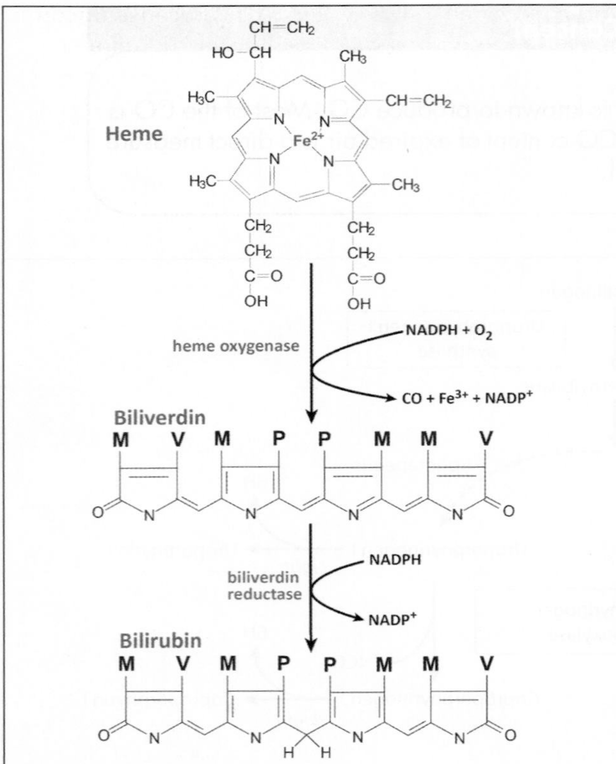

FIGURE 33-5: Heme catabolism initiated by the action of heme oxygenase. The heme ring is cleaved by heme oxygenase yielding biliverdin. Biliverdin is then converted to bilirubin via the action of bilverdin reductase. The side groups on bilverdin and bilirubin are abbreviated: M, methyl; V, vinyl, P, propyl. Reproduced with permission of themedicalbiochemistrypage, LLC.

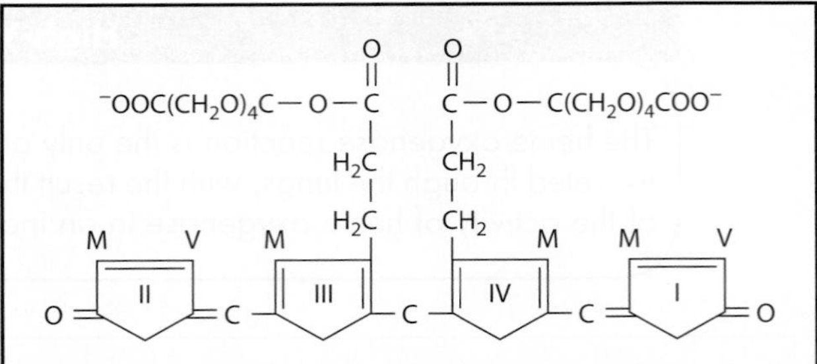

FIGURE 33-6: Structure of bilirubin diglucuronide (conjugated, "direct-reacting" bilirubin). Glucuronic acid is attached via ester linkage to the two propionic acid groups of bilirubin to form an acylglucuronide. Murray RK, Bender DA, Botham KM, Kennelly PJ, Rodwell VW, Weil PA. *Harper's Illustrated Biochemistry*, 29th ed. New York: McGraw-Hill; 2012.

The oxidation produces the linear tetrapyrrole biliverdin, ferric iron (Fe^{3+}), and carbon monoxide (CO).

The next reaction is catalyzed by biliverdin reductase, producing bilirubin. Bilirubin is significantly less conjugated than biliverdin causing a change in the color of the molecule from blue-green (biliverdin) to yellow-red (bilirubin). The latter catabolic processes are responsible for the progressive changes in the color of a hematoma, or bruise, in which the damaged tissue changes its color from an initial dark blue to a red-yellow and finally to a yellow color before all the pigment is transported out of the affected tissue. Peripherally arising bilirubin is transported to the liver in association with albumin, where the remaining catabolic reactions take place.

In hepatocytes, bilirubin-UDP-glucuronyltransferase (bilirubin-UGT) adds 2 equivalents of glucuronic acid to bilirubin to produce the more water-soluble bilirubin diglucuronide derivative (Figure 33-6). Bilirubin-UGT is encoded by the *UGT1A* gene, and several UGT1A enzymes including bilirubin-UGT (identified as UGT1A1) are encoded by the *UGT1A* gene complex. The increased water solubility facilitates its excretion with bile. In the intestines, bilirubin and its catabolic products, generated by bacterial metabolism, are collectively known as the bile pigments. The overall process of bilirubin transport, conjugation, and excretion in the bile is summarized in Figure 33-7.

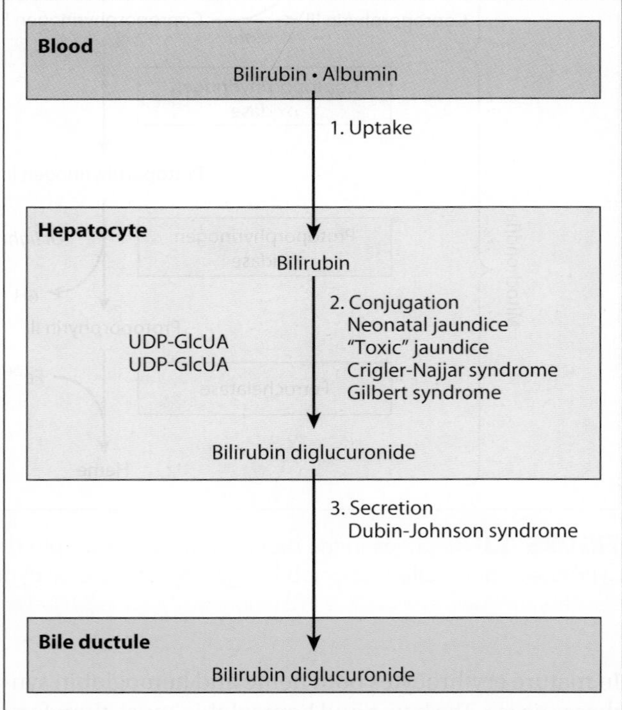

FIGURE 33-7: Diagrammatic representation of the three major processes (uptake, conjugation, and secretion) involved in the transfer of bilirubin from blood to bile. Certain proteins of hepatocytes, such as ligandin (a member of the glutathione *S*-transferase family of enzymes) and Y protein, bind intracellular bilirubin and may prevent its efflux into the blood stream. The process affected in a number of conditions causing jaundice is also shown. Murray RK, Bender DA, Botham KM, Kennelly PJ, Rodwell VW, Weil PA. *Harper's Illustrated Biochemistry*, 29th ed. New York: McGraw-Hill; 2012.

The sites in this process where defects are known to cause various disorders of bilirubin metabolism resulting in hyperbilirubinemias are also indicated.

Abnormalities in Heme Metabolism

Excess circulation and accumulation of bilirubin (hyperbilirubinemia) results jaundice. There are 2 major classes of hyperbilirubinemias: unconjugated and conjugated (Clinical Box 33-1). Because unconjugated bilirubin is not water soluble and therefore much more toxic, the clinical symptoms of unconjugated hyperbilirubinemias can be severe and even fatal. Several inherited disorders in bilirubin metabolism have been identified. Gilbert syndrome (Clinical Box 33-2) and the Crigler-Najjar syndromes (Clinical Box 33-3) result from predominantly unconjugated hyperbilirubinemia. Dubin-Johnson syndrome and Rotor syndrome result from conjugated hyperbilirubinemia.

CLINICAL BOX 33-1: HYPERBILIRUBINEMIA CLASSIFICATIONS

There are 2 major classes of hyperbilirubinemias: unconjugated and conjugated. Bilirubin levels are measured in the serum by an assay utilizing Ehrlich diazo reagent and results in the formation of an azobilirubin product. Conjugated bilirubin does not require addition of alcohol to promote the azotization reaction, and thus this is referred to as measurement of **direct bilirubin**. The reaction with unconjugated bilirubin requires the addition of alcohol, and thus is referred to as the measurement of **indirect bilirubin**. Normal bilirubin measurements are 0.3 to 1.2 mg/dL for total (indirect + direct). Direct type bilirubin does not exist in the plasma; however, a small portion of indirect type bilirubin may present as direct reacting type and thus the serum measurement may show a direct bilirubin, but this is never above 0.3mg/dL in a normal individual. The mildest form of this condition is jaundice which is caused by a yellow-orange discoloration of the tissues and is most easily visible as icteric discoloration in the sclera of the eyes. Bilirubin toxicity (bilirubin encephalopathy) can be life threatening in neonates. Bilirubin encephalopathy is characterized by yellow discoloration of the basal ganglia in babies with intense jaundice and is termed **kernicterus**. Any increase in plasma bilirubin above 20 mg/dL is considered dangerous in neonates. However, individual differences in bilirubin sensitivity can result in kernicterus at lower bilirubin levels. Kernicterus occurs in infants with severe unconjugated hyperbilirubinemia and in young adults with high serum levels of unconjugated bilirubin, with the latter the result of inherited deficiencies in bilirubin-UGT. Bilirubin has been shown to inhibit DNA synthesis, uncouple oxidative phosphorylation, and inhibit ATPase activity in brain mitochondria. Bilirubin also inhibits a variety of different classes of enzymes including dehydrogenases, electron transport proteins, hydrolases, and enzymes of RNA synthesis, protein synthesis, and carbohydrate metabolism. All of these toxic effects of bilirubin are reversed by binding to albumin. In fact, albumin plays a vital role in the disposition of bilirubin in the body by keeping the compound in solution and transporting it from its sites of production (primarily bone marrow and spleen) to its site of excretion which is the liver.

CLINICAL BOX 33-2: GILBERT SYNDROME

Gilbert syndrome results from mutations in the TATA-box of the promoter region upstream of exon 1 in the *UGT1A* gene which results in reduced levels of expression of a normal bilirubin-UGT enzyme. The normal sequence of the UGT1A TATA-box is $A(TA)_6TAA$, whereas in Gilbert syndrome individuals it is $A(TA)_7TAA$. Gilbert syndrome is also referred to as constitutional hepatic dysfunction and familial nonhemolytic jaundice. The syndrome is characterized by mild chronic, unconjugated hyperbilirubinemia. Almost all afflicted individuals have a degree of icteric discoloration in the eyes typical of jaundice. Serum bilirubin levels in Gilbert syndrome patients are usually less than 3 mg/dL. Many patients manifest with fatigue and abdominal discomfort, symptoms that are ascribed to anxiety, but are not due to bilirubin metabolism. Expression of the Gilbert phenotype requires a relatively high level of bilirubin production. This is evident from the fact that persons homozygous for the UGT1A TATA-box mutation do not exhibit hyperbilirubinemia. Presentation of Gilbert syndrome symptoms also occurs more frequently in men than in women because the production of bilirubin is higher in males.

CLINICAL BOX 33-3: CRIGLER-NAJJAR SYNDROMES

There are two forms of Crigler-Najjar syndrome: type I results from mutations in the bilirubin-UGT gene that result in complete loss of enzyme activity, whereas type II is the result of mutations that cause incomplete loss of enzyme activity.

Type I: In patients with very high levels of unconjugated bilirubin, but with normal liver function tests, Crigler-Najjar syndrome type I is indicated. Almost all afflicted infants manifest with severe nonhemolytic icterus within the first few days of life. The jaundice in these patients is characterized by increased concentrations of indirect-reacting bilirubin in the plasma. The advent of phototherapy has allowed for greater survival in type I patients; in fact without this therapy infants will succumb to kernicterus by the age of 15 months. Use of phototherapy and intermittent plasmapheresis has allowed many type I infants to survive until puberty without significant brain damage. The risk for kernicterus persists following puberty, however, because phototherapy is less effective at this age. Liver transplantation is considered the only definitive treatment for type I Crigler-Najjar syndrome.

Type II: The clinical manifestations of type II disease are similar to those of type I except that serum bilirubin levels are much lower, generally below 20 mg/dL. The prognosis for type II patients is also much better than for type I patients. Induction of bilirubin-UGT by drugs such as phenobarbitol can lead to reductions in serum bilirubin levels in type II patients. Given that type I Crigler-Najjar results from complete loss of functional bilirubin-UGT it is not surprising that phenobarbitol has no effect in those patients. Type II Crigler-Najar syndrome was first described by I.M. Arias and thus, this form of the disease is also sometimes referred to as Arias syndrome.

TABLE 33-1: Summary of Major Findings in the Porphyrias[1]

Enzyme Involved	*Type, Class, and OMIM Number*	*Major Signs and Symptoms*	*Results of Laboratory Tests*
ALA synthase 2, ALAS2 synthase (erythroid form)	X-linked sideroblastic anemia[2] (erythropoietic) (OMIM 301300)	Anemia	Red cell counts and hemoglobin decreased
ALA dehydratase	ALA dehydratase deficiency (hepatic) (OMIM 125270)	Abdominal pain, neuropsychiatric symptoms	Urinary ALA and coproporphyrin III increased
Uroporphyrinogen I synthase[3]	Acute intermittent porphyria (hepatic) (OMIM 176000)	Abdominal pain, neuropsychiatric symptoms	Urinary ALA and PBG increased
Uroporphyrinogen III synthase	Congenital erythropoietic (erythropoietic) (OMIM 263700)	Photosensitivity	Urinary, fecal, and red cell uroporphyrin I increased
Uroporphyrinogen decarboxylase	Porphyria cutanea tarda (hepatic) (OMIM 176100)	Photosensitivity	Urinary uroporphyrin I increased
Coproporphyrinogen oxidase	Hereditary coproporphyria (hepatic) (OMIM 121300)	Photosensitivity, abdominal pain, neuropsychiatric symptoms	Urinary ALA, PBG, and coproporphyrin III and fecal coproporphyrin III increased
Protoporphyrinogen oxidase	Variegate porphyria (hepatic) (OMIM 176200)	Photosensitivity, abdominal pain, neuropsychiatric symptoms	Urinary ALA, PBG, and coproporphyrin III and fecal protoporphyrin IX increased
Ferrochelatase	Protoporphyria (erythropoietic) (OMIM 177000)	Photosensitivity	Fecal and red cell protoporphyrin IX increased

[1]Only the biochemical findings in the active stages of these diseases are listed. Certain biochemical abnormalities are detectable in the latent stages of some of the above conditions. Conditions 3, 5, and 8 are generally the most prevalent porphyrias. Condition 2 is rare.
[2]X-linked sideroblastic anemia is not a porphyria but is included here because ALA synthase is involved.
[3]This enzyme is also called PBG deaminase or hydroxymethylbilane synthase.
Abbreviations: ALA, δ-aminolevulinic acid; PBG, porphobilinogen.
Murray RK, Bender DA, Botham KM, Kennelly PJ, Rodwell VW, Weil PA. *Harper's Illustrated Biochemistry*, 29th ed. New York: McGraw-Hill; 2012.

The porphyrias are both inherited and acquired disorders in heme synthesis. These disorders are classified as either erythroid or hepatic, depending upon the principal site of expression of the enzyme defect. Eight different porphyrias have been classified encompassing defects in each of the enzymes of heme synthesis (Table 33-1). The most commonly occurring hepatic porphyria is acute intermittent porphyria (AIP) (Clinical Box 33-4), which is caused by a defect in PBG deaminase. This enzyme is also called hydroxymethylbilane synthase or rarely uroporphyrinogen I synthase. All of the porphyrias lead to excretion of heme biosynthetic by-products that turn the

CLINICAL BOX 33-4: ACUTE INTERMITTENT PORPHYRIA, AIP

Acute intermittent porphyria (AIP) is an autosomal dominant disorder that results from defects in PBG deaminase (PBGD) resulting in 50% of normal activity. AIP is classified as an acute hepatic porphyria and is the most common hepatic type porphyria. AIP is prevalent in Swedish populations, particularly northern Swedes where the frequency approaches 100 cases per 100,000 population. Because of this prevalence, AIP is also known as Swedish porphyria. Using immunological assays for the presence of PBGD activity, mutations in the PBGD gene have been classified into 3 distinct categories. Type I mutations result in about 50% detectable PBGD protein and enzyme activity. These mutations are referred to as CRIM-negative mutations where CRIM means "cross-reactive immunologic material." Type I mutations represent the largest percentage of mutations in AIP patients, consisting of approximately 85% of mutations. Type II mutations are also CRIM-negative and result in absence of the house-keeping form of the enzyme but normal amounts of the erythroid-specific isozyme. These mutations are found in less than 5% of AIP patients. Type III mutations are CRIM-positive and result in decreased PBGD activity but do not alter the stability of the mutant enzyme. The clinical manifestations of AIP are related to the visceral, autonomic, peripheral, and central nervous system involvement of the disease. In fact almost all of the symptoms of AIP result from neurological dysfunction; however, the exact mechanism leading to neural cell damage is not clearly understood. The pain associated with the neurological dysfunction can be so severe as to require treatment with opiates. The symptoms of AIP result from a dramatic increase in the production and excretion of porphyrin precursors. A reduced ability to synthesize heme in a state of increased demand results in loss of heme-mediated control of the rate-limiting enzyme of heme synthesis, ALAS1. In this circumstance, unregulated ALAS1 results in large increases in synthesis of ALA. The large increases in ALA drive the ALA dehydratase reaction to produce large amounts of PBG. With the block in heme synthesis at the PBGD reaction the resulting increases in ALA and PBG synthesis leads to marked increases in urinary excretion of both compounds resulting in deep red urine, a hallmark of AIP. Clinical manifestation in AIP becomes apparent in the event of an increased demand for hepatic heme production. This most often occurs due to drug exposure or some other precipitating factor such as an infection. In fact, an infection is the leading cause of attacks of acute porphyria. If a drug is the cause of an attack its use should be discontinued immediately. The neurovisceral signs and symptoms of AIP are nonspecific and highly variable resulting in patients being diagnosed with an unrelated illness. Because certain factors such as hormonal or nutritional influences or drug interactions can affect the clinical manifestation of AIP, as well as other hepatic porphyrias, these diseases are referred to as ecogenetic or pharmacogenetic disorders. Numerous drugs are known to lead to acute attacks of porphyria, in particular barbiturates. Other drugs include ACE inhibitors and calcium channel blockers, the sulfonylureas used by type 2 diabetics, and the sulfonamide class of antibiotic. The most common symptom (occurring in 85%-95% of cases) during an acute attack is diffuse, poorly localized abdominal pain which can be quite severe. The abdominal pain is usually accompanied by constipation, nausea, and vomiting. The most common physical sign that is observed in up to 80% of AIP cases is tachycardia which may be due to sympathetic nervous system overactivity. Additional symptoms of AIP are pain in the limbs, head, neck, or chest; muscle weakness; and sensory loss. Often, without any precipitating influences, AIP remains latent and there may be no family history of the disease. The symptoms of AIP are almost never observed in prepubescent children and are seen more frequently in women than in men. Treating the symptoms of AIP involves a high-carbohydrate diet and during a severe attack, an infusion of 10% glucose is highly recommended. Panhematin, a form of alkaline heme, is used to treat attacks of porphyria as it acts like heme to inhibit ALAS, thereby reducing the production of ALA and subsequently PBG.

urine red and when deposited in the teeth turn them reddish brown. Accumulation of these by-products in the skin renders it extremely sensitive to sunlight causing ulceration and disfiguring scars. Increased hair growth (hypertrichosis) is also a symptom of the porphyrias leading to appearance of fine hairs over the entire face and on the extremities. This latter symptom lends to the description of "werewolf syndrome" in many porphyria patients.

REVIEW QUESTIONS

1. A-18-year-old woman presented with 1-week of history of fever and malaise. She had mild jaundice and elevated temperature. Hemoglobin was 13.8 g/dL, leukocyte count 13 x 10^9/L. Serum bilirubin was elevated (42 mmol/L) and contained 95% unconjugated bilirubin. Liver enzyme tests were normal. Which of the following is the most likely cause of these signs and symptoms?

A. alcohol poisoning
B. decreased glucuronyl transferase
C. increased lactate dehydrogenase
D. excessive hemolysis
E. obstruction of bile flow

Answer B: Glucuronyl transferase is the enzyme that conjugates bilirubin in the liver, after which it is excreted in bile or urine. A hereditary defect in glucuronyl transferase concentration, or activity, is called Gilbert syndrome. It may lead to mild jaundice and general discomfort with typical onset in childhood or early adulthood. Alcohol poisoning leads to liver damage, and an elevation of conjugated bilirubin. Abnormalities of liver enzyme tests would be expected. Lactate dehydrogenase catalyzes the conversion of lactate to pyruvate as part of cellular energy production. Since many cells including red blood cells are rich in LDH, increased serum LDH levels could point toward excessive hemolysis, but would not be a cause for it. Although hemolysis that exceeds the capacity of the liver to clear bilirubin from serum would lead to increased unconjugated bilirubin, it is not the best choice due to the woman's normal hemoglobin (12-16 g/dL for females). Obstruction of bile flow leads to backup of largely conjugated bilirubin in the blood stream.

2. An 11-month-old male infant is presented with failure to thrive and a persistence of anemia. Blood analysis revealed levels of lead to be twice the level deemed toxic. Additional laboratory results reveal high levels of coproporphyrinogen III in the urine. In order to rapidly lower the levels of lead in the child's blood, he is placed on chelation therapy. The child recovers fully following this treatment. The symptoms observed in this child are due to the lead-induced inhibition of which of the following enzymes of heme biosynthesis?

A. δ-aminolevulinic acid (ALA) dehydratase
B. δ-aminolevulinic acid (ALA) synthase
C. ferrochelatase
D. porphobilinogen (PBG) deaminase
E. uroporphyrinogen decarboxylase

Answer C: The enzymes ferrochelatase, ALA synthase, and ALA dehydratase are highly sensitive to inhibition by heavy metal poisoning. Indeed, a characteristic of lead poisoning is an increase in ALA in the circulation in the absence of an increase in porphobilinogen. The appearance of coproporphyrinogen III in the urine of this patient indicates that the inhibition of ferrochelatase is profound, whereas ALA synthase and ALA dehydratase are minimally inhibited.

3. In carrying out an assay using cultured hepatocytes you find that addition of hemin (Fe^{3+} heme) does not have the expected consequence of reduced protoporphyrin IX synthesis. This result suggests that your hepatocytes harbor a mutant form of one of the heme-regulated enzymes of porphyrin biosynthesis. Which of the following represents the likely enzyme?

A. ALA dehydratase
B. ALA synthase
C. ferrochelatase
D. heme oxygenase
E. PBG deaminase

Answer B: In the liver, hemin acts as a feedback inhibitor on ALA synthase reducing its activity. In addition, hemin acts to repress transport of ALA synthase into the mitochondria as well as repressing synthesis of the enzyme. Therefore, a continued synthesis of protoporphyrin IX in the presence of hemin indicates that ALA synthase is active but nonresponsive to the inhibitory action of hemin.

4. A 32-year-old man has suffered from chronic blistering and scarring of his skin following periods of unprotected exposure to sunlight. In the course of taking a history from the patient his doctor learns that the symptoms that occur following sun exposure are worse when he has been drinking heavily and smoking. The doctor orders blood and urine tests which show a high accumulation of uroporphyrin. Which of the following disorders would best explain the symptoms and clinical signs manifesting in this patient?

A. acute intermittent porphyria (AIP)
B. hereditary coproporphyria (HCP)
C. porphyria cutanea tarda (PCT)
D. variegate porphyria
E. X-linked sideroblastic anemia

Answer C: PCT is the most common porphyria. Symptoms of PCT include cutaneous involvement and liver abnormalities. Cutaneous features include chronic blistering lesions on sun-exposed skin. These lesions lead to skin thickening, scarring, and calcification. Symptoms usually develop in adults and are exacerbated by excess hepatic iron, alcohol consumption, and induction of cytochrome P450 (CYP) enzymes as occurs in smokers.

5. Acute intermittent porphyria (AIP) is the major autosomal dominant acute hepatic porphyria. This disease is caused by a deficiency in porphobilinogen deaminase, an enzyme of heme biosynthesis. Patients afflicted with this disease would be expected to excrete excess amounts of which of the following?
A. δ-aminolevulinic acid (ALA)
B. coproporphyrinogen III
C. hydroxymethylbilane
D. protoporphyrin IX
E. type III uroporphyrinogen

Answer A: Porphobilinogen (PBG) deaminase (also called hydroxymethylbilane synthase) catalyzes the heme biosynthesis reaction involving the head-to-tail condensation of 4 molecules of porphobilinogen to produce the linear tetrapyrrole intermediate, hydroxymethylbilane. Hydroxymethylbilane can nonenzymatically cyclize into uroporphyrinogen I which is why PBG deaminase is also known as uroporphyrinogen I synthase. δ-aminolevulinic acid (ALA) is the precursor for porphobilinogen, thus a defect in PBG deaminase would lead to excess ALA excretion.

6. There is but a single enzyme-catalyzed reaction in the human body known to generate carbon monoxide (CO) as one of its products. Which of the following enzymes represents the one that catalyzes this CO-producing reaction?
A. biliverdin reductase
B. coproporphyrinogen oxidase
C. heme oxygenase
D. protoporphyrinogen oxidase
E. uroporphyrinogen decarboxylase

Answer C: Heme is oxidized, with the heme ring being opened by the endoplasmic reticulum enzyme, heme oxygenase (see Figure 33-5). The oxidation step requires heme as a substrate, and any hemin (Fe^{3+}) is reduced to heme (Fe^{2+}) prior to oxidation by heme oxygenase. The oxidation occurs on a specific carbon producing the linear tetrapyrrole biliverdin, ferric iron (Fe^{3+}), and CO. This is the only reaction in the body that is known to produce CO. Most of the CO is excreted through the lungs, with the result that the CO content of expired air is a direct measure of the activity of heme oxidase in an individual.

7. A 9-month-old infant who suffered bouts of jaundice and was diagnosed with severe nonhemolytic icterus shortly after birth has died of kernicterus. During the periods of jaundice, serum analysis showed an increased concentration of indirect-reacting bilirubin with no detection of conjugated bilirubin. The premature death and early clinical findings in this infant suggest which of the following disorders?
A. acute intermittent porphyria
B. Crigler-Najjar syndrome, type 1
C. Dubin-Johnson syndrome
D. Gilbert syndrome
E. Rotor syndrome

Answer B: Jaundice is caused by an elevation in the circulating levels of bilirubin, the heme degradation by-product. Bilirubin, which is toxic, is rendered harmless by binding to albumin in the serum and by conjugation to glucuronate in the liver. Profound hyperbilirubinemia leads to encephalopathy (kernicterus), which results in death if untreated. The hepatic conjugation of bilirubin to glucuronate is catalyzed by bilirubin-UDP-glucuronyltransferase (UGT). The conjugated form of bilirubin is less toxic due to its increased solubility. Hyperbilirubinemia can be of 2 types, unconjugated or conjugated. Defects in UGT will lead to unconjugated hyperbilirubinemia. The deficiency of UGT in Crigler-Najjar syndrome type I is complete (due to loss of coding exons in the UGT gene) and as a consequence affected individuals will die from the profound kernicterus.

8. An 18-month-old boy was referred to the pediatrics clinic because of persistent anemia and associated failure to thrive. Laboratory analysis confirmed a microcytic anemia and revealed blood lead levels of 50 mg/dL (2 times normal levels) and high levels of coproporphyrinogen III in the urine. The child was put on chelation therapy and recovered uneventfully. The cause of the child's difficulty was most likely due to the effects of the lead. The findings in this patient most closely reflect lead inhibition of which of the following enzymes of heme biosynthesis?
A. δ-aminolevulinic acid (ALA) dehydratase
B. ferrochelatase
C. porphobilinogen (PBG) deaminase
D. proporphyrinogen III cosynthase
E. uroporphyrinogen decarboxylase

Answer B: Three enzymes of the heme biosynthesis pathway are targets of the toxic effects of lead.

These include ferrochelatase, ALA dehydratase, and ALA synthase. Ferrochelatase sensitivity to lead is the greatest of the 3 and thus the most significant in lead poisoning. The ability to distinguish between inhibition of ferrochelatase and ALA dehydratase is the fact that high levels of coproporphyrinogen III were found in the urine. Since this heme biosynthetic intermediate is downstream of the ALA dehydratase catalyzed reaction, inhibition of this enzyme would not result in the observed urine analysis result.

9. Which of the following represents the enzyme of porphyrin biosynthesis whose activity is negatively affected by hemin?

A. δ-aminolevulinic acid dehydratase (ALA dehydratase)
B. δ-aminolevulinic acid synthase (ALA synthase)
C. porphobilinogen deaminase (PBG deaminase)
D. porphobilinogen synthase
E. protoporphyrinogen IX oxidase

Answer B: The enzyme ALA synthase is the rate-limiting enzyme of heme biosynthesis. In hepatocytes, heme is required for incorporation into the cytochromes, in particular, the P450 class of cytochromes that are important for detoxification. In addition, numerous cytochromes of the oxidative-phosphorylation pathway contain heme. The Fe^{3+} oxidation product of heme is termed hemin. Hemin acts as a feedback inhibitor on ALA synthase. Hemin also inhibits transport of ALA synthase from the cytosol (its site of synthesis) into the mitochondria (its site of action), as well as represses synthesis of the enzyme.

10. An elderly homeless woman is brought to the hospital with yellowish color of her skin. From her somewhat incoherent story, it can be determined that she has consumed substantial amounts of alcohol over the past 3 decades. The physician made the diagnosis of alcoholic liver cirrhosis, associated with extensive liver fibrosis. Which of the following changes in plasma and urinary levels of bilirubin are most likely?

	Unconjugated bilirubin in plasma	Conjugated bilirubin in plasma	Conjugated bilirubin in urine
A.	decrease	decrease	decrease
B.	decrease	no change or increase	increase
C.	increase	decrease	increase
D.	increase	no change	increase
E.	no change or increase	increase	increase

Answer E: Jaundice occurs from buildup of bilirubin metabolites, which are products of hemoglobin degradation. During degradation, first unconjugated bilirubin is generated, which is then taken up from the plasma by the liver. The liver conjugates bilirubin with glucuronic acid and releases it via bile into the GI tract. Excessive and long-term alcohol consumption damages hepatocytes and leads to increased total bilirubin, mostly conjugated, in plasma. Although the mechanism is not fully defined, the increase in conjugated plasma bilirubin might be due to release from damaged hepatocytes, reduced disposition within hepatocytes, and reduced secretion from hepatocytes. It is also possible that the liver damage resulted in obstruction of bile flow, which leads to a backup of largely conjugated bilirubin in the blood stream. Conjugated bilirubin is eventually removed by the kidneys and results in increased conjugated bilirubin in urine. Alcoholism might also lead to an increase in unconjugated plasma bilirubin, in the case that the ability of hepatocytes to remove unconjugated bilirubin from plasma is grossly impaired. As with all chronic diseases, alcoholism may present with a wide spectrum of symptoms.

11. A 37-year-old woman visits her primary care physician after developing jaundice and scleral icterus. She is diagnosed with paroxysmal nocturnal hemoglobinuria. Which of the following metabolites would you expect to be increased in her urine?

A. bile
B. conjugated bilirubin
C. stercobilin
D. unconjugated bilirubin
E. urobilinogen

Answer E: Paroxysmal nocturnal hemoglobinuria is a hemolytic anemia in which an acquired cell membrane defect increases red blood cell susceptibility to lysis by endogenous complement. Intravascular hemolysis overwhelms hepatic enzyme conjugation capability and leads to an increase in unconjugated bilirubin (water-insoluble) in serum. The liver enzyme glucuronyl transferase converts unconjugated bilirubin into conjugated bilirubin (now water-soluble), which is then excreted by hepatocytes into the bile. After secretion of bile into the intestine, ileal and colonic bacteria convert conjugated bilirubin into urobilinogen. A fraction of urobilinogen is oxidized to stercobilin and directly excreted in feces (and hence, would not be a urinary metabolite). The remaining urobilinogen is reabsorbed from the intestine and reenters the portal circulation where a portion is taken up by the liver and reexcreted into bile, while the rest bypasses the liver and is excreted by the kidney. Therefore, in hemolytic anemias, increased liver excretion of conjugated bilirubin will lead to an increase in urinary urobilinogen levels. Note that this is in contrast to biliary tract obstruction in which failure of conjugated bilirubin to enter the intestine would lead to decreased levels of both fecal and urinary urobilinogen.

12. A 20-year-old woman admits herself to the emergency room with a yellow discoloration of the whites of her eyes. She says that she does not drink and that she has not experienced any changes in her stool. Her liver enzyme profile and direct serum bilirubin levels are normal, while total bilirubin is elevated. What is the most likely cause for her jaundice?
A. defect in hepatocytes
B. defect in Kupffer cells
C. gallstones
D. hemolysis
E. tumor obstructing bile duct

Answer D: Rupture of large numbers of red blood cells can result in jaundice in the absence of any liver disease. The capacity of the liver to clear released heme metabolites such as bilirubin is temporarily exceeded. Since the liver will not perform its normal function to conjugate bilirubin before excretion in bile and urine, unconjugated bilirubin backs up in serum. This is the reason for the increase in total bilirubin, while conjugated bilirubin, also called direct bilirubin, is not affected.

13. You are attending to a 47-year-old male patient who complains of chronic fatigue and persistent abdominal discomfort. Examination of the patient shows mildly icteric sclera and blood work indicates that serum bilirubin levels are 3 mg/dL. The bilirubin is predominantly unconjugated. The signs and symptoms in this patient are most likely due to which of the following disorders?
A. acute intermittent porphyria
B. Crigler-Najjar syndrome, type 1
C. Dubin-Johnson syndrome
D. Gilbert syndrome
E. Rotor syndrome

Answer D: Gilbert syndrome is characterized by mild, chronic unconjugated hyperbilirubinemia. Almost all afflicted individuals have a degree of icteric discoloration in the eyes typical of jaundice. Serum bilirubin levels in Gilbert syndrome patients are usually less than 3 mg/dL. Many patients manifest with fatigue and abdominal discomfort. Presentation of Gilbert syndrome symptoms occurs more frequently in men than in women because the production of bilirubin is higher in men.

14. You are treating a 5-day-old infant who is suffering from severe jaundice with serum indirect bilirubin levels of 21 mg/dL. Given the age of onset and the severity of the hyperbilirubinemia in this infant, which of the following would represent the most likely diagnosis?
A. acute intermittent porphyria
B. Crigler-Najjar syndrome, type 1
C. Dubin-Johnson syndrome
D. Gilbert syndrome
E. Rotor syndrome

Answer B: There are 2 forms of Crigler-Najjar syndrome: type I results from mutations in the bilirubin-UDP-glucuronyltransferase gene that result in complete loss of enzyme activity, whereas type II is the result of mutations that cause incomplete loss of enzyme activity. In patients with very high levels of indirect-reacting (unconjugated) bilirubin in the plasma, but with normal liver function tests, Crigler-Najjar syndrome type I is indicated. Almost all afflicted infants manifest with severe nonhemolytic icterus within the first few days of life.

15. A 35-year-old male patient goes to the ER because he is troubled by his chronic fatigue and persistent abdominal discomfort. Additional signs in this patient are mildly icteric sclera. The ER attending calls for blood workup for bilirubin which shows the predominantly unconjugated form at a level of 2 mg/dL. The physician suspects the patient has Gilbert syndrome. Which of the following enzymes would be expected to be found at reduced levels if this is the correct diagnosis?
A. δ-aminolevulinic acid synthase (ALA synthase)
B. ferrochelatase
C. heme oxygenase
D. porphobilinogen deaminase (PBG deaminase)
E. UDP-glucuronyltransferase

Answer E: Gilbert syndrome is characterized by mild, chronic unconjugated hyperbilirubinemia. The disorder results from mutations in the TATA-box of the promoter region upstream of exon 1 in the *UGT* gene which results in reduced levels of expression of a normal bilirubin UDP-glucuronyltransferase enzyme. The normal sequence of the UGT1A TATA-box is $A(TA)_6TAA$, whereas in Gilbert syndrome individuals it is $A(TA)_7TAA$. Almost all afflicted individuals have a degree of icteric discoloration in the eyes typical of jaundice. Serum bilirubin levels in Gilbert syndrome patients are usually less than 3 mg/dL. Many patients manifest with fatigue and abdominal discomfort. Presentation of Gilbert syndrome symptoms occurs more frequently in men than in women because the production of bilirubin is higher in men.

16. Which of the following represents the most common form of hepatic porphyria?

A. acute intermittent porphyria
B. ALA dehydratase–deficient porphyria
C. hereditary coproporphyria
D. porphyria cutanea tarda type I
E. variegate porphyria

Answer A: The most commonly occurring hepatic porphyria is acute intermittent porphyria, which is caused by a defect in porphobilinogen deaminase.

17. A 23-year-old man is seen by his physician complaining of weakness, abdominal pain, nausea, and hair loss. Laboratory studies indicate hypochromic and microcytic anemia and iron overload. Histological examination of the patients' blood shows iron deposits around perinuclear mitochondria. Which of the following is the correct diagnosis for this patient?

A. acute intermittent porphyria
B. erythropoietic porphyria
C. porphyria cutanea tarda type I
D. variegate porphyria
E. X-linked sideroblastic anemia

Answer E: X-linked sideroblastic anemia (XLSA) is a disorder that results from deficiencies in the erythroid-specific form of δ-aminolevulinc acid synthase, ALAS2. As a result of defective ALAS2, activity iron accumulates in the erythroid marrow. People with X-linked sideroblastic anemia have mature red blood cells that are smaller than normal (microcytic) and appear pale (hypochromic) because of the shortage of hemoglobin which also results in iron accumulation in the cells. The excess iron deposits as nonferritin iron in the mitochondria that surround the nuclei. These deposits give the cells a distinctive pathologic appearance referred to as ring sideroblasts.

18. A 7-year-old boy is being examined to determine the cause of his severe skin blistering upon mild exposure to the sun. His parents also note that when he doesn't flush the toilet after urinating, his urine turns a very dark reddish-orange. Physical examination shows the child has darkly stained teeth and fine hairs over his entire face, arms, and legs. Blood and urine studies show high levels of uroporphyrinogen I in both and high coproporphyrinogen I in the blood. Which of the following most likely explains the signs and symptoms in the child?

A. defective bilirubin UDP-glucuronyltransferase
B. deficiency in ALA synthase
C. deficiency in uroporphyrinogen III synthase
D. enhanced activity of PBG deaminase
E. lead-induced inhibition of ALA dehydratase

Answer C: A deficiency in uroporphyrinogen synthase III (the fourth enzyme of heme synthesis) results in the accumulation of its substrate, hydroxymethylbilane. Hydroxymethylbilane can nonenzymatically cyclize forming uroporphyrinogen I and coproporphyrinogen I. These heme biosynthetic by-products turn the urine red to reddish-orange and when deposited in the teeth turn them yellow to reddish brown. Accumulation of these by-products in the skin renders it extremely sensitive to sunlight causing ulceration and disfiguring scars. Increased hair growth (hypertrichosis) is also a symptom of the porphryias leading to appearance of fine hairs over the entire face and on the extremities.

19. Hemin is heme with oxidized ferric (Fe^{3+}) iron. This compound is known to interfere with the synthesis of the porphyrins and heme. Which of the following enzymes is inhibited by the presence of hemin?

A. ALA dehydratase
B. ALA synthase
C. ferrochelatase
D. PBG deaminase
E. uroporphyrinogen III synthase

Answer B: The rate-limiting step in hepatic heme biosynthesis occurs at the ALA synthase catalyzed step, which is the committed step in heme synthesis. The Fe^{3+} oxidation product of heme is hemin which acts as a feedback inhibitor on ALA synthase. Hemin also inhibits transport of ALA synthase from the cytosol into the mitochondria (its site of action) as well as represses synthesis of the enzyme.

20. A 28-year-old pregnant woman is concerned about the yellowing of her eyes and skin and goes to see her obstetrician. Blood work shows mildly elevated levels of direct-reacting bilirubin. Analysis of her urine shows significant amounts of coproporphyrin I. Which of the following disorders most likely explains the signs and symptoms in this patient?

A. acute intermittent porphyria
B. Crigler-Najjar syndrome, type 1
C. Dubin-Johnson syndrome
D. Gilbert syndrome
E. Rotor syndrome

Answer C: Dubin-Johnson syndrome is inherited as an autosomal recessive disorder characterized by mild, predominantly conjugated hyperbilirubinemia. The syndrome results from mutations in the bile canalicular multispecific organic anion transporter (*CMOAT*). The *CMOAT* gene is also referred to as the ATP-binding cassette, subfamily C, member 2 gene (*ABCC2*), and the multidrug resistance-associated protein 2 gene (*MRP2*). This transporter is involved in the excretion of many nonbile organic anions by an ATP-requiring process.

The defect-causing Dubin-Johnson syndrome leads to an abnormality in porphyrin metabolism such that more than 80% of the urinary compound from this pathway is coproporphyrin I, whereas in a normal individual it is usually less than 35%. Jaundice is usually the only physical symptom detected in this disease. Women may exhibit overt symptoms for the first time when taking oral contraceptives or when pregnant.

21. A 2-year-old boy is brought to the physician because he developed blistering sunburn after a 15-miute exposure. His parents say that he has always burned easily. Examination shows photophobia, anemia, and splenomegaly. The urine stains in his diaper are pink to dark brown. The most likely cause of these symptoms is a defect in which of the following biosynthetic pathways?

A. cholesterol
B. ganglioside
C. glycogen
D. porphyrin
E. ubiquinone

Answer D: The porphyrias constitute a family of disorders resulting from deficiencies in the various enzymes of heme biosynthesis which is also called the porphyrin pathway. The porphyrias lead to excretion of heme biosynthetic by-products that turn the urine red and when deposited in the teeth turn them reddish brown. Accumulation of these by-products in the skin renders it extremely sensitive to sunlight causing ulceration and disfiguring scars. Increased hair growth (hypertrichosis) is also a symptom of the porphryias leading to appearance of fine hairs over the entire face and on the extremities. This latter symptom lends to the description of "werewolf syndrome" in many porphyria patients.

22. The rate-limiting step in the biosynthesis of heme is catalyzed by the mitochondrial enzyme δ-aminolevulinic acid synthase (ALAS) from which of the following substrates?

A. acetyl-CoA and alanine
B. acetyl-CoA and glycine
C. adenine and glycine
D. succinyl-CoA and glycine
E. succinyl-CoA and GTP

Answer D: The first reaction in heme biosynthesis takes place in the mitochondrion and involves the condensation of 1 glycine and 1 succinyl-CoA by the pyridoxal phosphate-containing enzyme, δ-aminolevulinic acid synthase (ALAS).

23. Which of the following is a product of heme degradation?

A. hemin
B. porphobilinogen
C. protoporphyrin
D. urobilinogen
E. uroporphyrinogen III

Answer C: Urobilinogen is a colourless product of bilirubin catabolism formed in the intestines by bacterial action. It is one of the many bile pigments. Each of the other compounds represents intermediates in heme synthesis or heme derivatives.

24. A 3-day-old full-term male newborn is brought to the physician by his mother because of a 24-hour history of yellow skin. He appears healthy. Physical examination shows mild jaundice. Laboratory studies show a hemoglobin concentration of 17 g/dL and a total serum bilirubin concentration of 10 mg/dL, with an indirect component of 8 mg/dL. The jaundice resolves 5 days later. A deficiency of which of the following is the most likely cause of the jaundice in this patient?

A. erythrocyte glucose6-phosphate dehydrogenase activity
B. erythrocyte pyruvate kinase activity
C. glutathione synthetase activity
D. hepatic excretion of bilirubin
E. hepatic UDP-glucuronyltransferase activity

Answer E: Excess circulation and accumulation of bilirubin (hyperbilirubinemia) results in a yellow-orange discoloration of the tissues and is most easily visible as icteric (yellowish) discoloration in the sclera of the eyes. These symptoms are referred to as jaundice. There are several causes of jaundice including defects in the enzyme responsible for bilirubin conjugation to glucuronic acid, bilirubin UDP-glucuronyltransferase (bilirubin-UGT).

25. Bilirubin, the degradation product of heme, is only mildly water-soluble. The solubility of bilirubin in water is increased by forming a conjugate with which of the following?

A. bile acids
B. glucuronic acid
C. glycine
D. sialic acid
E. taurine

Answer B: In hepatocytes, bilirubin-UDP-glucuronyltransferase (bilirubin-UGT) adds 2 equivalents of glucuronic acid to bilirubin to produce the more water-soluble, bilirubin diglucuronide derivative. The increased water solubility of the tetrapyrrole facilitates its excretion with the remainder of the bile as the bile pigments.

Checklist

✓ Heme-containing proteins include hemoglobin, cytochromes of the electron transport chain, and the cytochrome P450 enzymes. Heme is composed of iron and the tetrapyrrole compound protoporphyrin IX.

✓ Protoporphyrin IX is synthesized via the porphyrin biosynthetic pathway that takes place in the mitochondria and the cytosol utilizing glycine and succinyl-CoA. The initial reaction is catalyzed by the rate-limiting and highly regulated enzyme δ-aminolevulinic acid synthase (ALAS).

✓ Iron is inserted into protoporphyrin IX by ferrochelatase.

✓ Defects in enzymes of porphyrin synthesis result in a family of disorders called the porphyrias. The porphyrias can be divided into erythroid and hepatic forms dependent upon the tissue most affected by the deficiency. Common symptoms of the porphyrias are photosensitivity and variable levels of neurological deficit.

✓ The major site of heme utilization is in erythrocytes. Erythrocytes are in continual flux, dying after approximately 120 days in the circulation. The turnover of erythrocytes creates a significant demand for the degradation of the heme in hemoglobin. Heme degradation occurs primarily in the liver and is initiated via the action of heme oxygenase, the only enzyme in the body to produce carbon monoxide.

✓ The by-product of heme catabolism is bilirubin. Bilirubin is insoluble in the aqueous environment so the liver conjugates it to glucuronic acid to increase its solubility. This reaction is catalyzed by bilirubin DP-glucuronyltransferase.

✓ Elevated levels of bilirubin in the blood (hyperbilirubinemia) and tissues is the cause of jaundice, characterized by yellowing skin and sclera of the eyes. Conjugated hyperbilirubinemias are not as toxic as the unconjugated hyperbilirubinemias due to its increased solubility. Excessive hyperbilirubinemia, especially in the neonate, can lead to the potential for severe neurological impairment; this is referred to as kernicterus (bilirubin encephalopathy).

✓ There are numerous causes of hyperbilirubinemia including anemias and hepatic dysfunction. Several hyperbilirubinemias are due to inherited defects in bilirubin metabolism and include Crigler-Najjar syndrome, Gilbert syndrome, Dubin-Johnson syndrome, and Rotor syndrome.

CHAPTER 34 Nitrogen: Metabolic Integration

CHAPTER OUTLINE

High-Yield Terms

Ischemia: refers to a condition caused by restricted blood flow to a tissue, resulting in a shortage of oxygen and glucose needed for continued metabolism

Hypoxia: a condition where a tissue, or the entire body, is restricted or deprived of the flow of oxygen

Pasteur effect: strictly speaking, this refers to the inhibition of bacterial fermentation by oxygen; with respect to eukaryotic metabolism it refers to an increased rate of glycolysis in response to hypoxia

Anorexigenic: causing a suppression of appetite

Orexigenic: causing an increase in appetite

Major Organ Integration of Metabolism

All tissues of the body carry out metabolic processes for survival and growth but not all of the major metabolic pathways are operational at the same time, nor at the same level in all tissues. Changes in nutritional, hormonal, physiological, and pathological status lead to alterations in metabolism in each tissue. In addition, and critical to an understanding of *metabolic integration*, is that changes in metabolic function in one tissue can, and often do, have potentially profound impacts on the metabolic processes of other tissues.

In the context of overall tissue integration, it is most important to demonstrate how the metabolic processes of the brain, liver, adipose tissue, gastrointestinal tract, and skeletal muscle are interconnected. Within the context of organ integration of metabolism, the pathways that are involved include glycogen synthesis (glycogenesis) and breakdown (glycogenolysis), glycolysis, gluconeogenesis, TCA cycle, lipid synthesis (lipogenesis) and breakdown (lipolysis), lipid oxidation, ketogenesis, amino acid catabolism, urea cycle, protein synthesis, and proteolysis. Each of these processes is most often discussed, as in this text, as isolated metabolic pathways. However, in order to fully appreciate how normal and abnormal physiology and pathology affect the status of the human organism, it is imperative to fully understand their interconnection.

With respect to metabolic integration, the best way to gain an understanding of the processes involved is to examine how these major metabolic pathways respond to everyday feeding and then fasting between meals. Prolonged absence of food results in death within a very short period of time. This fact explains why humans have evolved a complex system of regulatory circuits that were evolutionarily designed to stimulate our desire to seek and consume food. These circuits involve both neuroendocrine (Chapters 43 and 44) and endocrine (Chapters 46, 49, and 50) functions throughout the body. These regulatory pathways allow humans to survive periods of fasting by stimulating energy storage after meal intake and precisely controlling the release of this energy when needed. Unfortunately, humans have not evolved with an equally exquisite means to control the storage of energy. Caloric excess ultimately results in obesity (Chapter 45) and its many associated pathologies including diabetes (Chapter 47), cardiovascular disease (Chapter 48), and cancer (Chapter 52).

Although overall metabolic regulation across multiple tissues as a result of various physiological states involves many different factors (hormones, neuroendocrine factors, enzymes, etc), the most important global regulator is the enzyme, AMP-regulated protein kinase (AMPK). AMPK functions within all tissues to control the level of energy (ATP) consumption and production.

The Master Metabolic Integrator: AMPK

AMPK was first discovered as an activity that inhibited acetyl-CoA carboxylase (ACC) and HMG-CoA reductase (HMGR) and whose activity was induced by increasing AMP concentration. AMPK induces a cascade of events within cells in response to the ever-changing energy charge of the cell. The role of AMPK in regulating cellular energy charge places this enzyme at a central control point in maintaining energy homeostasis. The significance of AMPK activity to overall metabolic integration is that it can also be regulated by physiological stimuli (including nutrients and hormones), independent of the energy charge of the cell.

Once activated, AMPK-mediated phosphorylation events switch cells from active ATP consumption (eg, fatty acid and cholesterol biosynthesis) to active ATP production (eg, fatty acid and glucose oxidation). These events are rapidly initiated and are referred to as short-term regulatory processes. The activation of AMPK also exerts long-term effects at the level of both gene expression and protein synthesis. Other important activities attributable to AMPK are regulation of insulin synthesis and secretion in pancreatic β-cells and modulation of hypothalamic functions involved in the regulation of satiety. How these latter 2 functions impact obesity and diabetes are discussed in Chapters 45 and 46, respectively.

Structure of AMPK

Mammalian AMPK is a trimeric enzyme composed of a catalytic α-subunit and the noncatalytic β- and γ-subunits. There are 2 genes encoding isoforms of both the a- and β-subunits (α_1, α_2, β_1, and β_2) and 3 genes encoding isoforms of the γ-subunit (γ_1-γ_3) allowing for the formation of 12 different isoforms of AMPK. The α_2-isoform is the subunit of AMPK found predominantly within skeletal and cardiac muscle, whereas, approximately equal distribution of both the α_1 and α_2 isoforms are present in hepatic AMPK. Within pancreatic islet β-cells, the α_1 isoform predominates, which is also the case for white adipose tissue (WAT). The expression of specific γ-subunits also exhibits tissue specificity with the γ_3-subunit found almost exclusively in glycolytic skeletal muscle.

The *N*-terminal half of the α-subunits contains a typical serine/threonine kinase catalytic domain. Interaction with the β- and γ-subunits occurs via the *C*-terminal half of the α-subunits. The core of the β-subunits have a

High-Yield Concept

Mutations in nucleotide-binding domains of the γ_2-subunit (gene symbol *PRKAG2*) are associated with Wolff-Parkinson-White syndrome and familial hypertrophic cardiomyopathy. An additional inherited disorder associated with mutations in the *PRKAG2* gene is a severe cardiac condition called lethal congenital glycogen storage disease of the heart.

glycogen-binding domain (GBD) and the resulting close proximity of AMPK to cellular glycogen stores allows it to rapidly effect changes in glycogen metabolism in response to changes in metabolic demands. The γ-subunits of AMPK bind both regulatory AMP and catalytic ATP and their binding occurs in a mutually exclusive manner. Binding of ATP keeps the activity of AMPK low and when AMP levels rise, the exchange of AMP for ATP results in a 5-fold increase in kinase activity.

Regulation of AMPK

In the presence of AMP, the activity of AMPK is increased approximately 5-fold. However, more importantly is the role of AMP in regulating the level of phosphorylation of AMPK. An increased AMP:ATP ratio leads to a conformational change in the γ-subunit, leading to increased phosphorylation and decreased dephosphorylation of AMPK. The regulatory phosphorylation sites of AMPK reside in the α-subunit. The phosphorylation of AMPK results in activation by at least 100-fold. AMPK is phosphorylated by at least 3 different upstream AMPK kinases (AMPKKs). The activity of AMPK is also regulated by allosteric effectors and by the actions of several hormones, in particular those secreted by adipose tissue (eg, leptin and adiponectin).

As the name implies, AMPK is also regulated by AMP. The effects of AMP are 2-fold: a direct allosteric activation and making AMPK a poorer substrate for dephosphorylation. Because AMP affects both the rate of AMPK phosphorylation in the positive direction and dephosphorylation in the negative direction, the cascade is ultrasensitive. This means that a very small rise in AMP levels can induce a dramatic increase in the activity of AMPK. The activity of adenylate kinase, catalyzing 2ADP to ATP and AMP, ensures that AMPK is highly sensitive to small changes in the intracellular ATP:ADP ratio.

The kinase, LKB1 (also called serine-threonine kinase 11, STK11), which is encoded by the Peutz-Jeghers syndrome tumor suppressor gene (see Chapter 52), is required for activation of AMPK in response to stress. The active LKB1 kinase is actually a complex of 3 proteins: LKB1, Ste20-related adaptor (STRAD), and mouse protein 25 (MO25). LKB1 is widely expressed and is the primary AMPK-regulating kinase.

Calcium-calmodulin–dependent kinase kinase-β (CaMKK-β) phosphorylates and activates AMPK in response to increased intracellular calcium. The distribution of CaMKK-β expression is primarily in the brain. An increased release of intracellular stores of Ca^{2+} occurs simultaneously with a subsequent demand for ATP. Activation of AMPK, in response to Ca^{2+} fluxes, thus provides a mechanism for cells to anticipate the increased demand for ATP.

Targets of AMPK

The signaling cascades initiated by the activation of AMPK exert effects on glucose and lipid metabolism, gene expression, and protein synthesis. These effects are most important for regulating integrative metabolism in the liver, skeletal muscle, heart, adipose tissue, and pancreas (Figure 34-1).

The uptake, by skeletal muscle, accounts for greater than 70% of the glucose removal from the serum in humans. Therefore, this process is extremely important for overall glucose homeostasis. An important fact related to skeletal muscle glucose uptake is that this process is markedly impaired in individuals with Type 2 diabetes. The uptake of glucose increases dramatically in response to stress (such as ischemia) and exercise and is stimulated by insulin-induced recruitment of glucose transporters to the plasma membrane, primarily GLUT4. Insulin-independent recruitment of GLUT4 also occurs in skeletal muscle in response to contraction (exercise). The ability of AMPK to stimulate GLUT4 translocation to the plasma membrane in skeletal muscle occurs via a mechanism distinct from that stimulated by insulin since together, insulin and AMPK effects are additive. AMPK activation also results in increased expression of the *GLUT4* gene. Increased glucose uptake will result in an increase in glycolysis and ATP production.

Under ischemic/hypoxic conditions in the heart, the activation of AMPK leads to the phosphorylation and activation of the kinase activity of PFK-2 (6-phosphofructo-2-kinase). The activation of PFK-2 kinase activity results in increased production of fructose-2,6-bisphosphate (F2,6BP), which in turn potently stimulates PFK-1 activity and increased glycolysis. In liver, the

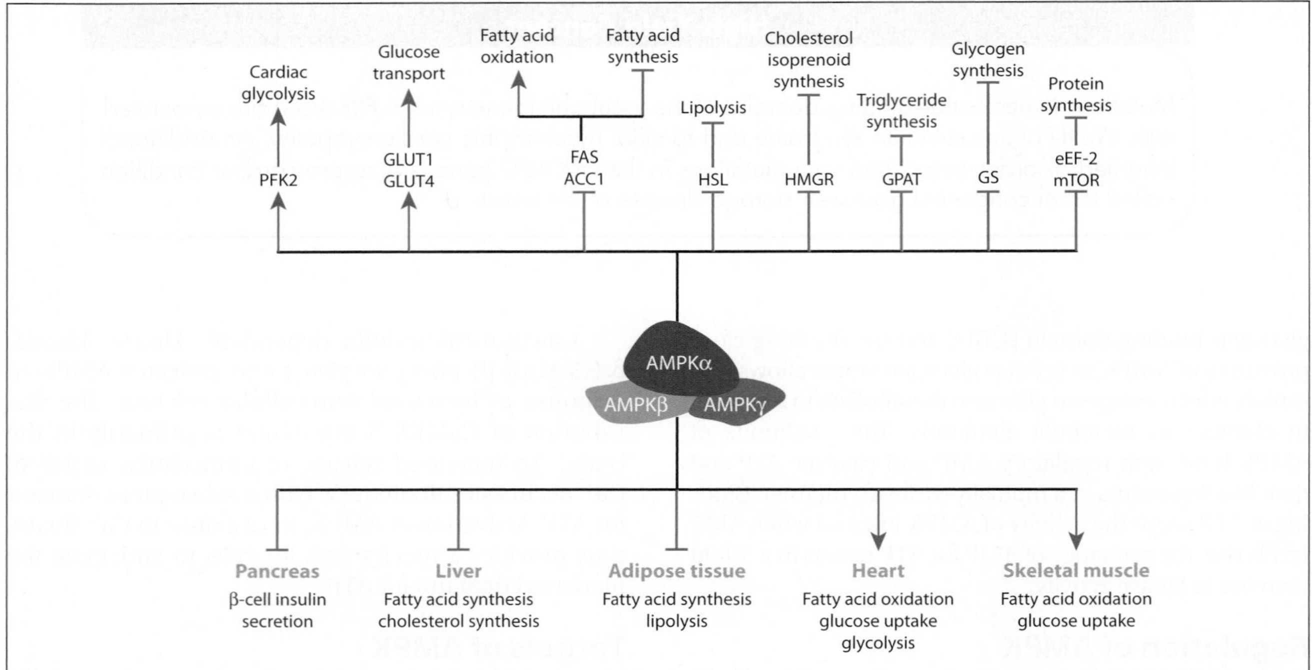

FIGURE 34-1: Demonstration of the central role of AMPK in the regulation of metabolism in response to events such as nutrient- or exercise-induced stress. Several of the known physiologic targets for AMPK are included and several pathways as well whose flux is affected by AMPK activation. Arrows indicate positive effects of AMPK, whereas, T-lines indicate inhibitory effects. (See text for definition of enzyme abbreviations.)

PKA-mediated phosphorylation of PFK-2 results in conversion of the enzyme from a kinase to a phosphatase, opposite the effects exerted by AMPK in the heart. There are 4 isoforms of PFK-2 and neither the liver nor the skeletal muscle isoforms contain the AMPK phosphorylation sites that are found in cardiac PFK-2 (see Chapter 10).

Within skeletal and cardiac muscles, activation of AMPK leads to the phosphorylation and inhibition of both isoforms of acetyl-CoA carboxylase (ACC1 and ACC2). This inhibition results in a drop in the level of malonyl-CoA, which itself is an inhibitor of carnitine palmitoyltransferase I (CPTI). With a drop

High-Yield Concept

The ability to activate the kinase activity by phosphorylation of PFK-2 in cardiac tissue in response to ischemic conditions allows these cells to continue to have a source of ATP via anaerobic glycolysis. This phenomenon is recognized as the *Pasteur effect*: an increased rate of glycolysis in response to hypoxia.

High-Yield Concept

The activity of the inducible form of PFK-2 (iPFK2) is also regulated by AMPK like that of the cardiac isoform. Of pathological significance is the fact that iPFK2 is commonly expressed in many tumor cells and this may allow AMPK to play an important role in protecting tumor cells from hypoxic stress. Indeed, the techniques for depleting AMPK in tumor cells have shown that these cells become sensitized to nutritional stress upon loss of AMPK activity.

High-Yield Concept

When HSL is phosphorylated in response to the activation of PKA, it actively removes fatty acids from adipose tissue triglycerides. In contrast, phosphorylation of HSL by AMPK inhibits its activity. This inhibition may seem paradoxical since the release of stored fatty acids would seem necessary to promote the production of ATP via fatty acid oxidation. This paradigm can be explained if one considers that if the fatty acids that are released from triglycerides are not consumed, they will be recycled back into triglycerides at the expense of ATP consumption. The inhibition of HSL by AMPK is, therefore, likely to be a mechanism to ensure that the rate of fatty acid release does not exceed the rate at which they are utilized either by export or oxidation.

in the inhibition of CPTI, a concomitant increase in β-oxidation of fatty acids will occur within the mitochondria. An increase in fatty acid oxidation, like increases in glycolysis, will lead to increases in ATP production. In addition to ACC, AMPK has been shown to phosphorylate and thus regulate the activities of HMG-CoA reductase (HMGR); hormone-sensitive lipase (HSL); glycerol-3-phosphate acyltransferase (GPAT); malonyl-CoA decarboxylase (MCD); glycogen synthase (GS), and creatine kinase (CK). Therefore, the effects of AMPK activation are exerted on not only glucose and fatty acid metabolism but overall energy homeostasis, including glycogen metabolism, cholesterol metabolism, and phosphocreatine metabolism.

Additional cardiovascular effects exerted by activation of AMPK include phosphorylation and activation of endothelial nitric oxide synthase, eNOS, in cardiac endothelium. AMPK-mediated phosphorylation of eNOS leads to increased activity and consequent NO production and provides a link between metabolic stresses and cardiac function. In platelets, insulin action leads to an increase in eNOS activity as a result of AMPK activity. Activation of NO production in platelets leads to a decrease in thrombin-induced aggregation, thereby, limiting the procoagulant effects of platelet activation. The response of platelets to insulin function clearly indicates why disruption in insulin action is a major contributing factor in the development of the cardiovascular defects in the metabolic syndrome (see Chapter 48).

AMPK activity also leads to changes in the expression of numerous metabolic regulatory genes in the liver and adipose tissue, including the liver isoform of pyruvate kinase (L-PK), fatty acid synthase (FAS), and ACC. Activation of AMPK leads to a reduction in the levels of transcription factors, SREBP (see Chapter 26), and hepatocyte nuclear factor 4α, HNF-4α. Both of these transcription factors are key regulators of the expression of numerous lipogenic enzymes. Of clinical significance is that mutations in HNF-4α are responsible for maturity-onset diabetes of the young, MODY-1 (see Chapter 47).

AMPK activation, in response to hypoxia, exerts negative effects on rates of protein synthesis. Hepatic translation elongation factor 2 (eEF2) is a target for phosphorylation in response to AMPK activation. AMPK phosphorylates and activates the kinase that phosphorylates eEF2 (eEF2K), leading to inhibition of protein synthesis. Another indirect substrate for AMPK that plays a role in protein synthesis is the mammalian target of rapamycin, mTOR (see Chapter 37).

AMPK and Hypothalamic Functions

The activity of AMPK in the hypothalamus is critical in the control of appetite, food intake, and other neuroendocrine functions. The level of active AMPK in the hypothalamus rises during periods of fasting and then decreases in response to refeeding. Pharmacologic activation of hypothalamic AMPK, by the purine nucleotide intermediate AICAR (5-aminoimidazole-4-carboxamide ribotide), leads to increased appetite and a consequent increase in food consumption.

Within the hypothalamus, actions of leptin, GLP-1, and insulin (anorexigenic hormones) result in inhibition of AMPK activation, whereas, actions of adiponectin and ghrelin (orexigenic hormones) result in activation of AMPK activity. Of significance to the tissue-specific distribution of AMPK isoforms, as well as to the differing roles of AMPK in various tissues, the actions of leptin in adipose tissue and liver result in activation of AMPK, while in the heart leptin inhibits AMPK activation as in the hypothalamus. Detailed information on the effects of these peptides and hormones on hypothalamic function is covered in Chapter 44.

Relevance of AMPK to Type 2 Diabetes

Impairment in fuel metabolism occurs in obesity and this impairment is a leading pathogenic factor in the development of Type 2 diabetes. The insulin resistance

High-Yield Concept

Cells of the gut will see the highest doses of metformin and, therefore, they will experience the greatest level of inhibited complex I activity. This may explain the gastrointestinal side effects (nausea, diarrhea, and anorexia) associated with metformin that limit its utility in many patients.

associated with Type 2 diabetes is most profound at the level of skeletal muscle as this is the primary site of glucose and fatty acid utilization. Therefore, an understanding of how to activate AMPK in skeletal muscle would offer significant pharmacologic benefits in the treatment of Type 2 diabetes. As indicated earlier, it has already been shown that metformin and the thiazolidinedione drugs exert some of their effects via activation of AMPK. In the nonpharmacologic context, activation of AMPK occurs in response to exercise, an activity known to have significant benefit for Type 2 diabetics.

In skeletal muscle, AMPK phosphorylates the transcription coactivator, PGC1α (peroxisome proliferator-activated receptor-γ coactivator 1α), leading to increased mitochondrial biogenesis and fatty acid oxidation. In addition, AMPK-activated PGC1α results in increased GLUT4 presentation in skeletal muscle cell membranes resulting in increased glucose uptake.

In the liver, AMPK activity enhances fatty acid oxidation via activation of PGC1α in addition to the effects on enzyme activity described earlier. Simultaneously, hepatic cholesterol synthesis is inhibited by AMPK actions at the level of SREBP and HMGR. During fasting AMPK activation results in the inhibition of hepatic gluconeogenesis while simultaneously increasing fatty acid oxidation. The negative effect of AMPK on gluconeogenesis does not involve PGC1α regulation. When fasting, the pancreas releases glucagon which increases hepatic glycogenolysis and gluconeogenesis. The effects of glucagon, on hepatic gluconeogenesis, involve PGC1α and these effects are inhibited by AMPK activity. The effects of hepatic AMPK activation, therefore, override the inductive signals elicited through glucagon.

Several of the current therapies for the treatment of Type 2 diabetes-induced hyperglycemia involve effects on AMPK activity. The thiazolidinedione (TZD) class of drug functions via the activation of peroxisome proliferator-activated receptor γ, PPAR-γ, which is also a target for the action of AMPK. PPAR-γ is primarily expressed in adipose tissue. The TZDs stimulate the expression and release of the adipocyte hormone, adiponectin. Adiponectin stimulates glucose uptake and fatty acid oxidation in skeletal muscle. In addition, adiponectin stimulates fatty acid oxidation in liver while inhibiting expression of gluconeogenic enzymes in this tissue. These responses to adiponectin are exerted via activation of AMPK.

The most widely prescribed Type 2 diabetes drug is metformin. Metformin has a mild inhibitory effect on complex I of oxidative phosphorylation, has antioxidant properties, and activates both glucose 6-phosphate dehydrogenase (G6PDH) and AMPK. The activation of AMPK by metformin is likely related to the inhibitory effects of the drug on complex I of oxidative phosphorylation. This results in a reduction in ATP production and, therefore, an increase in the level of AMP and as a result activation of AMPK.

Energy Requirements and Reserves

The energy needs of any given individual can vary considerably from another due to age, sex, physiological status, and due to various disease states. However, in general, a normal adult of approximately 70 kg (155 lb) requires between 1600 and 2400 calories per day in order to carry out basic metabolic functions. As the level of exertion increases, so too, will the need for caloric intake. The energy reserves in a typical adult are found in the form of carbohydrate (glycogen), fat (triglycerides), and amino acids, primarily as skeletal muscle protein (Table 34-1). As indicated in Table 43-5, the energy contained in fat is on the order of 9 kcal/g and that contained in protein and carbohydrate is approximately 4 kcal/g. These reserves of energy are called upon during fasting and starvation and replenished following feeding. Because glucose can be oxidized for energy, even in the absence of oxygen, it is the most readily utilizable energy source of the body. Fatty acids are released between meals but at high rates only when glycogen reserves are depleted during prolonged fasting. Protein serves as a source of energy because the amino acids can be released and oxidized. It is important to appreciate, though, that protein energy is not readily available like that of glycogen and triglyceride and is, therefore, generally utilized only as a last resort during periods of protracted fasting and starvation.

The 2 major hormones that control the use and storage of energy are the pancreatic hormones, insulin,

TABLE 34-1: Energy Reserves of a Typical 70-kg Human

Fuel Type	Tissue	Fuel Amount (g)	Fuel Amount (kcal)
Glycogen	Skeletal muscle	120	480
Glycogen	Liver	70	280
Glucose	Body fluids	20	80
Fat	Adipose tissue	15,000	135,000
Protein	Skeletal muscle	6,000	24,000

and glucagon. These 2 hormones serve as counter-regulatory hormones in that they oppose the primary actions of each other. Insulin is released following food intake to prepare the organs to absorb, utilize, and store the energy of the food. Conversely, glucagon is released during fasting in response to falling levels of blood glucose. Glucose levels also fall in stress situations, which also result in release of glucagon. Many other peptide and steroid hormones influence overall energy homeostasis through their actions on various tissues and within the central nervous system. Adipose tissue hormones, such as leptin and adiponectin have important metabolic regulatory functions particularly in the liver and skeletal muscle (see Chapter 45). The adrenal medullary hormones, epinephrine and norepinephrine, and the adrenal cortical steroid hormone, cortisol, each can control energy mobilization in response to various physiological states and due to different types of stress. Gut hormones and neuroendocrine peptides, primarily hypothalamic peptides, control behaviors related to energy homeostasis such as appetite and feeding (see Chapter 44). These same hypothalamic neuropeptides also affect tissue metabolic processes to ensure adequate energy storage and release.

Organ Interrelationships in Well-Fed State

The consumption of food triggers a series of global changes in the disposition of the carbon and nitrogen atoms contained in the carbohydrates, fats, and proteins present in the digested material. The redistribution is determined by the current physiological state and controlled by both endocrine and neuroendocrine functions throughout the body (Figure 34-2). Food intake allows for the replenishment of energy (ATP) used during the period between meals and for the storage of excess carbon to be accessed during the next fast.

The primary hormonal response to the intake of food is the release of insulin from the pancreas. The action of insulin, on its primary target tissues, skeletal muscle, and adipose tissue, is to ensure that glucose is readily absorbed from the blood and that the enzymes necessary for utilization and storage of the incoming carbon atoms (carbohydrates, fats, amino acids) are fully active.

Following consumption of food, the stomach and intestines digest the complex polymeric molecules into smaller monomeric units so that fatty acids, monoglycerides, amino acids, and monosaccharides can be absorbed. These processes are discussed in detail in Chapter 43. Within the intestines, glucose, amino acids, and fats can be utilized for the energy needs of this tissue. The primary source of carbon for ATP generation in the intestines is the absorbed amino acids.

Free fatty acids (FFAs) are not transported to the portal circulation from the intestines. They are first incorporated into triglycerides and phospholipids and then packaged into the lipoprotein particles called chylomicrons (see Chapter 28) and delivered to the lymphatic system. The intestinal lymphatics feed into the thoracic duct and then into the left subclavian vein for distribution throughout the body. The action of lipoprotein lipase (LPL) on endothelial cells of the vasculature allows dietary fatty acids to be absorbed by the tissues. Skeletal and cardiac muscle prefer fatty acid oxidation as a means to acquire ATP energy. Adipose tissue will incorporate the fatty acids into triglycerides for storage and future release during periods of fasting and starvation.

The primary dietary monosaccharides are glucose, fructose, and galactose. When delivered to the portal circulation, the high K_m of hepatic glucokinase ensures that the vast majority of the glucose passes through this organ to be utilized by other tissues. The brain is almost completely dependent on glucose oxidation for energy, so delivery of this carbohydrate to the brain is especially important during refeeding. In addition, erythrocytes and kidney medullary cells are absolutely dependent upon glucose oxidation for ATP production. Insulin released in response to food intake stimulates the uptake of glucose by skeletal muscle and adipose tissue. Within muscle cells, the glucose is stored as

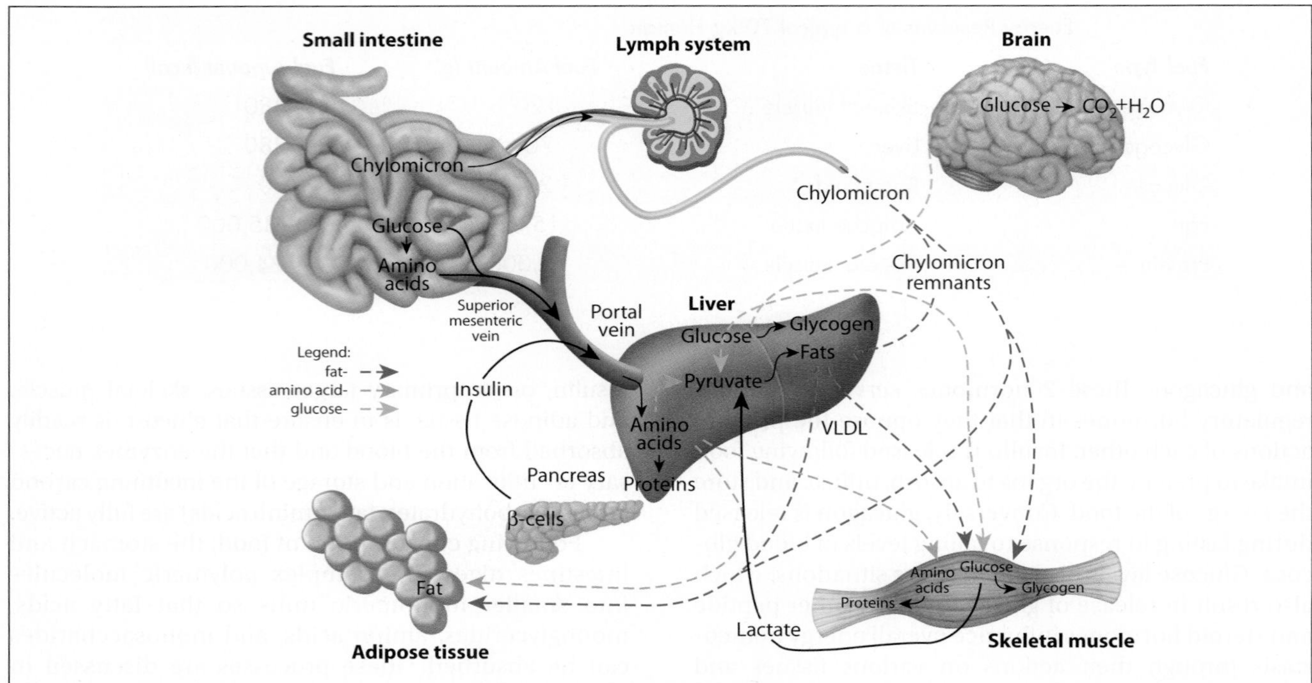

FIGURE 34-2: Interrelationships of major organs during well-fed state. Following the consumption of food, the intestines deliver the dietary lipid to the body in the form of chylomicrons via the lymphatic system to the left subclavian vein. Dietary glucose and amino acids enter the circulation via the superior mesenteric vein to the portal vein that enters the liver. Food intake stimulates pancreatic secretion of insulin, which enters the portal vein and then the overall circulation of the body where it activates various processes in tissues such as adipose tissue and skeletal muscle. Dietary fatty acids and fatty acids from the liver (in VLDL) are taken up by numerous tissues, where they are oxidized and/or stored as triglycerides. In the well-fed state, insulin increases lipoprotein lipase (LPL) density on endothelial cells, promoting fatty acid uptake and GLUT4 density in adipose tissue and skeletal muscle, promoting glucose uptake. Reproduced with permission of themedicalbiochemistrypage, LLC.

glycogen or oxidized for ATP production. Some of the ATP is used to phosphorylate creatine, generating creatine phosphate that is a rapidly utilizable source of phosphate for skeletal muscle ATP generation. Adipose tissue carries out glycolysis for both ATP production as well as diversion of the glucose carbons into the glycerol backbone of triglycerides. This latter function results from glycolytic DHAP being converted to glycerol 3-phosphate via the action of glycerol-3-phosphate dehydrogenase. Given that adipocytes do not express glycerol kinase, the use of DHAP demonstrates the absolute requirement for glycolysis in adipose tissue for fat storage as triglycerides. As the level of glucose rises in the blood, the liver will begin to trap some for use and storage in this tissue through the increased activity of glucokinase. The release of insulin alters the metabolic processes of the liver so that the glucose is stored as glycogen or oxidized to pyruvate. The pyruvate can either be reduced to lactate or oxidized to acetyl-CoA. The resulting acetyl-CoA is then utilized for fatty acid and cholesterol synthesis or completely oxidized to CO_2 and water in the TCA cycle.

In the well-fed state, lactate produced by glycolysis in erythrocytes, skeletal muscle, and other tissues is taken up by the liver and oxidized to pyruvate. The pyruvate generated in this way experiences the same fate as hepatic glycolysis-derived pyruvate; complete oxidation or the resulting acetyl-CoA diverted to fat and cholesterol synthesis. Due to the hormonal states following feeding, high insulin and low glucagon, the liver is not actively carrying out gluconeogenesis, so little, if any, lactate is utilized in this latter pathway. Therefore, the Cori cycle is minimally active in the well-fed state.

Dietary amino acids delivered to the portal circulation generally pass through the liver as a consequence of the high K_m of amino acid catabolic enzymes. This ensures that dietary amino acid, particularly essential amino acids, can be acquired by peripheral tissue for oxidation and/or protein synthesis. When oxidized in the liver, or for that matter in other tissues, the waste nitrogen is incorporated into urea and excreted. Within the liver, as well as peripheral tissues, the K_m of the aminoacyl-tRNA synthetases are low, ensuring that protein synthesis is able to occur, especially in the well-fed state when the load of amino acids is high.

As chylomicrons move through the vasculature and are acted upon by LPL, they lose fatty acids and become chylomicron remnants. The remnants are taken up by the liver and degraded in lysosomes. The released fatty acids are re-esterified to glycerol 3-phosphate (derived from glycolysis) and the triglycerides are packaged into VLDL. The VLDLs are then released to the circulation where the action of LPL exerts the same effects on these lipoprotein particles as in the case of chylomicrons.

Organ Interrelationships During Fasting or Starvation

The primary, whole-body response to the periods between feeding occurs due to the shift in pancreatic hormone secretion. These changes in hormone release result primarily from falling serum glucose levels. As serum glucose levels drop, the rate of insulin secretion falls and the rate of glucagon secretion increases. The major responses of the tissues to glucagon occur at the level of adipose tissue and the liver, triggering release of energy and conversion of carbon into glucose. Although the kidneys and the small intestines can contribute to overall endogenous glucose production, the liver is the most important organ controlling blood glucose levels, particularly during periods of fasting and starvation (Figure 34-3).

Within the liver, lactate, pyruvate, and alanine provide the carbon atoms necessary for hepatic gluconeogenesis. Within the kidney and intestines, gluconeogenesis is fueled by the carbon atoms from glutamine and glutamate. Since the process of gluconeogenesis is energetically expensive, the liver requires an adequate source of oxidizable carbon to provide the necessary ATP. This energy comes in the form of fatty acids released from adipose tissue triglycerides in response to the actions of glucagon. Lactate that arrives in the liver from skeletal muscle, erythrocyte, and adrenal medulla glycolysis is oxidized to pyruvate and then diverted into glucose. This glucose is then delivered to

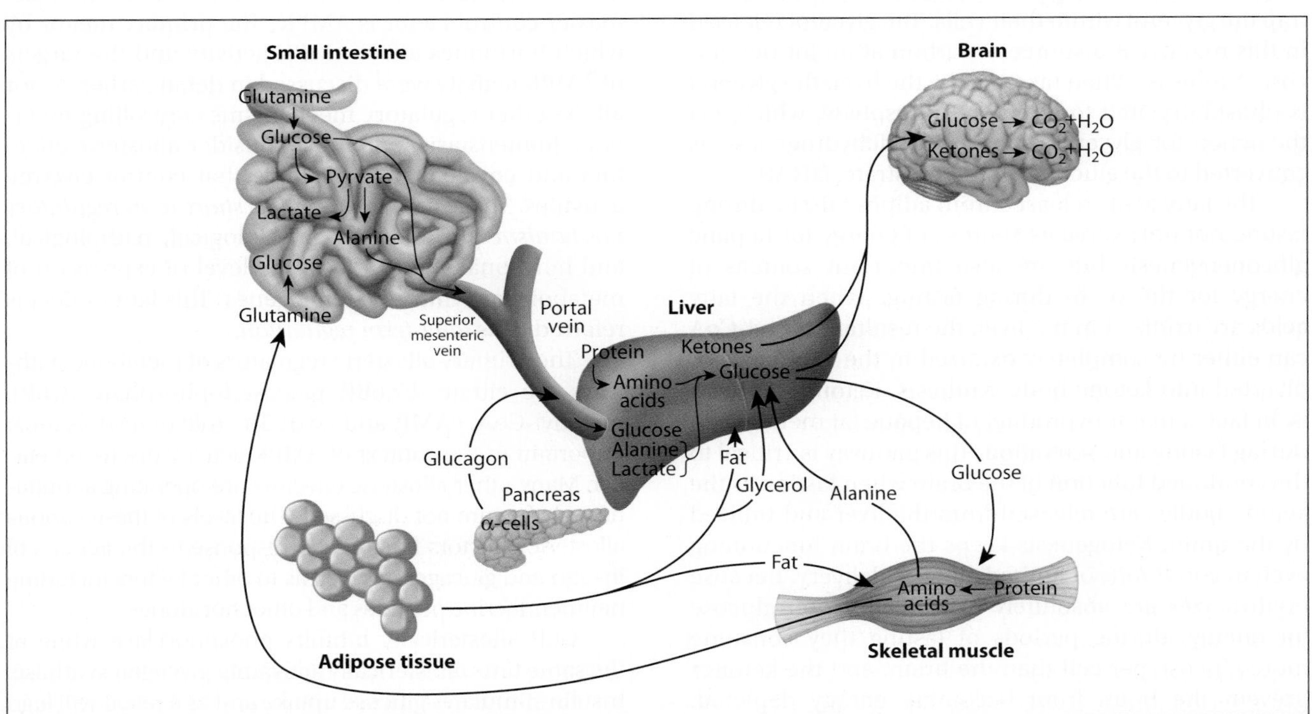

FIGURE 34-3: Interrelationships of major organs during fasting state. During fasting the blood glucose level falls, prompting the pancreas to secrete glucagon which stimulates the liver to undertake gluconeogenesis and glycogenolysis to provide glucose to the blood. Glucagon also stimulates adipose tissue to release fatty acids so that tissues such as the heart and skeletal muscles have adequate energy. The fatty acids released from adipose tissue are also oxidized by the liver to provide the energy necessary for gluconeogenesis. In addition, hepatic fatty acid oxidation provides the major source of acetyl-CoA for ketone synthesis, which is necessary to provide the brain with an energy source during periods of glucose restriction. In addition to gluconeogenesis in the liver, the kidneys and the duodenum carry out gluconeogenesis to contribute to endogenous glucose production during fasting. Reproduced with permission of themedicalbiochemistrypage, LLC.

the blood where these tissues can reoxidize the glucose, generating more lactate. This cycling of lactate and glucose carbons between the liver and peripheral tissues is referred to as the *Cori cycle*. During periods of fasting, skeletal muscle protein is degraded to release the amino acids so that they can be oxidized for ATP production. The waste nitrogen is transferred to pyruvate forming alanine that is then delivered to the liver via the blood. The alanine is deaminated and the nitrogen incorporated into urea for excretion. As a consequence, the levels of urea excretion can increase dramatically in fasting. The deaminated alanine is pyruvate, which is a substrate for gluconeogenesis. As for lactate, the glucose is then delivered back to peripheral tissues for oxidation. This cycling of alanine and glucose carbons between the liver and peripheral tissues is referred to as the *glucose-alanine cycle*. Because pyruvate and alanine carbons are derived from glucose and then diverted back into glucose, there is no net production of glucose via the Cori and glucose-alanine cycles.

When glucagon stimulates fatty acid release from adipose tissue triglycerides, the glycerol that is also released enters the blood. This is due to the fact that adipose tissue lacks glycerol kinase and thus cannot trap the glycerol within their cells. The glycerol released in this manner is a source of carbon atom for net glucose synthesis. When taken up by the liver, the glycerol is phosphorylated to glycerol 3-phosphate, which, via the action for glycerol 3-phosphate dehydrogenase, is converted to the gluconeogenic substrate, DHAP.

The fatty acids released from adipose tissue during fasting not only serve as sources of energy for hepatic gluconeogenesis but are also important sources of energy for the brain during fasting. When the fatty acids are oxidized in the liver, the resultant acetyl-CoA can either be completely oxidized in the TCA cycle or diverted into ketone body synthesis. Ketone synthesis is, in fact, a major byproduct of hepatic fat metabolism during fasting and starvation. This pathway is critical to the continued function of the brain when fasting as the ketone bodies are released from the liver and utilized by the brain. Ketogenesis keeps the brain functioning even in conditions of limited glucose delivery. Because erythrocytes are absolutely dependent upon glucose for energy, during periods of fasting they consume more glucose per cell than the brain, and the ketones prevent the brain from becoming energy depleted. Fatty acids released during fasting are also absorbed by skeletal and cardiac muscles to be used for ATP synthesis. Indeed, as indicated, these tissues prefer to oxidized fatty acids over carbohydrate, and this is true under all conditions excluding anaerobic metabolism.

In addition to serving as sources of energy for intestinal cells, both glucose and glutamine acquired from the diet (as well as from the arterial circulation) serve as important carbon skeletons for eventual hepatic gluconeogenesis, particularly during periods of fasting or when the liver is compromised in some way. Intestinal glycolysis converts glucose carbons into pyruvate, which can then be reduced to lactate or transaminated to alanine. Both enter the portal circulation for delivery into the liver. Dietary and arterial glutamine is deaminated to glutamate by glutaminase and the glutamate serves as the amino donor during pyruvate transamination by ALT. The resulting α-ketoglutarate enters the TCA cycle where eventually the OAA can be diverted into gluconeogenesis, yielding glucose for delivery into the portal circulation for supplying to the liver and importantly, the brain.

Controlling the Metabolic Regulatory Switches

As indicated, hormones and neuroendocrine peptides are the primary mechanism for regulating the switch in metabolic activity between the fed state and the fasting state. At the level of enzyme activity, the master control factor is AMPK. The primary means by which hormones affect AMPK activity and the targets of AMPK activity were discussed in detail earlier. As for all the other regulatory mechanisms controlling metabolic homeostasis, one must consider allosteric effectors and covalent modifications that control enzyme activities. These are referred to as *short-term regulatory mechanisms*. In addition, physiological, pathological, and hormonal status affects the level of expression of metabolic enzyme–encoding genes. This latter effect is referred to as *long-term regulation*.

The primary allosteric regulators of metabolic pathways are citrate, F2,6BP, glucose-6-phosphate (G6P), malonyl-CoA, cAMP, and AMP. The role of AMP is most important in the context of AMPK activity discussed earlier. Many other allosteric effectors are operating simultaneously but are not discussed. The levels of these various allosteric effectors fluctuate in response to the actions of insulin and glucagon, as well as to other factors including neuroendocrine peptides and other hormones.

G6P allosterically inhibits phosphorylase while at the same time allosterically activating glycogen synthase. Insulin stimulates glucose uptake and as a result will lead to increased G6P. The net effect, at the level of carbohydrate storage, will be reduced glycogen breakdown and increased glycogen synthesis. Citrate inhibits the rate-limiting enzyme of glycolysis (PFK-1) while simultaneously activating the rate-limiting enzyme of fatty acid synthesis (ACC). Inhibited glycolysis drives more glucose into glycogen, which is already highly active due to the allosteric effects of G6P. Fructose-6-phosphate (F6P) also plays a role in the regulation of hepatic glucose disposal, albeit indirectly and not through allosteric means. As glycogen stores reach their maximum and while glycolysis is inhibited, F6P levels begin to increase. The increased F6P levels indirectly inhibit glucokinase that results in the diversion of blood glucose from the liver to other peripheral tissues. Increasing ACC activity results in increased levels of malonyl-CoA, necessary both for fatty acid synthesis as well as to serve as an allosteric inhibitor of carnitine palmitoyltransferase I (CPTI). Inhibition of CPTI prevents newly synthesized fats from being taken up by the mitochondria and oxidized.

Covalent modification is a major mechanism controlling the activity of many enzymes, in particular those involved in metabolic pathways. Covalent modifications are necessary in many cases to regulate the proper localization of an enzyme. These types of modifications are permanent and do not change in the context of altering enzyme activity. The most important covalent modification used to regulate enzyme activity rapidly and interchangeably is phosphorylation. As a consequence, the effects of hormones such as insulin and glucagon, on metabolic homeostasis, are exerted almost exclusively as a result of altering the activity of the kinases and phosphatases that introduce and remove, respectively, regulatory phosphate. As indicated earlier, one of the most important kinases regulating metabolism is AMPK. Glucagon exerts almost all of its effects on metabolism by activating PKA, which then phosphorylates a number of substrates. Although insulin activates many different kinases, with respect to the major metabolic effects of this hormone, it is the activation of phosphodiesterase (PDE) that is most significant. Activation of PDE results in hydrolysis of cAMP, which is required to activate PKA. Loss of PKA activity results in termination of the effects of glucagon. As a result of this effect of insulin, in the well-fed state in the liver, most metabolic regulatory enzymes are dephosphorylated, including glycogen synthase (less active), phosphorylase (more active), PFK-2 (phosphatase [high activity]), phosphorylase kinase (more active), and ACC (more active). Conversely, in the fasted state these same enzymes are phosphorylated.

Adipose tissue enzymes also undergo changes in phosphorylation state in response to insulin and glucagon as a result of the well-fed and fasted states, respectively. The most important metabolic regulatory enzymes in this tissue are also dephosphorylated in the well-fed state including ACC (more active), pyruvate kinase (PK, more active), PDHc (more active), and hormone sensitive lipase (HSL, less active). In response to insulin action in adipose tissue, GLUT4 transporters migrate to the plasma membrane to allow for increased glucose uptake. The oxidation of this glucose is necessary to generate DHAP, which the tissue needs for the synthesis of triglycerides. Under these conditions, adipose tissue can effectively divert incoming carbon into storage material (triglycerides).

Skeletal muscle enzyme modification is also important for the regulation of metabolic activity in the fed and fasting states. In the well-fed state, muscle glycogen synthase (less active), phosphorylase (more active), PDHc (more active), ACC (more active), and malonyl-CoA decarboxylase (MCD, less active) are all dephosphorylated. In the well-fed state, the increased levels of insulin will trigger GLUT4 recruitment to the plasma membranes just as in the case of adipose tissue. This allows skeletal muscle to take up more glucose and given the status of the various metabolic enzymes, the glucose will be diverted into glycogen or would be completely oxidized. The differing activities of ACC and MCD ensure that the fatty acids are synthesized and not oxidized since there is adequate glucose in the well-fed state.

Long-term metabolic integration results from changes in the overall level of expression of many of the critical pathway regulatory enzymes. The changes in gene expression that occur in response to the well-fed and the fasting states are the result of several transcription factors and coactivators. Two of the most important transcription factors that regulate metabolic enzymes are SREBP (SREBP-1c and SREBP-2) and ChREBP. Important transcriptional coactivators include members of the PPAR family, PPAR-α and PPAR-γ. The activity of both PPAR-α and PPAR-γ is enhanced by the presence of another coactivator, PGC-1α. The mechanisms of the transcription factors and the principal genes and metabolic pathways regulated by their transcriptional regulatory activities are discussed throughout the text.

REVIEW QUESTIONS

1. A 33-year-old female patient presented complaining of a tender abdomen and fever. Examination revealed marked abdominal distension, acidosis, and leukocytosis. Laparoscopy revealed that large parts of the small intestine were necrotic and as a consequence, the entire ileum and the proximal portion of her colon were resected. Due to the resulting loss of a particular set of enteroendocrine cells, this patient is most likely to experience which of the following?
   A. increased fatty acid content of the feces
   B. increased gastric acid secretion

C. increased hypoglycemia during periods of fasting
D. loss of cholecystokinin-induced release of protein tyrosine tyrosine (PYY)
E. loss of ghrelin-mediated appetite induction

Answer D: PYY is produced by, and secreted from, intestinal enteroendocrine L-cells of the ileum and colon. Within the gastrointestinal tract, the highest detectable levels of PYY are found in the rectum with low levels found in the duodenum and jejunum. Within the central nervous system (CNS), PYY is detectable in the hypothalamus, medulla, pons, and spinal cord. The signals associated with the response of the proximal gut to food intake that lead to PYY release are the result of CCK and gastrin activity.

2. A 14-year-old boy presents with weight loss and diarrhea. His tongue becomes sore and blistery after eating oatmeal or rye bread, which leads to the diagnosis of celiac disease. The boy and his parents are advised to be sensitive to symptoms of malabsorption of calcium. Which of the following would be a most likely symptom of which the parents should be aware?
   A. dysostosis multiplex
   B. large muscle tetany
   C. megaloblastic anemia
   D. methylmalonic acidemia
   E. telangiectasias

Answer B: In patients with celiac disease, the protein gluten, which is found in bread, oats, and many other foods containing wheat, barley, or rye, triggers an autoimmune response that causes damage to the small intestine, leading to widespread manifestations of malabsorption. Calcium is difficult to absorb, so patients frequently experience symptoms of hypocalcemia such as muscle cramping, tetanic contractions, numbness, and tingling sensations. For sensory and motor nerves, calcium is a critical second messenger involved in normal cell function, neural transmission, and cell membrane stability. The nerves respond to a lack of calcium with hyperexcitability.

3. As a physician on a mission to treat patients in sub-Saharan Africa you encounter numerous children with a common cluster of signs and symptoms. These include chronic diarrhea, dizziness, fatigue, delayed wound healing, and muscle wasting. Given the constellation of symptoms in your patients, you make a diagnosis of marasmus. Which of the following is the principal cause of the observed symptoms?
   A. adequate carbohydrate and fat but lack of protein
   B. adequate caloric intake but a lack of essential fatty acids
   C. adequate protein but deficiency in carbohydrate and fat
   D. high concentration of total protein causing kidney failure
   E. total caloric intake of protein, carbohydrate, and fat far below necessary needs for growth

Answer E: The children you are treating are suffering from marasmus. Marasmus is a form of severe malnutrition caused by a deficiency of nearly all nutrients, especially protein and carbohydrates. A typical child with marasmus looks emaciated and has a body weight less than 60% of that expected for the age. Treatment of marasmus is normally divided into 2 phases. The initial acute phase of treatment involves restoring electrolyte balance, treating infections, and reversing the hypoglycemia and hypothermia. This is followed by refeeding and ensuring that sufficient caloric and nutrient intake is maintained to enable catch-up growth in order to restore a healthy normal body mass.

4. You are treating a 12-year-old male patient exhibiting severe episodes of hypoglycemia. Measurement of circulating insulin and glucagon levels indicate that they are normal and responsive to cycles of feeding and fasting. The hypoglycemia can most easily be explained as a defect in which of the following processes?
   A. adipose tissue HSL activation
   B. hepatic gluconeogenesis
   C. intestinal gluconeogenesis
   D. renal gluconeogenesis
   E. skeletal muscle GLUT4 translocation to plasma membrane

Answer B: The hepatic form of hexokinase (glucokinase), in this patient, most likely harbors a mutation that results in a significantly reduced K_m relative to normal glucokinase. Hepatic glucokinase normally has a K_m significantly higher than that of the hexokinase that is expressed in other insulin-responsive tissues such as adipose tissue and skeletal muscle. This prevents the liver from trapping glucose, thereby ensuring that peripheral tissues such as the brain and muscle have easy access to dietary carbohydrate. In the case of this patient, the expression of a variant glucokinase with a K_m similar to that of muscle hexokinase would result in significant trapping of glucose inside hepatocytes. The outcome would be expected to be periods of hypoglycemia as observed in this patient.

5. A healthy 35-year-old man exhibits a peak serum glucose concentration of 215 mg/dL within 30 minutes of participating in a glucose tolerance test involving the consumption of 60 g of glucose. Two hours after

ingestion, measurement of his serum glucose concentration shows it to be to 85 mg/dL. The observed decrease is due to the normal responses of tissues to insulin. In addition, part of the reduction is due to uptake and trapping of glucose within the liver cells, which is facilitated by which of the following enzymes?
A. galactokinase
B. glucokinase
C. phosphoenolpyruvate carboxykinase (PEPCK)
D. phosphofructokinase-1 (PFK1)
E. pyruvate dehydrogenase

Answer B: Hepatic glucokinase has a high K_m for glucose in order to ensure that the liver does not trap glucose before sufficient levels are obtained in the blood. This allows dietary carbohydrate to pass through the liver so that tissues such as the brain, skeletal muscle, erythrocytes, and kidney medulla can have access to the glucose. As the level of blood glucose increases, glucokinase will become more active, resulting in phosphorylation of more glucose thereby, trapping it in the hepatocyte.

6. A 9-month-old child is presented to the emergency room by his parents who report that he has been vomiting and has severe diarrhea. The episodes of vomiting began when the mother stopped breastfeeding and switched to the use of child cow's milk. The infant exhibits signs of failure to thrive, weight loss, hepatomegaly, and jaundice. Laboratory tests show elevated blood galactose, hypergalactosuria, and metabolic acidosis with coagulation deficiency characteristic of classic galactosemia. Which of the following is most likely to occur if this child continues to consume cow's milk?
A. anemia
B. blindness
C. hypercoagulopathy
D. renal failure
E. tetanic contractions

Answer E: Type 1 galactosemia occurs as a consequence of mutations in the gene encoding GALT. Classic galactosemia manifests by a failure of neonates to thrive. Vomiting and diarrhea occur following ingestion of milk, hence individuals are termed *lactose intolerant*. Clinical findings include impaired liver function (which if left untreated leads to severe cirrhosis), elevated blood galactose, hypergalactosemia, hyperchloremic metabolic acidosis, urinary galactitol excretion, and hyperaminoaciduria. Unless controlled by exclusion of galactose from the diet, these patients can go on to develop blindness and fatal liver damage. Blindness is due to the conversion of circulating galactose to the sugar alcohol galacitol, by an NADPH-dependent aldose reductase that is present in neural tissue and in the lens of the eye.

7. Prolonged ethanol consumption and subsequent metabolism ultimately leads to a condition referred to as steatohepatitis or more commonly, "fatty liver syndrome." The increased fat deposition in hepatocytes in response to chronic alcohol consumption is the result of which of the following?
A. decreased CYP7A1 activity
B. decreased malonyl-CoA decarboxylase activity
C. increased branched-chain ketoacid dehydrogenase (BCKD) activity
D. increased glycerol-3-phosphate dehydrogenase activity
E. increased HMG-CoA reductase activity

Answer D: The metabolism of ethanol by the liver leads to a large increase in NADH. This increase in NADH disrupts the normal processes of metabolic regulation such as hepatic gluconeogenesis, TCA cycle function, and fatty acid oxidation. Concomitant with reduced fatty acid oxidation is enhanced fatty acid synthesis and increased triacylglycerol production by the liver. In the mitochondria, the production of acetate from acetaldehyde leads to increased levels of acetyl-CoA. Since the increased generation of NADH also reduces the activity of the TCA cycle, the acetyl-CoA is diverted to fatty acid synthesis. The reduction in cytosolic NAD^+ leads to reduced activity of glycerol-3-phosphate dehydrogenase (in the glycerol 3-phosphate to DHAP direction), resulting in increased levels of glycerol 3-phosphate, which is the backbone for the synthesis of the triglycerides. Both of these 2 events lead to fatty acid deposition in the liver, leading to fatty liver syndrome and excessive levels of lipids in the blood, referred to as *hyperlipidemia*.

8. Shortly after birth, an infant presents with severe lactic acidemia, hyperammonemia, citrullinemia, and hyperlysinemia with the presence of α-ketoglurate in the urine. Tests are performed to determine where the defect lies that is causing this cluster of symptoms. These tests indicate that the infant does not have a urea cycle defect, nor a defect in fatty acid oxidation. A defect in which of the following metabolic pathways is most likely the cause of this infants symptoms?
A. bile acid synthesis
B. branched-chain amino acid catabolism
C. gluconeogenesis
D. glycogen synthesis
E. glycolysis

Answer C: The infant is experiencing symptoms associated with a defect in pyruvate carboxylase.

Pyruvate carboxylase is the first enzyme in the gluconeogenic conversion of pyruvate carbons into glucose. A defect in pyruvate carboxylase would restrict the conversion of lactate into pyruvate and then subsequently to glucose. This would lead to severe lactic academia. The other symptoms are primarily the result of liver damage due to impaired gluconeogenesis.

9. Which of the following statements concerning total body energy storage is correct?
   A. most of the body's energy store is held as carbohydrate
   B. most of the body's energy store is held as lipid
   C. most of the body's energy store is held as plasma glucose
   D. most of the body's energy store is held as protein
   E. total body energy storage approximately equals resting metabolic rate

Answer B: Lipid is the most concentrated form of energy storage, holding 9.4 kcal/g. For a typical 70-kg human, over 130,000 kcal is typically stored as fat. Storage of energy as available protein is about 20,000 kcal while storage as carbohydrate is about 3000 kcal.

10. During early fasting, glycogen is used as a source of glucose for the blood. After liver glycogen is depleted, which of the following is most likely to contribute to the maintenance of endogenous serum glucose levels?
   A. amino acids of muscle proteins are used to synthesize glucose in the brain
   B. fatty acids of adipose tissue are converted into glucose in the liver
   C. intestinal glutamine is used as a gluconeogenic substrate
   D. liver fatty acids are degraded as precursors for blood glucose
   E. skeletal muscle glycogen is broken down and the glucose delivered to the blood

Answer C: During periods of fasting and starvation, when liver glycogen levels are depleted, the major source of carbon atom for hepatic gluconeogenesis is from the amino acids released due to protein degradation within skeletal muscle. However, the kidneys and the small intestine do contribute to endogenous glucose production via the use of glutamine as a carbon source for gluconeogenesis in these 2 tissues.

11. You are treating a patient who is suffering from the glycogen storage disease known as von Gierke disease. Although the primary defect in this disease is in glucose homeostasis, which of the following other metabolic abnormalities is expected to be found in patients with this disease?
   A. hyperammonemia
   B. hyperuricemia
   C. hypokalemia
   D. hypophosphatemia
   E. ketoacidosis

Answer B: The metabolic consequences of the hepatic glucose-6-phosphate deficiency of von Gierke disease extend well beyond just the obvious hypoglycemia that results from the deficiency in liver in being able to deliver free glucose to the blood. The inability to release the phosphate from glucose 6-phopsphate results in diversion into glycolysis and production of pyruvate as well as increased diversion onto the pentose phosphate pathway. The production of excess pyruvate, at levels above the capacity of the TCA cycle to completely oxidize it, results in its reduction to lactate leading to lactic acidemia. In addition, some of the pyruvate is transaminated to alanine, leading to hyperalaninemia. Some of the pyruvate will be oxidized to acetyl-CoA, which cannot be fully oxidized in the TCA cycle. So the acetyl-CoA will end up in cytosol, where it will serve as a substrate for triglyceride and cholesterol synthesis resulting in hyperlipidemia. The oxidation of glucose 6-phophate via the pentose phosphate pathway leads to increased production of ribose-5-phosphate, which then activates the de novo synthesis of the purine nucleotides. In excess of the need, these purine nucleotides will ultimately be catabolized to uric acid, resulting in hyperuricemia and consequent symptoms of gout.

12. Following a minor respiratory illness, a seemingly healthy, developmentally normal 15-month-old girl exhibited repeated episodes of severe lethargy and vomiting in the middle of the night. The parents brought the infant to the ER following a seizure. The child was hypoglycemic and was administered 10% dextrose, but remained lethargic. Blood ammonia was high, liver enzymes were slightly elevated, and urine ketones were only barely detectable. A diagnosis of medium-chain acyl-CoA dehydrogenase (MCAD) deficiency is made. Measurement of which of the following would also be expected in this infant given the current diagnosis?
   A. decreased serum urea
   B. elevated serum carnitine
   C. elevated serum dicarboxylic acids
   D. hyperalaninemia
   E. hyperuricemia

Answer C: Deficiency in MCAD is the most common inherited defect in the pathways of mitochondrial fatty acid oxidation. The most common presentation of infants with this disorder is episodic hypoketotic hypoglycemia following periods of fasting. Although the first episode may be fatal, and incorrectly ascribed to sudden infant death syndrome, patients with MCAD deficiency are normal between episodes and are treated by avoidance of fasting and treatment of acute episodes with intravenous glucose. Accumulation of acylcarnitines (dicarboxylic acids), in particular octanoylcarnitine, is diagnostic.

13. A 7-year-old boy is examined by his pediatrician because of complaints of severe cramping pain in his legs whenever he rides his bike. In addition, he experiences nausea and vomiting during these attacks. The child has noted that the severity of the cramps is most intense after dinners that include baked potatoes or pasta and sometimes bread. Clinical studies undertaken following a treadmill test demonstrate myoglobinuria and hyperuricemia. Given these symptoms, it seems clear that the boy is suffering from Tarui disease. With which of the following symptoms would this disease also be expected to be associated?

A. ataxia
B. decreased creatinine clearance
C. hypercoagulopathy
D. jaundice
E. methylmalonic acidemia

Answer D: Tarui disease (GSD7) is a glycogen storage disease, resulting from mutations in the gene encoding muscle and erythrocyte PFK1. The symptoms of this disease are very similar to those observed in patients suffering from McArdle disease (GSDV), in particular the presentation of exercise-induced pain and myoglobinuria. However, since Tarui disease also involves a defect in erythrocyte PFK1, there are associated mild forms of jaundice, resulting from accelerated destruction of erythrocytes.

14. A 6-month-old who is failing to thrive is brought to your clinic. Tests reveal hepatosplenomegaly, muscle weakness and atrophy, hypotonia, and decreased deep tendon reflexes. Biopsy of the liver reveals initial stages of cirrhosis due to the accumulation of an abnormal glycogen whose structure resembles amylopectin. These results indicate the child is suffering from Andersen disease. Which of the following would also be expected in this child?

A. aminoaciduria
B. hyperglycemia
C. hyperlipidemia
D. hypoglycemia
E. normal glycemia

Answer E: Andersen disease or glycogen storage disease type IV (GSDIV) is also known as amylopectinosis. The disease results from defects in the gene encoding glycogen branching enzyme, also called amylo-(1,4 to 1,6) transglycosylase. The disease manifests with progressive hepatosplenomegaly along with the storage of an abnormal glycogen that exhibits poor solubility in the liver. The abnormal glycogen is characterized by few branch points with long outer chains containing more α-1,4-linked glucose than normal glycogen. Due to this structure of glycogen, the presence of normal activities of glycogen phosphorylase and glucose 6-phosphatase, patients with Andersen disease manifest the above symptoms but in the presence of normal serum glucose regulation.

15. A 4-month-old white male infant with a temperature of 38.4°C is examined by his pediatrician. His mother indicates that he has had the fever for the past 4 days, been listless, vomiting, and has watery stools. Blood work indicates the infants' blood pH is slightly acidic and shows reduced bicarbonate. Other untoward blood chemistry includes elevated liver enzymes. The child has a protuberant abdomen, thin extremities, and a doll-like face indicative of von Gierke disease. Given this diagnosis, what other deleterious symptom would be expected in this infant?

A. defective hepatic bile acid synthesis
B. defective hepatic fatty acid synthesis
C. depressed respiration rate
D. severe hyperglycemia
E. severe hypoglycemia

Answer E: von Gierke disease (GSDI) results from the absence of glucose-6-phosphatase activity. Patients with von Gierke disease can present during the neonatal period with lactic acidosis and hypoglycemia. The hallmark features of this disease are severe hypoglycemia, lactic acidosis, hyperuricemia, and hyperlipidemia. The severity of the hypoglycemia and lactic acidosis can be such that in the past affected individuals died in infancy. Infants often have a doll-like facial appearance due to excess adipose tissue in the cheeks. The metabolic consequences of the hepatic glucose-6-phosphate deficiency of von Gierke disease extend well beyond just the obvious hypoglycemia that results from the deficiency in liver being able to deliver free glucose to the blood. The inability to release the phosphate from glucose 6-phopsphate results in diversion into glycolysis and production of pyruvate as well as increased diversion onto the pentose phosphate pathway. The production of excess pyruvate, at levels above the capacity of the TCA cycle to completely oxidize it, results in its reduction to lactate, leading to lactic acidemia. In addition, some of the pyruvate is transaminated to alanine, leading to hyperalaninemia. Some of the pyruvate, which cannot be fully oxidized in the TCA cycle, will be oxidized to acetyl-CoA and so the acetyl-CoA will end up in the cytosol, where it will serve as a substrate for triglyceride and cholesterol synthesis resulting in hyperlipidemia. The oxidation of glucose 6-phophate via the pentose phosphate pathway leads to increased production of ribose 5-phosphate, which then activates the de novo synthesis of the purine nucleotides. In excess of the need, these purine nucleotides will ultimately be catabolized to uric acid, resulting in hyperuricemia and consequent symptoms of gout.

16. You are studying fatty acid synthesis in a cell line isolated from a hepatic cancer patient. You discover that addition of glucose 6-phosphate does not lead to an increase in the rate of palmitic acid synthesis as is the situation for normal hepatic cells. This indicates there is a defect in the allosteric regulation of fatty acid synthase (FAS). Which of the following would most likely also be observed in these cells?

A. decreased cholesterol synthesis
B. decreased ketone synthesis
C. decreased protein synthesis
D. increased amino acid oxidation
E. increased glycogen synthesis

Answer E: Regulation of de novo fatty acid synthesis by phosphorylated sugars takes place via allosteric activation of the activity of FAS. Addition of glucose 6-phosphate (G6P) to cells would also result in changes in the level of allosteric regulation of phosphorylase and glycogen synthase. G6P is an allosteric inhibitor of phosphorylase and an activator of glycogen synthase, the net result therefore, would be an increased ability to store glycogen.

17. The *Randle hypothesis* was proposed to explain the correlation between carbohydrate and lipid metabolic homeostasis and the effect of disruptions in both processes on diabetes and obesity. Which of the following statements best reflects the basis of the Randle hypothesis?

A. an increase in adipocyte volume due to increased lipid storage causes adipocytes to lose their responsiveness to insulin
B. increased circulating free fatty acids in obese individuals impair the ability of insulin to stimulate skeletal muscle cell glucose uptake
C. long-term hyperlipidemia leads to permanent elevation in pancreatic insulin secretion that ultimately causes downregulation of insulin receptors
D. the high level of circulating free fatty acids stimulates the liver to shut off gluconeogenesis that then impairs pancreatic sensing of the need for insulin release
E. the hyperglycemia prevalent in obese individuals activates insulin release from the pancreas, leading to increased adipocyte lipolysis

Answer B: The Randle hypothesis states that elevations in circulating free fatty acids (FFAs) interfere with insulin action in liver and skeletal muscle. Increased FFA uptake and metabolism by the liver results in an increased production of acetyl-CoA. All of the acetyl-CoA cannot be oxidized completely in the TCA cycle. The elevated acetyl-CoA levels result in inhibition of the PDHc, resulting in increased citrate transport to the cytosol. Increased cytosolic citrate inhibits PFK1, resulting in reduced glucose oxidation and an increase in glucose-6-phosphate levels. Increases in glucose-6-phosphate lead to inhibition of skeletal muscle hexokinase, resulting in reduced glucose utilization. In addition, the elevated plasma FFAs impair insulin receptor tyrosine phosphorylation of IRS1, leading to defects in insulin-mediated signaling events in target cells, primarily skeletal muscle. Loss of insulin signaling in skeletal muscle prevents glucose transporter (GLUT4) mobilization to the cell surface with a resultant block to glucose uptake. The overall consequences of a high-fat diet are a progressive impairment in hepatic glucose homeostasis, impairment of insulin-mediated glucose uptake by skeletal muscle, and pancreatic β-cell decompensation. The latter leads to reduced insulin secretion and, thus, further impairment of the role of insulin in regulation of blood glucose.

18. You are treating 46-year-old man who has suffered a heart attack. Measurement of his serum cholesterol level indicates it is 500 mg/dL. His father died at 37 years of age from a massive heart attack, and one of his 2 younger siblings also has an increased serum concentration of total cholesterol. This patient most likely has a defect in LDL receptor function associated with familial hypercholesterolemia (FH). Which of the following additional signs is characteristic in patients with FH?

A. arcus cornea
B. dysostosis multiplex
C. hyperammonemia
D. hypoglycemia
E. renal lithiasis

Answer A: The clinical characteristics of FH include elevated concentrations of plasma LDL and deposition of LDL-cholesterol in the arteries, tendons, and skin. Fat deposits in the arteries are called *atheromas* and in the skin and tendons they are called *xanthomas*. Xanthomas and the characteristic arcus cornea (whitish ring on the peripheral cornea) begin to appear in the second decade in heterozygotes, but will appear in childhood in homozygotes.

19. You are treating a 38-year-old man whose chief complaint is occasional right upper quadrant pain. Analysis of blood samples shows elevated aspartate transaminase (AST) and alanine transaminase (ALT). History indicates that these same enzymes have shown elevated levels each of the past 3 years during routine blood work in conjunction with his annual physical examination. His history also indicates reflux esophagitis, hypertension, and hyperlipidemia. You order tests for serologic and biochemical markers for viral hepatitis and autoimmune liver disease and other metabolic liver diseases, but these results are negative. The patient has gained 50 lb since the age of 18. He consumes less than 5 standard alcoholic drinks per week. Which of the following is the most likely diagnosis in this case?

A. familial hypercholesterolemia
B. medium-chain acyl-CoA dehydrogenase deficiency
C. nonalcoholic fatty liver disease
D. Refsum disease
E. type 2 diabetes

Answer C: Nonalcoholic fatty liver disease (NAFLD) is the most common liver disease in the Western world. NAFLD is characterized by fatty infiltration of the liver in the absence of alcohol consumption. One of the most significant contributing factors to the development of NAFLD is insulin resistance in the liver. Additional pathophysiology includes an enhanced state of hepatic oxidative stress and lipid peroxidation, decreased antioxidant defenses, early mitochondrial dysfunction, and iron accumulation.

20. A 59-year-old male is found unconscious in an alley and rushed to the emergency room (ER). He is disheveled, clad in dirty torn clothing, has filthy hair, and smells of urine and decaying trash. Emanating from the patient is a strong odor of alcohol. From information contained in his wallet, family are contacted and a history reveals that the man has been living on the streets for several years and that he suffers from severe post-traumatic stress disorder (PTSD). Upon entry into the ER he was administered an iv drip of 5% dextrose. Unfortunately the patient never regained consciousness and died within hours of admission to the hospital. Given the patient's condition and history, which of the following was the most likely cause of his death?

A. alcohol poisoning
B. hyperlipidemia
C. protein malnutrition
D. sepsis
E. severe lactic acidosis

Answer E: Chronic alcoholics have a tendency to very poor dietetic habits particularly those who are homeless or choose to live on the streets. The chronic poor nutritional intake in these individuals usually leads to severe vitamin deficiencies, in particular thiamine deficiency. Lack of adequate thiamine, especially in alcoholics, leads to Wernicke-Korsakoff syndrome, WKS. WKS is associated with significant deficit in the activity of dehydrogenases that require thiamine pyrophosphate (TPP) as a cofactor such as pyruvate dehydrogenase (PDH). In these individuals the capacity to carry out gluconeogenesis is severely impaired due primarily to excess alcohol metabolism and the resultant negative effects on liver function. Giving a person in this state an iv bolus of glucose (5% dextrose) results in massive increases in lactate production due to the lack of PDH activity. This increases an already lactic acidotic state to a potentially lethal acidosis.

21. During the course of normal cellular metabolism, the body generates large quantities of acid. Despite this, normal blood pH is maintained at a slightly alkaline pH of 7.4. Removal of which of the following is most responsible for the maintenance of the alkalinity of extracellular fluids?

A. ammonia
B. carbon dioxide
C. ketones such as acetoacetate
D. lactic acid
E. phosphoric acid

Answer B: The vast majority of metabolic acid excretion is in the form of the volatile acid, CO_2, which is removed via the lungs. Much smaller quantities of nonvolatile acids must be excreted in the urine. Within erythrocytes, metabolically produced CO_2 is combined with H_2O forming carbonic acid, which then ionizes to form a bicarbonate ion and a proton. The protons bind to hemoglobin displacing O_2, which not only provides the necessary oxygen for metabolism but also results in increased CO_2 removal. During periods of increased acidity, referred to as metabolic acidosis, chemoreceptors sense a deranged acid-base balance and compensate by increasing respiration rate, hyperventilation, to increase the rate of CO_2 removal.

Checklist

✓ *Metabolic integration* refers to the processes by which events occurring within one tissue can impact overall metabolism in one or more peripheral tissues.

✓ Metabolic integration affects all tissues of the body, but is most important within the context of the liver, brain, intestines, adipose tissue, and muscle.

✓ Carbohydrate and fat metabolism are the most intimately interrelated metabolic processes in the body. In the liver, skeletal muscle, and adipose tissue, the intake and metabolism of glucose exerts a negative impact on fatty acid utilization and vice versa. This represents a major foundation of the *Randle hypothesis*, which defines how disruptions in carbohydrate and fat metabolism contribute to insulin insensitivity, eventually leading to Type 2 diabetes.

✓ Metabolic integration is coordinated by a complex series of covalent protein modifications and transcriptional regulatory controls exerted on the expression of critical metabolic regulatory enzymes.

✓ Disorders such as obesity and diabetes are major causes of total body metabolic disruption and represent 2 of the most significant pathological conditions affecting persons in the developed world.

CHAPTER 35 Chromatin: DNA Structure and Replication

CHAPTER OUTLINE

High-Yield Terms

Phosphodiester bond: chemical bond between the 5′-phosphate of one base and the 3′-hydroxyl of an adjacent base in a nucleic acid

Watson-Crick base-pair: refers to the normal hydrogen bonding that occurs in a duplex of DNA, or an RNA-DNA duplex, where A bonds to T and G bonds to C

Annealing: with respect to nucleic acids this refers to DNA or RNA pairing by hydrogen bonds to a complementary sequence, forming a double-stranded polynucleotide

Nucleosome: a structure formed by DNA and protein interaction that consisting of an octamer protein structure composed of 2 subunits each of histones H2A, H2B, H3, and H4

Chromatin: the combination of DNA and proteins that make up the contents of the nucleus of a cell

High-Yield Terms

Heterochromatin: densely packed region of a chromosome often found near the centromeres, is generally transcriptionally silent

Euchromatin: loosely packed regions of a chromosome where active gene transcription can occur

Telomere: a region of repetitive nucleotide sequences at each end of a chromatid

Cyclin: any of a number of proteins whose levels fluctuate during the eukaryotic cell cycle; these proteins regulate the activity of a family of kinases involved in controlling passage through the cell cycle

Proof-reading: in the process of DNA replication this refers to the $3' \rightarrow 5'$ exonuclease activity of DNA polymerase, which allows it to remove an incorrectly incorporated nucleotide, recognized by non–Watson-Crick base-pairing

Okazaki fragment: short stretches of newly synthesized DNA representing the lagging strand

Topoisomerase: enzymes that cleave the DNA strand, thereby relieving torsional stresses incurred during the process of DNA replicaiton

Epigenetics: defines the mechanism by which changes in the pattern of inherited gene expression occur in the absence of alterations or changes in the nucleotide composition of a given gene

Imprinting: refers to the fact that the expression of some genes depends on whether or not they are inherited maternally or paternally

Trinucleotide repeat: sequences of 3 nucleotides repeated in tandem on the same chromosome a number of times, abnormal expansion of the repeat is associated with the genesis of disease

DNA Structure

DNA is a specialized form of polynucleotides. Polynucleotides are formed by the condensation of 2 or more nucleotides. The condensation most commonly occurs between the alcohol of a 5′-phosphate of one nucleotide and the 3′-hydroxyl of a second, with the elimination of H_2O, forming a phosphodiester bond. The formation of phosphodiester bonds in DNA and RNA exhibits directionality. The primary structure of DNA and RNA (the linear arrangement of the nucleotides) proceeds in the $5' \rightarrow 3'$ direction (Figure 35-1). The common representation of the primary structure of DNA or RNA molecules is to write the nucleotide sequences from left to right synonymous with the $5' \rightarrow 3'$ direction.

Within cells, DNA exists as a helix of 2 complementary antiparallel strands, wound around each other in a rightward direction and stabilized by hydrogen bonding (H-bonds) between nucleobases (bases) in adjacent strands (Figure 35-2). The bases are in the interior of the helix aligned at a nearly 90-degree angle relative to the axis of the helix. Due to the fact that purine bases form H-bonds with pyrimidines, in any given molecule of DNA the concentration of adenine (A) is equal to thymine (T) and the concentration of cytidine (C) is equal to guanine (G). This means that A will only base-pair with T, and C with G. According to this pattern, known as **Watson-Crick base-pairing**, the base-pairs composed of G and C contain 3 hydrogen bonds, whereas those of A and T contain 2 hydrogen bonds (Figure 35-3). This makes G-C base-pairs more stable than A-T base-pairs.

The antiparallel nature of the helix stems from the orientation of the individual strands. From any fixed position in the helix, one strand is oriented in the $5' \rightarrow 3'$ direction and the other in the $3' \rightarrow 5'$ direction. On its exterior surface, the double helix of DNA contains 2 deep grooves between the ribose-phosphate chains. These 2 grooves are of unequal size and termed the major and minor grooves (see Figure 35-2). The difference in their size is due to the asymmetry of the deoxyribose rings and the structurally distinct nature of

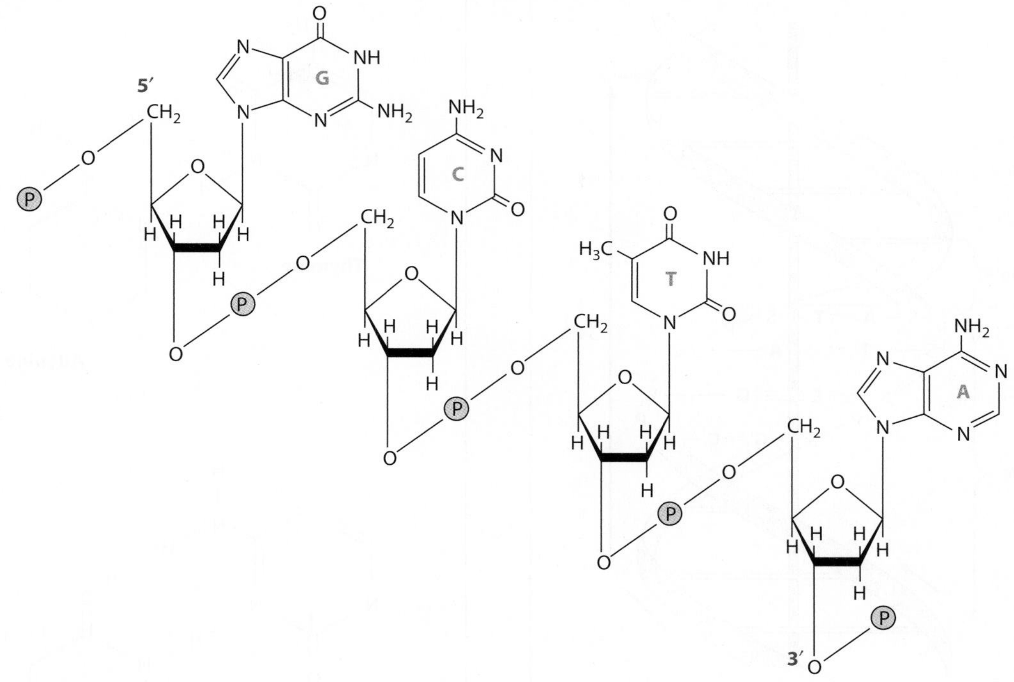

FIGURE 35-1: A segment of one strand of a DNA molecule in which the purine and pyrimidine bases guanine (G), cytosine (C), thymine (T), and adenine (A) are held together by a phosphodiester backbone between 2′-deoxyribosyl moieties attached to the nucleobases by an *N*-glycosidic bond. Note that the backbone has a polarity (ie, a direction). Convention dictates that a single-stranded DNA sequence is written in the 5′ to 3′ direction (ie, pGpCpTpA, where G, C, T, and A represent the 4 bases and p represents the interconnecting phosphates). Murray RK, Bender DA, Botham KM, Kennelly PJ, Rodwell VW, Weil PA. *Harper's Illustrated Biochemistry.* 29th, ed. New York: McGraw-Hill; 2012.

the upper surface of a base-pair relative to the bottom surface.

The double helix of DNA has been shown to exist in several different forms, depending upon sequence content and ionic conditions of crystal preparation. The B-form of DNA prevails under physiological conditions of low ionic strength and a high degree of hydration. Regions of the helix that are rich in pCpG dinucleotides can exist in a novel left-handed helical conformation termed Z-DNA. This conformation results from a 180-degree change in the orientation of the bases relative to that of the more common A- and B-DNA.

Thermal Properties of DNA

As cells divide, it is a necessity that the DNA be copied (replicated) in such a way that each daughter cell acquires the same amount of genetic material. In order for this process to proceed the 2 strands of the helix must first be separated in a process termed **denaturation**. DNA denaturation can also be accomplished experimentally by subjecting it to high temperature. Under these conditions the H-bonds between bases become unstable and the strands of the helix separate in a process of **thermal denaturation**. When thermally melted DNA is cooled, the complementary strands will again re-form the correct base-pairs in a process termed **annealing** or **hybridization**. The rate of annealing is dependent upon the nucleotide sequence of the 2 strands of DNA.

Regions of DNA that have predominantly A-T base-pairs will be less thermally stable than those rich in G-C base-pairs. In the process of thermal denaturation, the temperature required for 50% of the DNA molecule to exist single stranded is referred to as the melting temperature (T_m). The T_m is a characteristic of the base composition of that DNA molecule and the conditions of the solution containing the DNA.

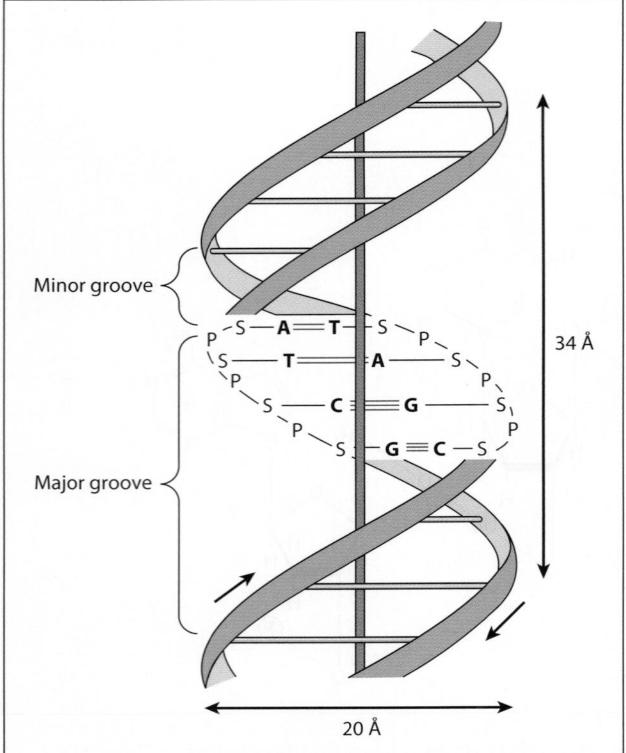

FIGURE 35-2: A diagrammatic representation of the Watson and Crick model of the double-helical structure of the B form of DNA. The horizontal arrow indicates the width of the double helix (20 Å), and the vertical arrow indicates the distance spanned by one complete turn of the double helix (34 Å). One turn of B-DNA includes 10 base pairs (bp), so the rise is 3.4 Å per bp. The central axis of the double helix is indicated by the vertical rod. The short arrows designate the polarity of the antiparallel strands. The major and minor grooves are depicted. (A, adenine; C, cytosine; G, guanine; P, phosphate; S, sugar [deoxyribose]; T, thymine.) Hydrogen bonds between A/T and G/C bases indicated by short, red, horizontal lines. Murray RK, Bender DA, Botham KM, Kennelly PJ, Rodwell VW, Weil PA. *Harper's Illustrated Biochemistry*, 29th ed. New York: McGraw-Hill; 2012.

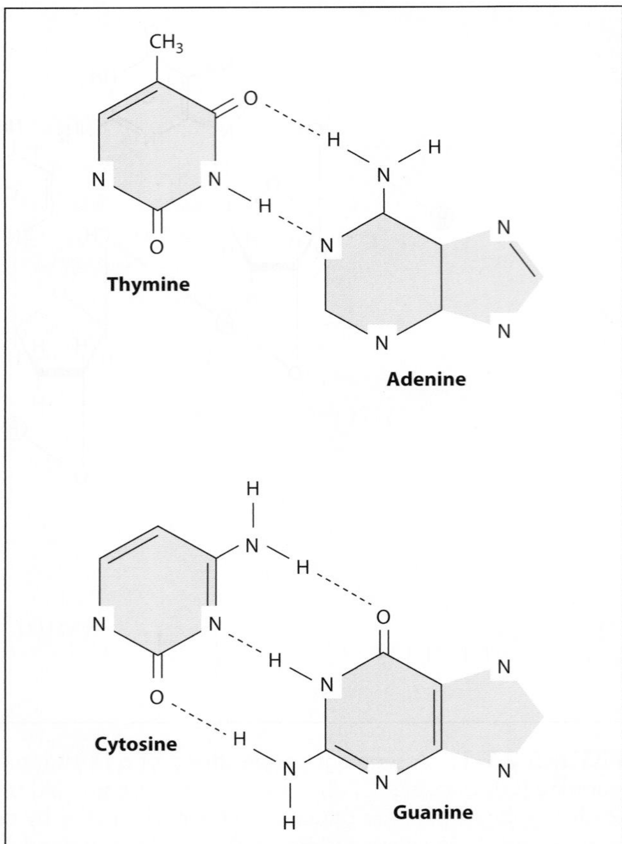

FIGURE 35-3: DNA base pairing between adenine and thymine involves the formation of 2 hydrogen bonds. Three such bonds form between cytidine and guanine. The broken lines represent hydrogen bonds. Murray RK, Bender DA, Botham KM, Kennelly PJ, Rodwell VW, Weil PA. *Harper's Illustrated Biochemistry*, 29th ed. New York: McGraw-Hill; 2012.

Chromatin Structure

Chromatin is a term designating the structure in which DNA exists within cells. The structure of chromatin is determined and stabilized through the interaction of the DNA with DNA-binding proteins. There are 2 classes of DNA-binding proteins. The histones are the major class of DNA-binding proteins involved in maintaining the compacted structure of chromatin. There are 5 different histone proteins identified as H1, H2A, H2B, H3, and H4.

The other class of DNA-binding proteins is a diverse group of proteins called simply, nonhistone proteins. This class of proteins includes the various transcription factors, polymerases, hormone receptors, and other nuclear enzymes. In any given cell there are greater than 1000 different types of nonhistone proteins bound to the DNA.

The binding of DNA by the histones generates a structure called the nucleosome (Figure 35-4). The nucleosome core contains an octamer protein structure consisting of 2 subunits each of H2A, H2B, H3, and H4. Histone H1 occupies the inter-nucleosomal DNA and is identified as the linker histone. The nucleosome core contains approximately 150 bp of DNA. The nucleosomes would appear as "beads-on-a-string" if the DNA were pulled into a linear structure and observed under an electron microscope.

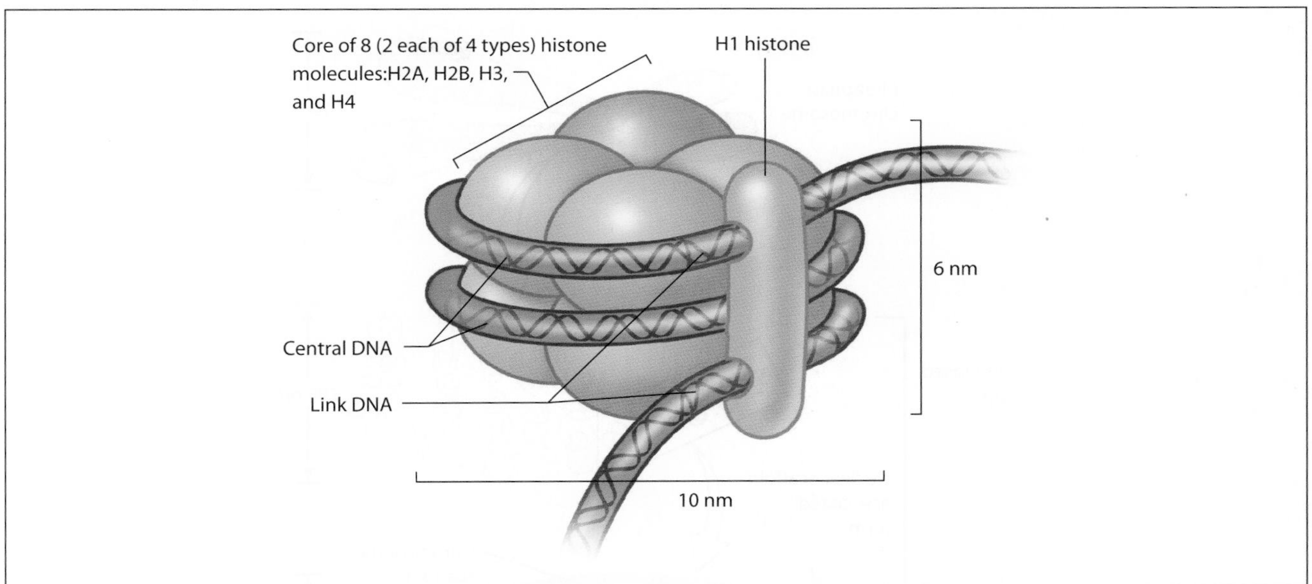

FIGURE 35-4: Components of a nucleosome. Nucleosome is a structure that produces the initial organization of free double-stranded DNA into chromatin. Each nucleosome has an octomeric core complex made up of 4 types of histones, 2 copies each of H2A, H2B, H3, and H4. Around this core is wound DNA approximately 150 bp in length. One H1 histone is located outside the DNA on the surface of each nucleosome. DNA associated with nucleosomes in vivo thus resembles a long string of beads. Nucleosomes are very dynamic structures, with H1 loosening and DNA unwrapping at least once every second to allow other proteins, including transcription factors and enzymes, access to the DNA. Mescher AL. *Junqueira's Basic Histology Text and Atlas,* 13th ed. New York: McGraw-Hill; 2013.

The nucleosome cores themselves coil into a solenoid shape which itself coils to further compact the DNA. These final coils are compacted further into the characteristic chromatin structure seen in a metaphase karyotype analysis (Figure 35-5).

In a broad consideration of chromatin structure there are 2 forms: **heterochromatin** and **euchromatin**. Heterochromatin is more densely packed than euchromatin and is often found near the centromeres of the chromosomes. Heterochromatin is generally transcriptionally silent. Euchromatin on the other hand is more loosely packed and is where active gene transcription can occur.

Histone Modifications and Chromatin Structure

Histone acetylation is known to result in a more open chromatin structure and these modified histones are found in regions of the chromatin that are transcriptionally active. Proteins are known to interact with acetylated histones that together lead to a more open chromatin structure. Proteins that bind to acetylated lysines in histones contain a domain called a **bromodomain**. Conversely, underacetylation of histones is associated with closed chromatin and transcriptional inactivity. A direct correlation between histone acetylation and transcriptional activity was demonstrated when it was discovered that protein complexes, previously known to be transcriptional activators, were found to have histone acetylase activity. And as expected, transcriptional repressor complexes were found to contain histone deacetylase activity (Chapter 36).

Another histone modification known to affect chromatin structure is methylation. However, with histone methylation there is not a direct correlation between the modification and a specific effect on transcription. Some histone methylations promote an open chromatin structure and thereby, lead to transcriptional activation, whereas other methylations are known to be associated with transcriptionally inactive genes. Proteins that bind to methylated histones contain a domain called **chromodomain**. The chromodomain is also found in the RNA-induced transcriptional silencing (RITS) complex which involves small interfering RNA (siRNA) and microRNA (miRNA)-mediated downregulation of transcription (Chapter 36).

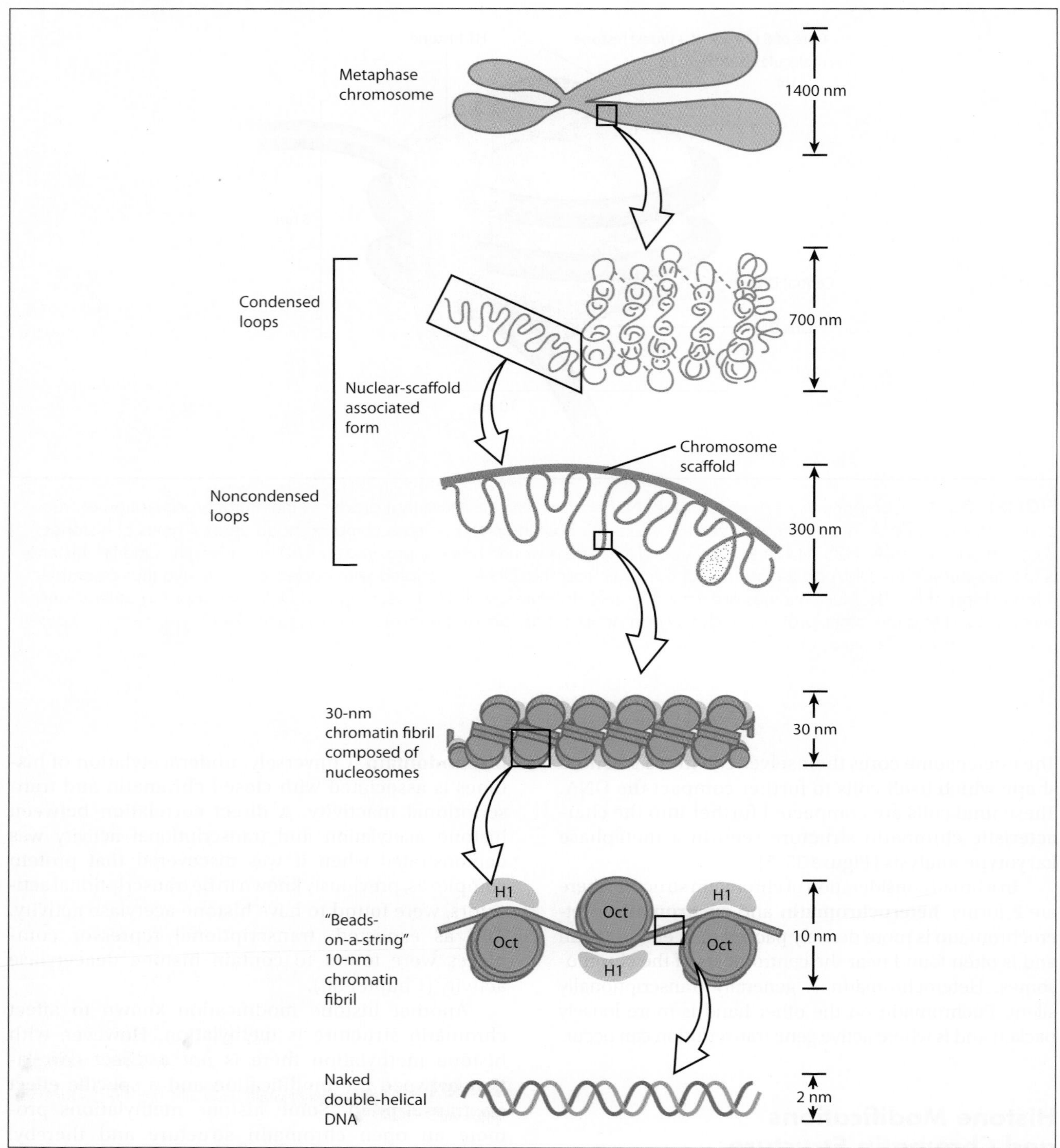

FIGURE 35-5: Levels of DNA packing in a typical metaphase chromosome (top) down to a naked duplex of DNA (bottom). The "beads-on-a-string" structure, formed as histones form nucleosomes and become wrapped by the DNA, is visible as such under electron microscopy. The DNA-protein complex within the cell is attached to a scaffold composed of highly specialized DNA-binding proteins that aid in the condensation of the chromosome to the metaphase stage. Murray RK, Bender DA, Botham KM, Kennelly PJ, Rodwell VW, Weil PA. *Harper's Illustrated Biochemistry*, 29th ed. New York: McGraw-Hill; 2012.

High-Yield Concept

There are 2 primary mechanisms operating in a dynamic manner to alter chromatin. These mechanisms are methylation of cytidine residues in specific locations in the DNA (see below) and histone modification. Histone modifications include acetylation, methylation, phosphorylation, and ubiquitination (Table 35-1).

TABLE 35-1: Possible Roles of Modified Histones

1. Acetylation of histones H3 and H4 is associated with the activation or inactivation of gene transcription.
2. Acetylation of core histones is associated with chromosomal assembly during DNA replication.
3. Phosphorylation of histone H1 is associated with the condensation of chromosomes during the replication cycle.
4. ADP-ribosylation of histones is associated with DNA repair.
5. Methylation of histones is correlated with activation and repression of gene transcription.
6. Monoubiquitylation is associated with gene activation, repression, and heterochromatic gene silencing.
7. Sumoylation of histones (SUMO; small ubiquitin-related modifier) is associated with transcription repression.

Murray RK, Bender DA, Botham KM, Kennelly PJ, Rodwell VW, Weil PA. *Harper's Illustrated Biochemistry*, 29th ed. New York, NY: McGraw-Hill; 2012.

Eukaryotic Cell Cycles

Most eukaryotic cells will proceed through an ordered series of events in which the cell duplicates its contents and then divides into two cells. This cycle of duplication and division is called the **cell cycle**. In order to maintain the fidelity of the developing organism this process of cell division in multicellular organisms must be highly ordered and tightly regulated. The loss of control will lead to abnormal development and is the cause of cancer. The eukaryotic cell cycle is composed of four steps, or phases identified as G_1, S, G_2, and M (Table 35-2). Not all cells continue to divide during the life span of an organism. Many cells undergo what is referred to as **terminal differentiation** and become quiescent and no longer divide and reside in a cell cycle phase termed G_0. Under certain conditions, such as that resulting from an external signal stimulating cell growth, cells can exit the quiescent state and reenter the cell cycle.

During M-phase there is an ordered series of events that leads to the alignment and separation of the duplicated chromosomes (called sister chromatids). The steps of mitosis are termed prophase, prometaphase, metaphase, anaphase, and telophase. Although cytokinesis is the process by which the parental cell is physically separated into 2 new daughter cells, it actually begins during anaphase. During prophase the duplicated chromosomes condense while outside the nucleus the mitotic spindle assembles between the 2 centrosomes. The centrosome is an organelle that serves as the main microtubule-organizing center that is involved in the attachment of microtubules to the sister chromatids. During prometaphase the nuclear membrane breaks apart and the chromosomes can attach to spindle microtubules and begin active movement. During metaphase the chromosomes are aligned at the equator of the spindle midway between the spindle poles. The sister chromatids are attached to opposite poles of the spindle. During anaphase the sister chromatids synchronously separate to form the 2 sets of daughter chromosomes. Each sister chromatid is slowly pulled toward the spindle pole it faces. During telophase the 2 daughter chromosomes arrive at the spindle poles and decondense. A new nuclear envelope forms around each set of chromosomes which forms the 2 new nuclei. This process marks the end of mitosis and sets the stage for cytokinesis.

Checkpoints and Cell Cycle Regulation

The processes that drive a cell through the cell cycle must be highly regulated so as to ensure that the resultant daughter cells are viable and each contains the complement of DNA found in the original parental cell. Many important genes involved in the regulation of cell cycle transit have been identified and are referred to as

TABLE 35-2: Overview of the Cell Cycle

	Phase	*Description*
Interphase	G_0	Period of no cell replication/division, usually entered from G_1 restriction checkpoint. Cell cycle progression is halted by an inhibitory protein cyclin-dependent kinase inhibitor 2A that blocks the interaction of CDK4 with cyclin D. G_0 cells lose cell cycle proteins, including cyclins and CDKs.
	G_1	Period of high rate of cell growth/protein production in preparation for DNA synthesis. Entry into G_1 relies on the G_1 restriction checkpoint in which binding of CDK4 to cyclin D leads to phosphorylation of the tumor suppressor retinoblastoma (Rb) protein. Phosphorylated Rb dissociates from the E2F transcription promoter, leading to the expression of cyclin E. Cyclin E activates CDK2, allowing progression into S-phase. These checks prepare the cell for DNA synthesis and cell cycle continuation.
	S	Synthesis phase during which DNA replication occurs. RNA transcription is very low except for that involved in histone production.
	G_2	Second period of cell growth between DNA synthesis and cell division (mitosis), mainly involving synthesis of microtubules for the mitotic spindle and chromosome condensation. The G_2 checkpoint prepares the cell for cell division and cell cycle continuation. This process is controlled by dephosphorylation of tyrosine residues in the maturation/mitosis-promoting factor complex, made of cyclin B (or A) and CDK1. CDK1 is activated, causing irreversible progression to mitosis. When the cell is unprepared for mitosis, Cdc25 can be inactivated by phosphorylation by a protein kinase.
Cell Division	M	No cell growth. Alignment of the replicated chromosomes and the tension created by the protein attachment of the mitotic spindle to the centromeres and the mitotic plate initiate mitosis. When the tension is sufficient, cyclin B is degraded, allowing activity of the anaphase-promoting complex (APC). Activated APC leads to degradation of the kinetichore structural protein securin, releasing its inhibition on separase, the protein that leads to the separation of the sister chromatids.

CDK, cyclin-dependent kinase; DNA, deoxyribonucleic acid.
(Used with permission from Janson LW, Tischler ME. *The Big Picture: Medical Biochemistry*, p. 114, 2012, New York: McGraw-Hill.)

cell division cycle genes (or ***cdc*** genes). Many of these genes encode proteins that control progression through the phases of a cell cycle at specific points called checkpoints or restriction points.

In addition to cell cycle checkpoints there is the need for cell cycle control mechanisms to exert their influences at specific times during each transit through a cell cycle. The heart of this timing control is the responsibility of a family of protein kinases that are called **cyclin-dependent kinases, CDK** (Table 35-3). The kinase activity of these enzymes rises and falls as the cell progresses through a cell cycle. Different CDK operate at different points in the cell cycle. The oscillating changes in the activity of CDK leads to oscillating changes in the phosphorylation of various intracellular proteins. These phosphorylations alter the activity of the modified proteins which then effect changes in events of the cell cycle. The cyclical activity of each CDK is controlled by a complex series of proteins, the most important of which are the **cyclins**, hence the name of the enzymes as cyclin-dependent kinases. The cyclins are so called because their levels cycle up and down as the cell progresses through the phase of the cell cycle. Four different classes of cyclins have been defined on the basis of the stage of the cell cycle in which they bind and activate CDKs. These 4 classes are G_1-cyclins, G_1/S-cyclins, S-cyclins, and M-cyclins.

TABLE 35-3: Cyclins and Cyclin-Dependent Kinases Involved in Cell-Cycle Progression

Cyclin	*Kinase*	*Function*
D	CDK4, CDK6	Progression past restriction point at G_1/S boundary
E, A	CDK2	Initiation of DNA synthesis in early S phase
B	CDK1	Transition from G_2 to M

Murray RK, Bender DA, Botham KM, Kennelly PJ, Rodwell VW, Weil PA. *Harper's Illustrated Biochemistry*, 29th ed. New York: McGraw-Hill; 2012.

In addition to control of CDK kinase activity by cyclin binding, control is exerted to inhibit CDK activity through interaction with inhibitory proteins as well as by inhibitory phosphorylation events. Thus, there is extremely tight control on the overall activity of each CDK. Proteins that bind to and inhibit cyclin-CDK complexes are called **CDK inhibitory proteins** (CKI, for cyclin-kinase inhibitor). Mammalian cells express 2 classes of CKI. These are called CIP for CDK inhibitory proteins and INK4 for inhibitors of kinase 4. The CIP bind and inhibit CDK1, CDK2, CDK4, and CDK6 complexes, whereas the INK4 bind and inhibit only the CDK4 and CDK6 complexes. There are at least 3 CIP proteins (p21, p27, and p57) and 4 INK proteins (p15, p16, p18, and p19) in mammalian cells. Working in concert, each of these proteins plays a critical role in controlling entry of cells into the cell cycle in response to mitogenic stimuli and to restrict entry in the presence of DNA damage (Figure 35-6).

The cyclical degradation of the cyclins is effected through the action of several different ubiquitin ligase complexes (Chapter 37). There are 2 important ubiquitin ligase complexes that control the turnover of cyclins and other cell cycle regulating proteins. One is the SCF complex which functions to control the transit from G_1 to S-phase and the other is called **anaphase-promoting complex (APC),** which controls the levels of the M-phase cyclins as well as other regulators of mitosis.

Tumor Suppressors and Cell Cycle Regulation

Tumor suppressors (Chapter 52) are so called because cancer ensues as a result of a loss of their normal function, that is, these proteins suppress the ability of cancer to develop. Several tumor suppressor proteins are required for regulation of cell cycle progression. Following the isolation and characterization of 2 tumor suppressor genes in particular it was found that they function to control the ability of cells to progress beyond important checkpoints in the cell cycle. The protein encoded by the retinoblastoma susceptibility gene (*pRB*) and the p53 protein are both tumor suppressors. The function of pRB is to prevent cells from exiting G_1 (see Figure 52-3) and that of p53 is to inhibit progression from G_1 to S-phase as well as from S-phase to M-phase (see Figure 52-4).

DNA Replication

As pointed out above, replication of DNA occurs during S-phase of normal cell division cycles. Because the genetic complement of the resultant daughter

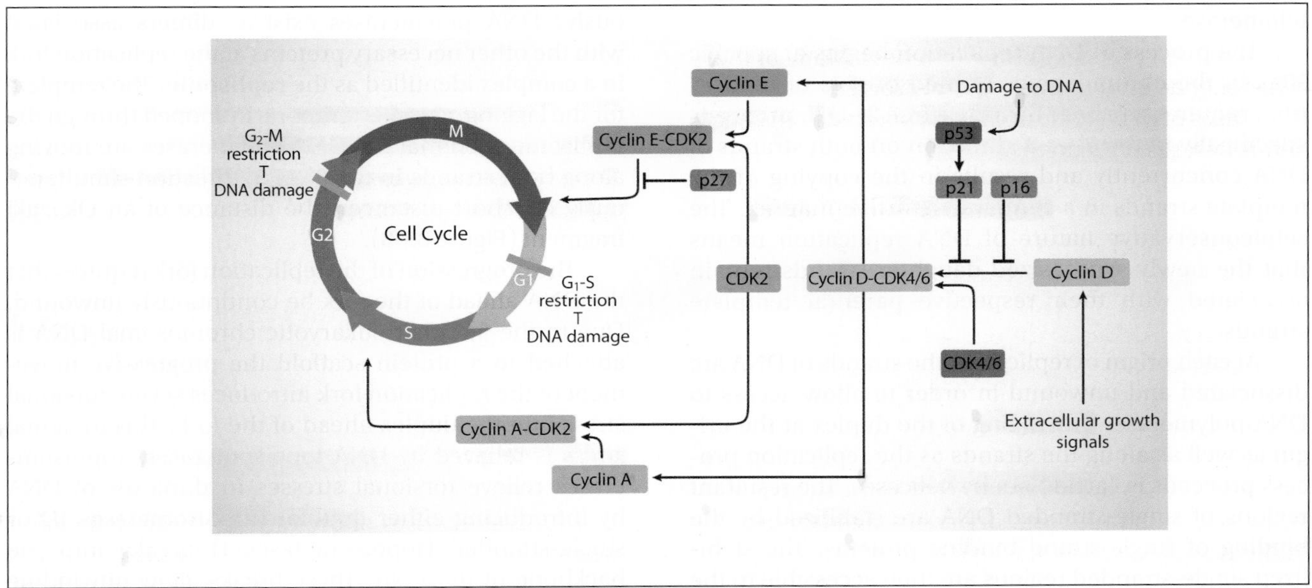

FIGURE 35-6: Overview of cell cycle control. Cells enter the cell cycle in response to various growth and mitogenic signals. These signals activate the modification of preexisting regulatory proteins and also induce the expression of genes encoding regulatory proteins. If a cell sustains DNA damage, cell cycle inhibitors can be activated to ensure that the cell does not enter S-phase until the damage has been repaired. Reproduced with permission of themedicalbiochemistrypage, LLC.

TABLE 35-4: Classes of Proteins Involved in Replication

Protein	*Function*
DNA polymerases	Deoxynucleotide polymerization
Helicases	Processive unwinding of DNA
Topoisomerases	Relieve torsional strain that results from helicase-induced unwinding
DNA primase	Initiates synthesis of RNA primers
Single-strand binding proteins	Prevent premature reannealing of dsDNA
DNA ligase	Seals the single strand nick between the nascent chain and Okazaki fragments on lagging strand

Murray RK, Bender DA, Botham KM, Kennelly PJ, Rodwell VW, Weil PA. *Harper's Illustrated Biochemistry*, 29th ed. New York: McGraw-Hill; 2012.

cells must be the same as the parental cell, DNA replication must possess a very high degree of fidelity. The entire process of DNA replication is complex and involves multiple enzymatic activities with the actual replication being catalyzed by DNA polymerases (Table 35-4).

Eukaryotic cells express several DNA polymerases that function in distinct types of DNA replication. These DNA polymerases are divided into 4 large families designated A, B, X, and Y (Table 35-5). In addition, there is a reverse transcriptase activity associated with telomerase.

The process of DNA replication begins at specific sites in the chromosomes termed origins of replication, requires a primer bearing a free 3′-OH, proceeds specifically in the 5′ → 3′ direction on both strands of DNA concurrently and results in the copying of the template strands in a **semiconservative** manner. The semiconservative nature of DNA replication means that the newly synthesized daughter strands remain associated with their respective parental template strands.

At each origin of replication the strands of DNA are dissociated and unwound in order to allow access to DNA polymerase. Unwinding of the duplex at the origin as well as along the strands as the replication process proceeds is carried out by helicases. The resultant regions of single-stranded DNA are stabilized by the binding of single-strand binding proteins. The stabilized single-stranded regions are then accessible to the enzymatic activities required for replication to proceed. The site of the unwound template strands is termed the **replication fork** (Figure 35-7).

In order for DNA polymerases to synthesize DNA they must encounter a free 3′-OH which is the substrate for attachment of the 5′-phosphate of the incoming nucleotide. During repair of damaged DNA the 3′-OH can arise from the hydrolysis of the backbone of one of the two strands. During replication the 3′-OH is supplied through the use of an RNA primer, synthesized by the primase activity which is DNA polymerase α.

Synthesis of DNA proceeds in the 5′ → 3′ direction through the attachment of the 5′-phosphate of an incoming dNTP to the existing 3′-OH in the elongating DNA strands with the concomitant release of pyrophosphate. While incorporating dNTP into DNA in the 5′ → 3′ direction DNA plymerases move in the 3′ → 5′ direction with respect to the template strand. Synthesis proceeds bidirectionally, with one strand in each direction being copied continuously and one strand in each direction being copied discontinuously. The strand of DNA synthesized continuously is termed the **leading strand** and the discontinuous strand is termed the **lagging strand**. The lagging strand of DNA is composed of short stretches of RNA primer plus newly synthesized DNA approximately 100- to 200-base long. The lagging strands of DNA are also called **Okazaki fragments**. The gaps that exist between the 3′-OH of one leading strand and the 5′-phosphate of another as well as between one Okazaki fragment and another are repaired by DNA ligases, thereby completing the process of replication.

How is it that DNA polymerase can copy both strands of DNA in the 5′ → 3′ direction simultaneously? DNA polymerases exist as dimers associated with the other necessary proteins at the replication fork in a complex identified as the **replisome**. The template for the lagging strand is temporarily looped through the replisome such that the DNA polymerases are moving along both strands in the 3′ → 5′ direction simultaneously for short distances, the distance of an Okazaki fragment (Figure 35-8).

The progression of the replication fork requires that the DNA ahead of the fork be continuously unwound. Due to the fact that eukaryotic chromosomal DNA is attached to a protein scaffold the progressive movement of the replication fork introduces severe torsional stress into the duplex ahead of the fork. This torsional stress is relieved by DNA topoisomerases. Topoisomerases relieve torsional stresses in duplexes of DNA by introducing either double- (topoisomerases II) or single-stranded (topoisomerases I) breaks into the backbone of the DNA. These breaks allow unwinding of the duplex and removal of the replication-induced torsional strain. The nicks are then resealed by the topoisomerases.

TABLE 35-5: Eukaryotic DNA Polymerases

Polymerase Family	*Common Nomenclature*	*Enzyme Function, Comments*
A	γ (gamma)	Mitochondrial DNA replication; encoded by the *POLG* gene
A	θ (theta)	DNA repair; encoded by the *POLQ* gene
B	α (alpha)	Initiation of chromosomal DNA replication, Okazaki fragment priming, also involved in double-strand break repair; encoded by the *POLA* gene
B	δ (delta)	Chromosomal DNA replication elongation, nucleotide excision repair, double-strand break repair, mismatch repair; consists of a multisubunit complex that includes the 4 subunit polymerase complex encoded by the *POLD1, POLD2, POLD3,* and *POLD4* genes as well as the multisubunit replication factor C protein (RFC1) and proliferating cell nuclear antigen (PCNA)
B	ε (epsilon)	Chromosomal DNA replication elongation, nucleotide excision repair, double-strand break repair, mismatch repair; consists of a 261-kDa catalytic subunit encoded by the *POLE* gene and a 55-kDa accessory protein encoded by the *POLE2* gene, additional proteins in the epsilon complex include 2 histone-fold proteins encoded by the *POLE3* and *POLE4* genes
B	ζ (zeta)	Bypass (translesion) DNA synthesis; encoded by the *POLZ* gene; also known as REV3; enzyme responsible for essentially all DNA damage-induced mutagenesis as well as the majority of spontaneous mutagenesis
X	β (beta)	Base-excision repair, required for DNA replication and maintenance, recombination, and drug-resistance; encoded by the *POLB* gene
X	λ (lambda)	Base-excision repair; encoded by the *POLL* gene
X	μ (mu)	Nonhomologous end joining (NHEJ); encoded by the *POLM* gene
X	σ (sigma)	Sister chromatid cohesion; encoded by the *POLS* gene; also known as topoisomerase-related function protein 4 (TRF4) and poly(A) polymerase-associated domain-containing protein 7 (PAPD7)
Y	η (eta)	Bypass (translesion) DNA synthesis; encoded by the *POLH* gene; required for replication through UV-induced cyclobutane pyrimidine dimers (CPD); mutations in *POLH* result in Xeroderma pigmentosum variant (XP-V)
Y	ι (iota)	Bypass (translesion) DNA synthesis; encoded by the *POLI* gene; also known as RAD30B
Y	κ (kappa)	Bypass (translesion) DNA synthesis; encoded by the *POLK*
Y	Rev1L	Bypass (translesion) DNA synthesis; interacts with *POLK* and is essential for *POLK* function

Additional Activities of DNA Polymerases

The main enzymatic activity of DNA polymerases is the 5′ → 3′ synthetic activity. However, DNA polymerases possess 2 additional activities of importance for both replication and repair. These additional activities include a 5′ → 3′ exonuclease function and a 3′ → 5′ exonuclease function. The 5′ → 3′ exonuclease activity allows the removal of ribonucleotides of the RNA primer, utilized to initiate DNA synthesis, along with their simultaneous replacement with deoxyribonucleotides by the 5′ → 3′ polymerase activity. The 5′ → 3′ exonuclease activity is also utilized during the repair of damaged DNA. The 3′ → 5′ exonuclease function is utilized during replication to allow DNA polymerase to remove mismatched bases, termed **"proof-reading."** These mismatched bases are recognized by the polymerase immediately due to the lack of Watson-Crick base-pairing.

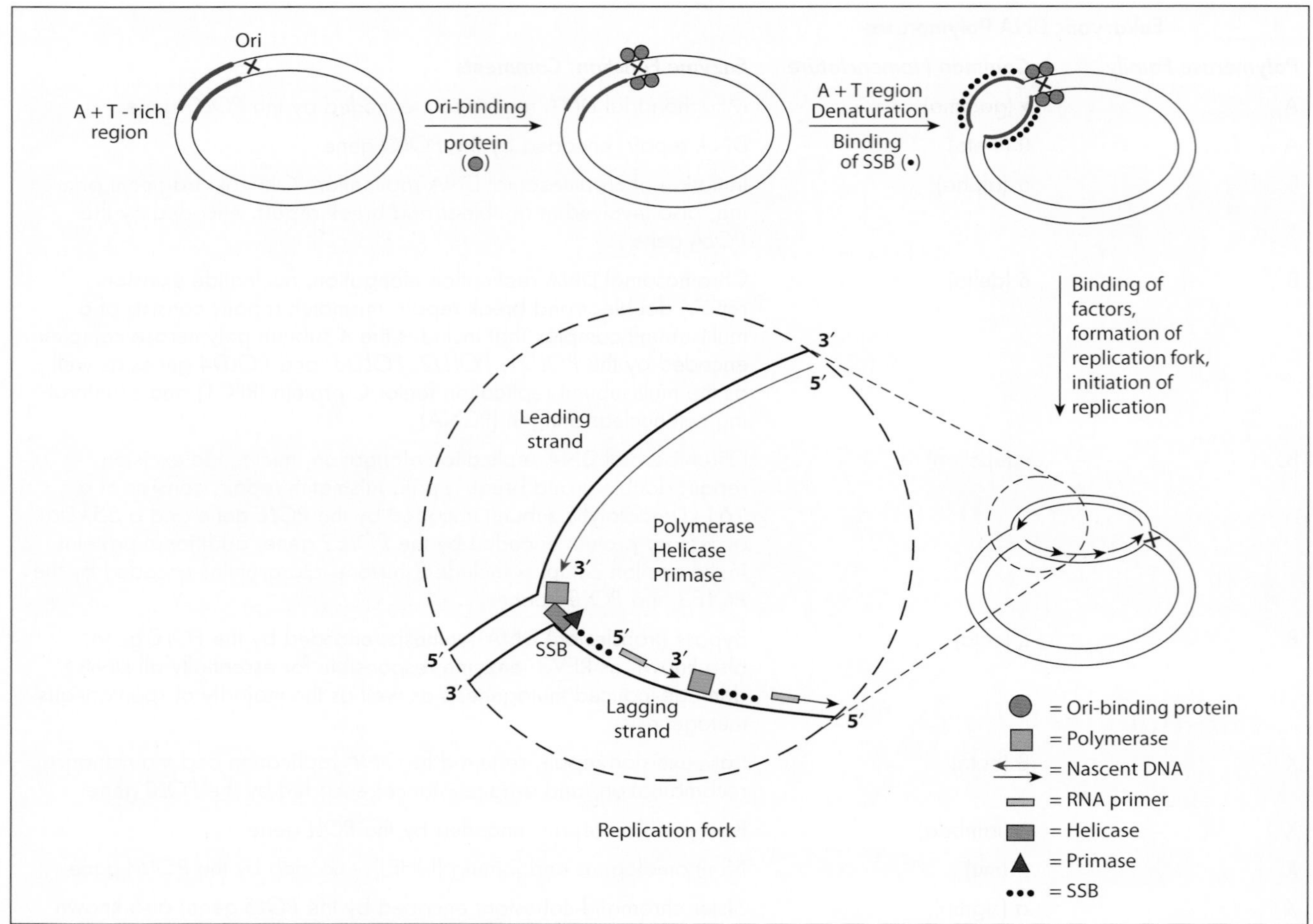

FIGURE 35-7: Steps involved in DNA replication. This figure describes DNA replication in an *Escherichia coli* cell, but the general steps are similar in eukaryotes. A specific interaction of a protein to the origin of replication (Ori) results in local unwinding of DNA at an adjacent A+T-rich region. The DNA in this area is maintained in the single-strand conformation (ssDNA) by single-strand–binding proteins (SSBs). This allows a variety of proteins, including helicase, primase, and DNA polymerase to bind and to initiate DNA synthesis. The replication fork proceeds as DNA synthesis occurs continuously (long red arrow) on the leading strand and discontinuously (short black arrows) on the lagging strand. The nascent DNA is always synthesized in the 5′ to 3′ direction, as DNA polymerases can add a nucleotide only to the 3′ end of a DNA strand. Murray RK, Bender DA, Botham KM, Kennelly PJ, Rodwell VW, Weil PA: *Harper's Illustrated Biochemistry*, 29th ed. New York: McGraw-Hill; 2012.

Telomere Replication: Implications for Aging and Disease

Telomeres are the specialized DNA structures at the ends of all chromosomes. Telomeres consist of repetitive DNA sequences and nucleoproteins, the overall structure of which is referred to as a nucleoprotein cap. The telomere sequence on the lagging strand is composed of the repeat 5′-TTAGGG-3′. The telomeric repeat sequence spans up to several kilobases and is involved in protecting the ends of the chromosomes from exonuclease activity.

The telomeric ends of the lagging strand of each chromosome require a unique method of replication which involves the activity of the enzyme complex called **telomerase**. Telomerase is complex composed of several proteins, an RNA with sequence complimentary to the telomeric repeats, and a reverse transcriptase activity that extends the 3′-end of the lagging strands using the telomerase RNA as the template (Figure 35-9). The reverse transcriptase activity of telomerase is encoded by the *TERT* gene (**te**lomerase **r**everse **t**ranscriptase) and the RNA component is encoded by the *TERC* gene (**te**lomerase **R**NA **c**omponent). The TERC RNA contains a repeating hexanucleotide sequence, 3′-AAUCCC-5′,

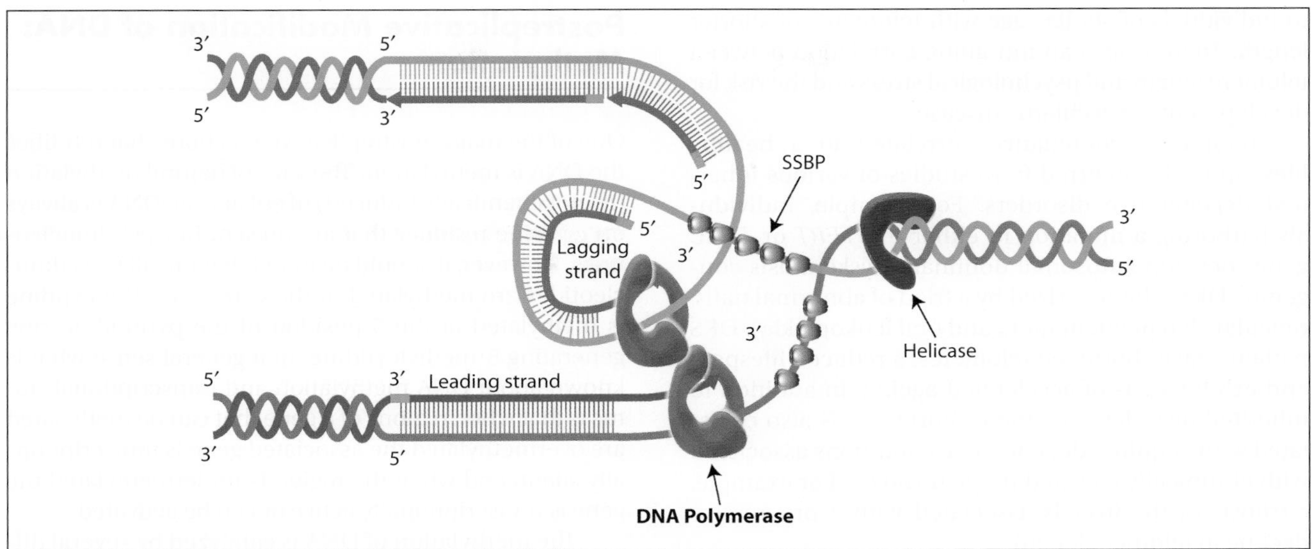

FIGURE 35-8: Details of the mechanism by which both strands of DNA are replicated simultaneously in the same direction. A portion of the lagging strand is looped around through the DNA polymerase holoenzyme complex such that short stretches of 500–1000 can be continuously replicated in the same direction as the leading strand. Eventually torsional stress will result in disassociation of the enzyme complex and the looping process will need to begin again. This is what results in the average length of the Okasaki fragments generated from the lagging strand. Only DNA helicase, single-strand binding proteins (SSBPs), and the DNA polymerase complex are shown. Reproduced with permission of themedicalbiochemistrypage, LLC.

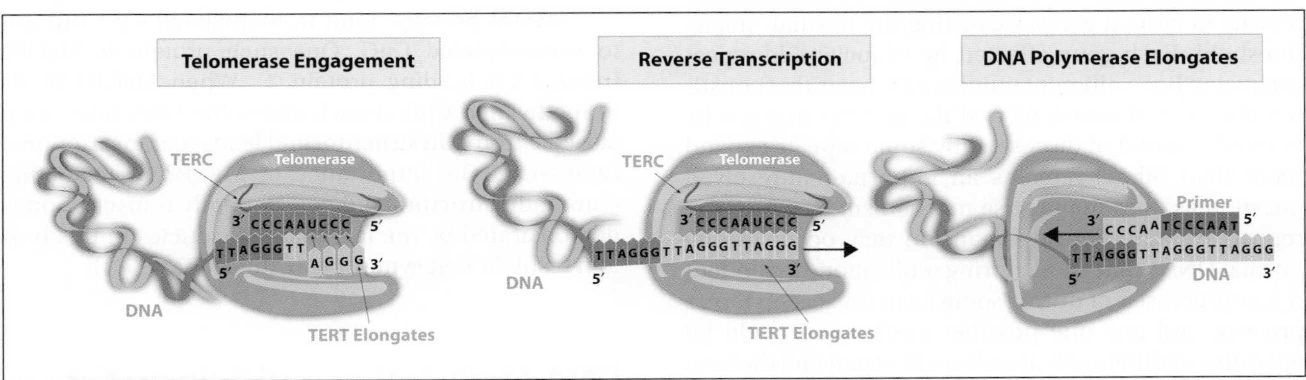

FIGURE 35-9: Steps in telomere replication by telomerase. Reproduced with permission of themedicalbiochemistrypage, LLC.

that spans between 3 and 20 kilobases. This sequence in the TERC RNA forms a duplex with the lagging DNA strand at the ends of the chromosomes. The 3′-end of the lagging strand then serves as the primer for the reverse transcriptase activity (TERT) which extends the 3′-end of the chromosome using the TERC RNA as a template. The telomerase process extends the end of the lagging strand that can then be replicated by normal DNA polymerase, thereby preserving the length of the chromosome.

Telomere shortening is associated with the activation of programmed cell death (apoptosis), loss of tissue stem cells, disease progression, and the overall processes of aging. Decreased telomere length in peripheral blood leukocytes has been shown to correlate with higher mortality rates in older (> 60 years of age) individuals. This is contrasted by studies in centenarians and their offspring that have shown a positive link between telomere length and longevity. Individuals with longer telomeres exhibit an overall healthier profile relative to individuals of similar age with telomeres of shorter length. There is also an intriguing correlation between telomere length and psychological stress and the risk for development of psychiatric disease.

Telomere maintenance correlated to a healthy lifespan is also inferred from studies of various inherited degenerative disorders. For example, individuals harboring a mutation in either the *TERT* or *TERC* genes develop autosomal dominant dyskeratosis congenita, DKS (characterized by a triad of abnormal nails, reticular skin pigmentation, and oral leukoplakia). DKS patients have shortened telomeres, a reduced lifespan, and exhibit signs of accelerated ageing. In addition to inherited disorders, telomere shortening is also correlated with acquired degenerative conditions associated with chronically elevated tissue turnover. For example, cirrhosis of the liver is associated with a progressive decline in telomere length.

Trinucleotide Repeat Expansion

The trinucleotide repeat disorders (also known as trinucleotide repeat expansion disorders or triplet repeat expansion disorders) are a set of genetic disorders caused by an increase in the number of trinucleotide repeats in certain genes exceeding the normal, stable, threshold. Each gene affected by trinucleotide repeat expansion has a different number of repeats that constitute the normal threshold and the number that results in manifestation of disease. Why some repeats expand more than others remains an important unresolved question as does the precise mechanism by which the repeats expand. Repeat expansion may occur during normal DNA replication, during replication-dependent repair processes, or during some form of excision repair process, and any one possible mechanism could be operative in different types of repeat expansion disease. Currently, repeat expansion is thought to occur through the formation of looped intermediates which are then incorporated into DNA.

The trinucleotide repeat disorders are divided into 2 categories determined by the type of repeat. The most common repeat is the triplet CAG which when present in the coding region of a gene codes for the amino acid glutamine (Q). Therefore, these disorders are referred to as the **polyglutamine (polyQ) disorders** with the best known disorder of this type being Huntington disease (Clinical Box 35-1). The remaining disorders, either do not involve the CAG triplet, or the CAG triplet is not in the coding region of the gene and are, therefore, referred to as the **nonpolyglutamine disorders**. Fragile X syndrome (Clinical Box 35-2) is the best known form of a nonpolyglutamine expansion disorder.

Postreplicative Modification of DNA: Methylation

One of the major postreplicative reactions that modifies the DNA is methylation. The sites of natural methylation (ie, not chemically induced) of eukaryotic DNA is always on cytosine residues that are present in CpG dinucleotides. However, it should be noted that not all CpG dinucleotides are methylated at the C residue. The cytidine is methylated at the 5 position of the pyrimidine ring generating 5-methylcytidine. In a general sense what is known about DNA methylation and transcriptional status is that when regions of a gene that can be methylated are overmethylated the associated gene is transcriptionally silent, and when the region is undermethylated the gene is transcriptionally active or can be activated.

The methylation of DNA is catalyzed by several different DNA methyltransferases (DNMT). When cells divide the DNA contains 1 strand of parental DNA and 1 strand of the newly replicated DNA (the daughter strand). If the DNA contains methylated cytidines in CpG dinucleotides the daughter strand must undergo methylation in order to maintain the parental pattern of methylation. This "maintenance" methylation is catalyzed by DNMT1, and thus this enzyme is called the maintenance methylase (Figure 35-10).

Several proteins bind to methylated CpG but not to unmethylated CpG. One such protein is MeCP2 (methyl Cp binding protein 2). When MeCP2 binds to methylated CpG dinucleotides the DNA takes on a closed chromatin structure and leads to transcriptional repression. The importance of MeCP2 in regulating chromatin structure and consequently transcription is demonstrated by the fact that deficiencies in this protein result in Rett syndrome (Clinical Box 35-3).

DNA Methylation and Epigenetics

The term epigenetics is used to define the mechanism by which changes in the pattern of inherited gene expression occur in the absence of alterations or changes in the nucleotide composition of a given gene. Several different types of epigenetic events have been identified and include DNA methylation. DNA methylation is likely to be the most important epigenetic event controlling and maintaining the pattern of gene expression during development.

Whereas epigenesis plays a vital role in the regulation, control, and maintenance of gene expression leading to the many differentiation states of cells in an organism, recent evidence has identified a linkage between epigenetic processes and disease. Most significant is

CLINICAL BOX 35-1: HUNTINGTON DISEASE

Huntington disease (HD) is an autosomal dominantly inherited disease characterized by slowly progressive neurodegeneration associated with choreic movements (abnormal involuntary movements) and dementia. The pathology of HD reveals neurodegeneration in the corpus striatum and shrinkage of the brain. HD is caused by expansion of a CAG trinucleotide repeat in the first exon of the huntingtin gene. The CAG repeat resides 17 codons downstream of the initiator AUG codon. The range of CAG repeat size in normal individuals is 6 to 34 and in affected individuals it is 36 to 121. Repeat growth from a premutation length (29–35) to the disease range (>35) occurs almost exclusively through paternal transmission. The longer the length of the CAG repeat, the earlier is the onset of symptoms. However, there is a wide degree of variation in age of onset for any given length of CAG repeat. Thus, the CAG repeat number itself is not predictive for age of onset. The variation in age of onset is related to the effects of other modifying genes, the environment, and the length of the CAG repeat. In addition, HD exhibits a genetic phenomenon termed "**anticipation**" which means that the symptoms of the disease appear earlier and are more severe in subsequent generations. This phenomenon is explained by meiotic instability which increases the CAG repeat number and is greater in spermatogenesis than in oogenesis. Therefore, anticipation is mainly observed when the mutation is inherited through the paternal line. Wild-type huntingtin protein is found primarily in the cytoplasm with a small percentage being intranuclear. The protein is associated with the plasma membrane, the ER, the Golgi apparatus, endocytic vesicles, the mitochondria, and microtubules. Although the exact function of Huntingtin is still poorly defined, it is known that the protein is essential for early embryonic development, is important in adult neurons and testes for cellular viability, and has a role in regulation of transcription through its interaction with numerous transcription factors and other proteins involved in the regulation of mRNA production. The classical symptoms of Huntington disease consist of progressive dementia, evolving involuntary movements and psychiatric disturbances that include personality changes and mood disorder. Choreic movements are the most prominent physical abnormality in HD and as such the disease was early on referred to as Huntington's chorea. The earliest indications of HD are the appearance of spasmodic twitching of the extremities, generally beginning with the fingers. Additional early physical manifestations of HD are clumsiness, hyperreflexia, and eye movement disturbances. Positron-emission tomography (PET scanning) is used to demonstrate a loss of uptake of glucose in the caudate nuclei and is a valuable indication of affectation in the presymptomatic period in HD patients. There is no cure for HD and all afflicted individuals will succumb to the disease. The age of death in HD is related to the age of onset, that is, the earlier the onset, the earlier an individual will die.

CLINICAL BOX 35-2: FRAGILE X SYNDROME

Fragile X syndrome is an X-linked dominant disorder representing the most common form of inherited mental retardation. The syndrome belongs to a family of disorders that are related to the relationship between fragile chromosomal sites and disease. Fragile chromosomal sites are only detectable in vitro when cells are exposed to chemical agents that disrupt the DNA replication process. Fragile X syndrome occurs with a frequency of approximately 1 in 4000 males and 1 in 8000 females. Affected males will exhibit moderate to severe mental retardation as well as a speech delay, hyperactivity, and behavioral and social difficulties. Fragile X syndrome results from the expansion of a CGG trinucleotide repeat in the *FMR1* gene which encodes the FMRP protein. The CGG repeat resides in the 5′-untranslated region (UTR) of the *FMR1* gene. Normal individuals have 6 to 60 CGG repeats and the premutation size is between 55 and 200 repeats. A full mutation in affected individuals is more than 200 repeats. Repeat expansion from the premutation length to a full-mutation length occurs almost exclusively through maternal transmission. Males with the premutation-sized expansion develop a late-onset neurodegenerative condition termed fragile X-associated tremor/ataxia syndrome (FXTAS). In females with the premutation expansion there is a 25% chance of their developing ovarian failure.

CLINICAL BOX 35-2: (*Continued*)

The encoded FMRP protein is an RNA-binding protein found in ribonucleoprotein complexes associated with polyribosomes. Early during human fetal development the *FMR1* gene is expressed at highest levels in cholinergic neurons of the nucleus basalis magnocellularis and in pyramidal neurons of the hippocampus which may contribute to the pathogenesis of the syndrome. One important pathway involving the activity of FMRP is the metabotropic glutamate receptor-(mGluR) dependent long-term depression (LTD) pathway. Glutamate functions in both the central and peripheral nervous systems are involved in memory, learning, anxiety, and the perception of pain. The characteristic symptoms of fragile X syndrome in males are moderate to severe mental retardation. In males with the full mutation (>200 repeats) the physical hallmarks of the disorder include a long narrow face, prominent ears, and macroorchidism (large testicles). These physical signs are most apparent in postpubertal males. Additional physical findings can include hyperextensible finger joints, flat feet, double jointed thumbs, and a high arched plate. Fragile X syndrome also manifests with distinct behavioral abnormalities that include hyperactivity, anxiety, extreme sensitivity to stimulation and sensations, hyperarousal, and occasionally aggressive tendencies. The behavioral anomalies overlap with those of autism such as impaired verbal and nonverbal communication, difficulty with social interactions, poor eye contact, tactile defensiveness, hand flapping, and hand biting. Females with a full mutation are less affected with respect to all aspects of the mental and physical characteristics of fragile X syndrome due to the process of X chromosome inactivation.

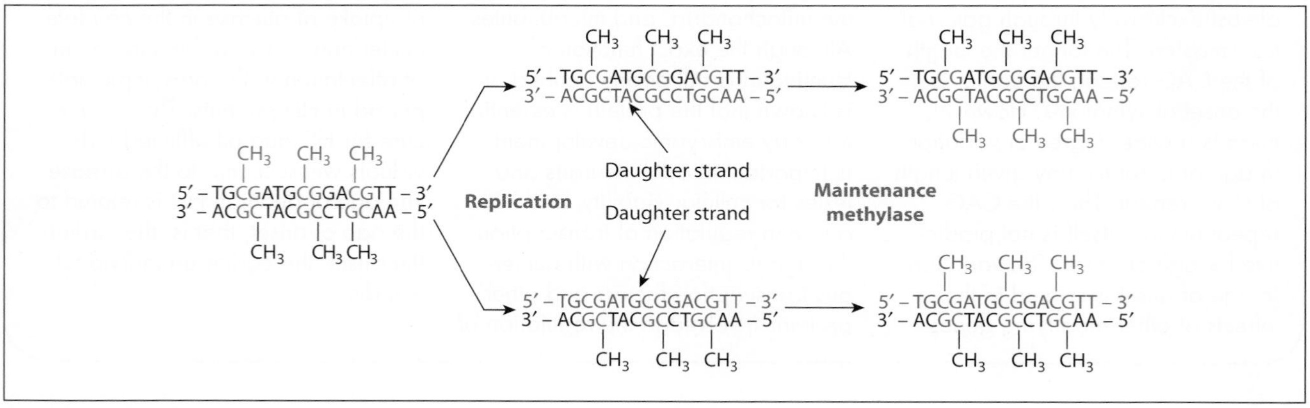

FIGURE 35-10: Process of maintenance methylation of DNA following replication. Reproduced with permission of themedicalbiochemistrypage, LLC.

the link between epigenesis and cancer which has been suggested to be a contributing factor in nearly half of all cancers. A clear demonstration has been made between changes in the methylation status of tumor suppressor genes and the development of many types of cancers.

DNA Methylation and Imprinting

The phenomenon of genomic imprinting refers to the fact that the expression of some genes depends on whether or not they are inherited maternally or paternally. Imprinted genes are "marked" by their state of methylation. At least 41 different imprinted loci have been identified in the human genome. Incorrect inheritance of, or mutations/deletions in, imprinted loci is associated with numerous disorders. These include Prader-Willi syndrome, Angelman syndrome, and Beckwith-Weidemann syndrome.

DNA Recombination

DNA recombination refers to the phenomenon whereby 2 parental strands of DNA are spliced together resulting in an exchange of portions of their respective strands.

CLINICAL BOX 35-3: RETT SYNDROME

Rett syndrome is one of the most common causes of complex disability in girls. It is characterized by early neurological regression that severely affects motor, cognitive, and communication skills; autonomic dysfunction, and often a seizure disorder, microcephaly, and arrested development. Characteristic of Rett syndrome is a delay in acquiring new skills, absence of speech, emergence of autistic features, loss of purposeful manipulation skills along with other motor abnormalities that includes abnormal muscle tone, ataxia, and apraxia. Rett syndrome is a monogenic X-linked dominant disorder resulting from mutations in the *MECP2* gene encoding the methyl-CpG-binding protein MeCP2. Seven point mutations account for around 70% of Rett syndrome cases. The MeCP2 protein is ubiquitously present but is most abundantly expressed in the brain. MeCP2 suppresses the transcription of other tissue-specific genes whose activity is not required. Loss of function of MeCP2 in differentiated postmitotic neurons likely results in the inappropriate overexpression of these other genes, with potentially damaging effect during central nervous system maturation. To date the only clear MeCP2 target gene is brain-derived neurotrophic factor, *BDNF*, which is an essential gene for learning and neural plasticity.

This process leads to new molecules of DNA that contain a mix of genetic information from each parental strand.

Homologous recombination is the most common type of DNA recombination occurring in eukaryotic cells. This involves a process of genetic exchange that occurs between any 2 molecules of DNA that share a region (or regions) of homologous DNA sequences (Figure 35-11). This form of recombination occurs frequently while sister chromatids are paired prior to mitosis. Indeed, it is the process of homologous recombination between the maternal and paternal chromosomes that imparts genetic diversity to an organism. Homologous recombination generally involves exchange of large regions of the chromosomes.

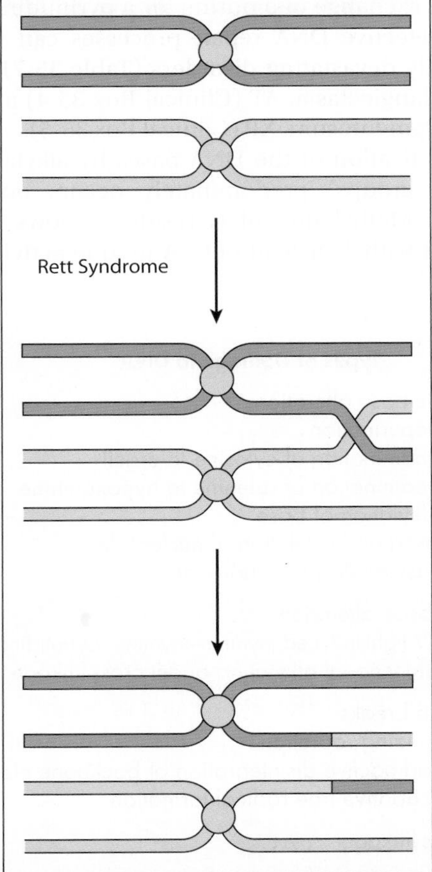

FIGURE 35-11: The process of crossing over between homologous metaphase chromosomes to generate recombinant chromosomes. Murray RK, Bender DA, Botham KM, Kennelly PJ, Rodwell VW, Weil PA. Harper's Illustrated Biochemistry, 29th ed. New York: McGraw-Hill; 2012.

DNA Transposition

Transposition is a unique form of recombination where mobile genetic elements can virtually move from one region to another within one chromosome or to another chromosome entirely. There is no requirement for sequence homology for a transpositional event to occur. Transposition does require an enzymatic activity encoded by the mobile genetic element called transposase. Because the potential exists for the disruption of a vitally important gene by a transposition event this process must be tightly regulated. The exact nature of how transpositional events are controlled is unclear.

The identification of the occurrence of transposition in the human genome resulted when it was found that certain processed genes were present in the genome. These processed genes are nearly identical to the mRNA encoded by the normal gene. The processed genes contain the poly(A) tail that would have been present in the RNA and they lack the introns of the normal gene. Since most of the processed genes that have been identified are nonfunctional they have been termed pseudogenes.

Repair of Damaged DNA

DNA damage (Table 35-6) can occur as the result of exposure to environmental stimuli such as alkylating chemicals, ultraviolet or radioactive irradiation, and free radicals generated spontaneously in the oxidizing environment of the cell. These phenomena can, and do, lead to the introduction of mutations in the coding capacity of the DNA. Single-nucleotide mutations in DNA are of 2 types. Transition mutations result from the exchange of one purine or pyrimidine for another purine or pyrimidine. Transversion mutations result from the exchange of a purine for a pyrimidine or visa versa. Defective DNA repair processes can result in potentially devastating disorders (Table 35-7) such as ataxia telangiectasia, AT (Clinical Box 35-4) and xeroderma pigmentosum, XP (Clinical Box 35-5).

Modification of the DNA bases by alkylation (eg, $-CHCH_3$ groups) predominately occurs on purine residues. Methylation of G residues allows them to base pair with T instead of C. A unique activity called O^6-alkylguanine transferase removes the alkyl group from G residues. The protein itself becomes alkylated and is no longer active, thus a single protein molecule can remove only 1 alkyl group.

TABLE 35-6: Types of Damage to DNA

I. Single-base alteration A. Depurination B. Deamination of cytosine to uracil C. Deamination of adenine to hypoxanthine D. Alkylation of base E. Insertion or deletion of nucleotide F. Base-analog incorporation
II. Two-base alteration A. UV light-induced thymine–thymine (pyrimidine) dimer B. Bifunctional alkylating agent cross-linkage
III. Chain breaks A. Ionizing radiation B. Radioactive disintegration of backbone element C. Oxidative free radical formation
IV. Cross-linkage A. Between bases in same or opposite strands B. Between DNA and protein molecules (eg, histones)

Murray RK, Bender DA, Botham KM, Kennelly PJ, Rodwell VW, Weil PA. *Harper's Illustrated Biochemistry*, 29th ed. New York: McGraw-Hill; 2012.

TABLE 35-7: Human Diseases of DNA Damage Repair

Defective Non homologous End Joining Repair (NHEJ) Severe combined immunodeficiency disease (SCID) Radiation sensitive severe combined immunodeficiency disease (RS-SCID)
Defective Homologous Repair (HR) AT-like disorder (ATLD) Nijmegen breakage syndrome (NBS) Bloom syndrome (BS) Werner syndrome (WS) Rothmund thomson syndrome (RTS) Breast cancer suspectibility 1 and 2 (BRCA1, BRCA2)
Defective DNA Nucleotide Exicision Repair (NER) Xeromderma pigmentosum (XP) Cockayne syndrome (CS) Trichothiodystrophy (TTD)
Defective DNA Base Excision Repair (BER) MUTYH-associated polyposis (MAP)
Defective DNA Mismatch Repair (MMR) Hereditary non-polyposis colorectal cancer (HNPCC)

Murray RK, Bender DA, Botham KM, Kennelly PJ, Rodwell VW, Weil PA. *Harper's Illustrated Biochemistry*, 29th ed. New York: McGraw-Hill; 2012.

The prominent by-product from UV irradiation of DNA is the formation of pyrimidine dimers (most often thymidine dimers) between two adjacent pyrimidines in the DNA. Thymine dimers are removed by several mechanisms. Specific glycohydrolases recognize the dimer as abnormal and cleave the *N*-glycosidic bond of the bases in the dimer. This results in the base leaving and generates an apyrimidinic site in the DNA. This is repaired by DNA polymerase and ligase. Glycohydrolases are also responsible for the removal of other abnormal bases, not just thymine dimers. Another, widely distributed repair activity is DNA photolyase or photoreactivating enzyme. This protein binds to thymine dimers in the dark and visible light stimulates the enzyme to cleave the pyrimidine rings.

Chemotherapies Targeting Replication and the Cell cycle

The class of compounds that have been used the longest as anticancer drugs are the alkylating agents. The major alkylating agents are derived from nitrogenous

CLINICAL BOX 35-4: ATAXIA TELANGIECTASIA

Ataxia telangiectasia (AT) syndrome represents a disorder that is characterized by hypersensitivity to ionizing radiation, progressive truncal ataxia affecting the gait with onset by 1 to 3 years of age, slurring of speech, oculocutaneous telangiectasias that begin to develop by age 6, frequent infections and cellular immunodeficiencies, and susceptibility to leukemias and lymphomas. Telangiectasias are areas of the skin under which there are dilated superficial vessels resulting in an appearance similar to that in patients with rosacea or scleroderma. In addition, as is common in AT, the telangiectasias can develop in the eye. The AT syndrome results from mutations in the ataxia telangiectasia–mutated (ATM) gene. There are at least 4 complementation groups comprising the AT syndrome identified as ATA, ATC, ATD, and ATE all of which result from mutations in the ATM gene. Expression of the ATM gene is seen in all tissues with multiple mRNAs being derived by alternative splicing. The ATM protein is a member of the large-molecular-weight protein kinase family. Specifically, ATM is a member of the phosphatidylinositol-3-kinase (PI3K) family of kinases. The ATM kinase responds to DNA damage by initiating the phosphorylation of numerous proteins involved in DNA repair and/or cell cycle control. In the presence of mutant ATM, cell cycle arrest does not occur and damaged DNA does not get repaired prior to replication leading to the propagation of potentially cancer causing mutations. ATM is known to phosphorylate the tumor suppressor p53 and also interacts with many other proteins involved in the control of cell cycle progression. AT is a highly pleiotropic disease reflecting the numerous pathways requiring the ATM kinase. The most striking and obvious clinical manifestations seen in AT is progressive cerebellar ataxia. Additional organ involvement is seen in the thymus which remains embryonic. The growth deficit in the thymus is responsible, in part, for the immunodeficiency seen in AT patients. Many other organs show nuclear changes resulting in nucleomegaly. An additional characteristic observation in 95% of AT patients is an elevation in serum α-fetoprotein (AFP). Children suffering from AT may begin to learn to walk but will shortly begin to stagger and eventually will be confined to a wheelchair by the age of 10. Two additional classic symptoms in AT patients are slurred speech and oculomotor apraxia (difficulty in moving the eyes from side to side). All teenage AT patients will need help with eating, getting dressed, and using the bathroom. Uncontrolled drooling is a frequent complaint with AT patients. Although neurological status may appear to improve between the ages of 3 and 7 years, it begins to progressively deteriorate again. Approximately 35% to 40% of AT patients will develop cancers within their shortened life spans and approximately 85% of these cancers are leukemias or lymphomas.

mustards that were originally developed for use by the military. Alkylating agents function by reacting with and disrupting the structure of DNA. Some agents react with alkyl groups in DNA resulting in fragmentation of the DNA as a consequence of the action of DNA repair enzymes. Some agents catalyze the cross-linking of bases in the DNA which prevents the separation of the 2 strands during DNA replication. Some agents induce mispairing of nucleotides resulting in permanent mutations in the DNA. Alkylating agents act upon DNA at all stages of the cell cycle, thus they are potent anticancer drugs. However, because of their potency, prolonged use of alkylating agents can lead to secondary cancers, particularly leukemias.

The class of anticancer drugs that interfere with aspects of nucleotide metabolism is known as the antimetabolites. There are 2 major types of antimetabolites used in the treatment of a broad range of cancers: compounds that inhibit thymidylate synthase and compounds that inhibit dihydrofolate reductase (DHFR). Both of these enzymes are involved in thymidine nucleotide biosynthesis (Chapter 32). Drugs that inhibit thymidylate synthase include 5-fluorouracil and 5-fluorodeoxyuridine. Those that inhibit DHFR are analogs of the vitamin folic acid and include methotrexate and trimethoprim.

The anticancer drugs of the **anthracycline** and the **camptothecin** class function through interference with the actions of the topoisomerases. The anthracyclines include doxorubicin and daunorubicin which have similar modes of action, although doxorubicin is the more potent of the 2 and is used in the treatment breast cancers, lymphomas, and sarcomas. The anthracyclines inhibit the actions of topoisomerase II. Anthracyclines also function by inducing the formation of oxygen-free radicals that cause DNA strand breaks resulting in

CLINICAL BOX 35-5: XERODERMA PIGMENTOSUM

Xeroderma pigmentosum defines a class of autosomal recessive inherited diseases that are characterized clinically by sun sensitivity that results in progressive degeneration of sun-exposed areas of the skin and eyes. Often these changes will result in neoplasia. Some XP patients also manifest with progressive neurological degeneration. There are currently 8 alleles whose mutations result in manifestation of XP. Seven of the genes are involved in processes of nucleotide excision repair, NER. These 7 complementation groups are identified as XPA, XPB, XPC, XPD, XPE, XPF, and XPG. An additional class of XP patients referred to as XP variants (XP-V) result from deficiencies in a gene involved in semiconservative replication of previously damaged sites in DNA. In most XP patients the initial symptoms are an abnormal reaction to sun exposure which includes severe sunburn with blistering and persistent erythema with minimal exposure to the sun. These symptoms most often manifest between 1 to 2 years, although some patients do not exhibit symptoms until the teens. Most XP patients will develop xerosis (dry skin) and poikiloderma (referring to areas of increased pigment alternating with areas of reduced pigment, atrophy, and telangiectasias). This constellation of skin manifestations gave rise to the name of this disease. The skin of affected patients will appear similar to that of a person exposed to the sun for many years, such as a farmer, even though they are very young. Additional benign lesions in the skin include actinic keratoses (scaly crusty bumps), keratoacanthomas (well-differentiated squamous cell carcinoma), angiomas (benign tumors composed of blood vessels at or near the surface of the skin), and fibromas (benign tumors of connective tissue). Patients with XP who are younger than 20 years old have a greater than 1000-fold increase in developing cancer at UV-exposed areas of the skin relative to unaffected individuals. In addition to photophobia, XP-related ocular symptoms are restricted to the sun exposed anterior portion of the eye. The anterior portion of the eye includes the lid, cornea, and conjunctiva and these protect the posterior eye (uveal tract and retina) from *uv* irradiation. The ocular symptoms include conjunctivitis, ectropion (eyelids that turn outward) due to atrophy of the skin of the eyelids, exposure keratitis, and benign and malignant neoplasms of the eyelids. In XP patients with neurological symptoms there is variation in age of onset and severity. However, all are characterized by progressive deterioration. Frequently observed symptoms are sensorineural deafness and diminished deep tendon reflexes. In some patients progressive mental retardation is evident but usually is not evident until the second decade of life

inhibition of replication. Etoposide is another anticancer compound that functions through inhibition of topoisomerase II Etoposide is isolated from the mandrake plant and is in a class of compounds referred to as epipodophyllotoxins. The camptothecins were originally found in the bark of the *Camptotheca acuminata* tree and include irinotecan and topotecan. Camptothecins inhibit the action of topoisomerase I.

Anticancer compounds that are extracted from the periwinkle plant, *Vinca rosea*, are called the vinca alkaloids. These compounds bind to tubulin monomers leading to the disruption of the microtubules of the mitotic spindle fibers that are necessary for cell division during mitosis. There are 4 major vinca alkaloids that are currently used as chemotherapeutics, vincristine, vinblastine, vinorelbine, and vindesine.

The taxanes are another class of plant-derived compounds that act via interference with microtubule function. These compounds are isolated from the Pacific yew tree, *Taxus brevifolia* and include paclitaxel and docetaxel. The taxanes function by hyperstabilizing microtubules which prevents cell division. These compounds are used to treat a wide range of cancers including head and neck, lung, ovarian, breast, bladder, and prostate cancers.

REVIEW QUESTIONS

1. When dividing cells are progressing through the cell cycle, many checks are imposed to ensure that the process is occuring with fidelity. A critical checkpoint in the cell cycle occurs in response to DNA damage, such as that induced by UV light. Which of the following cell-cycle proteins is involved in DNA damage–mediated cell-cycle arrest?

A. CDK2
B. cyclin A
C. cyclin D
D. E2F
E. p53

Answer E: One major function of the p53 protein is to serve as a component of the checkpoint that controls whether cells enter as well as progress through S-phase. The action of p53 is induced in response to DNA damage. Under normal circumstances p53 levels remain very low due to its interaction with a member of the ubiquitin ligase family called MDM2. In response to DNA damage, for instance, as a result of UV-irradiation or γ-irradiation, cells activate several kinases including checkpoint kinase 2 (CHK2) and ataxia telangiectasia mutated (ATM). One target of these kinases is p53. ATM also phosphorylates MDM2. When p53 is phosphorylated it is released from MDM2 and can carry out its transcriptional activation functions. One target of p53 is the cyclin inhibitor $p21^{Cip1}$ gene. Activation of $p21^{Cip1}$ leads to increased inhibition of the cyclin D1-CDK4 and cyclin E-CDK2 complexes, thereby halting progression through the cell cycle either prior to S-phase entry or during S-phase.

2. You are carrying out experiments to study DNA replication in a cell line derived from a breast cancer tumor. You discover that the replication process does not completely copy all of each chromosome. Examination of the process using electron microscopy indicates that replication ceases near to where the DNA strands are attached to the chromatin scaffold. Given these observations, which of the following activities is most likely to be defective in these cells?

A. DNA ligase
B. helicase
C. polymerase-α
D. single-stranded binding proteins
E. topoisomerase

Answer E: The progression of the replication fork requires that the DNA ahead of the fork be continuously unwound. Due to the fact that eukaryotic chromosomal DNA is attached to a protein scaffold the progressive movement of the replication fork introduces severe torsional stress into the duplex ahead of the fork. This torsional stress is relieved by DNA topoisomerases. Topoisomerases relieve torsional stresses in duplexes of DNA by introducing either double- (topoisomerases II) or single-stranded (topoisomerases I) breaks into the backbone of the DNA. These breaks allow unwinding of the duplex and removal of the replication-induced torsional strain. The nicks are then resealed by the topoisomerases.

3. You are involved in a clinical study aimed at examination of effects of telomere length on aging and disease. You experimentally determine the length of telomeric repeats in children and adults, including both groups with individuals of normal development and abnormal development. In addition, you have included a group of individuals suffering various cancers. Which of the following observations would most closely reflect the findings of your study?

A. longer telomeres in all the abnormal groups
B. longer telomeres in developmentally disabled and cancer groups
C. shorter telomeres in the older group and the developmentally disabled group
D. shorter telomeres in the older group only
E. shorter telomeres in only the young and developmentally normal individuals

Answer C: Numerous studies have demonstrated a correlation between telomere shortening and human aging, disease progression, and developmental delay. Decreased telomere length in peripheral blood leukocytes has been shown to correlate with higher mortality rates in older (>60 years of age) individuals. This is contrasted by studies in centenarians and their offspring that have shown a positive link between telomere length and longevity. There is also an intriguing correlation between telomere length and psychological stress and the risk for development of psychiatric disease. The level of telomerase activity in peripheral blood leukocytes has been shown to be lowest in individuals with the highest levels of stress, which also coincided with the highest levels of oxidative stress. This correlation between stress and telomerase activity and telomere length is quite intriguing given that it is known that individuals subject to chronic psychological stress show a shortened lifespan and more rapid onset of diseases that are more typical of an aged population such as cardiovascular disease.

4. You are treating a child who presents with short stature, hypotonia, small hands and feet, obesity, and mild to moderate retardation. An analysis for genomic anomalies reveals a deletion in chromosome 15 and it is determined that this deletion came from the paternal genome. The symptoms and genetic data indicate the child is suffering from which of the following disorders?

A. Angelman syndrome
B. Ataxia telangiectasia
C. Beckwith-Wiedemann syndrome
D. Prader-Willi syndrome
E. Rett syndrome

Answer D: Prader-Willi syndrome (PWS) is characterized by a failure to thrive in the neonatal period accompanied by muscular hypotonia. PWS results from the loss of a group of paternally inherited genes due to a deletion of a region of chromosome 15. During early childhood PWS patients exhibit hyperphagia (excessive hunger and abnormally large intake of solid foods), obesity, hypogonadism, sleep apnea, behavior problems, and mild to moderate mental retardation. Additionally, PWS children have small hands and feet. In prepubertal males, the hypogonadism results in sparse body hair, poor development of skeletal muscles, and delay in epiphyseal closure, which results in long arms and legs.

5. The camptothecins are an alkaloid class of anticancer drugs used in the treatment of colon and breast cancers. These compounds function by inhibiting the activity of which of the following enzymes?
- **A.** ATP-dependent DNA helicase
- **B.** DNA ligase
- **C.** DNA polymerase
- **D.** histone deacetylase
- **E.** topoisomerase I

Answer E: The camptothecins were originally found in the bark of the *Camptotheca accuminata* tree and include irinotecan (Campto, Camptosar) and topotecan (Hycamtin). Camptothecins inhibit the action of topoisomerase I, an enzyme that induces single-strand breaks in DNA during replication.

6. Addition of 5-azacytidine to cultures of growing cells would be expected to result in which of the following?
- **A.** decreased mutagenesis
- **B.** hypermethylation
- **C.** hypomethylation
- **D.** increased mutagenesis
- **E.** inhibition of replication

Answer C: The nucleotide analog, 5-azacytidine (5-azaC), is incorporated into replicating DNA when DNA polymerase would normally use deoxycytidine as the substrate. The incorporation of a nitrogen instead of carbon at position 5 of the nucleobase prevents subsequent methylation of 5-azaC in the DNA when it is inserted into positions where the template strand of DNA contains CpG methylation sites. Thus, the incorporation of 5-azaC prevents conservation of methylation status in newly synthesized DNA, that is, results in hypomethylation.

7. Which of the following statements reflects the process by which of the telomeric ends of chromosomes are replicated?
- **A.** a unique DNA molecule serves as the primer for synthesis
- **B.** a unique RNA molecule serves as the template for synthesis
- **C.** short template-independent blocks of DNA are ligated to the ends using a $5' \rightarrow 5'$ bond
- **D.** telomeres are replicated as short tandem repeated stretches of ribonucleotides instead of deoxyribonucleotides
- **E.** telomeres are replicated in a temple-independent process

Answer B: The telomeric end on the lagging strand of a replicating eukaryotic chromosome is synthesized by an enzymatic activity termed telomerase. Telomerase is complex composed of several proteins, an RNA with sequence complimentary to the telomeric repeats, and a reverse transcriptase activity that extends the 3′-end of the lagging strands using the telomerase RNA as the template. The reverse transcriptase activity of telomerase is encoded by the *TERT* gene (telomerase reverse transcriptase) and the RNA component is encoded by the *TERC* gene (telomerase RNA component). The TERC RNA contains a repeating hexanucleotide sequence, 3′–AAUCCC–5′, that spans between 3 and 20 kilobases. This sequence in the TERC RNA forms a duplex with the lagging DNA strand at the ends of the chromosomes. The 3′-end of the lagging strand then serves as the primer for the reverse transcriptase activity (TERT) which extends the 3′-end of the chromosome using the TERC RNA as a template.

8. The anticancer drug, Taxol, has been an effective chemotherapeutic agent in the fight against ovarian cancer. Which of the following represents the mechanism of action of Taxol?
- **A.** binds to the activated form of the RAS protein which in turn interferes with the signaling cascades involving this protein
- **B.** binds to microtubules, which stabilizes them preventing their shortening and interfering with cell division
- **C.** interacts with the tumor suppressor protein (pRB) encoded by the retinoblastoma susceptibility gene inducing its suppressive activity
- **D.** interacts with topoisomerase II preventing its role in DNA synthesis, which effectively terminates replication
- **E.** interferes with steroid hormone receptor interaction with DNA, thus preventing the growth induction by this class of hormone

Answer B: The compound paclitaxel (the generic name for Taxol) interferes with the normal function of microtubule growth leading to increased stability of the structure. This effect of Taxol destroys the cell ability to use its cytoskeleton in a flexible manner. Specifically, Taxol binds to the tubulin protein of microtubules and locks them in place. The resulting microtubule/Taxol complex does not have the ability to disassemble. This adversely affects cell function because the shortening and lengthening of microtubules (termed dynamic instability) is necessary for their function as a transportation highway for the cell. Chromosomes, for example, rely on this property of microtubules during mitosis. Therefore, the inability of cells to organize and undertake the necessary movements of mitosis prevents cell division. Since cancer cells are rapidly proliferating cells, the action of Taxol inhibits their growth.

9. The term "genomic imprinting" refers to the phenomenon of gene expression dependence on the mode of inheritance. A typical example of this phenomenon is the control of the expression of the growth factor IGF-II. Genomic imprinting is termed "epigenesist," which is defined by which of the following?

- **A.** gene expression results from regulated levels of DNA methylation
- **B.** gene expression that is restricted to a specific cell lineage
- **C.** gene regulation is exerted by sex-type specific factors
- **D.** genotype differences are not reflected by phenotype differences
- **E.** phenotype differences are independent of genotype variation

Answer E: The term epigenetics is used to define the mechanism by which changes in the pattern of inherited gene expression occur in the absence of alterations or changes in the nucleotide composition of a given gene. A literal interpretation is that epigenetics mean "in addition to changes in genome sequence."

10. Many effective anticancer drugs function as such by interfering with processes of DNA replication. The drug, doxorubicin, is useful in the treatment of lymphomas and breast cancers because of its ability to interfere with which of the following enzyme activities?

- **A.** DNA ligase
- **B.** DNA polymerase α
- **C.** primase
- **D.** topoisomerase II
- **E.** uracil *N*-glycosylase

Answer D: Doxorubicin is a drug of the class that functions by interfering with topoisomerases. In particular, doxorubicin inhibits topoisomerase II. During the process of DNA replication, the 2 strands of the DNA helix are separated. As the replication fork progresses toward sites of chromosomal attachment to the scaffold, there is an increase in the torsional stress on the helix due to supercoiling. These torsional stresses are relieved by the action of topoisomerases that introduce nicks into the DNA, which allows the strands to unwind the supercoils. Topoisomerase I introduces single-strand nicks, whereas topoisomerase II introduces double-strand nicks. Interference with the action of topoisomerases would thus impair the rate of DNA replication and this would be detrimental for rapidly proliferating cells such as cancer.

11. You are carrying out experiments to study DNA replication in a cell line derived from a breast cancer tumor. You discover that the DNA polymerase in these cells incorporates the incorrect nucleotide into the elongating strand approximately once every thousand bases. These errors suggest that the "proof-reading" capacity of the polymerase is defective. This would be indicative of the following processes not being correctly carried out by the defective polymerase?

- **A.** 3′ to 5′ exonuclease activity
- **B.** 5′ to 3′ exonuclease activity
- **C.** insertion of nucleotides in 5′ to 3′ orientation
- **D.** synthesis of ribonucleotide polymers
- **E.** topoisomerase-mediated cleavage of the DNA backbone

Answer A: The main enzymatic activity of DNA polymerases is the 5′—>3′ synthetic activity. However, DNA polymerases possess two additional activities of importance for both replication and repair. These additional activities include a 5′—>3′ exonuclease function and a 3′—>5′ exonuclease function. The 3′—>5′ exonuclease function is utilized during replication to allow DNA polymerase to remove mismatched bases and is referred to as the proof-reading activity of DNA polymerase. It is possible (but rare) for DNA polymerases to incorporate an incorrect base during replication. These mismatched bases are recognized by the polymerase immediately due to the lack of Watson-Crick base-pairing. The mismatched base is then removed by the 3′→5′ exonuclease activity and the correct base inserted prior to progression of replication.

12. Which of the following represents the correct composition of a eukaryotic nucleosome core?

- **A.** histone H1
- **B.** one copy each of histone H2A, H3, and H4
- **C.** one copy each of histone H1, H2A, and H2B
- **D.** two copies each of histone H2A, H2B, H3, and H4
- **E.** two copies each of histone H1, H2A, H3, and H4

Answer D: The binding of DNA by the histones generates a structure called the nucleosome. The nucleosome core contains an octamer protein structure consisting of 2 subunits each of H2A, H2B, H3, and H4. Histone H1 occupies the internucleosomal DNA and is identified as the linker histone. The nucleosome core contains approximately 150 bp of DNA.

13. Which of the following relates to the process of DNA replication?
A. is semiconservative
B. must begin with an incision step
C. requires a primer in eukaryotes but not in prokaryotes
D. requires only proteins with DNA polymerase activity
E. uses 5′→3′ polymerase activity to synthesize 1 strand and 3′→5′ polymerase activity to synthesize the complementary strand

Answer A: The process of DNA replication begins at specific sites in the chromosomes termed origins of replication, requires a primer bearing a free 3′-OH, proceeds specifically in the 5′ → 3′ direction on both strands of DNA concurrently and results in the copying of the template strands in a semiconservative manner. The semiconservative nature of DNA replication means that the newly synthesized daughter strands remain associated with their respective parental template strands.

14. An alteration in the structure of topoisomerase II that maintained its functional activity but prevented the action of inhibitory compounds would render useless the action of which of the following chemotherapeutic agents?
A. alkylating drugs
B. anthracyclins
C. antimetabolites
D. camptothecins
E. taxanes

Answer B: The anthracyclins were originally isolated from the fungus, *Streptomyces*. Doxorubicin (Adriamycin, Doxil, Rubex) and daunorubicin (Cerubidine, DaunoXome, Daunomycin, Rubidomycin) have similar modes of action, although doxorubicin is the more potent of the 2 and is used in the treatment of breast cancers, lymphomas, and sarcomas. The anthracyclins inhibit the actions of topoisomerase II.

15. The activation of histone deacetylases would be expected to have which of the following effects on DNA replication?
A. decreases the rate
B. destabilizes the double-helix allowing access for polymerases
C. enhances formation of new chromatin following completion of replication
D. increases the rate
E. will have no effect on replication activity

Answer E: Histone deacetylases are responsible for changing the state of histone acetylation. The consequences of reduced histone acetylation are altered chromatin structure making it difficult for the transcriptional machinery to engage the DNA. Thus, histone deacetylation is associated with reduced transcription but does not appreciably, or at all, affect DNA replication.

16. Which of the following class of compounds is known to inhibit topisomerse II and thus have shown utility as cancer chemotherapeutics?
A. anthracyclins
B. antimetabolites
C. camptothecins
D. taxanes
E. vinca alkaloids

Answer A: The anthracyclins were originally isolated from the fungus, *Streptomyces*. Doxorubicin (Adriamycin, Doxil, Rubex) and daunorubicin (Cerubidine, DaunoXome, Daunomycin, Rubidomycin) have similar modes of action, although doxorubicin is the more potent of the 2 and is used in the treatment of breast cancers, lymphomas, and sarcomas. The anthracyclins inhibit the actions of topoisomerase II.

17. Genomic imprinting is termed “epigenesist,” which is defined by which of the following?
A. gene expression results from regulated levels of DNA methylation
B. gene expression that is restricted to a specific cell lineage
C. gene regulation is exerted by sex-type specific factors
D. genotype differences are not reflected by phenotype differences
E. phenotype differences are independent of genotype variation

Answer E: The term epigenetics is used to define the mechanism by which changes in the pattern of inherited gene expression occur in the absence of alterations or changes in the nucleotide composition of a given gene. A literal interpretation is that epigenetics mean “in addition to changes in genome sequence.”

18. In analyzing a sample of double-stranded DNA, it has been determined that the molar amount of adenosine is 20%. Given this information, what is the content of cytidine?

A. 10
B. 20
C. 30
D. 40
E. 60

Answer C: The molar ratio of adenosine in any molecule of double-stranded DNA will be equivalent to that of thymidine, since these two nucleotides hydrogen bond to form base-pairs. Therefore, the total amount of the DNA accounted for in A-T base-pairs would be 40%. Since guanosine and cytidine hydrogen bond to form base-pairs, they too contribute an equivalent molar ratio in double-stranded DNA. In double-stranded DNA with 40% A-T composition, the molar ratio of cytidine would be half of the remaining 60% of the DNA, or 30%.

19. Chromatin remodeling is associated with alterations in the transcriptional activity of genes in the region of the remodeling. Which of the following statements is most correct concerning the events of chromatin remodeling?

A. chromatin remodeling occurs predominantly in regions enriched in CpG dinucleotides
B. histone acetylation tends to destabilize chromatin structure
C. methylation of guanine residues induces the remodeling event
D. methylation of histone H1 is sufficient to stimulate remodeling
E. remodeling is necessary to induce the property of genomic imprinting

Answer B: The posttranslational modification of histone proteins has considerable effect on numerous activities at the level of the chromatin. In particular, the acetylation and/or methylation of histones in the nucleosome (H2A, H2B, H3, and H4) results in an altered stability of the 30-nm chromatin fiber as well as other higher-order chromatin structure. Imprinting is regulated by the state of DNA methylation.

20. Genomic imprinting is a mechanism by which gene expression is regulated. Which of the following correctly defines this mechanism?

A. activation of expression by hypermethylation of genomic DNA sites
B. activation of expression by hypomethylation of genomic DNA sites
C. expansion of trinucleotide repeats in imprinted genes resulting in regulated expression
D. inhibition of expression by hypomethylation of genomic DNA sites
E. regulated expression dependent upon parental origin of regulated gene

Answer E: Genomic imprinting refers to a genetic phenomenon, whereby there is preferential expression of a gene from only 1 of the 2 parental alleles. This phenomenon of allele-specific expression results from allele-specific epigenetic modifications such as CpG dinucleotide methylation or histone methylation or histone acetylation. These modifications are referred to as epigenetic modifications (also referred to as epigenetic "marks"). In nonimprinted regions of the chromosomes, the parental epigenetic marks are erased in the germ cells only to be newly established in a parental-specific manner. Once the parental-specific epigenetic marks are established, they are maintained following fertilization.

21. Telomerase is the specialized activity that allows for replication of the telomeric ends of the chromosomes. In addition to an RNA that is complimentary to the telomeric repeat sequence what other component is required of this complex for its normal activity?

A. DNA-dependent DNA polymerase
B. DNA-dependent RNA polymerase
C. DNA helicase
D. RNA-dependent DNA polymerase
E. RNA-dependent RNA polymerase

Answer D: Telomerase is a complex composed of several proteins, an RNA with sequence complimentary to the telomeric repeats, and a reverse transcriptase activity that extends the 3′-end of the lagging strands using the telomerase RNA as the template. The reverse transcriptase activity of telomerase is encoded by the *TERT* gene (telomerase reverse transcriptase). Reverse transcriptases are RNA-dependent DNA polymerases.

22. The cyclin D-CDK4/6 complex is involved in the regulation of progression through the G_1 phase of the cell cycle. Which of the following represents a major target of this kinase complex?

A. cyclin E-CDK2
B. E2F
C. p27
D. p53
E. pRb

Answer E: In the context of cell cycle regulation, the transcription factor E2F activates the expression of cyclin A, cyclin E, and CDK2. The activity of E2F is itself controlled via interaction with pRB. When pRB binds

E2F it can no longer function as a transcription factor as it is sequestered in the cytosol. Interaction of pRB and E2F correlates to the state of phosphorylation of pRB and the affinity between the 2 proteins is highest when pRB is hypophosphorylated. Phosphorylation of pRB is maximal at the start of S-phase and lowest after mitosis and entry into G_1. When pRB is phosphorylated by G_1 cyclin-CDK complexes (cyclin D-CDK4/6), it releases E2F allowing E2F to transcriptionally activate its target genes.

23. You are examining the efficacy of a new potential anticancer drug. Addition of this drug to rapidly dividing cancer cells results in a blockade to progression through M-phase and the cells arrest at metaphase in the cell cycle. You determine that the drug targets a specific regulatory protein of cell cycle progression and show that it is which of the following proteins/complexes?

A. anaphase-promoting complex
B. cyclin D-CDK4/6
C. cyclin E-CDK2
D. E2F
E. securing

Answer A: The anaphase-promoting complex (APC) is a ubiquitin ligase that controls the levels of the M-phase cyclins as well as other regulators of mitosis. One important function of APC is to control the initiation of sister chromatid separation which begins at the metaphase-anaphase transition. The attachment of the sister chromatids to the opposite poles of the mitotic spindles occurs early during mitosis. The ability of the sister chromatids to be pulled apart is initially inhibited because they are bound together by a protein complex termed cohesin complex. The cohesin complex is deposited along the chromosomes as they are duplicated during S-phase. Anaphase can only begin with the disruption of the cohesin complex. The breakdown of the cohesin complex is brought about as a consequence of the activation of the ubiquitin ligase activity of the APC. APC targets a protein called securin. Securin functions to inhibit the protease called separase and the action of separase is to degrade the proteins of the cohesin complex, thus allowing sister chromatid separation.

24. You are carrying out experiments designed to ascertain the defect in a cell line derived from a breast cancer tumor. Your studies show that these cells likely arose due to an inability to control progress through the cell cycle in the presence of DNA damage. Exposure of the cells to a dose of γ-irradiation results in a significant propagation of mutated nucleotides into the DNA of daughter cells. Given these observations, which of the following proteins/complexes is most likely defective in your study cell line?

A. anaphase-promoting complex
B. CDK4/6
C. cohesin
D. p53
E. pRB

Answer E: One major function of the p53 protein is to serve as a component of the checkpoint that controls whether cells enter as well as progress through S-phase. The action of p53 is induced in response to DNA damage. Under normal circumstances p53 levels remain very low due to its interaction with a member of the ubiquitin ligase family called MDM2. In response to DNA damage, for instance, as a result of UV-irradiation or γ-irradiation, cells activate several kinases including checkpoint kinase 2 (CHK2) and ataxia telangiectasia mutated (ATM). One target of these kinases is p53. ATM also phosphorylates MDM2. When p53 is phosphorylated it is released from MDM2 and can carry out its transcriptional activation functions. One target of p53 is the cyclin inhibitor $p21^{Cip1}$ gene. Activation of $p21^{Cip1}$ leads to increased inhibition of the cyclin D1-CDK4 and cyclin E-CDK2 complexes, thereby halting progression through the cell cycle either prior to S-phase entry or during S-phase.

25. The tumor suppressor pRB functions in the cell cycle by regulating progression from G_1 to S-phase. In a cell line derived from a colon carcinoma it is found that the activity of pRB is defective. Which of the following proteins is most likely to be hyperactive in these tumor cells as a consequence of the defective function of pRB?

A. anaphase-promoting complex
B. E2F
C. p21
D. p53
E. securin

Answer B: In the context of cell cycle regulation, the transcription factor E2F activates the expression of cyclin A, cyclin E, and CDK2. The activity of E2F is itself controlled via interaction with pRB. When pRB binds E2F it can no longer function as a transcription factor as it is sequestered in the cytosol. Interaction of pRB and E2F correlates to the state of phosphorylation of pRB and the affinity between the 2 proteins is highest when pRB is hypophosphorylated. Phosphorylation of pRB is maximal at the start of S-phase and lowest after mitosis and entry into G_1. When pRB is phosphorylated by G_1 cyclin-CDK complexes (cyclin D-CDK4/6), it releases E2F allowing E2F to transcriptionally activate its target genes.

26. Control of specific steps in the cell cycle can be studied in cell culture by the use of cell fusion experiments. If cells that are currently in S-phase of the cell cycle are fused with cells that are in the G_1-phase of the cell cycle, which of the following would most correctly reflect the process of DNA synthesis?

A. it is induced in the G_1-phase nucleus
B. it is inhibited in the S-phase nucleus
C. it is stimulated in the S-phase nucleus
D. it is unaffected in the G_1-phase nucleus

Answer A: The cells that are already synthesizing DNA will have active S-phase CDK complexes as they will have been allowed to progress beyond the G_1-S checkpoint. Therefore, these active S-CDK complexes would trigger the activation of DNA synthesis in the cells that were in G_1 following cell fusion.

27. You are examining a 7-year-old girl brought to you by her parents because they are concerned about the severe skin blistering on her arms and back of her neck a few days after she played in the sun for 15 minutes without sunscreen. Physical examination shows the girl has numerous freckles on her face, neck, arms, and hands. In addition she has numerous telangiectasias on her arms as well as crusty and scaly patches of skin. You suspect the child may have xeroderma pigmentosum. Which of the following processes is most likely to be defective in this child if your diagnosis is correct?

A. DNA polymerase proof-reading activity
B. double-strand break repair during replication
C. photoactivatable thymine dimer removal
D. removal of uracil from DNA
E. reverse transcription of telomeric DNA

Answer C: Xeroderma pigmentosum is characterized clinically by sun sensitivity that results in progressive degeneration of sun-exposed areas of the skin and eyes. Often these changes will result in neoplasia. There are currently 8 alleles whose mutations result in manifestation of XP. Seven of the genes are involved in processes of nucleotide excision repair (NER) including pyrimidine dimer removal. In most XP patients the initial symptoms are an abnormal reaction to sun exposure which includes severe sunburn with blistering and persistent erythema with minimal exposure to the sun. These symptoms most often manifest between 1 and 2 years, although some patients do not exhibit symptoms until the teens. Most XP patients will develop xerosis (dry skin) and poikiloderma (referring to areas of increased pigment alternating with areas of reduced pigment, atrophy, and telangiectasias). Telangiectasias are areas of the skin under which there are dilated superficial vessels.

28. The anticancer drug etoposide functions because it inhibits the activity of topoisomerase. Which of the following represents the normal function of this enzyme?

A. introduce the primer onto the template of DNA prior to replication
B. remove mismatched nucleotides at the end of replication
C. remove the RNA primer from each Okasaki fragment
D. stabilize single-stranded regions of DNA at the replication fork
E. unwind the DNA duplex during replication

Answer E: Topoisomerases are enzymes that regulate the overwinding or underwinding of DNA. For example, during DNA replication, DNA becomes overwound ahead of a replication fork. This torsional stress would eventually halt DNA replication. Topoisomerases bind to either single-stranded or double-stranded DNA and cut the phosphate backbone of the DNA. This intermediate break allows the DNA to be untangled or unwound. When the stress is relieved, the DNA backbone is resealed again.

29. RNA and DNA molecules can form double-stranded structures just as in the case of DNA-DNA duplexes. Given this fact, hybridization of a DNA strand (5′-ACGTC-3′) with which of the following RNA molecules will result in the most stable RNA-DNA duplex?

A. 5′-AGUAC-3′
B. 5′-CAUGA-3′
C. 5′-GACGU-3′
D. 5′-GGCAG-3′
E. 5′-UGCAG-3′

Answer C: DND-DNA and RNA-DNA duplexes can form due to base paring between complimentary nucleotides. In the case of RNA-DNA duplexes, the U in an RNA molecule forms a base-pair with A in a DNA molecule. In addition, duplexes are formed with antiparallel orientation. Thus, the only RNA that can form a stable 1:1 duplex with the target DNA must have the antiparallel complimentary sequence.

30. You are studying the differences in a particular protein between normal and cancer cells. You find that in the cancer cells the protein is smaller than in the normal cells. Which of the following mutations in the gene encoding the protein would best explain your observations?

A. A to T change in the middle of a long intron in the gene
B. A to T change in the promoter of the gene

C. G to C change in an enhancer found in an intron of the gene
D. missense mutation in the middle of an exon of the gene
E. nonsense mutation in the middle of an exon of the gene

Answer E: A nonsense mutation is a point mutation that introduces a premature stop codon into the transcribed mRNA. This results in the synthesis of a truncated and usually nonfunctional protein. It differs from a missense mutation, which is a point mutation where a single nucleotide is changed to cause substitution of a different amino acid at that codon.

31. Various types of mutations have been found in DNA from damaged, defective, or diseased cells. Which of the following types of mutation will manifest a phenotype only as a consequence of specific circumstances (eg, increased temperature or oxidative stress)?
A. conditional
B. dominant negative
C. gain-of-function
D. lethal
E. null

Answer A: Conditional mutations are a type of mutation that manifest wild-type (or less severe) phenotype under certain permissive conditions (such as environmental), but manifest mutant phenotype under certain nonpermissive conditions. For example, a temperature-sensitive mutation can cause cell death at high temperature (nonpermissive condition), but might have no deleterious consequences at a lower temperature (permissive condition).

32. Environmental factors can result in the incorporation of mutations into DNA. Many mutagenic compounds and various forms of radiation lead to mutations through the activity of an error-prone DNA repair mechanism. Which of the following causes mutations by the process of dimerization of adjacent pyrimidines?
A. 5-bromouracil
B. hydroxylamine
C. nitrous acid
D. γ-radiation
E. ultraviolet light

Answer E: Pyrimidine dimers are formed from thymine or cytosine bases in DNA via photochemical reactions. Ultraviolet light induces the formation of covalent linkages generating cyclobutane pyrimidine dimers, CPDs (including thymine dimers). Pyrimidine dimers can be repaired by a process termed photoreactivation. This requires photolyase enzymes that directly reverse CPDs following the absorption of fluorescent light or sunlight. This absorption enables the photochemical reactions to occur, which results in the elimination of the pyrimidine dimer, returning it to its original state.

33. Within human chromosomes there are regions of highly concentrated GC content. Many of the cytosine residues that fall within CpG dinucleotide sequences are methylated at the 5 position (m^5CpG). Which of the following best explains why these methyl-CpG sequences are exceptionally prone to mutation?
A. deamination of m^5C produces T
B. histones bind less tightly to m^5C sequences than to other sequences
C. homologous recombination occurs preferentially at m^5C sequences
D. methylation of C directly changes its base-pairing properties
E. methylation of C directly interfere with base-pairing during DNA replication

Answer A: Cytosine in DNA can spontaneously deaminate generating uracil. This spontaneous deamination is corrected for by the removal of uracil by uracil-DNA glycosylase. Spontaneous deamination of 5-methylcytosine generates thymine. This is the most common single nucleotide mutation. In DNA, this reaction can be corrected by the enzyme thymine-DNA glycosylase.

34. Which of the following is the major role of the $3' \rightarrow 5'$ exonuclease activity of DNA polymerases?
A. cleaving Okasaki fragments
B. elongating DNA strands
C. excision of RNA primers
D. excision of thymine dimers
E. removing mismatched nucleotides

Answer E: The main enzymatic activity of DNA polymerases is the $5' \rightarrow 3'$ synthetic activity. However, DNA polymerases possess two additional activities of importance for both replication and repair. These additional activities include a $5' \rightarrow 3'$ exonuclease function and a $3' \rightarrow 5'$ exonuclease function. The $3' \rightarrow 5'$ exonuclease function is utilized during replication to allow DNA polymerase to remove mismatched bases and is referred to as the proof-reading activity of DNA polymerase. It is possible (but rare) for DNA polymerases to incorporate an incorrect base during replication. These mismatched bases are recognized by the polymerase immediately due to the lack of Watson-Crick base-pairing. The mismatched base is then removed by the 3′ → 5′ exonuclease activity and the correct base inserted prior to progression of replication.

35. You have isolated a gene that spans a total of 1800 nucleotides. The gene contains 400 nucleotides within 4 exons and 900 nucleotides are associated with the 3 introns. In addition there are 500 nucleotides associated with the regulatory sequences of the gene. Given this information, which of the following numbers most likely represents the number of amino acids encoded by this gene?
A. 130
B. 260
C. 400
D. 800
E. 1200

Answer A: The coding region of any given gene is contained within the exons. The introns are removed from the mRNA following processing. It is possible for all or a part of any given 5′ and 3′ exon to be noncoding, but this information was not provided. Therefore, the most likely number of encoded amino acids in this gene is determined from the number of nucleotides comprising the exons. Since each amino acid is encoded by 3 nucleotides, the closest number to that which could be encoded by 400 nucleotides is 130.

36. You are studying the characteristics of retroviral integration and replication in mouse cells. You find that in your cells the integrated retroviral genome is highly methylated and transcriptionally inactive. Given these findings, it is most likely that the retrovirus integrated into which of the following chromosomal structures?
A. euchromatin
B. heterochromatin
C. polytene DNA
D. puffed DNA
E. satellite DNA

Answer B: In a broad consideration of chromatin structure there are 2 forms: heterochromatin and euchromatin, which were originally designated based on cytological observations of how darkly the 2 regions were stained. Heterochromatin is more densely packed than euchromatin and is often found near the centromeres of the chromosomes. Heterochromatin is generally transcriptionally silent. Euchromatin on the other hand is more loosely packed and is where active gene transcription will be found to be taking place.

37. Reverse transcriptase is a specialized form of polymerase. Which of the following most correctly describes the function of this special polymerase?
A. 3′ → 5′ synthesis of DNA from an RNA template
B. 5′ → 3′ synthesis of DNA from an RNA template
C. 3′ → 5′ synthesis of RNA from a DNA template
D. 5′ → 3′ synthesis of RNA from a DNA template

Answer B: Reverse transcriptase is an RNA-dependent DNA polymerase that is used in the laboratory to generate complementary DNA (cDNA) from an RNA template. Like all DNA polymerases, reverse transcriptase moves along its template strand of RNA in the 3′ → 5′ direction while synthesizing DNA in the 5′ → 3′ direction.

38. The final step in the maturation of the newly synthesized lagging strand of DNA is the formation of phosphodiester bonds between the Okazaki fragments. Which of the following enzymes catalyzes this reaction?
A. DNA polymerase
B. helicase
C. ligase
D. primase
E. topoisomerase

Answer C: The RNA primers of the leading strands and Okazaki fragments are removed by the repair DNA polymerases, simultaneously replacing the ribonucleotides with deoxyribonucleotides. The gaps that exist between the 3′-OH of one leading strand and the 5′-phosphate of another as well as between one Okazaki fragment and another are repaired by DNA ligases.

39. The octomeric core of histones provides a structural framework for which of the following complexes?
A. ciliary axonemes
B. endosomes
C. mitochondrial ribosomes
D. nucleosomes
E. the fibrillar region of the nucleus

Answer D: The binding of DNA by the histones generates a structure called the nucleosome. The nucleosome core contains an octamer protein structure consisting of 2 subunits each of H2A, H2B, H3, and H4. Histone H1 occupies the internucleosomal DNA and is identified as the linker histone. The nucleosome core contains approximately 150 bp of DNA.

40. Functional eukaryotic chromosomes contain stretches of DNA harboring specialized nucleotide sequences. Which of the following represents the type of DNA sequence that prevents the strands from becoming shorter with each replication cycle?
A. centromere
B. intron

C. kinetochore
D. replication origin
E. telomere

Answer E: A telomere is a region of repetitive nucleotide sequences at the end of each chromosome. The telomere protects the end of the chromosome from deterioration or from fusion with neighboring chromosomes. Without telomeres, the chromosomes would progressively lose DNA and be truncated after each cell division because the synthesis of the lagging strands of the duplex requires RNA primers to be placed ahead of the synthesizing DNA. Over time, due to each cell division, the telomere ends become shorter.

41. You are carrying out experiments examining the DNase I digestion results in nuclei isolated from several different mammalian cells. Your results show that there is preferential digestion of a set of unique DNA sequences in each cell type. Which of the following characteristics of chromatin in these sequences best explains your observations?

A. deletion of the centromeric DNA
B. incorrect assembly into nucleosomes
C. presence of mutated base pairs
D. transcriptionally active
E. translocation to the nucleus

Answer D: DNase I is a versatile enzyme that nonspecifically cleaves DNA. DNA within chromosomes is complexed with a variety of different proteins including the histones. The protein-DNA complexes can restrict the access of DNase I to the DNA strand. Various types of chromatin structure exist across a wide range of DNA and the structure changes in a dynamic way. Transcriptionally active regions of the chromosomes are in a much more open configuration than transcriptionally silent regions. Therefore, the DNA in regions of the chromosomes from various cell types that are transcriptionally active will more likely be accessible to digestion by DNase I.

Checklist

- ✓ DNA present in eukaryotic cells is complexed with a variety of proteins forming a structure referred to as chromatin.
- ✓ The major proteins associated with DNA in chromatin are the histones. An octamer core composed of 2 copies of each of 4 different histone proteins is wrapped by approximately 150 bp of DNA.
- ✓ The histone proteins are subject to a wide variety of posttranslational modifications, the consequences of which dynamically alter the structure of chromatin. These dynamic changes result in variable access of the DNA to the transcriptional machinery.
- ✓ Transcriptional activity is controlled, in part, by the overall structure of chromatin, which itself is regulated by the state of histone modifications and DNA methylation. Histone acetylation is associated with activation of transcription, whereas deacetylation is associated with transcriptional silencing.
- ✓ Actively dividing eukaryotic cells progress through a highly order series of events referred to as the cell cycle. The cell cycle consists of an initial stage called G1, then DNA is synthesized in S-phase, the cell pauses again in G2, and then cytokinesis occurs in M-phase.
- ✓ The ability of cells to progress through the different phases of the cell cycle requires a specialized set of proteins known as cyclins. The cyclins regulate the family of kinases called cyclin-dependent kinases, CDKs. The cyclins are so called because their levels fluctuate during the cell cycle phases due to repeated ubiquitin-mediated degradation and transcription of the corresponding gene.

- ✓ DNA replication occurs during the S-phase of the cell cycle and involves a wide array of different protein activities including polymerases, various types of DNA-unwinding proteins, primer-synthesizing enzymes, single-strand stabilizing proteins, and DNA ligases.
- ✓ Replication is initiated at multiple locations in each chromosome termed origins of replication and proceeds along both strands simultaneously in both directions from the origin. The leading edge of the replication process is referred to as the replication fork.
- ✓ Given the restrictions on the process of DNA synthesis catalyzed by DNA polymerases, 1 of the 2 strands can be synthesized continuously (called the leading strand), the other discontinuously (called the lagging strand). The fragments of new DNA from the lagging strand of synthesis are called Okazaki fragments.
- ✓ Due to the process of replication the ends of the lagging strand of each chromosome cannot be replicated by DNA polymerase. The ends of the chromosomes are called telomeres and they contain highly repeated sequences that are recognized by the enzyme complex called telomerase. Telomerase aids in the extension of the lagging strand so that DNA polymerase can carry out replication. The process is never complete such that the telomeric ends of the chromosomes shorten with each cell cycle.
- ✓ DNA can be posttranscriptionally modified by DNA methyltransferases that methylate the 5-position of cytosine residues present in a CpG dinucleotide.
- ✓ The state of DNA methylation can affect chromatin structure and consequently the level of transcriptional activity. DNA methylation is also associated with the phenomenon of genomic imprinting.
- ✓ Remodeling of DNA can occur via the actions of recombination or transposition. The primary form of recombination in eukaryotic DNA is between regions of homology in sister chromatids.
- ✓ Several genes contain regions of trinucleotide repeats that can become abnormally expanded (amplified) resulting in the development of disease, such as is the case in Huntington disease. These diseases are all referred to as trinucleotide repeat diseases.
- ✓ Numerous events of the cell cycle, such as DNA synthesis and cytokinesis, are the targets of various chemotherapeutic drugs used to treat various forms of cancer.

CHAPTER

36 Transcription: RNA Synthesis, Processing, and Regulation

CHAPTER OUTLINE

High-Yield Terms

Transcription: describes the process by which the genetic information in a gene is converted into polyribonucleotides, the RNAs

Promoter: sequences in the gene that promote the ability of RNA polymerases to recognize the nucleotide at which initiation begins; must reside close to the gene and in a specific orientation for activity

Enhancer: sequences that act in *cis* by binding proteins that result in enhancement of transcription; can be located long distance from the gene or even on different chromosomes, also do not require orientation for activity

Splicing: the process whereby the introns are removed from heteronuclear RNA (hnRNA)

RNA editing: a novel enzymatic mechanism for the modification of nucleotide sequences of RNA, resulting in altered coding capacity

Small noncoding RNAs: includes the U small nuclear RNAs (snRNAs) of the splicing machinery, the microRNAs (miRNAs) derived from noncoding genes that are involved in processes of expression control, and the small interfering RNAs (siRNAs) responsible for the process of RNA-mediated interference (RNAi) in gene expression

ribozyme: an enzyme activity solely associated with an RNA molecule, such as the peptidyltransferase activity of the large ribosomal subunit

Classes of RNA and RNA Polymerases

Transcription is the mechanism by which a template strand of DNA is utilized by specific RNA polymerases to generate 1 of the 4 distinct classifications of RNA (Table 36-1).

In the eukaryotic cells, there are 3 distinct classes of RNA polymerase: RNA polymerase (pol) I, II, and III. Each polymerase is responsible for the synthesis of a different class of RNA. RNA pol I is responsible for rRNA synthesis (excluding the 5*S* rRNA). There are 4 major rRNAs in eukaryotic cells designated by their sedimentation size. The 28*S*, 5*S*, and 5.8*S* rRNAs are associated with the large ribosomal subunit and the 18*S* rRNA is associated with the small ribosomal subunit. The rRNAs are synthesized as long precursors termed *preribosomal RNAs* and the 45*S* preribosomal RNA serves as the precursor for the 18*S*, 28*S*, and 5.8*S* rRNAs. RNA pol II synthesizes the mRNAs and some of the small nuclear RNAs (snRNAs) and some of the miRNAs. RNA pol III synthesizes the tRNAs, the 5*S* rRNA, some snRNAs, and some miRNAs.

TABLE 36-1: Classes of Eukaryotic RNA

RNA	*Types*	*Abundance*	*Stability*
Ribosomal (rRNA)	28S, 18S, 5.8S, 5S	80% of total	Very stable
Messenger (mRNA)	~10^5 Different species	2-5% of total	Unstable to very stable
Transfer (tRNA)	~60 Different species	~15% of total	Very stable
Small RNAs			
Small nuclear (snRNA)	~30 Different species	≤1% of total	Very stable
Micro (miRNA)	100s-1000	<1% of total	Stable

Murray RK, Bender DA, Botham KM, Kennelly PJ, Rodwell VW, Weil PA. *Harper's Illustrated Biochemistry.* 29th ed. New York, NY: McGraw-Hill; 2012.

RNA Transcription

Synthesis of RNA exhibits several features that are synonymous with DNA replication. RNA synthesis requires accurate and efficient initiation, elongation proceeds in the 5′→3′ direction (ie, the polymerase moves along the template strand of DNA in the 3′→5′ direction), and RNA synthesis requires distinct and accurate termination. In contrast to DNA polymerases, RNA polymerases need not exhibit the same high level of fidelity. This is allowable since the aberrant RNA molecules can simply be turned over and new correct RNAs made.

Initiation of transcription, particularly the transcription of mRNA genes is tightly regulated. Sequences in the template DNA act in *cis* to stimulate the initiation of transcription (Figure 36-1). These sequence elements are termed *promoters*. Promoter sequences promote the ability of RNA polymerases to recognize the nucleotide at which initiation begins. Additional sequence elements are present within genes that act in *cis* to enhance polymerase activity even further. These sequence elements are termed *enhancers* (Table 36-2). Transcriptional promoter and enhancer elements are important sequences used in the control of gene expression.

The process of eukaryotic mRNA transcriptional initiation is an extremely complex event. There are numerous protein factors controlling initiation, some of which are basal factors (Figure 36-2) present in all cells and others are specific to cell type and/or the differentiation state of the cell. Two basal promoter elements that are found in essentially all eukaryotic *mRNA* genes are the TATA-box and the CAAT-box (Figure 36-1). These elements are so called because of the DNA sequences that constitute the promoter element. The TATA-box is found approximately 20-25 bases upstream of the start site for transcription and

High-Yield Concept

All RNA polymerases are dependent upon a DNA template in order to synthesize RNA. The resultant RNA is, therefore, complimentary to the template strand of the DNA duplex and identical to the nontemplate strand. The nontemplate strand is called the *coding strand* because its sequences are identical to those of the mRNA. However, in RNA, U is substituted for T.

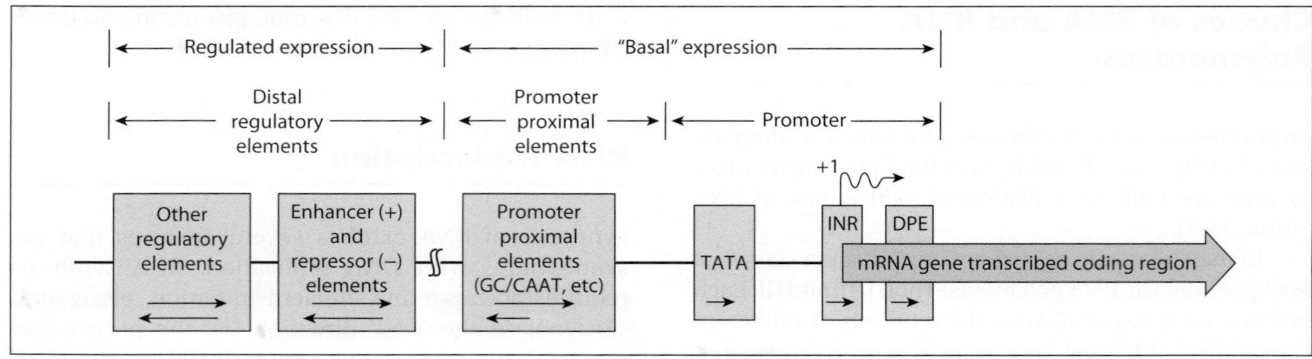

FIGURE 36-1: Schematic diagram showing the transcription control regions in a hypothetical mRNA-producing, eukaryotic gene transcribed by RNA polymerase II. Such a gene can be divided into its coding and regulatory regions, as defined by the transcription start site (**arrow**; +1). The coding region contains the DNA sequence that is transcribed into mRNA, which is ultimately translated into protein. The regulatory region consists of 2 classes of elements. One class is responsible for ensuring basal expression. The "promoter," is often composed of the TATA box and/or INR and/or DPE elements direct RNA polymerase II to the correct site (fidelity). However, in certain genes that lack TATA, the so-called TATA-less promoters, an initiator (INR) and/or DPE elements may direct the polymerase to this site. Another component, the upstream elements, specifies the frequency of initiation; such elements can either be proximal (50–200 bp) or distal (1000–10^5 bp) to the promoter as shown. Among the best studied of the proximal elements is the CAAT box, but several other elements (bound by the transactivator proteins Sp1, NF1, AP1, etc) may be used in various genes. The distal elements enhance or repress expression, several of which mediate the response to various signals, including hormones, heat shock, heavy metals, and chemicals. Tissue-specific expression also involves specific sequences of this sort. The orientation dependence of all the elements is indicated by the arrows within the boxes. For example, the proximal promoter elements (TATA box, INR, DPE) must be in the 5′–3′ orientation, while the proximal upstream elements often work best in the 5′–3′ orientation, but some can be reversed. The locations of some elements are not fixed with respect to the transcription start site. Indeed, some elements responsible for regulated expression can be located interspersed with the upstream elements or can be located downstream from the start site. Murray RK, Bender DA, Botham KM, Kennelly PJ, Rodwell VW, Weil PA. *Harper's Illustrated Biochemistry*. 29th ed. New York, NY: McGraw-Hill; 2012.

the CAAT-box is around 100 bases upstream. Many of the basal transcription factors are identified by the fact that they control the activity of RNA pol II. Thus, the nomenclature of these proteins is TFII, for transcription factor of RNA pol II (Figures 36-2 and 36-3).

TABLE 36-2: **Summary of the Properties of Enhancers**
• Work when located long distances from the promoter
• Work when upstream or downstream from the promoter
• Work when oriented in either direction
• Can work with homologous or heterologous promoters
• Work by binding one or more proteins
• Work by facilitating binding of the basal transcription complex to the *cis*-linked promoter
• Work by recruiting chromatin-modifying coregulatory complexes

Murray RK, Bender DA, Botham KM, Kennelly PJ, Rodwell VW, Weil PA. *Harper's Illustrated Biochemistry*. 29th ed. New York, NY: McGraw-Hill; 2012.

TFIID is the factor that binds to the TATA-box and its binding is facilitated by another factor called TFIIA.

Another critical TFII is TFIIH, which is in fact a complex of proteins. The TFIIH complex is not only involved in transcription but also in certain steps of DNA repair. The role of TFIIH in DNA repair can be seen as critical since defects in its function are responsible for certain forms of xeroderma pigmentosum (see Clinical Box 35-2). The critical role of TFIIH in transcription initiation is due to the fact that one of the proteins of the complex is a kinase that phosphorylates serine residues in the *C*-terminal domain (CTD) of the large subunit of RNA pol II. The CTD contains a tandem repeat sequence that is composed of the consensus heptad of amino acids: $Y_1S_2\ P_3T_4\ S_5P_6\ S_7$ which can be repeated from 25 to 52 times. It is Ser5 and Ser7 that become phosphorylated during transcriptional initiation. These serines are different from the serine (Ser2) phosphorylated in the CTD by pTEF-b involved in the capping process as discussed later.

Elongation involves the addition of the 5′ phosphate of ribonucleotides to the 3′–OH of the elongating RNA with the concomitant release of pyrophosphate.

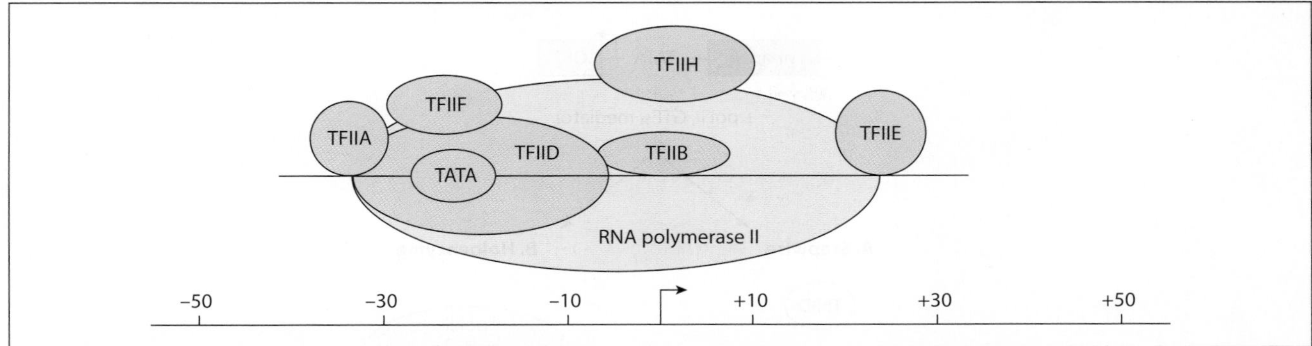

FIGURE 36-2: The eukaryotic basal transcription complex. Formation of the basal transcription complex begins when TFIID binds to the TATA box. It directs the assembly of several other components by protein-DNA and protein-protein interactions; TFIIA, B, E, F, H, and polymerase II (pol II). The entire complex spans DNA from position −30 to +30 relative to the transcription start site (TSS; +1, marked by bent arrow). The atomic level, x-ray-derived structures of RNA polymerase II alone and of the TBP subunit of TFIID bound to TATA promoter DNA in the presence of either TFIIB or TFIIA have all been solved at 3 Å resolution. The structures of TFIID and TFIIH complexes have been determined by electron microscopy at 30 Å resolution. Thus, the molecular structures of the transcription machinery are beginning to be elucidated. Much of this structural information is consistent with the models presented here. Murray RK, Bender DA, Botham KM, Kennelly PJ, Rodwell VW, Weil PA. *Harper's Illustrated Biochemistry.* 29th ed. New York, NY: McGraw-Hill; 2012.

Nucleotide addition continues until specific termination signals are encountered. Following termination, the core polymerase dissociates from the template (Figure 36-4).

Processing of RNAs

Eukaryotic RNAs undergo significant co- and post-transcriptional processing. Almost all *mRNA*, *tRNA*, and *rRNA* genes RNA are transcribed from genes that contain introns. The sequences encoded by the intronic DNA must be removed from the primary transcript prior to the RNAs being biologically active. The process of intron removal is called *RNA splicing*. In addition to intron removal in tRNAs, extra nucleotides at both the 5′ and 3′ ends are cleaved, the sequence 5′–CCA–3′ is added to the 3′ end of all tRNAs, and several nucleotides undergo modification. Additional processing occurs to mRNAs. The 5′ end of all eukaryotic mRNAs are capped with a unique 5′→5′ linkage to a 7-methylguanosine residue (Figure 36-5). The capped end of the mRNA is thus, protected from exonucleases and more importantly is recognized by specific proteins of the translational machinery (Chapter 37).

The capping process occurs after the newly synthesizing mRNA is around 20-30 bases long. At this point, RNA pol II pauses and the kinase, positive transcription elongation factor b (pTEF-b), phosphorylates RNA pol II on the serine-2 residues (Ser2) in the repeat unit of the CTD of the large subunit of the enzyme. The pTEF-b complex is also called *C*-terminal domain kinase 1 (CTDK1). This pausing and regulatory phosphorylation event allows for the potential of attenuation in the rate of transcription.

Most eukaryotic mRNAs are also polyadenylated at the 3′ end. A specific sequence, **AAUAAA**, is recognized by the endonuclease activity of polyadenylate polymerase, which cleaves the primary transcript approximately 11-30 bases 3′ of the sequence element. A stretch of 20-250 A residues is then added to the 3′ end by the polyadenylate polymerase activity.

Splicing of RNAs

Mammalian *mRNA* genes contain highly conserved consensus sequences that ultimately reside at the 5′ and 3′ ends of the introns in the mRNA (Figure 36-6). Intron removal from nascent RNA molecules involves a process termed *splicing* (Figure 36-7). The process of intron removal is catalyzed by a specialized RNA-protein complex called the *splicesome*. The splicesome is composed of small nuclear ribonucleoprotein particles (snRNPs, pronounced snurps) that contain proteins and several snRNAs identified as U1, U2, U4, U5, and U6. The U1 RNA has sequences that are complimentary to sequences near the 5′ end of the intron. The binding of U1 snRNA distinguishes the GU at the 5′ end of the

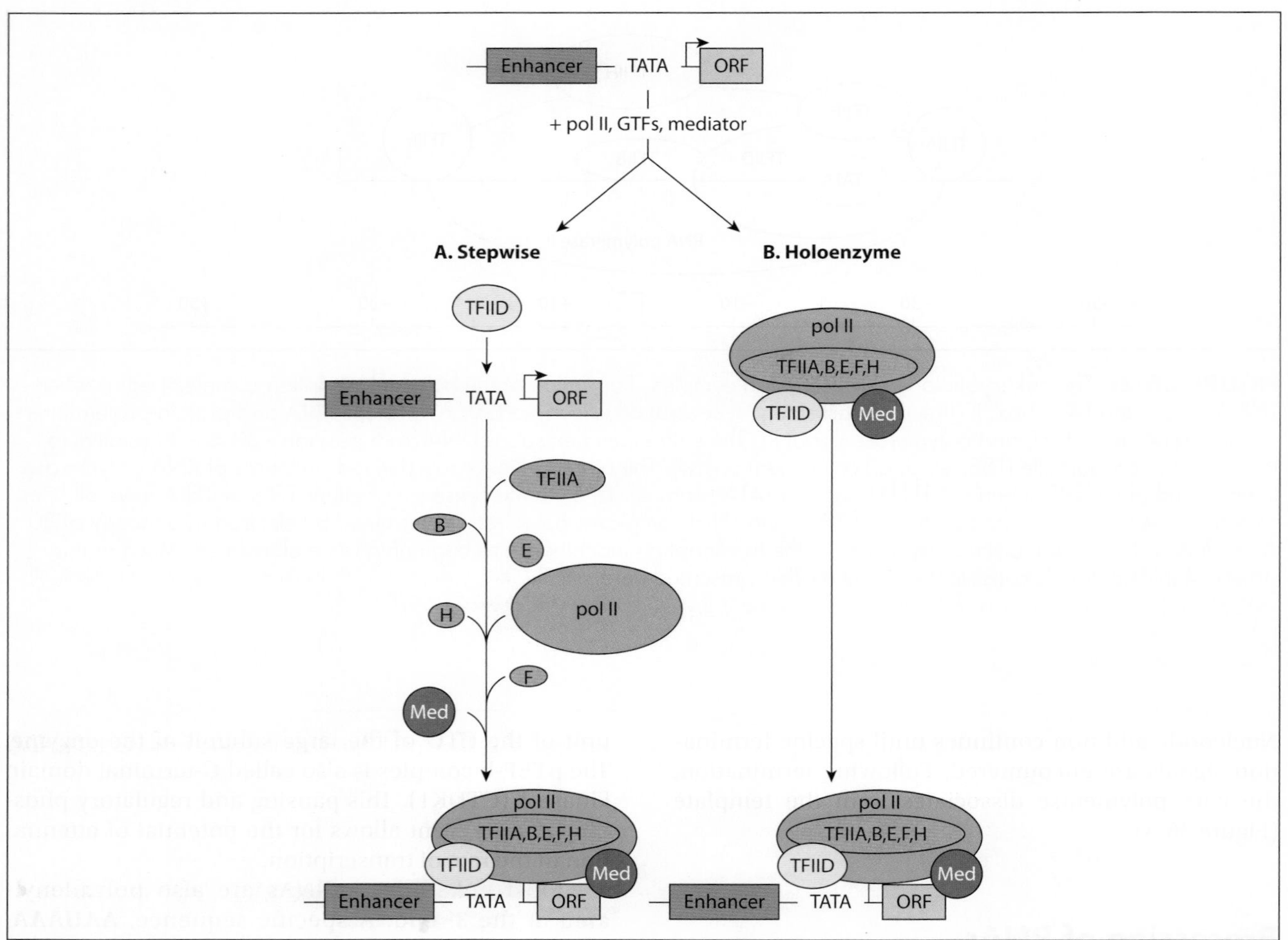

FIGURE 36-3: Models for the formation of an RNA polymerase II preinitiation complex. Shown at top is a typical mRNA encoding transcription unit: enhancer-promoter (TATA)-initiation site (bent arrow) and transcribed region (ORF; open reading frame). PICs have been shown to form by at least 2 distinct mechanisms: (A) the stepwise binding of GTFs, pol II, and mediator, or (B) by the binding of a single multiprotein complex composed of pol II, Med, and the 6 GTFs. DNA-binding transactivator proteins specifically bind enhancers and in part facilitate PIC formation (or PIC function) by binding directly to the TFIID-TAF subunits or Med subunits of mediator (not shown, see Figure 36-10); the molecular mechanism(s) by which such protein-protein interactions stimulate transcription remain a subject of intense investigation. Murray RK, Bender DA, Botham KM, Kennelly PJ, Rodwell VW, Weil PA. *Harper's Illustrated Biochemistry*. 29th ed. New York, NY: McGraw-Hill; 2012.

intron from other randomly placed GU sequences in mRNAs. The U2 RNA also recognizes sequences in the intron, in this case near the 3′ end.

Alternative Splicing

The presence of introns in RNAs allows for alternative splicing to occur, the result of which is the potential for an increase in phenotypic diversity without increasing the overall number of genes. By altering the pattern of exons that are spliced together, different proteins can arise from the processed mRNA from a single gene (Figure 36-8). Alternative splicing can occur either at specific developmental stages or in different cell types. Depending upon the site of transcription, the *calcitonin* gene yields an mRNA that synthesizes calcitonin (thyroid) or *calcitonin* gene–related peptide (CGRP, brain): 2 proteins with distinctly different functions. Even more complex alternative splicing occurs in the α-tropomyosin mRNA such that at least 8 different alternatively spliced α-tropomyosin mRNAs are formed.

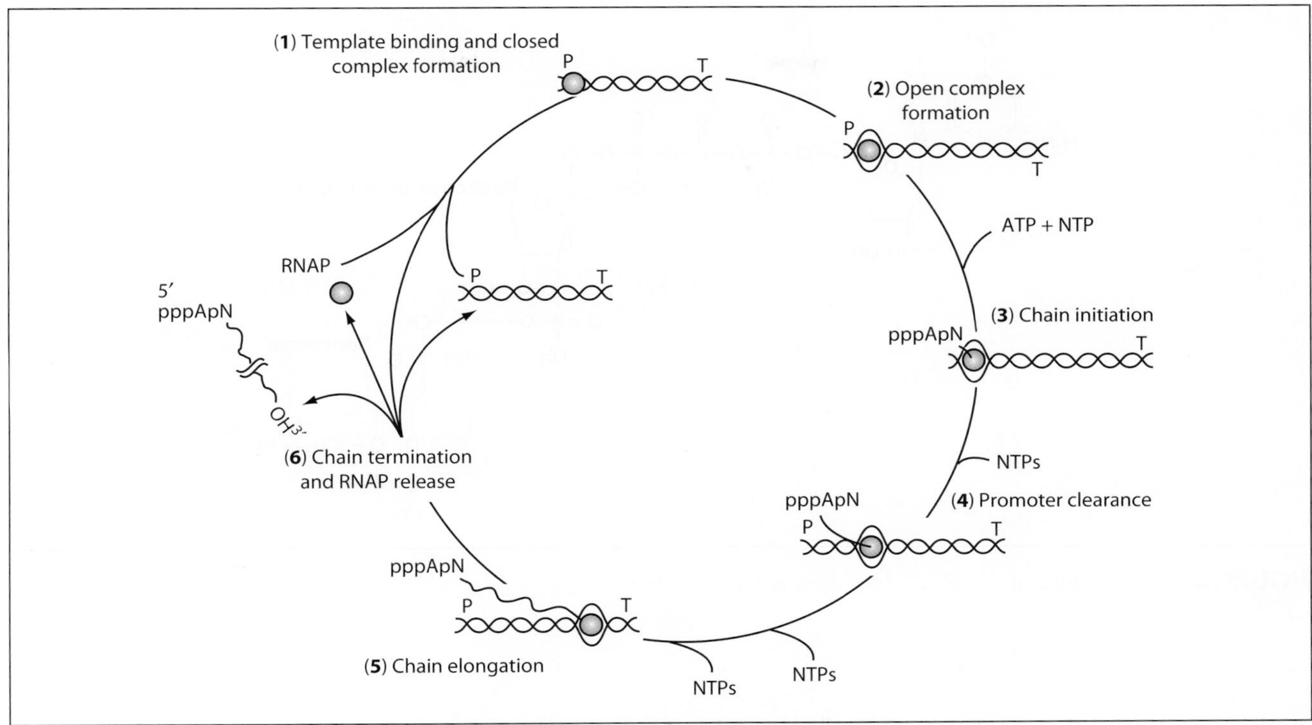

FIGURE 36-4: The transcription cycle. Transcription can be described in 6 steps: (1) Template binding and closed RNA polymerase promoter complex formation: RNA polymerase (RNAP) binds to DNA and then locates a promoter (**P**), (2) Open promoter complex formation: once bound to the promoter, RNAP melts the 2 DNA strands to form an open promoter complex; this complex is also referred to as the preinitiation complex or PIC. Strand separation allows the polymerase to access the coding information in the template strand of DNA, (3) Chain initiation: using the coding information of the template RNAP catalyzes the coupling of the first base (often a purine) to the second, template-directed ribonucleoside triphosphate to form a dinucleotide (in this example forming the dinucleotide 5′ pppApN$_{OH}$ 3′). (4) Promoter clearance: after RNA chain length reaches ~10–20 nt, the polymerase undergoes a conformational change and then is able to move away from the promoter, transcribing down the transcription unit. (5) Chain elongation: Successive residues are added to the 3′-OH terminus of the nascent RNA molecule until a transcription termination signal (**T**) is encountered. (6) Chain termination and RNAP release: Upon encountering the transcription termination site, RNAP undergoes an additional conformational change that leads to release of the completed RNA chain, the DNA template and RNAP. RNAP can rebind to DNA beginning the promoter search process and the cycle is repeated. Note that all of the steps in the transcription cycle are facilitated by additional proteins, and indeed are often subjected to regulation by positive and/or negative-acting factors. Murray RK, Bender DA, Botham KM, Kennelly PJ, Rodwell VW, Weil PA. *Harper's Illustrated Biochemistry*. 29th ed. New York, NY: McGraw-Hill; 2012.

Abnormalities in the splicing process can lead to various disease states. Many defects in the β-*globin* genes are known to exist leading to β-thalassemias. Some of these defects are caused by mutations in the sequences of the mRNA required for intron recognition and, therefore, result in abnormal processing of the β-globin primary transcript.

RNA Editing

RNA editing refers to a process by which there is post-transcriptional modification of nucleotide sequences of a given RNA transcripts via an enzymatic reaction. There are 2 types of RNA editing reactions that occur in mammalian cells. One involves the substitution of a uridine (U) for a cytidine (C) and the other involves the substitution of an inosine (I) for an adenosine (A). The C-to-U substitutions involve a cytidine deaminase that deaminates a cytidine base into a uridine base. The A-to-I substitutions involve an adenosine deaminase acting on RNA (ADAR). This enzyme is not the same as the adenosine deaminase involved in the salvage of purine nucleotides (Chapter 32).

An example of a physiologically and clinically significant C-to-U editing involves the apolipoprotein B (*apoB*) gene in humans (Figure 36-9). *ApoB-100* is expressed in the liver and *apoB-48* is expressed

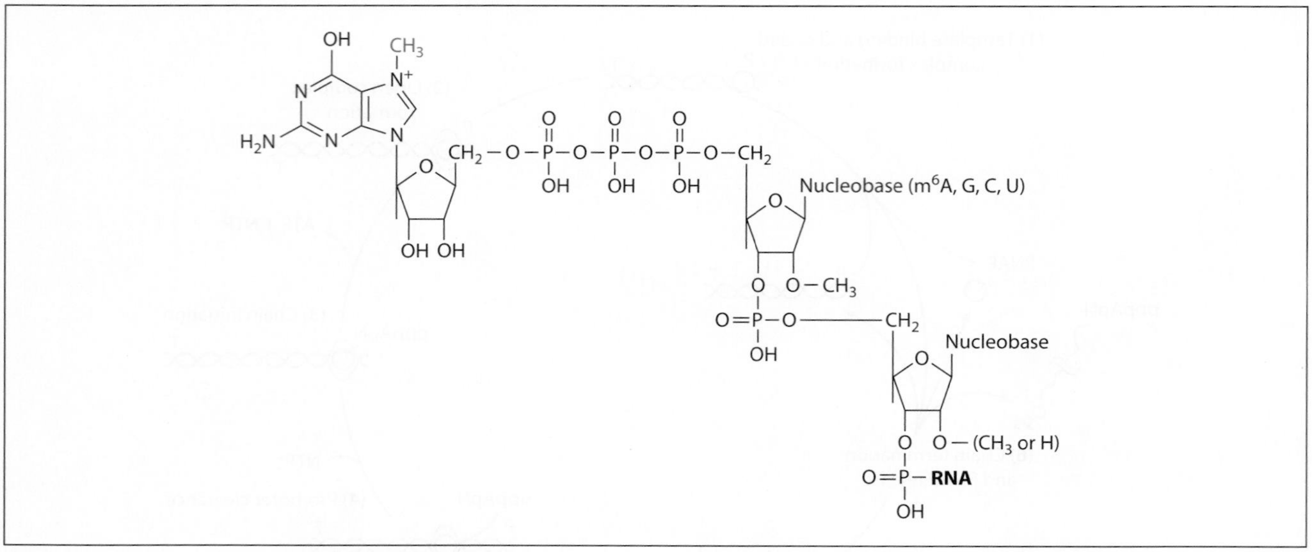

FIGURE 36-5: Structure of the 5′ cap found on eukaryotic mRNAs.

in the intestines. The *apoB-100* form has a CAA sequence that is edited to UAA, a stop codon, in the intestines but is left unedited in the liver. The process of A-to-I editing is the most common form of RNA editing in humans. Due to the fact that I behaves as if it is G both in translation and when forming secondary structures, the effects of these types of RNA edits include alteration of coding capacity, altered splicing, cytoplasmic sequestration, endonucleolytic cleavage, and inhibition of miRNA and siRNA processing.

Catalytically Active RNAs: Ribozymes

Ribozymes are RNAs with catalytic activity. The catalytic properties of ribozymes are exclusively due to the capacity of these RNA molecules to assume particular structures. Ribozymes function during protein synthesis, in RNA processing reactions, and in the regulation of gene expression. The processes of RNA-mediated catalysis were first identified by the discovery of self-splicing RNAs. Subsequently, numerous natural RNA motifs endowed with catalytic activity have been identified in mammalian tissues. Almost all ribozymes carry out a phosphoryl transfer reaction, catalyzing the cleavage or ligation of the RNA phosphodiester backbone. A notable exception is the peptidyl transferase activity of the ribozyme associated with the 28*S* subunit of the ribosome.

The mammalian cytoplasmic polyadenylation element-binding protein 3 (CPEB3) ribozyme is a self-cleaving noncoding RNA located in the second intron of the *CPEB3* gene. This ribozyme is involved in the process of mRNA polyadenylation. Other mammalian ribozymes have been characterized that are involved

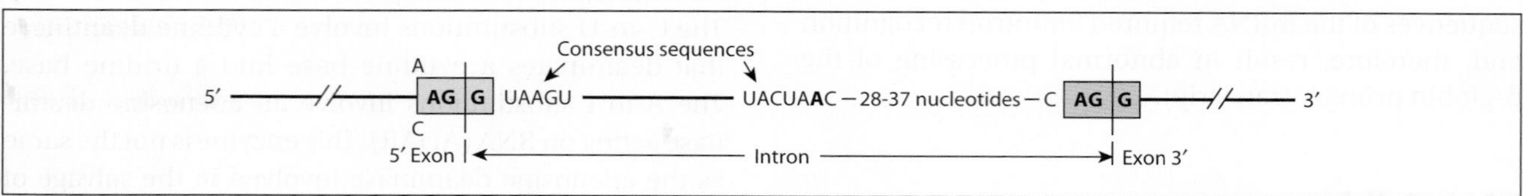

FIGURE 36-6: Consensus sequences at splice junctions. The 5′ (donor; left) and 3′ (acceptor; right) sequences are shown. Also shown is the yeast consensus sequence (UACUA **A** C) for the branch site. In mammalian cells, this consensus sequence is PyNPyPyPuAPy, where Py is a pyrimidine, Pu is a purine, and N is any nucleotide. The branch site is located 20-40 nucleotides upstream from the 3′ splice site. Murray RK, Bender DA, Botham KM, Kennelly PJ, Rodwell VW, Weil PA. *Harper's Illustrated Biochemistry*. 29th ed. New York, NY: McGraw-Hill; 2012.

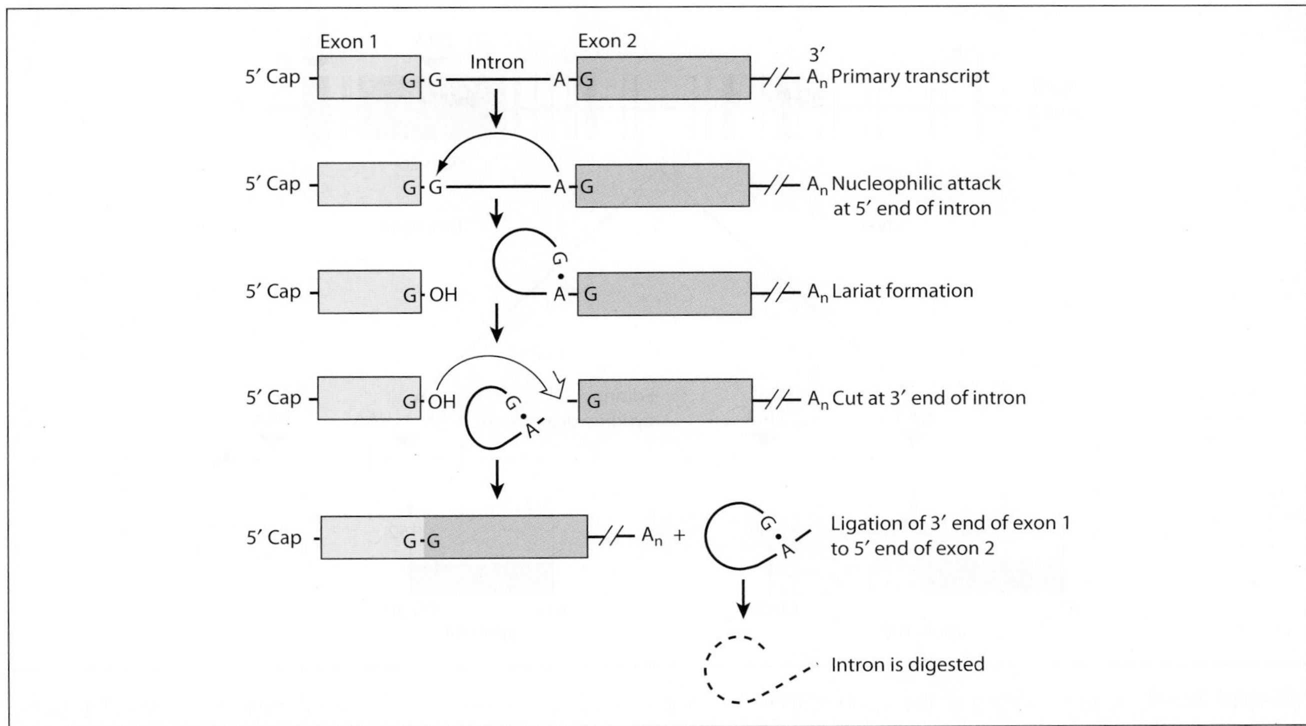

FIGURE 36-7: The processing of the primary transcript to mRNA. In this hypothetical transcript, the 5′ (left) end of the intron is cut (↓) and a lariat forms between the G at the 5′ end of the intron and an A near the 3′ end, in the consensus sequence UACUAAC. This sequence is called the branch site, and it is the 3′ most **A** that forms the 5′–2′ bond with the G. The 3′ (**right**) end of the intron is then cut (⇓). This releases the lariat, which is digested, and exon 1 is joined to exon 2 at G residues. Murray RK, Bender DA, Botham KM, Kennelly PJ, Rodwell VW, Weil PA. *Harper's Illustrated Biochemistry*. 29th ed. New York, NY: McGraw-Hill; 2012.

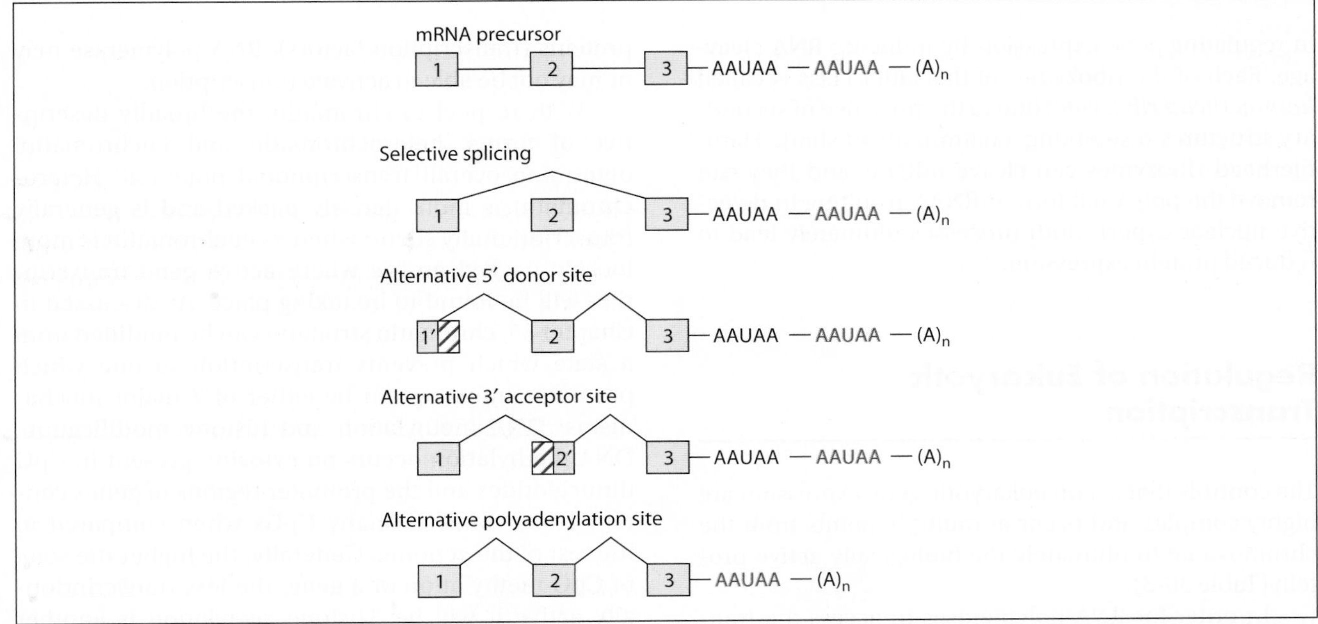

FIGURE 36-8: Mechanisms of alternative processing of mRNA precursors. This form of mRNA processing involves the selective inclusion or exclusion of exons, the use of alternative 5′ donor or 3′ acceptor sites, and the use of different polyadenylation sites. Murray RK, Bender DA, Botham KM, Kennelly PJ, Rodwell VW, Weil PA. *Harper's Illustrated Biochemistry*. 29th ed. New York, NY: McGraw-Hill; 2012.

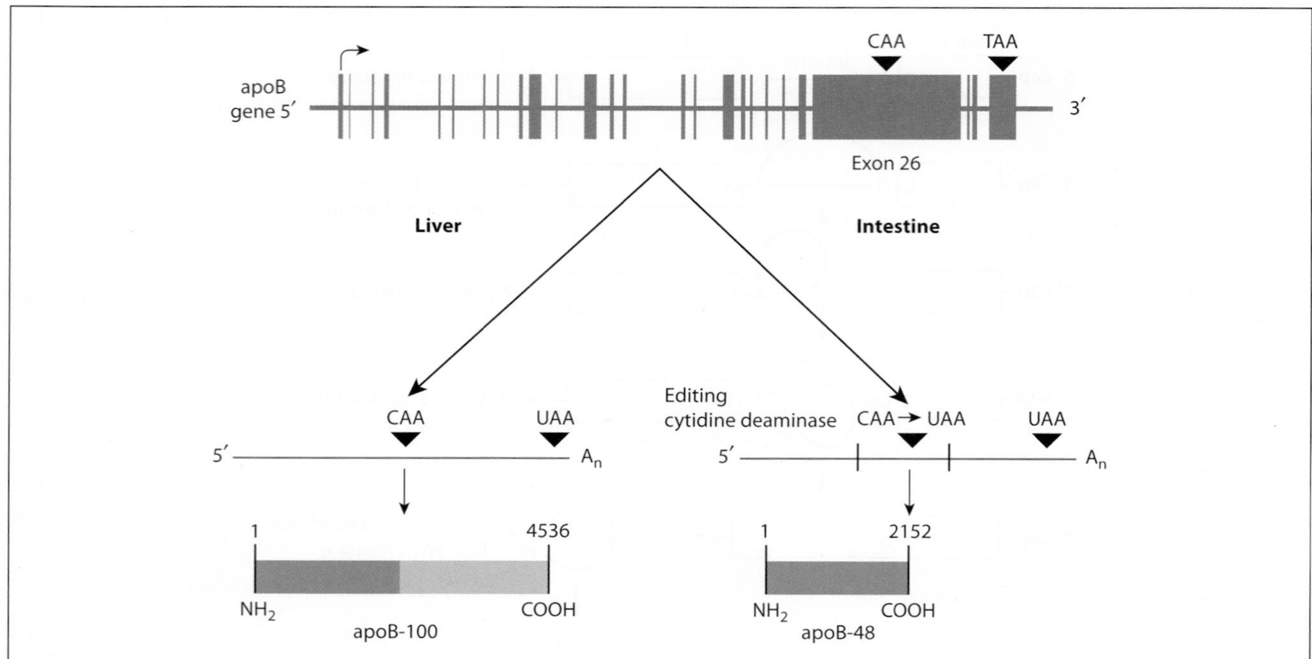

FIGURE 36-9: C-to-U editing of the apoB mRNA. In humans (and other mammals) the *apoB* gene is expressed in both hepatocytes and intestinal epithelial cells. In liver cells, the protein product is a 500-kD protein identified as apoB-100, whereas in intestinal cells the protein product is a smaller protein identified as apoB-48. The apoB-100 protein is translated from a nonedited mRNA, but the apoB-48 is translated from an edited mRNA. The C-to-U editing occurs in a CAA codon in exon 26 that results in the generation of a stop codon at that location in the edited mRNA, resulting in the truncation apoB-48 protein. The editing of the apoB mRNA is catalyzed by a cytidine deaminase. Reproduced with permission of themedicalbiochemistrypage, LLC

in regulating gene expression by inducing RNA cleavage. Each of the ribozymes of this latter class is called *hammerhead ribozymes* due to the presence of secondary structures resembling a hammerhead shark. Hammerhead ribozymes can cleave mRNAs and they can remove the polyA tail from mRNAs, resulting in defective nuclear export. Both processes ultimately lead to reduced protein expression.

Regulation of Eukaryotic Transcription

The controls that act on eukaryotic gene expression are highly complex and occur at multiple points from the chromosome to ultimately the biologically active protein (Table 36-3).

In order for RNA polymerases to access the transcriptional start site of a given gene, they must obtain access to the DNA template. Due to the organization of chromatin, the state of histone modification, and the presence or absence of transcriptional accessory proteins (transcription factors), RNA polymerase may or may not be able to activate transcription.

With respect to chromatin, the broadly descriptive of forms, heterochromatin and euchromatin, determine overall transcriptional potential. Heterochromatin is more densely packed and is generally transcriptionally silent; whereas euchromatin is more loosely packed and is where active gene transcription will be found to be taking place. As discussed in Chapter 35, chromatin structure can be modified from a state which prevents transcription to one which promotes transcription by either of 2 major mechanisms: DNA methylation and histone modification. DNA methylation occurs on cytosine present in CpG dinucleotides and the promoter regions of genes contain 10-20 times as many CpGs when compared to the rest of the genome. Generally, the higher the state of CpG methylation of a gene, the less transcriptionally active it will be. Histone acetylation is another major regulator of transcriptional initiation, where the presence of acetylation is associated with higher transcriptional activity. Many transcriptional activator complexes contain histone acetylase activity, whereas

TABLE 36-3: Gene Expression Control in Eukaryotes

Control point	*Properties*
Chromatin structure	The physical structure of chromatin can affect the ability of transcriptional regulatory proteins and RNA polymerases to find access to specific genes and to activate transcription
Epigenetic	Refers to changes in the pattern of gene expression that are not due to changes in the nucleotide composition of the genome, involves DNA methylation and histone modifications
Transcriptional initiation	Specific factors that exert control include the strength of promoter elements, the presence or absence of enhancer sequences, and the interaction between multiple activator and inhibitor proteins
RNA processing and modification	mRNAs are capped, polyadenylated, and the introns must be accurately removed from all RNA classes
RNA transport	A fully processed mRNA must leave the nucleus in order to be translated into protein
RNA stability	Certain mRNAs have sequences that are signals for rapid degradation
Small RNAs	Small RNA-mediated control can be exerted either at the level of the translatability of the mRNA, the stability of the mRNA, or via changes in chromatin structure
Translational initiation	Many mRNAs have multiple methionine codons, the ability of ribosomes to recognize and initiate synthesis from the correct AUG codon can affect the expression of a gene product
Posttranslational modification	Multiple types of modifications including glycosylation, acetylation, fatty acylation, disulfide bond formations, etc
Protein transport	To be biologically active, proteins must be transported to their site of action
Protein stability	Many proteins are rapidly degraded, whereas others are highly stable

transcriptional repressor complexes contain histone deacetylase activity.

The most complex controls observed in eukaryotic genes are those that regulate the expression of RNA pol II–transcribed genes, the *mRNA* genes. Eukaryotic *mRNA* genes contain a basic structure (see Figure 36-1) consisting of coding exons and noncoding introns and any number of different transcriptional regulatory domains (Table 36-4) that are sites for the interaction of various classes of transcription factor (Table 36-5). Several conserved structural motifs (Table 36-6) are found in most transcription factors including the helix-turn-helix, the zinc finger (Figure 36-10), and the leucine zipper (Figure 36-11).

The helix-loop-helix (HLH) domain is involved in protein homo- and heterodimerization. The HLH motif is composed of 2 regions of α-helix separated by a region of variable length, which forms a loop between the 2 α-helices. The HLH class of transcription factor most often contains a region of basic amino acids located on the *N*-terminal side of the HLH domain (termed bHLH proteins) that is necessary in order for the protein to bind DNA at specific sequences.

TABLE 36-4: Some of the Mammalian RNA Polymerase II Transcription Control Elements, Their Consensus Sequences, and the Factors That Bind to Them

Element	*Consensus Sequence*	*Factor*
TATA box	TATAAA	TBP/TFIID
CAAT box	CCAATC	C/EBP*, NF-Y*
GC box	GGGCGG	Sp1*
	CAACTGAC	Myo D
	T/CGGA/CN$_5$GCCAA	NF1*
Ig octamer	ATGCAAAT	Oct1, 2, 4, 6*
AP1	TGAG/CTC/AA	Jun, Fos, ATF*
Serum response	GATGCCCATA	SRF
Heat shock	(NGAAN)$_3$	HSF

Note: A complete list would include hundreds of examples. The asterisks mean that there are several members of this family.

Murray RK, Bender DA, Botham KM, Kennelly PJ, Rodwell VW, Weil PA. *Harper's Illustrated Biochemistry*. 29th ed. New York, NY: McGraw-Hill; 2012.

TABLE 36-5: Three Classes of Transcription Factors Involved in mRNA Gene Transcription

General Mechanisms	*Specific Components*
Basal components	RNA Polymerase II, TBP, TFIIA, B, D, E, F, and H
Coregulators	TAFs (TBP + TAFs) = TFIID; certain genes Mediator, Meds Chromatin modifiers Chromatin remodelers
Activators	SP1, ATF, CTF, AP1, etc

Murray RK, Bender DA, Botham KM, Kennelly PJ, Rodwell VW, Weil PA. *Harper's Illustrated Biochemistry*. 29th ed. New York, NY: McGraw-Hill; 2012.

The zinc finger domain is a DNA-binding motif consisting of specific spacing of cysteine and histidine residues that allow the protein to bind zinc atoms. The metal atom coordinates the sequences around the cysteine and histidine residues into a fingerlike domain. The finger domains can lie within the major groove of the DNA helix.

The leucine zipper domain is necessary for protein homo- and heterodimerization. It is a motif generated by a repeating distribution of leucine residues spaced 7 amino acids apart within α-helical regions of the protein. These leucine residues end up with their R groups protruding from the α-helical domain and are thought to interdigitate with leucine R groups of another

TABLE 36-6: Examples of Transcription Factors That Contain Various DNA Binding Motifs

Binding Motif	*Organism*	*Regulatory Protein*
Helix-turn-helix	*E coli* Phage Mammals	lac repressor CAP λcl, cro, and 434 repressors Homeobox proteins Pit-1, Oct1, Oct2
Zinc finger	*E coli a* Yeast *Drosophila* Xenopus Mammals	Gene 32 protein Gal4 Serendipity, Hunchback TFIIIA Steroid receptor family, Sp1
Leucine zipper	Yeast Mammals	GCN4 C/EBP, fos, Jun, Fra-1, CRE binding protein, *c-myc*, *n-myc*, *l-myc*

Murray RK, Bender DA, Botham KM, Kennelly PJ, Rodwell VW, Weil PA. *Harper's Illustrated Biochemistry*. 29th ed. New York, NY: McGraw-Hill; 2012.

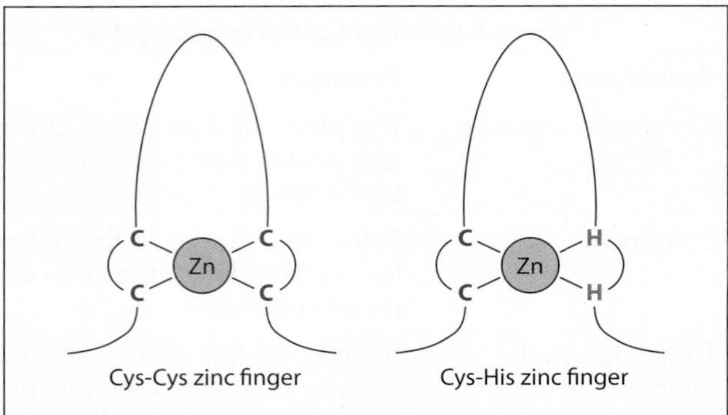

FIGURE 36-10: Zinc fingers are a series of repeated domains (two to nine) in which each is centered on a tetrahedral coordination with zinc. In the case of TFIIIA, the coordination is provided by a pair of cysteine residues (C) separated by 12–13 amino acids from a pair of histidine (H) residues. In other zinc finger proteins, the second pair also consists of C residues. Zinc fingers bind in the major groove, with adjacent fingers making contact with 5 bp along the same face of the helix. Murray RK, Bender DA, Botham KM, Kennelly PJ, Rodwell VW, Weil PA. *Harper's Illustrated Biochemistry*. 29th ed. New York, NY: McGraw-Hill; 2012.

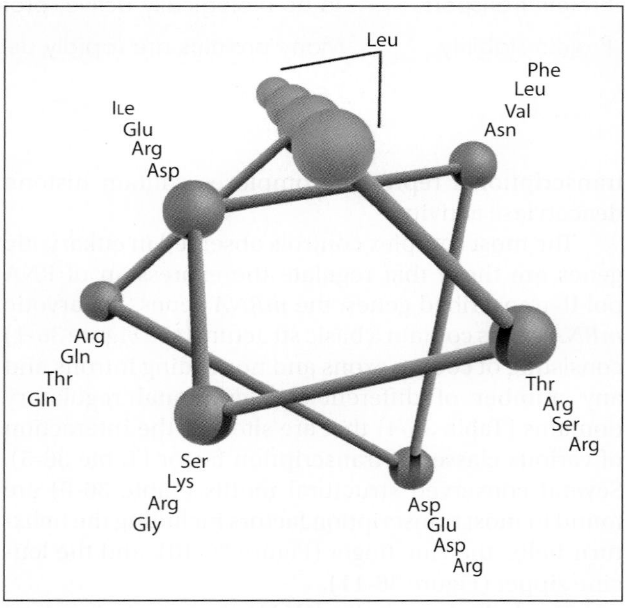

FIGURE 36-11: Helical wheel orientation of the backbone of the leucine zipper domain. Reproduced with permission of themedicalbiochemistrypage, LLC.

leucine zipper domain, thus stabilizing homo- or heterodimerization.

Small RNAs and Posttranscriptional Regulation

As recently as 15 years ago, it was believed that the only noncoding RNAs were the tRNAs and rRNAs of the translational machinery, and the U RNAs of the splicing machinery. However, in a landmark study published in 1993 on the control of developmental timing in the roundworm *Caenorhabditis elegans*, it was shown that the control of one gene was exerted by the small noncoding RNA product of another gene. This noncoding RNA was first identified in a large class of small regulatory RNAs called microRNAs or miRNAs that consist of approximately 22 nt. It is predicted that at least 250 *miRNA* genes are present in the human genome.

The processing and functioning of miRNAs is similar to that of the RNA silencing pathway, identified in plants as the posttranscriptional gene silencing (PTGS) pathway and in mammals as the RNA inhibitory (RNAi) pathway. The RNAi pathway involves the enzymatic processing of double-stranded RNA into small interfering RNAs (siRNAs) of approximately 22-25 nt that may have evolved as a means to degrade the RNA genomes of invading RNA viruses.

Micro-RNAs are transcribed by either RNA pol II or pol III as larger precursor RNAs that form a stem-loop structure while in the nucleus (Figure 36-12). The stem-loop of the primary *miRNA* gene transcript (pri-miRNA) is first cleaved through the action of the RNase III–related activity called *Drosha*, which takes place in the nucleus and generates the precursor miRNA

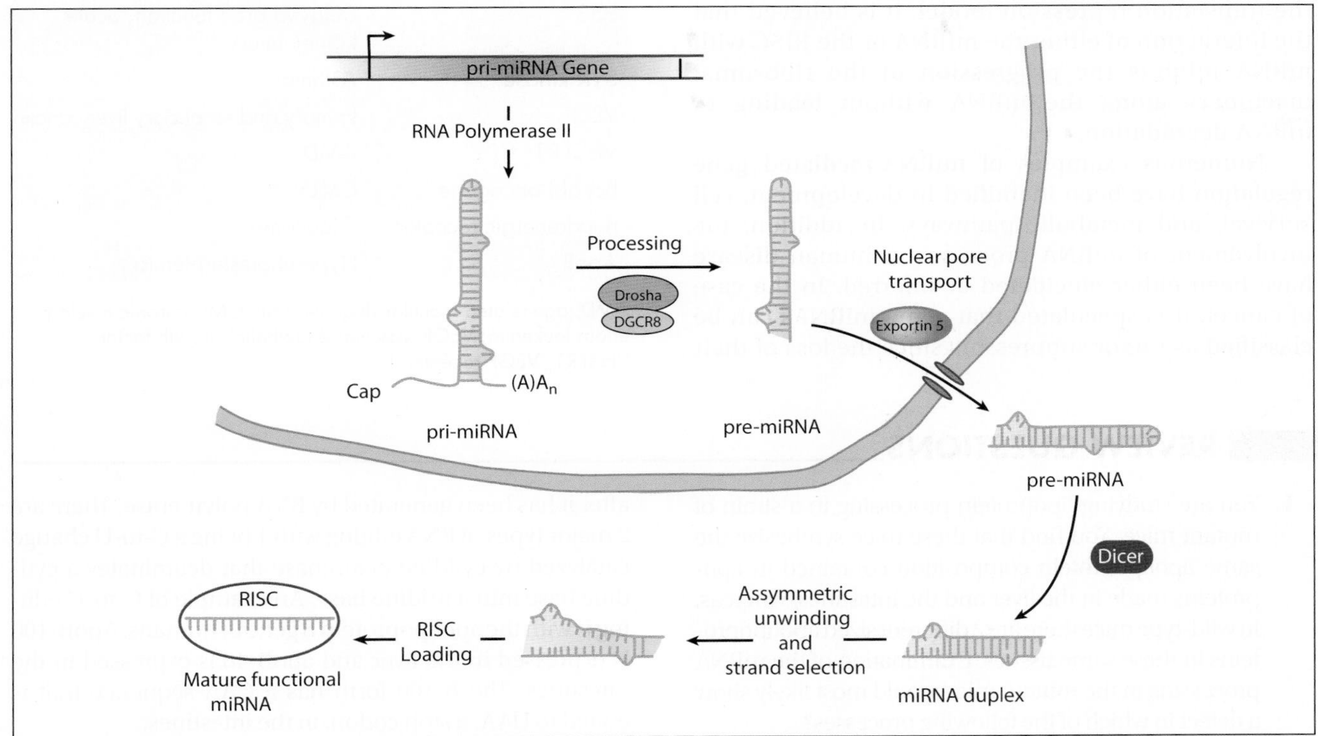

FIGURE 36-12: Biogenesis of miRNAs. miRNA-encoding genes are transcribed by RNA pol II into a primary miRNA transcript (pri-miRNA), which is 5′-capped and polyadenylated as is typical of mRNA coding primary transcripts. This pri-miRNA is subjected to processing within the nucleus by the action of the Drosha-DGCR8 nuclease, which trims sequences from both 5′ and 3′ ends, generating the pre-miRNA. This partially processed double-stranded RNA is transported through the nuclear pore by exportin-5. The cytoplasmic pre-miRNA is then trimmed further by the action of the multi-subunit nuclease termed Dicer, to form the miRNA duplex. One of the 2 resulting 21-22 nucleotide-long RNA strands is selected, the duplex unwound, and the selected strand loaded into the RISC complex, thereby generating the mature, functional miRNA. Murray RK, Bender DA, Botham KM, Kennelly PJ, Rodwell VW, Weil PA. *Harper's Illustrated Biochemistry*. 29th ed. New York, NY: McGraw-Hill; 2012.

(pre-miRNA). In the siRNA pathway, the duplex RNAs are cleaved into 22-25 nt pieces through the action of the enzyme Dicer in the cytosol. Processed miRNA stem-loop structures are transported from the nucleus to the cytosol via the activity of exportin 5. In the cytosol, the processed miRNA stem-loop is targeted by Dicer, which removes the loop portion. Ultimately, fully processed miRNAs and siRNAs are engaged by the RNA-induced silencing complex (RISC), which separates the 2 RNA strands. The active strand of RNA derived either from the miRNA or siRNA pathway is antisense to a region of the target mRNA.

Two models exist for how siRNAs and miRNAs interfere with the expression of target genes. These models include directed degradation of the target mRNA or interference with the translation of a target mRNA. In the case of miRNA-directed mRNA degradation, the proposed model involves the complimentary interaction of the miRNA with the mRNA and then the recruitment of the RISC, which ultimately leads to degradation of the target mRNA. In the translation repression model, it is believed that the interaction of either the miRNA or the RISC with mRNA inhibits the progression of the ribosomal machinery along the mRNA without leading to mRNA degradation.

Numerous examples of miRNA-mediated gene regulation have been identified in development, cell survival, and metabolic pathways. In addition, the involvement of miRNA processes in human disease have been either elucidated or inferred. In the case of cancer, it is speculated that some miRNAs can be classified as tumor suppressors since the loss of their activity is associated with cancer progression. A role for miRNAs in neurodegenerative diseases is also suggested by the example of fragile X syndrome. *Fragile X syndrome* is caused by expansion of a trinucleotide repeat in the *FMR1* gene, and the product of the *FMR1* gene, FMRP, is an RNA-binding protein that associates with miRNAs.

The role of RNAi in the inhibition of gene expression has allowed for the development of a whole new class of pharmaceuticals. The ability to introduce an RNAi-expressing construct or an RNAi-like molecule into the body could result in a significant reduction in the expression of abnormal proteins associated with certain disease states. Indeed, several therapeutic approaches involving RNAi are being developed and tested in human clinical trials (Table 36-7).

TABLE 36-7: Diseases Targeted for miRNA Therapy

Target RNA	*Disease Indication*
p53	Delayed graft function, acute kidney injury
SYK kinase	Asthma
VEGF	Primary and secondary liver cancer
VEGFR1	AMD
Bcr-abl oncogene	CML
β_2-adrenergic receptor	Glaucoma
ApoB	Hypercholesterolemia

AMD, age-related macular degeneration; CML, chronic myelogenous leukemia; VEGF, vascular endothelial growth factor; VEGFR1, VEGF receptor 1.

REVIEW QUESTIONS

1. You are studying lipoprotein processing in a strain of mutant mice. You find that these mice synthesize the same apolipoprotein composition contained in lipoproteins made in the liver and the intestines, whereas, in wild-type mice there are 2 different sized apolipoproteins in these same tissues. Examination of the mRNA processing in the mutant mice would most likely show a defect in which of the following processes?

A. alternative polyadenylation
B. alternative splicing
C. differential capping
D. posttranscriptional modification converting a U to a T residue
E. RNA editing

Answer E: RNA editing is a molecular process through which some cells can make discrete changes to specific nucleotide sequences within an mRNA molecule after it has been generated by RNA polymerase. There are 2 major types of RNA editing with 1 being a C-to-U change catalyzed by cytidine deaminase that deaminates a cytidine base into a uridine base. An example of C-to-U editing is with the apolipoprotein B gene in humans. ApoB-100 is expressed in the liver and apoB-48 is expressed in the intestines. The B-100 form has a CAA sequence that is edited to UAA, a stop codon, in the intestines.

2. You are studying the processes of RNA transcription in a cell-free system. You find that although the RNA polymerase II in your system initiates transcription as expected, it does not complete the process. Which of the following modifications to the enzyme is most likely not taking place, thereby, explaining the lack of complete transcription?

A. 5′ capping
B. acetylation

C. methylation
D. phosphorylation
E. ubiquitination

Answer D: In order for RNA pol II to initiate, as well as to continue, transcription it must be phosphorylated. The transcription factor complex TFIIH contains a kinase that phosphorylates serine residues in the *C*-terminal domain (CTD) of the large subunit of RNA pol II. This phosphorylation event allows transcription initiation to commence. The 5′ end of all eukaryotic mRNAs are capped and this process occurs after the newly synthesizing mRNAs are around 20-30 bases long. At this point, RNA pol II pauses and a different kinase phosphorylates additional residues in the CTD. This pausing and regulatory phosphorylation event allows for the potential of attenuation in the rate of transcription. Lack of phosphorylation would, therefore, prevent continued transcription.

3. Which of the following represents a characteristic feature of the cap structure on the 5′ end of most eukaryotic mRNAs?
A. it is a methylated adenine
B. it is a methylated cytidine
C. it is a methylated guanine
D. it is an adenine found attached to a cytidine dinucleotide in the context A-C-C
E. it is a guanine found attached to a cytidine dinucleotide in the context G-C-C

Answer C: The 5′ end of all eukaryotic mRNAs are capped with a unique 5′→5′ linkage to a 7-methylguanosine residue. The capped end of the mRNA is thus protected from exonucleases and more importantly is recognized by specific proteins of the translational machinery.

4. You are comparing the process of RNA splicing in an mRNA from normal and mutant cells of the same tissue. You find that the mutant mRNA is longer than the mRNA from the normal cells. Examination of the sequences of the gene encoding this mRNA reveals that there are nucleotide changes at the boundary of one of the exons in the mutant cell gene. Which of the following nucleotides would be expected to be found at the 3′ end of upstream donor exons and the 5′ end of downstream acceptor exons in the normal gene but not in the mutant gene?
A. AG–G
B. AG–AG
C. CA–GA
D. CG–G
E. G–AG

Answer A: Analysis of the human genome and the encoded mRNA have revealed highly conserved consensus sequences at the 5′ and 3′ ends of essentially all mRNA exons and introns. The 3′ end of all upstream exons contains AG with the G being the donor nucleotide attached to the 5′ end of the downstream exon. The 5′ end of the acceptor exon is always a G residue.

5. Which of the following relates to the transcription of a eukaryotic *mRNA* gene?
A. begins only when repressors are removed from nucleosomes in which the gene lies
B. occurs when the gene is in heterochromatin
C. requires binding of RNA polymerase II to the CCAAT box
D. requires binding of TFIID to the TATA box
E. requires eIF-2

Answer D: There are numerous protein factors controlling transcription initiation. Two basal promoter elements that are found in essentially all eukaryotic *mRNA* genes are the TATA box and the CAAT box. Many of the basal transcription factors are identified by the fact that they control the activity of RNA pol II. Thus, the nomenclature of these proteins is TFII, for transcription factor of RNA pol II. TFIID is the factor that binds to the TATA-box.

6. You are examining the process of RNA synthesis in a cell line derived from a pancreatic tumor. You discover that the cells do not contain any U1 small nuclear RNA (snRNA). The lack of this RNA species in these cells is most likely to have which of the following effects on overall RNA synthesis?
A defective polyA tail addition
B failure of capping mRNAs
C loss of intron splicing
D no synthesis of any mRNAs
E synthesis of only rRNAs

Answer C: Nuclear mRNA introns undergo a splicing reaction catalyzed by specialized RNA-protein complexes called small nuclear ribonucleoprotein particles (snRNPs, pronounced snurps). The RNAs found in snRNPs are identified as U1, U2, U4, U5, and U6. Lack of the U snRNPs would lead to a failure to properly splice mRNAs.

7. The process of RNA editing leads to sequence changes that are not reflective of the genetic information contained within the gene for an edited RNA. RNA editing occurs through the action of specific nucleotide deaminases that change either adenine to inosine or cytidine to uridine. These nucleotide changes can affect the coding or splicing capacity of the RNA. Which of the following proteins is an important example of the result of RNA editing?

A. apo-B48
B. calcitonin gene related peptide (CGRP)
C. ferritin
D. glutamate dehydrogenase
E. tissue factor (factor III)

Answer A: RNA editing in mammals involves the deamination of adenine (A) to produce inosine (I) in pre-mRNAs. The process of A to I editing is catalyzed by ADARs (ADAs acting on RNA). In some pre-mRNAs this alters splicing; in some it alters codon(s). RNA editing also occurs to convert C to U. A C-to-U edit in the gene for apolipoprotein B leads to tissue-specific generation of apoB-48 in intestines, whereas, the nonedited mRNA makes apoB-100 in liver.

8. If the DNA strand shown below is used as a template for RNA polymerase, what would be the sequence of the resultant mRNA following transcription?

5′-CATTCCATAGCATGT-3′

A. 5′-ACAUGCUAUGGAAUG-3′
B. 5′-CAUUCCAUAGCAUGU-3′
C. 5′-GUAAGGUAUCGUACA-3′
D. 5′-UGUACGAUACCUUAC-3′

Answer A: DNA template strands are used by RNA polymerases to direct the synthesis of an RNA. The nucleotides incorporated are ribonucleotides and they will be complimentary to the sequences of the template strand and oriented in the antiparallel direction. Whenever RNA polymerase encounters an adenosine, it will incorporate a uracil into the RNA molecule.

9. A mutation that resulted in the loss of histone deacetylation activity in a eukaryotic cell line would be expected to have what effect on transcription?

A. conversion of activators into repressors
B. conversion of repressors into activators
C. enhanced rate of transcription
D. no effect
E. reduced rate of transcription

Answer C: Histone deacetylases are responsible for changing the state of histone acetylation. The consequences of reduced histone acetylation are altered chromatin structure, making it difficult for the transcriptional machinery to engage the DNA. Thus, histone deacetylation is most often associated with reduced capacity for transcription initiation.

10. Which of the following best describes the role of proteins that contain a basic helix-loop-helix (bHLH) domain, such as in the MyoD protein involved in the determination of muscle lineages?

A. binds to specific regions of DNA
B. interacts with the splicesome
C. participates in the polyadenylation of mRNAs
D. participates in the splicing of mRNAs
E. promotes the transnuclear transport of processed mRNAs

Answer A: The helix-loop-helix domain is a protein interaction domain characteristic of numerous transcription factors. The basic region is required for the recognition of, and binding to, specific DNA sequences.

11. Which of the following is the sequence of the DNA strand that serves as the template strand for transcription of the following strand of RNA?

RNA: 5′-AAGCGUUUGGG-3′

A. 3′-AAGCGTTTGGG-5′
B. 5′-AAGCGTTTGGG-3′
C. 5′-CCCAAACGCTT-3′
D. 5′-GGGTTTGCGAA-3′
E. 5′-TTCGCAAACCC-3′

Answer C: DNA template strands are used by RNA polymerases to direct the synthesis of an RNA. The nucleotides incorporated are ribonucleotides and they will be complimentary to the sequences of the template strand and oriented in the antiparallel direction. Whenever RNA polymerase encounters an adenosine, it will incorporate a uracil into the RNA molecule.

12. You are studying RNA processing in a cell-free system. You find that incomplete RNA processing is occurring in your system and that the failure is most likely due to incomplete assembly of the splicesome complex. Which of the following RNA-processing events is most likely defective in your assay system?

A. addition of poly(A)
B. guiding ribosomes to the endoplasmic reticulum
C. modification of the 5′ end of hnRNA
D. removal of introns in hnRNA
E. transport of mRNA to the cytoplasm

Answer D: A spliceosome is a complex of small nuclear RNAs (snRNAs) and proteins, which is responsible for the catalytic removal of introns from a transcribed pre-mRNA in the process referred to as RNA splicing.

13. You have developed a strain of transgenic mice that express a human β-globin gene. Your transgenic construct includes all 3 exons of the human β-globin gene plus 500 nucleotides of both 5′- and 3′-flanking sequences. Examination of these transgenic mice shows that the human β-globin construct is expressed at levels about 10-fold lower than the endogenous mouse β-globin gene. Which of the following regulatory elements is most likely missing from your transgenic construct, thereby explaining the reduced level of expression?

A. enhancer elements
B. mRNA splicing signals
C. polyadenylation signals
D. promoter elements
E. silencer elements

Answer A: Enhancer elements are *cis*-acting–DNA sequences that can increase transcription of genes. Enhancers can usually function in either orientation and at various distances from a promoter. The β-globin construct used to create the transgenic mice most likely did not include the appropriate enhancer element(s) that are present in the endogenous mouse β-globin gene, thereby accounting for the reduced expression of the transgene.

14. The completion of the human genome project demonstrated that the human genome codes for approximately 25,000 genes. However, these limited numbers of genes actually encode several hundreds of thousands of different proteins. Which of the following processes provides the majority of the additional diversity of the protein products from these genes?

A. DNA transposition
B. mRNA splicing
C. mutagenesis
D. rRNA processing
E. tRNA modification

Answer B: The precise splicing outcome of a transcribed gene is controlled by complex interactions between *cis*-regulatory splicing signals and *trans*-acting regulators. Alternative splicing is a prevalent mechanism for generating transcriptome and proteome diversity. It can modulate gene function, affect organismal phenotype, and cause disease.

15. Many members of the nuclear family of receptors are prevented from activity through protein-protein interaction. The glucocorticoid receptor, for example, is released from hsp90 (a chaperone protein) following binding by the appropriate steroid hormone. Which of the following represents the next event for the localization of the receptor-hormone complex?

A. cytoplasmic surface of the plasma membrane
B. Golgi cisterna
C. specific DNA sequences
D. specific mRNA transcripts
E. 50*S* ribosomal subunit

Answer C: The steroid/thyroid hormone receptor superfamily is a class of proteins that reside in the cytoplasm and bind their lipophilic hormone ligands in this compartment as these hormones are capable of freely penetrating the hydrophobic plasma membrane. Upon binding ligand, the hormone-receptor complex translocates to the nucleus and binds to specific DNA sequences termed *hormone response elements* (HREs). The binding of the complex to an HRE results in altered transcription rates of the associated gene.

16. You are characterizing the expression of a gene suspected of causing a form of ovarian cancer. You have isolated the gene and found that it is approximately 35 kilobases (kb) in length. Transcriptional analysis reveals that there are several discrete mRNAs produced by this gene ranging in length from 2.0 to 5.5 kb in normal and cancerous cells. Which of the following processes is the most likely cause of the difference in size of the mRNAs produced by this gene?

A. poly(A) addition
B. posttranslational modification
C. recombination
D. RNA editing
E. splicing

Answer E: The precise splicing outcome of a transcribed gene is controlled by complex interactions between *cis*-regulatory splicing signals and *trans*-acting regulators. Alternative splicing is a prevalent mechanism for generating transcriptome and proteome diversity. Alternative splicing can modulate gene function, affect organismal phenotype, and cause disease.

17. You are studying the activities of the apolipoproteins, apoB-48 and apoB-100. Both of these proteins are encoded by the same gene; yet apoB-48 is primarily expressed in the intestine, while apoB-100 expression is restricted to the liver. Which of the following is the most likely molecular process accounting for this difference in gene expression?

A. different initiation codons
B. DNA methylation
C. gene duplication
D. reiterated sequences
E. RNA editing

Answer E: RNA editing in mammals involves the deamination of adenine (A) to produce inosine (I) in pre-mRNAs. The process of A-to-I editing is catalyzed by ADARs (ADAs acting on RNA). In some pre-mRNAs this alters splicing; in some it alters codon(s). RNA editing also occurs to convert C to U. A C-to-U edit in the gene for apolipoprotein B leads to tissue-specific generation of apoB-48 in intestines, whereas, the nonedited mRNA makes apoB-100 in liver.

18. You are isolating and characterizing the nucleic acids from a variety of different cell types. You fractionate and hydrolyze a specific sample of the nucleic acids. You find that the sample being analyzed contains pseudouridine. Which of the following is the most likely nucleic acid you have analyzed?
A. DNA
B. mtDNA
C. mRNA
D. rRNA
E. tRNA

Answer E: More than 300 different tRNAs have been characterized and shown to have extensive similarities. They vary in length from 60-95 nucleotides (18-28 kD) and exhibit a cloverleaf-like secondary structure that is composed of an anticodon loop, a D loop, and a TΨC loop. The D loop contains the modified nucleotide, dihydrouridine, and the TΨC loop contains pseudouridine, hence the derivation of the names for these loops.

19. You are carrying out experiments designed to characterize the structure-function relationships of tRNAs. You isolate an enzyme with tRNA nucleotidyltransferase activity and show that it adds a CCA sequence to the 3′ end of human tRNAs. Which of the following characteristics best distinguishes this enzyme from other RNA polymerases?
A. requires only a GG template
B. synthesizes a specific sequence without a template
C. uses both mRNA and tRNA as substrates
D. uses nucleoside monophosphate as substrates
E. works in a 3′→5′ direction

Answer B: Since all human tRNAs contain variable nucleotide sequence yet also have the CCA sequence added posttranscriptionally, there is no template-specific control for the activity of tRNA nucleotidyltransferase. The growing 3′ terminus of the tRNA progressively refolds to allow the solitary active site of the enzyme to reuse a single CTP-binding site. The ATP-binding site is then created collaboratively by the refolded *CC* terminus and the enzyme, and nucleotide addition to any tRNA ceases when the nucleotide-binding pocket of the enzyme is full. The template for CCA addition is, therefore, a dynamic ribonucleoprotein structure and not a typical nucleotide template as for other RNA polymerases.

20. You are studying the rRNA synthesis and processing in a mutant cell line. You find that these cells synthesize a correct precursor rRNA, but do not correctly process it into the expected 3 rRNAs that are found in normal cells. Which of the following organelles is likely to be missing or defective in these cells, thus accounting for the failed rRNA processing?
A. endoplasmic reticulum
B. Golgi complex
C. nuclear matrix
D. nucleolus
E. ribosome

Answer D: During or immediately following transcription of pre-rRNA from rDNA in the nucleolus, the ribosomal RNA precursor (pre-rRNA) is modified and associates with a few ribosomal proteins. In order to generate the mature 18*S*, 5.8*S*, and 28*S* rRNAs from the precursor 45*S* rRNA, the precursor rRNA goes through a series of cleavages in order to remove the external and internal spacers.

21. You are treating cultured cells with an experimental compound. You find that addition of the compound results in a 2-fold increase in the expression of a specific gene. However, you find that the addition of the test compound causes a 10-fold increase in the level of the protein derived from the gene. The major effect of this experimental compound is most likely to be a decrease in which of the following?
A. degradation of mRNA by nucleases
B. rate of mRNA translation
C. rate of ribosomes binding to mRNA
D. RNA polymerase II activity
E. splicing of nascent RNA transcripts

Answer A: The disconnect between the level of gene expression, which results in mRNA increases and the level of protein increases from the resultant mRNAs can be accounted for by numerous consequences. However, in this case the most likely cause of the dramatically elevated level of protein from a slight elevation in mRNA levels is increased mRNA stability. The more stable mRNA can be engaged by the translational machinery more often resulting in more protein being made. Therefore, the test compound is most likely inhibiting the degradation of mRNAs by ribonucleases.

22. A transcriptional promoter is required for which of the following processes?

A. cleavage and polyadenylation of mRNA
B. initiation of RNA synthesis
C. recognition of the 3′ boundary for mRNA splicing
D. recognition of the 5′ boundary for mRNA splicing
E. termination of RNA synthesis

Answer B: The promoter region is a specific sequence of DNA upstream of the transcription start site of a gene. Promoters stimulate the initiation of transcription. Promoters are located near the genes they transcribe, on the same strand and upstream on the DNA.

23. The most common mechanism for the regulated expression of human genes during fetal development occurs at which of the following levels?

A. degradation of the protein product
B. excision of introns from precursor RNA
C. initiation of protein synthesis
D. initiation of RNA synthesis
E. modification of the newly synthesized protein

Answer D: In eukaryotic cells, the ability to express biologically active proteins can be regulated at several different stages from the activity of the gene to the final functional protein. Transcriptional initiation is the most important mode for control of eukaryotic gene expression.

24. Transcription factor proteins bind to specific DNA sequences present in their target genes. These factors subsequently lead to increased transcription of target genes by which of the following processes?

A. blocking the effects of repressor molecules
B. bringing RNA nucleotides into contact with the DNA template
C. increasing the rate of initiation
D. increasing the speed of RNA polymerase transcription
E. preventing the pausing of RNA polymerase along the DNA template

Answer C: Transcription factors are proteins that bind to specific DNA sequences, thereby controlling the activity of the gene whose regulatory sequences they bind. Transcription factors perform this function alone or with other proteins in a complex, by promoting or blocking the recruitment of RNA polymerase to specific genes. A defining feature of transcription factors is that they contain one or more DNA-binding domains (DBDs), which recognize and bind to specific sequences of DNA adjacent to the genes that they regulate.

25. Which of the following mechanisms inhibits expression of imprinted genes?

A. capping of the genes' mRNA
B. deletion of the gene's promoter region
C. dissociation of RNA pol II from the gene
D. inhibition of mRNA splicing
E. methylation of cytosine residues within the gene

Answer E: Genomic imprinting refers to a genetic phenomenon whereby there is preferential expression of a gene from only 1 of the 2 parental alleles. This phenomenon of allele-specific expression results from allele-specific epigenetic modifications such as CpG dinucleotide methylation. These modifications are referred to as *epigenetic modifications* (also referred to as epigenetic "marks").

26. You are studying the changes that have occurred in the genomes of members of a family susceptible to an inherited form of liver cancer. You find that afflicted family members harbor a mutation in the zinc-finger motif of a cell-cycle regulatory gene. Which of the following is the most likely result of this mutation?

A. decreased binding of a transcription factor to a DNA sequence
B. enhanced binding of hormones to receptors
C. enhanced transport of a hormone receptor complex into the nucleus
D. stimulation of mRNA synthesis
E. "unzipping" of leucine-rich helices

Answer A: The zinc finger domain is a DNA-binding motif consisting of specific spacings of cysteine and histidine residues that allow the protein to bind zinc atoms. The metal atom coordinates the sequences around the cysteine and histidine residues into a fingerlike domain. The finger domains can interdigitate into the major groove of the DNA helix. The spacing of the zinc finger domain in this class of transcription factor coincides with a half turn of the double helix.

27. Homeobox (*HOX*) genes play a role in controlling events of embryogenesis. These genes exert their functions through which of the following processes?

A. allelic exclusion
B. alternate mRNA splicing
C. regulation of transcription
D. regulation of translation
E. signal transduction

Answer C: *HOX* genes are a group of related genes that control the body plan of the embryo. All of the proteins encoded by the *HOX* genes are transcription factors that contain a DNA-binding domain and function by binding to specific target genes and regulating their rate of transcription.

28. Classically it was considered that each gene encoded one protein, the so-called one gene-one enzyme hypothesis. However, this model was modified as a result of the discovery of which of the following?

A. alternative splicing of primary transcripts to produce different forms of a protein
B. enhancer elements located upstream or downstream of the transcriptional promoter site in the DNA
C. oncogene products that act as transcription factors
D. transcription attenuation that regulates gene expression
E. variable number tandem repeats generating alternative processed genes during meiosis

Answer A: The precise splicing outcome of a transcribed gene is controlled by complex interactions between *cis*-regulatory splicing signals and *trans*-acting regulators. Alternative splicing is a prevalent mechanism for generating transcriptome and proteome diversity. Alternative splicing can modulate gene function, affect organismal phenotype, and cause disease.

29. All cells contain the same compliment of DNA. However, adipose tissue cells and gastrointestinal epithelial cells are not composed of the same proteins. The differences in these cells, as well as all other cells, is most likely a result of differences in which of the following?

A. DNA sequences
B. mRNAs
C. quantity of DNA in their nuclei
D. rRNAs
E. tRNAs

Answer B: The differentiation of cells into specific types, such as adipocytes and intestinal enterocytes, is the result of the pattern of genes that are allowed to be expressed in each cell type. This means that each distinct type of cell contains a unique and distinct set of mRNAs, directing the synthesis of cell-type specific proteins.

30. You are studying the effects of exposure of mouse embryos to various concentration of retinoic acid. Your studies show that the developmental malformations you observe are due to retinoic acid–induced changes in the expression of several homeobox (*HOX*) genes. Both retinoic acid receptors and *HOX* gene products recognize and bind to specific DNA sequences at numerous sites on multiple chromosomes. Which of the following best describes the function of these molecules?

A. initiation factors
B. ligands
C. polymerases
D. signal recognition particles
E. transcription factors

Answer E: Retinoic acid binds to a family of nuclear receptors called the retinoic acid receptors (RARs). Like all nuclear receptors, the RARs are ligand- and DNA-binding transcription factors. All of the proteins encoded by the *HOX* genes are also transcription factors that contain a DNA-binding domain and function by binding to specific target genes and regulating their rate of transcription.

Checklist

✓ RNAs are synthesized from a template of DNA by the action of RNA polymerases in a process termed transcription.

✓ Mammalian cells contain 3 distinct RNA polymerases involved in the transcription of nuclear DNA, identified as pol I, pol II, and pol III. Each polymerase transcribes a unique set of genes.

✓ The rate of transcription is controlled by a series of basal transcription factors and the concerted actions of gene-specific transcriptional regulators (both activators and repressors).

- ✓ The basal transcription factors of RNA polymerase II are called TFII proteins. Two promoter elements that are present upstream of almost all *mRNA* genes (called the TATA-box and the CAAT-box) interact with members of the TFII family of basal factors.
- ✓ Transcription involves efficient, accurate, and regulated initiation, followed by elongation, and termination.
- ✓ Almost all eukaryotic RNAs (mRNA, tRNA, and rRNA) are synthesized as precursor molecules that undergo various posttranscriptional processing that includes intron removal (all classes), nucleotide modification (all tRNAs), capping, and polyadenylation (almost all mRNAs).
- ✓ Some mRNAs are edited following transcription, which is an enzymatic modification of some of the nucleotides, resulting in altered coding capacity of the edited RNA.
- ✓ Ribozymes are a highly specialized class of RNA that possess enzymatic activity.
- ✓ Regulation of gene expression is a term that relates to the multiple processes that control the ability of a gene to be converted into a biologically active protein. Regulation of eukaryotic transcription is the most important mechanism for the regulation of gene expression.
- ✓ Numerous small noncoding RNAs are involved in regulating the gene expression. These include the small nuclear RNAs (snRNAs) that are involved in mRNA splicing, the micro RNAs (miRNAs)–directed mRNA degradation and translation repression processes, and the small interfering RNAs (siRNAs) of the RNA interference (RNAi) pathway in mammals.

CHAPTER

37 Translation: Protein Synthesis and Modification

CHAPTER OUTLINE

High-Yield Terms

Genetic code: the genetic code defines the set of rules (the nucleotide triplets) by which information encoded within the genes is translated into proteins

Wobble hypothesis: explains the non–Watson-Crick base-pairing that can occur between the 3′-nucleotide of a codon and the 5′-nucleotide of an anticodon

Ternary complex: translational initiation complex composed of eIF-2 with GTP bound and the initiator methionine tRNA

Peptidyltransferase: an RNA-mediated (ribozyme) enzymatic activity of the 60S ribosome that catalyzes transpeptidation during protein elongation.

Selenoprotein: any of a family of proteins that contain a modified selenocysteine amino acid

Signal sequence: the *N*-terminal 15-25 hydrophobic amino acids in proteins that are destined for secretion of membrane insertion; the sequences are recognized by the signal recognition particle which assists in binding of the ribosome to the ER membrane

Prenylation: posttranslational modification by the isoprenoid molecules farnesyl or geranyl allowing proteins to associate with membranes

Ubiquitin: a 76-amino-acid peptide enzymatically attached to proteins which, in most cases, targets the modified protein for degradation in the proteosome

Proteosome: a large protein complex whose function is to proteolytically degrade damaged or unneeded proteins

Translation is the RNA-directed synthesis of proteins. The process requires not only the template RNA, the mRNA, but also the participation of the tRNAs and rRNAs. The tRNAs are necessary to carry activated amino acids into the ribosome which itself is composed of rRNAs and ribosomal proteins. Although the chemistry of peptide bond formation is relatively simple, the processes leading to the ability to form a peptide bond are exceedingly complex. During translation the ribosome is intimately associated with the mRNA ensuring correct access of activated tRNAs and the necessary enzymatic activities to catalyze peptide bond formation.

Translation proceeds in an ordered process. First, accurate and efficient **initiation** must take place, then peptide **elongation**, and finally accurate and efficient **termination** must occur. All three of these processes require specific proteins, some of which are ribosome associated and some of which are separate from the ribosome, but may be temporarily associated with it.

Determination of the Genetic Code

Early experiments, designed to ascertain how the information in the DNA of genes was transmitted via RNAs to proteins, demonstrated several key facts that resulted in the definition of the **genetic code**. In addition, it was determined that the genetic code is read in a sequential manner starting from a fixed point in the mRNA and that the 5′-end of the mRNA corresponded to the amino terminus of the encoded protein. This means that translation proceeds along the mRNA in the 5′ → 3′ direction which corresponds to the *N*-terminal to *C*-terminal direction of the amino acid sequences within proteins.

The code was shown to be a triplet of nucleotides and all 64 possible combinations of the 4 nucleotides could code for amino acids. This latter fact is defined as the degeneracy of the genetic code since there are only 20 different amino acids required for the synthesis of all the different proteins. The precise dictionary of the genetic code was originally determined from in vitro experiments which also established the identity of translational termination codons (Table 37-1).

In addition to the genetic code present in the mRNA, accurate translation requires 2 equally important recognition steps. The correct choice of amino acid needs to be made for attachment to the correspondingly correct tRNA and the subsequent selection of the correct amino acid–charged tRNA by the translational machinery so that the amino acid is incorporated in the correct location in the protein.

TABLE 37-1: The Genetic Code[1] (Codon Assignments in Mammalian Messenger RNAs)

First Nucleotide	Second Nucleotide				Third Nucleotide
	U	C	A	G	
U	Phe	Ser	Tyr	Cys	U
	Phe	Ser	Tyr	Cys	C
	Leu	Ser	Term	Term[2]	A
	Leu	Ser	Term	Trp	G
C	Leu	Pro	His	Arg	U
	Leu	Pro	His	Arg	C
	Leu	Pro	Gln	Arg	A
	Leu	Pro	Gln	Arg	G
A	Ile	Thr	Asn	Ser	U
	Ile	Thr	Asn	Ser	C
	Ile[2]	Thr	Lys	Arg[2]	A
	Met	Thr	Lys	Arg[2]	G
G	Val	Ala	Asp	Gly	U
	Val	Ala	Asp	Gly	C
	Val	Ala	Glu	Gly	A
	Val	Ala	Glu	Gly	G

[1]The terms first, second, and third nucleotide refer to the individual nucleotides of a triplet codon read 5′→3′, left to right. A, adenine nucleotide; C, cytosine nucleotide; G, guanine nucleotide; Term, chain terminator codon; U, uridine nucleotide. AUG, which codes for Met, serves as the initiator codon in mammalian cells and also encodes for internal methionines in a protein. (Abbreviations of amino acids are explained in Chapter 3.)
[2]In mammalian mitochondria, AUA codes for Met and UGA for Trp, and AGA and AGG serve as chain terminators.

Murray RK, Bender DA, Botham KM, Kennelly PJ, Rodwell VW, Weil PA. *Harper's Illustrated Biochemistry*. 29th ed. New York: McGraw-Hill; 2012.

Characteristics of tRNAs

More than 300 different tRNAs have been characterized and shown to have extensive similarities. They vary in length from 60 to 95 nucleotides (18-28 kD) and exhibit a cloverleaf-like secondary structure that is composed of an anticodon loop, a D-loop, and a TψC-loop (Figure 37-1). The D-loop contains the modified nucleotide, dihydrouridine, and the TΨC loop contains pseudouridine, hence the derivation of the names for these loops. All tRNAs also have the trinucleotide sequence, CCA, added to their 3′-ends posttranscriptionally. The A residue serves as the acceptor site for attachment of the appropriate amino acid.

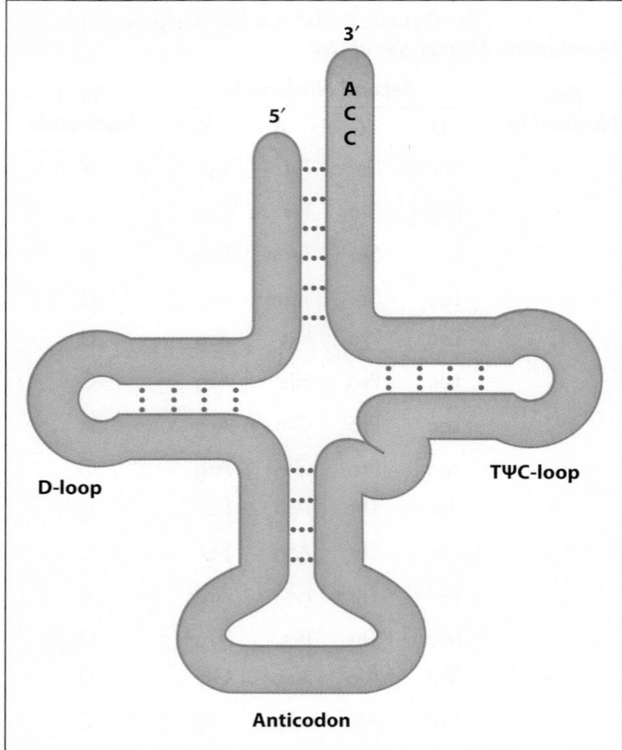

FIGURE 37-1: Two-dimensional structure of a typical tRNA. Reproduced with permission of themedicalbiochemistrypage, LLC.

Amino Acid Activation

Activation of amino acids is carried out by a 2-step process catalyzed by aminoacyl-tRNA synthetases (Figure 37-2). There are at least 21 different aminoacyl-tRNA synthetases since the initiator met-tRNA is distinct from noninitiator met-tRNAs. Accurate recognition of the correct amino acid as well as the correct tRNA is different for each aminoacyl-tRNA synthetase.

In the 2-step reaction the enzyme first attaches the amino acid to the α-phosphate of ATP with the concomitant release of pyrophosphate forming an aminoacyl-adenylate intermediate. In the second step the enzyme catalyzes transfer of the amino acid to either the 2′- or 3′-OH of the ribose portion of the 3′-terminal adenosine residue of the tRNA generating the activated aminoacyl-tRNA.

Most cells contain isoacceptor tRNAs, different tRNAs that are specific for the same amino acid; however, many tRNAs bind to 2 or 3 codons specifying their cognate amino acids (see Table 37-1). Given the high degree of nucleotide modifications that occur in tRNAs it is possible for non–Watson-Crick base-pairing to occur at the third codon position, that is, the 3′-nucleotide of the mRNA codon and the 5′-nucleotide of the tRNA anticodon. This phenomenon has been termed the **wobble hypothesis.**

Translation Initiation

Initiation of translation requires numerous components including an mRNA, a pool of amino acid charged tRNAs including a specific initiator tRNA, $tRNA_i^{met}$, the ribosome, and numerous nonribosomal proteins termed initiation factors (Table 37-2). Translational initiation factors are identified as eIFs (eukaryotic translation initiation factors).

Initiation of translation requires four specific steps: 1) a ribosome must dissociate into its' 40S and 60S subunits; 2) a ternary complex (termed the

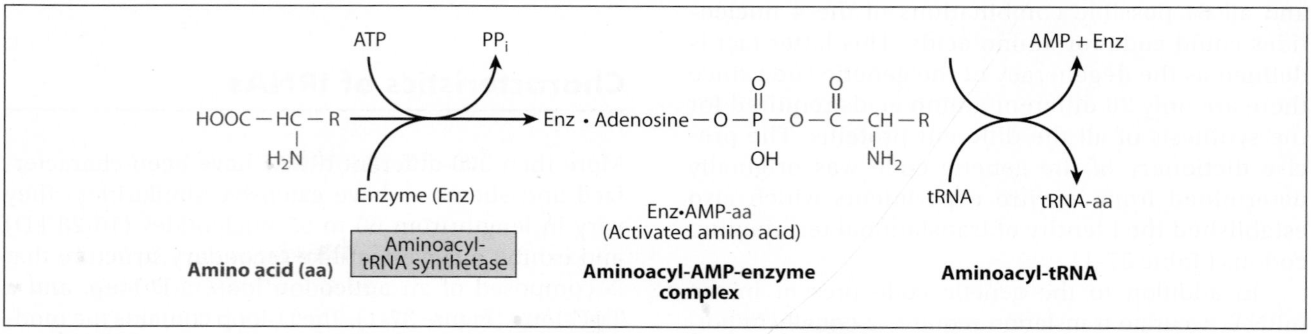

ATP → PP_i

HOOC—HC(—H_2N)—R → Enz • Adenosine—O—P(=O)(—OH)—O—C(=O)—CH(NH_2)—R

Enzyme (Enz)

tRNA → AMP + Enz, tRNA-aa

Enz•AMP-aa (Activated amino acid)

Amino acid (aa) | Aminoacyl-tRNA synthetase | **Aminoacyl-AMP-enzyme complex** | **Aminoacyl-tRNA**

FIGURE 37-2: Formation of aminoacyl-tRNA. A 2-step reaction involving the enzyme amino-acyl-tRNA synthetase results in the formation of aminoacyl-tRNA. The first reaction involves the formation of an AMP-amino acid–enzyme complex. This activated amino acid is next transferred to the corresponding tRNA molecule. The AMP and enzyme are released, and the latter can be reutilized. The charging reactions have an error rate (ie, esterifying the incorrect amino acid on $tRNA_x$) of less than 10^{-4}. Murray RK, Bender DA, Botham KM, Kennelly PJ, Rodwell VW, Weil PA. *Harper's Illustrated Biochemistry*. 29th ed. New York: McGraw-Hill; 2012.

High-Yield Concept

It is absolutely necessary that the discrimination of correct amino acid and correct tRNA be made by a given synthetase prior to release of the aminoacyl-tRNA from the enzyme. Once the product is released there is no further way to proof-read whether a given tRNA is coupled to its correspondingly correct tRNA.

pre-initiation complex) consisting of the initiator met-tRNA, eIF-2 and GTP must engage the dissociated 40S subunit; 3) the mRNA is then bound to the pre-initiation complex; 4) the 60S subunit must associate with the pre-initiation complex to form the 80S initiation complex (Figure 37-3).

The first step in the formation of the preinitiation complex is the binding of GTP to eIF-2 to form a binary complex. The binary complex then binds to the activated initiator tRNA, met-tRNA$_i^{met}$ forming a ternary complex that then binds to the 40S subunit forming the 43S preinitiation complex.

TABLE 37-2: Important Eukaryotic Translation Initiation Factors and Their Functions

Initiation Factor	*Activity*
eIF-1	Repositioning of met-tRNA to facilitate mRNA binding
eIF-2	Heterotrimeric G-protein composed of α, β, and γ subunits; formation of ternary complex consisting of eIF2-GTP plus initiator methionine tRNA (met-tRNA$_i^{met}$); AUG-dependent met-tRNA$_i^{met}$ binding to 40S ribosome
eIF-2B (also called GEF) guanine nucleotide exchange factor, composed of 5 subunits: α, β, γ, δ, ε	GTP/GDP exchange during eIF-2 recycling; genes encoding the subunits identified as EIF2B1–EIF2B5, mutations in any one of which causes the severe autosomal recessive neurodegenerative disorder called leukoencephalopathy with vanishing white matter (VWM)
eIF-3, composed of 13 subunits	Ribosome subunit antiassociation by binding to 40S subunit; eIF-3e and eIF-3i subunits transform normal cells when overexpressed; eIF-3A (also called eIF3 p170) overexpression has been shown to be associated with several human cancers
Initiation factor complex often referred to as eIF-4F composed of 3 primary subunits: eIF-4E, eIF-4A, eIF-4G and at least 2 additional factors: PABP, Mnk1 (or Mnk2)	mRNA binding to 40S subunit, ATPase-dependent RNA helicase activity, interaction between polyA tail and cap structure
PABP: polyA-binding protein	Binds to the polyA tail of mRNAs and provides a link to eIF-4G
Mnk1 and Mnk2 eIF-4E kinases	Phosphorylate eIF-4E increasing association with cap structure
eIF-4A	ATPase-dependent RNA helicase
eIF-4E	5′ cap recognition; frequently found overexpressed in human cancers, inhibition of eIF4E is currently a target for anticancer therapies
4E-BP (also called PHAS) 3 known forms	When dephosphorylated 4E-BP binds eIF-4E and represses its activity, phosphorylation of 4E-BP occurs in response to many growth stimuli leading to release of eIF-4E and increased translational initiation
eIF-4G	Acts as a scaffold for the assembly of eIF-4E and -4A in the eIF-4F complex, interaction with PABP allows 5′-end and 3′-ends of mRNAs to interact
eIF-4B	Stimulates helicase, binds simultaneously with eIF-4F
eIF-5	Releases eIF-2 and eIF-3, ribosome-dependent GTPase
eIF-6	Ribosome subunit antiassociation

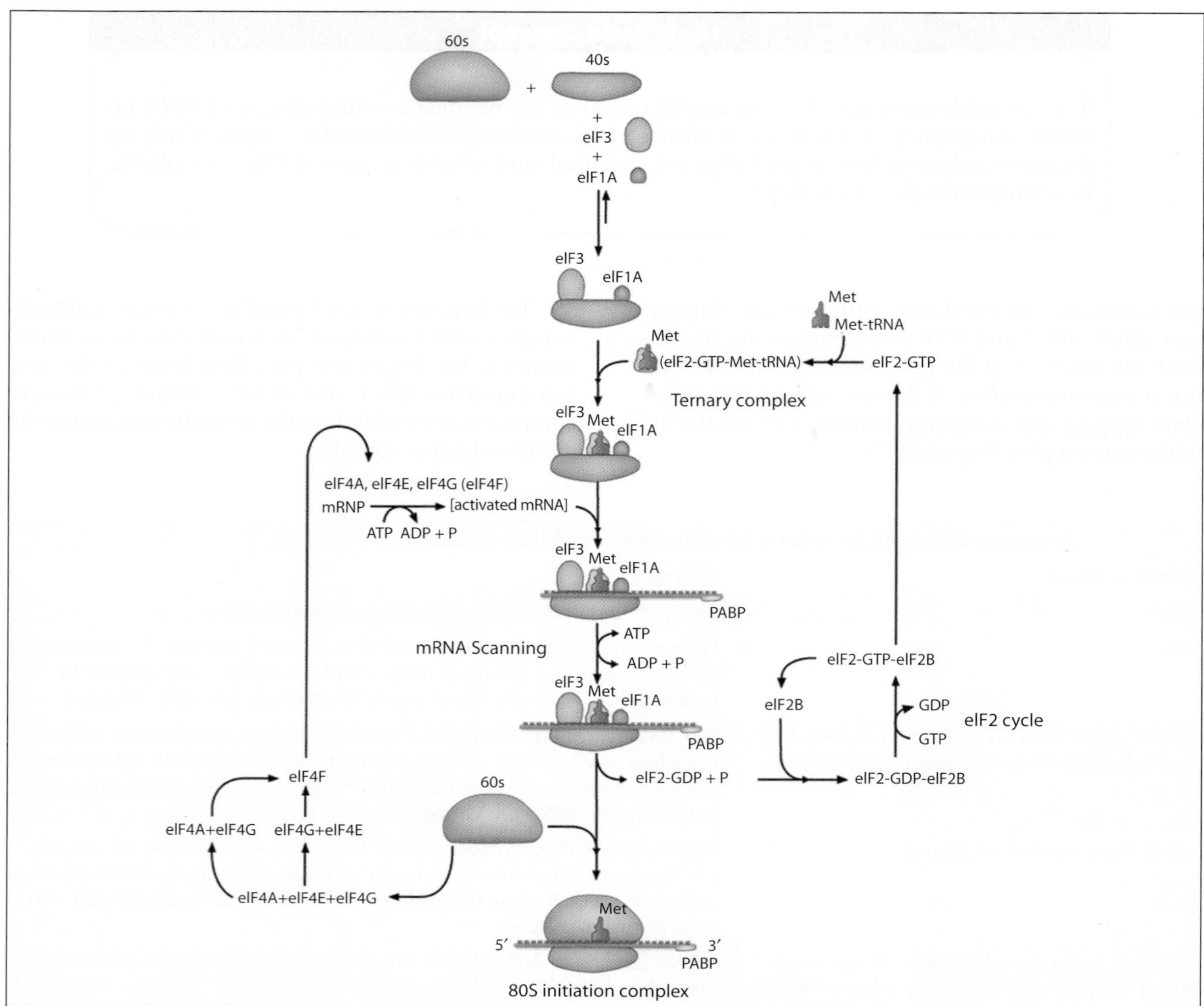

FIGURE 37-3: Details of the complex processes required for accurate and efficient initiation of translation. Several initiation factors (eg, eIF-1 and eIF-3) are required to ensure that the 60S and 40S ribosomal subunits remain separated (antiassociation) so that new rounds of translation can begin. The ternary complex, composed of GTP bound to the α-subunit of eIF2 and the initiator methionyl-tRNA^{met}, can engage the 40S subunit. The eIF-4F complex, which comprises the cap-binding factor, eIF-4E, the RNA helicase eIF-4A, and the scaffold subunit, eIF-4G, captures an mRNA and brings it to the 40S subunit and the ternary complex. Once the mRNA, 40S and 60S subunits, and the ternary complex are integrated, the resulting 80S initiation complex constitutes the completion of the process of translation initiation. PABP, polyA-binding protein. Reproduced with permission of themedicalbiochemistrypage, LLC.

High-Yield Concept

The cap structure of eukaryotic mRNAs is bound by eIF-4F prior to association with the preinitiation complex. This factor is actually a complex of 3 proteins; eIF-4E, eIF-4A, and eIF-4G. The protein eIF-4E physically recognizes and binds to the cap structure, eIF-4A binds and hydrolyzes ATP and exhibits RNA helicase activity to unwind mRNA secondary structure, and eIF-4G aids in binding of the mRNA to the 43S preinitiation complex.

CLINICAL BOX 37-1: eIF-2B MUTATIONS AND DISEASE

Leukoencephalopathy with vanishing white matter (VWM), also referred to as childhood ataxia with central hypomyelination and myelinopathia centralis diffusa, is one of the most prevalent inherited white matter disorders of childhood but it can affect people of all ages, including neonates and adults. Although other tissues are affected, VWM is primarily a brain disorder in which oligodendrocytes and astrocytes are selectively affected. VWM is a progressive disorder clinically dominated by cerebellar ataxia and in which minor stress conditions, such as fever or mild trauma, can induce major episodes of neurological deterioration. Typical pathological findings are diminishing white matter, the gross pathology that lends its name to this disorder. Additional pathology includes cystic degeneration, oligodendrocytosis with highly characteristic foamy oligodendrocytes, limited astrogliosis with dysmorphic astrocytes, and apoptotic loss of oligodendrocytes. VWM is caused by mutations in any of the 5 genes (*EIF2B1-EIF2B5*), encoding the subunits (α, β, γ, δ, and ε) of initiation factor 2B (eIF-2B). All identified mutations in these genes result in eIF-2B complexes with diminished activity and impair its function to couple protein synthesis to the cellular demands in basal conditions and during stress. The reduction in eIF-2B function results in a sustained inappropriate activation of the unfolded protein response (UPR). Sustained activation of the UPR triggers an apoptotic process leading to the observed apoptotic loss of oligodendrocytes.

Once the mRNA is properly aligned onto the preinitiation complex and the initiator met-$tRNA_i^{met}$ is bound to the initiator AUG codon (a process facilitated by eIF-1), the 60S subunit associates with the complex forming the 80*S* initiation complex. The energy needed to stimulate the formation of the 80S initiation complex comes from the hydrolysis of the GTP bound to eIF-2. The large ribosomal subunit contains domains termed the A-site, P-site, and E-site. The A-site resides over the next codon to be recognized in the mRNA and each incoming aminoacyl-tRNA enters the ribosome at this site. The P-site is where the elongating protein attached to a tRNA will reside following each round of elongation. The E-site is where the protein is ejected from the ribosome upon completion of translation.

The GDP bound form of eIF-2 then binds to eIF-2B which stimulates the exchange of GTP for GDP on eIF-2. The overall process of eIF-2B–mediated GTP for GDP exchange in eIF-2 is termed the eIF-2 cycle (see Figure 37-3). The activity called eIF-2B is actually a complex of 5 subunits identified as α, β, γ, δ, and ε, each encoded by a separate gene. Inherited mutations in any one of these 5 genes results in a severe neurodegenerative disorder termed leukoencephalopathy with vanishing white matter (Clinical Box 37-1).

Regulation of Translation Initiation: The eIF-2α Kinases

Regulation of initiation in eukaryotes is primarily affected by phosphorylation of Ser (S) residues in the α-subunit of eIF-2 (eIF-2α). Phosphorylated eIF-2, in the absence of eIF-2B, is just as active an initiator as nonphosphorylated eIF-2. However, when eIF-2 is phosphorylated the GDP-bound complex is stabilized and exchange for GTP is inhibited. Regulation of translational initiation, via phosphorylation of eIF-2α, occurs under a number of different conditions that include endoplasmic reticulum (ER) stress, nutrient stress (deprivation or restriction), viral infection, and in erythrocytes as a consequence of limiting heme. Each of these distinct regulatory pathways involves a unique eIF-2α kinase, and there are 4 of these related kinases known to exist in mammalian cells (Figure 37-4).

The first eIF-2α kinase identified and characterized was isolated from reticulocyte lysates and shown to be involved in the control of globin mRNA translation in response to deficiency in heme. This kinase is called the heme-regulated inhibitor (HRI). When heme levels are low HRI is active and phosphorylates eIF-2α to limit translational initiation until there is adequate heme to generate functional hemoglobin. When heme levels rise eIF-2α is protected from phosphorylation by a protein that associates with the γ-subunit of eIF-2. Removal of the phosphate from eIF-2α is catalyzed by a specific eIF-2 phosphatase, which is unaffected by heme.

Viral infection involving double-stranded RNA viruses activates the expression of the interferons which in turn activate the eIF-2α kinase known as PKR (RNA-dependent protein kinase). Proteins that are destined for secretory vesicles are translated while associated with endoplasmic reticulum (ER) membranes.

During translation secreted proteins are transported into the lumen of the ER in an unfolded state.

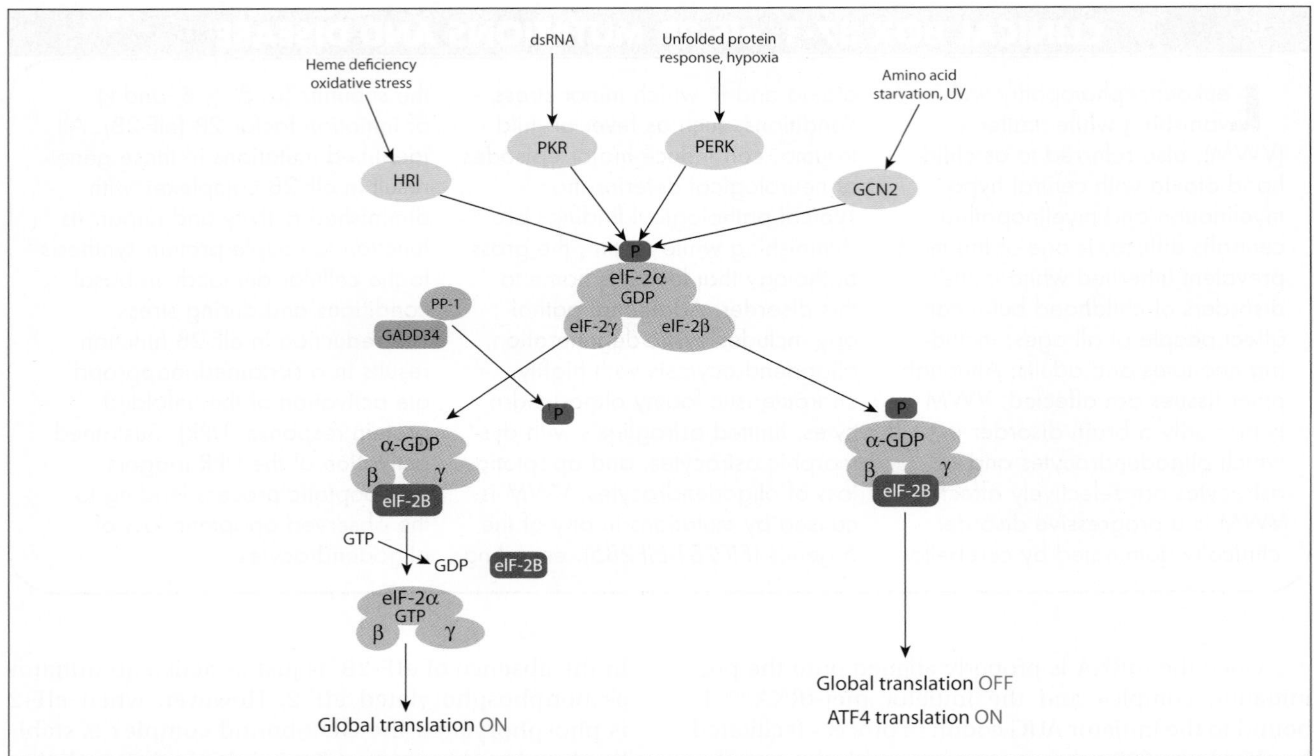

FIGURE 37-4: Each of the various eIF-2α kinases responds to different physiological and/or environmental stressors and induces the phosphorylation of the α-subunit of eIF-2. In the case of nutritional stress or the unfolded protein response (UPR), the phosphorylation of eIF-2α results in the preferential translation of transcription factors (eg, ATF4) that initiate a pattern of gene expression that allows the cell to respond to the stress or in the case of severe and damaging stress the apoptotic program is triggered. GADD34 is a regulatory subunit of protein phosphatase-1 (PP-1). Transcription of the GADD34 gene by ATF4 allows for a feedback control loop on the level of eIF-2α phosphorylation. Reproduced with permission of themedicalbiochemistrypage, LLC.

Proper folding occurs prior to the transfer of the protein to the Golgi apparatus. Under certain conditions the secretory responses of a cell can exceed the capacity of the folding processes of the ER. Accumulation of unfolded proteins triggers the unfolded protein response (UPR) which is a form of ER stress. The UPR activates an eIF-2α kinase termed PERK [RNA-dependent protein kinase (PKR)-like ER kinase]. Deficiencies in PERK result in the extremely rare autosomal recessive disorder known as Wolcott-Rallison syndrome, WRS (Clinical Box 37-2).

Nutritional deprivation, in particular amino acid deficiency, results in the activation of the eIF-2α kinase known as GCN2 (mammalian homolog of the general control nonderepressible-2 gene). In addition to nutritional deprivation, GCN2 is induced by UV irradiation, inhibition of proteosome function, and infection by certain viruses.

Regulation of eIF-4E Activity

At least 3 distinct mechanisms are known to exist that regulate the level and activity of eIF-4E. These include regulation of the level of transcription of the eIF-4E gene, posttranslational modification via phosphorylation, and inhibition by interaction with binding proteins. Although the exact effect of eIF-4E phosphorylation is not clearly defined, it may be necessary to increase affinity of eIF-4E for the mRNA cap structure and for eIF-4G. Of clinical significance is the observation that promiscuous elevation in the levels of eIF-4E can lead to tumorigenesis placing this translation factor in the category of a proto-oncogene.

The principal mechanism utilized in the regulation of eIF-4E activity is through its interaction with a family of binding/repressor proteins termed 4E-BPs (4E-binding proteins). Binding of 4E-BPs to eIF-4E

CLINICAL BOX 37-2: WOLCOTT-RALLINSON SYNDROME

Wolcott-Rallison syndrome (WRS) is a rare autosomal recessive disease, characterized by neonatal/early-onset nonautoimmune insulin-requiring diabetes associated with skeletal dysplasia and growth retardation. WRS is the most frequent cause of neonatal/early-onset diabetes in patients with consanguineous parents. WRS should be suspected as the cause of diabetes mellitus occurring neonatally or before 6 months of age and originating from a population where there is a high prevalence of consanguinity. Additional signs in these children are skeletal dysplasia and/or episodes of acute liver failure. Other symptoms show variability in their nature and severity between patients with WRS. These additional symptoms include frequent episodes of acute liver failure, renal dysfunction, exocrine pancreas insufficiency, intellectual deficit, hypothyroidism, neutropenia, and recurrent infections. WRS is caused by mutations in the gene encoding the eIF-2α kinase, PERK (PKR-like endoplasmic reticulum kinase). PERK plays a key role in translation control during the unfolded protein response (UPR). Indeed, ER dysfunction is central to the disease processes in WRS. Molecular genetic testing confirms the diagnosis in patients suspected of having WRS. Aggressive therapeutic monitoring and interventional treatment of the diabetes with an insulin pump is highly recommended because of the risk of acute episodes of hypoglycemia and ketoacidosis. The prognosis for WRS patients is poor and most patients die at a young age.

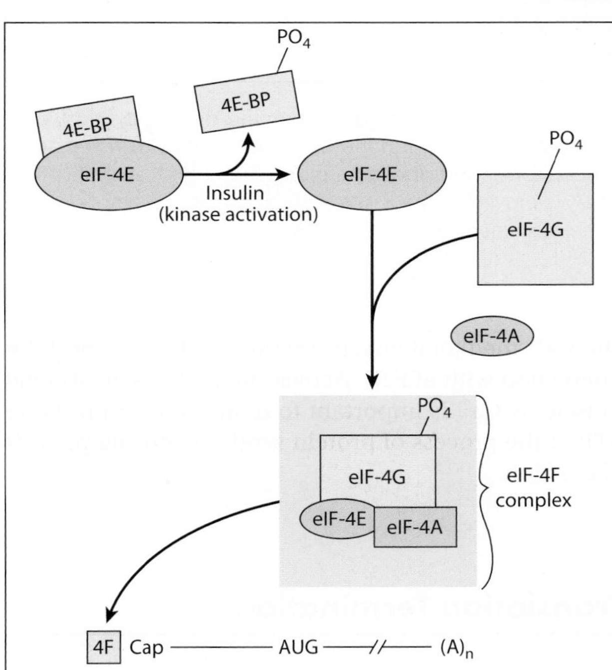

FIGURE 37-5: Activation of eIF-4E by insulin and its subsequent incorporation into the functional eIF-4F cap-binding complex. When 4E-BP is phosphorylated by insulin (as well as numerous other growth factors and mitogens), it dissociates from eIF-4E which allows the latter factor to interact with eIF-4G and then form the eIF-4F complex. Growth factors also induce phosphorylation of eIF-4G, generating a phosphorylated eIF-4F complex that interacts with the cap with higher affinity than nonphosphorylated eIF-4F. Murray RK, Bender DA, Botham KM, Kennelly PJ, Rodwell VW, Weil PA. *Harper's Illustrated Biochemistry*. 29th ed. New York: McGraw-Hill; 2012.

does not alter the affinity of eIF-4E for the cap structure but prevents the interaction of eIF-4E with eIF-4G which in turn suppresses the formation of the eIF-4F complex. The ability of 4E-BPs to interact with eIF-4E is controlled via their state of phosphorylation (Figure 37-5). When not phosphorylated, 4E-BP binds with high efficiency to eIF-4E but lose their binding capacity when phosphorylated. Numerous growth factors, such as insulin, lead to phosphorylation of 4E-BPs, thereby releasing eIF-4E to interact efficiently with the cap structure allowing for increased translational initiation.

Translation Elongation

The process of elongation like that of initiation requires specific nonribosomal proteins termed eEFs (elongation factors). Protein elongation occurs in a cyclic manner such that at the end of one complete round of amino acid addition the A-site will be empty and ready to accept the next incoming aminoacyl-tRNA dictated by the next codon of the mRNA (Figure 37-6). Each incoming aminoacyl-tRNA is brought to the ribosome by an eEF-1α-GTP complex. When the correct tRNA is deposited into the A-site, the GTP is hydrolyzed and the eEF-1α-GDP complex dissociates. In order for additional translocation events to occur, the GDP must be exchanged for GTP. This is carried out by eEF-1βγ similarly to the GTP exchange that occurs with eIF-2 catalyzed by eIF-2B.

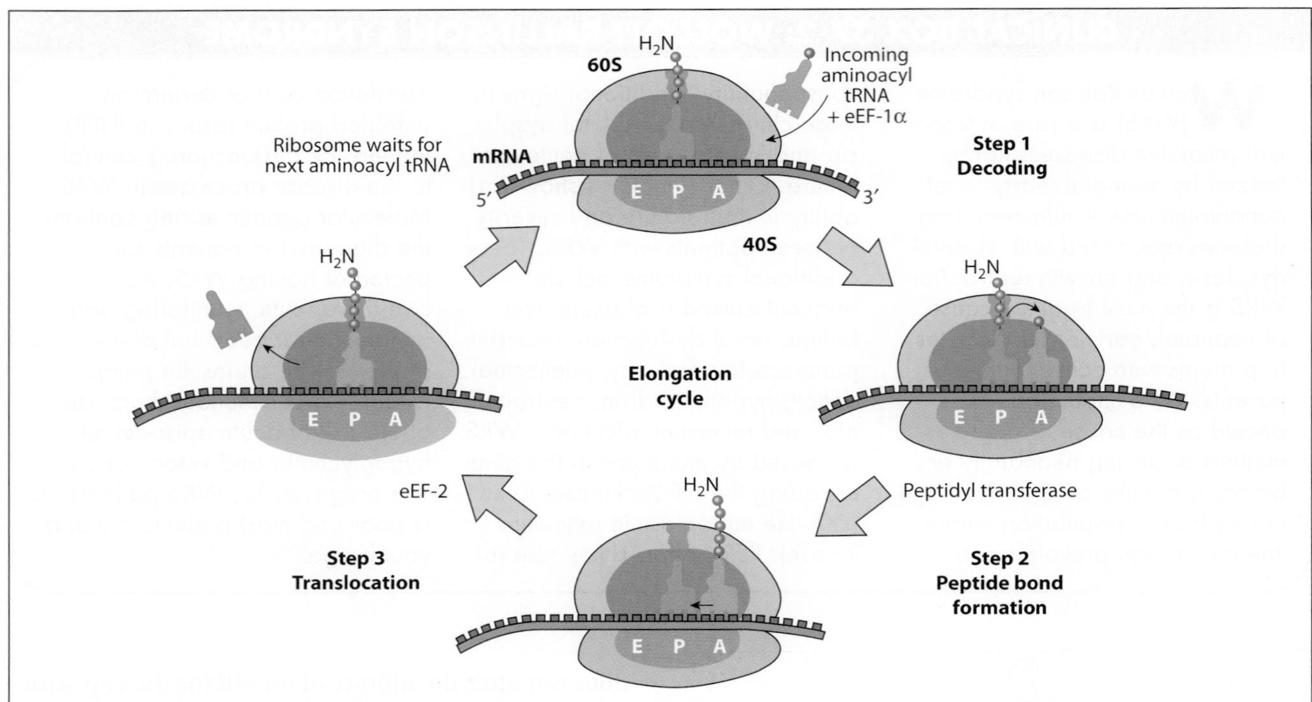

FIGURE 37-6: The cyclical steps of elongation. The elongation factor eEF-1α carries each incoming aminoacyl-tRNA to the A-site. The peptide in the P-site is transferred to the amino acid in the A-site through the action of peptidyltransferase. Following peptide transfer the elongation factor eEF-2 induces translocation of the ribosome along the mRNA such that the naked tRNA is temporarily within the E-site and the peptidyl-tRNA is moved to the P-site leaving the A-site empty and residing over the next codon of the mRNA. Reproduced with permission of themedicalbiochemistrypage, LLC.

The peptide attached to the tRNA in the P-site is transferred to the amino acid on the aminoacyl-tRNA in the A-site forming a new peptide bond. This reaction is catalyzed by peptidyltransferase activity which resides in what is termed the peptidyltransferase center (PTC) of the large ribosomal subunit (60S subunit). This enzymatic process is termed transpeptidation. This enzymatic reaction is not mediated by any ribosomal proteins but instead by a ribozyme (see Chapter 36) contained in the 60S subunit.

The elongated peptide now resides on a tRNA in the A-site. The process of moving the peptidyl-tRNA from the A-site to the P-site is termed translocation and is catalyzed by eEF-2 coupled to GTP hydrolysis. In the process of translocation the ribosome is moved along the mRNA such that the next codon of the mRNA resides under the A-site. Following translocation eEF-2 is released from the ribosome.

The ability of eEF-2 to carry out translocation is regulated by the state of phosphorylation of the enzyme; when phosphorylated the eEF-2 activity is inhibited. Phosphorylation of eEF-2 is catalyzed by the enzyme eEF-2 kinase (eEF2K). Regulation of eEF2K activity is normally under the control of insulin and Ca^{2+} fluxes. The Ca^{2+}-mediated effects are the result of calmodulin interaction with eEF2K. Activation of eEF2K in skeletal muscle by Ca^{2+} is important to reduce consumption of ATP in the process of protein synthesis during periods of exertion.

Translation Termination

Unlike initiation and elongation which require multiple protein activities, translational termination requires only 1 factor, termed eRF (for releasing factor). The signals for translation termination are the 3 termination codons, UAG, UAA, and UGA. The eRF binds to the A-site of the ribosome in conjunction with GTP (Figure 37-7). The binding of eRF to the ribosome stimulates the peptidyltransferase activity to transfer the peptidyl group to water instead of an aminoacyl-tRNA. The resulting uncharged tRNA left in the P-site is expelled with concomitant hydrolysis of GTP. The inactive ribosome then releases its mRNA and the 80S complex dissociates into the

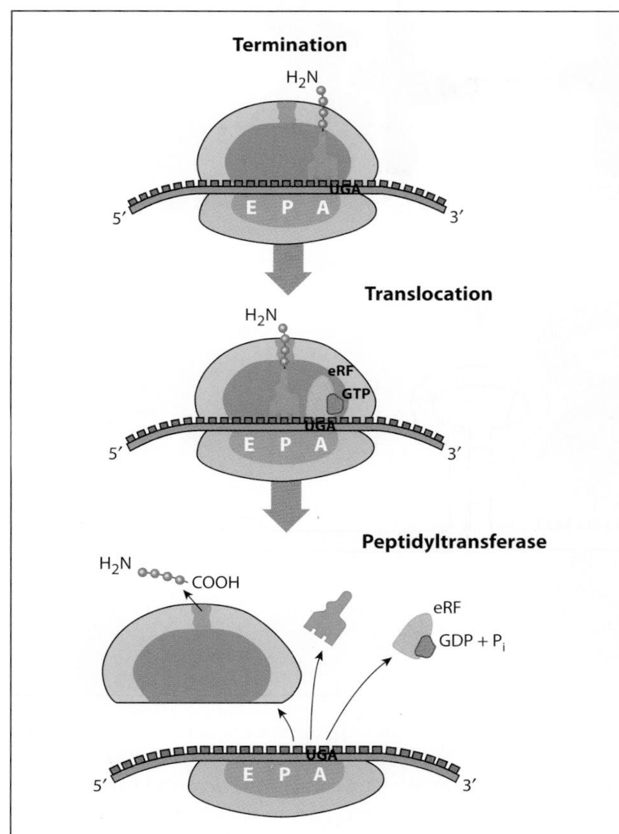

FIGURE 37-7: Translation termination occurs when a stop codon is encountered. The termination factor eRF, which binds GTP, then stimulates the peptidyltransferase to transfer the peptide, from the tRNA in the P-site to H_2O coupled with the hydrolysis of GTP. The peptide is released from the ribosome along with the naked tRNA and eRF-GDP complex. Reproduced with permission of themedicalbiochemistrypage, LLC.

40S and 60S subunits ready for another round of translation.

Selenoproteins

Selenium is a trace element and is found as a component of several enzymes that are involved in redox reactions such as glutathione peroxidase. The selenium in these selenoproteins is incorporated as a unique amino acid, selenocysteine, during translation. Selenocysteine incorporation in eukaryotic proteins occurs cotranslationally at UGA codons (normally stop codons) via the interactions of a number of specialized proteins and protein complexes (Figure 37-8). In addition, there are specific secondary structures in the 3′-untranslated regions (UTR) of selenoprotein mRNAs, termed SECIS elements that are required for selenocysteine insertion into the elongating protein. One of the complexes required for this important modification is comprised of a selenocysteinyl-tRNA [(Sec)-tRNA$^{(Ser)Sec}$] and its specific elongation factor identified as selenoprotein translation factor B (SelB).

Iron-Mediated Control of Translation

Regulation of the translation of certain mRNAs occurs through the action of specific RNA-binding proteins. Proteins of this class have been identified as those that bind to sequences in either 5′-UTR or 3′-UTR. Regulation of iron homeostasis (Chapter 42) involves RNA binding proteins that bind to the transferrin receptor and ferritin mRNAs (Figure 37-9). When iron levels are low the rate of synthesis of the transferrin receptor increases so that cells can take up more iron, whereas translation of the ferritin mRNA is inhibited in order to restrict intracellular storage of iron. This regulation occurs through the action of an iron-response element–binding protein (IRBP) that binds to specific iron-response elements (IRE) in the 3′-UTR of the transferrin receptor mRNA and the 5′-UTR of the ferritin mRNA. When iron levels are low, IRBP is free of iron and can, therefore, interact with the IREs. Conversely, when iron levels are high, IRBP binds to iron and then cannot interact with the IRE.

Protein-Synthesis Inhibitors

Many of the antibiotics utilized for the treatment of bacterial infections as well as certain toxins function through the inhibition of translation. Inhibition can be affected at all stages of translation from initiation to elongation to termination (Table 37-3).

Secreted and Membrane-Associated Proteins

Proteins that are membrane bound or are destined for excretion are synthesized by ribosomes associated with the membranes of the ER (Figure 37-10). The ER associated with ribosomes is termed rough ER (RER). This class of protein all contains an

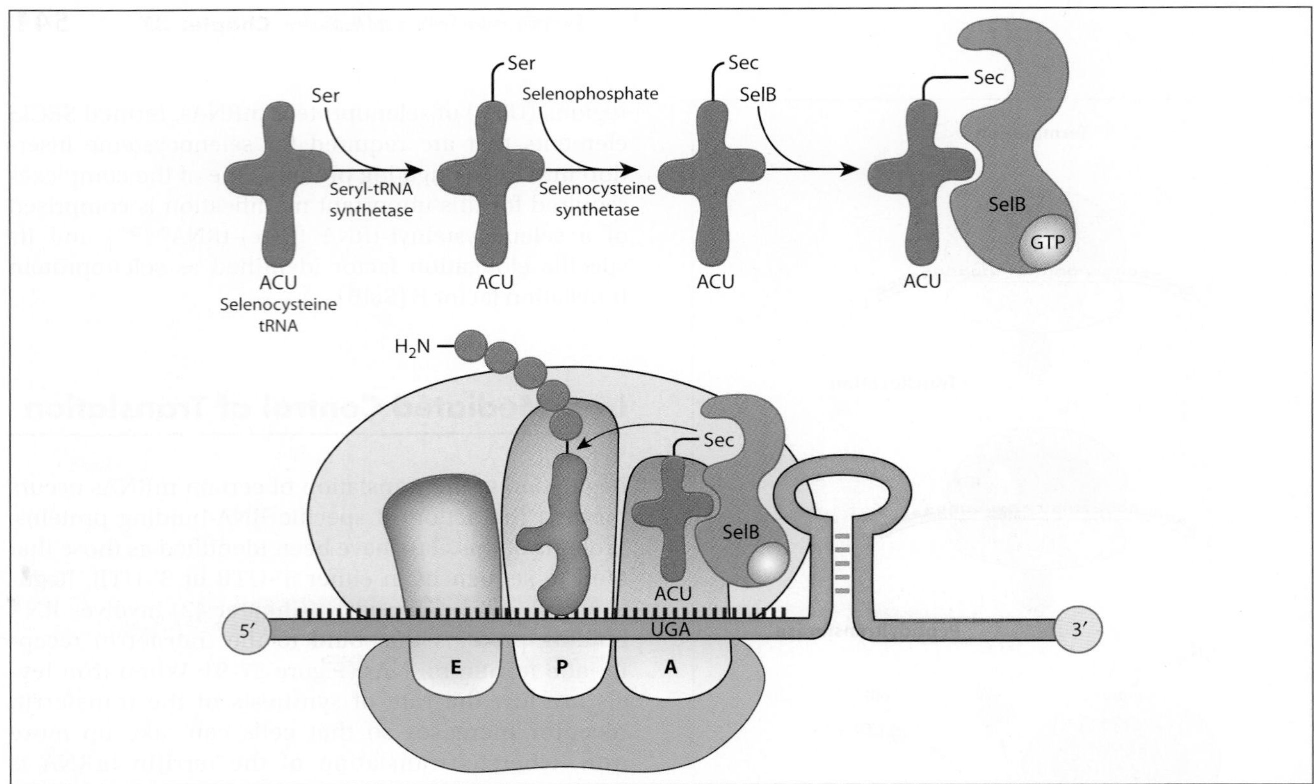

FIGURE 37-8: Selenocysteine biosynthesis and incorporation. The first steps involve the activation of serine onto the (Sec)-tRNA followed by enzymatic conversion to selenocysteine generating (Sec)-tRNA$^{(Ser)Sec}$. Next the (Sec)-tRNA$^{(Ser)Sec}$ is bound by SelB and the complex is incorporated into the translational machinery. The elongating protein is transferred to the selenocysteinyl-tRNA via the action of peptidyltransferase as for any other incoming amino acid and normal elongation continues. Reproduced with permission of themedicalbiochemistrypage, LLC.

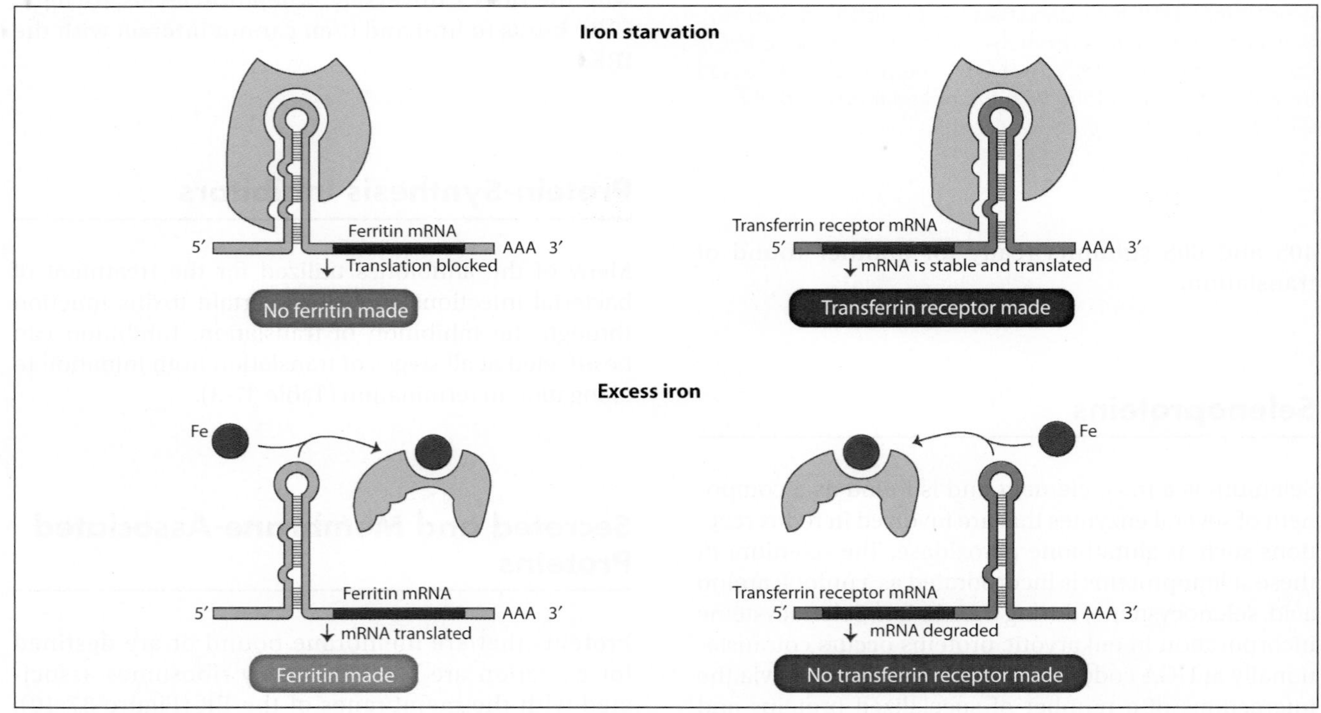

FIGURE 37-9: Iron-mediated regulation of translation of the ferritin and transferrin receptor mRNAs. Reproduced with permission of themedicalbiochemistrypage, LLC.

TABLE 37-3: **Antibiotic and Toxin Inhibitors of Translation**

Inhibitor	***Comments***
Chloramphenicol	Inhibits prokaryotic peptidyltransferase
Streptomycin	Inhibits prokaryotic peptide chain initiation, also induces mRNA misreading
Tetracycline	Inhibits prokaryotic aminoacyl-tRNA binding to the ribosome small subunit
Neomycin	Similar in activity to streptomycin
Erythromycin	Inhibits prokaryotic translocation through the ribosome large subunit
Fusidic acid	Similar to erythromycin only by preventing prokaryotic elongation factor G (EF-G, also called translocase) from dissociating from the large subunit
Puromycin	Resembles an aminoacyl-tRNA, interferes with peptide transfer resulting in premature termination in both prokaryotes and eukaryotes
Diphtheria (diphtheria) toxin	Protein from *Corynebacterium diphtheriae,* which causes diphtheria; catalyzes ADP-ribosylation and inactivation of eEF-2; eEF-2 contains a modified His residue known as **diphthamide** (it is this residue that is the target of the toxin)
Ricin	Found in castor beans, catalyzes cleavage of the eukaryotic large subunit rRNA
Cycloheximide	Inhibits eukaryotic peptidyltransferase

N-terminus termed a **signal sequence** or **signal peptide**. The signal peptide is usually 13-36 predominantly hydrophobic residues. The signal peptide is recognized by a multi-protein complex termed the signal recognition particle (SRP). This signal peptide is removed following passage through the ER membrane. The removal of the signal peptide is catalyzed by signal peptidase. Proteins that contain a signal peptide are called preproteins to distinguish them from proproteins. However, some proteins that are destined for secretion are also further proteolyzed following secretion and, therefore contain pro sequences. This class of proteins is termed preproproteins.

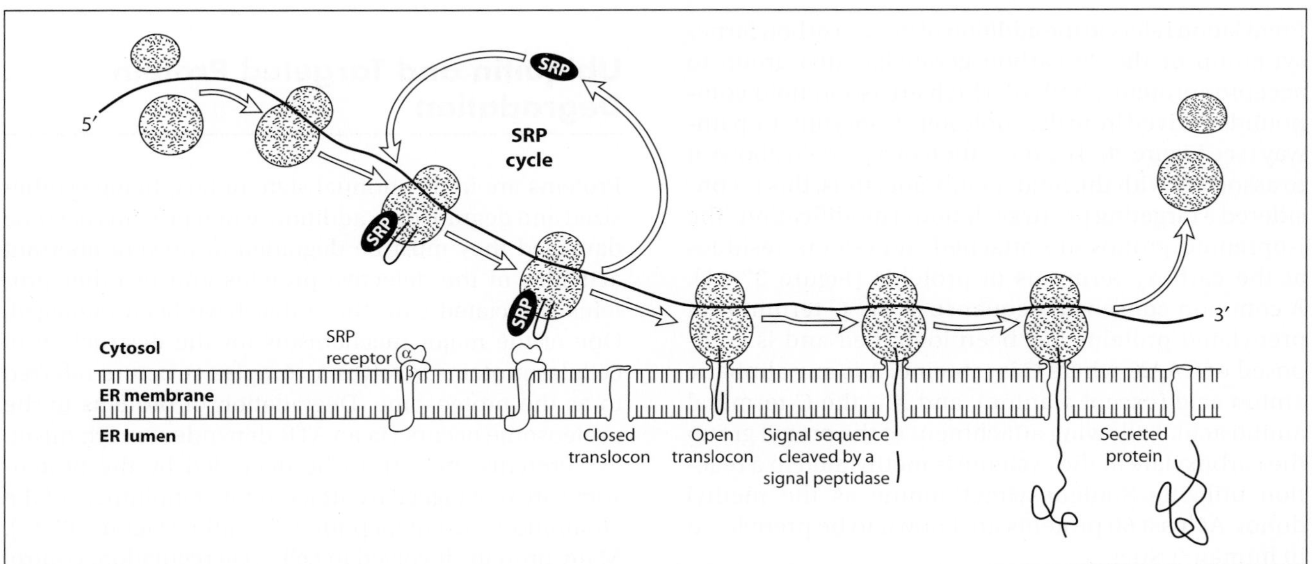

FIGURE 37-10: Mechanism of synthesis of membrane bound or secreted proteins. Ribosomes engage the ER membrane through interaction of the signal recognition particle (SRP) in the ribosome with the SRP receptor in the ER membrane. As the protein is synthesized the signal sequence is passed through the ER membrane into the lumen of the ER. After sufficient synthesis the signal peptide is removed by the action of signal peptidase. Synthesis will continue and if the protein is secreted it will end up completely in the lumen of the ER. If the protein is membrane associated a stop transfer motif in the protein will stop the transfer of the protein through the ER membrane. This will become the membrane-spanning domain of the protein. Reproduced with permission of themedicalbiochemistrypage, LLC.

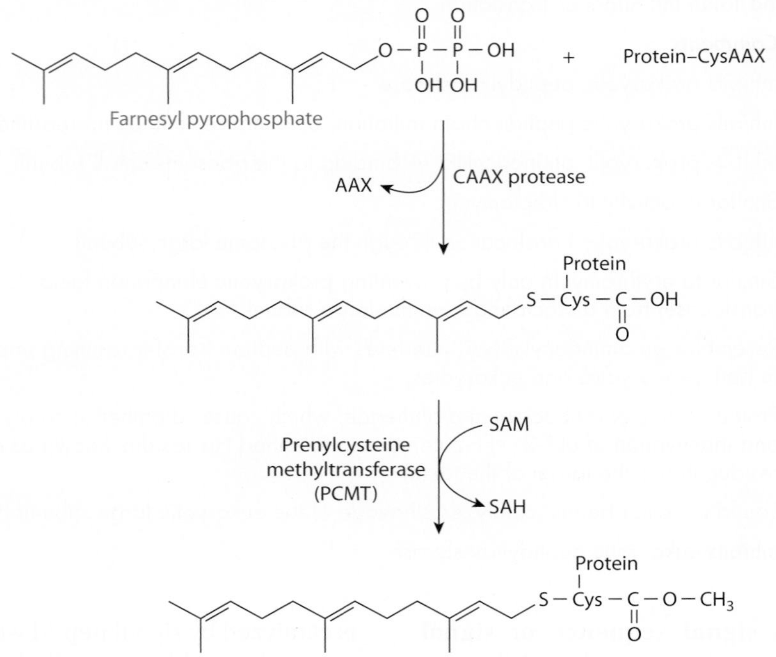

FIGURE 37-11: Mechanism of protein prenylation. Reproduced with permission of themedicalbiochemistrypage, LLC.

Membrane targeting by Prenylation

Prenylation refers to the addition of the 15-carbon farnesyl group or the 20-carbon geranylgeranyl group to acceptor proteins, both of which are isoprenoid compounds derived from the cholesterol biosynthetic pathway (see Figure 26-4). Prenylation of a protein allows it to associate with the lipid membrane; thus, this is considered a targeting posttranslational modification. The isoprenoid groups are attached to cysteine residues at the carboxy terminus of proteins (Figure 37-11). A common consensus sequence at the *C*-terminus of prenylated proteins has been identified and is composed of CAAX, where C is cysteine, A is any aliphatic amino acid (except alanine), and X is the *C*-terminal amino acid. Following attachment of the prenyl group the carboxylate of the cysteine is methylated in a reaction utilizing S-adenosylmethionine as the methyl donor. At least 60 proteins are known to be prenylated in human tissues.

Some of the most important proteins whose functions depend upon prenylation are those that modulate immune responses. It is these immune modulatory roles of many prenylated proteins that are the basis for a portion of the anti-inflammatory actions of the statin class of cholesterol synthesis-inhibiting drugs due to a reduction in the synthesis of farnesylpyrophosphate and geranylpyrophosphate and thus reduced extent of inflammatory events.

Ubiquitin and Targeted Protein Degradation

Proteins are in a continual state of flux, being synthesized and degraded. In addition, when proteins become damaged they must be degraded to prevent aberrant activities of the defective proteins and/or other proteins associated with those that have been damaged. One of the major mechanisms for the destruction of cellular proteins involves a complex structure referred to as the proteosome. Degradation of proteins in the proteosome occurs via an ATP-dependent mechanism.

Proteins that are to be degraded by the proteosome are first tagged by attachment of multimers of the 76-amino-acid-polypeptide ubiquitin (Figure 37-12). Many proteins involved in cell cycle regulation, control of proliferation and differentiation, programmed cell death (apoptosis), DNA repair, immune and inflammatory processes, and organelle biogenesis undergo regulated degradation via the proteosome. Of clinical significance is the fact that deregulation of the functions of the proteosome can contribute to the pathogenesis of various human diseases such as cancer, myeloproliferative diseases, and neurodegenerative diseases.

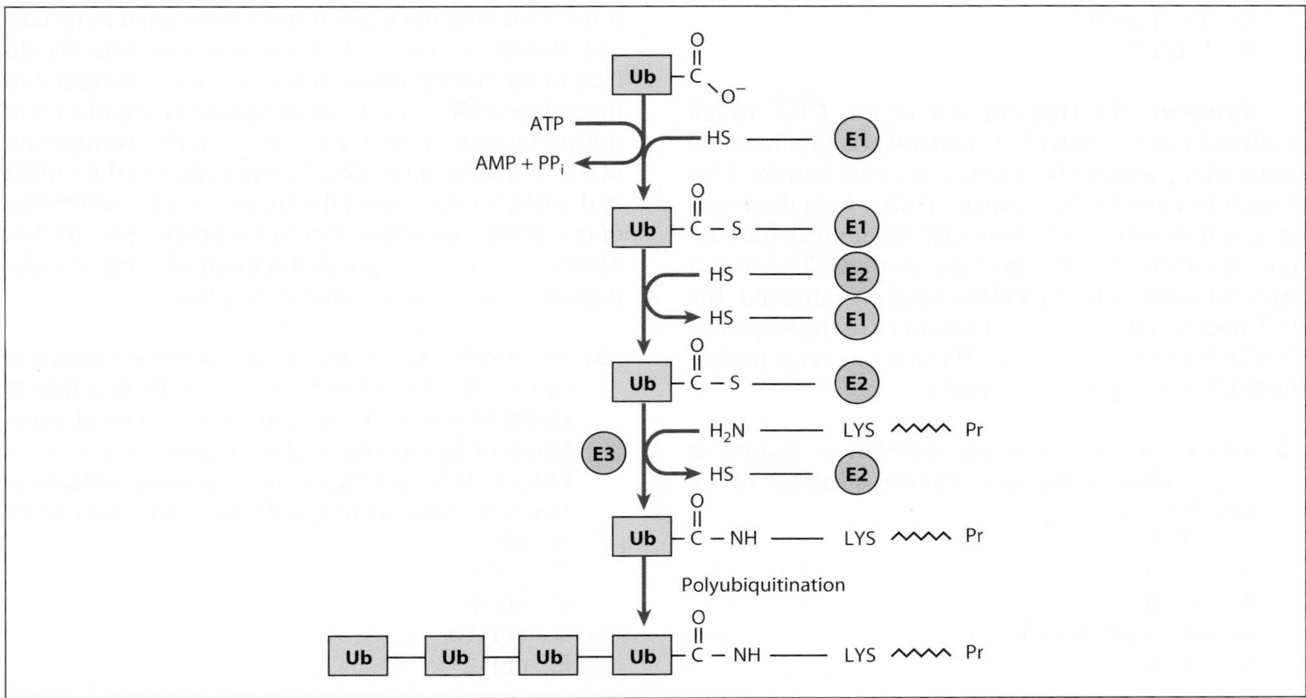

FIGURE 37-12: Reactions involved in the attachment of ubiquitin (Ub) to proteins. Three enzymes are involved. E1 is an activating enzyme, E2 a ligase, and E3 a transferase. While depicted as single entities, there are several types of E1, and over 500 types of E2. The terminal COOH of ubiquitin first forms a thioester. The coupled hydrolysis of PP_i by pyrophosphatase ensures that the reaction will proceed readily. A thioester exchange reaction now transfers activated ubiquitin to E2. E3 then catalyzes the transfer of ubiquitin to the ε-amino group of a lysyl residue of the target protein. Additional rounds of ubiquitination result in subsequent polyubiquitination. Murray RK, Bender DA, Botham KM, Kennelly PJ, Rodwell VW, Weil PA. *Harper's Illustrated Biochemistry*. 29th ed. New York: McGraw-Hill; 2012.

REVIEW QUESTIONS

1. During the process of protein synthesis the factor eEF-2 induces the hydrolysis of GTP. The energy of this hydrolysis is coupled to which of the following?

A. amino acid activation by attachment to a tRNA
B. correct alignment of the mRNA on the 40S ribosome
C. formation of the 80S initiation complex
D. formation of the peptide bond
E. translocation of the ribosome

Answer E: The process of moving the peptidyl-tRNA from the A-site to the P-site is termed translocation. Translocation is catalyzed by eEF-2 coupled to GTP hydrolysis. In the process of translocation the ribosome is moved along the mRNA such that the next codon of the mRNA resides under the A-site. Following translocation eEF-2 is released from the ribosome. The cycle can now begin again.

2. If the DNA shown was transcribed and then translated in a eukaryotic in vitro translation system, what would be the composition of the resultant peptide?

5′-CATTCCATAGCATGT-3′

ACA	threonine	(T)	CAU	histidine	(H)
ACG	threonine	(T)	CUA	leucine	(L)
AUG	methionine	(M)	CGU	arginine	(R)
AAU	asparagine	(N)	CCU	proline	(P)
AGG	arginine	(R)	UGC	cysteine	(C)
AUA	isoleucine	(I)	UGU	cysteine	(C)
GGA	glycine	(G)	UAU	tyrosine	(Y)
GUA	valine	(V)	UAC	tyrosine	(Y)
GCA	alanine	(A)	UCC	serine	(S)
UGG	tryptophan	(W)			

A. C-T-I-P-Y
B. H-S-I-A-C
C. M-L-W-N

D. T-C-Y-G-M
E. V-R-Y-R-T

Answer C: Transcription of the DNA would result in the generation of an antiparallel complimentary strand of RNA where U would be inserted into the RNA at each location in the template DNA where there was an A. Translation in eukaryotic cells begins with methionine. Therefore, translation of the synthetic RNA in this study will begin at the first AUG codon encountered. The RNA resulting from the DNA would have the sequence 5′-ACAUGCUAUGGAAUG-3′. The only correct peptide is the one beginning with methionine.

3. Which of the following translation factors is responsible for engaging the cap structure of the mRNA?
   A. eIF-2
   B. eIF-2B
   C. eIF-4E
   D. eIF-4EBP (4EBP)
   E. eIF-4G

Answer C: The cap structure of eukaryotic mRNAs is bound by specific eIFs prior to association with the preinitiation complex. Cap binding is accomplished by the initiation factor eIF-4F. This factor is actually a complex of 3 proteins: eIF-4E, eIF-4A, and eIF-4G. The protein eIF-4E is a 24-kDa protein, which physically recognizes and binds to the cap structure.

4. A hypothetical cell is exposed to a chemical agent that alters the structure of serine converting it to alanine but only when the serine is activated on an appropriate tRNA. What is the most likely outcome of this modification relative to protein synthesis?
   A. protein synthesis ceases and the mRNA is degraded
   B. the alanine is exchanged for serine by the appropriate aminoacyl-tRNA synthetase
   C. the alanine is incorporated because there is no mechanism for the translational machinery to detect the change
   D. the aminoacyl-tRNA is degraded and thus no effect is observable
   E. translation is halted temporarily due to recognition of the abnormal aminoacyl-tRNA, while the alanine is removed and serine replaced

Answer C: It is absolutely necessary that the discrimination of correct amino acid and correct tRNA be made by a given aminoacyl tRNA synthetase prior to release of the aminoacyl-tRNA from the enzyme. Once the product is released there is no further way to proof-read whether a given tRNA is coupled to its corresponding amino acid. Erroneous coupling would lead to the wrong amino acid being incorporated into the polypeptide since the discrimination of amino acid during protein synthesis comes from the recognition of the anticodon of a tRNA by the codon of the mRNA and not by recognition of the amino acid. Desulfuration of cys-$tRNA^{cys}$ with Raney nickel generates ala-$tRNA^{cys}$. Alanine is then incorporated into an elongating polypeptide where cysteine should have been.

5. The unfolded protein response is a stress response in the ER. This stress pathway results in a halt to global protein synthesis and the activation of translation of factors required to respond to the stress inducer. Which of the following proteins of translation is the primary target of the ER stress response?
   A. eIF-2
   B. eIF2B
   C. eIF-4E
   D. eEF-1α
   E. eEF-2

Answer A: Proteins that are destined for secretory vesicles are translated while associated with endoplasmic reticulum (ER) membranes. During translation secreted proteins are transported into the lumen of the ER in an unfolded state. Proper folding occurs prior to the transfer of the protein to the Golgi apparatus. Accumulation of unfolded proteins triggers the unfolded protein response (UPR) which is a form of ER stress. Among the proteins activated by the UPR is an eIF-2α kinase termed PERK (RNA-dependent protein kinase [**P**KR]-like **ER** **k**inase). The aim of PERK-mediated phosphorylation of eIF-2α is to reduce global protein synthesis allowing the cell time to correct the impaired process of protein folding.

6. Growth factor effects on the rate of translation are, for the most part, the consequence of the phosphorylation of which of the following factors?
   A. 4E-BP
   B. eEF-2
   C. eEF-1α
   D. eIF-2
   E. eIF-4A

Answer A: The principal mechanism utilized in the regulation of eIF-4E activity is through its interaction with a family of binding/repressor proteins termed 4EBPs (4E-binding proteins). Binding of 4E-BPs to eIF-4E does not alter the affinity of eIF-4E for the cap structure but prevents the interaction of eIF-4E with eIF-4G, which in turn suppresses the formation of the eIF-4F complex. The ability of 4EBPs to interact with eIF-4E is controlled via the phosphorylation of specific Ser and Thr residues in 4EBP. When hypophosphorylated, 4EBPs bind with high efficiency to eIF-4E but lose their binding capacity when phosphorylated. Numerous growth and signal transduction stimulating effectors lead to phosphorylation of 4EBP.

7. The immunosuppressant drug rapamycin exerts its function on processes of protein synthesis by interfering with the activity of mTOR. Which of the following translation factors is the protein that would normally be targeted for mTOR-mediated regulation in the absence of rapamycin?
   A. eIF-2
   B. eIF-2B
   C. eIF-4A
   D. eIF-4E
   E. eIF-4G

Answer D: The principal mechanism utilized in the regulation of eIF-4E activity is through its interaction with a family of binding/repressor proteins termed 4EBPs (4E-binding proteins). There are several signal transduction pathways, the activation of which leads to phosphorylation of 4EBP resulting in the release of eIF-4E. These include mTOR complexes. The mTOR protein is a kinase which is a component of 2 distinct multiprotein complexes termed mTORC1 and mTORC2. The activity of mTORC1 is sensitive to inhibition by rapamycin, whereas mTORC2 is not. Numerous growth factors activate the kinase activity of mTOR which then phosphorylates 4EBP allowing the release of eIF-4E and activation of protein synthesis.

8. Which of the following statements most closely reflects the actions of the translation factor eIF-4E?
   A. ATP-dependent unwinding of secondary structures in mRNAs
   B. exchange of GTP for GDP bound to eIF-2
   C. facilitation of the ternary complex (eIF-2/GTP/^{met}tRNA) binding to 40S ribosomal subunit
   D. interaction with eIF-4G in order to bind to the cap structure of the mRNA
   E. scaffold for the binding of eIF-4A

Answer D: The cap structure of eukaryotic mRNAs is bound by specific eIFs prior to association with the preinitiation complex. Cap binding is accomplished by the initiation factor eIF-4F. This factor is actually a complex of 3 proteins: eIF-4E, eIF-4A, and eIF-4G. The protein eIF-4E is a 24-kDa protein which physically recognizes and binds to the cap structure. In order to bind the cap, eIF-4E must interact with eIF-4G which serves as the scaffold for the formation of the complete eIF-4F complex.

9. Reticulocytes control the rate of globin synthesis as a consequence of the level of heme in the cell. This prevents globin protein from being made when there are insufficient amounts of heme. Which of the following best explains the effects of heme on protein synthesis in these cells?
   A. a heme-controlled phosphatase dephosphorylates cap-binding factor, which prevents recognition of globin mRNA by the ribosomes
   B. a tRNA degrading enzyme is active in the absence of heme
   C. heme normally activates peptidyltransferase in reticulocytes
   D. RNA polymerase activity is decreased in reticulocytes by low heme
   E. the initiation factor eIF-2 becomes phosphorylated, reducing its level of activity

Answer E: One mechanism by which initiation of translation in eukaryotes is effected is phosphorylation of a ser(S) residue in the α-subunit of eIF-2. The factor eIF-2 requires activation by interaction with GTP. The energy of GTP hydrolysis is used during translational initiation, thereby allowing eIF-2 to have GDP bound instead of GTP. In order to reactivate eIF-2, the GDP must be exchanged for GTP. This requires an additional protein of the GEF family known as eIF-2B. The phosphorylated form of eIF-2, in the absence of the eIF-2B, is just as active an initiator of translation as the nonphosphorylated form. However, when eIF-2 is phosphorylated, the GDP-bound complex is stabilized and exchange for GTP is inhibited. When eIF-2 is phosphorylated it binds eIF-2B more tightly, thus slowing the rate of exchange. It is this inhibited exchange that affects the rate of initiation. Within reticulocytes the phosphorylation of eIF-2 is the result of an activity called heme-controlled inhibitor (HCI). When the level of heme falls, HCI becomes activated, leading to the phosphorylation of eIF-2 and reduced globin synthesis.

10. Which of the following translation factors is the target of an interferon-mediated translational control mechanism?
   A. eEF-1α
   B. eEF-2
   C. eIF-2
   D. eIF-4A
   E. eIF-4E

Answer C: Regulation of translation in virally infected cells is accomplished by the induced synthesis of interferons (IFs). IFs are induced by dsRNAs and they induce a specific kinase termed RNA-dependent protein kinase (PKR) that phosphorylates the α-subunit of eIF-2, thereby shutting off translation in a similar manner to that of stress and heme control of translation.

11. You are utilizing a cell culture system derived from a breast cancer tumor to examine the process of protein synthesis. You discover that these cells do not effectively generate the GTP-bound form of the translation initiation factor, eIF-2. Which of the following translation factors is most likely to be defective in these cells, thereby impairing the GDP for GTP exchange in eIF-2?

A. eIF-1
B. eIF-2B
C. eIF-4A
D. eIF-4E
E. eIF-4G

Answer B: The eIF-2 cycle involves the regeneration of GTP-bound eIF-2 following the hydrolysis of GTP during translational initiation. When the 40S preinitiation complex is engaged with the 60S ribosome to form the 80*S* initiation complex, the GTP bound to eIF-2 is hydrolyzed providing energy for the process. In order for additional rounds of translational initiation to occur, the GDP bound to eIF-2 must be exchanged for GTP. This is the function of eIF-2B.

12. You are utilizing a cell culture system derived from a breast cancer tumor to examine the process of protein synthesis. You discover that short peptides are present in the P-site of the ribosome whenever there is an aminoacyl-tRNA in the A-site, but it takes several hours for new aminoacyl-tRNAs to enter the ribosome. These results are most likely to be the result of a highly defective form of which of the following proteins?

A. eIF-2
B. eIF-2
C. eEF-1α
D. eEF-1βγ
E. eEF-2

Answer E: Each step of protein elongation comprises movement of the mRNA through the ribosome so that the tRNA carrying the elongating polypeptide resides within a pocket of the 60S subunit termed the P-site (for peptide site). The elongation factor eEF-1α carries each incoming aminoacyl-tRNA to the A-site (for amino acid site) dependent upon the correct codon-anticodon interactions. The peptide in the P-site is transferred to the amino acid in the A-site through the action of the ribozyme activity known as peptidyltransferase. The elongation factor eEF-2 induces translocation of the ribosome along the mRNA such that the naked tRNA is temporarily within the E-site (for ejection site) of the 60S ribosome and the peptidyl-tRNA is moved to the P-site leaving the A-site empty and residing over the next codon of the mRNA.

13. Which of the following translation factors contains a modified amino acid recognized by a toxin produced by *Diphtheria*?

A. eIF-2B
B. eIF-4F
C. eEF-1α
D. eEF-2
E. eRF

Answer D: A protein from *Corynebacterium diphtheria* which causes diphtheria catalyzes the ADP-ribosylation and inactivation of eEF-2. eEF-2 contains a modified His residue known as diphthamide and it is this residue that is the target of the toxin.

14. A mutation that results in the loss of the formation of the iron response element (IRE) in the 5′-UTR of the ferritin mRNA will be expected to have what effect?

A. decreased translation of the mRNA in the presence of high iron
B. decreased translation of the mRNA when iron is low
C. increased translation of the mRNA in the presence of high iron
D. increased translation of the mRNA when iron is low
E. reduced stability of the mRNA

Answer D: Ferritin is an iron-binding protein that prevents toxic levels of ionized iron (Fe^{2+}) from building up in cells. When iron levels are high, the iron-response element–binding protein (IRBP) cannot bind to the IRE in the 5′-UTR of the ferritin mRNA. This allows the ferritin mRNA to be translated. Conversely, when iron levels are low, the IRBP binds to the IRE in the ferritin mRNA preventing its translation. Therefore, loss of the IRE in ferritin would result in increased translation even when iron levels are low since the IRBP would have nothing to which to bind.

15. A decrease in the amount of heme within erythrocytes activates the heme-controlled inhibitor leading to phosphorylation of which factor?

A. eIF-2
B. eIF-2B
C. eEF-4G
D. eEF-2
E. eIF-4E

Answer A: One mechanism by which initiation of translation in eukaryotes is affected is phosphorylation of a ser(S) residue in the α-subunit of eIF-2. Within reticulocytes the phosphorylation of eIF-2 is the result of an activity called heme-controlled inhibitor (HCI). When heme is limiting it would be a waste of energy for reticulocytes to make globin protein, since active hemoglobin could not be generated. Therefore, when the level of heme falls, HCI becomes activated, leading to the phosphorylation of eIF-2 and reduced globin synthesis. Removal of phosphate is catalyzed by a specific eIF-2 phosphatase which is unaffected by heme.

16. Some viruses, for example, poliovirus, contain a protease that cleaves one of the eukaryotic initiation factors allowing for cap-independent translational initiation of viral RNAs at internal ribosome entry site (IRES). Which of the following factors is the target of these viral proteases?

A. eIF-2
B. eIF-2B
C. eIF-4A
D. eIF-4E
E. eIF-4G

Answer E: Poliovirus is a member of the picornavirus family. The RNAs encoded by the viral genome contain internal ribosome entry sites (IRES) that do not require cap structure recognition for translational initiation. The polio virus carries with it a protease that cleaves the eIF-4E binding site on eIF-4G. Cleavage renders eIF-4E incapable of interaction with eIF-4G and as a consequence no active eIF-4F complex forms preventing cap binding and translational initiation of host mRNAs. Due to the presence of the IRES in the viral RNAs, translations take place with the host translational machinery.

17. Control of the rate of translational initiation can be exerted at the level of the activity of the GTP-binding and hydrolyzing initiation factor, eIF-2. The efficiency with which eIF-2 recycles between the active GTP-bound form and the inactive GDP-bound form is controlled by which of the following translation factors?

A. eIF-1
B. eIF-2B
C. eIF-4A
D. eIF-4E
E. eIF-4G

Answer B: The eIF-2 cycle consists of the translation initiation factors: eIF-2A and eIF-2B (also called guanine-nucleotide exchange factor, GEF). The cycle involves the binding of GTP by eIF-2A forming a complex that then interacts with the initiator methionyl-tRNA. When the initiator methionyl-tRNA is placed into the correct position of the 40S ribosomal subunit, the GTP is hydrolyzed (generating GDP and release of P_i) to provide the energy necessary to correctly position the incoming mRNA such that the initiator AUG codon and the initiator methionyl-tRNA anticodon are aligned. In order to regenerate an active eIF-2A for subsequent translation initiation events, the GDP must be exchanged for GTP. The exchange reaction is catalyzed by eIF-2B.

18. You are studying the effects of a novel compound on the processes of protein synthesis using a cell culture system. You find that addition of your compound results in premature termination of protein synthesis. Analysis of the compound reveals that it has structural characteristics of an aminoacyl-tRNA. Which of the following protein-synthesis inhibitors is most similar to your test compound?

A. erythromycin
B. puromycin
C. ricin
D. streptomycin
E. tetracyclin

Answer B: Puromycin has a chemical structure that resembles an aminoacyl-tRNA and it interferes with peptide transfer resulting in premature termination in both prokaryotes and eukaryotes.

19. You are examining the mutational changes that occurred in a breast cancer cell line. You discover that there is a mutation in the gene encoding selenoprotein translation factor B (SelB). Which of the following is most likely defective in these cells as a result of this mutation?

A. decreased bile acid synthesis
B. decreased glycogen synthesis
C. decreased reactive oxygen species generation by pancreatic mitochondria
D. increased fatty acid incorporation into triglycerides
E. increased rate of erythrocyte lysis

Answer E: Selenocysteine incorporation in eukaryotic proteins occurs cotranslationally at UGA codons (normally stop codons) via the interactions of a number of specialized proteins and protein complexes. One of the complexes required for this important modification is comprised of a selenocysteinyl tRNA [(Sec)-tRNA$^{(Ser)Sec}$] and its specific elongation factor identified as selenoprotein translation factor B (SelB).

A particularly important eukaryotic selenoenzyme is glutathione peroxidase, GPx. The main biological role for GPx is to protect cells from oxidative damage, particularly from membrane lipoid peroxidation. Since erythrocytes are exposed to a highly oxidizing environment, the loss of function GPx activity would lead to increased hemolysis.

20. You are studying the function of a protein isolated from a lung tumor cell line and comparing it to the same protein from normal tissue. You find that the protein derived from the cancer cells does not carry out its correct function as a result of improper folding of the protein. Which of the following, involved in the prevention of aggregation and improper folding of newly synthesized proteins, is most likely to be defective in the lung cancer cells?

A. chaperones
B. lysozymes
C. mitochondrial precursor proteins
D. ribosomal-binding proteins
E. zymogens

Answer A: Nearly all proteins of the organelles along the secretory pathway, as well as proteins that are expressed at the cell surface or secreted from the cell, are first cotranslationally translocated into the lumen of the endoplasmic reticulum (ER) as unfolded polypeptide chains. Immediately after entering the ER, they are often modified with *N*-linked glycans, folded into the appropriate secondary and tertiary structures, and finally in many cases are assembled into multimeric complexes. These processes are aided and monitored by ER chaperones and any loss of ER chaperone activity will result in misfolded and potentially aggregated proteins.

21. The RNA codon for methionine is 5′-AUG-3′. Which of the following is the anticodon in the correct methionyl-tRNA?

A. 5′-CAT-3′
B. 5′-CAU-3′
C. 5′-GAU-3′
D. 5′-TAC-3′
E. 5′-UAC-3′

Answer B: The correct anticodon for any given codon is the antiparallel complimentary sequence. Therefore, the anticodon for methionine would be 5′-CAU-3′.

22. Reading of the genetic code is dependent on recognition of a codon on which of the following?

A. DNA by an amino acid
B. DNA by an mRNA
C. mRNA by an amino acid
D. mRNA by an aminoacyl-tRNA
E. tRNA by an amino acid

Answer D: The codons in an mRNA must be faithfully recognized by the anticodon sequences of an aminoacyl-tRNA in order for the correct protein sequence to be generated during translation.

23. Which of the following is a function of codons in eukaryotic cells?

A. initiation of gene expression
B. recognition of complementary sequences in mRNA
C. recognition of specific mRNA sequences
D. specification of individual amino acids
E. used for directing the cap-binding complex to an mRNA

Answer D: The genetic code of an mRNA is contained within the triplet codons which dictate the amino acids to be incorporated during protein synthesis.

24. You are studying the process of protein synthesis and the effects of mutations introduced into tRNA genes. You alter the sequences of the anticodon of a tRNA from CAU into GUU. As a consequence of this change, which of the following, regarding the steps of translation, is most likely to occur?

A. increased translation rate
B. premature termination
C. shift of the reading frame
D. substitution of 1 amino acid
E. no effect

Answer D: A change in the anticodon sequences of a tRNA would most likely result in an amino acid substitution. The amino acid normally attached to the CAU-containing tRNA would now be incorporated at the codon (AAC) that the mutated anticodon now recognizes.

25. Which of the following best describes what happens when an 80S ribosome completes synthesis of a protein?

A. the entire ribosome is degraded by proteases and nucleases
B. the protein components of the ribosome are degraded by the proteasome, but the rRNAs are recycled
C. the ribosome dissociates into 60S and 40S subunits, which are then available for another round of protein synthesis

D. the 80S ribosome stays intact and is available for initiating another round of protein synthesis
E. the RNA components of the ribosome are degraded by nucleases, but the proteins are recycled

Answer C: Translation termination occurs when a stop codon is encountered within the context of the A-site of the 60S subunit. The termination factor eRF stimulates the peptidyltransferase ribozyme to transfer the peptide to H_2O. The peptide is released from the ribosome along with the naked tRNA and mRNA. The antiassociation factors then promote dissociation of the 80S ribosome into its 2 ribosomal subunits so the process can begin anew.

26. During the process of protein synthesis the elongating peptide is transferred to the incoming aminoacyl-tRNA by a peptidyltransferase activity. Which of the following components of the translational machinery is most likely to possess this enzymatic activity?
A. peptidase
B. ribosomal protein L11
C. ribosomal protein S16
D. 5S rRNA
E. 28S rRNA
F. tRNA nucleotidyltransferase

Answer E: During protein elongation, the peptide attached to the tRNA in the P-site is transferred to the amino group at the aminoacyl-tRNA in the A-site forming a new peptide bond. This reaction is catalyzed by peptidyltransferase activity which resides in what is termed the peptidyltransferase center (PTC) of the large ribosomal subunit (60S subunit). This enzymatic process is termed transpeptidation. This enzymatic activity is not mediated by any ribosomal proteins but instead by ribosomal RNA contained in the 60S subunit. This RNA-encoded enzymatic activity is referred to as a ribozyme. The 60S subunit contains the 28S rRNA as well as many other proteins.

27. Which of the following describes the direction of translation of mRNAs and synthesis of protein on ribosomes?

	Translation	*Synthesis*
A.	5′ → 3′	*C*-terminus → *N*-terminus
B.	3′ → 5′	*C*-terminus → *N*-terminus
C.	5′ → 3′	*N*-terminus → *C*-terminus
D.	3′ → 5′	*N*-terminus → *C*-terminus

Answer C: The ribosomes "read" the mRNA in the 5′ to 3′ direction and synthesis proceeds from the *N*-terminus to the *C*-terminus of the protein.

28. You are studying the processes of protein synthesis via the use of a cell-free system and synthetic RNAs. You have introduced the following RNA to this system:

5′-AUAUAAUGACUAAAUAU-3′

Table of codons

AAA	lysine
AAU	asparagine
ACU	threonine
AUA	isoleucine
AUG	methionine
UAU	tyrosine
CAU	leucine

Using the above indicated codons, which of the following is the most likely sequence of the peptide synthesized in this system?
A. isoleucine, methionine, threonine, lysine, tyrosine
B. methionine, isoleucine, asparagine
C. methione, threonine, leucine, threonine
D. methionine, threonine, lysine, tyrosine

Answer D: Translation in eukaryotic cells begins with methionine. Therefore, translation of the synthetic RNA in this study will begin at the first AUG codon encountered and result in the generation of a peptide with the sequence, M-T-K-Y.

29. You are a visiting physician treating patients at a clinic in Bangladesh. Your current patient is a 5-year-old girl complaining of a fever and sore throat for the past week. Physical examination shows a gray-white membrane on the tonsils and the pharyngeal wall. A swab of the membranes is taken and an infectious agent is characterized. Your studies of a toxin purified from this infectious agent demonstrate that it markedly inhibits protein synthesis. Which of the following is most likely to be the mechanism by which this toxin exerts its activity?
A. inhibition of GTP binding to aminoacyl-tRNA
B. inhibition of release of factor binding to the translational complex
C. inhibition of transcript initiation
D. inhibition of the translocation step in protein chain elongation
E. premature termination of the translated protein

Answer D: The child is most likely suffering from diphtheria. A protein from *Corynebacterium diphtheria* which causes diphtheria catalyzes the ADP-ribosylation and inactivation of eEF-2. eEF-2 contains a modified

His residue known as diphthamide and it is this residue that is the target of the toxin. The process of moving a peptidyl-tRNA from the A-site to the P-site is termed translocation. Translocation is catalyzed by eEF-2 coupled to GTP hydrolysis. In the process of translocation the ribosome is moved along the mRNA such that the next codon of the mRNA resides under the A-site.

30. Which of the following occurs to mRNA molecules during protein synthesis?
A. amplification in the cytoplasm to code for new proteins
B. conversion to DNA by reverse transcriptase
C. synthesis from individual ribonucleotides
D. transcription in a 3′ → 5′ direction
E. translation in a 5′ → 3′ direction

Answer E: The ribosomes "read" the mRNA in the 5′ to 3′ direction.

31. At which of the following sites on a eukaryotic mRNA is translation most likely to begin?
A. at the cap
B. at the 3′-end of the mRNA
C. at the 5′-end of the mRNA
D. first AUG codon
E. within 5 nucleotides of the Shine-Delgarno sequence

Answer D: In eukaryotes, initiator AUGs are generally, but not always, the first encountered by the translational machinery. A specific sequence context, surrounding the initiator AUG, aids ribosomal discrimination and is referred to as the Kozak consensus sequence.

32. Which of the following proteins or complexes involved in protein synthesis exhibits peptidyltransferase activity?
A. elongating peptide
B. elongation factor 2 (eEF-2)
C. mRNA
D. ribosome
E. tRNA

Answer D: During protein elongation, the peptide attached to the tRNA in the P-site is transferred to the amino group at the aminoacyl-tRNA in the A-site forming a new peptide bond. This reaction is catalyzed by peptidyltransferase activity which resides in what is termed the peptidyltransferase center (PTC) of the large ribosomal subunit (60S subunit). This enzymatic process is termed transpeptidation. This enzymatic activity is not mediated by any ribosomal proteins but instead by ribosomal RNA contained in the 60S subunit. This RNA-encoded enzymatic activity is referred to as a ribozyme.

33. The synthesis of all proteins in both prokaryotic and eukaryotic cells begins with which of the following amino acids?
A. alanine
B. glycine
C. leucine
D. methionine
E. tryptophan

Answer D: Initiation of translation in both prokaryotes and eukaryotes requires a specific initiator tRNA, $tRNA_i^{met}$, that is used to incorporate the initial methionine residue into all proteins.

34. You are studying the effects of chemical treatment of components of the translational machinery. You discover that one chemical in particular results in the conversion of the cysteine attached to a tRNA to alanine. Which of the following would best describe the results of this chemical-induced insertion of alanine into the resultant polypeptide?
A. it would not occur due to altered structure
B. it would occur randomly
C. it would occur where alanine is normally present
D. it would occur where cysteine is normally present

Answer D: It is absolutely necessary that the discrimination of correct amino acid and correct tRNA be made by a given aminoacyl tRNA synthetase prior to release of the aminoacyl-tRNA from the enzyme. Once the product is released, there is no further way to proofread whether a given tRNA is coupled to its corresponding amino acid. Erroneous coupling would lead to the wrong amino acid being incorporated into the polypeptide, since the discrimination of amino acid during protein synthesis comes from the recognition of the anticodon of a tRNA by the codon of the mRNA and not by recognition of the amino acid. Desulfuration of cys-$tRNA^{cys}$ with Raney nickel generates ala-$tRNA^{cys}$. Alanine is then incorporated into an elongating polypeptide where cysteine should have been.

35. You are studying the process of protein synthesis in cultures of hepatocytes. During an experiment, you observe that translation of certain mRNAs continues until a termination codon reside in the A-site of the ribosome. The liberation of the polypeptide chain at this point involves the eukaryotic releasing factor and hydrolysis of which of the following?
A. ATP
B. CTP
C. GTP
D. TTP
E. UTP

Answer C: Translation termination occurs when a stop codon is encountered within the context of the A-site of the 60S subunit. The termination factor eRF, which binds GTP, then stimulates the peptidyltransferase ribozyme to transfer the peptide, from the tRNA in the P-site, to H_2O coupled with the hydrolysis of GTP to GDP + P_i. The peptide is released from the ribosome along with the naked tRNA and eRF-GDP complex.

36. Which of the following determines the sequence of a polypeptide synthesized by the polyribosome complex?
A. aminoacyl-tRNA
B. aminoacyl-tRNA synthetase
C. elongation factor 1 (eEF-1)
D. mRNA
E. peptidyltransferase

Answer D: The genetic code that dictates the sequence of amino acids in a protein is contained within the codons of the mRNA.

37. You are studying the effects of insulin addition to cultures of eukaryotic cells at the level of protein synthesis. Your results demonstrate that addition of insulin stimulates protein synthesis concomitant with the phosphorylation of protein S6 of the 40S ribosomal subunit of the ribosome. Which of the following steps in protein synthesis is most likely stimulated when S6 is phosphorylated in this system?
A. aminoacyl-tRNA binding to the A-site of the ribosome
B. initiation
C. peptide bond formation
D. termination
E. translocation

Answer B: Translation initiation involves the interactions of eIF-2-GTP, an activated initiator tRNA (met-tRNA^{met}), and binding to the 40S subunit forming the 43S preinitiation complex. Phosphorylation of the 40S ribosome-associate protein S6 is therefore most likely to be associated with regulation of translation initiation.

38. During the development of B cells there is switch from the synthesis of membrane-bound immunoglobulin to a secreted form of immunoglobulin. This change occurs because the mRNA population encodes a protein missing which of the following sequence motifs?
A. anchor sequence
B. glycosylation sites
C. leucine zipper
D. signal sequence
E. zinc-binding domain

Answer A: Membrane-bound and secreted proteins are synthesized by ribosomes attached to the membranes of the ER. As synthesis of these types of proteins begins a complex on the ER called the signal recognition particle (SRP) engages the signal peptide of the newly synthesizing protein. The SRP then assists in the transfer of the elongating peptide through the ER membrane into the lumen of the ER. Proteins that are membrane bound contain a stretch of hydrophobic amino acids that constitutes the transmembrane domain(s). These hydrophobic amino acids stop the transfer of the protein into the ER lumen and are referred to as anchor sequences or stop-transfer sequences.

39. You are studying the translation of mRNAs derived from human erythrocytes in cell-free system derived from the *E coli* bacterium. You find the human globin mRNA is translated with extremely low efficiency in this system. Which of the following is the best explanation for these findings?
A. absence of methylated nucleotides
B. absence of more than 1 open-reading frame
C. absence of a Shine-Delgarno sequence
D. presence of intron
E. presence of a poly(a) tail

Answer C: Initiation of translation in both prokaryotes and eukaryotes requires a specific initiator tRNA and the recognition of an AUG codon in the mRNA. In the polycistronic prokaryotic RNAs this AUG codon is located adjacent to a Shine-Delgarno element in the mRNA. The Shine-Delgarno element is recognized by complimentary sequences in the small subunit rRNA. The lack of the Shine-Delgarno sequence in the globin RNA would restrict its translatability, as evidenced by the low efficiency of translation in the *E Coli*-derived system.

40. Many proteins contain a specialized stretch of amino acids that are recognized by a protein complex called the signal recognition particle. Which of the following best describes the function of this complex during the synthesis of secretory proteins?
A. anchors the ribosome to the Golgi membrane
B. enhances the rate of protein synthesis
C. interact with the amino terminus of the nascent polypeptide
D. interacts with glycosyltransferases within the endoplasmic reticulum
E. promotes the binding of specific mRNAs to ribosomes

Answer C: Membrane-bound and secreted proteins are synthesized by ribosomes attached to the membranes of the ER. As synthesis of these types of proteins begins a complex on the ER called the signal recognition particle (SRP) engages the signal peptide of the newly synthesizing protein. Since protein synthesis proceeds from the *N*-terminus to the *C*-terminus, the SRP is recognizing the signal sequence at the *N*-terminus of the protein.

41. Translocation of newly synthesized protein from the ribosome into the lipid bilayer of a membrane occurs most frequently at the level of which of the following?
   A. *cis* Golgi membrane
   B. nucleolus
   C. plasma membrane
   D. rough endoplasmic reticulum
   E. secretory vesicles

Answer D: Membrane-bound and secreted proteins are synthesized by ribosomes attached to the membranes of the ER. As synthesis of these types of proteins begins a complex on the ER called the signal recognition particle (SRP) engages the signal peptide of the newly synthesizing protein. The SRP then assists in the transfer of the elongating peptide through the ER membrane into the lumen of the ER.

42. You are studying the effects of a novel drug on the process of protein synthesis in a cell culture system. You discover that addition of the drug causes failure of ribosomes to attach to membranes of the ER. Which of the following is the most likely short-term consequence in the treated cells?
   A. general decrease in translation of all proteins
   B. increase in biogenesis of lysosomes
   C. increase in exocytosis
   D. no short-term consequences
   E. selective decrease in secretion of glycoproteins

Answer E: Membrane-bound and secreted proteins are synthesized by ribosomes attached to the membranes of the ER. Failure of the ribosomes to attach would, therefore, lead to reduced capacity to synthesis both secreted and membrane-bound proteins.

43. Ribosomal RNAs are synthesized and processed within the nucleolus. Which of the following molecular mechanisms best describes the method by which a newly assembled 60S ribosomal subunit is made available to the translational machinery in the cytoplasm?
   A. disassembled at the nuclear pore and reassembled in the cytoplasm
   B. transported by transcytosis
   C. transported out of the nucleus by active transport through the nuclear envelope
   D. transported out of the nucleus by passive diffusion through the nuclear envelope
   E. transported out of the nucleus through a nuclear pore complex

Answer E: The different RNA species that are produced in the nucleus are exported through the nuclear pore complexes via mobile export receptors. Large RNAs (such as ribosomal RNAs and mRNAs) assemble into complicated ribonucleoprotein (RNP) particles and recruit their exporters via class-specific adaptor proteins prior to transport through the pore complex.

Checklist

✓ Protein synthesis is the process whereby the genetic information, transferred from the DNA of the genes to the mRNAs, is translated into the correct order of amino acids in a protein.

✓ The genetic information in the mRNA is decoded in the tandem array of triplet nucleotide codons. Multiple different codons can encode the same amino acid and this phenomenon is referred to as the degeneracy of the genetic code.

✓ The process of protein synthesis occurs through the concerted actions of numerous proteins, tRNAs, and rRNA that form a functional ribosome. The ribosomal machinery travels down the template mRNA from the 5′-end where it will encounter a start codon (AUG) within the correct sequence context, and then proceed toward the 3′-end until it encounters a translational stop codon, synthesizing a protein from the N-terminal end to the C-terminal end.

✓ Translation consists of 3 highly ordered steps beginning with initiation, then elongation, followed by termination. Initiation is the most complex of the 3 processes and involves the largest number of translation factors.

✓ Several specialized enzymes involved in red-ox reactions require the incorporation of a modified amino acid, selenocysteine. These enzymes are called selenoproteins and their synthesis requires a dedicated selenocysteinyl-tRNA and a stem-loop structure in the mRNA that directs the incorporation of the modified amino acid at a codon that is normally a stop codon (UGA).

✓ Numerous antibiotics function through inhibition of various processes of protein synthesis.

✓ Numerous ribosomes can engage a single mRNA at the same time forming what are called polyribosomes, or polysomes. Polysomes associated with the endoplasmic reticulum (ER) form what is called the rough ER.

✓ All secreted and membrane-bound proteins are synthesized on rough ER. These proteins all have a signal sequenced recognized by a protein complex that directs the ribosomes to the ER.

✓ Many proteins undergo posttranslational modification. These modifications include cleavage, acetylation, methylation, lipid attachment (prenylation or acylation), phosphorylation, sulfation, hydroxylation, carboxylation, and glycosylation. Each of these modifications is necessary for any given protein to be targeted to its site of action and/or for its biochemical function.

✓ All proteins have a normal tertiary or quaternary structure for function, and all have a variable life span before begin turned over. Proteins that are misfolded and proteins that are destined for turnover are most often "tagged" by incorporation of polymers of the 76-amino-acid-peptide ubiquitin. Ubiquitination targets the protein for degradation in the proteosome.

CHAPTER

38 Glycoproteins

CHAPTER OUTLINE

High-Yield Terms

Sugar code: refers to the total complement of sugars in an organism and how it relates to normal and abnormal physiology and pathology, also called the *glycome*

***N*-glycans:** glycoprotein family with carbohydrate attachment to asparagine residues

***O*-glycans:** glycoprotein family with carbohydrate attachment to serine, threonine, or hydroxylysine hydroxyl groups

Lipid-linked oligosaccharide (LLO): refers to the core glycan structure attached to the lipid dolichol pyrophosphate prior to addition to an asparagine residue of an *N*-linked glycoprotein; the core glycan structure is also referred to as the *en bloc* oligosaccharide

Hexosamine biosynthesis pathway (HBP): pathway for conversion of glucose to *O*-GlcNAc, which is important for the carbohydrate modification of numerous cytoplasmic and nuclear proteins

Lectin: any of a family of proteins that contain a carbohydrate-binding domain; lectin is derived from the Latin word meaning "to select"

Mucin: any of a family of high molecular weight, heavily glycosylated proteins with the ability to form gels that lubricate and form chemical barriers

Congenital disorders of glycosylation (CDG): a family of diseases resulting from inherited defects in the synthesis, processing, and modification of both *N*-linked and *O*-linked glycoproteins and related glycan-modified molecules

High-Yield Concept

This significance underscores the relatively new field of study called *glycomics*, which analogous to genomics and proteomics, involves the analysis of the glycome (the total complement of sugars in an organism) and how it relates to normal and abnormal physiology and pathology. The glycome can be considered the **sugar code** of an organism.

Membrane-associated carbohydrate is exclusively in the form of oligosaccharides covalently attached to proteins, forming glycoproteins and to a lesser extent covalently attached to lipid, forming the glycolipids. Most proteins that are secreted, or bound to the plasma membrane, are modified by carbohydrate attachment. The posttranslational attachment of carbohydrate to proteins plays a critical role in overall biochemical complexity in humans. The importance of this protein modification can be emphasized by the fact that approximately 50% of all human proteins are known to be glycosylated and at least 1% of the human genome is represented by genes involved in glycan synthesis, processing, and homeostasis.

In addition to their critical roles in normal biochemical and physiological processes, the carbohydrate structures of many glycoproteins have been hijacked by pathogens and used as attachment sites for entry into host cells. HIV, poxviruses, parvoviruses, rhinoviruses, and herpes virus 6 all gain entry into cells by attaching to cell-surface glycoproteins. In addition, malarial parasite infection into erythrocytes involves recognition of cell-surface glycoproteins. Even bacteria utilize glycoproteins for attachment to host cells. *Helicobacter pylori*, the causative agent for one of the most common forms of cancer in humans, adenocarcinoma, adheres to gastric mucosal cells via glycoprotein recognition.

Glycoproteins

The predominant sugars found in glycoproteins are glucose (Glc), galactose (Gal), mannose (Man), fucose (Fuc), *N*-acetylgalactosamine (GalNAc), *N*-acetylglucosamine (GlcNAc), and *N*-acetylneuraminic acid (NANA). NANA is also called sialic acid (Sia) (Table 38-1). The distinction between proteoglycans (Chapter 39) and glycoproteins resides in the level and types of carbohydrate modification. Proteoglycans also contain the sugar glucuronic acid (GlcA) and the carbohydrate modifications found in glycoproteins are rarely as complex as that of proteoglycans.

The carbohydrates of glycoproteins are linked to the protein component through either *O*-glycosidic or *N*-glycosidic bonds (Figure 38-1). The *N*-glycosidic linkage is through the amide group of asparagine (*N*). In *N*-linked glycoproteins, the sugar attached to the *N* residue is always GlcNAc. The predominant carbohydrate attachment in glycoproteins of mammalian cells is via *N*-glycosidic linkage. The site of carbohydrate attachment to *N*-linked glycoproteins is found within a consensus sequence of amino acids, N-X-S/T (Asn-X-Ser/Thr), where X is any amino acid except Pro (P), Asp (D), or Glu (E). Analysis of the human protein database demonstrates that approximately 65% of all proteins contain at least one occurrence of the N-X-S/T consensus. The *O*-glycosidic linkage is to the hydroxyl of serine (S), threonine (T), or hydroxylysine (hLys). The linkage of carbohydrate to hLys is generally found only in the collagens. When attached to S or T, the sugar of *O*-linked glycoproteins is most often GalNAc. This most common *O*-glycoprotein type is also commonly referred to as a mucin-type glycan.

The protein component of all glycoproteins is synthesized from polyribosomes that are bound to the ER. The processing of the sugar groups occurs co- and posttranslationally in the lumen of the ER and continues in the Golgi apparatus for *N*-linked glycoproteins. Attachment of sugars in *O*-linked glycoproteins occurs posttranslationally in the Golgi apparatus. Sugars used for glycoprotein synthesis (both *N*-linked and *O*-linked) are activated by coupling to nucleotides.

Nucleotide Sugar Biosynthesis

The monosaccharides that are attached to proteins are first activated by coupling to a nucleotide. The synthesis of nearly all nucleotide-activated sugars occurs in the cytosol. The exception to this is the synthesis of CMP-activated NANA, which takes place in the nucleus. Since the nucleotide-activated sugars are synthesized in the cytosol, they must be translocated into the ER and Golgi before they can be used in the process of glycan synthesis. Since nucleotide-activated

TABLE 38-1: The Principal Sugars Found in Human Glycoproteins

Sugar	*Type*	*Abbreviation*	*Nucleotide Sugar*	*Comments*
Galactose	Hexose	Gal	UDP-Gal	Often found subterminal to NeuAc in *N*-linked glycoproteins. Also, found in the core trisaccharide of proteoglycans.
Glucose	Hexose	Glc	UDP-Glc	Present during the biosynthesis of *N*-linked glycoproteins but not usually present in mature glycoproteins. Present in some clotting factors.
Mannose	Hexose	Man	GDP-Man	Common sugar in *N*-linked glycoproteins.
N-Acetylneuraminic acid	Sialic acid (nine C atoms)	NeuAc	CMP-NeuAc	Often the terminal sugar in both *N*- and *O*-linked glycoproteins. Other types of sialic acid are also found, but NeuAc is the major species found in humans. Acetyl groups may also occur as *O*-acetyl species as well as *N*-acetyl.
Fucose	Deoxyhexose	Fuc	GDP-Fuc	May be external in both *N*- and *O*-linked glycoproteins or internal, linked to the GlcNAc residue attached to Asn in *N*-linked species. Can also occur internally attached to the OH of Ser (eg, in t-PA and certain clotting factors).
N-Acetylgalactosamine	Aminohexose	GalNAc	UDP-GalNAc	Present in both *N*- and *O*-linked glycoproteins.
N-Acetylglucosamine	Aminohexose	GlcNAc	UDP-GlcNAc	The sugar attached to the polypeptide chain via Asn in *N*-linked glycoproteins; also found at other sites in the oligosaccharides of these proteins. Many nuclear proteins have GlcNAc attached to the OH of Ser or Thr as a single sugar.
Xylose	Pentose	Xyl	UDP-Xyl	Xyl is attached to the OH of Ser in many proteoglycans. Xyl in turn is attached to two Gal residues, forming a link trisaccharide. Xyl is also found in t-PA and certain clotting factors.

Murray RK, Bender DA, Botham KM, Kennelly PJ, Rodwell VW, Weil PA. *Harper's Illustrated Biochemistry.* 29th ed. New York, NY: McGraw-Hill; 2012.

sugars cannot freely pass through the ER or Golgi membranes, specific transport systems are responsible for their translocation. There are 2 mechanisms for the importation of nucleotide-activated sugars into the ER and/or Golgi apparatus. The first mechanism involves dolichol phosphate and it is used to transport mannose and glucose. The second mechanism involves specific nucleotide sugar transporters (NST) all of which belong to the solute carrier 35 (SLC35) family of membrane transporters. When the nucleotide-activated sugar is transported into the lumen of the ER or Golgi, there is a concomitant equimolar exit of a corresponding nucleoside monophosphate to the cytosol. Following entry into the ER or Golgi, a glycosyltransferase will transfer the monosaccharide to a target glycan concomitant with removal of the nucleoside diphosphate.

Mechanism of *N*-Glycosylation

Synthesis of carbohydrate portions of *N*-linked glycoproteins requires a lipid intermediate, dolichol phosphate (Figure 38-2). The phosphate moiety of dolichol phosphate is attached to the –OH group.

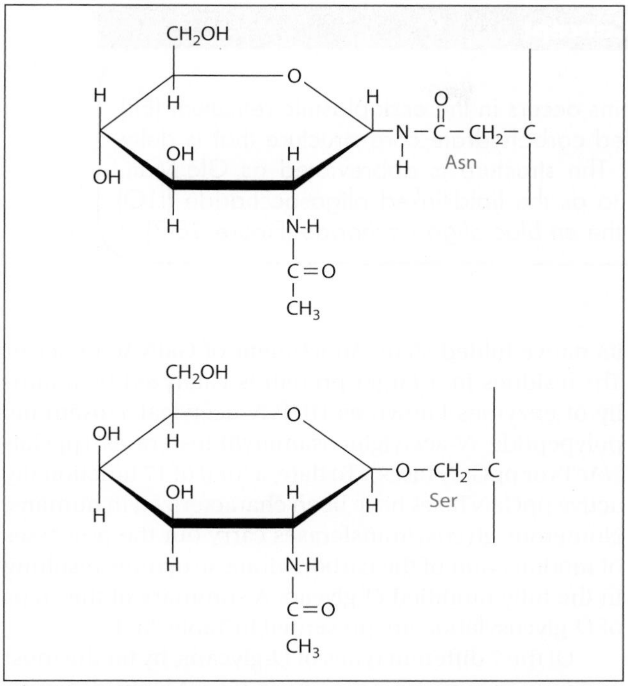

FIGURE 38-1: Representation of the *N*-glycosidic linkage of *N*-acetylglucosamine (GlcNAc) and the *O*-glycosidic linkage of *N*-acetylgalactosamine (GalNAc) to proteins. Reproduced with permission of themedicalbiochemistrypage, LLC.

Synthesis of the en bloc dolichol–PP–oligosaccharide unit (Figure 38-3) begins on the cytoplasmic face of the ER membrane and prior to transfer to the protein, the structure "flips" to the luminal side (Figure 38-4).

Immediately following transfer of the en bloc oligosaccharide unit to the protein, processing and alteration of the composition of the oligosaccharide ensues and continues as the protein passes through the ER and then into and through the Golgi apparatus. Initially, the terminal glucose is removed through the action of glucosidase I (GI), a membrane-bound enzyme recognizing α-1,2-linked glucose. The remaining 2 glucose residues are then removed by glucosidase II (GII), a soluble enzyme recognizing α-1,3-linked glucose. After removal of the glucose residues, the action of α-mannosidases removes several mannose residues as the protein progresses to the Golgi. The action of the various glucosidases and mannosidases leaves *N*-linked glycoproteins containing a common core of carbohydrate consisting of 3 mannose residues and 2 GlcNAc. Through the action of a wide range of glycosyltransferases and glycosidases, a variety of other sugars are attached to this core as the protein progresses through the Golgi ultimately generating 3 major families of *N*-linked glycoproteins (Figure 38-5). A summary of the steps of *N*-glycosylation are presented in Table 38-2.

O-Glycosylation and Mucin-Type *O*-Glycans

The attachment of carbohydrate to the hydroxyl group of serine (Ser, S) or threonine (Thr, T) residues in proteins, as well as hydroxylysine (hLys) in collagens, constitutes the bulk of *O*-linked glycans (*O*-glycans) found

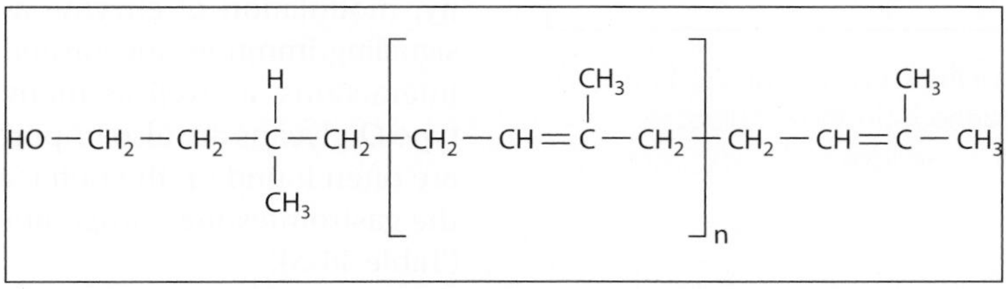

FIGURE 38-2: The structure of dolichol. The phosphate in dolichol phosphate is attached to the primary alcohol group at the left-hand end of the molecule. The group within the brackets is an isoprene unit (n = 17-20 isoprenoid units). Murray RK, Bender DA, Botham KM, Kennelly PJ, Rodwell VW, Weil PA. *Harper's Illustrated Biochemistry.* 29th ed. New York, NY: McGraw-Hill; 2012.

High-Yield Concept

The synthesis of nucleotide-activated sugars is under tight regulatory control such that the alteration in production of only a single nucleotide sugar can significantly impair glycosylation with potentially profound effects. That the disruption in the processes of nucleotide-activated sugar synthesis can result in severe clinical symptomatology is evident from the large number of disorders classified as congenital disorders of glycosylation, CDG (Clinical Box 38-2).

High-Yield Concept

The formation of the GlcNAc-β-N linkage in proteins occurs in the endoplasmic reticulum (ER) through cotranslational addition of a preassembled carbohydrate core structure that is delivered via the carbohydrate-dolichol intermediate. The structure is abbreviated as Glc_3Man_9 $GlcNAc_2$–PP–dolichol and is commonly referred to as the lipid-linked oligosaccharide (LLO) and the oligosaccharide structure itself is termed the *en bloc oligosaccharide* (Figure 38-3).

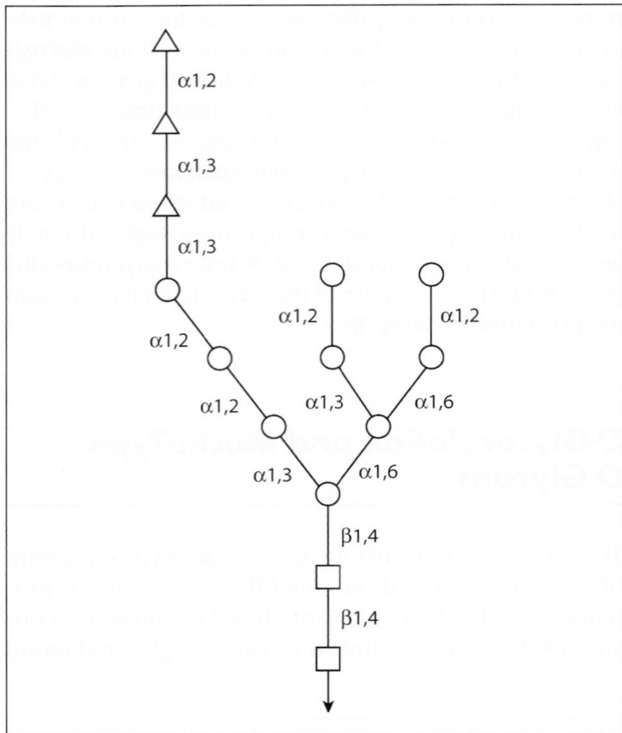

FIGURE 38-3: Structure of the en bloc oligosaccharide. Squares: GlcNAc; circles: mannose; triangles: glucose. Reproduced with permission of themedicalbiochemistrypage, LLC.

in the humans. Carbohydrate addition in *O*-glycans occurs via the stepwise addition of nucleotide-activated sugars as the modified proteins traverse the ER and the Golgi network. There are 7 major types of *O*-glycans in humans that are defined by the first sugar residue that is attached to Ser, Thr, or hLys (Table 38-3).

The process of *O*-GalNAc glycosylation occurs via 2 distinct steps that consist of initiation and processing. The initiation step controls the pattern and the density of the carbohydrate structures attached to the protein. The processing step determines the ultimate *O*-glycan structure that is present in the fully modified protein. The attachment of the initial GalNAc residue occurs in the Golgi network after the target protein has obtained its native folded state. Attachment of GalNAc to Ser or Thr residues in a target protein is catalyzed by a family of enzymes known as UDP-*N*-acetylgalactosamine: polypeptide *N*-acetylglucosaminyltransferases (ppGalNAcTs or ppGaNTases). To date, a total of 17 functionally active ppGaNTases have been characterized in humans. Numerous glycosyltransferases carry out the processes of modification of the carbohydrate structures resulting in the fully modified *O*-glycan. A summary of the steps of *O*-glycosylation are presented in Table 38-4.

Of the 7 different types of *O*-glycans, by far the most common in humans is the mucin type. Mucin glycoproteins are so called because of their abundance in the mucous secretions on cell surfaces and in body fluids. Mucin-type *O*-glycans all have the amino sugar GalNAc attached to the Ser or Thr residue of the modified protein. There are 8 mucin-type core structures, which are defined based upon the second sugar attached to the GalNAc and the linkage of that attachment.

The attachment of carbohydrates to proteins forming *O*-glycans serves multiple critical functions with respect to the structure and activity of the modified proteins. *O*-linked glycans are important for protein stability, modulation of enzyme activity, receptor-mediated signaling, immune function and immunity, protein-protein interactions, as well as many other functions. Mucin-type *O*-glycans are also important for binding water and are often found on the outer surfaces of tissues, such as the gastrointestinal, urogenital, and respiratory systems (Table 38-5).

O-Mannosylation

Incorporation of mannose into target proteins by attachment to Ser and/or Thr, referred to as *O*-mannosylation, serves a critical function in humans. *O*-mannosylation has been identified on α-dystroglycan (α-DG) from nerve and muscle, chondroitin sulfate proteoglycans, and several other proteins. Clinically, *O*-mannosylation of α-DG is the most significant as evidenced by the constellation of symptoms that result from defects in the processes of *O*-mannosylation.

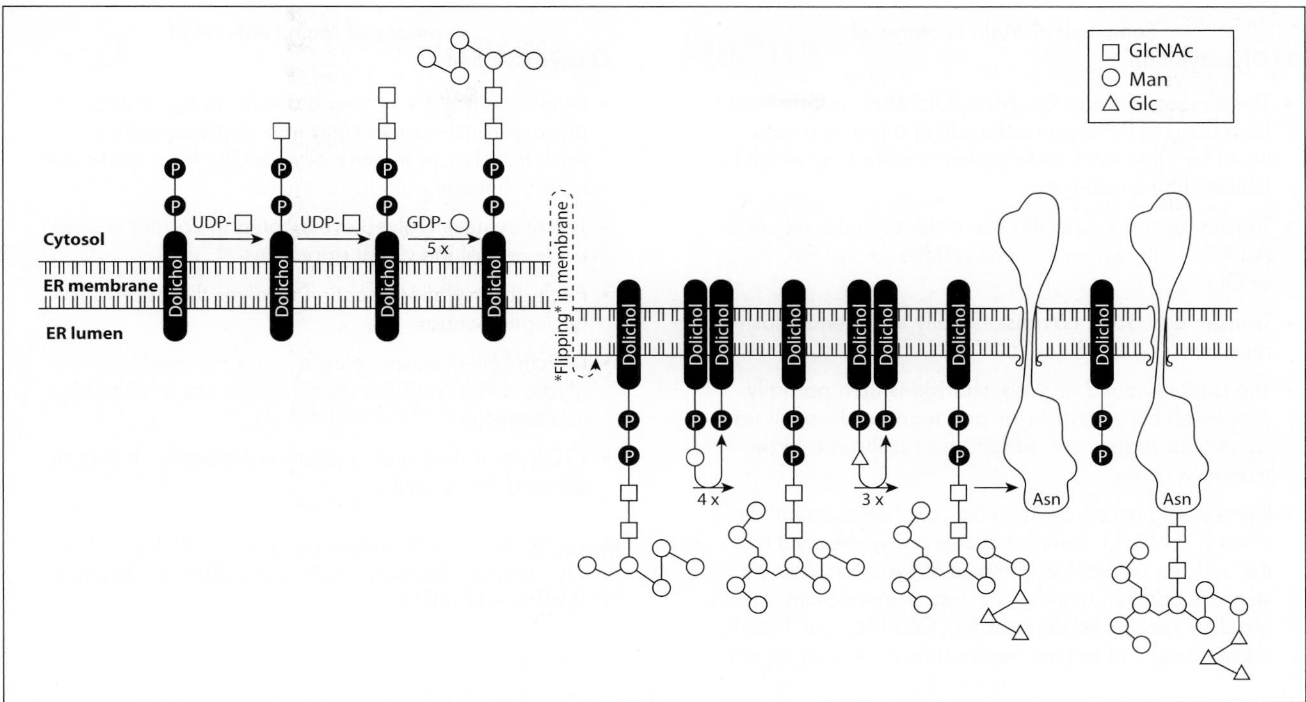

FIGURE 38-4: Synthesis and transfer of the LLO unit to a protein within the ER. The synthesis of the dolichol-coupled oligosaccharide complex (the lipid-linked oligosaccharide, LLO) begins on the cytosolic face of the ER membrane. When the dolichol-sugar complex contains the initial 2 GlcNAc residues and several mannose residues it is flipped such that the carbohydrate portion is moved to the luminal side of the ER membrane. Several more sugars are added to form the complete LLO. The sugars portion of the LLO is then transferred to an appropriate Asn residue in an acceptor protein, leaving the dolichol within the membrane. Reproduced with permission of themedicalbiochemistrypage, LLC.

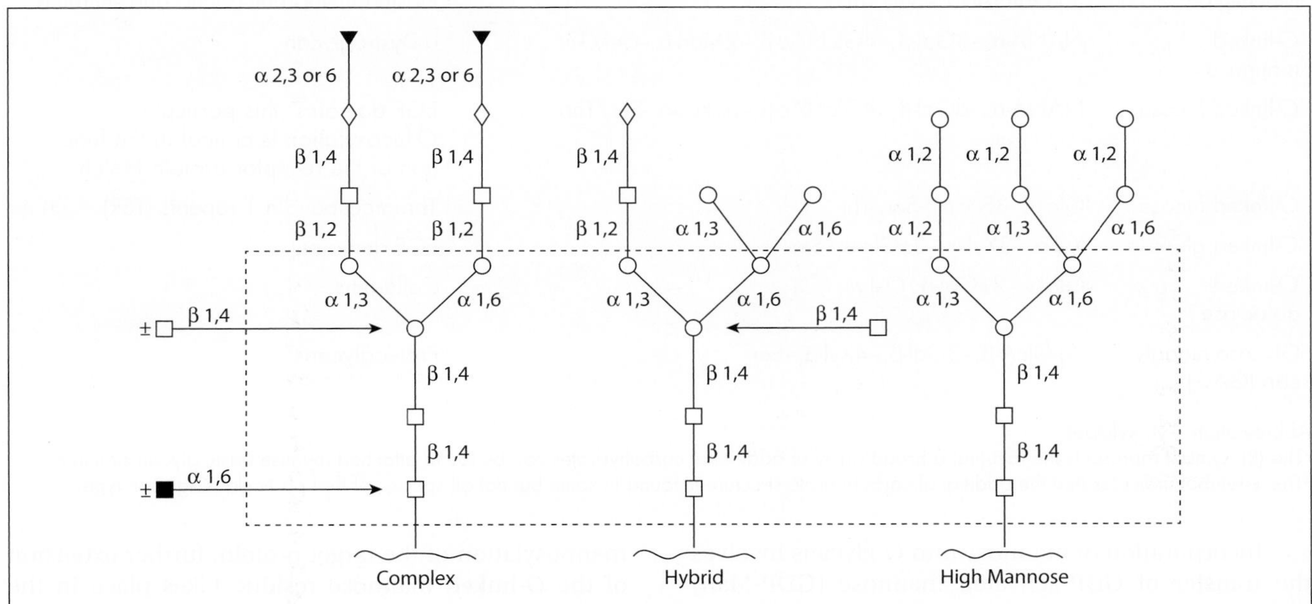

FIGURE 38-5: Structures of oligosaccharides found on the 3 major classes of *N*-glycoprotein. Open squares: GlcNAc; open circles: mannose; open diamonds: galactose; filled squares: fucose; filled triangles: sialic acid. Reproduced with permission of themedicalbiochemistrypage, LLC.

TABLE 38-2: Summary of Main Features of *N*-Glycosylation

- The oligosaccharide $Glc_3Man_9(GlcNAc)_2$ is transferred from dolichol-P-P-oligosaccharide in a reaction catalyzed by oligosaccharide:protein transferase, which is inhibited by tunicamycin.
- Transfer occurs to specific Asn residues in the sequence AsnX-Ser/Thr, where X is any residue except Pro, Asp, or Glu.
- Transfer can occur cotranslationally in the endoplasmic reticulum.
- The protein-bound oligosaccharide is then partially processed by glucosidases and mannosidases; if no additional sugars are added, this results in a high-mannose chain.
- If processing occurs down to the core heptasaccharide ($Man_5[GlcNAc]_2$), complex chains are synthesized by the addition of GlcNAc, removal of two Man, and the stepwise addition of individual sugars in reactions catalyzed by specific transferases (eg, GlcNAc, Gal, NeuAc transferases) that employ appropriate nucleotide sugars.

Murray RK, Bender DA, Botham KM, Kennelly PJ, Rodwell VW, Weil PA. *Harper's Illustrated Biochemistry.* 29th ed. New York, NY: McGraw-Hill; 2012.

TABLE 38-4: Summary of Main Features of *O*-Glycosylation

- Involves a battery of membrane-bound glycoprotein glycosyltransferases acting in a stepwise manner; each transferase is generally specific for a particular type of linkage.
- The enzymes involved are located in various subcompartments of the Golgi apparatus.
- Each glycosylation reaction involves the appropriate nucleotide sugar.
- Dolichol-P-P-oligosaccharide is not involved, nor are glycosidases; and the reactions are not inhibited by tunicamycin.
- *O*-Glycosylation occurs posttranslationally at certain Ser and Thr residues.

Murray RK, Bender DA, Botham KM, Kennelly PJ, Rodwell VW, Weil PA. *Harper's Illustrated Biochemistry.* 29th ed. New York, NY: McGraw-Hill; 2012.

TABLE 38-3: Description of the 7 Major Types of *O*-Glycans[1]

***O*-Glycan Type**	***Structure of Linkage***	***Glycoprotein Characteristics***
O-linked GlcNAc	GlcNAc-β_1–Ser/Thr	Nuclear and cytoplasmic
Mucin-type	(R)-GalNAc-α_1–Ser/Thr	Plasma membrane-bound and secreted
O-linked mannose	NANA-α_2–3Gal-β_1–4GlcNAc-β_1–2Man-α_1–Ser/Thr	α-Dystroglycan
O-linked fucose	NANA-α_2–6Gal-β_1–4GlcNAc-β_1–3±Fuc-α_1-Ser/Thr[2]	EGF domains; this particular *O*-fucosylation is critical in the function of the receptor protein Notch
O-linked fucose	Glc-β_1–3Fuc-α_1–Ser/Thr	Thrombospondin 1 repeats (TSR)
O-linked glucose	Xyl-α_1–3Xyl-α_1–3±Glc-β_1–Ser	EGF domains
O-linked galactose	Glc-α_1–2±Gal-β_1-*O*–Lys	Collagens
Glycosaminoglycan (GAG)	(R)-GlcA-β_1–3Gal-β_1–4Xyl-β_1–Ser	Proteoglycans

Abbreviation: Xyl, xylulose.
[1]The (R)- symbol represents the fact that a broad array of additional carbohydrates can be found attached to these basic glycan structures.
[2]The ± symbol indicates that the additional carbohydrate structure is found in some but not all species of that particular *O*-glycan type.

Incorporation of mannose into *O*-glycans involves the transfer of GDP-activated mannose (GDP-Man) to dolichol-phosphate forming Dol-P-Man. Since it occurs in the ER, the actual process of *O*-mannosylation is distinct from most other *O*-glycosylation reactions that take place exclusively in the Golgi apparatus. After mannosylation of the target protein, further extension of the *O*-linked mannose residue takes place in the Golgi apparatus.

The best-studied *O*-mannosylated protein in humans is α-DG. It comprises 2 globular domains separated by a Ser/Thr-rich mucin-like region that is

TABLE 38-5: Some Properties of Mucins
• Found in secretions of the gastrointestinal, respiratory, and reproductive tracts and also in membranes of various cells.
• Exhibit high content of *O*-glycan chains, usually containing NeuAc.
• Contain repeating amino acid sequences rich in serine, threonine, and proline.
• Extended structure contributes to their high viscoelasticity.
• Form protective physical barrier on epithelial surfaces, are involved in cell–cell interactions, and may contain or mask certain surface antigens.

Murray RK, Bender DA, Botham KM, Kennelly PJ, Rodwell VW, Weil PA. *Harper's Illustrated Biochemistry.* 29th ed. New York, NY: McGraw-Hill; 2012.

substantially *O*-mannosylated. α-DG is an essential component of the dystrophin-glycoprotein complex (DGC) in skeletal muscle. Highlighting the significance of *O*-mannosylated α-DG is the fact that most of the defects associated with impaired *O*-mannosylation can be explained by reduced function of α-DG. In humans, defective *O*-mannosylation is associated with a group of autosomal recessive muscular dystrophies termed *congenital muscular dystrophies (CMDs)*. The CMDs are also referred to as secondary α-dystroglycanopathies since their common pathological feature is the hypoglycosylation of α-DG. Mutations in 6 glycosyltransferase genes have been identified to cause various α-dystroglycanopathies. The most severe CMD is Walker-Warburg syndrome (WWS) and as a consequence of multiple malformations, WWS patients often die within the first year of life.

Hexosamine Biosynthesis Pathway

Numerous nuclear and cytoplasmic proteins are post-translationally modified on serine and threonine residues with β-*N*-acetylglucosamine (*O*-GlcNAc), in a process referred to as *O*-GlcNAcylation. The gamut of *O*-GlcNAcylated proteins includes enzymes involved in the metabolism of amino acids, nucleotides (eg, thymidine kinase), and carbohydrates (eg, glucose-6-phosphatase), general metabolic processes, cell growth and maintenance (eg, MYC, Sp1), DNA damage responses, intracellular transport, transcription (eg, RNA polymerase II), and translation (eg, eIF-5). The carboxy-terminal domain of a subpopulation of RNA polymerase II is extensively *O*-GlcNAcylated, and almost all RNA polymerase II transcription factors (TFII) are *O*-GlcNAcylated. Thus far, more than 600 proteins have been shown to be *O*-GlcNAcylated.

The synthesis of *O*-GlcNAc, which initiates with glucose, occurs via the metabolic pathway called the hexosamine biosynthesis pathway, HBP (Figure 38-6). Upon entering cells, most of the glucose is utilized for glycolysis or glycogen synthesis or in the pentose phosphate pathway; however, 2% to 5% will enter the HBP to generate uridine diphospho-*N*-acetylglucosamine (UDP-GlcNAc). The end product of the HBP, UDP-GlcNAc, is an essential intermediate in the synthesis of a wide array of complex glycans.

Whereas there are hundreds of different kinases and phosphatases that add and remove phosphate from serine and threonine residues, respectively, in various target proteins, the process of *O*-GlcNAc cycling is maintained by the action of only 2 enzymes. Addition of GlcNAc (*O*-GlcNAcylation) is catalyzed by the enzyme UDP-*N*-acetylglucosamine:polypeptide β-*N*-acetylglucosaminyltransferase or more commonly just *O*-GlcNAc transferase, OGT. Removal of the *O*-GlcNAc modification is catalyzed by β-*N*-acetylglucosaminidase or more commonly *O*-GlcNAcase, OGA.

The HBP integrates the nutrient status of the cell by utilizing glucose, acetyl-CoA, glutamine, and UTP to produce UDP-GlcNAc. In turn, OGT will transmit this nutrient information throughout the cell changing the level of GlcNAcylated target proteins. This means that the cycling of *O*-GlcNAc is a nutrient-responsive, post-translational modification that, like phosphorylation, impacts target protein activity. Additionally, disruption of the HBP has a profound impact on diseases of nutrient sensing, such as Type 2 diabetes. Numerous proteins involved in insulin signaling and the downstream targets of these signaling cascades have been shown

High-Yield Concept

Unlike all other sugar modification of proteins, *O*-GlcNAc modification at serine and threonine residues cycles between addition and removal throughout the life of a target protein. In this respect *O*-GlcNAcylation is a modification akin to protein phosphorylation and dephosphorylation.

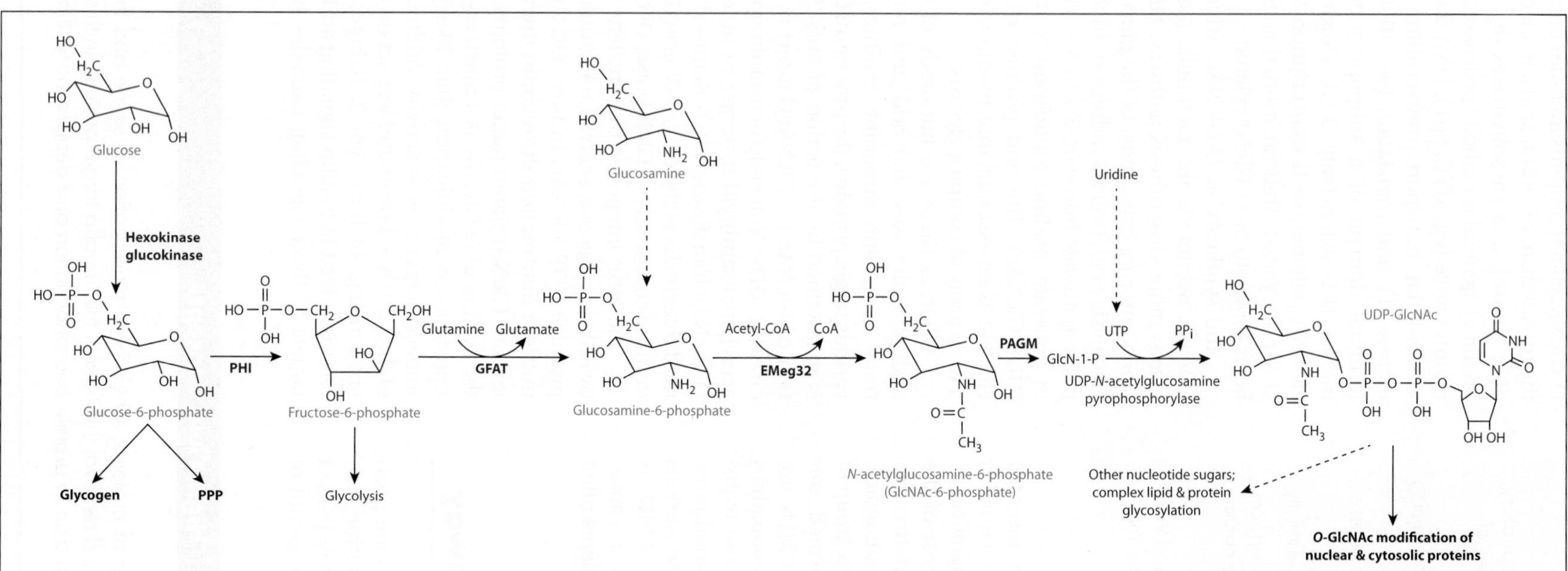

FIGURE 38-6: The hexosamine biosynthesis pathway (HBP). Although the majority of the glucose taken up by the cell is committed to glycolysis, glycogen synthesis, and the pentose phosphate pathway, in general about 2% to 5% of it enters the HBP for the formation of UDP-GlcNAc. The UDP-GlcNAc then serves as the substrate for a wide array of glycosylations, including *O*-GlcNAcylation. The first and rate-limiting enzyme in the HBP is glutamine:fructose 6-phosphate aminotransferase 1 (GFAT; also abbreviated GFPT1). Like other metabolic rate-limiting enzymes, GFAT is negatively regulated by the end product of the pathway, UDP-GlcNAc. Glucosamine can enter the HBP directly by conversion to GlcN6P via the action of hexokinase, thus bypassing the rate-limiting GFAT step. EMeg32 is glucosamine 6-phosphate *N*-acetyltransferase (also abbreviated GNPNAT1). The derivation EMeg32 is from the fact that the gene was originally isolated from a screen for genes specific for precursors of **E**rythroid and **Meg**akaryocytic lineages and was clone 32. PHI is phosphohexose isomerase. PAGM is phosphoacetylglucosamine mutase.

High-Yield Concept

Overexpression of the rate-limiting enzyme of the HBP, GFAT, leads to peripheral insulin resistance. In addition, overexpression of O-GlcNAc transferase (OGT) in skeletal muscle and adipose tissue results in elevated circulating insulin levels and insulin resistance.

to be *O*-GlcNAcylated. This modification of proteins involved in insulin signaling plays an important role in the development of insulin resistance under conditions of metabolic disruption (see Chapter 46).

O-GlcNAcylation and Glucose Homeostasis

Insulin resistance is a major contributing factor to the hyperglycemia typical of Type 2 diabetes, due in part, to the loss of GLUT4 presentation in the plasma membranes of skeletal muscle and adipose tissue. Aberrantly regulated hepatic gluconeogenesis also contributes to hyperglycemia. Several transcription factors (eg, FOXO1 and PGC-1α), that are involved in the regulated expression of gluconeogenic genes, can be modified by *O*-GlcNAcylation. The activity of OGT ultimately regulates gluconeogenesis through *O*-GlcNAcylation of PGC-1α that stabilizes the protein by inhibiting its ubiquitination. Stabilization of PGC-1α results in enhanced hepatic gluconeogenesis, allowing for more glucose to be delivered to the blood.

Lysosomal Targeting of Enzymes

Enzymes that are destined for the lysosomes (lysosomal enzymes) are directed there by a specific carbohydrate modification. During transit through the Golgi apparatus, a residue of GlcNAc-1-phosphate (GlcNAc-1-P) is added to the carbon-6 hydroxyl group of one or more specific mannose residues that have been added to these enzymes. The GlcNAc is transferred by UDP-GlcNAc:lysosomal enzyme GlcNAc-1-phosphotransferase (GlcNAc-phosphotransferase), yielding a phosphodiester intermediate: GlcNAc-1-P-6-Man-protein. The phosphotransferase is a hexameric complex whose protein subunits are encoded by 2 genes. The α- and β-subunits of the phosphotransferase are encoded by the *GNPTAB* gene. The second reaction (catalyzed by GlcNAc-1-phosphodiester-*N*-acetylglucosaminidase) removes the GlcNAc, leaving mannose residues phosphorylated in the 6 position: Man-6-P protein. A specific Man-6-P receptor (MPR) is present in the membranes of the Golgi apparatus. Binding of Man-6-P to this receptor targets proteins to the lysosomes. Defects in the process of mannose-6-phosphorylation result in several disorders referred to as mucolipidoses (eg, I-cell disease, Clinical Box 38-1).

Glycosylphosphatidylinositol-Anchored Proteins (GPI-Linkage)

Many membrane-associated glycoproteins are tethered to the outer leaflet of the plasma membrane via a glycosylphosphatidylinositol (GPI) linkage to their *C*-termini (Figure 38-7). These types of glycoproteins are termed *glypiated proteins*. The use of the GPI anchor has been found in a functionally diverse array of mammalian proteins that includes hydrolytic enzymes, adhesion molecules, complement regulatory proteins, and receptors. One clinically important glypiated protein is the erythrocyte surface glycoprotein, decay-accelerating factor (DAF; also known as CD55 = cluster of differentiation protein 55). DAF prevents erythrocyte lysis by complement. Other important GPI-linked proteins are the enzymes acetylcholinesterase, the cell adhesion molecule N-CAM-120 (neural cell adhesion molecule-120), and the T-cell markers Thy-1 and LFA-3 (lymphocyte function–associated antigen-3).

Glycoprotein Degradation

Degradation of glycoproteins occurs within lysosomes and requires specific lysosomal hydrolases, termed *glycosidases* (Figure 38-8). Exoglycosidases remove sugars sequentially from the nonreducing end and exhibit restricted substrate specificities. In contrast, endoglycosidases cleave carbohydrate linkages from within and exhibit broader substrate specificities. Several inherited disorders involving the abnormal

CLINICAL BOX 38-1: I-CELL DISEASE

I-cell disease *(also called mucolipidosis II α/β)* is an autosomal recessive disorder that results as a consequence of defective targeting of lysosomal hydrolases to the lysosomes. The disorder is so called because fibroblasts from afflicted patients contain numerous phase-dense inclusion bodies in the cytosol. The inclusion bodies seen in I-cell disease are also observed in pseudo-Hurler polydystrophy (mucolipidosis III α/β) that presents later and with milder symptoms compared to I-cell disease. The targeting of lysosomal enzymes to lysosomes is mediated by receptors that bind mannose 6-phosphate recognition markers on the enzymes. The recognition marker is synthesized in a 2-step reaction in the Golgi complex. The enzyme that catalyzes the first step is GlcNAc-phosphotransferase whose α- and β-subunits are encoded by the *GNPTAB* gene. Both I-cell disease and pseudo-Hurler polydystrophy result from defects in the *GNPTAB* gene. I-cell disease is characterized by severe psychomotor retardation that rapidly progresses, leading to death between 5 and 8 years of age. I-cell patients exhibit coarse facial features, craniofacial abnormalities, and severe skeletal abnormalities. These skeletal abnormalities include kyphoscoliosis (an abnormal curvature of the spine in both the coronal and sagittal planes), widening of the ribs, lumbar gibbus deformity (refers to a hump or swelling or enlargement on one side of a body surface), anterior beaking and wedging of the vertebral bodies, and proximal pointing of the metacarpals. Additional clinical symptoms of I-cell disease include hepatomegaly, cardiomegaly, umbilical hernias, and recurrent upper respiratory infections. The disease progresses rapidly with developmental delay and failure to thrive. Psychomotor retardation is evident in almost all patients by 6 months of age.

storage of glycoprotein degradation products have been identified in humans (Table 38-6). As a general class, such disorders are known as lysosomal storage diseases. Numerous proteins and sphingolipids harbor similar carbohydrate modifications. The enzymes that remove these sugar residues are the same for both glycoproteins and glycolipids and as such there is often overlapping phenotypes in diseases that were originally identified as being caused by defects in glycoprotein degradation or glycolipid degradation.

Carbohydrate Recognition: Lectins

The ability of certain proteins to recognize and bind to specific carbohydrate structures is of critical importance in overall cellular homeostasis. Proteins that recognize specific types of carbohydrates displayed on other proteins and/or lipids are referred to as *lectins*. All lectins contain a carbohydrate recognition domain, CRD. The lectin family of proteins does not include the immunoglobulins, which by themselves constitute a specialized class of carbohydrate-recognizing proteins. The clinical laboratory definition of lectins describes nonimmunoglobulins that are capable of differential agglutination (clumping: Latin for "to glue to") of erythrocytes (Table 38-7).

C-type Lectins

C-type lectin family is composed of 7 subfamilies where the designation of C-type relates to their dependence on Ca^{2+} ions for binding activity. C-type lectins recognize carbohydrate structures on many different forms of protein, including cell surface proteins and extracellular matrix (ECM) proteins and other ECM structures containing carbohydrate modifications, such as proteoglycans, glycosaminoglycans, and glycolipids. One of the most important functions for carbohydrate recognition by C-type lectins is the role that function plays in pathogen recognition by the innate immune system.

The collectins are subtype III C-type lectins defined by having an additional collagen-like domain. Mannan-binding lectin, MBL (also termed mannose-binding protein), is the best-characterized human collectin. The major function of the collectins is recognition of carbohydrate structures on microbial surfaces, leading to activation of the complement cascade and phagocytosis. MBL is synthesized by the liver and secreted into the circulation and is considered one of the **acute-phase proteins** synthesized by the liver. Upon binding to carbohydrate structures on microbial surfaces, MBL activates the complement system.

The selectins are subtype IV C-type lectins defined by the presence of the C-type lectin CRD, an epidermal

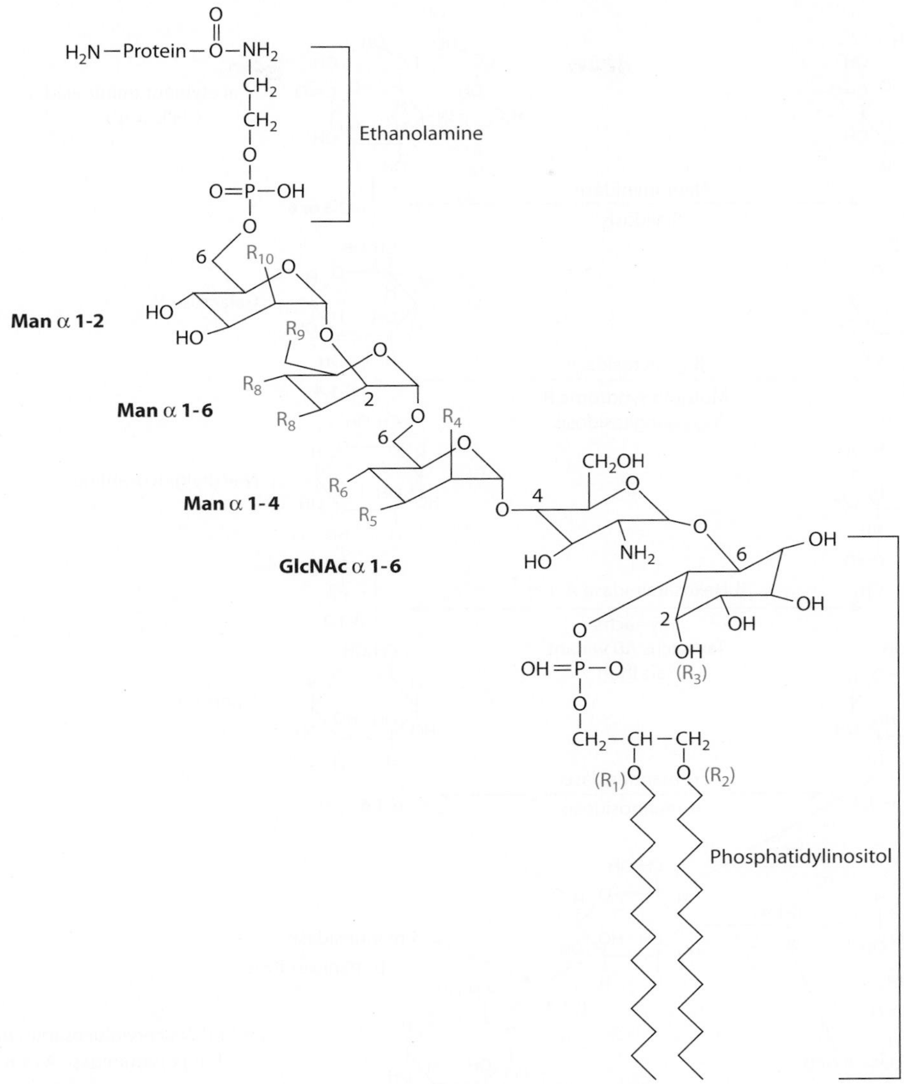

FIGURE 38-7: General structure of the GPI anchor. R_1 is most often an unsaturated fatty acid but can be just –OH; R_2 is either a fatty acid, alkyl or alkenyl group, can also be ceramide instead of glycerolipid, can also just be –OH; R_3 is most often palmitic acid attached to the C–2 carbon of inositol; R_4, R_9 are ethanolamine phosphate or –OH; R_5, R_6, R_7, R_8, R_{10} are carbohydrate substituents or –OH. Reproduced with permission of themedicalbiochemistrypage, LLC.

growth factor-like (EGF-like) domain, and a variable number of complement regulatory protein-like repeat domains. The selectins are also members of the cell adhesion family of proteins. There are 3 characterized selectins that were originally identified as the adhesion molecules: endothelial-leukocyte adhesion molecule-1 (ELAM-1), murine lymph node homing receptor, and platelet granule membrane protein-140. These 3 proteins are now referred to as E-selectin, L-selectin, and P-selectin, respectively. A major function of the selectins is the recruitment of neutrophils to sites of inflammation.

S-type Lectins: Galectins

The S-type lectins were so designated because the original family members exhibited a sulfhydryl dependence on carbohydrate binding. The S-type lectins are now

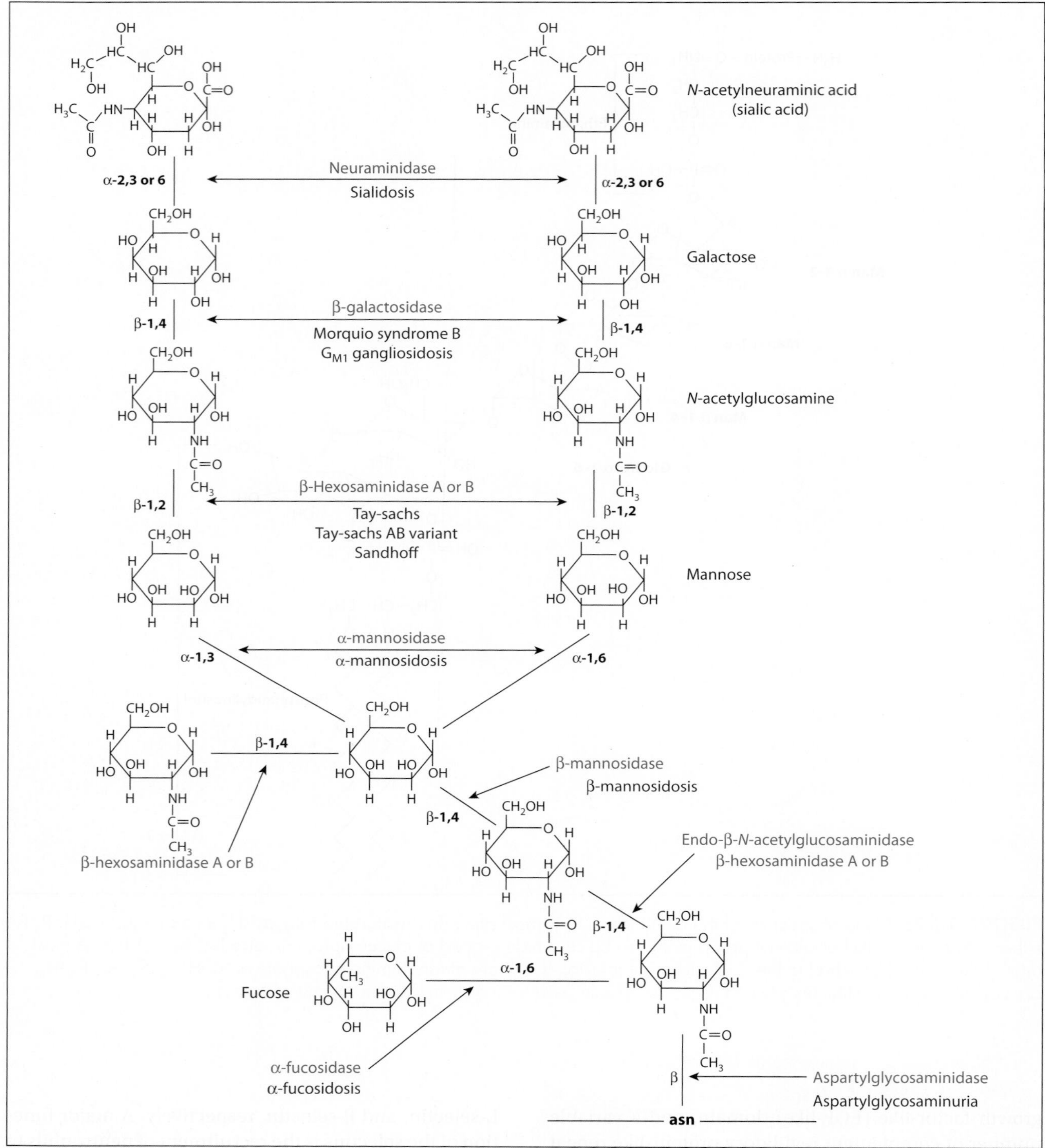

FIGURE 38-8: Locations of the actions of several glycosidases involved in glycoprotein metabolism. The structures of the carbohydrates in a typical complex oligosaccharide cluster are included (when linked as they would be by the indicated bonds, eg, α-2,3, or 6 indicated for sialic acid linkage to galactose, there would be loss of H_2O). The bonds are indicated for each linkage by the solid line between structures. Enzyme names are in green and the bonds hydrolyzed by each hydrolase are indicated by the arrows. Diseases associated with defects in the indicated enzymes are in blue. Note that as indicated, many lysosomal storage diseases (eg, Tay-Sachs) resulting from defective enzymes that metabolize both glycolipids and glycoproteins are defined by one or the other defective pathway (see Chapter 21 for more information).

TABLE 38-6: Disorders Resulting From Defects in Glycoprotein Degradation

Disease	*Enzyme Deficiency*	*Symptoms*
Aspartylglucosaminuria	Aspartylglycosaminidase (*N*-aspartyl-β-glucosaminidase)	Hallmark symptom is a global delay in psychomotor development that begins between 2 and 4 years of age, progressive severe mental retardation, delayed speech and motor development, coarse facial features
α-Mannosidosis	α-Mannosidase	Type I disease is more severe and is the infantile disease presenting between 3 and 12 months of age, rapid mental deterioration and pronounced hepatosplenomegaly lead to fatality between 3 and 8 years of age; Type II disease is the juvenile form; both types of disease exhibit mental retardation, coarse facial features, corneal opacities, enlarged skull, thickened calvarium, premature closure of lamboid and sagittal sutures, shallow orbits, anterior hypoplasia of the lumbar vertebrae, poorly formed pelvis, short clavicles; analysis for the presence of vacuolated lymphocytes is a useful diagnostic finding in α-mannosidosis patients
β-Mannosidosis	β-Mannosidase	Mental retardation, hearing loss, and respiratory infections, no corneal opacities, hepatosplenomegaly, or skeletal defects, definitive diagnosis by the measurement of β-mannosidase activity in leukocytes or fibroblasts
G_{M1} Gangliosidosis	β-Galactosidase	Type 1: arrest or delay in developmental milestones beginning between 3 and 6 months of age, severe psycho-motor retardation, frequent seizures, skeletal dysplasia, large low-set ears and hair on the forehead, death within a few years of onset; Type 2: symptoms as seen in type 1 disease absent or greatly reduced in severity, progressive deterioration occurring between 12 and 18 months; Type 3: symptoms not generally evident until at least 3 years of age but often not until the second decade, dystonia is the major neurological finding
Sandhoff disease	β-Hexosaminidases A and B	Infantile forms of Sandhoff disease indistinguishable from Tay-Sachs disease (Clinical Box 21-4), discrimination accomplished by enzyme assay
Sialidosis (also identified as mucolipidosis I)	Neuraminidase (sialidase)	Type I: walking difficulties and/or the loss of visual acuity; Type II: more severe and presents much earlier than type I; divided into congenital, infantile, and juvenile forms; congenital form is evident in utero, infantile form manifests between birth and 12 months of age, juvenile form manifests after 2 years of age, congenital form associated with hydrops fetalis and afflicted fetuses are stillborn, all patients with type II will develop a progressive severe phenotype including mental retardation and a constellation of skeletal abnormalities
Fucosidosis	α-Fucosidase	Type I: more severe infantile form, manifests between 3 and 1 8 months of age; Type II: milder form, manifests between 1 and 2 years of age, both forms are associated with mental retardation and coarse facial features, the major clinical symptom that distinguishes type II from type I is the presence of angiokeratoma corporis diffusum (hyperkeratinized deep red to blue-black skin lesions)

TABLE 38-7: Lectin Families and Their Carbohydrate Specificities

Lectin Family	*Characteristics*	*Binding Specificity*
C-type (7 subfamilies)	Require Ca^{2+} for activity	Variable
Collectins (C-type subfamily III)	C-type CRD with collagen-like domains	Variable, mannose
Galectins (S-type lectins)	Sulfhydryl-dependent or β-galactosidase binding	Strict for β-galactosides
Siglecs (I-type lectins)	Contain immunoglobulin-like domains	Sialic acid
Phosphomannosyl receptors (P-type lectins)	Recognize mannose 6-phosphate	Mannose 6-phosphate
Pentraxins	Quaternary structure composed of 5 identical polypeptides that form a ring with a central hole	Variable and can be noncarbohydrate
Calnexin and calreticulin	Recognition of properly folded glycoproteins in the ER	Glucose
Ficolins	Contain fibrinogen-like homology domain	Variable
Tachylectins	Distinct CRD but also contain fibrinogen-like domain	GlcNAc/GalNAc

more commonly referred to as the *galectins*. The galectins are all defined by a canonical CRD having an affinity for β-galactosides.

Galectin-1 is a potent inhibitor of activated T cell–mediated inflammatory responses. Using experimentally induced models of several autoimmune disorders (eg, myasthenia gravis, multiple sclerosis, and rheumatoid arthritis), it has been shown that administration of recombinant galectin-1 can significantly ameliorate the resultant clinical symptoms. Conversely, the presence of autoantibodies to galectin-1 has been identified in several neurodegenerative disorders.

Galectin-3 exhibits antiapoptotic effects in the same cell types in which galectin-1 promotes apoptosis. In addition, the levels of autoantibodies to galectin-3 are inversely associated with severity of Crohn disease (inflammatory bowel disease, IBD).

Congenital Disorders of Glycosylation

Congenital disorders of glycosylation (CDG) represent a constellation of diseases that result from defects in the synthesis of carbohydrate structures (glycans) and in the attachment of glycans to other compounds. These defective processes involve the *N*-linked and *O*-linked glycosylation pathways, GPI-linkage, biosynthesis of proteoglycans, and lipid glycosylation pathways.

The CDG encompassing *N*-glycosylation defects are clustered into 2 broad categories (Table 38-8). Group I CDG diseases are characterized by alterations/deficiencies in the synthesis and/or transfer of the lipid-linked oligosaccharide (LLO) to Asn residues in substrate proteins. Group II CDG diseases are characterized as those that result from defects in subsequent *N*-linked glycan processing.

High-Yield Concept

One of the most crucial functions of the galectins is in regulation of the inflammatory response. Galectin-1 is expressed by antigen-stimulated T cells, activated B cells, and by macrophages. The action of galectin-1 in these systems is to stimulate apoptosis resulting in cell death. Negative growth effects of galectin-1 are also seen in breast and prostate cancer cell lines.

TABLE 38-8: Congenital Disorders of Glycosylation Involving Defective *N*-Glycosylation

CDG: Original Name (proposed name)	*Affected Enzyme (gene symbol)*	*Major Symptoms*
CDG-Ia (PMM2-CDG)	Phosphomannomutase 2 (*PMM2*)	Psychomotor retardation, cerebellar hypoplasia, ataxia, axial hypotonia, strabismus, skeletal abnormalities, vomiting, anorexia, diarrhea
CDG-Ib (MPI-CDG)	Phosphomannose isomerase (*MPI*)	Protein-losing enteropathy (PLE), diarrhea, cyclical vomiting, hepatomegaly, coagulopathy, hypoglycemia
CDG-Ic (ALG6-CDG)	Glucosyltransferase I (*ALG6*)	Frequent seizures, mild psychomotor, pronounced axial hypotonia, strabismus, frequent intestinal viral infections
CDG-Id (ALG3-CDG)	Mannosyltransferase VI (*ALG4*)	Profound psychomotor retardation, intractable seizures, eye abnormalities, optic atrophy, postnatal microcephaly, hypsarrhythmia
CDG-Ie (DPM1-CDG)	Catalytic subunit of Dol-P-Man synthase I (*DPM1*)	Profound psychomotor retardation, intractable seizures, hypotonia, eye abnormalities, cortical blindness, failure to thrive
CDG-If (MPDU1-CDG)	Protein responsible for utilization of Dol-P-Man independent of DPM1 (*MPDU1*)	Dwarfism, hypotonia, frequent seizures, severe psychomotor retardation, cerebral atrophy
CDG-Ig (ALG12-CDG)	Mannosyltransferase VIII (*ALG12*)	Psychomotor retardation, facial dysmorphy, hypotonia, feeding problems, microcephaly, convulsions, frequent respiratory tract infections
CDG-Ih (ALG8-CDG)	Glucosyltransferase II (*ALG8*)	Moderate hepatomegaly, PLE, hypotonia, lung hypoplasia, anemia, thrombocytopenia
CDG-Ii (ALG2-CDG)	Mannosyltransferase II (*ALG2*)	Severe psychomotor retardation, spasms, hypsarrhythmia, irregular nystagmus
CDG-Ij (DPAGT1-CDG)	UDP-GlcNAc: Dol-P-GlcNAc-P phosphotransferase (*DPAGT1*)	Intractable spasms, hypotonia, sever psychomotor retardation, microcephaly, micrognathia, esotropia
CDG-Ik (ALG1-CDG)	Mannosyltransferase I (*ALG1*)	Seizures, severe psychomotor retardation, hypotonia, dysmorphy, microcephaly, liver dysfunction, severe infections, coagulation defects, early mortality
CDG-IL (ALG9-CDG)	Mannosyltransferase VII-IX (*ALG9*)	Psychomotor retardation, hypotonia, hepatomegaly, microcephaly, seizures
CDG-IIa (MGAT2-CDG)	UDP-*N*-acetylglucosamine:α-6-D-mannoside-β-1,2-*N*-acetylglucosaminyltransferase II (*MGAT2*)	Severe psychomotor retardation, hypotonia, coarse facial features, frequent infections; true incidence of human *MGAT2* defects may go undetected due to spontaneous fetal abortion or death shortly after birth
CDG-IIb (GCS1-CDG)	Glucosidase I (GCS1)	Dysmorphia, seizures, hypotonia, hepatomegaly, feeding difficulty
CDG-IIc (SLC35C1-CDG)	GDP-fucose transporter encoded by the *FUCT1* gene	Clinical Box: 38-2
CDG-IId (B4GALT1-CDG)	β-1,4-Galactosyltransferase (*B4GALT1*)	Psychomotor retardation, severe spontaneous bleeding, hydrocephalus, myopathy
CDG-IIe (COG7-CDG)	Oligomeric Golgi complex-7 subunit (*COG7*)	Growth retardation, progressive severe microcephaly, hypotonia, adducted thumbs, gastrointestinal pseudo-obstruction, failure to thrive, cardiac anomalies, wrinkled skin, episodes of extreme hyperthermia
CDG-IIf (SLC35A1-CDG)	CMP-sialic acid transporter (*SLC35A1*)	Marked thrombocytopenia and neutropenia, recurrent infections

CLINICAL BOX 38-2: LEUKOCYTE ADHESION DEFICIENCY SYNDROME II, LAD II

Congenital disorder of glycosylation IIc is more commonly referred to as *leukocyte adhesion deficiency syndrome II (LAD II)*. LAD II belongs to the class of disorders referred to as primary immunodeficiency syndromes as the symptoms of the disease manifest due to defects in leukocyte function. Symptoms of LAD II are characterized by unique facial features, recurrent infections, persistent leukocytosis, defective neutrophil chemotaxis, and severe growth and mental retardation. The genetic defect resulting in LAD II is in the pathway of fucose utilization leading to loss of fucosylated glycans on the cell surface. An additional feature of LAD II is that individuals harbor the rare Bombay (hh) blood type at the ABO locus as well as lack the Lewis blood group antigens. The Bombay blood type is characterized by a deficiency in the H (referred to as the O-type), A, and B antigens due to loss of the fucose residue. Each of these blood group antigens contains a Fuc-α-1,2-Gal modification that is the final carbohydrate addition to these antigens. These fucosylation reactions are catalyzed by α-1,2-fucosyltransferase, which is encoded by the *H* and *Se* loci (the *Se* locus is the secretor locus). The defective neutrophil chemotaxis is due to the loss of a specific ligand on these cells that is recognized by the selectins. This ligand is the sialylated Lewis X antigen. The recurrent infections seen in LAD II patients are the result of the defective neutrophil function. Neutrophils are involved in innate immunity responses to bacterial infection. To carry out their role in host defense mechanisms, neutrophils must adhere to the surface of the endothelium at the site of inflammation, which is an event mediated by cell surface adhesion molecules. Once neutrophils adhere to and roll along the surface of the endothelium, the integrin family of adhesion molecules allow for firm adherence followed by tissue penetration. The pathways to GDP-fucose synthesis or utilization by the fucosyltransferases in the Golgi are deficient in LAD II. The major defect causing LAD II is an impairment in the transport of GDP-fucose into the Golgi catalyzed by the GDP-fucose transporter, encoded by the *FUCT1* gene (also identified as solute carrier family 35, member C1: SCL35C1).

REVIEW QUESTIONS

1. I-cell disease (also identified as mucolipidosis type II) is characterized by the presence of inclusion bodies in fibroblasts (hence the derivation of the term I-cell), severe psychomotor retardation, corneal clouding, and dysostosis multiplex. These symptoms arise from a defect in the targeting of lysosomal enzymes due to an inability to carry out which of the following processes?

A. produce mannose-6-phosphate modifications in lysosomal enzymes
B. recycle the lysosomal receptor for mannose 6-phosphate present on lysosomal enzymes
C. remove mannose 6-phosphates from lysosomal enzymes prior to their transport to the lysosomes
D. synthesize the mannose 6-phosphate receptor found in lysosomes
E. transport mannose-6-phosphate receptors to lysosomes

Answer A: Enzymes that are destined for the lysosomes (lysosomal enzymes) are directed there by a specific carbohydrate modification. During transit through the Golgi apparatus, a residue of GlcNAc-1-phosphate (GlcNAc-1-P) is added to the carbon-6 hydroxyl group of one or more specific mannose residues that have been added to these enzymes. A specific Man-6-P receptor (MPR) is present in the membranes of the Golgi apparatus. Binding of Man-6-P to this receptor targets proteins to the lysosomes.

2. You are treating an 8-month-old female infant brought in by her parents because of seizures. Physical examination indicates microcephaly, microphthalmia with retinal detachment. and severe mental retardation. You suspect these symptoms are associated with a specific gene defect and order a test for the presence of mutations in α-dystroglycan. Test results are positive. A defect in which of the following, related to α-dystroglycan processing, is most likely in this patient?

A. *N*-glycosylation
B. *O*-GlcNAcylation
C. *O*-glycosylation mucin type
D. *O*-mannosylation

Answer D: *O*-mannosylation has been identified on α-dystroglycan (α-DG) from nerve and muscle, chondroitin sulfate proteoglycans and total glycopeptides from brain tissue. Clinically, *O*-mannosylation of α-DG is the most significant as evidenced by the constellation of symptoms that result from defects in the processes of *O*-mannosylation. Defective *O*-mannosylation is associated with a group of autosomal recessive muscular dystrophies termed congenital muscular dystrophies (CMDs). In addition to muscle dysfunction, these CMDs are also associated with variable brain and ocular abnormalities.

3. You are studying the responses of adipocytes in culture to insulin following addition of a test compound. In the absence of the compound, addition of insulin to your culture system results in increased glucose uptake. However, following addition of the test compound, the effects of insulin on glucose uptake are severely impaired. Analysis of components of the insulin-signaling pathway indicates that addition of the compound results in a dramatic increase in *O*-GlcNAcylation. Your test compound is likely to be most highly related to which of the following?

A. CTP
B. glucosamine
C. glucose
D. glucose-6-phosphate
E. UTP

Answer B: Numerous proteins involved in insulin signaling and the downstream targets of these signaling cascades have been shown to be *O*-GlcNAcylated. With respect to insulin receptor signaling proteins, IRS-1, PI3K, PKB/Akt, PDK1, and GSK-3β are all known to be *O*-GlcNAcylated. These modifications have all been observed in adipocytes, which are a major target for the actions of insulin. It is possible for glucosamine to enter the HBP directly by conversion to glucosamine-6-phosphate (GlcN6P) via the action of hexokinase. This reaction bypasses the rate-limiting step of the pathway catalyzed by GFAT and will lead to increased *O*-GlcNAcylation of proteins.

4. You are examining a 2-year-old girl brought in by her parents because they are concerned about her lack of any type of talking and she seems unusually clumsy. History reveals that the child has had numerous upper respiratory infections over the past 6 months. You suspect the child is suffering from a particular form of a lysosomal storage disease. Genetic testing reveals a missense mutation in the *N*-aspartyl-β-glucosaminidase gene. This child is most likely suffering from which of the following defects in glycoprotein metabolism?

A. aspartylglucosaminuria
B. fucosidosis
C. leukocyte adhesion deficiency syndrome II (LAD II)
D. Sandhoff disease
E. sialidosis

Answer A: *Aspartylglucosaminuria* belongs to a family of disorders identified as lysosomal storage diseases. This disorder is characterized by the lysosomal accumulation of glycoasparagines, primarily aspartylglycosamine. These glycoasparagines accumulate in the lysosomes as a consequence of defects in the lysosomal hydrolase, *N*-aspartyl-β-glucosaminidase. The hallmark symptom of aspartylglucosaminuria is a global delay in psychomotor development that begins between 2 and 4 years of age. There is a period of frequent upper respiratory infections followed by delayed speech and physical clumsiness. The disorder in speech development is a cardinal sign of mental retardation and is usually the first indication to parents that there is something amiss with their child.

5. E-selectin is a member of the lectin family of carbohydrate-binding proteins. The cell surface presentation of E-selectin is required for which of the following processes?

A. ability of monocytes to bind and phagocytose cholesterol
B. activation of platelet adhesion to subendothelial extracellular matrix proteins
C. binding of platelets to endothelial cells
D. binding of monocytes to platelets
E. interaction of neutrophils with endothelial cells

Answer E: The selectins are subtype IV C-type lectins defined by the presence of the C-type lectin CRD, an epidermal growth factor-like domain, and a variable number of complement regulatory protein-like repeat domains. The selectins are also members of the cell adhesion family of proteins. Each selectin is tethered to the plasma membrane via a single transmembrane domain. A major function of the selectins is the recruitment of neutrophils to sites of inflammation.

6. Patients with classic paroxysmal nocturnal hemoglobinuria (PNH) have clinical evidence of intravascular hemolysis typified by reticulocytosis, abnormally high concentration of serum lactate dehydrogenase, indirect bilirubin, and abnormally low concentration of serum haptoglobin. These symptoms are due to a lack of being able to carry out which of the following posttranslational modifications?

A. glipiated linkage
B. mannose 6-phosporylation
C. *N*-linked glycosylation
D. *O*-linked glycosylation
E. prenylation

Answer A: Many membrane-associated glycoproteins belong to neither the peripheral nor the transmembrane class. These glycoproteins are tethered to the outer leaflet of the plasma membrane via a glycosylphosphatidylinositol linkage to their *C*-termini. This type of membrane attachment is referred to as a GPI linkage and the glycoproteins are termed glypiated proteins. One clinically important glypiated protein is the glycoprotein present on the surface of erythrocytes, that is, decay-accelerating factor (DAF; also known as CD55 = cluster of differentiation protein 55). The normal function of DAF is to prevent erythrocyte lysis by complement.

7. A 4-year-old boy presents with persistent leukocytosis. Patient history reveals that the boy has suffered from recurrent infections. On physical examination, the physician notes severe growth and mental retardation. An additional feature of this child is that he harbors the rare Bombay (hh) blood type at the ABO locus. These findings are consistent with the child suffering from which of the following disorders?

A. congenital disorder of glycosylation Ia (CDG Ia)
B. I-cell disease
C. leukocyte adhesion deficiency syndrome II (LAD II)
D. pseudo-Hurler polydystrophy
E. Tay-Sachs disease

Answer C: The child is suffering from LAD II, which is a disease that belongs to the class of disorders referred to as primary immunodeficiency syndromes. Symptoms of LAD II are characterized by unique facial features, recurrent infections, persistent leukocytosis, defective neutrophil chemotaxis, and severe growth and mental retardation. The genetic defect resulting in LAD II is in the pathway of fucose utilization leading to loss of fucosylated glycans on the cell surface. An additional feature of LAD II is that individuals harbor the rare Bombay (hh) blood type at the ABO locus as well as lack the Lewis blood group antigens. The recurrent infections seen in LAD II patients are the result of the defective neutrophil function. Neutrophils are involved in innate immunity responses to bacterial infection. To carry out their role in host defense mechanisms, neutrophils must adhere to the surface of the endothelium at the site of inflammation, which is an event mediated by cell surface adhesion molecules. The selectin family (E-, L-, and P-selectins) of animal lectins are necessary to mediate the initial process of neutrophil adherence to the endothelium. The selectins recognize sialylated fucosylated lactosamines typified by the Lewis X antigen.

8. A 6-month-old infant presents with failure to thrive, obvious developmental delay, abnormal skeletal development, coarse facial features, and restricted joint movement. Cellular and biochemical analysis indicates the infant is suffering from a defect in protein modification. These clinical symptoms are most indicative of which of the following disorders?

A. congenital disorder of glycosylation Ia (CDG Ia)
B. I-cell disease
C. leukocyte adhesion deficiency syndrome II (LAD II)
D. pseudo-Hurler polydystrophy
E. Tay-Sachs disease

Answer B: I-cell disease (also called mucolipidosis II α/β, ML-II α/β) is an autosomal recessive disorder that results as a consequence of defective targeting of lysosomal hydrolases to the lysosomes. The disorder is so called because fibroblasts from afflicted patients contain numerous phase-dense inclusion bodies in the cytosol. I-cell disease is characterized by severe psychomotor retardation that rapidly progresses. leading to death between 5 and 8 years of age. I-cell patients exhibit coarse facial features, craniofacial abnormalities, and severe skeletal abnormalities. Additional clinical symptoms of I-cell disease include hepatomegaly, cardiomegaly, umbilical hernias, and recurrent upper respiratory infections.

9. A percentage of the population manifests the ABO blood group antigens in saliva and other mucous secretions and are thus referred to as "secretors," whereas those that do not are termed "nonsecretors." The difference between these 2 populations results from which of the following?

A. ABO antigens present on circulating lipids
B. ABO antigens present on circulating proteins
C. inappropriate activation of the ABO-specific glycosyltransferases in mucus-secreting tissues
D. mild hemolysis that releases cellular ABO antigens
E. presence of a mutant glycosyl hydrolase, which releases the ABO antigens from cell surfaces

Answer B: The ABO blood group antigens are the carbohydrate moieties of glycolipids on the surface of cells as well as the carbohydrate portion of serum glycoproteins. When the ABO carbohydrates are associated with protein in the form of glycoproteins, they are found in the serum and are referred to as the secreted forms. Some individuals produce the glycoprotein forms of the ABO antigens while others do not. This property distinguishes secretors from nonsecretors, a property that has forensic importance such as in cases of rape.

10. The correct targeting of newly synthesized hydrolytic enzymes to the lysosomes requires which of the following modifications?

A. attachment of mannose 6-phosphate to the enzymes
B. γ-Carboxylation of glutamate residues in the enzymes
C. *O*-linkage of carbohydrate to the enzymes
D. prenylation of the enzymes
E. proteolytic activation following transport to the lysosome

Answer A: Enzymes that are destined for the lysosomes (lysosomal enzymes) are directed there by a specific carbohydrate modification. During transit through the Golgi apparatus, a residue of GlcNAc-1-phosphate (GlcNAc-1-P) is added to the carbon-6 hydroxyl group of one or more specific mannose residues that have been added to these enzymes. A specific Man-6-P receptor (MPR) is present in the membranes of the Golgi apparatus. Binding of Man-6-P to this receptor targets proteins to the lysosomes.

11. You are examining a 2-year-old child who has begun having trouble walking and stumbles and falls frequently. Additional manifesting symptoms are developmental delay, muscle weakness, and speech and vision impairment. Muscle biopsy results indicate the patient has a deficiency in functional α-dystroglycan. The clinical signs in this patient would most likely be associated with a defect in which of the following pathway?

A. addition of sialic acid residues to α-dystroglycan
B. *O*-mannosylation of α-dystroglycan
C. processing of the lipid-linked oligosaccharide used in *N*-glycosylation of α-dystroglycan
D. regulation of the hexosamine biosynthesis pathway such that α-dystroglycan is abnormally *O*-GlcNAcylated
E. synthesis of *O*-linked hydroxylysine residues in collagens associated with α-dystroglycan

Answer B: *O*-mannosylation has been identified on α-dystroglycan (α-DG) from nerve and muscle, chondroitin sulfate proteoglycans, and total glycopeptides from brain tissue. Clinically, *O*-mannosylation of α-DG is the most significant as evidenced by the constellation of symptoms that result from defects in the processes of *O*-mannosylation. Defective *O*-mannosylation is associated with a group of autosomal recessive muscular dystrophies termed congenital muscular dystrophies (CMDs). In addition to muscle dysfunction, these CMDs are also associated with variable brain and ocular abnormalities.

12. Which of the following carbohydrate-modified molecules are enriched in the viscous gel that lines the pulmonary airways?

A. GlcNAcylated glycoproteins
B. glycosphingolipids
C. *N*-linked glycoproteins
D. *O*-linked glycoproteins
E. *O*-mannosylated glycoproteins

Answer D: *O*-linked glycans are important for protein stability, modulation of enzyme activity, receptor-mediated signaling, immune function and immunity, protein-protein interactions, as well as many other functions. Mucin-type *O*-glycans are also important for binding water and are often found on the outer surfaces of tissues such as the gastrointestinal, urogenital, and respiratory systems. The interaction of water with the mucin-type *O*-glycans results in the formation of a viscous solution or gel that forms a protective barrier harboring antibacterial properties.

13. The hexosamine biosynthesis pathway (HBP) is regulated at the level of the reaction catalyzed by glutamine:fructose-6-phosphate aminotransferase 1 (GFAT). However, excess availability of which of the following can lead to unregulated *O*-GlcNAc synthesis?

A. fructose 1-phosphate
B. glucosamine
C. glucose
D. glucose 6-phosphate
E. glutamine

Answer B: It is possible for glucosamine to enter the HBP directly by conversion to glucosamine 6-phosphate (GlcN6P) via the action of hexokinase. This reaction bypasses the rate-limiting step of the pathway catalyzed by GFAT.

14. You are studying the consequences of carbohydrate modification of proteins in hepatocyte cultures. Your studies reveal that addition of high levels of glucose to the culture system results in modification and activation of the transcription factor PGC-1α, leading to an increased rate of gluconeogenesis. Which of the following is the most likely modification that results in the observed activation of PGC-1α?

A. *N*-glycosylation
B. *O*-GlcNAcylation
C. *O*-glycosylation mucin type
D. *O*-mannosylation

Answer B: Hyperglycemia is associated with *O*-GlcNAcylation of transcription factors and cofactors such as FOXO1, FOXO3, CREB-regulated transcription coactivator 2 (CRTC2), and PGC-1α that are involved in the modulation of the expression of gluconeogenic genes. PGC-1α is a key transcriptional coactivator that regulates mitochondrial biogenesis as well as hepatic gluconeogenesis. Under euglycemic conditions, *O*-GlcNAc transferase (OGT) activation leads to *O*-GlcNAcylation of PGC-1α and expression of gluconeogenic genes.

15. The lectins are proteins that recognize and bind to specific types of carbohydrate structures displayed on other proteins and/or lipids. Perhaps the most important homeostatic function of the animal lectins is their roles in the regulation of immune responses and autoimmunity. Which of the following classes of lectins have a member that exhibits potent anti-inflammatory effects due to its ability to induce apoptosis in activated T cells?
A. collectins
B. ficolins
C. galectins (S-type lectins)
D. pentraxins
E. siglecs (I-type lectins)

Answer C: The galectins are all defined by a canonical carbohydrate recognition domain (CRD), having an affinity for β-galactosides. One of the most crucial functions of the galectins is in the regulation of the inflammatory response. Galectin-1 is expressed by antigen-stimulated T cells, activated B cells, and macrophages. The action of galectin-1 in these systems is to stimulate apoptosis resulting in cell death. Negative growth effects of galectin-1 are also seen in the breast and prostate cancer cell lines. Although the collectins, ficolins, pentraxins, and siglecs all have roles in modulating immune responses, none have been shown to have the potent apoptosis-inducing effect of galectin-1.

16. You are studying the process of protein glycosylation utilizing cells isolated from a breast cancer tumor. Analysis of the cells reveals that they are incapable of incorporating glucose into glycoproteins. Which of the following is most likely not synthesized, thereby preventing glycosyltransferases from incorporating glucose into the oligosaccharide portion of glycoproteins in these cells
A. AMP 1-glucose
B. CDP 6-glucose
C. glucose 1-phosphate
D. glucose 1,6-bisphosphate
E. UDP 1-glucose

Answer E: The monosaccharides that are attached to proteins (as well as lipids in the formation of glycolipids) are first activated by coupling to a nucleotide. These nucleotide-activated sugars are derived from dietary sources and salvage pathways. Nucleotide-activated glucose is found as UDP-1-glucose synthesized via the activity of UDP-glucose pyrophosphorylase.

17. Which of the following features of the carbohydrate portion of glycoproteins determines their uptake into lysosomes?
A. multiple galactose residues
B. *N*-acetylneuraminic acid residues
C. *O*-linked oligosaccharides
D. terminal fucose residues
E. terminal mannose 6-phosphate residues

Answer E: Enzymes that are destined for the lysosomes (lysosomal enzymes) are directed there by a specific carbohydrate modification. During transit through the Golgi apparatus, a residue of GlcNAc-1-phosphate (GlcNAc-1-P) is added to the carbon-6 hydroxyl group of 1 or more specific mannose residues that have been added to these enzymes. A specific Man-6-P receptor (MPR) is present in the membranes of the Golgi apparatus. Binding of Man-6-P to this receptor targets proteins to the lysosomes.

18. An oligosaccharide unit is transferred from dolichol pyrophosphate to an asparagine moiety of a protein in which of the following structures?
A. endosomes
B. lysosomes
C. mitochondria
D. nuclei
E. rough endoplasmic reticulum

Answer E: The formation of *N*-linked glycoproteins occurs in the endoplasmic reticulum (ER) through cotranslational addition of a preassembled carbohydrate core structure that is delivered via the carbohydrate-dolichol lipid intermediate. The preassembled carbohydrate core structure comprises 3 terminal residues of glucose attached to a branched cluster of 9 mannose residues that are in turn attached to 2 GlcNAc residues attached to dolichol pyrophosphate.

19. A 6-month-old boy is brought to his pediatrician by his mother for a follow-up examination. When born, the infant had a low birth weight, coarse facial features, and restricted motion of the extremities. Serum and urine analysis at this time indicated the presence of lysosomal enzyme activity. Physical examination today shows psychomotor retardation and hepatomegaly. A biopsy of skin is taken and analysis of the fibroblasts indicates that they contain multiple intracellular cytoplasmic inclusions. A deficiency in which of the following

posttranslational modifications is most likely present in this infant?
A. acetylation of galactosamine
B. acetylation of glucosamine
C. phosphorylation of galactose
D. phosphorylation of mannose
E. phosphorylation of sialic acid

Answer D: Enzymes that are destined for the lysosomes (lysosomal enzymes) are directed there by the presence of mannose-6-phosphate residues in these enzymes. A specific Man-6-P receptor (MPR) is present in the membranes of the Golgi apparatus. Binding of Man-6-P to this receptor targets proteins to the lysosomes. Lack of this modification results in increased levels of lysosomal enzymes in the blood and urine.

20. You are studying the processes of glycoprotein synthesis using a cell culture system. Your experiments are focused on the attachment of oligosaccharides to asparagine residues in proteins as they transit the ER. Your experiments detect that the cells you are using are incapable of the initial transfer of nucleotide-activated sugars. Given these results, which of the following is most likely deficient in these cells?
A. arachidonic acid
B. asparagine
C. dolichol pyrophosphate
D. glucose 6-phosphate
E. serine

Answer C: The formation of *N*-linked glycoproteins occurs in the endoplasmic reticulum (ER) through cotranslational addition of a preassembled carbohydrate core structure that is delivered via the carbohydrate-dolichol lipid intermediate. The preassembled carbohydrate core structure comprises 3 terminal residues of glucose attached to a branched cluster of 9 mannose residues that are in turn attached to 2 GlcNAc residues attached to dolichol pyrophosphate. Lack of dolichol pyrophosphate would prevent the ability to incorporate oligosaccharides onto appropriate asparagine residues in normally *N*-linked glycoproteins.

Checklist

✓ Glycoproteins represent a diverse family of widely distributed proteins that contain from one to many covalently linked carbohydrate structures. Essentially all plasma proteins, secreted proteins, and membrane-attached proteins are modified with carbohydrate attachment.

✓ Approximately 50% of all human proteins are known to be glycosylated and at least 1% of the human genome is represented by genes involved in glycan processing.

✓ There are 2 broad categories of glycoprotein: those that have carbohydrate attached to asparagine residues (*N*-linked glycoproteins) and those with carbohydrate attached to the hydroxyl of serine, threonine, or hydroxylysine (*O*-linked glycoproteins).

✓ Glycoproteins are synthesized as they transit the endoplasmic reticulum (ER) and the Golgi apparatus.

✓ Sugars attached to glycoproteins are all activated by nucleotide addition prior to incorporation into proteins via the actions of a family of glycosyltransferases.

✓ Glycosidases are responsible for removal of carbohydrates and are involved in the remodeling of the sugar composition of glycoproteins.

✓ Synthesis of *N*-linked glycoproteins involves the initial attachment of a core glycan structure to the lipid dolichol pyrophosphate, followed by transfer to the acceptor protein.

✓ *N*-linked glycoproteins are represented by 3 distinct families termed high mannose, complex, and hybrid each of which is determined by the glycan composition of the functional protein.

- ✓ Most lysosomal hydrolases are modified with mannose 6-phosphate, which is recognized by a specific receptor in the membranes of the lysosome. Defective production of this modification results in defective lysosome function, resulting in a family of disorders termed lysosomal storage disease, many of which have devastating clinical consequences.
- ✓ Synthesis of *O*-linked glycoproteins involves direct attachment of the sugar from a nucleotide-activated intermediate through the action of glycosyltransferases.
- ✓ The most common family of *O*-linked glycoproteins is the mucins. These high molecular weight, heavily glycosylated proteins form gels that lubricate and form chemical barriers on the surfaces of epithelial cells in the gastrointestinal, respiratory, and reproductive systems.
- ✓ *O*-mannosylation is a specialized form of *O*-linkage that is clinically most significant with respect to modification of α-dystroglycan, as evidenced by the fact that the major symptoms associated with defects in *O*-mannosylation are reflective of α-dystroglcan dysfuntion.
- ✓ The hexosamine biosynthesis pathway is responsible for the synthesis of *O*-GlcNAc, which is an important glycan modification of cytoplasmic and nuclear proteins. Numerous proteins involved in the regulation of insulin function and glucose homeostasis are *O*-GlcNAcylated. Defects in regulation of *O*-GlcNAcylation can lead to insulin resistance with consequent disruption in glucose homeostasis.
- ✓ A number of important proteins are tethered to the plasma membrane via a unique glycan attachment to membrane phospholipid: a glycophosphatidylinositol (GPI) linkage. These proteins are termed *glipiated proteins*.
- ✓ Many viruses and pathogens gain entry into human cells by recognition of the carbohydrate structures on membrane proteins.
- ✓ Lectins are a family of proteins that all contain a carbohydrate recognition domain.
- ✓ Inherited deficiencies in many of the enzymes responsible for *N*-linkage and *O*-linkage can result in clinically severe disorders. This family of diseases is called the congenital disorders of glycosylation, CDG. Leukocyte adhesion deficiency syndrome II (LAD II) is a primary immunodeficiency resulting from a defect in fucosylation of critical proteins involved in immune homeostasis.

CHAPTER

39 Extracellular Matrix: Glycosaminoglycans and Proteoglycans

CHAPTER OUTLINE

High-Yield Terms

Basement membrane: a thin sheet of fibers that underlies the epithelium, which lines the cavities and surfaces of organs including skin, or the endothelium lining the interior surface of blood vessels

Basal lamina: one of the layers of the basement membrane

Ground substance: the noncellular components of the extracellular matrix (ECM) composed of a complex mixture of glycosaminoglycans (GAGs), proteoglycans, and glycoproteins

Glycosaminoglycan: a family of large polymers containing a repeat disaccharide structure, most often attached to a core protein forming a proteoglycan

Mucopolysaccharidosis: any of a large family of inherited diseases that result from defects in lysosomal hydrolases responsible for the degradation of GAGs

The Extracellular Matrix

A substantial portion of the volume of tissues is extracellular space, which is largely filled by an intricate network of macromolecules constituting ECM. The ECM is composed of 2 major classes of biomolecules: glycosaminoglycans (GAGs), most often covalently linked to protein forming the proteoglycans, and fibrous proteins which include collagen, elastin, fibronectin, and laminin. These components are secreted locally and assembled into the organized meshwork that is the ECM.

Connective tissue (Figure 39-1) refers to the matrix composed of the ECM, cells (primarily fibroblasts), and **ground substance** that is tasked with holding other tissues and cells together forming the organs. Ground substance is a complex mixture of GAGs, proteoglycans, and glycoproteins (primarily laminin and fibronectin), but generally does not include the collagens. In most connective tissues, the matrix constituents are secreted principally by fibroblasts, but in certain specialized types of connective tissues, such as cartilage and bone, these components are secreted by chondroblasts and osteoblasts, respectively.

Collagens

Collagens, the major protein comprising the ECM, were introduced in Chapter 5. There are at least 30 different collagen genes dispersed through the human genome (Table 39-1). These 30 genes generate proteins that combine in a variety of ways to create over 28 different types of collagen fibrils. Types I, II, and III collagens are the most abundant, accounting for nearly 90% of all the collagen in the body. Type IV collagen forms a 2-dimensional reticulum and is a major component of the basal lamina. Collagens are predominantly synthesized by fibroblasts but epithelial cells also synthesize these proteins. Given the abundance and complexity of the collagens it is not surprising that a number on inherited disorders in connective tissue result from defects in any of the collagen genes. The Ehlers-Danlos syndromes (EDS) and the various types of osteogenesis imperfect (OI) are the most common forms of connective tissue disorders resulting from defective collagen genes (see Clinical Box 5-1).

The nomenclature for collagens involves the chain composition and the numbering of the collagen gene encoding that particular α-chain. For example,

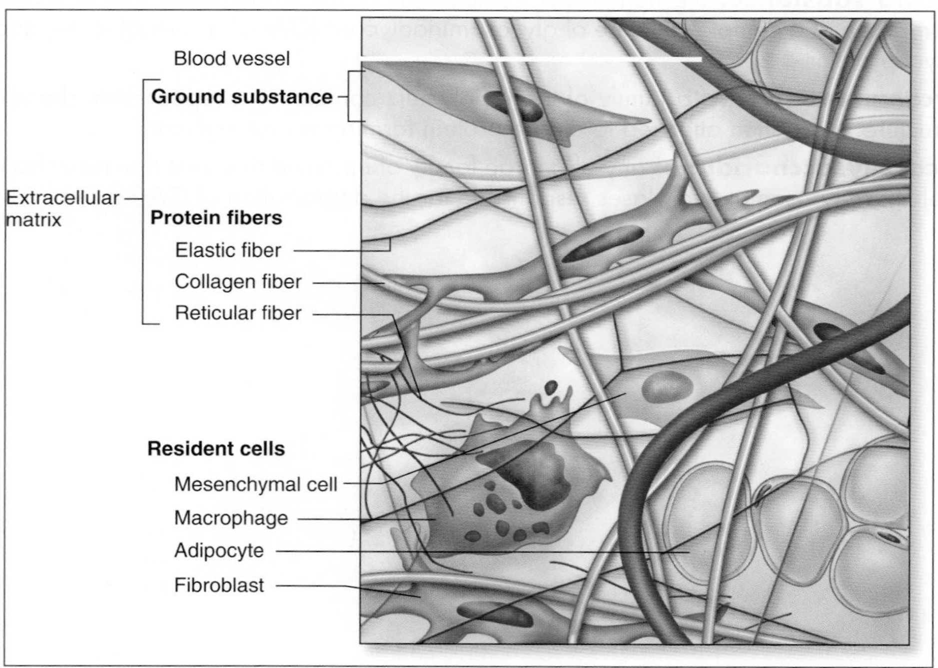

FIGURE 39-1: Components of typical connective tissue. In addition to the extracellular matrix, typical connective tissues contain cells (primarily fibroblasts) all of which is surrounded by ground substance. Mescher AL. *Junqueira's Basic Histology Text and Atlas*. 13th ed. New York: McGraw-Hill; 2013.

High-Yield Concept

The ECM is not only critical for connecting cells together to form the tissue, but it is also a substrate upon which cell migration is guided during the process of wound healing as well as during embryonic development. In addition, the ECM is responsible for the relay of environmental signals to the cell surface.

type I collagen proteins are encoded by the *COL1A1* and *COL1A2* genes with 2 of the triple helix proteins encoded by one gene and 1 by the other. Therefore, type I collagen fibrils are denoted $[\alpha1(I)]_2[\alpha(I)]$, where the Roman numeral designates the fibril as type I.

The fundamental higher-order structure of collagens is a long and thin-diameter rod-like protein (Figure 39-2). Type I collagen, for instance, is 300-nm long, 1.5-nm in diameter, and consists of 3 coiled subunits composed of two α1(I) chains and one α2(I) chain. Each chain consists of 1050 amino acids wound around each other in a characteristic right-handed triple helix. Collagen proteins are rich in glycine, proline, and lysine, with many of the proline and lysine R-groups being modified. A characteristic feature of collagens is the spacing of glycine residues within the triple helical portion of the protein. There is a repeating sequence containing the glycine, denoted as $(Gly\text{-}X\text{-}Y)_n$ where *X* and *Y* can be any amino acid but many of the *X* position amino acids are proline and many of the *Y* positions are hydroxyproline.

TABLE 39-1: Composition and Characteristics of Various Collagen Fibers

Type	*Chain Composition*	*Gene Symbol(s)*	*Structural Details*	*Localization*
I	$[\alpha1(I)]_2[\alpha(I)]$	*COL1A1*, *COL1A2*	300-nm, 67-nm banded fibrils	Skin, tendon, bone, etc
II	$[\alpha1(II)]_3$	*COL2A1*	300-nm, small 67-nm fibrils	Cartilage, vitreous humor
III	$[\alpha1(III)]_3$	*COL3A1*	300-nm, small 67-nm fibrils	Skin, muscle, frequently with type I
IV	$[\alpha1(IV)]_2[\alpha2(IV)]$	*COL4A1* thru *COL4A6*	390-nm *C*-term globular domain, nonfibrillar	All basal lamina
V	$[\alpha1(V)][\alpha2(V)][\alpha3(V)]$	*COL5A1*, *COL5A2*, *COL5A3*	390-nm *N*-term globular domain, small fibers	Most interstitial tissue, associates with type I
VI	$[\alpha1(VI)][\alpha2(VI)][\alpha3(VI)]$	*COL6A1*, *COL6A2*, *COL6A3*	150-nm, *N*- and *C*-terminal globular domains, microfibrils, 100-nm banded fibrils	Most interstitial tissue, associates with type I
VII	$[\alpha1(VII)]_3$	*COL7A1*	450-nm, dimer	Epithelia
VIII	$[\alpha1(VIII)]_3$	*COL8A1*, *COL8A2*		Some endothelial cells
IX	$[\alpha1(IX)][\alpha2(IX)][\alpha3(IX)]$	*COL9A1*, *COL9A2*, *COL9A3*	200-nm, *N*-term, globular domain, bound proteoglycan	Cartilage, associates with type II
X	$[\alpha1(X)]_3$	*COL10A1*	150-nm, *C*-term, globular domain	Hypertrophic and mineralizing cartilage
XI	$[\alpha1(XI)][\alpha2(XI)][\alpha3(XI)]$	*COL11A1*, *COL11A2*	300-nm, small fibers	Cartilage
XII	α1(XII)	*COL12A1*		Interacts with types I and III

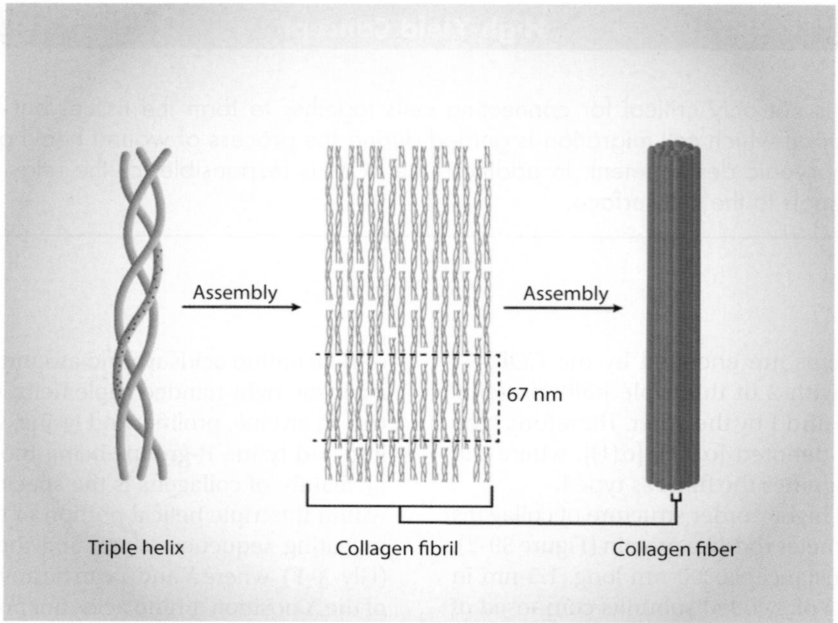

FIGURE 39-2: Higher-order structural features of a typical collagen fibril. Each individual polypeptide chain is twisted into a left-handed triple helix comprising the Gly-X-Y residues. The triple helical structure of processed collagen is formed by right-handed coiling of 3 polypeptides into a superhelix. Reproduced with permission of themedicalbiochemistrypage, LLC.

All collagens are synthesized as longer precursor alpha (α) proteins called procollagens (Figure 39-3). Type I procollagen contains an additional 150 amino acids at the *N*-terminus and 250 at the *C*-terminus. These prodomains are globular and form multiple intrachain disulfide bonds. The disulfides stabilize the proprotein allowing the triple helical section to form. Collagen fibers begin to assemble in the ER and Golgi complexes. The signal sequence is removed and numerous modifications take place in the collagen chains. Specific proline residues are hydroxylated by prolyl 4-hydroxylase and prolyl 3-hydroxylase. Specific lysine residues also are hydroxylated (hLys) by lysyl hydroxylase. Both prolyl hydroxylases are absolutely dependent upon vitamin C as a cofactor. Glycosylations of the *O*-linked type also occurs on many of the hLys residues during Golgi transit. Following completion of the processing, the procollagens are secreted into the extracellular space where extracellular enzymes remove the prodomains. The collagen molecules then polymerize to form collagen fibrils. Accompanying fibril formation is the oxidation of certain lysine residues by the extracellular enzyme lysyl oxidase forming reactive aldehydes. These reactive aldehydes form specific cross-links between 2 chains, thereby stabilizing the staggered array of the collagens in the fibril.

Overall, the various collagens are grouped according to the major structures formed through subunit interactions. These groupings consist of the fibril-forming, the sheet-forming, and the anchoring (or linking) collagens. For example, type I collagen, the most abundant collagen, is a member of the fibril-forming group and forms large fibrils that constitute the framework for the dermis, tendons, and organ capsules. Although there are 28 known different types of collagen, those that have been best characterized either by structure or by the three main classifications are outlined in Table 39-2.

Elastin and Fibrillin

The ECM of tissues that undergo significant stretching and/or bending contains significant quantities of the protein elastin found in a specialized type of fibril called elastic fibers. Elastic fibers are composed of large masses of cross-linked elastin interspersed with another ECM protein called fibrillin. The walls of large arteries are particularly abundant with elastin (and thus elastic fibers) which allows them to undergo continual deformation and reformation during changes in intravascular pressure. The lungs and the skin are additional organs whose tissues are rich in elastin and elastic fibers.

Elastin is synthesized as the precursor, tropoelastin. Tropoelastin has 2 major types of alternating domains. One domain is hydrophilic and rich in Lys (K) and Ala (A), while the other domain is hydrophobic and rich in Val (V), Pro (P), and Gly (G) where these amino acids are frequently contained in repeats of either VPGVG or VGGVG.

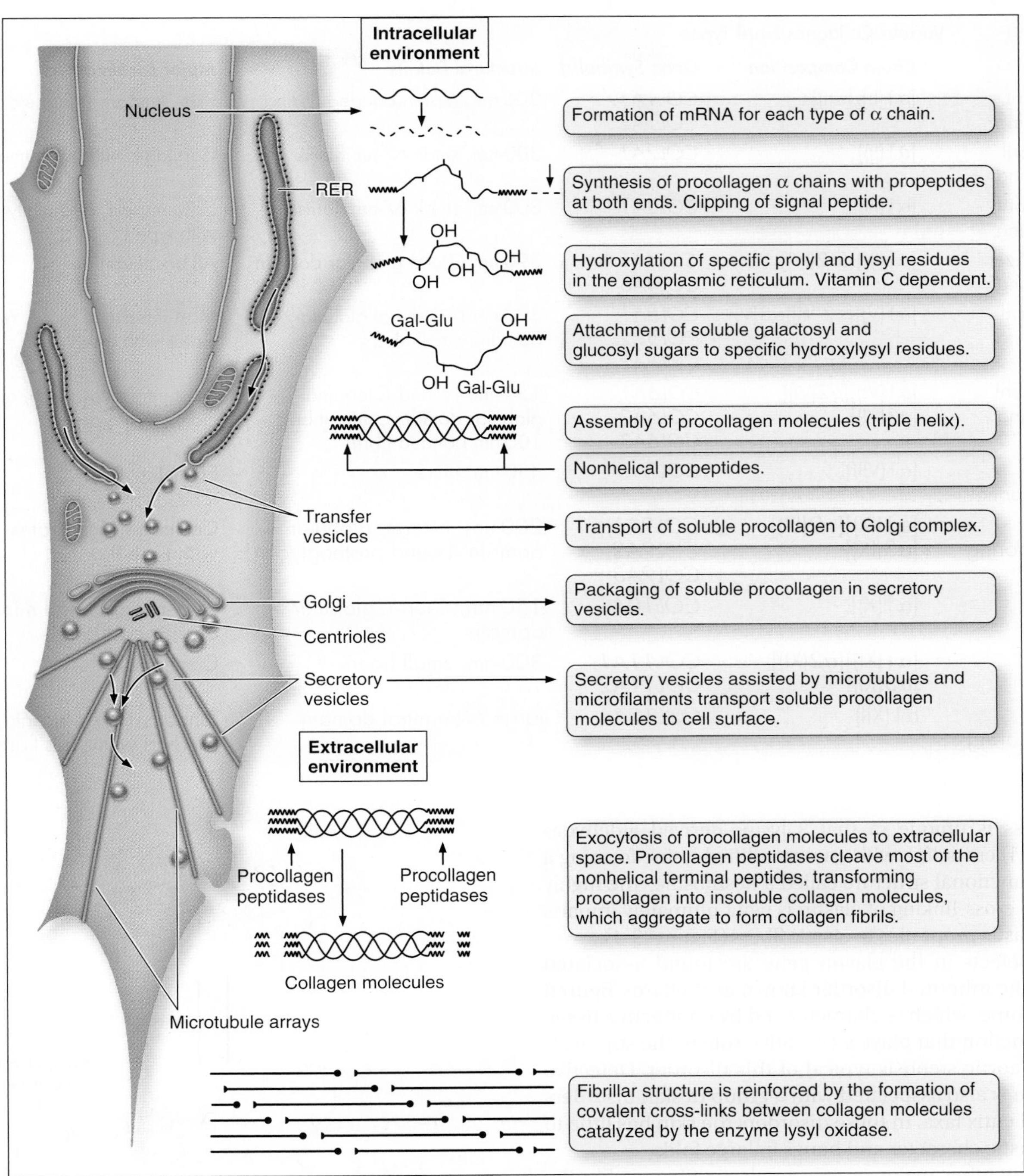

FIGURE 39-3: Synthesis of collagen. Each collagen is composed of a α-chain encoded by 1 of the 30 different α-collagen genes. Synthesis, hydroxylation, and glycosylation of the procollagen protein occurs during transit through the ER. Final assembly into structural fibrils occurs after procollagen is secreted into the ECM. Mescher AL. *Junqueira's Basic Histology Text and Atlas*. 13th ed. New York: McGraw-Hill; 2013.

The hydrophobic domains of elastin are responsible for its elastic character. Tropoelastin is expressed, then secreted as a mature protein into the extracellular matrix and accumulates at the surface of the cell. After secretion and alignment with ECM fibrils, numerous K residues are oxidized by lysyl oxidases, a reaction which initiates cross-linking of elastin monomers. This process of elastin cross-linking, induced by lysyl oxidases, is the same as occurs in the cross-linking of collagens. Although lysyl oxidase activity promotes elastin cross-linking, the

TABLE 39-2: Various Collagens Fibril Types

Type	*Chain Composition*	*Gene Symbol(s)*	*Structural Details*	*Major Localizations*
I: fibril forming	$[\alpha 1(I)]_2[\alpha(I)]$	*COL1A1, COL1A2*	300-nm, 67-nm banded fibrils	Skin, tendon, bone, etc
II: fibril forming	$[\alpha 1(II)]_3$	*COL2A1*	300-nm, small 67-nm fibrils	Cartilage, vitreous humor
III: fibril forming	$[\alpha 1(III)]_3$	*COL3A1*	300-nm, small 67-nm fibrils	Skin, muscle, frequently with type I
IV: sheet forming	$[\alpha 1(IV)_2[\alpha 2(IV)]$	*COL4A1* thru *COL4A6*	390-nm *C*-term globular domain	All basal lamina
V: fibril forming	$[\alpha 1(V)][\alpha 2(V)][\alpha 3(V)]$	*COL5A1, COL5A2, COL5A3*	390-nm *N*-terminal globular domain, small fibers	Most interstitial tissue, associates with type I
VI: fibril forming	$[\alpha 1(VI)][\alpha 2(VI)][\alpha 3(VI)]$	*COL6A1, COL6A2, COL6A3*	150-nm, *N*- and *C*-terminal globular domains, microfibrils, 100-nm banded fibrils	Most interstitial tissue, associates with type I
VII: anchoring	$[\alpha 1(VII)]_3$	*COL7A1*	450-nm, dimer	Epithelia
IX: anchoring	$[\alpha 1(IX)][\alpha 2(IX)][\alpha 3(IX)]$	*COL9A1, COL9A2, COL9A3*	200-nm, *N*-term. globular domain, bound proteoglycan	Cartilage, associates with type II
X	$[\alpha 1(X)]_3$	*COL10A1*	150-nm, *C*-term. globular domain	Hypertrophic and mineralizing cartilage
XI	$[\alpha 1(XI)][\alpha 2(XI)][\alpha 3(XI)]$	*COL11A1, COL11A2*	300-nm, small fibers	Cartilage
XII: anchoring	$\alpha 1(XII)$	*COL12A1*	large *N*-terminal domain	Tendons, skin, placenta, interacts with types I and III

process is unique in that 3 lysine-derived aldehydes (allysyl) cross-link with an unmodified lysine forming a tetrafunctional structure called a desmosine. The highly stable cross-linking of elastin is what ultimately imparts the elastic properties to elastic fibers (Figure 39-4).

Defects in the elastin gene are found associated with the inherited disorder known as Williams-Beuren syndrome, which is characterized by connective tissue dysfunction that plays a causative role in the supravalvular aortic stenosis typical of this disorder. Defective elastin is also associated with a group of skin disorders called cutix laxa. In these disorders the skin has little to no elastic character and hangs in large folds.

The other major protein in elastic fibers is fibrillin 1. Fibrillin 1 serves as the scaffold in elastic fibers upon which cross-linked elastin is **deposited.** Inherited defects in the fibrillin 1 gene result in the connective tissue disorder called Marfan syndrome, MFS (Clinical Box 39-1).

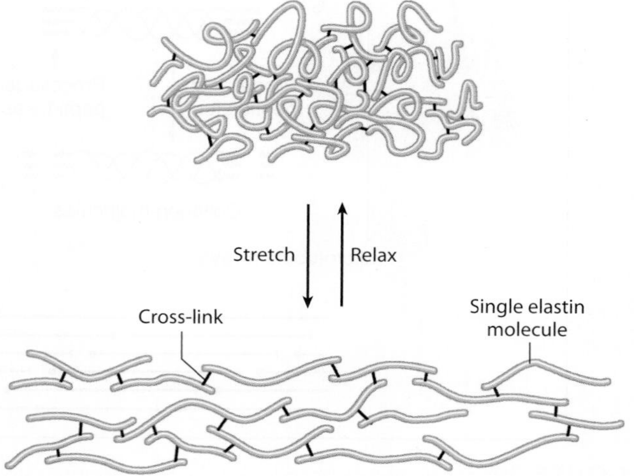

FIGURE 39-4: Molecular basis of elasticity. Subunits of the glycoprotein elastin are joined by covalent bonds formed among lysine residues of different subunits, catalyzed by lysyl oxidase. This produces an extensive and durable cross-linked network of elastin. (Such bonds give rise to the unusual amino acids desmosine and isodesmosine.) Each elastin molecule in the network has multiple random-coil domains which expand and contract; this allows the entire network to stretch and recoil like a rubber band. Mescher AL. *Junqueira's Basic Histology Text and Atlas.* 13th ed. New York: McGraw-Hill; 2013.

Fibronectin

Fibronectin is a major fibrillar glycoprotein of the ECM where its role is to attach cells to a variety of ECM types. Fibronectin is also found in a soluble compact

CLINICAL BOX 39-1: MARFAN SYNDROME

Marfan syndrome (MFS) is an autosomal dominant disorder affecting the connective tissue. The symptoms of MFS are the result of inherited defects in the extracellular matrix glycoprotein fibrillin 1. The fibrillin 1 gene (symbol FBN1) is composed of 65 exons encoding a profibrillin protein of 2871 amino with a processed molecular weight of approximately 350,000 Da. There are 5 distinct structural regions in the fibrillin 1 protein. The largest of these structural regions comprises 75% of the total protein and is composed of 46 EGF-like repeats. These EGF-like repeats are cysteine-rich domains that were first identified in the epidermal growth factor (EGF) protein. Almost all of the EGF-like domains are encoded by individual exons. There are 8 additional cysteine motifs that share homology to a domain first identified in transforming growth factor–β1-binding protein (TGFBR1) called a TB domain. The fibrillin protein has also been shown to bind calcium. In addition to the defects in connective tissue, there are systemic effects in the cardiovascular, musculoskeletal, and ophthalmic systems and the integument in MFS patients. There are certain diagnostic criteria that allow for differentiating MFS from several related disorders such as congenital contractural arachnodactyly, which is caused by mutations in a highly homologous gene identified as *FBN2* encoding the fibrillin 2 protein. The cardinal manifestations of MFS are tall stature with dolichostenomelia (condition of unusually long and thin extremities) and arachnodactyly (abnormally long and slender fingers and toes), joint hypermobility and contracture, deformity of the spine and anterior chest, mitral valve prolapse, dilatation and dissection of the ascending aorta, pneumothorax, and ectopia lentis (displacement of the crystalline lens of the eye). Correct diagnosis of MFS relies on the presence of a combination of manifestations in skeletal, cardiovascular, pulmonary, and ocular organ systems. Individuals with MFS are taller at all ages than would be predicted based on their kinship. The tall stature is the result of overgrowth of the long bones, which leads to the characteristic features of MFS such as disproportionately long legs, arms, and digits. As indicated above, this phenotype is called dolichostenomelia where one diagnostic feature is that the arm span will exceed the body height. The overgrowth of the tubular bones leads to deformity of the anterior chest. This can result in the ribs pushing the ribs either in (pectus excavatum) or out (pectus carinatum) or in on one side and out on the other. The skull is often elongated (termed dolichocephaly), the mandible underdeveloped with the palate narrow and highly arched, and the face is long and narrow. Because of ligament laxity the joints are hypermobile and there is often joint pain. Mitral valve prolapse (MVP) is the most common finding in children with MFS. The prolapse is due to redundancy of the valve tissue, elongation of the valve annulus (valve ring), and elongation of the chordae tendineae (these are the tendons that connect the papillary muscles to the tricuspid and mitral valves). MVP will progress to severe mitral regurgitation which requires surgical intervention usually before 10 years of age. Progressive dilation of the proximal portions of both the aorta and main pulmonary arteries occurs in MFS and are highly important diagnostic and prognostic indicators. The combination of the deformity of the anterior chest and pectus excavatum results in a reduction in lung volume, which can lead to severe restrictive pulmonary deficits. Spontaneous pneumothorax occurs in 4% to 5% of MFS patients. Obstructive sleep apnea is a common symptom in MFS. The ocular hallmark of MFS is displacement of the lens from the center of the pupil (ectopia lentis). Because of the presence of this symptom in a high percentage of MFS patients, displacement of the lens in the absence of any traumatic event should lead to a consideration of MFS. Later in life many MFS patients will suffer from cataracts and/or glaucoma.

nonfunctional form in the blood. The transformation from the compact form to the extended fibrillar form of fibronectin is referred to as fibrillogenesis. This transformation requires the application of mechanical forces generated by cells. This occurs as cells bind and exert forces on fibronectin through transmembrane receptor proteins of the integrin family (Figure 39-5).

Fibronectin attaches cells to all matrices except type IV that involves laminin as the adhesive molecule. Fibronectin is functional as a dimer of 2 similar peptide chains. Each chain is 60 to 70 nm long and 2 to 3 nm thick. At least 20 different fibronectin chains have been identified that arise by alternative RNA splicing of the primary transcript from a single fibronectin gene. Fibronectin consists of a multimodular structure composed predominantly of 3 different repeats termed FN-I, FN-II, and FN-III. Each of the 2 fibronectin subunits consists of 12 FN-I, 2 FN-II, and 15 to 17 FN-III modules, respectively. These functional modules are responsible for fibronectin binding to fibrin, collagen, DNA, and the integrins in plasma membranes. The primary sequence motif of fibronectin that binds to integrin is a tripeptide, Arg-Gly-Asp (RGD).

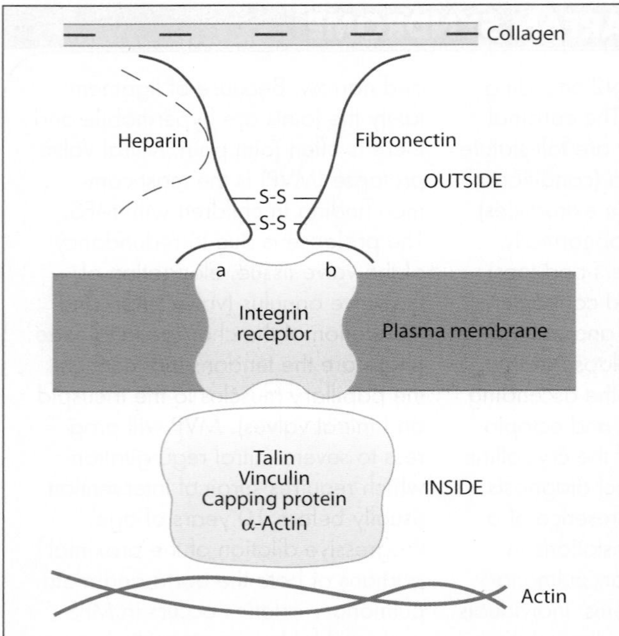

FIGURE 39-5: Representation of fibronectin interaction with an integrin receptor. Extracellular fibronectin interacts with an integrin present in the plasma membrane. The interaction of fibronectin with an integrin triggers activation of intracellular protein complexes that are associated with the actin microfilaments that control cell shape and movement. Murray RK, Bender DA, Botham KM, Kennelly PJ, Rodwell VW, Weil PA. *Harper's Illustrated Biochemistry*. 29th ed. New York: McGraw-Hill; 2012.

Laminin

All basal laminas contain a common set of proteins and GAGs. These are type IV collagen, heparan sulfate proteoglycans (HSPGs), entactin, and glycoproteins of the laminin family. The basal lamina is often referred to as the type IV matrix. Each of the components of the basal lamina is synthesized by the cells that rest upon it. The laminins anchor cell surfaces to the basal lamina.

Laminins are heterotrimeric proteins that contain an α-chain, a β-chain, and a γ-chain. There are 5 genes encoding the α-chains, 4 encoding the β-chains, and 3 encoding the γ-chains. The different laminin proteins have been found to form at least 15 different types of heterotrimers. Laminin heterotrimers are quite large, ranging from under 500,000 to nearly a 1,000,000 Da in mass. Laminins contain common structural features that include a tandem distribution of globular, rod-like, and coiled-coil domains. The coiled-coil domains are responsible for joining the 3 chains into the characteristic heterotrimeric structure called **merosin**.

Glycosaminoglycans

The most abundant heteropolysaccharides in the body are the glycosaminoglycans (GAGs). These molecules are long unbranched polysaccharides containing a repeating disaccharide unit. The disaccharide units contain either of 2 modified sugars, *N*-acetylgalactosamine (GalNAc) or *N*-acetylglucosamine (GlcNAc), and a uronic acid such as glucuronate or iduronate. GAGs are highly negatively charged molecules, with extended conformations that impart high viscosity to a solution in which they are found. GAGs are located primarily on the surface of cells or in the ECM. Along with the high viscosity of GAGs comes low compressibility, which makes these molecules ideal for a lubricating fluid in the joints. At the same time, their rigidity provides structural integrity to cells and provides passageways between cells, allowing for cell migration.

The specific GAGs of physiological significance are hyaluronic acid, dermatan sulfate, chondroitin sulfate, heparin, heparan sulfate, and keratan sulfate (Table 39-3). Although each of these GAGs has a predominant disaccharide component, heterogeneity does exist in the sugars present in the makeup of any given class of GAG; for example, the keratan I and keratin II forms of keratan GAGs.

Hyaluronic acid (also called hyaluronan) is unique among the GAGs in that it does not contain any sulfate and is not found covalently attached to proteins as a proteoglycan. It is, however, a component of noncovalently formed complexes with proteoglycans in the ECM. Hyaluronic acid polymers are very large (with molecular weights of 100,000-10,000,000 Da) and can displace a large volume of water. This property makes them excellent lubricators and shock absorbers.

One well-defined function of the GAG heparin is its role in preventing coagulation of the blood. Heparin is abundant in granules of mast cells that line blood vessels. The release of heparin from these granules, in response to injury, and its subsequent entry into the serum leads to an inhibition of blood clotting. Free heparin complexes with antithrombin III and activates it, which in turn inhibits all the serine proteases of the coagulation cascade (see Chapter 51). This phenomenon has been clinically exploited in the use of heparin injection for anticoagulation therapies.

Each of the GAGs serves a distinct function in the formation of the various types of ECM (Table 39-4).

Proteoglycans

The majority of GAGs in the body are linked to core proteins, forming proteoglycans (also called **mucopolysaccharides**). The linkage of GAGs to the protein core

TABLE 39-3: Composition of the Disaccharide Units of the Major Glycosaminoglycans

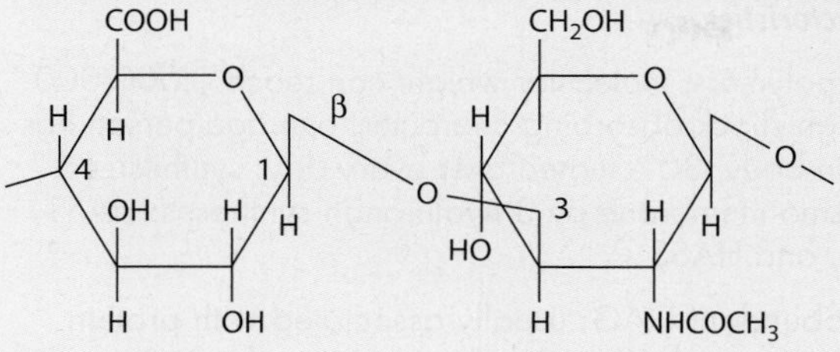 D-glucuronate β N-acetyl-D-glucosamine	**Hyaluronates** Composed of d-glucuronate + GlcNAc Linkage is β(1, 3)
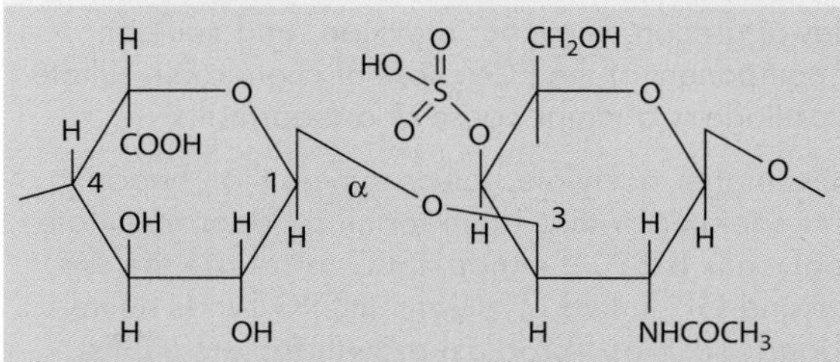 L-iduronate α N-acetyl-D-galactosamine-4-sulfate	**Dermatan sulfates** Composed of L-iduronate (many are sulfated) + GalNAc-4-sulfate Linkages is α(1, 3)
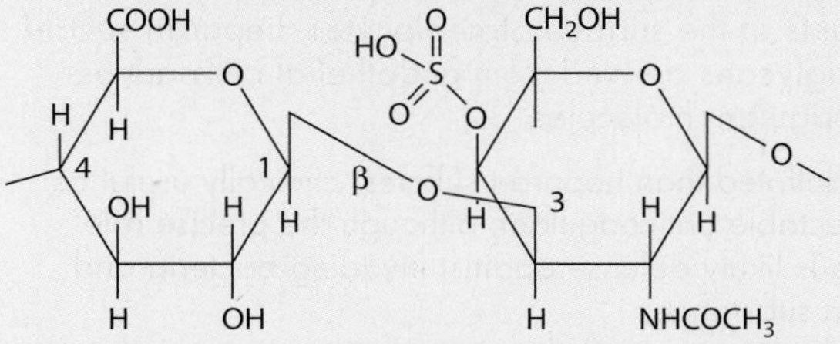 D-glucuronate β N-acetyl-D-glalactosamine-4-sulfate	**Chondroitin 4- and 6-sulfates** Composed of d-glucuronate and GalNAc-4- or 6-sulfate Linkage is β(1, 3) (the figure contains GalNAc 4-sulfate)
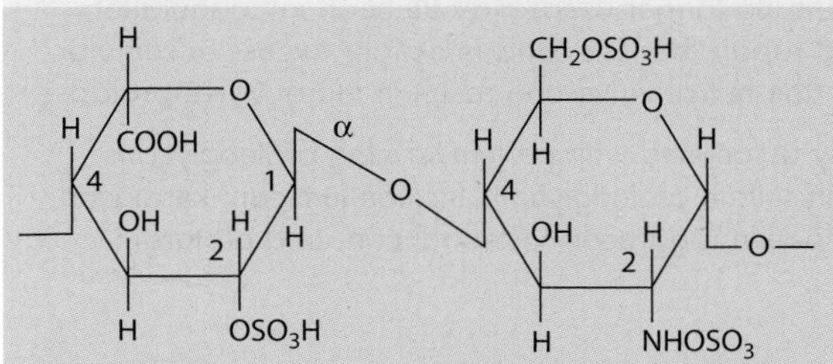 L-iduronate-2-sulfate α N-sulfo-D-glucosamine-6-sulfate	**Heparin and heparan sulfates** Composed of iduronate-2-sulfate (D-glucuronate-2-sulfate) and N-sulfo-D-glucosamine-6-sulfate Linkage is α(1, 4) (heparans have less sulfate than heparins)
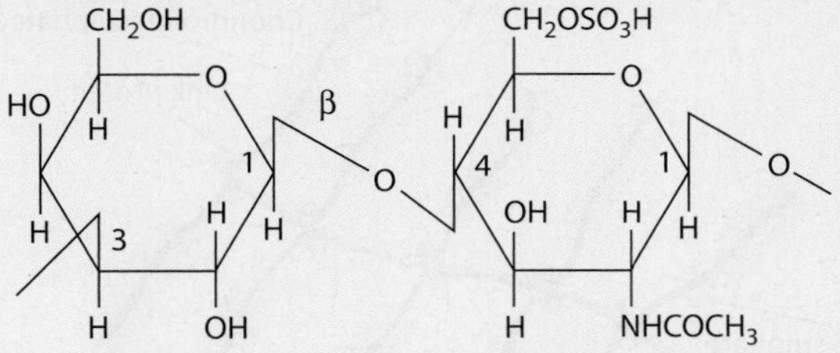 D-galactose β N-acetyl-D-glucosamine-6-sulfate	**Keratan sulfates** Composed of galactose + GlcNAc-6-sulfate Linkage is β(1, 4)

involves a specific trisaccharide composed of 2 galactose residues and a xylose residue, GAG-GalGalXyl-O-CH_2-protein (Figure 39-6). The trisaccharide linker is coupled to the protein core through an *O*-glycosidic bond to a Ser residue in the protein. Some forms of keratan sulfates are linked to the protein core through an *N*-asparaginyl bond. The protein cores of proteoglycans are rich in Ser and Thr residues, which allows for multiple GAG attachments forming a brush-like structure (Figure 39-7).

TABLE 39-4: Characteristics of the Various Glycosaminoglycans

GAG	*Localization*	*Characteristics*
Hyaluronate	Synovial fluid, articular cartilage, skin, vitreous humor, ECM of loose connective tissue	Large polymers, molecular weight can reach 1,000,000 Da; high shock absorbing character; average person has 15 g in body, 30% turned over every day; synthesized in plasma membrane by 3 hyaluronan synthases: HAS1, HAS2, and HAS3
Chondroitin sulfate	Cartilage, bone, heart valves	Most abundant GAG; usually associated with protein to form proteoglycans; the chondroitin sulfate proteoglycans form a family of molecules called lecticans and includes aggrecan, versican, brevican, and neurcan; major component of the ECM; loss of chondroitin sulfate from cartilage is a major cause of osteoarthritis
Heparan sulfate	Basement membranes, components of cell surfaces	Contains higher acetylated glucosamine than heparin; found associated with protein forming heparan sulfate proteoglycans (HSPG); major HSPG forms are the syndecans and GPI-linked glypicans; HSPG binds numerous ligands such as fibroblast growth factors (FGFs), vascular endothelial growth factor (VEGFs), and hepatocyte growth factors (HGFs), also binds chylomicron remnants at the surface of heptocytes; heparan sulfate proteoglycans derived from endothelial cells act as anticoagulant molecules
Heparin	Component of intracellular granules of mast cells, lining the arteries of the lungs, liver, and skin	More sulfated than heparan sulfates; clinically useful as an injectable anticoagulant, although the precise role in vivo is likely defense against invading bacteria and foreign substances
Dermatan sulfate	Skin, blood vessels, heart valves, tendons, lung	Was originally referred to as chondroitin sulfate B which is a term no longer used; may function in coagulation, wound repair, fibrosis, and infection; excess accumulation in the mitral valve can result in mitral valve prolapse
Keratan sulfate	Cornea, bone, cartilage aggregated with chondroitin sulfates	Usually associated with protein-forming proteoglycans; keratan sulfate proteoglycans include lumican, keratocan, fibromodulin, aggrecan, osteoadherin, and protargin

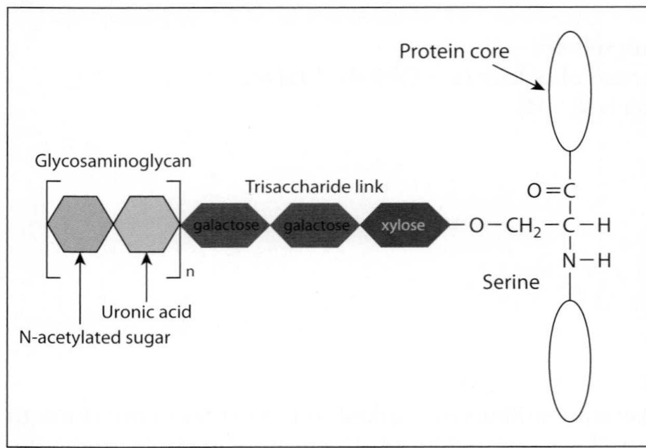

FIGURE 39-6: Structure of the GAG linkage to protein in a typical proteoglycan. Reproduced with permission of themedicalbiochemistrypage, LLC.

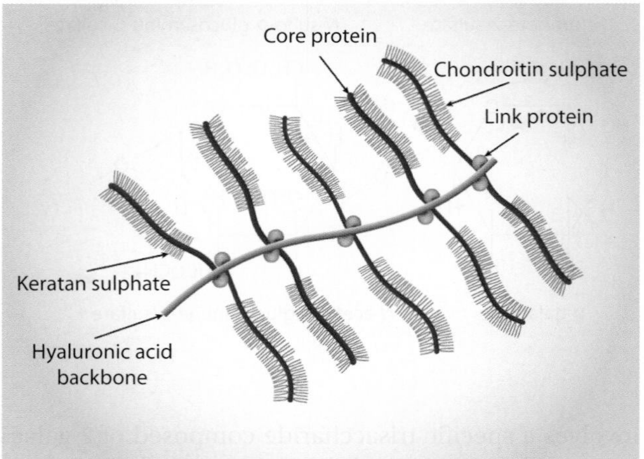

FIGURE 39-7: Structure of typical hyaluronic acid-based proteoglycan. Reproduced with permission of themedicalbiochemistrypage, LLC.

Different types of proteoglycans are classified based not only on the type(s) of GAG attached to the protein core but also on the basis of the core protein of the different proteoglycans. The various proteoglycan families (Table 39-5) consist of the lecticans, the small leucine-rich proteoglycan family (SLRP), keratin sulfate proteoglycan family, and the heparin sulfate proteoglycan (HSPG) family.

TABLE 39-5: Vertebrate Proteoglycan Types

Proteoglycan	***Comments***
Aggrecan	Belongs to the lectican family; a chondroitin sulfate proteoglycan; protein core encoded by the *ACAN* gene; forms a complex with hyaluronan; major component of articular cartilage
Brevican	Belongs to the lectican family; a chondroitin sulfate proteoglycan; protein core encoded by the *BCAN* gene; predominantly expressed in the central nervous system; brevican protein devoid of glycosaminoglycan chains is also found within the brain
Decorin	Is a member of the small leucine-rich proteoglycan (SLRP) family; protein core encoded by the *DCN* gene; binds to type I collagen fibrils; also interacts with fibronectin, thrombospondin, the epidermal growth factor receptor (EGFR), and transforming growth factor-beta (TGF-β); may play a role in epithelial/mesenchymal interactions during organ development
Keratocan	A keratan sulfate proteoglycan; protein core encoded by the *KERA* gene; is a member of the small leucine-rich proteoglycan (SLRP) family; important to the transparency of the cornea
Lumican	Major keratan sulfate proteoglycan; the protein core encoded by the *LUM* gene; is a member of the small leucine-rich proteoglycan (SLRP) family, also referred to as the small interstitial proteoglycan gene (*SIPG*) family; present in large quantities in the corneal stroma and in interstitial collagenous matrices of the heart, aorta, skeletal muscle, skin, and intervertebral discs; interacts with collagen fibrils; may regulate collagen fibril organization, corneal transparency, and epithelial cell migration and tissue repair
Neurocan	Belongs to the lectican family; a chondroitin sulfate proteoglycan; a nervous system proteoglycan; protein core encoded by the *NCAN* gene; is a susceptibility factor for bipolar disorder, absence of the *NANC* gene in mice results in a variety of manic-like behaviors which can be normalized by administration of lithium
Perlecan	More commonly called heparan sulfate proteoglycan of basement membrane; protein core encoded by the *HSPG2* gene; possesses angiogenic and growth-promoting properties primarily by acting as a coreceptor for fibroblast growth factor 2 (FGF2)
Syndecans	A family of cell surface heparan sulfate proteoglycans (HSPGs) that act as transmembrane cell surface receptors; consists of 4 members: syndecan-1, -2, -3, and -4; aberrant syndecan regulation plays a critical role postnatal tissue repair, inflammation and tumour progression; syndecan-1 expression is prevalent in differentiating plasma cells and its expression can serve as a marker for cells that are secreting immunoglobulin; syndecan-2 (also referred to as the original HSPG) prevalent on endothelial cells; strong expression of syndecan-3 found in many regions of the brain; syndecan-4 prevalently expressed in epithelial and fibroblastic cells; protein core of syndecan-1 encoded by the *SDC1* gene; syndecan-2 protein core encoded by the *SDC2* gene; protein core of syndecan-3 encoded by the *SDC3* gene; protein core of syndecan-4 encoded by the *SDC4* gene
Versican	Belongs to the lectican family; a chondroitin sulfate proteoglycan; protein core encoded by the *VCAN* gene; alternative splicing generates 3 versican species designated V0, V1, and V2 that differ in the length of the attached glycosaminoglycans; one of the main components of the ECM; significant proteoglycan in vitreous body of the eye; participates in cell adhesion, proliferation, migration, and angiogenesis; contributes to the development of atherosclerotic vascular diseases, cancer, tendon remodeling, hair follicle cycling, central nervous system injury, and neurite outgrowth; Wagner syndrome is caused by mutation in the *VCAN* gene, causes vitreoretinal degeneration

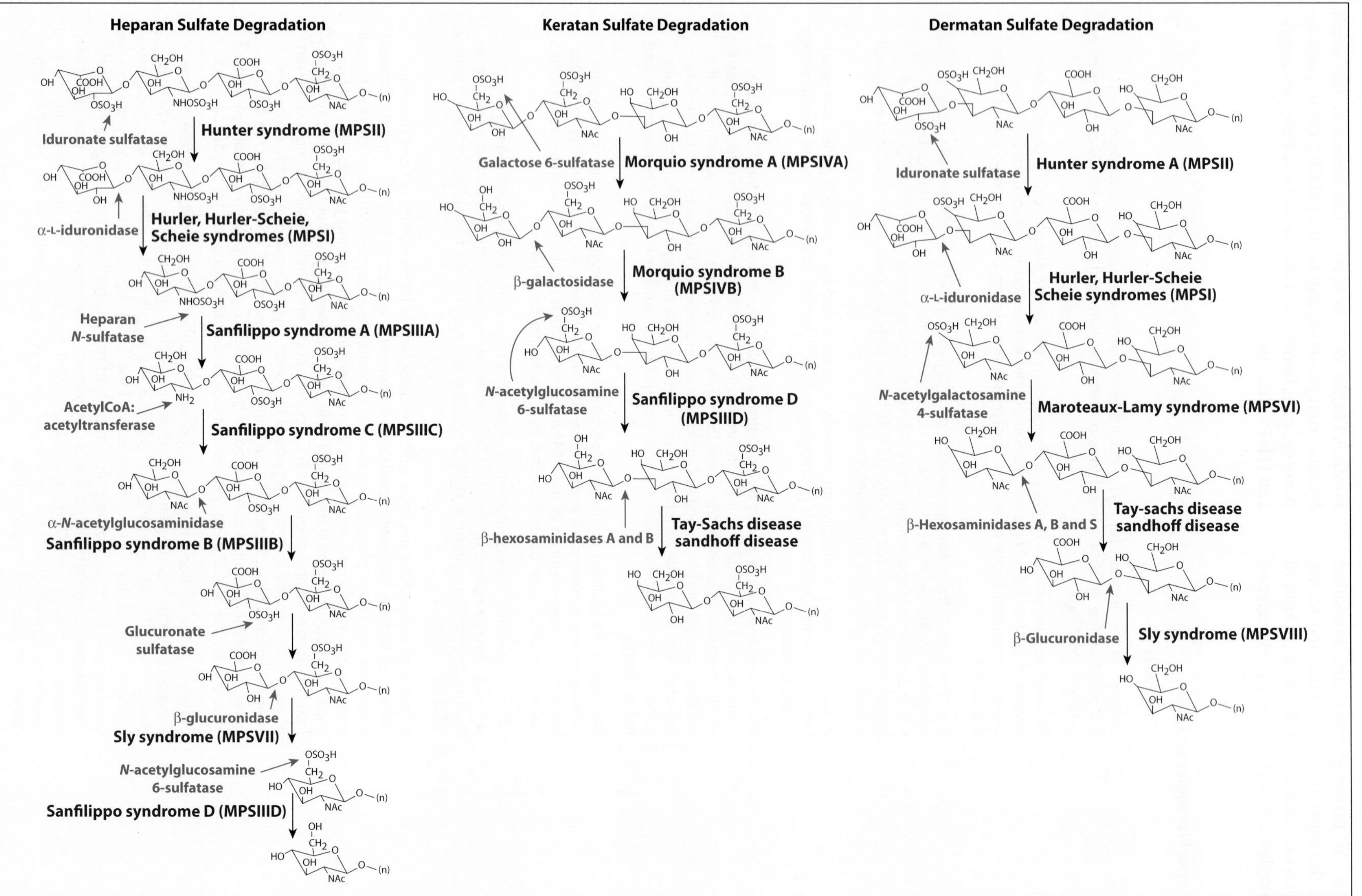

FIGURE 39-8: Degradation of heparan, keratan, and dermatan sulfates. The pathway for degradation of chondroitin sulfates (not shown) is similar to that of the dermatan sulfates, given that their compositions are somewhat similar (they both contain GalNAc-sulfates). The removal of iduronate and iduronate sulfates is unique to the dermatan sulfates, since chondroitin sulfates contain glucuronate residues which are removed by glucuronidase. Chondroitin sulfates containing GalNAc 6-sulfates are hydrolyzed by *N*-acetylgalactosamine 6-sulfatase (also called galactose 6-sulfatase), which is defective in Morquio syndrome type A. Enzyme names are shown in green. Defective enzyme activity leads to the disorders indicated in blue. Note, for example, that although Tay-Sachs disease is a lysosomal storage disease it is not considered an MPS, since a deficiency in β-hexosaminidase A results in symptoms that are principally due to defective sphingolipid degradation (see Chapter 21).

Glycosaminoglycan Degradation

Several genetically inherited diseases, for example the lysosomal storage diseases, result from defects in the lysosomal hydrolases responsible for the metabolism of complex membrane-associated GAGs (Figure 39-8). These specific diseases are historically termed the **mucopolysaccharidoses** (MPS) in reference to the earlier term, mucopolysaccharide, used for glycosaminoglycans. There are at least 14 known lysosomal storage diseases that are the result of defective GAG catabolism (Table 39-6).

TABLE 39-6: Lysosomal Storage Diseases Caused by Defective Glycosaminoglycan Degradation

Type: Syndrome	*Enzyme Defect*	*Affected GAG*	*Major Symptoms*
Hurler MPSIH (MPS1H)	α-L-iduronidase	Dermatan sulfate, heparan sulfate	Corneal clouding, dysostosis multiplex, organomegaly, heart disease, dwarfism, mental retardation; early mortality
Scheie MPSIS (MPS1S)	α-L-iduronidase	Dermatan sulfate, heparan sulfate	Corneal clouding; aortic valve disease; joint stiffening; normal intelligence and life span
Hurler-Scheie MPSIHS (MPS1HS)	α-L-iduronidase	Dermatan sulfate, heparan sulfate	Intermediate between I H and I S
Hunter MPSII (MPS2)	L-iduronate-2-sulfatase	Dermatan sulfate, heparan sulfate	Mild and severe forms, only X-linked MPS, dysostosis multiplex, organomegaly, facial and physical deformities, no corneal clouding, mental retardation, death before 15 except in mild form, then survival to 20-60
Sanfilippo A MPSIIIA (MPS3A)	heparan *N*-sulfatase	Heparan sulfate	Profound mental deterioration, hyperactivity, skin, brain, lungs, heart and skeletal muscle are affected in all 4 types of MPS-III
Sanfilippo B MPSIIIB (MPS3B)	α-*N*-acetyl-D-glucosaminidase	Heparan sulfate	Phenotype similar to III A
Sanfilippo C MPSIIIC (MPS3C)	acetyl-CoA:α-glucosaminide-acetyltransferase	Heparan sulfate	Phenotype similar to III A
Sanfilippo D MPSIIID (MPS3D)	*N*-acetylglucosamine-6-sulfatase	Heparan sulfate	Phenotype similar to III A
Morquio A MPSIVA (MPS4A)	Galactose 6-sulfatase	Keratan sulfate, chondroitin 6-sulfate	Corneal clouding, odontoid hypoplasia, aortic valve disease, distinctive skeletal abnormalities
Morquio B MPSIVB (MPS4B)	β-Galactosidase	Keratan sulfate	Severity of disease similar to IV A
MPS V, a designation no longer used			
Maroteaux-Lamy MPSVI (MPS6)	Arylsulfatase B; also called *N*-acetylgalactosamine-4-sulfatase	Dermatan sulfate	3 distinct forms from mild to severe, aortic valve disease, dysostosis multiplex, normal intelligence, corneal clouding, coarse facial features
Sly MPSVII (MPS7)	β-Glucuronidase	Heparan sulfate, dermatan sulfate, chondroitin 4,6-sulfates	Hepatosplenomegaly, dysostosis multiplex, wide spectrum of severity, hydrops fetalis
MPS VIII, a designation no longer used			

REVIEW QUESTIONS

1. A male infant, delivered at 38 weeks' gestation, presents with severe bowing of long bones, blue sclera, and craniotabes at birth. Radiographs show severe generalized osteoporosis, a broad and crumpled long bones, beading ribs, and a poorly mineralized skull. Histologic examination of the long bones revealed the trabeculae of the calcified cartilage with an abnormally thin layer of osteoid, and the bony trabeculae are thin and basophilic. The symptoms observed in the infant are characteristic of which disease?
   A. Ehlers-Danlos syndrome
   B. Hunter syndrome
   C. Hurler syndrome
   D. Marfan syndrome
   E. osteogenesis imperfecta

Answer E: Osteogenesis imperfecta consists of a group of at least 4 types (mild, extensive, severe, and variable). The disorder is characterized by brittle bones and abnormally thin sclerae, which appear blue owing to the lack of connective tissue. The symptoms arise due to defects in two α-collagen genes, the *COL1A1* and *COL1A2* genes. There have been over 100 mutations identified in these 2 genes. The mutations lead to decreased expression of collagen or abnormal pro1 proteins. The abnormal proteins associate with normal collagen subunits, which prevents the triple helical structure of normal collagen to form. The result is degradation of all the collagen proteins, both normal and abnormal.

2. A 30-month-old child presents with coarse facial features, corneal clouding, hepatosplenomegaly, and exhibiting disproportionate short-trunk dwarfism. Radiographic analysis indicates enlargement of the diaphyses of the long bones and irregular metaphyses, along with poorly developed epiphyseal centers. Other skeletal abnormalities typify the features comprising dysotosis multiplex. The child's physical stature and the analysis of bone development indicate the child is suffering from which of the following disorders?
   A. Ehlers-Danlos syndrome
   B. Hunter syndrome
   C. Hurler syndrome
   D. Marfan syndrome
   E. osteogenesis imperfecta

Answer C: Although multiorgan involvement, liver and spleen enlargement, and skeletal abnormalities are common to all the mucopolysaccharidotic (MPS) diseases, each encompasses features that allow for specific diagnosis. Hurler syndrome is characterized by progressive multiorgan failure and premature death. Hallmark features include enlargement of the spleen and liver, severe skeletal deformity, and coarse facial features (which are associated with the constellation of defects referred to as dysotosis multiplex). The disease results from a defect in α-L-iduronidase activity, which leads to intracellular accumulations of heparan sulfates and dermatan sulfates. The accumulation of these GAGs (glycosaminoglycan) in Hurler syndrome patients severely affect development of the skeletal system leading, primarily, to defective long bone growth plate disruption.

3. A 12-month-old female infant exhibits severe developmental delay with associated macrocephaly, dysmorphic facies, hypotonia, and hepatosplenomegaly. Clouding of the corneas is not evident. A pebbly ivory-colored lesion is present over the infant's back. The activity of iduronate sulfatase in the plasma is not detectable. These symptoms are indicative of which type of mucopolysaccharidosis?
   A. Ehlers-Danlos syndrome
   B. Hunter syndrome
   C. Hurler syndrome
   D. Marfan syndrome
   E. osteogenesis imperfecta

Answer B: Although multiorgan involvement, liver and spleen enlargement, and skeletal abnormalities are common to all the mucopolysaccharidotic (MPS) diseases, each encompasses specific and unique features. Each different MPS is caused by defects in different enzymes which allows for specific diagnosis. Hunter syndrome is characterized by progressive multiorgan failure and premature death. Hallmark features include enlargement of the spleen and liver, severe skeletal deformity, and coarse facial features (which are associated with the constellation of defects referred to as dysotosis multiplex). Unlike Hurler syndrome, whose symptoms are similar (but more severe), Hunter syndrome does not cause corneal opacities. Hunter syndrome results from a defect in iduronidate sulfatase activity and this activity can be measured in the plasma.

4. The migration of cancer cells from a solid tumor to another location in the body is referred to metastasis. This process requires the activity of which of the following enzymes?
   A. glycosylhydrolases
   B. glycosyltransferases
   C. lysosomal hydrolases
   D. lysyl hydroxylases
   E. matrix metalloproteinases

Answer E: Cell migration requires the hydrolysis of the extracellular matrix (ECM) holding the cells into a tissue or a tumor. The primary enzymes responsible for the degradation and remodeling of the ECM are the matrix metalloproteinases.

5. You are examining a 5-year-old girl with severe psychomotor retardation. Physical examination shows distinct hepatosplenomegaly, corneal clouding, coarse facial features, and short stature. Suspecting a lysosomal storage disease you order a test for lysosomal enzyme activity in a skin biopsy. Results of the test shows deficiency in arylsulfatase B and accumulation of dermatan sulfates in the biopsy cells. Given these symptoms and lab studies, this child is most likely suffering from which of the following disorders?

A. Ehlers-Danlos syndrome
B. Maroteaux-Lamy syndrome
C. Hurler-Scheie syndrome
D. Marfan syndrome
E. Morquio syndrome type B

Answer B: Maroteaux-Lamy syndrome is characterized by the lysosomal accumulation of dermatan sulfates as a consequence of deficiencies in the lysosomal hydrolase *N*-acetylgalactosamine 4-sulfatase (arylsulfatase B). Although mental development proceeds normally in Maroteaux-Lamy patients, the progression of physical and visual impairments ultimately impedes psychomotor abilities. The clinical features and severity in Maroteaux-Lamy patients is variable, but usually include short stature, hepatosplenomegaly, stiff joints, corneal clouding, cardiac abnormalities, facial dysmorphism, and dysotosis multiplex. Hepatosplenomegaly is always present in Maroteaux-Lamy patients after the age of 6. In patients with the most severe forms of the disease there is a shortened trunk, protuberant abdomen, and prominent lumbar lordosis.

6. You are studying the production of an extracellular matrix by cultures of fibroblasts isolated from a melanoma. Histological studies demonstrate an absence of merosin. Based upon this finding, which of the following ECM components is most likely not being synthesized or processed appropriately in your cell culture system?

A. collagen
B. elastin
C. fibrillin
D. fibronectin
E. laminin

Answer E: Laminins are heterotrimeric proteins that have been found to form at least 15 different types of heterotrimers. Laminin heterotrimers are quite large, ranging from under 500,000 to nearly a 1,000,000 Da in mass. Laminins contain common structural features that include a tandem distribution of globular, rod-like, and coiled-coil domains. The coiled-coil domains are responsible for joining the 3 chains into the characteristic heterotrimeric structure called merosin.

7. Some types of malignant cells lack expression of fibronectin. The loss of fibronectin by these cells would most likely be associated with which of the following?

A. decreased production of GAGs found in fibroblast proteoglycans
B. increased adherence of the cells to the basement membrane
C. inhibition of matrix metalloproteinase activation
D. loss of collagen processing in the extracellular matrix
E. reduced integrin-mediated cell adhesion

Answer E: Fibronectin is an ECM glycoprotein that is responsible for interaction with integrins present in the plasma membrane of cells, as well as interactions with collagens and glycosaminoglycans. The loss of functional fibronectin would result in inappropriate intracellular signaling, cell shape changes, and cell movements.

8. A female infant, delivered at 37 weeks' gestation, presents with severe bowing of long bones. Physical examination shows blue sclera and x-rays show broad and crumpled long bones. As the attending physician, you suspect a disorder in connective tissues and order an evaluation of collagen gene defects. Results demonstrate the infant harbors a mutation in the *COL1A1* gene. The presenting symptoms and molecular analysis indicate this child is suffering from which of the following disorders?

A. Ehlers-Danlos syndrome
B. Maroteaux-Lamy syndrome
C. Hurler-Scheie syndrome
D. Marfan syndrome
E. osteogenesis imperfecta

Answer E: Osteogenesis imperfecta consists of a group of at least 4 types (mild, extensive, severe, and variable). The disorder is characterized by brittle bones and abnormally thin sclerae, which appear blue owing to the lack of connective tissue. The symptoms arise due to defects in 2 α-collagen genes, the *COL1A1* and *COL1A2* genes. There have been over 100 mutations identified in these 2 genes. The mutations lead to decreased expression of collagen or abnormal pro1 proteins. The abnormal proteins associate with normal collagen subunits, which prevents the triple helical structure of normal collagen to form. The result is degradation of all the collagen proteins, both normal and abnormal.

9. You are examining a 10-month-old male infant who exhibits severe developmental delay. The infant also shows macrocephaly, dysmorphic facies, and

hepatosplenomegaly. Clouding of the corneas is not evident, so you suspect the infant has a particular form of a lysosomal storage disease and order a test for the activity of iduronate sulfatase in the blood. Results of this test confirm that the enzyme activity is absent. Which of the following would you expect to find at elevated levels in fibroblasts from a skin biopsy from this patient?
A. chondroitin sulfates
B. dermatan sulfates
C. hyaluronates
D. keratin sulfate I
E. keratin sulfate II

Answer B: The infant is suffering from Hunter syndrome. This disorder is characterized by the lysosomal accumulation of dermatan and heparan sulfates as a consequence of deficiencies in the lysosomal hydrolase iduronate sulfatase. Iduronate sulfatase (also called iduronate 2-sulfatase) hydrolyzes sulfates from the 2-position of L-iduronate present in dermatan and heparan sulfates.

10. You are examining a 2-year-old child presenting with disproportionate short-trunk dwarfism. Additional physical signs are coarse facial features, corneal clouding, and hepatosplenomegaly. You suspect the child is suffering from a lysosomal storage disease and order a test for α-iduronidase activity and find that it is severely impaired. Which of the following would you expect to find at elevated levels in fibroblasts from a skin biopsy from this patient?
A. chondroitin sulfates
B. heparan sulfates
C. hyaluronates
D. keratin sulfate I
E. keratin sulfate II

Answer B: The child is most likely suffering from Hurler syndrome. This disorder is characterized by the lysosomal accumulation of dermatan and heparan sulfates as a consequence of defects in the lysosomal hydrolase α-L-iduronidase.

11. A 12-month-old girl is referred for genetic evaluation because of coarse facial features, an enlarged tongue, hepatosplenomegaly, joint stiffness, and delayed growth and development. She appeared normal at birth except for an umbilical hernia. Urine screening shows increased concentrations of dermatan sulfate and heparan sulfate. The child most likely has a disorder in the lysosomal metabolism of which of the following substances?
A. cholesterol esters
B. glycogen
C. glycosaminoglycans
D. glycosphingolipids
E. spingomyelins

Answer C: The child is most likely suffering from Hurler or Hunter syndrome. These disorders are characterized by the lysosomal accumulation of the glycosaminoglycans, dermatan sulfate, and heparan sulfate as a consequence of defects in the lysosomal hydrolases α-L-iduronidase or iduronate sulfatase, respectively.

12. An 18-month-old girl is brought to the physician by her parents because of developmental delays since the age of 9 months. She has a history of recurrent otitis media. She underwent bilateral inguinal hernia repair at the age of 12 months. Her vocabulary consists of 2 single words, and she is starting to walk with assistance. She is at the 10th percentile for length and the 25th percentile for weight. Physical examination shows generalized hirsutism, a prominent forehead with full cheeks, cloudy corneas, a depressed nasal bridge, and rhinorrhea. There is moderate hepatomegaly. The catabolism of which of the following is most likely abnormal in this patient?
A. branched-chain amino acids
B. coproporphyrins
C. glycogen
D. glycosaminoglycans
E. phospholipids

Answer D: The symptoms present in this child are most closely associated with a deficiency in the β-galactosidase-1 gene (GLB1) which is a lysosomal enzyme involved in the degradation of keratin sulfates, G_{M1} gangliosides (G_{A1}), and glycoprotein-derived oligosaccharides.

13. A 5-year-old girl has had numerous childhood fractures. She is also found to have blue sclera, hearing abnormalities, and misshapen teeth. Which of the following is the most likely cause of these findings?
A. abnormal intestinal receptors for calcium
B. an inability to metabolize vitamin D
C. inadequate mineralization of bone matrix
D. renal inability to conserve phosphorous
E. synthesis of abnormal type I collagen

Answer E: Osteogenesis imperfecta type I is a genetic disorder characterized by synthesis of an abnormal type I collagen. Frequent childhood fractures, blue sclera, poor hearing, and misshapen teeth may all occur clinically because of the abnormal collagen synthesis.

Checklist

✓ The extracellular matrix (ECM) provides the structural support that holds cells together to form the various tissues.

✓ The ECM is composed of structural proteins (primarily collagens and elastin), specialized proteins (such as fibronectin and laminin), and a variety of proteoglycans.

✓ Collagen is the most abundant protein in the human body. There are 28 different types of collagen all derived from 30 different α-collagen genes. Functional collagens comprise 3 polypeptides wound around each other to form a triple helix. The collagen monomers in the triple helix are held together by cross-linking between the chains. Each collagen protein contains a highly repeating sequence of $(Gly\text{-}X\text{-}Y)_n$.

✓ Numerous disorders in collagen synthesis and processing are known and include the various types of osteogenesis imperfect and Ehlers-Danlos syndrome.

✓ Elastin forms cross-linked fibers via a mechanism similar to that in collagen but is unique in that 3 lysine-derived aldehydes (allysyl) cross-link with an unmodified lysine forming a tetrafunctional structure called a desmosine. The highly stable cross-linking of elastin is what ultimately imparts its elastic properties.

✓ Fibrillin is found interspersed in cross-linked elastin fibers and plays a role in the elastic character of elastic fibers. Deficiencies in fibrillin result in the connective tissue disorder called Marfan syndrome.

✓ Fibronectin is a major ECM glycoprotein that interacts with cell surface receptors of the integrin family, connecting the ECM to intracellular signaling pathways.

✓ Laminin are heterotrimeric ECM proteins that are quite large, ranging from under 500,000 to nearly a 1,000,000 Da in mass. Laminins contain common structural features that include a tandem distribution of globular, rod-like, and coiled-coil domains. The coiled-coil domains are responsible for joining the 3 chains into the characteristic heterotrimeric structure called merosin.

✓ Glycosaminoglycans (GAGs) are composed of various repeating disaccharides that consist of a uronic acid (glucuronic or iduronic acid) and a hexose or hexosamine (galactose, galactosamine, or glucosamine). Many GAGs also have varying degrees of sulfate addition.

✓ The major GAGs in human tissues are hyaluronic acid, chondroitin sulfate, keratin sulfate, dermatan sulfate, heparin and heparan sulfate.

✓ Proteoglycans are heavily glycosylated ECM proteins composed of 1 or more GAGs attached to serine residues. The GAGs extend perpendicularly from the core protein forming a brush-like structure. Proteoglycans are extremely large and confer lubricating and shock-absorbing properties to the tissues.

✓ Inherited deficiencies in the enzymes responsible for lysosomal degradation of GAGs result in a class of lysosomal storage diseases commonly referred to as the mucopolysaccharidoses.

CHAPTER

40 Mechanisms of Signal Transduction

CHAPTER OUTLINE

High-Yield Terms

Signal transduction: refers to the movement of signals from outside the cell to inside, resulting in a change in the "state" of the cell

Growth factor: any of a family of proteins that bind to receptors with the primary result of activating cellular proliferation and/or differentiation

Cytokine: any of unique family of growth factor proteins primarily secreted from leukocytes

Chemokine: a subfamily of cytokines (**chemo**tactic cyto**kines**) that is capable of inducing chemotaxis

Interleukin: any of a family of multifunctional cytokines that are produced by a variety of lymphoid and nonlymphoid cells

Serpentine receptors: any of a family of G-protein–coupled receptors (GPCRs) so called because they span the plasma membrane 7 times

G-protein: any of a large family of proteins that bind and hydrolyze GTP in the act of transmitting signals, includes the heterotrimeric and the monomeric G-protein families

Nuclear receptors: intracellular receptors that bind lipophilic ligands and then bind to specific DNA sequences in target genes regulating their expression

Mechanisms of Signal Transduction

Signal transduction at the cellular level refers to the movement of signals from outside the cell to inside. The movement of signals can be simple, like that associated with receptor molecules of the acetylcholine class: receptors that constitute channels which, upon ligand interaction, allow signals to be passed in the form of small ion movement, either into or out of the cell. These ion movements result in changes in the electrical potential of the cells that, in turn, propagates the signal along the cell. More complex signal transduction involves the coupling of ligand-receptor interactions to many intracellular events. These events include phosphorylations by tyrosine kinases and/or serine/threonine kinases. Protein phosphorylations change enzyme activities and protein conformations. The eventual outcome is an alteration in cellular activity and changes in the program of genes expressed within the responding cells.

Growth Factors

Growth factors are classified as substances that bind to receptors with the primary result of activating cellular proliferation and/or differentiation. The vast majority of growth factors are proteins that bind to extracellular ligand-binding domains of transmembrane receptors (Table 40-1). However, some steroid hormones have growth factor activity. Steroid hormones bind

TABLE 40-1: Representative List of Well-Characterized Growth Factors

Factor	*Principal Source*	*Primary Activity*	*Comments*
PDGF	Platelets, endothelial cells, placenta	Promotes proliferation of connective tissue, glial and smooth muscle cells	Two different protein chains form 3 distinct dimer forms: AA, AB, and BB
EGF	Submaxillary gland, Brunner gland	Promotes proliferation of mesenchymal, glial, and epithelial cells	Numerous proteins with very different activities contain 1 or more domains first identified in EGF and thus referred to as EGF-like domains
TGF-α	Common in transformed cells, macrophages, keratinocytes	May be important for normal wound healing	Is a member of the EGF family of proteins
FGF	Wide range of cells; protein is associated with the ECM	Promotes proliferation of many cells; inhibits some stem cells; induces mesoderm to form in early embryos	At least 18 family members, 5 distinct receptors
NGF	Mast cells, eosinophils, bone marrow stromal cells, keratinocytes	Promotes neurite outgrowth and neural cell survival	Member of a family of proteins termed *neurotrophins* that promote proliferation and survival of neurons; neurotrophin receptors are a class of related proteins first identified as proto-oncogenes: TrkA ("trackA"), TrkB, TrkC
Erythropoietin	Kidney	Promotes proliferation and differentiation of erythrocytes	
TGF-β	Activated Th1 cells (T-helper) and natural killer (NK) cells	Anti-inflammatory (suppresses cytokine production and class II MHC expression), promotes wound healing, inhibits macrophage and lymphocyte proliferation	At least 100 different family members
IGF-1	Primarily liver	Promotes proliferation of many cell types	Related to IGF-2 and proinsulin, also called somatomedin C
IGF-2	Variety of cells	Promotes proliferation of many cell types primarily of fetal origin	Related to IGF-1 and proinsulin

High-Yield Concept

Cytokines that are secreted from lymphocytes are termed *lymphokines*, whereas those secreted by monocytes or macrophages are termed *monokines*. A large family of cytokines is produced by various cells of the body. Many of the lymphokines are more commonly known as *interleukins (ILs)*, since they are not only secreted by leukocytes but are also able to affect the cellular responses of leukocytes.

intracellular receptors (see later). Many growth factors are quite versatile, stimulating cellular division in numerous different cell types; while others are specific to a particular cell type. Individual growth factor proteins tend to occur as members of larger families of structurally and evolutionarily related proteins. For example, there are at least 18 members of the fibroblast growth factor (FGF) family of proteins.

Cytokines and Chemokines

Cytokines are a unique family of growth factors (Table 40-2). Secreted primarily from leukocytes, cytokines stimulate both the humoral and cellular immune responses, as well as the activation of phagocytic cells.

Specifically, interleukins are growth factors targeted to the cells of hematopoietic origin. Several growth factors are also considered members of the cytokine family, such as the members of the colony-stimulating factor (CSF) family of proteins that stimulate the proliferation of specific pluripotent stem cells of the bone marrow, and TNF-α and some members of the large TGF-β family.

Proteins are classified as chemokines according to shared structural characteristics such as small size and the presence of 4 cysteine residues in conserved locations that are key to forming their 3-dimensional shape. The nomenclature for cytokines and chemokines is a mix of the widely accepted, but slightly misleading,

TABLE 40-2: Representative Well Characterized Cytokines

Interleukins	*Principal Source*	*Primary Activity*
IL-1α and -1β	Macrophages and other antigen-presenting cells (APCs)	Costimulation of APCs and T-cells, inflammation and fever, acute phase response, hematopoiesis
IL-2	Activated Th1 cells, NK cells	Proliferation of β-cells and activated T-cells, NK functions
IL-6	Activated Th2 cells, APCs, other somatic cells such as hepatocytes and adipocytes	Acute-phase response, β-cell proliferation, thrombopoiesis, synergistic with IL-1β and TNF on T-cells
IL-8	Macrophages, other somatic cells	Chemoattractant for neutrophils and T-cells
IL-10	Activated Th2 cells, CD8$^+$ T and B cells, macrophages	Inhibits cytokine production, promotes β-cell proliferation and antibody production, suppresses cellular immunity, mast cell growth
IL-12	β-cells, T-cells, macrophages, dendritic cells	Proliferation of NK cells, INF-γ production, promotes cell-mediated immune functions
IL-17: 6 isoforms all from different genes; IL-17A, B, C, D, E, and F (IL-17E also called IL-25)	A and F forms only expressed in a subset of T-cells; B expressed in leukocytes and peripheral tissues; C upregulated during inflammation; D expressed in nervous system and skeletal muscle; E expressed in peripheral tissues	Increases production of inflammatory cytokines, angiogenesis, affects endothelial and epithelial cells
IL-18	Macrophages	Increases NK cell activity, induces production of INF-γ

High-Yield Concept

Chemokines represent a subfamily of cytokines whose name is derived from **chemo**tactic cyto**kines**. These proteins are capable of inducing chemotaxis in nearby responsive cells.

designations. For example, interleukin-8 (IL-8) is actually a chemokine but the interleukin name remains in common usage.

Like the protein family of growth factors, cytokines and chemokines elicit their effects through interaction with the ligand-binding domain of transmembrane receptors.

Classifications of Signal-Transducing Receptors

Signal-transducing receptors are of 3 general classes:

1. Receptors that penetrate the plasma membrane and have intrinsic enzymatic activity. Receptors that have intrinsic enzymatic activities include those that are tyrosine kinases (eg, PDGF, insulin, EGF, and FGF receptors), tyrosine phosphatases (eg, CD45 [cluster determinant-45] protein of T cells and macrophages), guanylate cyclases (eg, natriuretic peptide receptors), and serine/threonine kinases (eg, activin and TGF-β receptors). Receptors with intrinsic tyrosine kinase activity are capable of autophosphorylation as well as phosphorylation of other substrates. Additionally, several families of receptors lack intrinsic enzyme activity, yet are coupled to intracellular tyrosine kinases by direct protein-protein interactions.
2. Receptors that are coupled, inside the cell, to GTP-binding and hydrolyzing proteins (termed G-proteins). Receptors of the class that interact with G-proteins have a structure that is characterized by 7 transmembrane spanning domains. These receptors are termed *serpentine receptors*. Examples of this class are the adrenergic receptors, odorant receptors, and certain hormone receptors (eg, glucagon, angiotensin, vasopressin, and bradykinin).
3. Receptors that are found intracellularly and upon ligand binding migrate to the nucleus, where the ligand-receptor complex directly affects gene transcription. Because this class of receptors is intracellular and functions in the nucleus as transcription factors, they are commonly referred to as the *nuclear receptors*. Receptors of this class include the large family of steroid and thyroid hormone receptors. Receptors in this class have a ligand-binding domain, a DNA-binding domain, and a transcriptional regulatory domain.

Receptor Tyrosine Kinases

The receptor tyrosine kinase (RTK) family of transmembrane ligand-binding proteins is comprised of 59 members in the human genome. Each of the RTKs exhibit similar structural and functional characteristics. Most RTKs are monomers and their domain structure includes an extracellular ligand-binding domain, a transmembrane domain, and an intracellular domain possessing the tyrosine kinase activity (Figure 40-1). The insulin and insulin-like growth factor receptors are the most complex in the RTK family, being disulfide-linked heterotetramers.

The amino acid sequences of the tyrosine kinase domains of RTKs are highly conserved with those of cAMP-dependent protein kinase (PKA) within the ATP-binding and substrate-binding regions. RTK proteins are classified into families based upon structural features in their extracellular portions, as well as the presence or absence of a kinase domain insert. The extracellular domains include the cysteine-rich domains, immunoglobulin-like domains, leucine-rich domains, Kringle domains, cadherin domains, fibronectin type III repeats, discoidin I–like domains, acidic domains, and EGF-like domains. Based upon the presence of these various extracellular domains, the RTKs have been subdivided into at least 20 different families (Table 40-3).

Many receptors that have intrinsic tyrosine kinase activity as well as the tyrosine kinases that are associated with cell surface receptors contain tyrosine residues that, upon phosphorylation, interact with other proteins of the signaling cascade. These other proteins contain a domain of amino acid sequences that are homologous to a domain first identified in the kinase encoded by the SRC proto-oncogene. These domains are termed SH2 domains (SRC homology domain 2).

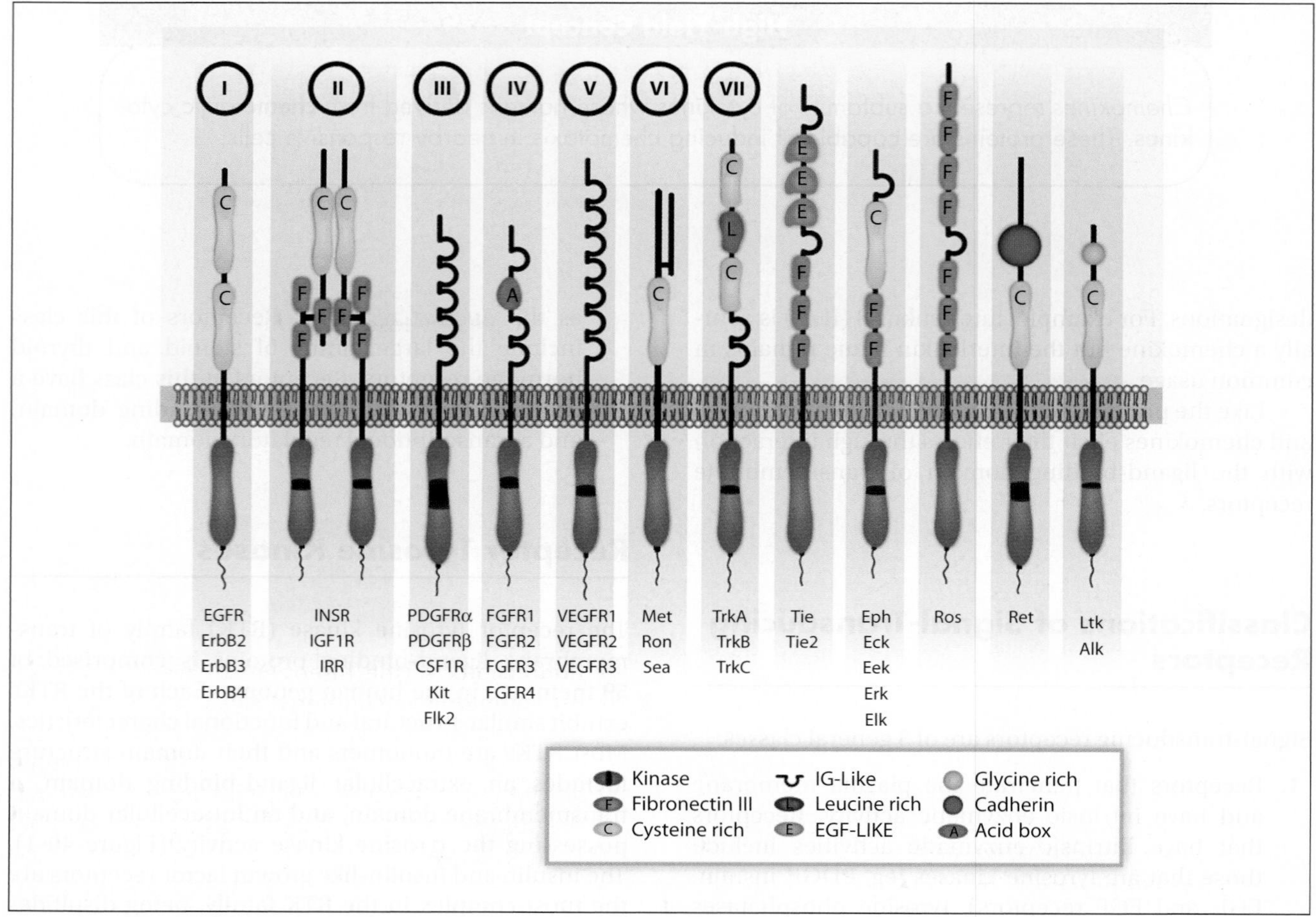

FIGURE 40-1: A diagrammatic representation of several members of the receptor tyrosine kinase (RTK) family. Several members of each receptor subfamily are indicated below each representative. The Roman numerals above the first 7 subtypes correspond to those subtypes described in Table 40-3. These RTK subtypes do not represent the entire RTK family. Reproduced with permission of themedicalbiochemistrypage, LLC.

TABLE 40-3: Characteristics of the Common Classes of RTKs

Class	*Examples*	*Structural Features of Class*
I	EGF receptor, NEU/HER2, HER3	Cysteine-rich sequences
II	Insulin receptor, IGF-1 receptor	Cysteine-rich sequences; characterized by disulfide-linked heterotetramers
III	PDGF receptors, c-kit	Contain 5 immunoglobulin-like domains; also contain the kinase insert
IV	FGF receptors	Contain 3 immunoglobulin-like domains as well as the kinase insert; acidic domain
V	Vascular endothelial cell growth factor (VEGF) receptor	Contain 7 immunoglobulin-like domains as well as the kinase insert domain
VI	Hepatocyte growth factor (HGF) and scatter factor (SF) receptors	Heterodimeric, like the class II receptors except that 1 of the 2 protein subunits is completely extracellular. The HGF receptor is a proto-oncogene that was originally identified as the MET oncogene
VII	Neurotrophin receptor family (TRKA, TRKB, TRKC) and NGF receptor	Contain no or few cysteine-rich domains; NGFR has leucine-rich domain

Another conserved protein-protein interaction domain identified in many signal-transduction proteins is related to a third domain in SRC identified as the SH3 domain.

The interactions of SH2 domain–containing proteins with RTKs, or receptor-associated tyrosine kinases, leads to tyrosine phosphorylation of the SH2-containing proteins. Phosphorylation of SH2-containing proteins that have enzymatic activity results in an alteration (either positively or negatively) in that activity. Several SH2-containing proteins that have intrinsic enzymatic activity include phospholipase C-γ (PLC-γ), the proto-oncogene RAS-associated GTPase-activating protein (rasGAP), phosphatidylinositol-3-kinase (PI3K), protein phosphatase-1C (PTP1C), as well as members of the SRC family of protein tyrosine kinases (PTKs).

Nonreceptor Protein Tyrosine Kinases

There are numerous intracellular protein tyrosine kinases (PTKs) that are responsible for phosphorylating a variety of intracellular proteins on tyrosine residues following activation of cellular growth and proliferation signals. There are 2 distinct families of nonreceptor PTKs. The archetypal PTK family is related to the SRC protein. The SRC protein is a tyrosine kinase first identified as the transforming protein in Rous sarcoma virus. The second family is related to the Janus kinase (JAK). Most proteins in these 2 families couple to transmembrane receptors that do not themselves have intrinsic enzymatic activity. This class of receptors includes all of the cytokine receptors.

Receptor Serine/Threonine Kinases

The receptors for the TGF-β superfamily of ligands have intrinsic serine/threonine kinase (RSK) activity. There are more than 30 multifunctional proteins of the TGF-β superfamily, which also includes the activins, inhibins, and the bone morphogenetic proteins (BMPs). This superfamily of proteins can induce and/or inhibit cellular proliferation or differentiation and regulate migration and adhesion of various cell types.

At least 17 RSTKs have been isolated and can be divided into 2 subfamilies identified as the type I and type II receptors. Ligand first binds to a type II receptor, which then leads to interaction with a type I receptor. When the complex between ligand and the 2 receptor subtypes forms, the type II receptor phosphorylates the type I receptor, leading to initiation of the signaling cascade.

Nonreceptor Serine/Threonine Kinases

There are more than 500 different types of kinases in the human genome and at least 125 of those are members of the serine/threonine kinase family, many of which are nonreceptor serine/threonine kinases (STKs). The 2 most commonly encountered STKs in the context of metabolic biochemistry are cAMP-dependent protein kinase (PKA) and protein kinase C (PKC). Additional serine/threonine kinases important for signal transduction are the MAP kinases, whose designation refers to mitogen-activated protein kinase. MAP kinases are also called ERKs for extracellular signal-regulated kinases.

G-Proteins

G-proteins are so called because their activities are regulated by binding and hydrolyzing GTP. When a G-protein is bound to GTP, it is in the active state and when the GTP is hydrolyzed to GDP the protein is in the inactive state.

There are 2 major classes of G-protein: the heterotrimeric (or simply the trimeric) family that are composed of 3 distinct subunits (α, β, and γ), and the monomeric class that are related to the archetypal

High-Yield Concept

The G-proteins possess intrinsic GTPase activity that is regulated by interaction with membrane-associated signal-transducing receptors (termed G-protein–coupled receptors, GPCRs) or with intracellular effector proteins.

member Ras (originally identified as the **ra**t **s**arcoma oncogene). This latter class of G-protein is also referred to as the Ras superfamily or the small GTPase family of G-proteins. The structure and function of the monomeric G-proteins is similar to that of the α-subunit of the trimeric G-proteins.

Trimeric G-Proteins

All the known cell surface receptors that are of the G-protein–coupled receptor class interact with trimeric G-proteins. The α-subunit of the trimeric class of G-proteins is responsible for the binding of GDP/GTP. When G-proteins are activated by receptors or intracellular effector proteins, there is an exchange of GDP for GTP turning on the G-protein which enables it to transmit the original activating signal to downstream effector proteins. In the trimeric class of G-protein, when associated receptor activation stimulates the GDP/GTP exchange in the α-subunit, the protein complex dissociates into separate α- and βγ-activated complexes (Figure 40-2). The released and activated βγ-complex serves as a docking site for interaction with downstream effectors of the signal-transduction cascade. Once the α-subunit hydrolyzes the bound GTP to GDP, it reassociates with the βγ complex thereby terminating its activity.

The GTPase activity of G-proteins is augmented by GTPase-activating proteins (GAPs) and the GDP/GTP exchange reaction is catalyzed by guanine nucleotide exchange factors (GEFs). Within the small GTPase family (Ras family) of G-proteins there are guanosine nucleotide dissociation inhibitors (GDIs) that maintain the G-protein in its inactive state.

The G_α-subunits are a family of 39-52 kDa proteins that share 45% to 80% amino acid similarity. The distinction of the different types of α-subunits found in trimeric G-proteins is based upon the downstream signaling responses activated or inhibited as a result of G-protein activation. These classifications include G_s (since it is the α-subunit, these designations can also be written $G_{\alpha s}$), G_i, G_q, and G_{12} (Table 40-4).

Monomeric G-proteins

The Ras superfamily of monomeric G-proteins comprises well over 100 different proteins. This superfamily is divided into 8 main families with each of these major families being comprised of several subfamilies. The 8 major families are Ras (33 members), Rho (20 members), Rab (70 members), Rap (5 members), Ran, Rheb (2 members), Rad, Rit (2 members), and Arf (30 members). The Ras subfamily is primarily responsible for regulation of events of cell proliferation, while the Rho subfamily is involved in the regulation of cell morphology through control of cytoskeletal dynamics. The Rab subfamily is involved in membrane-trafficking events and the Rap subfamily is involved in control of cell adhesion. While the Ran subfamily is responsible for the regulation of nuclear transport, the Rheb subfamily gets its name from the original member identified as **R**as **h**omolog **e**xpressed in **b**rain. The Rheb proteins are

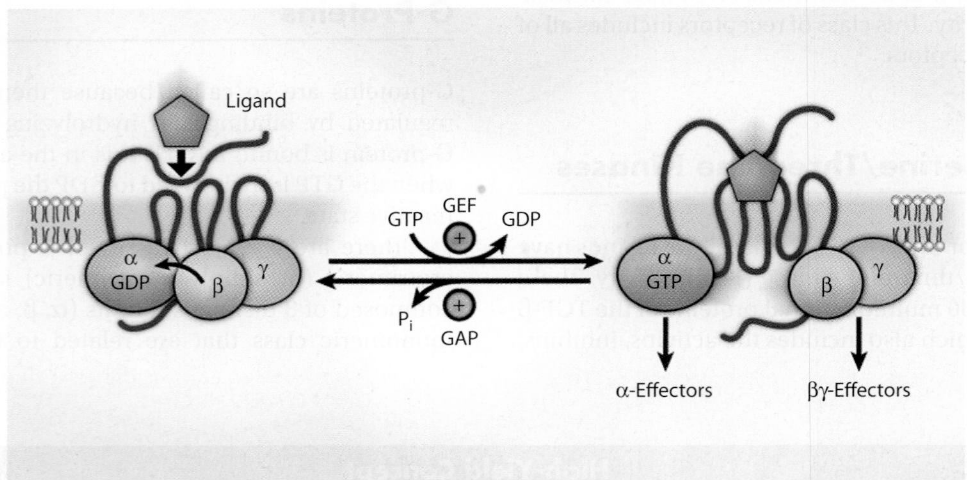

FIGURE 40-2: A diagrammatic representation of the activation of trimeric G-proteins upon ligand binding to typical G-protein–coupled receptors. Upon ligand binding to a GPCR, there is an activated exchange of GDP bound to the α-subunit for GTP catalyzed by an associated guanine nucleotide exchange factor (GEF). The resultant GTP-associated α-subunit can then activate downstream effector proteins. In some cases, G-protein βγ-subunits also regulate the activity of downstream effectors. Hydrolysis of GTP to GDP during the G-protein activation of effectors as a result of the action of GTPase-activating proteins (GAPs) results in termination of the activity of the α-subunit. Reproduced with permission of themedicalbiochemistrypage, LLC.

TABLE 40-4: Trimeric G-Protein G_α Subtypes

G_α-type	Members	Stimulated Activities
$G_{\alpha s}$ (G_s)	$G_{\alpha s}$ and $G_{\alpha olf}$	Stimulate the activity of adenylate cyclase resulting in increased production of cAMP, which then results in the activation of PKA. $G_{\alpha olf}$ was originally identified as being involved in **olf**action.
$G_{\alpha i}$ (G_i)	$G_{\alpha i}$, $G_{\alpha o}$, $G_{\alpha z}$, $G_{\alpha t}$, and $G_{\alpha gust}$	α-Subunits either inhibit adenylate cyclase, thereby inhibiting the production of cAMP ($G_{\alpha i}$, $G_{\alpha o}$, $G_{\alpha z}$) or activate phosphodiesterase ($G_{\alpha t}$, $G_{\alpha gust}$), leading to increased hydrolysis of cyclic nucleotides; the βγ-subunits that are associated with $G_{\alpha i}$ and $G_{\alpha o}$ function to open K^+ channels; $G_{\alpha t}$ is the α-subunit of transducin involved in night vision; $G_{\alpha gust}$ is the α-subunit in gustducin which is involved in the gustatory system
$G_{\alpha q}$ (G_q)	$G_{\alpha q}$, $G_{\alpha 11}$, $G_{\alpha 14}$, $G_{\alpha 15}$, and $G_{\alpha 16}$	Activates membrane-associated PLC-β, resulting in increased production of the intracellular messengers IP_3 and DAG
$G_{\alpha 12}$ (G_{12})	$G_{\alpha 12}$ and $G_{\alpha 13}$	Involved in the activation of the Rho family of monomeric G-protein

involved in the regulation of mTOR (**m**ammalian **t**arget **o**f **r**apamycin, see Chapter 46). The Arf subfamily is involved in intracellular vesicle transport.

G-Protein Regulators

The activity state of G-proteins is regulated both by the rate of GTP exchange for GDP and by the rate at which the GTP is hydrolyzed to GDP. The former process is catalyzed by guanine nucleotide exchange factors GEFs. The activity of G-proteins with respect to GTP hydrolysis is regulated by a family of proteins termed *GTPase-activating proteins, GAPs*. Both of these G-protein regulatory protein classes are termed *regulators of G-protein signaling, RGS*. Two clinically important proteins of the GAP family are the neurofibromatosis type-1 (NF1) susceptibility locus protein and the BCR locus (break point cluster region gene). The *NF1* gene is a tumor suppressor and the BCR locus is rearranged in the Philadelphia chromosome (Ph^+) observed with high frequency in chronic myelogenous leukemias (CMLs) and acute lymphocytic leukemias (ALLs).

G-Protein–Coupled Receptors

There are several different classifications of receptors that couple signal transduction through G-proteins. These classes of receptor are termed G-protein–coupled receptors (GPCRs).

There are at least 791 identified GPCRs in the human genome. Many do not have known ligands and are referred to as orphan GPCRs. The GPCR superfamily consists of 3 defined families or classes (class A, B, and C) as well as a group termed "others." The latter group consists of at least 92 GPCRs that include the adhesion, frizzled, and taste type-2 receptors.

Class A family: The class A GPCR family is referred to as the rhodopsin family. Class A contains the largest number of members compiled into at least 19 subclasses (subfamilies). Class A GPCRs include opsins, the vast majority of the odorant receptors (at least 290 receptors), and receptors for monoamines, purines, opioids, chemokines, some small peptide hormones, and the large glycoprotein hormones that consist of thyroid-stimulating hormone (TSH), luteinizing hormone (LH), and follicle-stimulating hormone (FSH).

Class B family: The class B GPCR family is referred to as the secretin-like receptor class. Class B is composed of 34 subclasses (subfamilies) and members include receptors for peptide hormones, such as parathyroid hormone (PTH), parathyroid hormone-related protein (PTHrP), and calcitonin.

High-Yield Concept

All GPCRs are composed of a similar structure that includes 7 membrane-spanning helices connected by 3 intracellular loops and 3 extracellular loops with an extracellular amino terminus and an intracellular carboxy terminus (Figure 40-3).

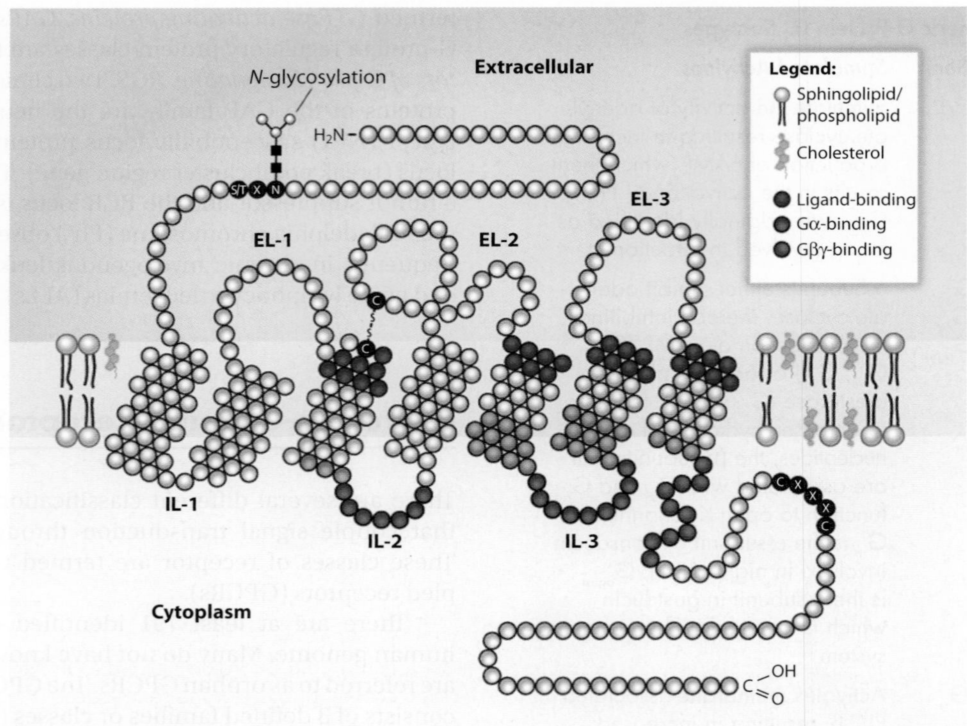

FIGURE 40-3: A diagrammatic representation of a typical member of the serpentine class of G-protein–coupled receptor. White, red, blue, and green spheres represent amino acids. Serpentine receptors are so called because they pass through the plasma membrane 7 times. Structural characteristics include the 3 extracellular loops (EL-1, EL-2, EL-3) and 3 intracellular loops (IL-1, IL-2, IL-3). Most GPCRs are modified by carbohydrate attachment to the extracellular portion of the protein. Shown is typical *N*-linked carbohydrate attachment. The different-colored spheres are involved in ligand binding and associated G-protein binding as indicated in the legend. Reproduced with permission of themedicalbiochemistrypage, LLC.

The class B family also contains the vast majority of the orphan GPCRs.

Class C family: The class C family is referred to as the metabotropic receptor or glutamate receptor-like family. Class C is composed of 8 subclasses (subfamilies) and all members form dimers and include the metabotropic glutamate receptors (mGluR), extracellular Ca^{2+}-sensing receptors, taste (gustatory) receptors, and several odorant receptors, as well as the pheromone receptors.

A characteristic feature of GPCR activity following ligand binding is a progressive loss of receptor-mediated signal transduction. This process is referred to as *desensitization* or *adaptation*. The events that reflect desensitization of a G-protein–coupled signaling system can involve the receptor itself, the G-protein associated with the receptor, and/or the downstream effector(s). In the majority of cases, it is impairment of the receptors' ability to activate its G-protein that accounts for most desensitization. This process involves phosphorylation of the GPCRs on one or more intracellular domains. On a longer time scale (several hours after ligand binding), the short-term desensitization is augmented by receptor downregulation, which involves the loss of membrane-associated receptor through a combination of protein degradation, transcriptional, and posttranscriptional mechanisms.

Heterologous desensitization involves phosphorylation of GPCRs by second-messenger–dependent kinases, such as PKA and PKC. Homologous desensitization of GPCRs involves a family of kinases termed G-protein–coupled receptor kinases (GRKs). The GRKs constitute a family of 6 mammalian serine/threonine kinases that phosphorylate ligand-activated GPCRs as their primary substrates. These 6 kinases are identified as GRK1 (originally called rhodopsin kinase); GRK2 (originally called β-adrenergic receptor kinase-1, βARK1); GRK3 (originally called β-adrenergic receptor kinase-2, βARK2); GRK4 (originally called IT-11); GRK5; and GRK6.

Upon receptor phosphorylation by a GRK, there is binding to one of a family of cytoplasmic inhibitory

TABLE 40-5: Diseases/Disorders Associated with GPCR Defects

Disease	*Affected Receptor*	*Comments*
Central hypogonadism	Gonadotropin-releasing hormone receptor, GNRHR	Impairment of pubertal maturation and reproductive function; loss-of-function mutation, autosomal recessive inheritance
Central hypothyroidism	Thyrotropin-releasing hormone receptor, TRHR	Characterized by insufficient TSH secretion resulting in low levels of thyroid hormones; loss-of-function mutation, autosomal recessive inheritance
Color blindness	Cone opsins	Loss-of-function mutation, autosomal recessive inheritance, X-linked
Congenital hypothyroidism	Thyroid-stimulating hormone receptor, TSHR	Increased levels of plasma TSH and low levels of thyroid hormone; loss-of-function mutation, autosomal recessive inheritance
Familial ACTH resistance	Adrenocorticotropic hormone, ACTH	Loss-of-function mutation, autosomal recessive inheritance
Hirschsprung disease susceptibility type 2	Endothelin receptor type B	Classic Hirschsprung disease (type 1) is caused by defects in the *RET* gene, which encodes a receptor tyrosine kinase receptor; type 2 Hirschsprung is also known as Waardenburg syndrome type 4A; involves loss-of-function mutation, complex mode of inheritance
Morbid obesity	Melanocortin 4 receptor, MC4R	Mutations in this gene are the most frequent genetic cause of severe obesity; MC4R binds α-melanocyte–stimulating hormone (α-MSH); results in loss-of-function mutation, codominant inheritance
Nephrogenic diabetes insipidus	Vasopressin V2 receptor, AVPR2	Symptoms include vomiting and anorexia, failure to thrive, fever, and constipation, caused by the inability of the renal-collecting ducts to absorb water in response to antidiuretic hormone (ADH), which is also known as arginine vasopression (AVP); loss-of-function mutation, X-linked inheritance
Retinitis pigmentosa	Rhodopsin	Loss-of-function mutation, autosomal dominant and recessive modes of inheritance

proteins called the *arrestins*. In the rhodopsin system, this inhibitory protein is referred to as arrestin. In nonretinal tissues, there are 2 related inhibitory proteins known as β-arrestin-1 and β-arrestin-2. As a result of arrestin or β-arrestin binding, the GPCR is prevented from activating its G-protein and, therefore, its downstream effector(s).

There are at least 25 known disorders that are the result of defects in a variety of different GPCRs; some of these are described in Table 40-5.

Intracellular Hormone Receptors

Upon binding ligand, the hormone-receptor complex binds to specific DNA sequences termed *hormone response elements* (*HREs*).

The nuclear receptors all contain a ligand-binding domain (LBD), a DNA-binding domain (DBD), and 2 activation function domains (AF-1 and AF-2). In addition to these critical functional domains, the nuclear

High-Yield Concept

The steroid and thyroid hormone family of receptors are proteins that effectively bypass all of the signal-transduction pathways described thus far by residing within the cytoplasm or the nucleus. Additionally, all of the hormone receptors are trifunctional. They are capable of binding hormone, binding DNA, and directly altering the transcription of target genes. Because these receptors bind ligand intracellularly and then interact with DNA directly, they are more commonly called the *nuclear receptors*.

receptors contain a total of 6 structural domains identified A through F. The AF domains are identified as the A/B domains, the DBD is the C domain, and the LBD is the E domain. Each receptor has a hinge region called the D domain and the *C*-terminus of each protein is identified as the F domain.

Based upon the sequences of the DBD and the LBD, the nuclear receptor family is divided into 6 subfamilies. Some members of the family bind to DNA as homodimers such as is the case for subfamily III receptors, which comprises the steroid receptors such as the estrogen receptor (ER), mineralocorticoid receptor (MR), progesterone receptor (PR), androgen receptor (AR), and the glucocorticoid receptor (GR). Other family members, such as all subfamily I members, bind to DNA as heterodimers through interactions with the retinoid X receptors (RXRs) (Figure 40-4).

In addition to the steroid hormone and thyroid hormone receptors, there are numerous additional family members that bind lipophilic ligands and are capable of forming heteromeric complexes with other members of the nuclear receptor family. These include the retinoid X receptors (RXRs), the liver X receptors (LXRs), the farnesoid X receptors (FXRs), and the peroxisome proliferator-activated receptors (PPARs). Many of the members of these latter families are referred to as coactivators.

RXRs: The RXRs represent a class of receptors that were originally defined by their ability to bind the retinoid, 9-*cis*-retinoic acid. There are 3 isotypes of the RXRs: RXRα, RXRβ, and RXRγ and each isotype is composed of several isoforms. The RXRs serve as obligatory heterodimeric partners for numerous members of the nuclear receptor family including the PPARs, LXRs, and FXRs. In the absence of a heterodimeric-binding partner, the RXRs are bound to hormone response elements (HREs) in DNA and are complexed with corepressor proteins that include a histone deacetylase (HDAC) and silencing mediator of retinoid and thyroid hormone receptor (SMRT) or nuclear receptor corepressor 1 (NCoR).

PPARs: The PPAR family is composed of 3 family members: PPARα, PPARβ/δ, and PPARγ. Each of these receptors forms a heterodimer with the RXRs. The first family member identified was PPARα and it was found by virtue of the fibrate class of anti-hyperlipidemic drugs binding to it and resulting in the proliferation of peroxisomes in hepatocytes, hence the derivation of the name of the protein. Although PPARγ and PPARδ are related to PPARα, they do not stimulate peroxisome proliferation. Subsequently, it was shown that PPARα is the endogenous receptor for polyunsaturated fatty acids (PUFAs). The principal function of PPARα is to induce hepatic peroxisomal fatty acid oxidation during periods of fasting. PPARγ is a master regulator of adipogenesis and is most abundantly expressed in adipose tissue. PPARγ was identified as the target of the thiazolidinedione (TZD) class of insulin-sensitizing drugs (see Chapter 46). PPARβ/δ (more commonly just PPARδ) is expressed in most

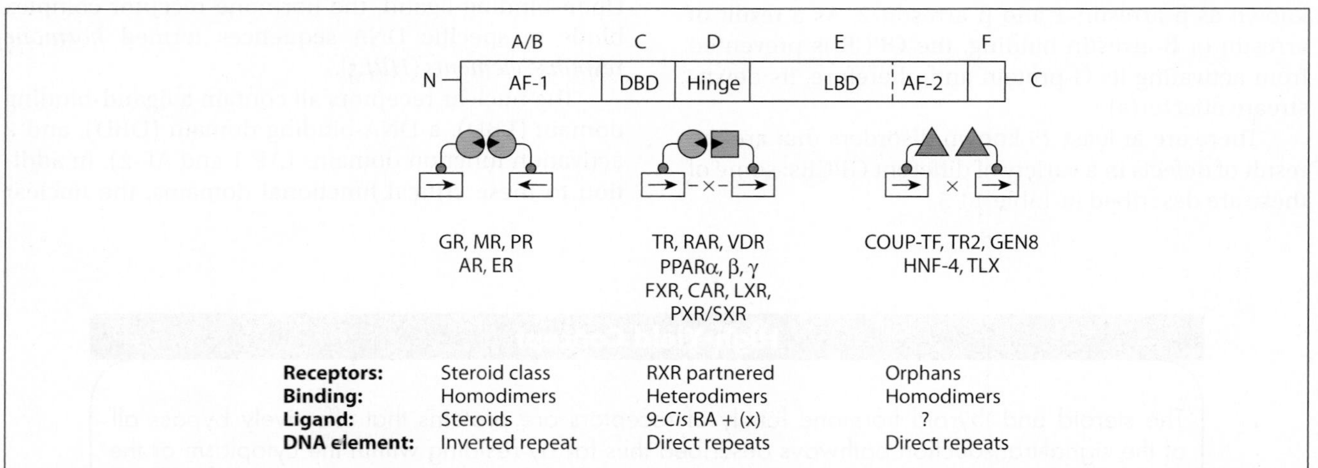

FIGURE 40-4: Structure of the nuclear receptor superfamily. Top: The 6 structural domains described in the text are indicated. Several classes of nuclear receptor are indicated (abbreviations are described in the text) along with ligand type, binding characteristics, and type of DNA element bound. Orphan nuclear receptors are so called because the ligand or ligands that are specific to those receptors have not yet been fully characterized. Murray RK, Bender DA, Botham KM, Kennelly PJ, Rodwell VW, Weil PA. *Harper's Illustrated Biochemistry*, 29th ed. New York, NY: McGraw-Hill; 2012.

tissues and is involved in the promotion of mitochondrial fatty acid oxidation, energy consumption, and thermogenesis.

LXRs: There are 2 forms of the LXRs: LXRα and LXRβ. The LXRs form heterodimers with the RXRs and as such can regulate gene expression either upon binding oxysterols (eg, 22R-hydroxycholesterol) or 9-*cis*-retinoic acid. Because the LXRs bind oxysterols, they are important in the regulation of cholesterol levels in the whole body. The primary function of LXRs in the liver is to mediate cholesterol metabolism by inducing the expression of SREBP-1c, which itself is a transcription factor involved in the control of the expression of numerous genes, including several involved in cholesterol synthesis (see Chapter 26).

FXRs: The FXRs were originally identified by their ability to bind farnesol metabolites. However, they were subsequently shown to be receptors for bile acids and bile acid metabolites. There are 2 genes encoding FXRs identified as FXRα and FXRβ. In humans, at least 4 FXR isoforms have been identified as being derived from the FXRα gene as a result of activation from different promoters and the use of alternative splicing: FXRα1, FXRα2, FXRα3, and FXRα4. FXR forms a heterodimer with members of the RXR family. Following heterodimer formation, the complex binds to specific sequences in target genes resulting in regulated expression. One major target of FXR is the small heterodimer partner (*SHP*) gene. Activation of SHP expression by FXR results in inhibition of transcription of *SHP* target genes. Of significance to bile acid synthesis, SHP represses the expression of the cholesterol 7-hydroxylase gene (CYP7A1). CYP7A1 is the rate-limiting enzyme in the synthesis of bile acids from cholesterol (see Chapter 27).

PXR: *The pregnane X receptor (PXR)* is involved in mediating drug-induced multidrug clearance. For this reason, PXR is important in protecting the body from harmful metabolites and xenobiotics. An additional physiologically significant function of PXR is in the regulation of bile acid synthesis. PXR is a recognized receptor for lithocholic acid and other bile acid precursors.

Phospholipases and Phospholipids in Signal Transduction

Protein Kinase C

Phospholipases and phospholipids are involved in the processes of transmitting ligand-receptor–induced signals from the plasma membrane to intracellular proteins. The primary protein affected by GPCR-mediated activation of phospholipases is PKC. PKC is maximally active in the presence of calcium ion and diacylglycerol (DAG). The generation of DAG occurs in response to agonist activation of various phospholipases. The principal mediators of PKC activity are receptors coupled to the activation of phospholipase C isoforms (PLCβ and PLGγ). Activation of PLC leads primarily to the hydrolysis of membrane-associated phosphatidylinositol-4,5-bisphosphate (PIP_2), leading to an increase in intracellular DAG and inositol trisphosphate (IP_3). The released IP_3 interacts with intracellular membrane receptors, leading to an increased release of stored calcium ions. Together, the increased DAG and intracellular free calcium ion concentrations lead to increased activity of PKC.

Phosphatidylinositol-3-Kinase

Phosphatidylinositol-3-Kinase (PI3K) is tyrosine phosphorylated, and subsequently activated, by various RTKs and receptor-associated PTKs. PI3K is a heterodimeric protein containing an 85-kDa and 110-kDa subunits. PI3K associates with and is activated by the PDGF, EGF, insulin, IGF-1, HGF, and NGF receptors. PI3K phosphorylates various membrane-associated phosphatidylinositols at the 3 position of the inositol ring. This activity generates additional substrates for PLC-γ, allowing a cascade of DAG and IP_3 to be generated by a single activated RTK or other protein tyrosine kinases.

Lysophospholipids

Lysophospholipids (LPLs) are minor lipid components compared to the major membrane phospholipids such as phosphatidylcholline (PC), phosphatidylethanolamine (PE), and sphingomyelin.

High-Yield Concept

Although considered minor lipid components of the cells, the lysophospholipids (LPLs) exhibit biological properties resembling those of extracellular growth factors or signaling molecules.

The most biologically significant LPLs are lysophosphatidic acid (LPA), lysophosphatidylcholine (LPC), lysophosphatidylinositol (LPI), sphingosine 1-phosphate (S1P), and sphingosylphosphorylcholine (SPC). The details of LPL activity are discussed in Chapter 23.

Phosphatases in Signal Transduction

Since activation of many signal-transduction events is controlled by addition of phosphate, removal of the incorporated phosphates must be a necessary event in order to turn off the proliferative signals. There are 2 classes of kinase, the serine/threonine and the tyrosine kinases. Thus, there are 2 classes of phosphatase necessary for phosphate removal, the serine/threonine and the tyrosine phosphatases.

Protein Tyrosine Phosphatases

There are 2 broad classes of protein tyrosine phosphatases (PTPs). One class comprises transmembrane enzymes, which contain the phosphatase activity domain in the intracellular portion of the protein. This class of PTP is commonly called the receptor (R) class of PTP. The other class includes intracellularly localized enzymes that are referred to as NT PTPs (for non-transmembrane). Currently, over 40 genes have been characterized as encoding one or the other class of PTP. The clearest studies of a role for transmembrane PTPs in signal transduction have involved the CD45 protein, which regulates tyrosine kinase activity in T-cells. One of the most important intracellular PTPs is PTP1B, which removes the tyrosine phosphates from the insulin receptor, thereby, negatively affecting the activity of the insulin receptor.

Protein Serine/Threonine Phosphatases

Phosphatases that recognize serine and/or threonine-phosphorylated proteins are referred to as *protein serine phosphatases* (*PSPs*). The PSPs are grouped into 3 major families: phosphoprotein phosphatases (PPPs), metal-dependent protein phosphatases (PPMs), and the aspartate-based phosphatases represented by FCP/SCP. This latter family name is derived from transcription factor IIF (TFIIF)–associating component of RNA polymerase II ***C***-terminal domain (CTD) ***p***hosphatase/***s***mall ***C***TD ***p***hosphatase.

Protein phosphatase 1 (PP1) is a major PSP and various isoforms of PP1 are expressed in all cells. PP1 plays an important role in a wide range of cellular processes, including protein synthesis, metabolism, regulation of membrane receptors and channels, cell division, apoptosis, and reorganization of the cytoskeletal architecture. The phosphatase activity of PP1 is regulated by a number of inhibitory proteins such as inhibitor-1 (I-1; more commonly known as PPI-1). Pyruvate dehydrogenase phosphatase is an important member of the PPM family. There is currently only 1 known substrate for FCP/SCP and as the name implies it is the *C*-terminal domain (CTD) of RNA polymerase II, which becomes phosphorylated during the course of transcription (see Chapter 36).

REVIEW QUESTIONS

1. You are studying the responses of adipocytes in culture following their exposure to γ-irradiation. In comparison to normal adipocytes you find that when glucagon is added, the normal cells release free fatty acids to the medium but the irradiated cells do not. Binding studies show that both cell populations bind the same amount of glucagon with the same dissociation kinetics, indicating the receptors on the irradiated cells are unchanged. Given these results, which of the following proteins is most likely to be defective in the irradiated cells?

A. a G_q-type G-protein
B. a G_s-type G-protein
C. phosphatidic acid phosphatase
D. phosphatidylinositol-3-kinase (PI3K)
E. protein kinase C (PKC)

Answer B: When glucagon binds its receptor on adipocytes, it activates an associated G_s-type G-protein. The activated G-protein in turn activates adenylate cyclase, which catalyzes the synthesis of cAMP from ATP. The cAMP binds to the regulatory subunits of protein kinase A (PKA), resulting in release of the catalytic subunits. One of the targets of PKA is the enzyme, hormone-sensitive lipase, HSL, which is activated by PKA-mediated phosphorylation. Activation of HSL results in increased release of fatty acid from stored triglycerides.

2. You are studying the responses of myocytes in culture following their exposure to γ-irradiation. In a comparison to normal myocytes you find that when insulin is added, the normal cells actively take up glucose but the irradiated cells do not. Binding studies show that both cell populations bind the same amount of insulin with the same dissociation kinetics, indicating the receptors on the irradiated cells are unchanged. Given these results, which of the following proteins is most likely to be defective in the irradiated cells?

A. a G_q-type G-protein
B. a G_s-type G-protein
C. phosphatidic acid phosphatase
D. phosphatidylinositol-3-kinase (PI3K)
E. protein kinase A (PKA)

Answer D: In most nonhepatic tissues, insulin increases glucose uptake by increasing the number of plasma membrane glucose transporters, specifically GLUT4 in muscle cells. Insulin action leads to an increase in the activity of PI3K, which in turn phosphorylates membrane phospholipids generating phosphatidylinositol-3,4,5-trisphophate (PIP_3) from phosphatidylinositol-4,5-bisphosphate (PIP_2). PIP_3 then activates the kinase PDK1, which in turn phosphorylates and activates a protein kinase C isoform (PKC-ζ) involved in the mobilization of GLUT4 to the plasma membrane. Loss of PI3K activation or activity would, therefore, result in reduced capacity to mobilize GLUT4-containing vesicles to the membrane.

3. Lysophospholipids (LPLs) exhibit biological properties resembling those of extracellular growth factors or signaling molecules. One of the most important LPLs is sphingosine-1-phosphate (S1P). Which of the following proteins is responsible for transmitting the signal-transduction processes of S1P?
A. a G_i-type G-protein coupled receptor (GPCR)
B. a nuclear receptor
C. a receptor serine/threonine kinase
D. a receptor tyrosine kinase
E. a receptor tyrosine phosphatase

Answer A: S1P functions via interaction with specific GPCRs. The first GPCR shown to bind S1P was called $S1P_1$. Currently, there are 5 characterized S1P receptors. The biological activities attributed to S1P interaction with any of the 5 identified receptors are broad. These activities include involvement in vascular system and central nervous system development, viability and reproduction, immune cell trafficking, cell adhesion, cell survival and mitogenesis, stress responses, tissue homeostasis, angiogenesis, and metabolic regulation.

4. You are studying the signaling pathways suspected to be altered in a colonic carcinoma. You are particularly focused on the activity of the G-protein RAS in these cells. Your studies reveal that the RAS protein can bind GTP and become activated with the same efficiency as the RAS from normal cells. However, the rate at which the cancer cell RAS activity is decreased is 10 times slower than in normal cells. Which of the following proteins is most likely to be defective in the carcinoma cells, resulting in abnormal RAS signaling?
A. a G_i-type G-protein
B. a G_q-type G-protein
C. a G_s-type G-protein
D. a GTPase-activating protein
E. a guanine nucleotide exchange factor

Answer D: The activity state of G-proteins is regulated both by the rate of GTP exchange for GDP and by the rate at which the GTP is hydrolyzed to GDP. The activity of G-proteins with respect to GTP hydrolysis is regulated by a family of proteins termed GTPase-activating proteins (GAPs). The proto-oncogenic protein, RAS, is a G-protein involved in the genesis of numerous forms of cancer (when the protein sustains specific mutations). Of particular clinical significance is the fact that oncogenic activation of RAS occurs with higher frequency than any other gene in the development of colorectal cancers.

5. Steroid hormones are able to penetrate the plasma membrane following which they bind to specific receptors inside the cell termed *intracellular* or *nuclear receptors*. If a cell line that normally were able to respond to the presence of a particular steroid hormone sustained a mutation in the ligand-binding domain of the receptor, which of the following processes would most likely be impaired?
A. posttranscriptional processing of specific mRNAs
B. posttranslational processing of specific proteins
C. replication of DNA
D. transcription of specific genes
E. translation of specific mRNAs

Answer D: Steroid hormones are lipophilic and hence freely penetrate the plasma membrane of all cells. Within target cells, steroid hormones interact with specific receptors. These receptor proteins are composed of 2 domains: a hormone-binding domain and a DNA-binding domain. Following hormone-receptor interaction, the complex is activated and enters the nucleus. The DNA-binding domain of the receptor interacts with specific nucleotide sequences termed *hormone response elements* (*HREs*). The binding of steroid-receptor complexes to HREs results in an altered rate of transcription of the associated gene(s). The effects of steroid-receptor complexes on specific target genes can be either stimulatory or inhibitory with respect to the rate of transcription.

6. In an examination of the signaling events in a myocyte cell line in culture, you find that addition of an α_1-adrenergic agonist does not lead to the expected release of stored intracellular calcium into the cytoplasm. You ascertain that the receptors for the agonist are present and that the agonist does indeed bind to the receptor. Given these results, which of the following proteins is most likely to be defective in these cells?

A. a G_s-type G-protein
B. a G_q-type G-protein
C. phosphatidic acid phosphatase
D. phosphatidylinositol-3-kinase (PI3K)
E. protein kinase A (PKA)

Answer B: The normal response of muscle cells to an α_1-adrenergic agonist binding to a receptor is the activation of an associated G_q-type G-protein. The activation of this G-protein results in the consequent activation of phospholipase Cβ (PLC-β) and the hydrolysis of membrane phosphoinositides. The released inositol trisphosphate (IP_3) binds to receptors on the sarcoplasmic reticulum, resulting in release of stored calcium into the cytosol.

7. In a comparative study of 2 related cell lines, you find that one responds normally to insulin while the other has an impaired response. You discover that both cell lines bind insulin with equal affinity, but that the impaired response is manifest in an inability to recruit the insulin response substrate-1 (IRS-1) protein to the receptor. This would most likely be due to which of the following?

A. inability of the receptor to phosphorylate the RAS G-protein
B. loss of activation of phospholipase C-β (PLC-β)
C. mutation in the tyrosine phosphate recognition site of IRS-1
D. serine phosphorylation of the insulin receptor preventing IRS-1 binding
E. tyrosine phosphorylation of the insulin receptor, leading to the loss of the IRS-1–binding site

Answer C: Binding of insulin to its receptors triggers activation of the intrinsic tyrosine kinase activity of the receptor. In addition to the incorporation of phosphate on tyrosine residues of several target proteins, the receptor autophosphorylates tyrosine residues on itself. These receptor-associated tyrosine phosphates serve as docking site for several signaling proteins including IRS-1. A loss in the ability of IRS-1 to bind to the phosphorylated tyrosine due to a mutation in the recognition motif would impair insulin-mediated signaling through IRS-1.

8. You are examining the characteristics of a cell line isolated from tumor tissue and comparing it to normal tissue cells. You find that addition of a particular growth factor to the normal cells results in increased gluconeogenesis, but that in the tumor-derived cells this effect is absent. You suspect that there is a defect in receptor-mediated signaling and surmise that there is altered G-protein–coupled activity in the tumor cells. Which type of G-protein is likely to be defective?

A. G_{12}
B. G_i
C. G_q
D. G_s

Answer D: When glucagon binds its receptor on cells, it activates an associated G_s-type G-protein. The activated G-protein in turn activates adenylate cyclase, which catalyzes the synthesis of cAMP from ATP. The cAMP binds to the regulatory subunits of protein kinase A (PKA), resulting in release of the catalytic subunits. The activation of PKA results in the activation of the normal responses of cells to glucagon.

9. Examination of cells from a tumor demonstrates that there is a defect in receptor-mediated activation of protein kinase C, PKC. You assume that this defect is due to the receptor-coupled G-protein. Which of the following G-protein classes is likely to be defective?

A. G_{12}
B. G_i
C. G_q
D. G_s

Answer C: Several members of the G-protein–coupled receptor (GPCR) family are coupled to the G_q class of G-proteins that activate membrane-associated PLC-β. Active PLC-β hydrolyzes membrane-associated phosphatidylinositol-4,5-bisphosphate, PIP_2, resulting in increased production of the intracellular messengers IP_3 and DAG. IP_3 binds to a receptor on the ER membrane and triggers the release of stored calcium ion into the cytosol. The calcium ions and the DAG serve to act as second messengers in the activation of PKC.

10. The frizzled proteins are a class of G-protein–coupled receptor (GPCR) that serves as receptors for the Wnt family of growth factors. Which of the following signal-transduction proteins is downstream of the frizzled receptors?

A. β-catenin
B. mitogen-activated protein kinase (MAPK)
C. phospholipase C-β (PLC-β)
D. protein kinase C (PKC)
E. $SMAD_4$

Answer A: The frizzled receptors couple the activity of Wnt binding to activation of a family of G-proteins called *Disheveled*. Activation of Disheveled results in inhibition of the kinase, glycogen synthase kinase 3β (GSK-3β). The consequences of Wnt-induced inhibition of GSK-3β activity is that the next protein identified in the cascade, β-catenin, is stabilized.

11. The regulatory subunit of a mutant protein kinase A (PKA) contains an amino acid substitution that prevents the binding of cAMP. As a consequence of this mutation, which of the following hormone responses is most likely to be decreased?

A. 1,25-dihydroxycholecalciferol
B. estrogen
C. glucagon
D. insulin
E. thyroxine (T_4)

Answer C: When glucagon binds its receptor on cells, it activates an associated G_s-type G-protein. The activated G-protein in turn activates adenylate cyclase, which catalyzes the synthesis of cAMP from ATP. The cAMP binds to the regulatory subunits of protein kinase A (PKA), resulting in release of the catalytic subunits. The activation of PKA results in the activation of the normal responses of cells to glucagon.

12. Phospholipase-catalyzed hydrolysis of which of the following compounds results in an increased cytosolic concentration of calcium ions in response to ligand binding to members of serotonin receptor family?

A. phosphatidylcholine
B. phosphatidylethanolamine
C. phosphatidylgylcerol
D. phosphatidylinositol bisphosphate
E. phosphatidylserine

Answer D: Several members of the serotonin receptor family are coupled to the G_q class of G-proteins that activate membrane-associated PLC-β. Active PLC-β hydrolyzes membrane-associated phosphatidylinositol-4,5-bisphosphate, PIP_2), resulting in increased production of the intracellular messengers IP_3 and DAG. IP_3 binds to a receptor on the ER membrane and triggers the release of stored calcium ion into the cytosol. The calcium ions and the DAG serve to act as second messengers in the activation of PKC.

13. Which of the following intracellular signal molecules regulates the catalysis of the conversion of GTP to cGMP?

A. cAMP
B. ceramide
C. diacylglycerol
D. inositol trisphosphate
E. nitric oxide

Answer E: Within smooth muscle cells, nitric oxide (NO) reacts with the heme moiety of a soluble guanylyl cyclase, resulting in activation of the latter and a consequent conversion of GTP to cGMP. The net effect is the activation of cGMP-dependent protein kinase (PKG) and the phosphorylation of substrates leading to smooth muscle cell relaxation.

14. You are studying the signal-transduction pathways in a cell line derived from a breast cancer. Your studies identify a novel protein that specifically binds a phosphorylated tyrosine residue on the cytoplasmic aspect of a protein kinase–linked receptor. This binding anchors the protein near the cell surface. Which of the following domains is most likely to be responsible for this binding property?

A. α-helix
B. helix-loop-helix
C. β-pleated sheets
D. SH2
E. zinc finger

Answer D: Many receptors that have intrinsic tyrosine kinase activity as well as the tyrosine kinases that are associated with cell surface receptors contain tyrosine residues that, upon phosphorylation, interact with other proteins of the signal-transduction cascade. These other proteins contain a domain of amino acid sequences that are homologous to a domain first identified in the SRC proto-oncogene. These domains are termed SH2 domains (SRC homology domain 2).

15. The pathogen, *Vibrio cholera*, secretes cholera toxin, which in turn leads to G-protein–mediated activation of adenylate cyclase in intestinal enterocytes, resulting in massive elevation in the kinase activity of protein kinase A (PKA). The phosphorylation of which of the following proteins, by PKA, results in the induction of watery diarrhea in individuals infected with this pathogen?

A. glucagon receptor
B. inositol 1,4,5-trisphosphate receptor
C. phosphorylase
D. plasma membrane chloride channel
E. tyrosine kinase

Answer D: The toxin protein from *Vibrio cholera* catalyzes the ADP ribosylation of the α-subunit of G_s G-proteins in the intestines. The ADP ribosylation causes the $G_{\alpha s}$ subunit to lose its catalytic activity in hydrolyzing GTP, so it remains activated longer than normal. Increased $G_{\alpha s}$ activation leads to increased adenylate cyclase activity, which increases the intracellular concentration of cAMP to more than 100-fold over the normal and overactivates PKA. The activated PKA then phosphorylates the cystic fibrosis transmembrane conductance regulator (CFTR) chloride channel proteins, which leads to ATP-mediated efflux of chloride ions and leads to secretion of H_2O and other ions into the intestinal lumen.

16. You are studying the activation of the enzyme adenylate cyclase in response to the addition of glucagon to myocytes in culture. You find that this activation involves the activity of a member of the G-protein family. Which of the following most closely describes the properties of this G-protein?
A. integral membrane protein
B. protein associated with the mitochondrial membrane
C. protein localized on the inner surface of the plasma membrane
D. soluble protein within the cytoplasm
E. transmembrane protein that binds a ligand at the outer surface of the plasma membrane

Answer C: The G_s family of G-proteins stimulates the activity of adenylate cyclase, resulting in increased production of cAMP from ATP. These G-proteins are localized to the inner surface of the plasma membrane in close proximity to G-protein–coupled receptors that activate the G_s protein in response to ligand binding.

17. You are studying the activity of the G-protein RAS in a cell line derived from a colonic adenoma. You find that the signal-transduction pathway induced by the activation of RAS is continuously active in these cells and that this correlates to a mutation in the *RAS* gene. This mutation in RAS most likely results in the inhibition of which of the following activities of this G-protein?
A. GTPase activity
B. guanylate cyclase activity
C. guanine nucleotide binding
D. phosphoprotein phosphatase activity
E. protein kinase activity

Answer A: The activity state of G-proteins is regulated both by the rate of GTP exchange for GDP and by the rate at which the GTP is hydrolyzed to GDP. The activity of G-proteins with respect to GTP hydrolysis is regulated by a family of proteins termed GTPase-activating proteins, GAPs. The inability to hydrolyze GTP bound to a G-protein, such as RAS, results in constant activation of the G-protein leading to inappropriate continuous activation of the growth signals transmitted by that G-protein. This can result in aberrant cell growth associated with cancer.

18. Activation of protein kinase C by epidermal growth factor requires a product of the reaction catalyzed by which of the following enzymes?
A. adenylate cyclase
B. guanylate cyclase
C. phospholipase C-γ
D. phosphoprotein phosphatase
E. protein kinase A

Answer C: When the EGF binds to its cell surface receptor, it triggers activation of the phospholipase C-γ (PLC-γ) isoform of PLC. PLC-γ hydrolyzes membrane-associated phosphatidylinositol-4,5-bisphosphate (PIP_2) into inositol trisphosphate (IP_3) and diacylglycerol (DAG). IP_3 binds to a receptor on the ER membrane and triggers the release of stored calcium ion into the cytosol. The calcium ions and the DAG serve to act as second messengers in the activation of PKC.

19. T-cells are activated when antigen-MHC complexes bind to the T-cell receptor on the cell membrane. This process activates second messengers that in turn activate protein kinase C (PKC), leading to induction of transcription factors and subsequent gene expression. Which of the following most likely represents the second messenger of this signal transduction?
A. calcium ions
B. cAMP
C. cGMP
D. diacylglycerol
E. interleukin-2 (IL-2)

Answer D: The activation of the T-cell receptor results in activation of the phospholipase C-γ (PLC-γ) isoform of PLC. PLC-γ hydrolyzes membrane-associated phosphatidylinositol-4,5-bisphosphate (PIP_2) into inositol trisphosphate (IP_3) and diacylglycerol (DAG). IP_3 binds to a receptor on the ER membrane and triggers the release of stored calcium ion into the cytosol. The calcium ions and the DAG serve to act as second messengers in the activation of PKC.

20. Cyclic AMP (cAMP) activates protein kinase A (PKA) by doing which of the following?
A. binding noncovalently to the regulatory subunit
B. binding to the receptor protein that moves to the nucleus
C. causing conformational changes in nuclear histones
D. modification of enzyme conformation by adenylation of a tyrosine residue
E. promoting proper conformation of the substrate

Answer A: cAMP binds to the regulatory subunits of PKA, resulting in release of the catalytic subunits.

Checklist

✓ Signal transduction refers to the cellular process in which a signal is conveyed to trigger a change in the activity or state of a cell.

✓ Signal transduction involves cell surface receptors and intracellular receptors, both of which bind specific ligands and become activated by this binding, resulting in a triggering of all of the resultant downstream events.

✓ Signal-transducing receptors are represented by 3 broad families, 2 of which are cell surface receptors and 1 is intracellular receptor.

✓ Cell surface receptors of one group possess intrinsic enzymatic activity while the other class is coupled to the activation of a family of GTP-hydrolyzing proteins termed G-proteins.

✓ Intracellular receptors bind lipophilic ligands and upon ligand binding the complexes binds to specific DNA sequences, resulting in regulated transcription of target genes.

✓ Receptors with intrinsic enzymatic activity generally span the plasma membrane once.

✓ The G-protein–coupled receptors (GPCR) span the membrane 7 times and are also referred to as the serpentine receptors.

✓ The GPCRs are classified into 3 distinct families (A, B, and C) and another diverse group termed "other." The human genome possesses over 791 GPCR-encoding genes. Many have unknown ligands and are referred to as "orphan" receptors.

✓ GPCRs are coupled to a family of heterotrimeric G-proteins composed of α, β, and γ subunits. The α subunits bind and hydrolyze GTP, a process that regulates the activity of the G-protein.

✓ There are 4 distinct families of G-proteins that are classified based upon the subsequent proteins whose activities they influence. This includes G-proteins that activate adenylate cyclase (G_s), those that inhibit adenylate cyclase (G_i), those that activate phospholipase C-γ (G_q), and those that activate a family of monomeric G-proteins (G_{12}).

✓ The activity state of G-proteins is regulated by the rate of GTP hydrolysis and the rate of exchange of GDP for GTP. The former involves a family of proteins called GTPase-activating proteins (GAPs) and the latter is regulated by a family of guanine nucleotide exchange factor (GEF) proteins.

✓ The intracellular receptors are all members of the steroid hormone– and thyroid hormone–binding receptors. These receptors all bind ligand inside the cell via a ligand-binding domain (LBD), possess a DNA-binding domain (DBD), and 1 or 2 activation function domains (AF-1, AF-2) that regulate the transcription of the target genes.

✓ Many signal-transduction pathways involve the phosphorylation of proteins and therefore, in order to terminate the signals there are numerous phosphatases that remove the activating phosphates. The phosphorylation events involve both tyrosine kinases and serine/threonine kinases, thus there are tyrosine phosphatases and serine/threonine phosphatase to terminate the signaling.

✓ Many plasma membrane receptors signal via the hydrolysis of membrane polyphosphoinositides (eg, phosphatidylinositol-4,5-bisphposphate, PIP_2) and the resultant products of this hydrolysis act as signaling molecules in the cascade.

CHAPTER 41 Molecular Biology Tools

CHAPTER OUTLINE

High-Yield Terms

Restriction endonuclease: any of a large family of enzymes that recognize, bind to, and hydrolyze specific nucleic acid sequences in double-stranded DNA

Cloning: in molecular biology this term refers to the production of large quantities of identical DNA molecules

Blotting: a molecular biological technique that involves the transfer of proteins, DNA, or RNA, out of the size-separating gel onto a solid support such as filter paper

DNA sequencing: the process of determining the precise order of nucleotides within a DNA molecule

Microarray: commonly known as DNA chip, is a collection of microscopic DNA spots attached to a solid surface

Gene chip: is the solid medium of a microarray containing the DNA spots

Transgenesis: the process of inserting a gene from one source into a living organism that would not normally contain it

Gene therapy: a technique involving the insertion of genes into an individual's cells and tissues to treat a disease, such as a hereditary disease in which a deleterious mutant allele is replaced with a functional one

Introduction

Modern molecular medicine encompasses the utilization of many molecular biological techniques in the analysis of disease, disease genes, and disease gene function. The study of disease genes and their function in an unaffected individual has been possible by the development of recombinant DNA and cloning techniques. The basis of the term recombinant DNA refers to the recombining of different segments of DNA. Cloning refers to the process of preparing multiple copies of an individual type of recombinant DNA molecule. The classical mechanisms for producing recombinant molecules involves the insertion of exogenous fragments of DNA into either bacterially derived plasmid (circular double-stranded autonomously replicating DNAs found in bacteria) vectors or bacteriophage (viruses that infect bacteria)-based vectors. The term vector refers to the DNA molecule used to carry or transport DNA of interest into cells.

The technologies of molecular biology are critical to modern medical diagnosis and treatment. For example, cloning allows large quantities of therapeutically beneficial human proteins to be produced in pure form. In addition the cloning of genes allows for the utilization of the DNA for treatments referred to as gene therapy which involves the introduction of a normal copy of a gene into an individual harboring a defect gene. These molecular biology techniques involve the use of a wide array of different enzymes, many of which are purified from bacteria (Table 41-1).

Restriction Endonucleases

Restriction endonucleases are enzymes that will recognize, bind to, and hydrolyze specific nucleic acid sequences in double-stranded DNA (Table 41-2).

The key to the in vitro utilization of restriction endonucleases is their strict nucleotide sequence specificity. The different enzymes are identified by being given a name indicating the bacterium from which they were isolated; for example, the enzyme EcoRI, which recognizes the sequences, 5′-GAATTC-3′, was isolated from *Escherichia coli*. One unique feature of restriction enzymes is that the nucleotide sequences they recognize are palindromic, that is, they are the same sequences in the 5′ → 3′ direction of both strands. Some restriction endonucleases make staggered symmetrical cuts away from the center of their recognition site within the DNA duplex; some make symmetrical cuts in the middle of their recognition site while still others cleave the DNA at a distance from the recognition sequence. Enzymes that make staggered cuts leave the resultant DNA with cohesive or sticky ends (Figure 41-1). Enzymes that cleave the DNA at the center of the recognition sequence leave blunt-ended fragments of DNA.

Any 2 pieces of DNA containing the same sequences within their sticky ends can anneal together and be covalently ligated together in the presence of DNA ligase. Any 2 blunt-ended fragments of DNA can be ligated together irrespective of the sequences at the ends of the duplexes.

Cloning DNA

Any fragment of DNA can be cloned once it is introduced into a suitable vector for transforming an applicable host cell. Cloning refers to the production of large quantities of identical DNA molecules and usually involves the use of a bacterial cell as a host for the DNA, although cloning can be done in eukaryotic cells as well. cDNA cloning refers to the production of a library of cloned DNAs that represent all mRNAs present in a particular cell or tissue. Genomic cloning refers to the production of a library of cloned DNAs representing the entire genome of a particular organism. From either of these types of libraries one can isolate (by a variety of screening protocols) a single cDNA or a gene clone.

In order to clone either cDNAs or copies of genes a vector is required to carry the cloned DNA. Vectors used in molecular biology are of 2 basic classes. One class of vectors is derived from bacterial plasmids (Figure 41-2). Plasmids are circular DNAs found in bacteria that replicate autonomously from the host genome. These DNAs were first identified because they harbored genes that conferred antibiotic resistance to the bacteria. The antibiotic resistance genes found on the original plasmids are used in modern in vitro engineered plasmids to allow selection of bacteria that have taken up the plasmids containing the DNAs of interest. Plasmids are limited in that in general fragments of DNA less than 10,000 base pairs (bp) can be cloned (Table 41-3).

The second class of vector is derived from the bacteriophage (bacterial virus) lambda. The advantage to lambda-based vectors is that they can carry fragments of DNA up to 25,000 bp. In the analysis of the human genome even lambda-based vectors are limiting and a yeast artificial chromosome (YAC) vector system has been developed for the cloning of DNA fragments from 500,000 bp to 3,000,000 bp.

TABLE 41-1: Common Enzymes Used in Molecular Biology

Enzyme(s)	*Activity*	*Comments*
Restriction endonucleases	Recognize specific nucleotide sequences and cleaves the DNA within or near to the recognition sequences	See Table 41-2
Reverse transcriptase (RT)	Retrovirally encoded RNA-dependent DNA polymerase	Used to convert mRNA into a complimentary DNA (cDNA) copy for the purpose of cloning cDNAs
RNase H	Recognizes RNA-DNA duplexes and randomly cleaves the phosphodiester backbone of the RNA	Used primarily to cleave the mRNA strand that is annealed to the first strand of cDNA generated by reverse transcription
DNA polymerase	Synthesis of DNA	Used during most procedures where DNA synthesis is required, also used in in vitro mutagenesis
Klenow DNA polymerase	Proteolytic fragment of DNA polymerase that lacks the $5' \rightarrow 3'$ exonuclease activity	Used to incorporate radioactive nucleotides into restriction enzyme generated ends of DNA, also can be used in place of DNA polymerase
DNA ligase	Covalently attaches a free 5′ phosphate to a 3′ hydroxyl	Used in all procedures where molecules of DNA need to be covalently attached
Alkaline phosphatase	Removes phosphates from 5′ ends of DNA molecules	Used to allow 5′ ends to be subsequently radiolabeled with the γ-phosphate of ATP in the presence of polynucleotide kinase, also used to prevent self-ligation of restriction enzyme digested plasmids and lambda vectors
Polynucleotide kinase	Introduces γ-phosphate of ATP to 5′ ends of DNA	See above for alkaline phosphatase
DNase I	Randomly hydrolyzes the phosphodiester bonds of double-stranded DNA	Is used in the identification of regions of DNA that are bound by protein and thereby protected from DNase I digestion, also used to identify transcriptionally active regions of chromatin since they are more susceptible to DNase I digestion
S_1 Nuclease	Exonuclease that recognizes single-stranded regions of DNA	Used to remove regions of single strandedness in DNA or RNA-DNA duplexes
Exonuclease III	Exonuclease that removes nucleotides from the 3′ end of DNAs	Used to generate deletions in DNA for sequencing, or to map functional domains of DNA duplexes
Terminal transferase	DNA polymerase that requires only a 3′-OH, lengthens 3′ ends with any dNTP	Used to introduce homopolymeric (same dNTP) tails onto the 3′ ends of DNA duplexes, also used to introduce radiolabeled nucleotides on the 3′ ends of DNA
T3, T7, and SP6 RNA polymerases	Bacterial virus–encoded RNA polymerase, recognizes specific nucleotide sequences for initiation of transcription	Used to synthesize RNA *in vitro*
Taq and Vent DNA polymerase	thermostable DNA polymerases	Used in PCR

High-Yield Term

The term restriction endonuclease was given to this class of bacterially derived enzymes since they were identified as being involved in restricting the growth of certain bacteriophages via a process referred to as **modification and restriction**.

TABLE 41-2: Selected Restriction Endonucleases and Their Sequence Specificities

Endonuclease	***Sequence Recognized Cleavage Sites Shown***	***Bacterial Source***
BamHI	↓ GGATCC CCTACC ↑	*Bacillus amyloliquefaciens* H
BglII	↓ AGATCT TCTAGA ↑	*Bacillus glolbigii*
EcoRI	↓ GAATTC CTTAAC ↑	*Escherichia coli* RY13
EcoRII	↓ CCTGG GGACC ↑	*Escherichia coli* R245
HindIII	↓ AAGCTT TTCGAA ↑	*Haemophilus influenzae* R_d
HhaI	↓ GCGC CGCG ↑	*Haemophilus haemolyticus*
HpaI	↓ GTTAAC CAATTC ↑	*Haemophilus parainfluenzae*
MstII	↓ CCTnAGG GGAnTCC ↑	*Microcoleus strain*
PstI	↓ CTGCAG GACGTC ↑	*Providencia stuartii* 164
TaqI	↓ TCGA AGCT ↓	*Thermus aquaticus* YTI

Abbreviations: A, adenine; C, cytosine; G, guanine; T, thymine. Arrows show the site of cleavage; depending on the site, the ends of the resulting cleaved double-stranded DNA are termed sticky ends (*BamHI*) or blunt ends (*HpaI*). The length of the recognition sequence can be 4 bp (*TaqI*), 5 bp (*EcoRII*), 6 bp (EcoRI), or 7 bp (*MstII*) or longer. By convention, these are written in the 5′ to 3′ direction for the upper strand of each recognition sequence, and the lower strand is shown with the opposite (ie, 3′ to 5′) polarity. Note that most recognition sequences are palindromes (ie, the sequence reads the same in opposite directions on the two strands). A residue designated (n) means that any nucleotide is permitted.
Murray RK, Bender DA, Botham KM, Kennelly PJ, Rodwell VW, Weil PA. *Harper's Illustrated Biochemistry.* 29th ed. New York: McGraw-Hill; 2012.

cDNA Cloning

cDNAs are made from the mRNAs of a cell by any number of related techniques (Figure 41-3). Each technique consists of first reverse transcription of the mRNA followed by synthesis of the second strand of DNA and insertion of the double-stranded cDNA into either a plasmid or lambda vector for cloning. This process creates a library of cloned cDNA representing each mRNA species. Screening of the library for a particular cDNA clone is accomplished using nucleic acid or protein-based (proteins or antibodies) probes. cDNA libraries can also be screened by biological assay of the products produced by the cloned cDNAs. Screening with proteins, antibodies, or by biological assay are mechanisms for analysis of the expression of proteins from cloned cDNAs and is given the term **expression cloning**. Nucleic acids probes can be generated from DNA (including synthetic oligonucleotides, oligos) or RNA. Nucleic acid probes can be radioactively labeled or labeled with modified nucleotides that are recognizable by specific antibodies and detected by colorimetric or chemiluminescent assays.

Genomic Cloning

The majority of genomic cloning utilizes lambda-based vector systems. These vector systems are capable of carrying 15,000 to 25,000 bp of DNA. Still larger genomic DNA fragments can be cloned into YAC vectors (see below). Genomic DNA can be isolated and cloned from any nucleated cell. The genomic DNA is first digested with restriction enzymes to generate fragments in the size range that are optimal for the vector being utilized for cloning. Given that some genes encompass many more base pairs than can be inserted into a given vector, the clones that are present in a genomic library must be overlapping (Figure 41-4). In order to generate overlapping clones, the DNA is only partially digested with restriction enzymes. This means that not every restriction site, present in all the copies of a given gene in the preparation of DNA, is cleaved. The partially digested DNA is then size-selected by a variety of techniques (eg, gel electrophoresis or gradient centrifugation) prior to cloning. Screening of genomic libraries is accomplished primarily with nucleic acid-based probes. However, they can be screened with proteins that are known to bind specific sequences of DNA (eg, transcription factors).

Cloning Genomic DNA in YAC Vectors

YAC vectors allow the cloning, within yeast cells, fragments of genomic DNA that approach 3,000,000 bp (Figure 41-5). These vectors contain several elements of typical yeast chromosomes, hence the term YAC.

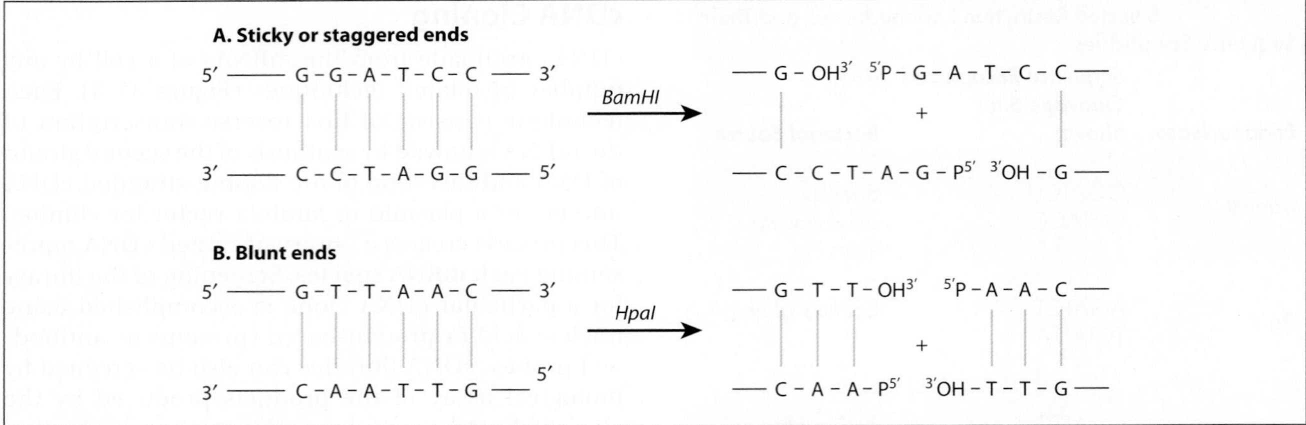

FIGURE 41-1: Results of restriction endonuclease digestion. Digestion with a restriction endonuclease can result in the formation of DNA fragments with sticky, or cohesive, ends **(A)** or blunt ends **(B)**; phosphodiester backbone, black lines; interstrand hydrogen bonds between purine and pyrimidine bases, blue. This is an important consideration in devising cloning strategies. Murray RK, Bender DA, Botham KM, Kennelly PJ, Rodwell VW, Weil PA. *Harper's Illustrated Biochemistry*. 29th ed. New York: McGraw-Hill; 2012.

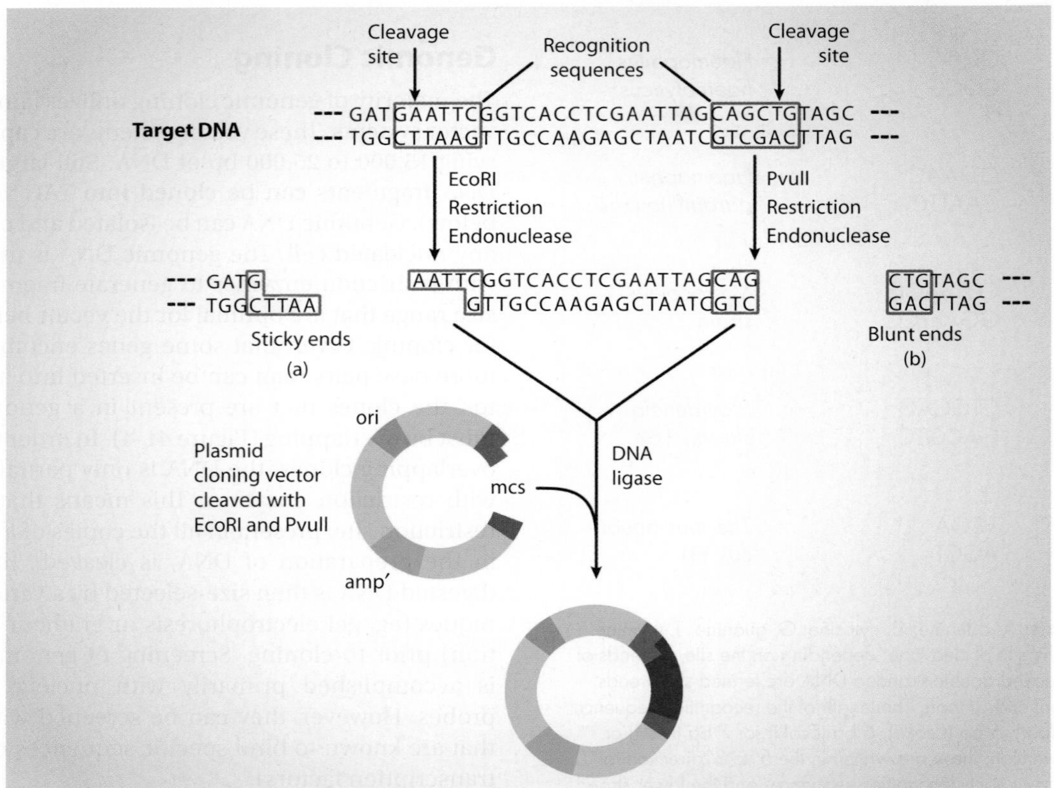

FIGURE 41-2: Typical plasmid vector cloning. A plasmid cloning vector is digested with the same enzymes (EcoRI and PvuII) as the target DNA. Most cloning plasmids have a section of unique restriction endonuclease sites called the multicloning site (MCS). The target DNA is ligated into the plasmid with DNA ligase with the result being a recombinant plasmid that can be used to transfect bacteria. Reproduced with permission of themedicalbiochemistrypage, LLC.

TABLE 41-3: Cloning Capacities of Common Cloning Vectors

Vector	*DNA Insert Size (kb)*
Plasmid pUC19	0.01-10
Lambda charon 4A	10-20
Cosmids	35-50
BAC, P1	50-250
YAC	500-3000

Murray RK, Bender DA, Botham KM, Kennelly PJ, Rodwell VW, Weil PA. *Harper's Illustrated Biochemistry*. 29th ed. New York: McGraw-Hill; 2012.

The YAC vectors contain a yeast centromere (CEN), yeast telomeres (TEL), and a yeast autonomously replicating sequence (ARS). Yeast ARS are essentially origins of replication that function in yeast cells autonomously from the replication of yeast chromosomal replication origins. YAC vectors also contain genes (eg, URA3, a gene involved in uracil synthesis) that allow selection of yeast cells that have taken up the vector. In order to propagate the vector in bacterial cells, prior to insertion of genomic DNA, YAC vectors contain a bacterial replication origin and a bacterial selectable marker such as the gene for ampicillin resistance.

Analysis of Cloned Products

The analysis of cloned cDNAs and genes involves a number of techniques. The initial characterization usually involves mapping of the number and location of different restriction enzyme sites. This information is useful for DNA sequencing since it provides a means to digest the clone into specific fragments for subcloning, a process involving the cloning of fragments of a particular cloned DNA. Once the DNA is fully characterized cDNA clones can be used to produce RNA in vitro and the RNA translated in vitro to characterize the encoded protein. Clones of cDNAs also can be used as

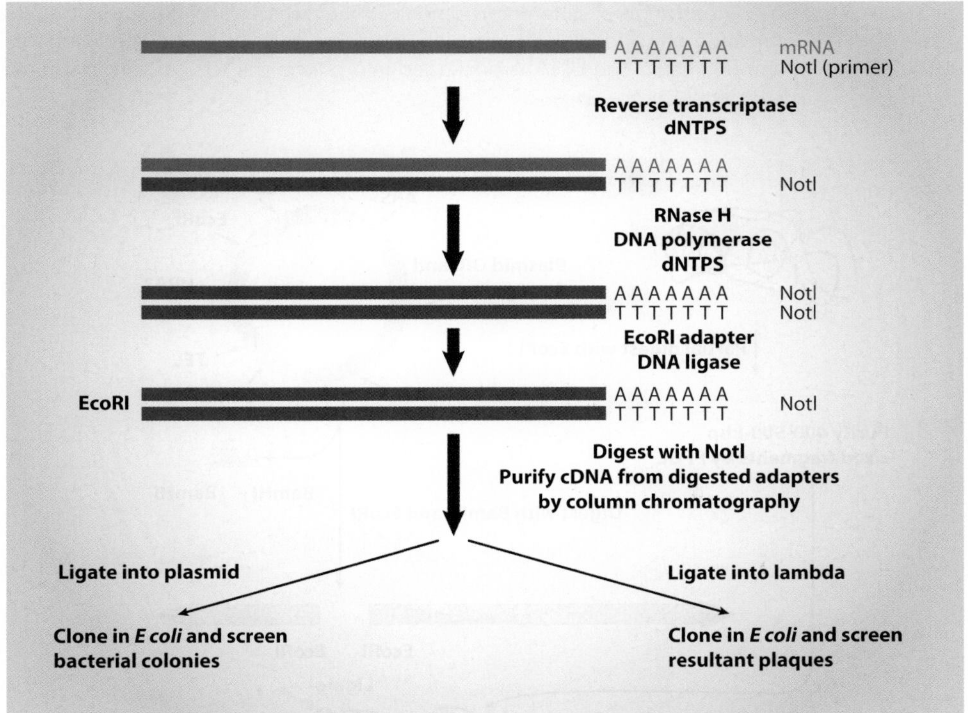

FIGURE 41-3: Typical process for production and cloning of cDNA. This example shows the use of a specific primer-adapter containing the sequences for the restriction enzyme NotI in addition to the poly(T) for annealing to the poly(A) tail of the RNA. It is possible to use only poly(T) or poly(T) with other restriction sites or random primers (a mixture of oligos that contain random sequences) to initiate the first strand cDNA reaction. In some cases poly(T) priming does not allow for extension of the cDNA to the 5′-end of the RNA, the use of random primers can overcome this problem since they will prime first strand synthesis all along the mRNA. This technique shows the ligation of EcoRI adapters followed by EcoRI and NotI digestion. This process allows the cDNAs to all be cloned in one direction, termed directional cloning.

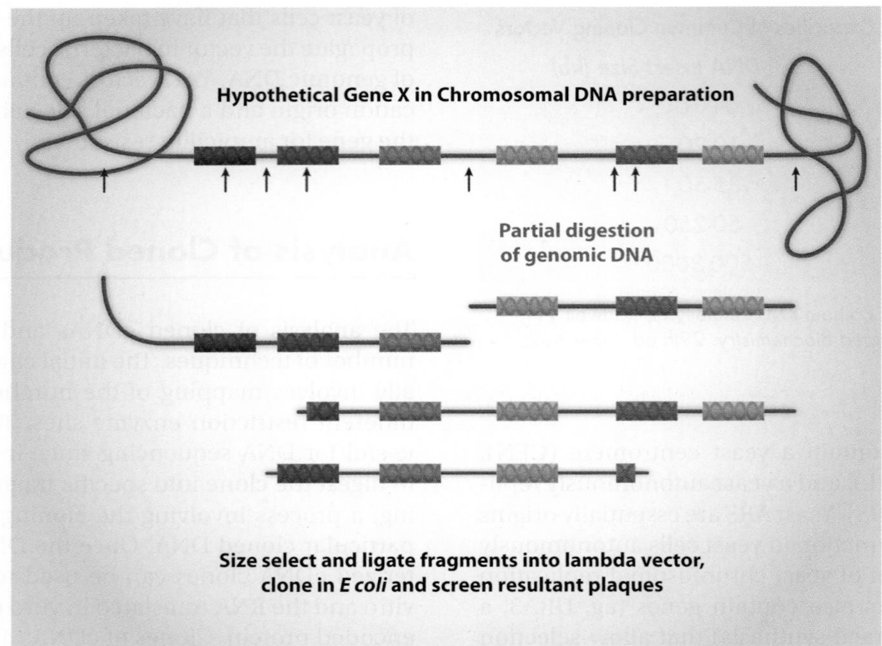

FIGURE 41-4: Diagrammatic representation of cloning genomic DNA. The boxes indicate exons and the lines separating the boxes represent introns. The bold arrows indicate the positions of restriction enzyme sites, for example, Sau3AI. Following partial enzyme digestion a wide range of different fragments of the gene will be generated; 4 possible fragments are indicated. Fragments in the size range of 15 to 25 kilobase pairs (kbp) are purified by gel electrophoresis or gradient centrifugation and ligated into a lambda vector. The DNA is packaged into phage particles in vitro and used to infect *E coli*. Reproduced with permission of themedicalbiochemistrypage, LLC.

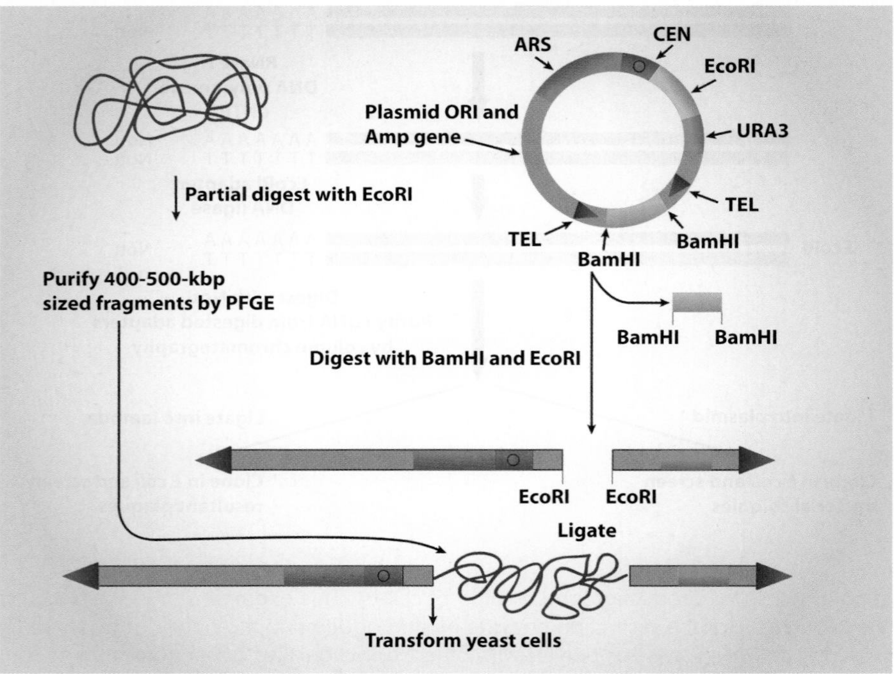

FIGURE 41-5: Diagrammatic representation of a typical YAC vector used to clone genomic DNA. The vector contains yeast telomeres (TEL), a centromere (CEN), a selectable marker (URA3), and autonomously replicating sequences (ARS) as well as bacterial plasmid sequences for antibiotic selection and replication in *E coli*. PFGE, pulsed field gel electrophoresis. Reproduced with permission of themedicalbiochemistrypage, LLC.

probes to analyze the structure of a gene by **Southern blotting** or to analyze the size of the RNA and pattern of its expression by **Northern blotting** (Figure 41-6). Northern blotting is also a useful tool in the analysis of the exon-intron organization of gene clones since only fragments of a gene that contain exons will hybridize to the RNA on the blot. Proteins in tissues or those expressed by cloned cDNA can be analyzed by the technique of **Western blotting**.

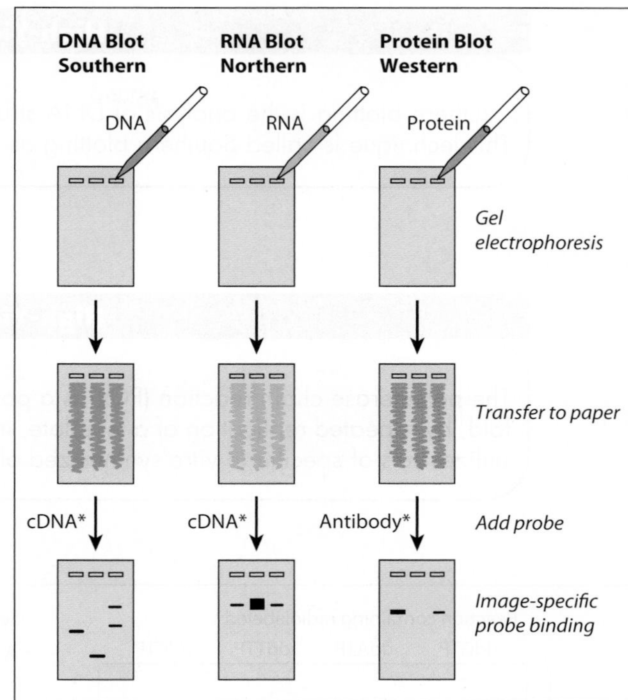

FIGURE 41-6: The blot transfer procedure. In a Southern, or DNA blot transfer, DNA isolated from a cell line or tissue is digested with one or more restriction enzymes. This mixture is pipetted into a well in an agarose or polyacrylamide gel and exposed to a direct electrical current. DNA, being negatively charged, migrates toward the anode; the smaller fragments move the most rapidly. After a suitable time, the DNA within the gel is denatured by exposure to mild alkali and transferred to nitrocellulose or nylon paper, resulting in an exact replica of the pattern on the gel, by the blotting technique devised by Southern. The DNA is bound to the paper by exposure to heat or UV, and the paper is then exposed to the labeled cDNA probe, which hybridizes to complementary strands on the filter. After thorough washing, the paper is exposed to x-ray film or an imaging screen, which is developed to reveal several specific bands corresponding to the DNA fragment that recognized the sequences in the cDNA probe. The RNA, or Northern, blot is conceptually similar. RNA is subjected to electrophoresis before blot transfer. This requires some different steps from those of DNA transfer, primarily to ensure that the RNA remains intact, and is generally somewhat more difficult. In the protein, or Western, blot, proteins are electrophoresed and transferred to special paper that avidly binds proteins and then probed with a specific antibody or other probe molecule. (Asterisks signify labeling, either radioactive or fl uorescent.) In the case of Southwestern blotting (see the text; not shown), a protein blot similar to that shown above under "Western" is exposed to labeled nucleic acid, and protein-nucleic acid complexes formed are detected by autoradiography or imaging. Murray RK, Bender DA, Botham KM, Kennelly PJ, Rodwell VW, Weil PA. *Harper's Illustrated Biochemistry*. 29th ed. New York: McGraw-Hill; 2012.

Southern Blotting

The DNA to be analyzed is first digested with a given restriction enzyme, then the resultant DNA fragments are separated in an agarose gel. The DNA is transferred from the gel to a solid support, such as a nylon filter, by either capillary diffusion or under electric current. The DNA is fixed to the filter by baking or ultraviolet light treatment. The filter can then be probed for the presence of a given fragment of DNA by various radioactive or nonradioactive means.

Northern Blotting

Northern blotting involves the analysis of RNA following its attachment to a solid support. The RNA is sized by gel electrophoresis then transferred to nitrocellulose or nylon filter paper as for Southern blotting. Probing the filter for a particular RNA is done similarly to probing of Southern blots.

Western Blotting

Western blotting involves the analysis of proteins following attachment to a solid support. The proteins are separated by size SDS-PAGE and electrophoretically transferred to nitrocellulose or nylon filters. The filter is then probed with antibodies raised against a particular protein or they can be probed with DNA probes if analyzing DNA-binding proteins.

DNA Sequencing

Sequencing of DNA can be accomplished by either chemical or enzymatic means. The original technique for sequencing, Maxam-Gilbert sequencing, relies on the nucleotide-specific chemical cleavage of DNA and is not routinely used any more. The enzymatic technique, Sanger sequencing, involves the use of dideoxynucleotides (2′,3′-dideoxy) that terminate DNA synthesis and is, therefore, also called dideoxy chain termination sequencing (Figure 41-7).

High-Yield Concept

Southern blotting is the analysis of DNA structure following its attachment to a solid support. This technique is called Southern blotting as it was developed by Edwin Southern.

High-Yield Concept

The polymerase chain reaction (PCR) is a powerful technique used to amplify DNA millions of fold, by repeated replication of a template, in a short period of time (Figure 41-8). The process utilizes sets of specific *in vitro* synthesized oligonucleotides to prime DNA synthesis.

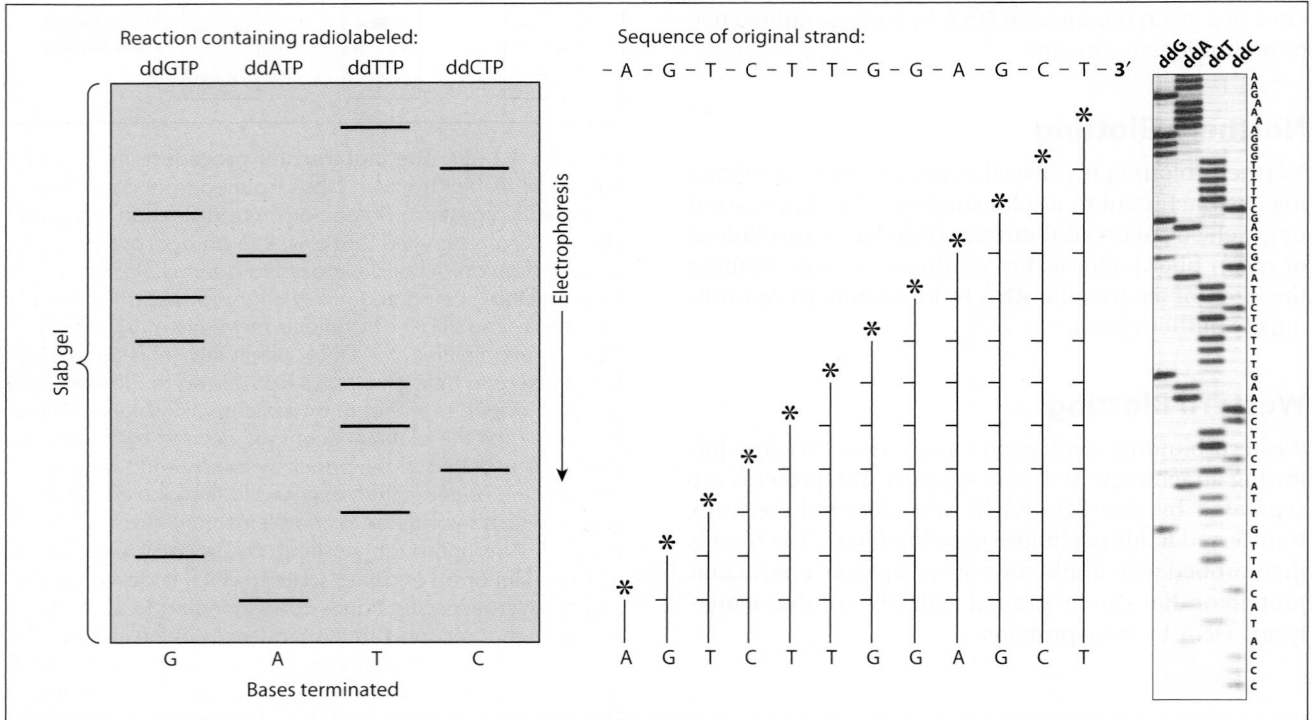

FIGURE 41-7: Sequencing of DNA by the chain termination method devised by Sanger. The ladder-like arrays represent from bottom to top all of the successively longer fragments of the original DNA strand. Knowing which specific dideoxynucleotide reaction was conducted to produce each mixture of fragments, one can determine the sequence of nucleotides from the unlabeled end toward the labeled end (*) by reading up the gel. The base-pairing rules of Watson and Crick (A-T, G-C) dictate the sequence of the other (complementary) strand. (Asterisks signify the site of radiolabeling.) Shown (left, middle) are the terminated synthesis products of a hypothetical fragment of DNA, sequence shown. An autoradiogram (right) of an actual set of DNA sequencing reactions that utilized the four ^{32}P-labeled dideoxynucleotides indicated at the top of the scanned autoradiogram (ie, dideoxy(dd)G, ddA, ddT, ddC). Electrophoresis was from top to bottom. The deduced DNA sequence is listed on the right side of the gel. Note the log-linear relationship between distance of migration (ie, top to bottom of gel) and DNA fragment length. Current state-of-the-art DNA sequencers no longer utilize gel electrophoresis for fractionation of labeled synthesis products. Moreover in the NGS sequencing platforms, synthesis is followed by monitoring incorporation of the four fluorescently labeled dNTPs. Murray RK, Bender DA, Botham KM, Kennelly PJ, Rodwell VW, Weil PA. *Harper's Illustrated Biochemistry*. 29th ed. New York: McGraw-Hill; 2012.

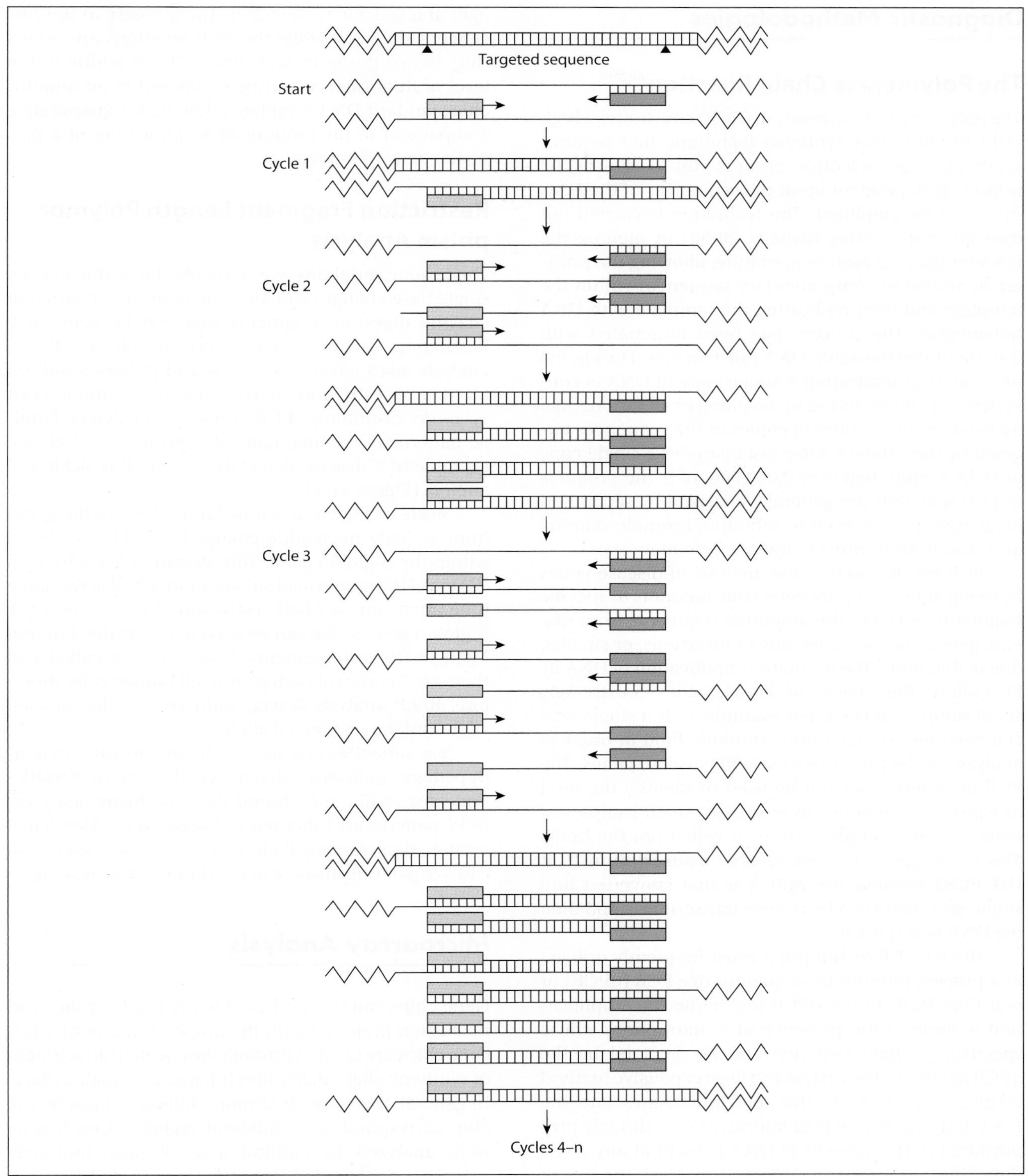

FIGURE 41-8: The polymerase chain reaction is used to amplify specific gene sequences. Double-stranded DNA is heated to separate it into individual strands. These bind two distinct primers that are directed at specific sequences on opposite strands and that define the segment to be amplified. DNA polymerase extends the primers in each direction and synthesizes 2 strands complementary to the original 2. This cycle is repeated several times, giving an amplified product of defined length and sequence. Note that the 2 primers are present in vast excess. Murray RK, Bender DA, Botham KM, Kennelly PJ, Rodwell VW, Weil PA. *Harper's Illustrated Biochemistry.* 29th ed. New York: McGraw-Hill; 2012.

Diagnostic Methodologies

The Polymerase Chain Reaction

The polymerase chain reaction (PCR) constitutes a high yield in vitro DNA synthesis technique that requires synthetic oligonucleotide primers. The design of the primers is dependent upon the sequences of the DNA that is to be amplified. The technique is carried out through many cycles (usually 20-50) of melting the DNA template at high temperature, allowing the primers to anneal to complimentary sequences within the template and then replicating the template with DNA polymerase. The process has been automated with the use of thermostable DNA polymerases. During the first round of replication a single copy of DNA is converted to 2 copies and so on resulting in an exponential increase in the number of copies of the sequences targeted by the primers. After just 20 cycles a single copy of DNA is amplified over 2,000,000 fold. The products of PCR reactions are generally analyzed by separation in agarose gels followed by ethidium bromide staining and visualization with UV transillumination.

PCR can be used in the analysis of disease genes by being able to amplify detectable amounts of specific fragments of DNA. The amplified fragments from disease genes may be larger, due to insertions, or smaller, due to deletions. The dramatic amplification of DNA by PCR allows the analysis of disease genes in extremely small samples of DNA. For example, only a single fetal cell need be extracted from amniotic fluid in order to analyze for the presence of specific disease genes. The PCR technique also can be used to identify the level of expression of genes in extremely small samples of material, for example, tissues or cells from the body. This technique is termed **reverse transcription-PCR (RT-PCR)** because the mRNA is first converted into single-stranded DNA by reverse transcriptase and then the DNA is amplified.

The RT-PCR technique is most frequently utilized in a process referred to as quantitative PCR (qPCR) or real-time PCR. In the qPCR technique the amplification is done in the presence of a fluorophore whose spectrum of light emission can be detected by the qPCR machine. The easiest and least expensive method involves a fluorescent dye that intercalates into the DNA and thus the level of fluorescence is directly proportional to the amount of DNA present at any given time. The more sensitive method involves the use of an oligo with a fluorophore attached but is unable to emit light in this form. The oligo is designed to hybridize to sequences between the 2 amplification primers. During DNA synthesize the fluorophore-tagged oligo is degraded and when released the fluorophore emits light at a specific wavelength. The increase in fluorescence is detected while the PCR reactions are occurring, hence the term real-time PCR. In addition, the level of fluorescence can be compared to an amplifiable standard DNA template allowing for quantitative comparison of the amount of amplification of a particular gene of interest.

Restriction Fragment Length Polymorphism Analysis

The genetic variability at a particular locus due to even single base changes can alter the pattern of restriction enzyme digestion fragments that can be generated. Restriction fragment length polymorphism (RFLP) analysis takes advantage of this and utilizes Southern blotting of restriction enzyme digested genomic DNA or more commonly, PCR products, to detect familial patterns of the fragments of a given gene. A classic example of a disease detectable by RFLP is sickle cell anemia (Figure 41-9).

Sickle cell anemia results (at the level of the gene) from a single nucleotide change (A to T) at codon 6 within the β-globin gene. This alteration leads to a glu (G) to val (V) amino acid substitution, while at the same time abolishing a MstII restriction site. As a result, a β-globin gene probe can be used to detect the different MstII restriction fragments. It should be recalled that there are 2 copies of each gene in all human cells, therefore, RFLP analysis detects both copies: the affected allele and the unaffected allele.

Size variability in detectable fragments within a family pedigree indicates differences in the pattern of restriction sites within and around the gene being analyzed. RFLP patterns are inherited and segregate in Mendelian fashion, thus allowing their use in genotyping such as in cases of paternity dispute or in criminal investigations.

Microarray Analysis

Gene chips can be purchased ready-made or they can be custom prepared with the proper equipment. Most gene chips are created through the covalent attachment of synthetic oligonucleotides (oligos) to a small surface. In general, there are 20 or more different oligos on the chip corresponding to different regions of each gene to be analyzed. In addition, a set of oligos that each contain a nucleotide mismatch are included as negative controls for each gene. The technology of creating gene chips is such that there can be tens of thousands of different genes represented on a single chip approximately 2 cm^2. Many custom gene arrays are created by robotic spotting of DNA onto glass slides.

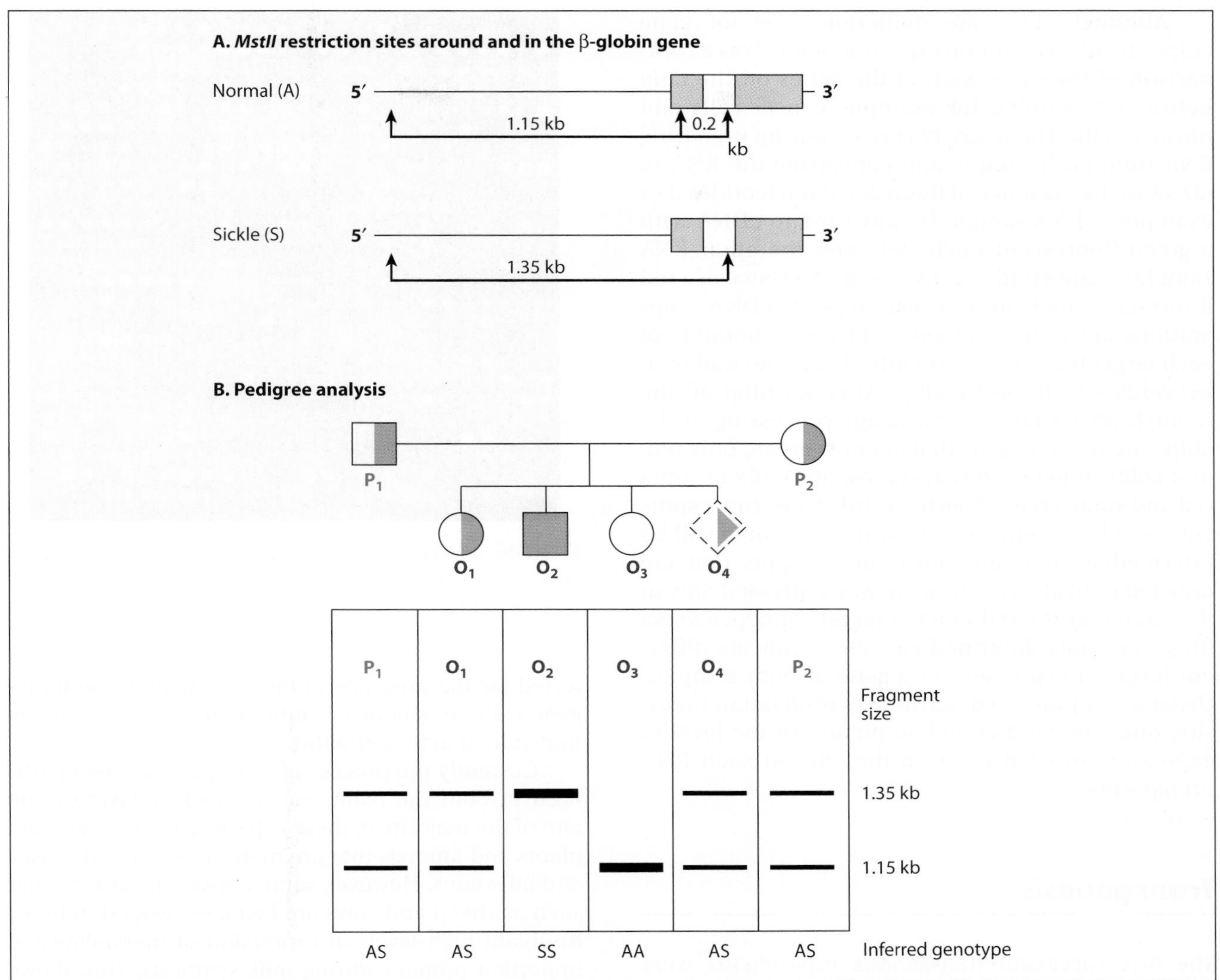

FIGURE 41-9: Pedigree analysis of sickle cell disease. The top part of the figure **(A)** shows the first part of the β-globin gene and the *MstII* restriction enzyme sites in the normal (A) and sickle-cell (S) β-globin genes. Digestion with the restriction enzyme *MstII* results in DNA fragments 1.15 kb and 0.2 kb long in normal individuals. The T-to-A change in individuals with sickle cell disease abolishes 1 of the 3 *MstII* sites around the β-globin gene; hence, a single restriction fragment 1.35 kb in length is generated in response to *MstII*. This size difference is easily detected on a Southern blot. (The 0.2-kb fragment would run off the gel in this illustration.) **(B)** Pedigree analysis shows 3 possibilities: AA = normal (open circle); AS = heterozygous (half-solid circles, half-solid square); SS = homozygous (solid square). This approach can allow for prenatal diagnosis of sickle-cell disease (dash-sided square). Murray RK, Bender DA, Botham KM, Kennelly PJ, Rodwell VW, Weil PA. *Harper's Illustrated Biochemistry*. 29th ed. New York: McGraw-Hill; 2012.

High-Yield Concept

Microarray analysis involves the use of what are commonly called "**gene chips**" to determine the expression of a large set of genes at the same time in a single experiment.

Although there are numerous uses for gene chips, the most common experiment involves a comparison of the expression of the genes on the chip between 2 samples, for example, cancer cells and normal cells. The assay is carried out by preparing RNA from each sample and converting the RNA to cDNA in the presence of fluorescent nucleotides. For example, 1 RNA sample is converted to cDNA with a green fluorescent nucleotide and the other RNA sample is converted to cDNA in the presence of a red fluorescent nucleotide. These "tagged" cDNA preparations are called "targets" and equal amounts of each target preparation are mixed together and then hybridized to the gene chip. After washing off the nonhybridized targets and image processing of the chip, one will see spots that are only green, only red, or a color in between that represents a mix of some red and some green (Figure 41-10). Thus, some spots will be yellow, some will be orange, or some will be intermediate (combination) colors. Spots that are only red indicate that the gene was expressed only in the source of the red labeled targets and vice versa for green spots. Intermediate colors indicate different levels of expression of a gene in both samples. Using a computer to determine hybridization intensity, one will get a complete picture of the level of expression of each gene on the chip in each RNA preparation.

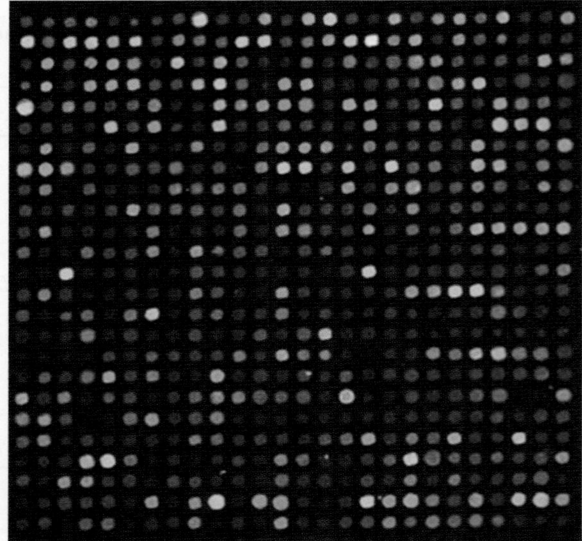

FIGURE 41-10: Example results from a spotted DNA array screen. Reproduced with permission of themedicalbiochemistrypage, LLC.

Transgenesis

The first successful transgenesis experiments were carried out in mice. To create a transgenic animal the gene of interest must be passed from generation to generation, that is, it must be inherited in the germ line. To accomplish this with mice or livestock animals, vectors containing the gene of interest with appropriate regulatory elements (eg, the β-lactoglobulin promoter if expression of the transgene in the milk is desired) are injected into the nucleus of fertilized eggs. The eggs are then transplanted into the uterus of receptive females for development of the potential transgenic offspring. In order to determine germ line transmission of the transgene, the chromosomal DNA of their offspring is tested for the presence of the transgene. If the transgene exhibits Mendelian inheritance, then it is being transmitted in the germ line.

Currently the process of transgenesis is being utilized in both the plant and livestock industries. The aim of the majority of these experiments is to generate plants and animals that are more resistant to diseases and infections. However, some transgenic farm animal such as sheep and cows are being developed in order to obtain high levels of expression of therapeutically important proteins during milk synthesis. This allows large amounts of the protein of interest to be purified from the milk of the transgenic animals.

Gene Therapy

Transgenesis with humans would allow for the elimination of disease genes in a population of offspring; however, technical as well as ethical issues likely will prevent any transgenic experiments to be carried out with human eggs. Therefore, the ability to replace known

High-Yield Concept

Transgenesis refers to the process of introducing exogenous genes into the germ line of an organism.

disease genes with normal copies in afflicted humans is the ultimate goal of gene therapy. Human gene therapy protocols aim to introduce correcting copies of disease genes into somatic cells of the affected individual. Expression of a correct copy of an affected gene in somatic cells prevents transmission through the germ line, thereby avoiding many of the ethical issues of transgenesis. This is analogous to treatment of individuals by organ or tissue transplantation.

The most common techniques utilized in gene therapy studies are the introduction of the corrected gene into bone marrow cells, skin fibroblasts, or hepatocytes. The vectors most commonly utilized are derived from modified retroviruses. The advantage of retroviral-based vector systems is that expression occurs in most cell types. A number of human inherited disorders have been corrected in cultured cells, and several diseases (eg, malignant melanoma and severe combined immunodeficiency disease, SCID) are currently being treated by gene therapy techniques indicating that gene therapy is likely to be a powerful therapeutic technique against a host of diseases in coming years (Table 41-4).

TABLE 41-4: Human Disorders Treated in Cultured Cells by Gene Therapy

Disorder	*Affected Gene*
SCID	Adenosine deaminase (ADA)
SCID	Purine nucleoside phosphorylase (PNP)
Lesch-Nyhan syndrome	Hypoxanthine-guanine phosphoribosyltransferase (HGPRT)
Gaucher disease	Acid β-glucosidase (glucocerebrosidase)
Familial hypercholesterolemia (FH)	LDL receptor
Phenylketonuria (PKU)	Phenylalanine hydroxylase
β-Thalassemia	β-Globin
Hemophilia B	Factor IX

REVIEW QUESTIONS

1. You are carrying out experiments designed to utilize DNA encoding a wild-type gene to treat a disease resulting from inheritance of a defective gene. Which of the following techniques would be the most useful in pursuit of the goal of these studies?
   A. gene therapy
   B. polymerase chain reaction, PCR
   C. restriction fragment length polymorphism, RFLP
   D. RNAi
   E. transgenesis

Answer A: Transgenesis with humans would allow for the elimination of disease genes in a population of offspring; however, technical as well as ethical issues likely will prevent any transgenic experiments to be carried out with human eggs. Therefore, the ability to replace known disease genes with normal copies in afflicted humans is the ultimate goal of gene therapy. Human gene therapy protocols aim to introduce correcting copies of disease genes into somatic cells of the affected individual. Expression of a correct copy of an affected gene in somatic cells prevents transmission through the germ line, thereby avoiding many of the ethical issues of transgenesis. This is analogous to treatment of individuals by organ or tissue transplantation.

2. You wish to analyze the pattern of genes expressed in a breast cancer in order to identify potential differences to normal breast tissue cells. Which of the following enzymes is most useful to you in your anticipated studies?
   A. DNA ligase
   B. DNase I
   C. polynucleotide kinase
   D. reverse transcriptase
   E. restriction endonucleases

Answer D: One of the most effective ways to ascertain gene expression differences between 2 different cell types is to analyze the mRNA differences. This can be done by a number of different techniques, the most rapid of which would be with the use of gene microarrays. In order to successfully utilize gene microarrays requires that the mRNAs first be converted into cDNAs with the use of reverse transcriptase.

3. You wish to incorporate radioactive phosphate onto the 5′-ends of a fragment of DNA so that it can be used as a probe on a Southern blot of genomic DNA. Which of the following enzymes is required in order for you to carry out the labeling of the DNA with radioactive phosphate?
   A. DNA ligase
   B. DNA polymerase

C. polynucleotide kinase
D. reverse transcriptase
E. terminal transferase

Answer C: Polynucleotide kinase introduces γ-phosphate of ATP to 5′-ends of DNA. In order for this reaction to take place the phosphate must first be removed and this is accomplished with the use of alkaline phosphatase.

4. You are testing the activity of an enzyme you have isolated from bovine pancreas. You find that when this enzyme is added to nuclei isolated from adipocytes and the products are subsequently analyzed by gel electrophoresis that the DNA in the nuclei is degraded into relatively discrete sizes approximately 150 bp in length. Which of the following most likely represents the enzyme activity in your pancreatic preparation?
A. a restriction endonuclease
B. DNA ligase
C. DNA polymerase
D. DNase I
E. reverse transcriptase

Answer D: DNase I randomly hydrolyzes the phosphodiester bonds of double-stranded DNA. The enzyme is used in the identification of regions of DNA that are bound by protein, and thereby protected from DNase I digestion. Since the nucleosomes would protect regions of DNA of approximately 150 bp in length, DNase I digestion would result in the generation of a high-proportion DNA fragments of that length. Although restriction enzymes digest DNA at discrete sequence motifs, the distribution of these motifs is essentially randomly distributed, and therefore would not result in most of the DNA being found as 150-bp fragments.

5. Which of the following is a means to identify all of the genes that are active in any given cell under any given set of conditions?
A. cDNA cloning
B. genomic cloning
C. polymerase chain reaction, PCR
D. Southern blotting
E. restriction fragment length polymorphism, RFLP

Answer A: Any fragment of DNA can be cloned once it is introduced into a suitable vector for transforming a bacterial host. Cloning refers to the production of large quantities of identical DNA molecules and usually involves the use of a bacterial cell as a host for the DNA, although cloning can be done in eukaryotic cells as well. cDNA cloning refers to the production of a library of cloned DNAs that represent all mRNAs present in a particular cell or tissue.

6. You are examining a 7-year-old female who suffers from recurrent vasculo-occlusive episodes. Her parents report that she complains often of severe bone pain. You suspect the patient is suffering from sickle cell anemia. Which of the following tests would be appropriate to the confirmation of this diagnosis?
A. cDNA cloning
B. genomic cloning
C. polymerase chain reaction, PCR
D. Southern blotting
E. restriction fragment length polymorphism, RFLP

Answer E: Sickle cell anemia results (at the level of the gene) from a single nucleotide change (A to T) at codon 6 within the β-globin gene. This alteration leads to a glu (G) to val (V) amino acid substitution, while at the same time abolishing a MstII restriction site. As a result a β-globin gene probe can be used to detect the different MstII restriction fragments. It should be recalled that there are 2 copies of each gene in all human cells; therefore, RFLP analysis detects both copies: the affected allele and the unaffected allele.

7. Which of the following enzymes is required in order to acquire templates for the process of quantitative PCR?
A. DNA I
B. DNA ligase
C. restriction endonuclease
D. reverse transcriptase
E. RNase H

Answer D: Reverse transcription-PCR (RT-PCR) is a rapid and quantitative procedure for the analysis of the level of expression of genes. This technique utilizes the ability of reverse transcriptase (RT) to convert RNA into single-stranded cDNA and couples it with the PCR-mediated amplification of specific types of cDNAs present in the RT reaction. The cDNAs that are produced during the RT reaction represent a window into the pattern of genes that are being expressed at the time the RNA was extracted.

8. In the technique of cDNA cloning, an enzyme is often used that recognizes duplexes formed between DNA and RNA. Which of the following is the enzyme in question?
A. DNA polymerase
B. polynucleotide kinase

C. reverse transcriptase
D. RNase H
E. terminal transferase

Answer D: RNase H recognizes RNA-DNA duplexes and randomly cleaves the phosphodiester backbone of the RNA. The enzyme is primarily used to cleave the mRNA strand that is annealed to the first strand of cDNA generated by reverse transcription.

9. A 47-year-old man is being examined by his personal physician because of a progressive dementia, evolving involuntary movements, and changes to his affect. History indicates that he noticed frequent uncontrolled spasmodic twitching of his fingers beginning about 1 year ago. Physical examination indicates clumsiness, hyperreflexia, and eye movement disturbances. You make a diagnosis and suggest that the patient is an ideal candidate for a new form of therapy. Which of the following techniques is most likely associated with the therapy for the suspected disease?
A. gene therapy
B. polymerase chain reaction, PCR
C. restriction fragment length polymorphism, RFLP
D. RNAi
E. transgenesis

Answer D: The patient is suffering from Huntington disease which results from a trinucleotide expansion in the gene encoding the huntingtin protein. Since this is an abnormal protein it is an amenable target for RNAi therapy. RNAi involves a mechanism of RNA-directed regulation of gene expression principally at the level of the mRNA product of the targeted gene. Interference can involve mRNA degradation or a block to translation or both.

10. In order to generate a genomic library which of the following enzymes is required?
A. DNase I
B. DNA polymerase
C. polynucleotide kinase
D. restriction endonuclease
E. reverse transcriptase

Answer D: Genomic DNA can be isolated from any cell or tissue for cloning. The genomic DNA is first digested with restriction enzymes to generate fragments in the size range that are optimal for the vector being utilized for cloning.

11. In an assay for the presence of a specific disease gene allele in several individuals, you isolate genomic DNA from each and perform polymerase chain reaction (PCR) using gene-specific primers. The PCR product is expected to have a recognition site for the restriction endonuclease BamHI. Following PCR and BamHI digestion, the products are separated by gel electrophoresis and the results are shown in the figure below. Which lane corresponds to the individual demonstrating heterozygosity for the BamHI site?

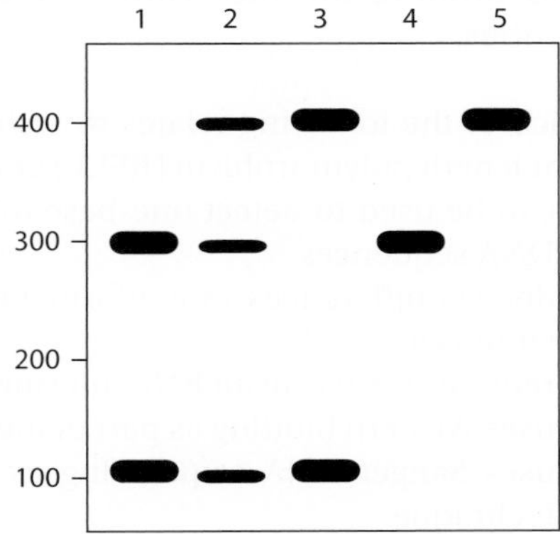

A. 1
B. 2
C. 3
D. 4
E. 5

Answer B: Someone who exhibits heterozygosity would harbor 2 distinct alelles. In the case of this analysis they would be identified as containing a copy of the gene that does not harbor the BamHI site and a copy that does harbor the site. The presence of the BamHI site in the PCR product in this example would result in the generation of 300 and 100 bp fragments. The lack of the site would yield a product of 400 bp. Thus, following PCR amplification and BamHI digestion of DNA from a heterozygote, one would be able to observe 3 bands of equal intensity.

12. The forensic analytical technique identified as DNA fingerprinting refers to which of the following processes?
A. the establishment of a complete collection of cloned fragments of DNA
B. the identification of sequences of DNA to which specific proteins bind, thereby rendering them resistant to digestion by DNA degrading nucleases
C. the specific association of complimentary strands of DNA to one another
D. the synthetic oligonucleotide-directed enzymatic amplification of specific sequences of DNA
E. the use of repeat sequences to establish a unique pattern of fragments for any given individual

Answer E: DNA fingerprinting refers to the process of using polymorphic repeat sequences to establish a unique pattern of DNA fragments for any given individual. The polymorphic repeats that are identifiable by the fingerprinting technique are hypervariable repeats such as variable number tandem repeats (VNTRs). The bands are detected by Southern blotting enzyme-digested chromosomal DNA and probing the blot with various different VNTR probes.

13. Which of the following relates to restriction fragment length polymorphism (RFLP) analysis?
- A. can be used to detect one-base differences in DNA sequences
- B. detects differences in conformation of single strands of DNA
- C. requires the use of an RNA intermediate
- D. uses Western blotting as part of the technique
- E. uses Sanger DNA sequencing as part of the technique

Answer A: Pathogenic alterations to the genotypic can be due to deletions or insertions within the gene being analyzed or even single nucleotide substitutions that can create or delete a restriction enzyme recognition site. RFLP analysis takes advantage of this and utilizes Southern blotting of restriction enzyme digested genomic DNA to detect familial patterns (polymorphisms) of the fragments of a given gene, detectable by screening the Southern blot with a probe corresponding to the gene of interest.

14. Restriction endonucleases are powerful enzymes used in molecular biological experimentation. Which of the follwing chemical bonds do these enzymes target?
- A. disulfide
- B. *N*-glycosidic
- C. *O*-glycosidic
- D. peptide
- E. phosphodiester

Answer E: Restriction endonucleases are enzymes that cut DNA at or near specific recognition nucleotide sequences. The "cutting" involves the hydrolysis of the phosphodiester bond in the DNA strands.

15. Clinical trials are assessing a new treatment for age-related macular degeneration by the targeting vascular endothelial cell growth factor receptor (VEGFR) using RNAi technology. Which of the following statements most closely describes the characteristics of RNAi that make it useful as a therapeutic approach to disease?
- A. RNAi activates phosphodiesterase, thus interfering with the cAMP signaling mediated by VEGFR activation
- B. RNAi molecules trigger the interferon response preventing translation of the VEGFR mRNA
- C. RNAi molecules will act as competitive inhibitors by interacting with the VEGFR protein
- D. RNAi treatment will prevent replication of the VEGFR gene during S-phase of the cell cycle
- E. RNAi treatment will specifically target the VEGFR mRNA for degradation

Answer E: The RNA inhibitory (RNAi) pathway in mammals involves the enzymatic processing of double-stranded RNA into small interfering RNAs (siRNAs) of approximately 22 to 25 nucleotides that may have evolved as a means to degrade the RNA genomes of RNA viruses such as retroviruses. Since RNAi reduces the level of the target mRNA the encoded protein is consequently reduced. Therefore, the RNAi technique can prove useful in treating diseases where expression of a mutant or aberrant protein is the cause of the symptoms such as the VEGFR in the progression of age-related macular degeneration.

16. The technique referred to as RNA interference (RNAi) involves the targeted destruction of mRNAs leading to reduced levels of bioactive protein. Using RNAi could be expected to have a pharmacological benefit in which of the following disorders?
- A. Huntington disease
- B. PKU
- C. retinoblastoma
- D. Tay-Sachs disease
- E. von Hippel-Lindau syndrome

Answer A: RNA interference (RNAi) involves a mechanism of RNA-directed regulation of gene expression principally at the level of the mRNA product of the targeted gene. Interference can involve mRNA degradation or a block to translation or both. The RNAi pathway is initiated by the enzyme dicer, which cleaves double-stranded RNA (dsRNA) to short double-stranded fragments of 20 to 25 bp. One of the 2 strands of each fragment, known as the guide strand, is then incorporated into the RNA-induced silencing complex (RISC) and base-pairs with complementary sequences. When the guide-strand base-pairs with an mRNA molecule, it induces degradation of the mRNA by argonaute, the catalytic component of the RISC complex. The short RNA fragments are known as small interfering RNA (siRNA) when they derive from exogenous sources and microRNA (miRNA) when they are produced from RNA-coding genes in the cell's own genome. Since

RNAi reduces the level of the target mRNA the encoded protein is consequently reduced. Therefore, the RNAi technique can prove useful in treating diseases where expression of a mutant or aberrant protein is the cause of the symptoms such as in Huntington disease.

17. A number of DNA diagnostic tests rely on the Southern blot, a method in which DNA samples are made single-stranded by brief exposure to high pH. Which of the following best accounts for separation of the DNA strands under these conditions?
- A. cleavage of phosphodisester bonds
- B. deamination of adenine, guanine, and cytosine residues
- C. disruption of hydrogen-bonding between bases
- D. loss of charges on the phosphate groups
- E. hydrolysis of *N*-glycosidic linkages between the sugars and the bases

Answer C: Southern blotting is the analysis of DNA structure following its attachment to a solid support. The DNA to be analyzed is first digested with a given restriction enzyme, then the resultant DNA fragments are separated in an agarose gel. The gel is treated with NaOH to denature the DNA, then the NaOH is neutralized. The DNA is transferred from the gel to nitrocellulose or nylon filter paper by either capillary diffusion or under electric current. The DNA is fixed to the filter by baking or ultraviolet light treatment.

18. The ability to incorporate restriction fragments with blunt ends into plasmid vectors linearized with similar enzymes is particularly dependent upon which of the following enzymes?
- A. DNA ligase
- B. DNA polymerase
- C. micrococcal nuclease
- D. polynucleotide kinase
- E. terminal transferase

Answer A: DNA ligase covalently attaches a free 5′-phosphate to a 3′-hydroxyl and it is, therefore, used in all procedures where the molecules of DNA need to be covalently attached.

19. The polymerase chain reaction (PCR) requires which of the following enzymes?
- A. DNA ligase
- B. DNA polymerase
- C. DNase I
- D. ribonuclease
- E. RNA polymerase

Answer B: The PCR is a powerful technique used to amplify DNA millions of fold, by repeated replication of a template, in a short period of time. The process normally utilizes thermostable DNA polymerases.

20. Which of the following is the function of restriction endonucleases in bacteria?
- A. degradation of foreign DNA
- B. enhancement of transcription
- C. participation in DNA repair
- D. participation in synthesis of lagging strand DNA
- E. stimulation of recombination

Answer A: Restriction endonucleases are enzymes that will recognize, bind to, and hydrolyze specific nucleic acid sequences in double-stranded DNA. The term restriction endonuclease was given to this class of bacterially derived enzymes since they were identified as being involved in restricting the growth of certain bacteriophages. Bacteria are capable of modifying specific sequences within their genomes by methylation, which prevents their own DNA from being recognized by the restriction enzymes encoded by their genomes. This process is termed modification and restriction.

21. A 27-year-old woman, who is 10-weeks into her second pregnancy, is being tested by a molecular genetics clinic. She and her husband's first child has a transfusion-dependent form of β-thalassemia. The prenatal diagnostic test used to determine if the fetus is affected is based upon the polymerase chain reaction method. Which of the following reagents is needed to carry out this test?
- A. chain-terminating dideoxynucleotides
- B. cloned copies of the child's β-globin genes
- C. DNA ligase
- D. oligonucleotides complementary to sequences in the β-globin gene
- E. restriction endonucleases

Answer D: The PCR is a powerful technique used to amplify DNA millions of fold, by repeated replication of a template, in a short period of time. The process utilizes sets of specific in vitro synthesized oligonucleotides to prime DNA synthesis. The design of the primers is dependent upon the sequences of the DNA that is desired to be analyzed and in this case would need to be complimentary to sequences of the β-globin gene.

22. Which of the following techniques is the most accurate in showing that 2 RNAs are identical?
- A. hybridization
- B. nucleotide sequencing
- C. polymerase chain reaction
- D. restriction endonuclease analysis
- E. Western blotting

Answer B: In order to accurately determine the identity of any given RNA it is necessary to determine the nucleotide sequences of the encoding gene or to generate cDNA clones of the RNAs and compare their nucleotide sequences. Blotting and hybridization of 2 different RNAs might demonstrate that they are identical in size, but that is all the information one would be able to use from that analysis.

23. The accuracy of DNA restriction maps in demonstrating changes in the DNA sequence of a specific gene reflects the ability of restriction endonucleases to do which of the following?

A. bind to transcription sites
B. degrade viral DNA introduced into bacteria
C. recognize a specific short DNA sequence in double-stranded DNA
D. remove bases from DNA within a sequence in a precise 5′ → 3′ direction from the middle of a sequence
E. repair DNA damaged by ultraviolet light by selectively destroying the modified bases

Answer C: Restriction endonucleases are enzymes that will recognize, bind to, and hydrolyze specific nucleic acid sequences in double-stranded DNA.

24. You are studying the characteristics of DNA isolated from a mutant strain of *E coli*. Your data show that it can be digested into numerous smaller fragments with a restriction endonuclease that is known to cleave at a GGATCC motif. In comparison, DNA from the wild-type parental strain is resistant to digestion with this restriction endonuclease. The mutation that causes this type of phenotype is most likely to occur in the gene encoding which of the following activities?

A. DNase
B. gyrase
C. helicase
D. ligase
E. methylase

Answer E: Restriction endonucleases are enzymes that will recognize, bind to, and hydrolyze specific nucleic acid sequences in double-stranded DNA. The term restriction endonuclease was given to this class of bacterially derived enzymes, since they were identified as being involved in restricting the growth of certain bacteriophages. Bacteria are capable of modifying specific sequences within their genomes by methylation, which prevents their own DNA from being recognized by the restriction enzymes encoded by their genomes.

25. You are carrying out experiments to insert fragments of the human genome into an appropriate vector and using the vector to transform bacterial cells. Which of the following is most likely to be used to transfer cloned human genetic material to bacteria?

A. DNA complexed with bacterial histones
B. human chromosomal fragments
C. naked DNA
D. purified euchromatin
E. purified heterochromatin

Answer C: Genomic DNA can be isolated from any cell or tissue for cloning. Following purification of the DNA, it is digested with restriction enzymes to generate fragments in the size range that are optimal for the vector being utilized for cloning.

Checklist

- ✓ Molecular biology is a technical field that involves the study of genes and the control of their expression in the elaboration of cellular and organismal function.
- ✓ A variety of enzymes, most isolated from bacteria, are utilized in the molecular study of DNA and genes.
- ✓ Cloning refers to the production of large quantities of identical DNA molecules and usually involves the use of a bacterial cell as a host for the DNA, although cloning can be done in eukaryotic cells as well.

✓ Reverse transcriptase is an RNA-dependent DNA polymerase that is used to generate complimentary DNA (cDNA) copies of the mRNAs present in a cell or tissue. The resultant cDNAs are generally inserted into an appropriate vector to generate a library of cDNA clones.

✓ Genomic cloning refers to the process of digesting the genome of an organism and inserting it into an appropriate vector system for the generation of a library of gene clones.

✓ The techniques that involve the cloning of DNA are used as a means to identify the chromosomal location of genes, to determine the nucleotide sequences of genes, to identify and characterize genes that cause disease, to understand how inappropriate regulation of genes results in disease, to diagnose genetic diseases, and to develop gene-based methods of treating disease.

✓ Gene therapy is a term used to describe a technique designed to introduce a functional gene into the cells or tissues of an individual in order to treat a disease resulting from an inherited gene defect.

CHAPTER 42 Iron and Copper Metabolism

CHAPTER OUTLINE

High-Yield Terms

Ferrous iron: iron with an oxidation state of +2 (Fe^{2+} or Fe[II])

Ferric iron: iron with an oxidation state of +3 (Fe^{3+} of Fe[III])

Cuprous copper: copper with an oxidation state of +1 (Cu^{1+} or Cu[I])

Cupric copper: copper with an oxidation state of +2 (Cu^{2+} or Cu[II])

Ferroxidase: any of a class of enzyme that oxidizes ferrous (Fe^{2+}) iron to ferric (Fe^{3+}) iron

Ferrireductase: any of a class of enzyme that reduces ferric (Fe^{3+}) iron to ferrous (Fe^{2+}) iron

Reticuloendothelial cells: comprise phagocytic cells located in different organs of the body, responsible for engulfing, bacteria, viruses, other foreign substances, and abnormal body cells

Hemosiderin: an intracellular complex of iron, ferritin, denatured ferritin and other material, most commonly found in macrophages, accumulates in conditions of hemorrhage and iron excess

Ceruloplasmin: is a ferroxidase that is also a major copper-requiring protein of the blood

Metallothioneins: a family of cysteine-rich proteins that bind a variety of metals and are thought to provide protection against metal toxicities

Role of Iron

Iron serves numerous important functions in the body relating to the metabolism of oxygen, not the least of which is its role in hemoglobin transport of oxygen. Within the body iron exists in 2 oxidation states: ferrous (Fe^{2+}) or ferric (Fe^{3+}). Because iron has an affinity for electronegative atoms such as oxygen, nitrogen, and sulfur, these atoms are found at the heart of the iron-binding centers of macromolecules.

Under conditions of neutral or alkaline pH, iron is found in the Fe^{3+} state and at acidic pH the Fe^{2+} state is favored. When in the Fe^{3+} state, iron will form large complexes with anions, water, and peroxides. These large complexes have poor solubility and upon their aggregation lead to pathological consequences. In addition, iron can bind to and interfere with the structure and function of various macromolecules. For this reason the body must protect itself against the deleterious effects of iron. This is the role served by numerous iron-binding and transport proteins.

Aside from its importance as the prosthetic group of hemoglobin and a number of enzymes (eg, redox cytochromes and the P450 class of detoxifying cytochromes), heme is important because a number of genetic disease states are associated with deficiencies of the enzymes used in its biosynthesis. Some of these disorders are readily diagnosed because they cause δ-aminolevulinic acid (ALA) and other abnormally colored heme intermediates to appear in the circulation, the urine, and in other tissues such as teeth and bones.

Iron Metabolism

Iron is associated with proteins either by incorporation into protoporphyrin IX (forming heme) or by binding to other ligands. There are a number of heme containing proteins involved in the transport of oxygen (hemoglobin), oxygen storage (myoglobin), and enzyme catalysis such as nitric oxide synthase (NOS) and prostaglandin synthase (cyclooxygenase). A number of non-heme iron–containing proteins are also known such as the iron-sulfur proteins of oxidative phosphorylation and the iron transport and storage proteins, transferrin and ferritin, respectively.

Iron, consumed in the diet, is either free iron or heme iron. Free iron in the intestines is reduced from the ferric (Fe^{3+}) to the ferrous (Fe^{2+}) state on the luminal surface of intestinal enterocytes and transported into the cells through the action of the divalent metal transporter 1 (DMT1) (Figure 42-1). Intestinal uptake of heme iron occurs through the interaction of dietary heme with the heme carrier protein (HCP1). The iron in the heme is then released within the enterocytes via the action the heme catabolizing enzyme heme oxygenase (see Figure 33-5). The iron can be stored within intestinal enterocytes bound to ferritin. Iron is transported across the basolateral membrane of intestinal enterocytes into the circulation, through the action of the transport protein ferroportin (also called IREG1 = iron-regulated gene 1). Associated with ferroportin is the enzyme hephaestin (a copper-containing ferroxidase with homology to ceruloplasmin) which oxidizes the ferrous form back to the ferric form. Once in the circulation, ferric iron is bound to transferrin and passes through the portal circulation of the liver. The liver is the major storage site for iron. The major site of iron utilization is the bone marrow where it is used in heme synthesis (see Chapter 33).

Transferrin, made in the liver, is the serum protein responsible for the transport of iron. Although several metals can bind to transferrin, the highest affinity is for the ferric (Fe^{3+}) form of iron. The ferrous form of iron does not bind to transferrin. Transferrin can bind 2 moles of ferric iron. Cells take up the transported iron through interaction of transferrin with cell-surface receptors (Figure 42-2). Internalization of the iron-transferrin-receptor complexes is initiated following receptor phosphorylation by protein kinase C (PKC). Following internalization, the iron is released due to the acidic nature of the endosomes. The transferrin receptor is then recycled back to the cell surface.

Ferritin is the major protein used for intracellular storage of iron. Ferritin without bound iron is referred to as apoferritin. Apoferritin is a large polymer of 24 polypeptide subunits. This multimeric structure of apoferritin is able to bind up to 2000 iron atoms in the form of ferric-phosphate. The majority of intracellularly stored iron is found in the liver, skeletal muscle, and reticuloendothelial cells. If the storage capacity of the ferritin is exceeded, iron will deposit adjacent to the ferritin-iron complexes in the cell. Histologically these amorphous iron deposits are referred to as hemosiderin. Hemosiderin is composed of ferritin, denatured ferritin, and other materials and its molecular structure is poorly defined. The iron present in hemosiderin is not readily available to the cell and thus cannot supply iron to the cell when it is needed. Hemosiderin is found most frequently in macrophages and is most abundant following hemorrhagic events.

In humans approximately 70% of total body iron is found in hemoglobin (Table 42-1). Because of storage and recycling very little (1-2 mg) iron will need to be replaced from the diet on a daily basis. Any excess dietary iron is not absorbed or is stored in intestinal enterocytes. Regulation of iron absorption, recycling, and release from intracellular stores is controlled

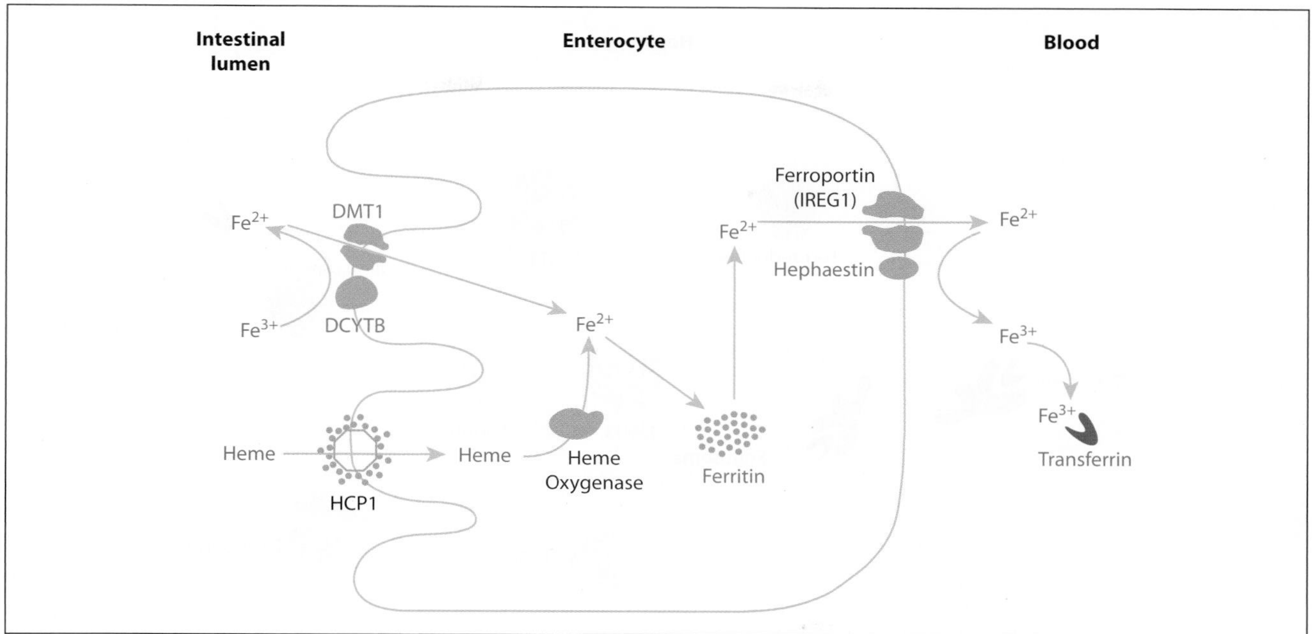

FIGURE 42-1: Dietary iron in the form of non-heme iron or heme iron is absorbed in the duodenum. Non-heme iron occurs primarily in the ferric state in the gut and is reduced to the ferrous state through the action of ferrireductases. In the duodenum this reduction is carried out primarily by duodenal cytochrome *b* (DCYTB). There are additional intestinal brush border ferrireductases since it has been shown in mice that loss of DCYTB does not impair iron absorption. Ferrous iron is then taken up by duodenal enterocytes through the action of divalent metal transporter 1 (DMT1). DMT1 is a member of the solute carrier protein family and is thus, also known as SLC11A2. Heme iron is taken up through the action of heme carrier protein 1 (HCP1). Once in the enterocyte heme is degraded through the action of heme oxygenase releasing the ferrous iron. Ferrous iron can be stored in the enterocyte bound to ferritin or released to the circulation through the action of ferroportin (also called IREG1). Ferroportin is also a member of the solute carrier protein family and has the designation SLC11A3. Iron is transported in the blood bound to transferrin but does so only in the ferric state so during the transport through ferroportin, ferrous iron is oxidized by the ferroxidase called hephaestin. Reproduced with permission of themedicalbiochemistrypage, LLC.

through the actions of the hepatic iron regulatory protein, hepcidin.

Hepcidin functions by inhibiting the presentation of one or more of the iron transporters (eg, DMT1 and IREG1) in intestinal membranes. With a high iron diet the level of hepcidin mRNA increases and conversely its levels decrease when dietary iron is low. This is occurring simultaneous to reciprocal changes in the levels of the transporters.

The regulation of iron homeostasis in the body is primarily controlled via iron-mediated regulation of mRNA translation (see Chapter 37). Both the transferrin receptor and the ferritin mRNAs contain stem-loop structures termed iron responsive elements, IREs. These IREs are recognized by an iron-binding protein containing an iron-sulfur center similar to that of the tricarboxylic acid (TCA) cycle enzyme aconitase. Other IRE-containing mRNAs include those encoding the erythrocyte protoporphyrin synthesis enzyme, ALA synthase, mitochondrial aconitase, and IREG1 (ferroportin).

Abnormal Iron Metabolism

Iron can bind to and form complexes with numerous macromolecules. Excess intracellular iron results in formation and deposition of hemosiderin which can lead to cellular dysfunction and damage. Thus, the consequences of excess iron intake and storage can have profound consequences, the most significant of which is hemochromatosis (Clinical Box 42-1). However, a reduction in iron intake can also lead to untoward consequences. Most notably, a reduced iron level negatively affects the function of oxygen transport in erythrocytes. Defects in iron metabolism can result from impaired intestinal absorption, excess loss of heme iron due to bleeding, as well as to mutations in the iron response elements of iron-regulated mRNAs.

Iron-deficiency anemia is characterized by microcytic (small) and hypochromic (low-pigment) erythrocytes. Reduced iron intake and/or excess iron excretion results in decreased globin protein content

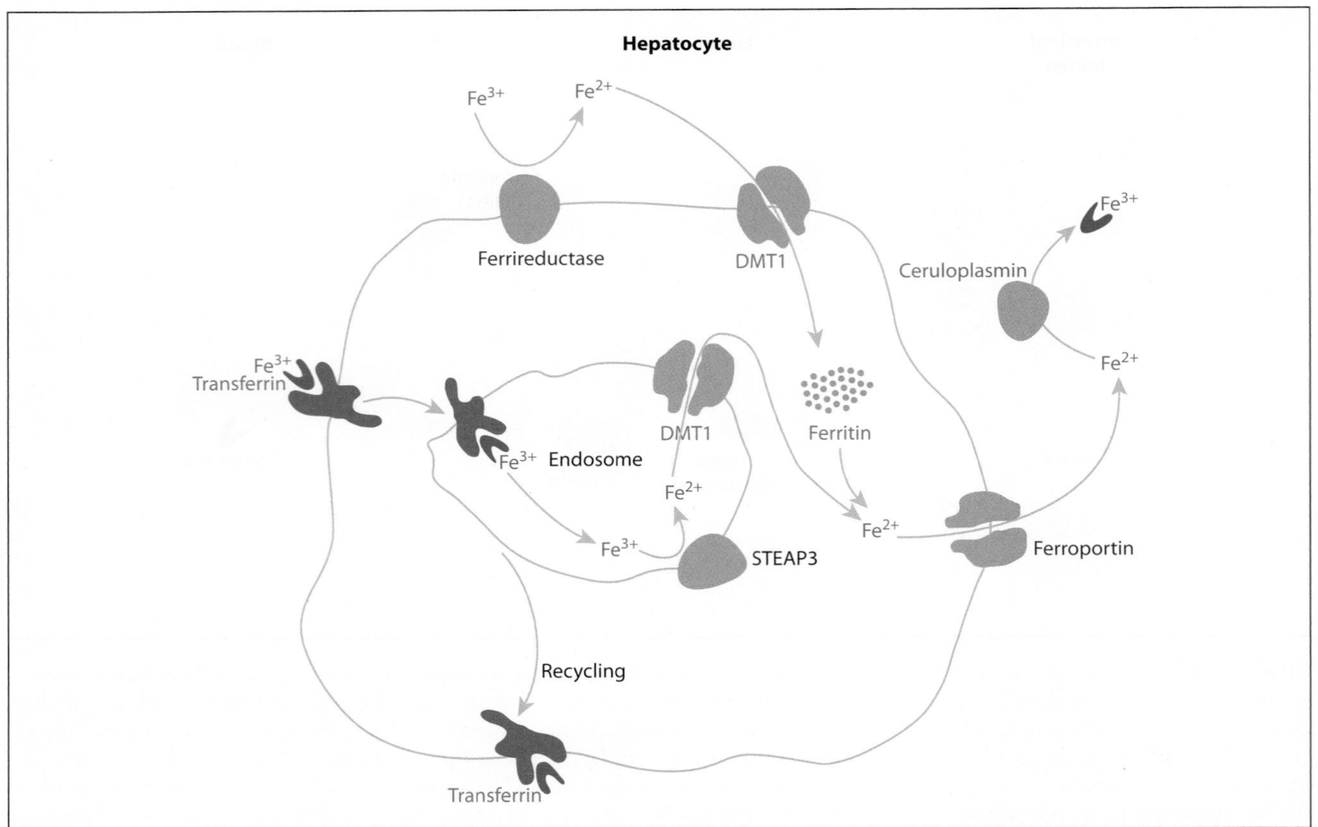

FIGURE 42-2: The main cellular site of iron storage is the liver, specifically in hepatocytes. Iron bound to transferrin is taken up from the blood by hepatocytes due to the binding of transferrin to the transferrin receptor. Free iron (called non-transferrin–bound iron, NTBI) in the plasma can also be absorbed by hepatocytes via the action of DMT1. However, the ferric form predominates in the blood and must first be reduced by ferrireductases prior to DMT1 transport. Upon binding transferrin, the transferrin receptor is internalized via receptor-mediated endocytosis. The acidic environment of the endosome results in the release of ferric iron from transferrin. The ferric iron is reduced in the endosome to the ferrous form via the action of an endosomal ferrireductase, most likely 6-transmembrane epithelial antigen of prostate protein 3 (STEAP3). The ferrous iron is transported out of the endosome via DMT1 action and can then be stored in the hepatocyte bound to ferritin as in intestinal enterocytes. The transferrin-transferrin receptor complexes are recycled back to the surface of the hepatocyte and the transferrin is released to the blood where it can bind more ferric iron in the circulation. Ferrous iron is released from hepatocytes to the circulation through the action of ferroportin. When in the circulation ferrous iron is oxidized to the ferric form by the plasma ferroxidase known as ceruloplasmin. The ferric iron can then be bound by transferrin and delivered to other tissues of the body. Reproduced with permission of themedicalbiochemistrypage, LLC.

TABLE 42-1: **Distribution of Iron in a 70-kg Adult Male**[1]	
Transferrin	3-4 mg
Hemoglobin in red blood cells	2500 mg
In myoglobin and various enzymes	300 mg
In stores (ferritin)	1000 mg
Absorption	1 mg/d
Losses	1 mg/d

[1]In an adult female of similar weight, the amount in stores would generally be less (100-400 mg) and the losses would be greater (1.5-2 mg/d).
Murray RK, Bender DA, Botham KM, Kennelly PJ, Rodwell VW, Weil PA. *Harper's Illustrated Biochemistry.* 29th ed. New York, NY: McGraw-Hill; 2012.

in erythrocytes as a consequence of the heme control of globin synthesis (see Chapter 37 for details). Table 42-2 shows the most common laboratory test results for determination of iron-deficiency anemia. The most common causes of iron-deficiency anemia are excess menstrual flow or gastrointestinal (GI) bleeding. Causes of GI bleeding can include the use of medications that lead to ulceration or erosion of the gastric mucosa, peptic ulcer disease, gastric tumors, hiatal hernia, or the gastritis associated with chronic alcohol consumption. Treatment of iron-deficiency anemia is to first determine the cause and source of the excess bleeding. Oral administration of ferrous sulfate is commonly used to supplement the iron loss; however, intravenous iron therapy may be called for

CLINICAL BOX 42-1: HEMOCHROMATOSIS

Hemochromatosis is defined as a disorder in iron metabolism that is characterized by excess iron absorption, saturation of iron-binding proteins, and deposition of hemosiderin in the tissues. The primary affected tissues are the liver, pancreas, and skin. Iron deposition in the liver leads to cirrhosis and in the pancreas causes diabetes. The excess iron deposition leads to bronze pigmentation of the organs and skin. The bronze skin pigmentation seen in hemochromatosis, coupled with the resultant diabetes lead to the designation of this condition as *bronze diabetes*. Primary hemochromatosis is referred to as type 1 hemochromatosis. The mutant locus causing type 1 hemochromatosis has been designated the HFE1 locus and it is a major histocompatibility complex (MHC) class 1 gene. Hemochromatosis, that is associated with the HFE1 locus, is one of the most common inherited genetic defects. Manifestation of the symptoms of the disease is modified by several environmental influences. Dietary iron intake and alcohol consumption are especially significant to hemochromatosis. Menstruation and pregnancy can also influence symptoms. Hemochromatosis occurs about 5 to 10 times more frequently in men than in women. Symptoms usually appear between the ages of 40 and 60 in about 70% of individuals. The *HFE1* gene encodes an α-chain protein with 3 immunoglobulin-like domains. This α-chain protein associates with β_2-microglobulin, typical of MHC class 1 encoded proteins. Normal *HFE1* has been shown to form a complex with the transferrin receptor thus, regulating the rate of iron transfer into cells. A mutation in *HFE1* will therefore, lead to increased iron uptake and storage. The majority of hereditary hemochromatosis patients have inherited a mutation in *HFE1* that results in the substitution of Cys 282 for a Tyr (C282Y). Another mutation found in certain forms of hereditary hemochromatosis also affects the HFE1 locus and causes a change of His 63 to Asp (H63D). This latter mutation is found along with the more common *C282Y* mutation resulting in a compound heterozygosity. As a result of the *C282Y* mutation the HFE1 protein remains trapped in the intracellular compartment. Because it cannot associate with the transferrin receptor there is a reduced uptake of iron by intestinal crypt cells. It is thought that this defect in intestinal iron uptake results in an increase in the expression of the DMT1 on the brush border of the intestinal villus cells. Excess DMT1 expression leads to an inappropriate increase in intestinal iron absorption. In hemochromatosis the liver is usually the first organ to be affected. Hepatomegaly will be present in more than 95% of patients manifesting symptoms. Initial symptoms include weakness, abdominal pain, change in skin color, and the onset of symptoms of diabetes mellitus. In advanced cases of hemochromatosis there will likely be cardiac arrhythmias, congestive heart failure, testicular atrophy, jaundice, increased pigmentation, spider angiomas, and splenomegaly. Diagnosis of the disease is usually suggested when there is the presence of hepatomegaly, skin pigmentation, diabetes mellitus, heart disease, arthritis, and hypogonadism. Treatment of hemochromatosis before there is permanent organ damage can restore life expectancy to normal. Treatment involves removal of the excess body iron. This is accomplished by twice-weekly phlebotomy at the beginning of treatment. Alcohol consumption should be curtailed and preferably eliminated in hemochromatosis patients. Iron-chelating agents, such as deferoxamine, can be used to remove around 10 to 20 mg of iron per day. However, phlebotomy is more convenient and safer for most patients.

Non-HFE Hemochromatosis: There are several additional causes of hemochromatosis, although none are as common as classic hemochromatosis. There are at least 4 additional genetic loci, that when defective lead to hemochromatosis. Two of which are juvenile forms identified as type 2A and 2B and 2 additional forms identified as type 3 and type 4.

Juvenile hemochromatosis (JH) type 2A (sometimes called HFE2A) is the result of defects in the gene encoding hemojuvelin (HJV). The function of hemojuvelin is to regulate the expression of the hepcidin gene (*HAMP*). As suggested by the juvenile nomenclature, this disorder manifests in patients under the age of 30. Cardiomyopathy and hypogonadism are prevalent symptoms with type 2A hemochromatosis. Type 2A hemochromatosis is inherited as an autosomal recessive disorder.

JH type 2B (sometimes called HFE2B) results from defects in the gene encoding hepcidin (*HAMP*). As with type 2A disease, symptoms of type 2B disease appear in patients under 30 years of age and include cardiomyopathy and hypogonadism. Type 2B hemochromatosis is inherited as an autosomal recessive disorder.

Type 3 hemochromatosis (sometimes called HFE3) is caused by mutations in the transferrin receptor 2 gene (*TFR2*). TFR2 is a homolog of the classic transferrin receptor (identified as TFR1). Unlike the ubiquitous expression of TFR1, TFR2 expression is almost exclusively found in the liver. The function of TFR2 in the liver is not to act in the uptake of transferrin-bound iron but to sense iron levels and to act as a regulator of hepcidin function. The clinical features of type 3 hemochromatosis are similar to those of classic type 1 disease. Type 3 hemochromatosis is inherited as an autosomal recessive disorder.

Type 4 hemochromatosis (sometimes called HFE4) is also called ferroportin disease because it is caused by mutations in the ferroportin gene. Ferroportin is highly expressed in the liver, duodenum, and reticuloendothelial cells. The major function of ferroportin is to transport dietary iron across the basolateral membranes of intestinal enterocytes into the blood and to recycle iron via the reticuloendothelial system. Symptoms of type 4 hemochromatosis are similar to those of classic type 1 disease but are generally milder. The unique aspect of type 4 hemochromatosis is that it is inherited as an autosomal dominant disease.

TABLE 42-2: Changes in Various Laboratory Tests Used to Assess Iron-Deficiency Anemia

Parameter	*Normal*	*Negative Iron Balance*	*Iron-Deficient Erythropoiesis*	*Iron-Deficiency Anemia*
Serum ferritin (μg/dL)	50-200	Decreased <20	Decreased <15	Decreased <15
Total iron-binding capacity (TIBC) (μg/dL)	300-360	Slightly increased >360	Increased >380	Increased>400
Serum iron (μg/dL)	50-150	Normal	Decreased <50	Decreased <30
Transferrin saturation (%)	30-50	Normal	Decreased <20	Decreased <10
RBC protoporphyrin (μg/dL)	30-50	Normal	Increased	Increased
Soluble transferrin receptor (μg/L)	4-9	Increased	Increased	Increased
RBC morphology	Normal	Normal	Normal	Microcytic Hypochromic

Modified, with permission, from Figure 98-2, page 630, Harrison's Principles of Internal Medicine, 17th ed. Fauci AS, et al (editors). McGraw-Hill, 2008.
Murray RK, Bender DA, Botham KM, Kennelly PJ, Rodwell VW, Weil PA. *Harper's Illustrated Biochemistry*. 29th ed. New York, NY: McGraw-Hill; 2012.

in some cases. Severe iron-deficiency anemia may necessitate transfusion with packed red blood cells.

Role of Copper

Copper is an essential trace element which plays a pivotal role in cell physiology as it constitutes a core part of copper-containing enzymes termed cuproenzymes. Like iron, copper exists in 2 oxidation states, cuprous (Cu^{1+} or Cu^{+}) and cupric (Cu^{2+}). Some important copper-containing enzymes include cytochrome oxidase of the electron transport chain and copper-zinc-superoxide dismutase (SOD1) involved in the detoxification of the reactive oxygen species, superoxide. Copper is required for respiration, connective tissue formation, iron metabolism, and many other processes. In human cells, copper is utilized in several cellular compartments, and the intracellular distribution of copper is regulated in response to metabolic demands and changes in cell environment. Although copper is an essential micronutrient, it can be potentially toxic when present in excessive amounts. Copper can also bind with high affinity to histidine, cysteine, and methionine residues of proteins which can result in their inactivation. Copper ions can also readily interact with oxygen leading to the production of the highly damaging hydroxyl radical. The need to provide copper to essential enzymes without causing cellular toxicity has resulted in the evolution of tightly regulated copper homeostatic mechanisms that involve regulated uptake, intracellular transport and efflux, and storage.

Copper Metabolism

Like iron, dietary copper is taken up by intestinal enterocytes via the action of a specific transport protein, copper transporter 1 (CTR1) as well as by the divalent metal transporter 1 (DMT1) which is not specific for any particular divalent metal. CTR1 is responsible for transport of cuprous (Cu^{+}) copper into cells. CTR1 is a member of the solute-carrier family of transporters and as such is also identified as SLC31A1. Uptake by other tissues (primarily the liver and kidneys) also involves CTR1. In the blood 65% to 90% of copper is transported bound to ceruloplasmin, and the rest of copper loosely binds with albumin, transcuprein, and amino acids. In the liver, kidney, placenta, and mammary gland, CTR1 is found mainly in the basolateral membrane where it is responsible for uptake of copper from the blood.

Dietary copper is found primarily in the cupric state (Cu^{2+}) and is reduced to cuprous (Cu^{+}) prior to duodenal uptake. Potential intestinal reductants include ascorbate and the ferrireductase DCYTB (see Figure 42-1). In cells, CTR1 is found at the plasma membrane and in intracellular vesicles. When CTR1 binds copper it is internalized and moves to endocytic vesicles. Copper-transporting P-type ATPases (Cu-ATPases) maintain intracellular copper levels. A low-affinity copper transporter, CTR2, is present intracellularly and functions to release copper from the lysosome or lysosome-like compartments for reutilization. In intestine, CTR1 has an additional role in making dietary copper available for further utilization by facilitating its release from intracellular vesicles. Consistent with this role, a significant fraction of CTR1 in intestinal enterocytes is intracellular and is located in the vicinity of the apical membrane.

Within cells, copper is escorted to specific compartments through the actions of several chaperones referred to as metallochaperones. Copper chaperone for superoxide dismutase (CCS) directly interacts with thereby delivering copper to this enzyme. Cytochrome oxidase assembly protein 17 (COX17) delivers copper to additional chaperones within the mitochondria for synthesis of cytochrome *c* oxidase. A third chaperone, ATOX1, delivers copper to the secretory pathway by docking with 2 Cu-ATPases, ATP7A and ATP7B. ATP7A is required for cuproenzyme biosynthesis, and in intestinal enterocytes it is required for copper efflux to the portal circulation. ATP7B is mainly expressed in the liver where it is required for copper incorporation into ceruloplasmin and for excretion of copper into the biliary circulation. Mutations in *ATP7A* result in Menkes disease (Clinical Box 42-2) and mutations in *ATP7B* are the cause of Wilson disease (Clinical Box 42-3). Other proteins involved in copper homeostasis include the metallothioneins and amyloid precursor protein.

CLINICAL BOX 42-2: MENKES DISEASE

Menkes disease is inherited as an X-linked disorder of copper homeostasis. The disorder is associated with an inability to absorb copper from the gastrointestinal tract. As a consequence of the reduced delivery of copper to the brain, Menkes patients exhibit severe mental and developmental impairment. In addition, because there is a need for copper as a cofactor in numerous enzymes (eg, lysyl oxidases) Menkes patients also exhibit connective tissue abnormalities and twisting of blood vessels where there are normally supposed to be turns. The vessel twisting can lead to blockages if it is severe. Menkes disease is so named because it was originally described in 1962 by Dr. John H. Menkes. The incidence of Menkes disease ranges from 1:40,000 to 1:360,000 live births. Menkes disease is the result of defects in the P-type ATPase protein that is responsible for the translocation of copper across the intestinal basal-lateral membrane into the blood, thus allowing for uptake of dietary copper. This protein is encoded by the ATPase, Cu^{2+}-transporting, α-polypeptide (*ATP7A*) gene. The *ATP7A* gene is located on the X chromosome (Xq12-q13) and is composed of 23 exons spanning 150 kbp encoding a 1500 amino acid protein. The ATP7A protein contains an ATPase domain, a hinge domain, a phosphorylation site, and 6 copper-binding sites. The structure of the *ATP7A* gene is highly similar to that of the *ATP7B* gene which is disrupted in another copper-transport defect disease called Wilson disease. *ATP7A* has 2 important activities related to copper homeostasis. It delivers copper to several copper-requiring enzymes and is required for the ATP-driven efflux of copper from cells. *ATP7A* is expressed in numerous tissues except the liver. Copper homeostasis affected by the liver is the function of the ATP7B protein. When carrying out its function to supply copper-dependent enzymes with copper, the ATP7A protein is localized to the *trans*-Golgi network where it transports copper into the lumen of the Golgi. When copper levels rise, *ATP7A* is translocated to vesicular compartments closely associated with the plasma membrane where it can transport copper into these compartments. The copper in these vesicles can then be released by exocytosis. Numerous mutations have been identified in the *ATP7A* gene resulting in Menkes disease. To date at least 357 different mutations have been characterized. The most frequently occurring mutations, accounting for 22% of all cases, are insertion or deletion of a few base pairs. Additional alterations include missense mutations, partial gene deletions, splice site mutations, and mutations leading to premature termination of translation. The clinical spectrum associated with Menkes disease includes progressive neurodegeneration, connective tissue abnormalities, and wiry brittle hair. The distinctive clinical features of Menkes disease are usually present by 3 months of age. Infants will lose, or fail to demonstrate, specific developmental milestones and failure to thrive. Most patients with Menkes disease do not survive beyond early childhood; however, there is phenotypic variability and some mildly affected patients have been reported to survive for longer periods. Because of the phenotypic variations Menkes disease has been divided into 3 classifications. Classic Menkes disease which results in early death, mild Menkes disease with longer survival times (accounting for 6% of all patients), and occipital horn syndrome, OHS (accounting for 3% of all patients). OHS was previously called X-linked cutis laxa, or Ehlers-Danlos syndrome type IX. In the classic form of Menkes disease infants have cherubic faces, sagging jowls, and no or scant eyebrows. Their hair is gray or white due to the lack of tyrosinase activity and has the appearance and feel of steel wool.

CLINICAL BOX 42-2: MENKES DISEASE (*Continued*)

The deficiency in lysyl oxidase activity accounts for most of the skeletal abnormalities present in Menkes infants. These anomalies include osteoporosis, metaphyseal dysplasia, wormian skull bones, and rib fractures. Progressive cerebral degeneration occurs primarily due to loss of cytochrome *c* oxidase, peptidyl α-amidating monooxygenase, and dopamine β-hydroxylase in the central nervous system. Unfortunately there is no effective treatment for Menkes disease and severely afflicted infants will not survive more than a few months after birth. In mildly afflicted patients there is some benefit to parenteral administration of various forms of copper such as copper histidine, copper chloride, and copper sulfate. Although this treatment can correct the hepatic copper deficiency, normalize serum copper, and ceruloplasmin levels it has not been shown to ameliorate the progressive neurological deterioration.

CLINICAL BOX 42-3: WILSON DISEASE

Wilson disease (WD) is inherited as an autosomal recessive disorder of copper homeostasis. The disease is characterized by excessive copper deposition primarily in the liver and brain. These sites of copper deposition are reflective of the major manifestations of Wilson disease. Wilson disease is named after Dr. Samuel Alexander Kinnier Wilson who first described the disorder in 1912. The frequency of Wilson disease ranges from 1:5000 to 1:30,000 live births. Wilson disease is the result of defects in the P-type ATPase protein that is primarily responsible for copper homeostas is effected by the liver. This protein is encoded by the ATPase, Cu^{2+}-transporting, β-polypeptide (*ATP7B*) gene. The *ATP7B* gene is located on chromosome 13q14.3-q21.1 and is composed of 21 exons spanning 80 kbp encoding a 1411 amino acid protein. The ATP7B protein contains an ATPase domain, a hinge domain, a phosphorylation site, and 6 copper-binding sites. The *ATP7B* gene is expressed predominantly in the liver, but also in the kidney and placenta. Lower levels of expression are also detectable in the brain, heart, and lungs. The structure of the *ATP7B* gene is highly similar to that of the *ATP7A* gene which is disrupted in another copper-transport defect disease called Menkes disease. The ATP7B protein is localized to the *trans*-Golgi network where it transports copper into the lumen of the Golgi. When copper levels rise, ATP7B is translocated to vesicular compartments closely associated with the plasma membrane where it can transport copper into these compartments. The copper in these vesicles can then be released by exocytosis. When copper is transferred from intestinal enterocytes to the plasma, through the action of the ATP7A protein, it is bound to albumin and delivered to the liver. In the liver the copper is transferred to intracellular storage sites by the chaperone ATOX1 (see later). Copper is stored intracellularly bound to the protein metallothionein. Any copper in excess of the binding capacity of metallothionein is excreted into the biliary canaliculi through the transport action of ATP7B. ATP7B also facilitates the transfer of copper to the major plasma copper transport protein, ceruloplasmin. Ceruloplasmin that does not have bound copper is referred to apoceruloplasmin. Ceruloplasmin is then released to the blood. More than 90% of the copper in the blood is bound to ceruloplasmin and this functions in the transport of copper to peripheral organs such as the brain and kidneys. Deficiencies in ATP7B result in increased levels of apoceruloplasmin and a toxic buildup of copper in hepatocytes due to defective transfer to the biliary canaliculi. Numerous mutations have been identified in the *ATP7B* gene resulting in Wilson disease. The majority of these mutations are clustered in the transmembrane domains of the encoded protein. In Europeans and North Americans 2 mutations account for 38% of the observed mutations in this disease. These 2 mutations are a substitution of glutamine for histidine at amino acid 1069 (H1069Q) and arginine for glycine at amino acid 1267 (G1267R). The molecular basis for the observed phenotypic variations in Wilson disease is complex and involves both environmental influences and the effects of modifier genes such as copper metabolism MURR1 domain-containing protein 1 (*COMMD1*). The MURR1 domain was first identified in a murine protein and refers to mouse U2af1-rs1 region. An additional ATP7B modifier protein is the chaperone protein ATOX1 (antioxidant protein 1). An additional locus affecting the phenotype of Wilson disease is apolipoprotein E (apoE) ε3/3. Individuals harboring this particular apoE allele have

CLINICAL BOX 42-3: WILSON DISEASE (*Continued*)

a delayed onset in the presentation of Wilson disease symptoms. The majority of patients with Wilson disease present with hepatic or neuropsychiatric symptoms. All other patients, representing about 20% of all Wilson disease cases, manifest with symptoms that are attributable to involvement of other organs. Hepatic presentation in Wilson disease occurs in late childhood or adolescence. The symptoms in these patients include hepatic failure, acute hepatitis, or progressive chronic liver disease. Patients that manifest neurological symptoms of Wilson disease present in the second to third decade of life. In these patients there will be extrapyramidal, cerebellar and cerebral-related symptoms such as parkinsonian tremors, diminished facial expressions and movement, dystonia, and choreoathetosis. About 30% of Wilson disease patients will exhibit psychiatric disturbances that include changes in behavior, personality changes, depression, attention deficit hyperactivity disorder, paranoid psychosis, suicidal tendencies, and impulsivity. As the disease progresses copper deposition leads to vacuolar degeneration in the proximal tubular cells of the kidneys which causes a Fanconi syndrome (substances that are normally absorbed by the kidney are excreted in the urine). Acute release of copper into the circulation results in damage to red blood cells resulting in hemolysis. The most significant sign in the diagnosis of Wilson disease results from the deposition of copper in Descemet's membrane of the cornea. These golden-brown deposits can be seen with a slit-lamp and are Kayser-Fleischer rings (Figure 42-3).

Treatment of Wilson disease is aimed at reducing the toxic concentration of copper. This can be accomplished with copper-chelating agents such as trientine and D-penicillamine. Once the copper levels have been reduced the chelating agents can be reduced or eliminated and zinc salt can be used to prevent systemic absorption of copper. Patients with progressive liver failure will require liver transplantation. Liver transplantation is also required in patients that do not respond to copper-chelation therapy.

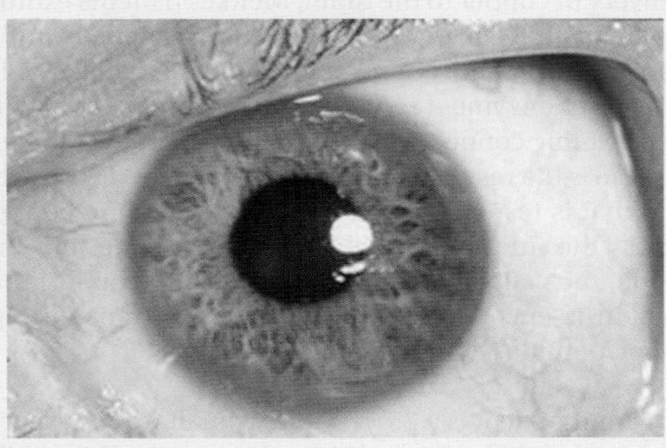

FIGURE 42-3: Kayser-Fleischer ring.

REVIEW QUESTIONS

1. A 3-month-old infant is brought to the doctor by distraught parents who indicate that they feel there is something seriously wrong with the child. The baby is not thriving, demonstrates clear neurodegenerative deficit, and has a cherubic face with sagging jowls and no eyebrows. The infant's hair is gray and has the appearance and feel of steel wool. This constellation of symptoms is associated with which of the following disorders?

A. acute intermittent porphyria (AIP)
B. hemochromatosis type 1
C. Menkes disease
D. porphyria cutanea tarda (PCT)
E. Wilson disease

Answer C: Menkes disease is inherited as an X-linked disorder of copper homeostasis. The disorder is associated with an inability to absorb copper from the gastrointestinal tract. As a consequence of the reduced delivery of copper to the brain, Menkes patients exhibit severe mental and developmental impairment. In addition, because there is a need for copper as a cofactor in numerous enzymes (eg, lysyl oxidases) Menkes patients also exhibit connective tissue abnormalities. Menkes disease is the result of defects in the P-type ATPase protein that is responsible for the translocation of copper across the intestinal basal-lateral membrane into the blood, thus allowing for uptake of dietary copper. This protein is encoded by the ATPase, Cu^{2+}-transporting, α-polypeptide (*ATP7A*) gene.

2. A 3-month-old infant who otherwise appeared normal during the first 2 months of life except for a bout of hyperbilirubinemia is now clearly exhibiting developmental delay. In addition, the infant's hair has become grayish and dull and there is a stubble of broken hair over the occiput and temporal regions. The facial appearance has also changed such that the infant has very pudgy cheeks, abnormal eyebrows, and sagging jowls. The occurrence of frequent convulsions was the stimulus for the parents to bring their child to the emergency room. These rapidly deteriorating symptoms are indicative of which of the following disorders?

A. Crigler-Najjar syndrome type I
B. Gilbert syndrome
C. hemochromatosis
D. Menkes disease
E. Refsum disease

Answer D: Menkes disease is inherited as an X-linked disorder of copper homeostasis. The disorder is associated with an inability to absorb copper from the gastrointestinal tract. As a consequence of the reduced delivery of copper to the brain, Menkes patients exhibit severe mental and developmental impairment. In addition, because there is a need for copper as a cofactor in numerous enzymes (eg, lysyl oxidases) Menkes patients also exhibit connective tissue abnormalities. Menkes disease is the result of defects in the P-type ATPase protein that is responsible for the translocation of copper across the intestinal basal-lateral membrane into the blood, thus allowing for uptake of dietary copper. This protein is encoded by the ATPase, Cu^{2+}-transporting, α-polypeptide (*ATP7A*) gene.

3. Your patient is a 25-year-old woman who is experiencing difficulty speaking, clumsiness while walking, uncontrolled twitching in her arms, fatigue, and depression. Physical examination shows distinct jaundice in skin and the eyes as well as a discoloration in the periphery of the cornea. These signs and symptoms are most likely indicative of which of the following disorders?

A. acute intermittent porphyria (AIP)
B. hemochromatosis type 1
C. Menkes disease
D. porphyria cutanea tarda (PCT)
E. Wilson disease

Answer E: Wilson disease is the result of defects in the P-type ATPase protein that is primarily responsible for copper homeostasis within the liver. This protein is encoded by the ATPase, Cu^{2+}-transporting, β-polypeptide (*ATP7B*) gene. *ATP7B* facilitates the transfer of copper to the major plasma copper transport protein, ceruloplasmin. In the liver, copper is stored intracellularly bound to the protein metallothionein. Any copper in excess of the binding capacity of metallothionein is excreted into the biliary canaliculi through the transport action of *ATP7B*. The majority of patients with Wilson disease present with hepatic or neuropsychiatric symptoms. The most significant sign in the diagnosis of Wilson disease results from the deposition of copper in Descemet's membrane of the cornea. These golden-brown deposits can be seen with a slit-lamp and are Kayser-Fleischer rings.

4. You are tending to a 40-year-old male patient complaining of severe abdominal pain, lack of energy, diminished sex drive, weight loss, and generalized weakness. You note a general darkening of the skin making it look bronze in color. Suspecting an iron overload, you prescribe addition tests because you believe the patient is most likely suffering from which of the following disorders?

A. type 1 hemochromatosis (*HFE1* gene defect)
B. type 2A hemochromatosis (hemojuvelin gene defect)
C. type 2B hemochromatosis (hepcidin gene defect)
D. type 4 hemochromatosis (ferroportin gene defect)

Answer A: Hemochromatosis is defined as a disorder in iron metabolism that is characterized by excess iron absorption, saturation of iron-binding proteins, and deposition of hemosiderin (amorphous iron deposits) in the tissues. Primary hemochromatosis is referred to as type 1 hemochromatosis and it is caused by the inheritance of an autosomal recessive allele. The locus causing type 1 hemochromatosis has been designated the HFE1 locus and is a major histocompatibility complex (MHC) class 1 gene.

5. You are tending to a 27-year-old male patient presenting with hypogonadism and cardiomyopathy. Additional testing has confirmed that the patient is suffering from juvenile hemochromatosis type 2A. This disorder results from a defect in the gene encoding the hemojuvelin protein. The expression of which of the following proteins would likely be unregulated in this patient?

A. ceruloplasmin
B. ferroportin
C. hephaestin
D. hepcidin
E. transferrin receptor

Answer D: Juvenile hemochromatosis (JH) type 2A is the result of defects in the gene encoding hemojuvelin (HJV). The function of hemojuvelin is to regulate the expression of the hepcidin gene. Unregulated expression of hepcidin allows for increased iron uptake resulting in the iron overload typical in hemochromatosis.

6. You are treating a 30-year-old patient for acute hepatitis and progressive chronic liver disease.

Your patient also shows parkinsonian tremors, diminished facial muscle movement, and choreoathetosis. In taking the patient history you learn that he has become progressively more depressed and paranoid. Which of the following disorders most likely explains the signs and symptoms observed in this patient?

A. aceruloplasminemia
B. GRACILE syndrome
C. hemochromatosis
D. Menkes disease
E. Wilson disease

Answer E: Wilson disease is the result of defects in the P-type ATPase protein that is primarily responsible for copper homeostasis within the liver. This protein is encoded by the ATPase, Cu^{2+}-transporting, β-polypeptide (*ATP7B*) gene. *ATP7B* facilitates the transfer of copper to the major plasma copper transport protein, ceruloplasmin. In the liver, copper is stored intracellularly bound to the protein metallothionein. Any copper in excess of the binding capacity of metallothionein is excreted into the biliary canaliculi through the transport action of *ATP7B*. The majority of patients with Wilson disease present with hepatic or neuropsychiatric symptoms. The most significant sign in the diagnosis of Wilson disease results from the deposition of copper in Descemet's membrane of the cornea. These golden-brown deposits can be seen with a slit-lamp and are Kayser-Fleischer rings.

7. Transport of iron from within intestinal enterocytes to the circulation requires that it be oxidized from the ferrous to the ferric form. This oxidation is catalyzed by which of the following proteins?

A. ceruloplasmin
B. DMT1
C. ferroportin
D. heme oxygenase
E. hephaestin

Answer E: Iron is transported across the basolateral membrane of intestinal enterocytes into the circulation, through the action of the transport protein ferroportin (also called IREG1 = iron-regulated gene 1). Associated with ferroportin is the enzyme hephaestin (a copper-containing ferroxidase with homology to ceruloplasmin) which oxidizes the ferrous form back to the ferric form. Once in the circulation, ferric form of iron is bound to transferrin and passes through the portal circulation of the liver.

8. Hemochromatosis, a disorder that is the result of excess iron accumulation, is caused by deficiencies in which of the following proteins?

A. divalent metal transporter 1 (DMT1)
B. HLA complex iron protein (HFE)
C. ferritin
D. ferroportin
E. transferrin

Answer B: Hemochromatosis is defined as a disorder in iron metabolism that is characterized by excess iron absorption, saturation of iron-binding proteins, and deposition of hemosiderin (amorphous iron deposits) in the tissues. Primary hemochromatosis is referred to as type 1 hemochromatosis and it is caused by the inheritance of an autosomal recessive allele. The locus causing type 1 hemochromatosis has been designated the HFE1 locus and is a major histocompatibility complex (MHC) class 1 gene.

9. Loss of the hepatic protein hepcidin can lead to severe iron overload with symptoms resembling those of hemochromatosis. Which of the following functions of hepcidin accounts for the iron overload when the protein is deficient?

A. activates the expression of the iron-response element binding protein that regulates transferring receptor and ferritin mRNA translation
B. decreases the level of intestinal membrane iron transporters, resulting in reduced iron uptake
C. facilitation of the interaction of transferrin with the transferrin receptor
D. forms a complex with ferritin allowing for higher intracellular storage
E. promotes the formation of hemosiderin, thus detoxifying iron

Answer B: Regulation of iron absorption, recycling, and release from intracellular stores is effected primarily as a consequence of the actions of the hepatic iron regulatory protein hepcidin. Hepcidin functions by inhibiting the presentation of one or more of the iron transporters (eg, DMT1 and ferroportin) in intestinal membranes. With a high iron diet the level of hepcidin mRNA increases and conversely its levels decrease when dietary iron is low. This is occurring simultaneous to reciprocal changes in the levels of the transporters.

10. The level of iron in the body must be tightly regulated due to the severe toxicity associated with elevated levels in the circulation and within cells. Which of the following proteins is primarily responsible for iron homeostasis?

A. ceruloplasmin
B. haptoglobin
C. metallothionein
D. α_2-macroglobulin
E. transferrin

Answer E: Transferrin, made in the liver, is the serum protein responsible for the transport of iron. Cells take up the transported iron through interaction of transferrin with cell-surface receptors. Internalization of the iron-transferrin-receptor complexes is initiated following receptor phosphorylation by PKC. Following internalization, the iron is released due to the acidic nature of the endosomes. The transferrin receptor is then recycled back to the cell surface.

11. Regulation of iron homeostasis occurs by controlling the amount that circulates in the serum as well as the amount contained within cells. One mechanism that plays a role in this homeostasis is iron-mediated control of the level of the intracellular iron-binding protein ferritin. Which of the following represents the mechanism of iron regulation of ferritin levels?

A. binding of iron to ferritin leads to secretion of the complex from cells and subsequent excretion in the urine
B. ferritin exists as a tetramer and when iron binds, the affinity for additional iron atoms increases
C. iron binds an additional protein that acts as a regulator of ferritin mRNA translation, high iron leads to increased translation and thus increased iron-binding capacity
D. when excess iron binds to ferritin it decreases the half-life of the protein allowing the iron to be released to the plasma and excreted

Answer C: An important regulatory scheme related to iron metabolism encompasses RNA binding proteins that bind to mRNA encoding ferritin. This regulation occurs through the action of an iron response element binding protein (IRBP) that binds to specific iron response elements (IREs) in the 5′-UTR of the ferritin mRNA. When iron levels are high, IRBP cannot bind to the IRE in the 5′-UTR of the ferritin mRNA. This allows the ferritin mRNA to be translated. Conversely, when iron levels are low, the IRBP binds to the IRE in the ferritin mRNA preventing its translation.

12. A 29-year-old man is being examined by his physician to determine the cause of his progressing tremors. His physician notes that the man has a diminished capacity to move his facial muscles and that the tremors in his arms are indicative of choreoathetosis. Serum analysis shows significantly elevated AST and ALT. Ophthalmic examination indicates that the patient has Keyser-Fleischer rings in his corneas suggesting he is suffering from Wilson disease. The lack of which of the following processes would most likely be found in this patient?

A. copper incorporation into ceruloplasmin
B. copper storage in renal tubule cells
C. copper transfer into the brain
D. copper transport from within intestinal enterocytes into the portal circulation
E. copper uptake by intestinal enterocytes

Answer A: Wilson disease is the result of defects in the P-type ATPase protein that is primarily responsible for copper homeostasis within the liver. This protein is encoded by the ATPase, Cu^{2+}-transporting, β-polypeptide (*ATP7B*) gene. *ATP7B* facilitates the transfer of copper to the major plasma copper transport protein, ceruloplasmin. In the liver, copper is stored intracellularly bound to the protein metallothionein. Any copper in excess of the binding capacity of metallothionein is excreted into the biliary canaliculi through the transport action of *ATP7B*. The majority of patients with Wilson disease present with hepatic or neuropsychiatric symptoms. The most significant sign in the diagnosis of Wilson disease results from the deposition of copper in Descemet's membrane of the cornea. These golden-brown deposits can be seen with a slit-lamp and are Kayser-Fleischer rings.

13. The parents of a 4-month-old infant bring their child to his pediatrician because they are concerned about his difficulty in feeding, irritability, and his overall floppiness. The pediatrician notes that the infant has pudgy, rosy, cheeks and brittle, easily broken hair. The doctor suspects the child is suffering from Menkes disease. Given that the physician is correct in her diagnosis, the lack of which of the following would likely be found in this patient?

A. copper incorporation into ceruloplasmin
B. copper storage in hepatocytes
C. copper transfer into the biliary circulation
D. copper transport from within intestinal enterocytes into the portal circulation
E. copper uptake by intestinal enterocytes

Answer E: Menkes disease is inherited as an X-linked disorder of copper homeostasis. The disorder is associated with an inability to absorb copper from the gastrointestinal tract. As a consequence of the reduced delivery of copper to the brain, Menkes patients exhibit severe mental and developmental impairment. In addition, because there is a need for copper as a cofactor in numerous enzymes (eg, lysyl oxidases) Menkes patients also exhibit connective tissue abnormalities. Menkes disease is the result of defects in the P-type ATPase protein that is responsible for the translocation of copper across the intestinal basal-lateral membrane into the blood, thus allowing for uptake of dietary copper.

This protein is encoded by the ATPase, Cu^{2+}-transporting, α-polypeptide (*ATP7A*) gene.

14. You are examining a patient manifesting symptoms typically seen in one suffering from severe hemochromatosis including slurred speech, memory impairment, ataxia, and dementia as well as bronze diabetes. Genetic analysis and examination of plasma proteins indicate the patient does not have the typical causes of iron overload. Which of the following proteins is most likely absent or defective in this patient that would explain the observed symptoms?

A. ceruloplasmin
B. ferritin
C. ferroportin
D. hephaestin
E. transferrin

Answer A: Ceruloplasmin is a copper-binding protein that serves not only to transport copper but also is a plasma ferroxidase that oxidizes ferrous iron to ferric iron which can then be bound by transferrin and transported in the blood. Aceruloplasminemia is a rare, recessively inherited neurodegenerative disorder characterized by a lack of ceruloplasmin in the circulation. The lack of ceruloplasmin results in abnormal iron use in the body and leads to iron deposits in various body tissues such as the brain, pancreas, and liver. The iron overload results a neurodegeneration, diabetes, and numerous other symptoms.

15. Loss or deficiency in which of the following proteins would result in the inability of transferrin bind and transport iron in the blood?

A. duodenal cytochrome *b* (DCYTB)
B. ferritin
C. ferroportin
D. heme oxygenase
E. hephaestin

Answer E: Transferrin can only bind the ferric form of iron within the circulation. Within the cells iron is stored, bound to ferritin in the ferrous form. Iron is transported across the basolateral membrane of intestinal enterocytes into the circulation, through the action of the transport protein ferroportin (also called IREG1 = iron-regulated gene 1). Associated with ferroportin is the enzyme hephaestin (a copper-containing ferroxidase with homology to ceruloplasmin) which oxidizes the ferrous form back to the ferric form. Once in the circulation, ferric form of iron is bound to transferrin and passes through the portal circulation of the liver.

16. You are examining a 44-year-old male patient who appears anemic. Blood work indicates his hemoglobin level is 12.2 g/dL (normal is 15.5 g/dL) and his erythrocytes are microcytic (mean corpuscular volume [MCV] = 70 fL, with normal MCV = 80-100 fL). Given these findings, which of the following would most likely be present in this patient?

A. acute bleeding
B. folate deficiency
C. iron deficiency
D. vitamin B_{12} deficiency
E. vitamin K deficiency

Answer C: Microcytic anemia can often be associated with defective hemoglobin synthesis. In the case of iron-deficiency anemia, heme synthesis is impaired due to the lack of iron. The most common causes of iron-deficiency anemia are insufficient dietary intake of the metal or chronic bleeding, most often due to gastrointestinal bleeding. Iron-deficiency anemia is characterized by skin, fatigue, light-headedness, and weakness.

17. Delivery of iron to cells by receptor-medicated endocytosis requires which of the following?

A. albumin
B. cytochrome a_1
C. ferredoxin
D. ferritin
E. transferrin

Answer E: Transferrin, made in the liver, is the serum protein responsible for the transport of iron. Cells take up the transported iron through interaction of transferrin with cell-surface receptors. Following internalization, the iron is released due to the acidic nature of the endosomes. The transferrin receptor is then recycled back to the cell surface.

18. The primary iron storage molecule in cells is which of the following?

A. albumin
B. ferredoxin
C. ferritin
D. haptoglobin
E. transferrin

Answer C: Ferritin is the major protein used for intracellular storage of iron. Ferritin without bound iron is referred to as apoferritin. Apoferritin is a large polymer of 24 polypeptide subunits. This multimeric structure of apoferritin is able to bind up to 2000 iron atoms in the form of ferric phosphate. The majority of intracellularly stored iron is found in the liver, skeletal muscle, and reticuloendothelial cells.

19. A 3-month-old infant who was born at 34 weeks' gestation is being breast-fed. Mean corpuscular volume

(MCV) is 70 μm³ (normal = 80-100), and mean corpuscular hemoglobin concentration (MHC) is 28% (normal = 30-34). The infant should receive an oral supplement of which of the following?

A. copper
B. fluoride
C. folate
D. iron
E. selenium

Answer D: The symptoms in this infant are indicative of iron-deficiency anemia which is characterized by microcytic (small) and hypochromic (low-pigment) erythrocytes. Oral administration of ferrous sulfate is commonly used to supplement iron loss causing the anemia, however, intravenous iron therapy may be called for in some cases. Severe iron-deficiency anemia may necessitate transfusion with packed red blood cells.

Checklist

✓ Iron serves numerous important functions in the body. These include its role in heme binding of oxygen in hemoglobin and as a significant functional part of heme and iron-sulfur centers in numerous other proteins.

✓ Iron will form large complexes with anions, water, and peroxides. These large complexes have poor solubility and upon their aggregation lead to pathological consequences. In addition, iron can bind to and interfere with the structure and function of various macromolecules necessitating the need for tight regulation of iron homeostasis.

✓ Iron consumed in the diet is either free iron or heme iron. Free iron in the intestines is reduced from the ferric (Fe^{3+}) to the ferrous (Fe^{2+}) state on the luminal surface of intestinal enterocytes and transported into the cells through the action of the divalent metal transporter, DMT1. Intestinal uptake of heme iron occurs through the interaction of dietary heme with the heme carrier protein (HCP1).

✓ Iron is transported out of intestinal enterocytes into the circulation, through the action of the transport protein ferroportin (also called IREG1 = iron-regulated gene 1). Associated with ferroportin is the enzyme hephaestin (a copper-containing ferroxidase with homology to ceruloplasmin) which oxidizes the ferrous form back to the ferric form.

✓ Within the circulation the ferric form of iron is bound to transferrin and passes through the portal circulation of the liver. Cells take up iron through interaction of iron-transferrin complexes with the transferrin receptor. The iron-transferrin-receptor complexes are internalized, the iron is released due to the acidic nature of the endosomes and the transferrin receptor is returned to the cell surface.

✓ Iron can be stored within cells bound to ferritin in the ferrous state.

✓ If the storage capacity of the ferritin is exceeded, iron will deposit adjacent to the ferritin-iron complexes in the cell in amorphous iron deposits called hemosiderin.

✓ Regulation of iron absorption, recycling, and release from intracellular stores occurs through the actions of the hepatic iron regulatory protein hepcidin. Hepcidin functions by inhibiting the presentation of one or more of the iron transporters (eg, DMT1 and ferroportin) in intestinal membranes.

✓ Defects in iron homeostasis can result from impaired intestinal absorption, excess loss of heme iron due to bleeding as well as to mutations in the iron response elements of iron-regulated mRNAs resulting in iron overload. Hemochromatosis is defined as a disorder in iron metabolism that is characterized by excess iron absorption, saturation of iron-binding proteins, and deposition of hemosiderin in the tissues. The primary affected tissues are the liver, pancreas, and skin.

- ✓ Copper is an essential trace element which plays a pivotal role in cell physiology as it constitutes a core part of copper-containing enzymes termed cuproenzymes. Copper exists in 2 oxidation states, cuprous (Cu^{1+} or Cu^{+}) and cupric (Cu^{2+}).
- ✓ Copper can be toxic when present in excessive amounts as it binds with high affinity to histidine, cysteine, and methionine residues of proteins which can result in their inactivation and it also readily interacts with oxygen leading to the production of hydroxyl radical.
- ✓ Dietary copper is found primarily in the cupric state (Cu^{2+}) and is reduced to cuprous (Cu^{+}) prior to uptake which is effected by copper transport protein 1, CTR1.
- ✓ In cells, CTR1 is found at the plasma membrane and in intracellular vesicles. When CTR1 binds copper it is internalized and moves to endocytic vesicles. Copper-transporting P-type ATPases (Cu-ATPases) maintain intracellular copper levels.
- ✓ Two critical Cu-ATPases are ATP7A and ATP7B. ATP7A is required for cuproenzyme biosynthesis, and in intestinal enterocytes it is required for copper efflux to the portal circulation. ATP7B is mainly expressed in the liver where it is required for copper incorporation into ceruloplasmin and for excretion of copper into the biliary circulation.
- ✓ Mutations in *ATP7A* result in Menkes disease and mutations in *ATP7B* are the cause of Wilson disease.

CHAPTER

43 Digestion: Anatomy, Biochemistry, and Physiology

CHAPTER OUTLINE

High-Yield Terms

Serous fluid: a watery pale yellow transparent fluid enriched in proteins and water produced by cells of serous glands

Mucus: a viscous mixture covering mucus membranes, produced and secreted by cells of mucus membranes, consists of glycoproteins termed mucins, water, and several other proteins such as antiseptic enzymes and immunoglobulins

Chyme: represents the semifluid mass of partially digested food expelled by the stomach into the duodenum

Enterocytes: columnar epithelial cells of the intestines responsible for nutrient uptake

Goblet cell: glandular epithelial cells that secrete the glycoproteins termed mucins

Chief cell: gastric chief cells are those cells in the stomach that secrete the zymogen and pepsinogen; the parathyroid gland also contains chief cells

Parietal cell: stomach glandular epithelial cells that secrete gastric acid in response to histamine, acetylcholine, and gastrin stimulation

Oxyntic cell: another name for parietal cells

Duct cell: specialized cells lining the pancreatic ducts that secrete bicarbonate

Acinar cell: a cell of an acinus which is any cluster of cells that resembles a many-lobed berry-like structure that is the terminus of an exocrine gland; acinar cells of pancreas are the duct cells that secrete bicarbonate and digestive enzymes

Enteroendocrine cell: specialized endocrine cells found in the intestines and pancreas that produce various gastrointestinal hormones and bioactive peptides

Enterochromaffin-like cell (ECL): neuroendocrine cells that secrete histamine and are found in gastric glands of the gastric mucosa

Gut microbiota: refers to the complex mixture of microorganisms (bacteria, fungi, viruses) that reside within the gastrointestinal tract

Prebiotic: refers to any nondigestible substance in food that stimulates the growth and/or activity of intestinal system bacteria

Probiotic: refers to live bacteria that can be consumed in order to confer a health benefit

Overview of Digestive System

The gastrointestinal (GI) system, with respect to the processes of food ingestion and digestion, comprises the hollow organs that include the oral cavity, the esophagus, the stomach, and the small and large intestines (Table 43-1). In addition to these hollow organs, ingestion and digestion of food requires several accessory glands and other organs that add secretions to the hollow organs of the GI. The primary accessory organs necessary for digestion are the salivary glands present within the oral cavity, the pancreas, and the liver.

The GI organs are separated from each other at key locations by specialized structures termed sphincters. Entry of food from the oral cavity to the esophagus requires passage through the upper esophageal sphincter. The bolus of food then enters the stomach by passage through the lower esophageal sphincter. When food is propelled from the stomach into the duodenum of the small intestine, it passes through the pyloric sphincter. Upon leaving the small intestines at the level of the ileum, digested food passes through the ileocecal valve into the large intestine, also referred to as the colon. Within the colon, waste is stored until it reaches the rectum which triggers nerve impulses to initiate defecation.

Each portion of the GI performs a specialized task in the overall process of digestion. The mouth begins the process by chopping and grinding the food into small pieces while simultaneously lubricating it and initiating the process of fat and carbohydrate digestion. When we swallow, the food is propelled by muscles in the esophagus past the lower esophageal sphincter into the stomach. The process of swallowing food is completely voluntary but all the rest of the events of digestion are carried out via involuntary processes. The primary function of the esophagus is to serve as a conduit from the mouth to the stomach. Once food enters the stomach it can be stored temporarily (in the upper stomach or fundus) or continued to be digested by stomach contractions that churn the food and mix it with acid and proteases in the lower stomach. Digestion continues in the small intestine after food is propelled from the stomach past the pyloric sphincter. The small intestine is also the major site for the absorption of nutrients in the food. The principal function of the large intestine is to reabsorb fluids and electrolytes and to store fecal matter prior to expulsion from the body (Figure 43-1).

TABLE 43-1: Major Anatomic Locations in the Overall Digestive Process

Organ	***Function***
Salivary glands	Fluid and digestive enzymes
Stomach	HCl and proteases
Pancreas	$NaHCO_3$ and enzymes for intraluminal digestion
Liver	Bile acids
Gallbladder	Storage and concentration of bile
Small intestine	Terminal digestion of food, absorption of nutrients and electrolytes
Large intestine	Absorption of water and electrolytes, storage of waste

Mouth and Esophagus

Even before we place food in our mouth our visual and olfactory senses trigger the release of salivary fluids in preparation for mixing with the food. The primary contents of saliva include water, enzymes, and electrolytes (Table 43-2). Saliva is secreted from the parotid, submandibular, and sublingual glands within the oral cavity. There is a pair of parotid glands and these are the largest of the salivary glands. These glands are located posterior to the mandibular ramus and in front of the mastoid process of temporal bone. The parotid gland secretes saliva through Stensen ducts into the oral cavity. Parotid secretions are mainly serous in nature and facilitate mastication and swallowing. Enzymes present in saliva are also responsible for the digestion of starches.

The submandibular glands are also a pair of glands. These glands are located beneath the lower jaw and

High-Yield Concept

On the gross level, the GI system can be divided into the upper GI and the lower GI. The upper GI includes the mouth, esophagus, and the stomach. The lower GI includes the small and large intestines and the rectum.

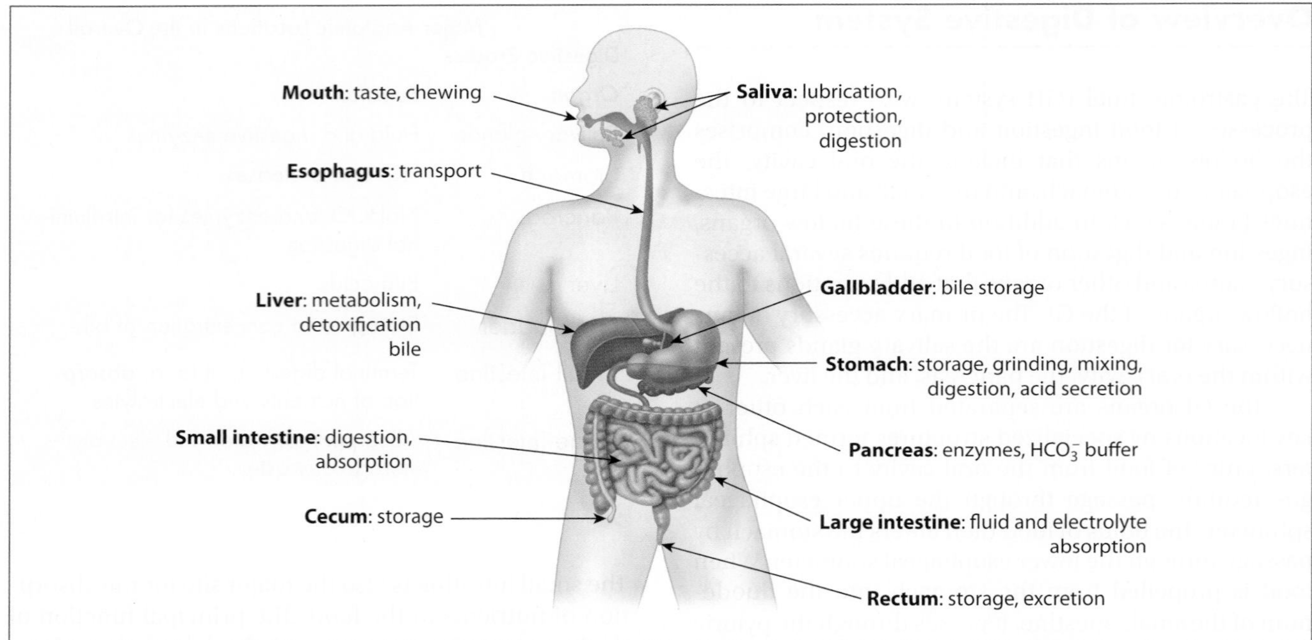

FIGURE 43-1: Digestive system overview. Reproduced with permission of themedicalbiochemistrypage, LLC.

superior to the digastric muscles which lie below the body of the mandible. Submandibular secretions are a mixture of both serous fluid and mucus that enters the oral cavity via Wharton's ducts. Roughly 70% of the saliva present in the oral cavity is derived from the submandibular glands.

The sublingual glands are also a pair of glands that reside beneath the tongue and anterior to the submandibular glands. The salivary secretion produced by the sublingual glands is mainly mucus in nature. The sublingual glands do not have striated ducts like the parotid and submandibular ducts. Sublingual fluid is released from 8 to 20 excretory ducts and this fluid constitutes approximately 5% of saliva entering the oral cavity.

Chewing food is designed to chop, mash, and mix the contents of the mouth. The mixing of food and saliva represents the initial process of digestion. The action of α-amylase, on starch, releases glucose into the mouth. Glucose is sweet tasting which enhances the flavor of the food making it much more palatable and rewarding.

When we swallow, the food is passed through the pharynx past the upper esophageal sphincter into the esophagus. Muscles in the esophagus then propel the food past the lower esophageal sphincter and into the stomach. The esophagus passes through the posterior mediastinum in the thorax and enters the abdomen through a hole in the diaphragm at the level of the tenth thoracic vertebrae. The esophagus is divided into three distinct sections referred to as cervical, thoracic, and abdominal. As a consequence of the actions of the inferior pharyngeal constrictor muscle, entry to the esophagus occurs only when swallowing or vomiting.

Stomach

The role of the stomach in overall digestive processes is complex and unique. The unique digestive functions of the stomach are related to its structure and to the types of

High-Yield Concept

The process of swallowing food is a completely voluntary event. Once food enters the rest of the GI system all of the subsequent events of digestion occur via completely involuntary processes that are controlled by the enteric, parasympathetic, and sympathetic nervous systems.

TABLE 43-2: Contents of Saliva

Component(s)	*Functions/Comments*
Water	Major component comprising almost 99% of the volume
Electrolytes	Sodium, potassium, phosphate, chloride, bicarbonate, calcium, magnesium
Mucus	A mixture of mucopolysaccharides and glycoproteins high in sialic acid and sulfated sugars, mixes with water to form a lubricant for ease of swallowing
α-Amylase	Secreted by acinar cells of the parotid and submandibular glands, digests starch into glucose
Lingual lipase	An acid lipase secreted by acinar cells of von Ebner glands, remains inactive until entering the acidic environment of the stomach
Lysozyme	Antibacterial enzyme that hydrolyzes β-1,4-glycosidic linkages between *N*-acetylmuramic acid and *N*-acetyl-D-glucosamine in cell wall peptidoglycans
Kallikrein	Secreted by acinar cells of all 3 major salivary glands, cleaves high-molecular-weight kininogen (HMWK) releasing the vasodilator, bradykinin
Antimicrobial components	Immunoglobulin, lactoperoxidase, lactoferrin, H_2O_2, thiocyanate
Opiorphin	Pain killing member of the endogenous opioid family
Haptocorrin	Binds vitamin B_{12} to protect it from degradation in the stomach before it is bound to intrinsic factor

secretory products produced by various specialized exocrine cells. The major secretory product of the stomach is gastric acid, HCl. In addition to acid, specialized cells of the stomach secrete the hormone ghrelin, water, mucus, bicarbonate, numerous anions and cations, intrinsic factor, and the zymogen pepsinogen. The stomach is tasked with storing ingested food, mixing ingested material with digestive juices and gastric acid, and then slowly emptying its contents past the pyloric sphincter into the duodenum.

In addition to being responsible for digesting food, the stomach also absorbs water-soluble and lipid-soluble substances. The digested contents of the stomach are referred to as chyme. Chyme is the semifluid material produced by the conversion of large solid particles into smaller particles via the combined peristaltic movements of the stomach and contraction of the pyloric sphincter. Chyme is generated by the propulsive, grinding, and retropulsive movements associated stomach peristalsis. The combination of the grinding action of the antrum, the retropulsion, and the squeezing of the chime through the pyloric sphincter into the duodenum is required for the emulsification of dietary fat and this plays an important role in the overall digestion and absorption of fat.

The stomach is anatomically divided into 3 major segments termed the fundus, the corpus (body), and the antrum (Figure 43-2). In addition, the stomach comprises two functional areas, the oxyntic gland and the pyloric gland areas. The oxyntic gland area comprises 80% of the stomach, encompassing both the fundus and the corpus. The pyloric gland area encompasses the antrum. An area of the stomach just distal to the lower esophageal sphincter is sometimes referred to as the cardia but whether it represents a normal or pathophysiological domain is an area of debate. The upper region of the stomach is called the fundus and this is where the bolus of food can be temporarily stored for up to an hour. The corpus is the largest segment of the stomach and the mucosa of this region contain many distinct exocrine and enteroendocrine cell types. The mucosal secretory cells of the fundus and corpus include mucus cells, parietal (oxyntic) cells, chief cells, and enteroendocrine cells. Chief cells are also called zymogen or peptic cells and are the cells that secrete the digestive enzymes, the pepsins. The primary function of mucus secretion by stomach epithelial cells is to protect the epithelium against shear stress and gastric acid. There are five or six distinct types of enteroendocrine cells in the mucosal layer of the stomach which includes enterochromaffin-like cells (ECL) that secrete histamine.

The last segment of the stomach is the antrum. The antrum is devoid of oxyntic glands and thus the acid secreting parietal cells. The antrum (also called the pyloric antrum) contains both exocrine and

High-Yield Concept

In addition to digestion, the stomach also plays a critical role in the sensations of appetite and satiety. These latter functions are related to the hormone ghrelin as well as to vagal nerve responses to the stomach stretching in response to uptake of the bolus of food from the esophagus.

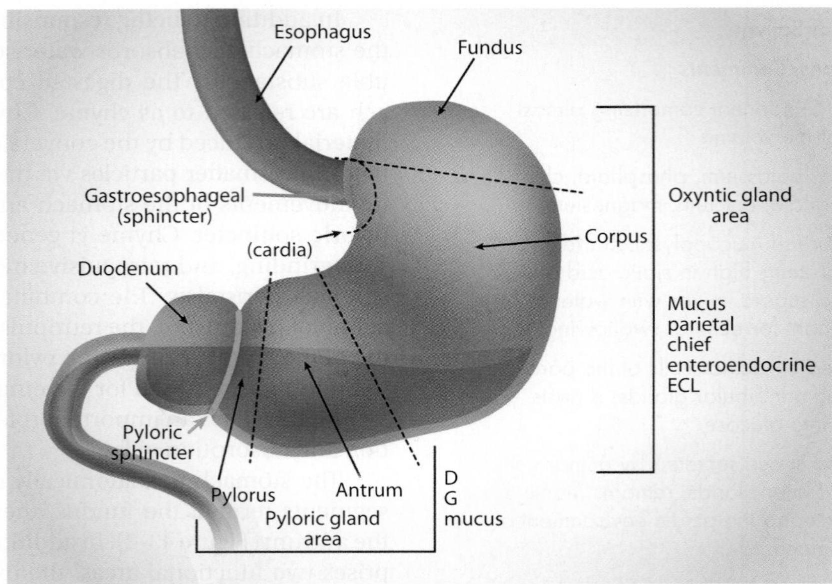

FIGURE 43-2: Organization of the major stomach segments. The 3 major structural areas are denoted by the dashed lines. The cardia is indicated in parentheses due to the fact that there is controversy as to whether or not this constitutes a normal functional region of the stomach. The 2 major functional areas, the oxyntic gland area and the pyloric gland area, are denoted in the large brackets. The major cell types in these 2 functional domains are also indicated. ECL, enterochromaffin-like cells that secrete histamine; D, D cells that secrete somatostatin; G, G cells that secrete gastrin. Reproduced with permission of themedicalbiochemistrypage, LLC.

enteroendocrine cells. The antrum enteroendocrine cells include G cells which secrete gastrin and D cells which secrete somatostatin. Both of these hormones are involved in regulated gastric acid production and secretion. Gastrin stimulates gastric acid secretion, whereas somatostatin inhibits gastrin release and, therefore, parietal cell acid secretion.

The wall of the stomach is composed of 4 distinct layers. The gastric mucosa is the layer that lines the inside of the stomach. The subsequent layers include the submucosa, the muscularis externa, and then the serosa. The mucosal layer of the stomach is composed of an epithelium that harbors the various secretory glands. The submucosa consists of fibrous connective tissue that separates the mucosa from the muscularis externa. The muscularis externa of the stomach contains 3 layers of smooth muscle, whereas the rest if the GI tract contains only 2 layers of smooth muscle. The serosa is the outer layer of the stomach consisting of connective tissue that is continuous with the peritoneum.

The mucosal lining of the corpus of the stomach contains 2 major types of specialized glands, the pyloric and oxyntic glands. The oxyntic glands are composed of parietal cells that secrete gastric acid, exocrine cells (chief) that secrete pepsinogen, and mucus secreting cells. The acid secreting parietal cells are also called oxyntic cells. In addition, parietal cells of the fundus and corpus secrete intrinsic factor. Intrinsic factor is a glycoprotein that binds to vitamin B_{12} within the small intestine allowing it to be absorbed. Initially vitamin B_{12} is protected from gastric acid by binding salivary haptocorrin. After passing into the duodenum the haptocorrin is degraded by pancreatic proteases and the vitamin is then bound to intrinsic factor. The pyloric glands are located in the antrum segment of the stomach and contain cells that are responsible for secretion of gastrin (G cells), somatostatin (D cells), and mucus.

Gastric acid production and secretion is the major exocrine function of the stomach (Figure 43-3). The production and secretion of gastric acid (HCl), by oxyntic cells, as well as the zymogen pepsinogen, by chief cells, is controlled by both hormonal- and nerve-mediated processes. The nervous system components that impact the gastrointestinal tract (see below) are complex and consist of autonomic, parasympathetic (vagus), sympathetic (prevertebral ganglia), and enteric nerve fibers possessing both efferent (motor) and afferent (sensory) neurons. The enteric nervous system functions autonomously all along the GI tract as well as interacting with the CNS via vagal and prevertebral ganglia.

The principal stimulants for acid secretion are histamine, gastrin, and acetylcholine (ACh) released from postganglionic enteric neurons. Each of the 3 stimulators of acid secretion has different levels of functional

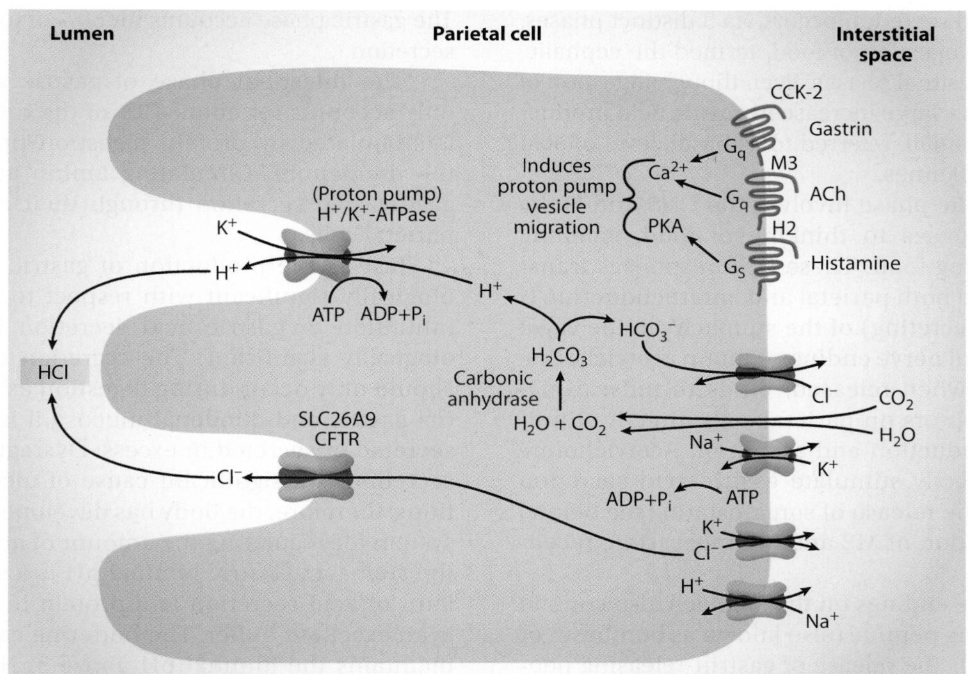

FIGURE 43-3: Gastric acid secretion by oxyntic cells. Stimulation of parietal cells by acetylcholine or gastrin binding triggers the release of intracellular calcium which in turn triggers the fusion of tubulovesicles containing the H^+,K^+-ATPase (proton pump) with the parietal cell membrane allowing transport of protons into the canaliculus of the cell and out into to lumen of the stomach. Histamine binding to parietal cells activates adenylate cyclase resulting in increased cAMP and activation of PKA which also triggers tubulovesicle fusion to the parietal cell membrane. CCK-2, cholecystokinin-2 (and gastrin) receptor; M3, muscarinic acetylcholine (ACh) receptor 3; H2, histamine receptor 2; CFTR, cystic fibrosis transmembrane conductance regulator. Reproduced with permission of themedicalbiochemistrypage, LLC.

importance, but histamine is thought to be the primary stimulus. Histamine is synthesized from the amino acid histidine via the action of histidine decarboxylase (see Chapter 30). Histamine is released from ECL cells in response to gastrin binding to these cells in fundal glands. The released histamine then binds to H_2 receptors on parietal cells. The H_2 receptor is a G_s-type GPCR that activates adenylate cyclase, leading to elevation of intracellular cAMP concentrations and activation of PKA. With respect to gastric acid production, PKA activation leads to phosphorylation of cytoskeletal proteins involved in transport of the H^+/K^+-ATPase (proton pump) from the cytoplasm to the apical plasma membrane of the parietal cell.

The gastric H^+/K^+-ATPase is a member of the P-type ATPase family (see Chapter 7). The H^+K^+-ATPase is the molecular pump of gastric acid secretion and it is solely responsible for the secretion of hydrogen ions into the lumen of the gastric glands and ultimately the stomach. The H^+/K^+-ATPase transports one hydrogen ion (H^+) out of the cytoplasm of the parietal cell in exchange for one potassium ion (K^+) obtained from the lumen of the gastric gland. The concentration of hydrogen ion in the lumen of gastric glands is such that the pH is on the order of 0.8, making it the most acidic environment in the human body.

The hydrogen ions are generated within the parietal cell from the dissociation of water. Water and CO_2 are combined to form carbonic acid via the action of carbonic anhydrase. Carbonic acid rapidly ionizes to H^+ and bicarbonate ion. This bicarbonate is then transported to the blood, across the parietal cell basolateral membrane, in exchange for chloride ion. The chloride ions are transported into the lumen of the gastric glands via the action of anion exchangers of the solute carrier family. The gastric chloride exchanger is encoded by the SLC26A9 gene. Within the lumen of the gastric gland the hydrogen ions and chloride ions combine to form gastric acid (HCl).

Like all P-type ATPase's, the H^+/K^+-ATPase is able to transport ions against a concentration gradient by utilizing the energy derived from the hydrolysis of ATP. During ATP hydrolysis a phosphate is transferred to the H^+/K^+-ATPase resulting in a conformational change in the pump. The conformational changes that occur to the H^+/K^+-ATPase in response to phosphorylation and dephosphorylation ensure that ion transport can only occur unidirectionally at any given point in time.

Gastric acid secretion occurs via 3 distinct phases, in response to ingestion of food, termed the cephalic, gastric, and intestinal phases. Even though ingestion of food stimulates a large increase in gastric acid production, there is a small, referred to as basal, level of acid production at all times.

The cephalic phase involves the CNS and is the result of responses to thinking of food, smelling food, and tasting food. These CNS responses transmit impulses to both parietal and enteroendocrine G cells (gastrin secreting) of the stomach via the vagal nerve. The vagal nerve endings contain acetylcholine (ACh) which, when released, binds to muscarinic-type (M3) receptors on parietal cells directly stimulating acid production and secretion. Acetylcholine can also indirectly stimulate gastric acid secretion by inhibiting the release of somatostatin (see below) through activation of M2 and M4 muscarinic receptors on D cells.

Vagal nerve endings on the stomach also contain gastrin-releasing peptide (also known as bombesin or neuromedin B). The release of gastrin-releasing peptide triggers G cells to release gastrin. Gastrin then binds to receptors on parietal cells indirectly stimulating acid secretion. Gastrin exists in 2 major forms: little gastrin (17 amino acids) and big gastrin (34 amino acids), both of which result from a single precursor protein of 101 amino acid. Both forms of gastrin function by binding to the cholecystokinin-2 receptor (CCK2 or CCK_B). The *C*-terminal tetrapeptide of both gastrins and cholecystokinin (CCK) are identical and possess all the biological activities of both gastrin and CCK. The cephalic phase accounts for 40% of total gastric acid secretion.

The distension (stretching) of the stomach as a result of food intake represents the gastric phase. The gastric phase of acid production is also stimulated by digestive products such as peptides. The distension of the stomach results in the stimulation of mechanoreceptors. Mechanoreceptor activation then causes parietal cell stimulation via both enteric (direct) and vagal nerve reflexes. Afferent and efferent impulses from the vagus nerve in the stomach mediate vago-vagal reflexes within the brain via the dorsal vagal complex. The gastric phase accounts for 50% of total gastric acid secretion.

The intestinal phase of gastric acid secretion only accounts for about 10% of the total. This phase is stimulated by protein digestion products within the duodenum. Circulating amino acids stimulate gastric acid secretion through their actions on the parietal cells.

Just as the production of gastric acid is physiologically significant with respect to digestion, the inhibition of gastric acid secretion is also physiologically significant. The secretion of gastric acid should only occur during digestion as it can damage the gastric and duodenal mucosa if inappropriately secreted or secreted in excess. Dysregulation of acid secretion is a significant cause of ulcerative conditions, therefore, the body has developed an elaborate system for regulating the amount of acid secreted by the stomach. Gastric luminal pH is a sensitive regulator of acid secretion and protein in digested food is an excellent buffer. The buffering capacity of food maintains the luminal pH above 3. However, when the stomach is empty, or if acid production is excessive gastric pH can fall below 3. When the pH falls, enteroendocrine D cells of the antrum secrete somatostatin which inhibits gastrin release from oxyntic cells. Acidification of the duodenal lumen also triggers mechanisms to inhibit gastric acid production. Under low pH conditions duodenal enteroendocrine S cells release secretin which inhibits the release of gastrin (Clinical Box 43-1).

Pancreas

The pancreas is a highly specialized organ found behind the stomach and it is surrounded by the small intestine, liver, and spleen (Figure 43-4). The organ is about six inches long and is largest at the end attached to the duodenum. This widest part is called the head of the pancreas, the middle section is called the neck and the body of the pancreas, and the thin end is called the tail.

High-Yield Concept

The response of the stomach to the effects of ACh, gastrin, and histamine occur via a phenomenon referred to as potentiation. Potentiation is the effect observed where the response to 2 stimulants is greater than the effect of either stimulant alone.

CLINICAL BOX 43-1: DISTURBANCES IN GASTRIC ACID HOMEOSTASIS

Increases in both basal and stimulated gastric acid production are the leading causes of ulcers in the mucosal lining of the gastrointestinal tract. These ulcers are collectively referred to as peptic ulcers. Four times as many peptic ulcers arise in the duodenum (called duodenal ulcers) versus the stomach itself (called gastric ulcers). The major cause of disrupted gastric acid homeostasis (accounting for as much as 70%-90% of such ulcers) is infection with *Helicobacter pylori* (*H pylori*), a helical-shaped bacterium that lives in the acidic environment of the stomach. Around 4% of all gastric ulcers are caused by malignant tumors called gastrinomas. Stress ulcers are most often found in the proximal stomach and result from mucosal ischemia and altered mucosal defense. Although duodenal ulcers are the result of increased acid secretion, gastric ulcers are more often associated with normal or decreased basal and stimulated acid production. Gastric ulcers are, therefore, most often caused by altered gastric mucosal defense which explains the propensity for NSAID (nonsteroidal anti-inflammatory drug)-induced ulcers to occur in the stomach. Gastric ulcers are classified into four groups according to their location and concomitant association with duodenal ulcer. Type I ulcers are found in the corpus and are generally characterized by low acid secretion, particularly at night. Type II ulcers occur in the antrum and are characterized by low, normal, or high acid secretion. Type III ulcers occur in close proximity to the pylorus and are associated with high acid output and duodenal ulcers. Type IV ulcers occur in the cardia and are characterized by low acid secretion. Treatment for gastric ulcers involves removing the injurious agent (e.g., NSAIDs or *H pylori*) and inhibiting acid secretion. Antacids were the first therapeutic approach for ulcers. Unfortunately in order to neutralize luminal acid adequately, they need to be taken frequently which results in noncompliance and adverse effects. Although antacids with high neutralizing capacity, given after meals and at bedtime, can accelerate ulcer healing, pain is not significantly. The histamine H_2 receptor antagonist (H2RA), cimetidine, was the first in this class of new peptic ulcer treatments. H2RAs block both histamine-stimulated acid secretion and that induced by gastrin, which functions via stimulation of histamine release from ECL cells. The development of H^+/K^+-ATPase inhibitors (proton pump inhibitors, PPIs), such as omeprazole, revolutionized the therapeutic management of gastric acid. PPIs directly inhibit the acid pump and therefore, they are capable of reducing both basal and stimulated gastric acid secretion independent of stimulus. PPIs are much more effective than H2RAs at reducing gastric pH as well as being more effective in aiding the healing of duodenal ulcers and preventing their recurrence. In addition to these more common conditions that cause abnormal gastric acid production resulting in ulcers, there are several uncommon conditions. The best characterized of these latter conditions is Zollinger-Ellison syndrome, ZES. ZES results from gastrin-producing tumors (gastrinomas) that result in hypersecretion of gastric acid. In any patient manifesting with refractory erosive esophagitis, multiple peptic ulcers, ulcers in the distal duodenum or jejunum, and recurrent ulcers after acid-reducing surgery the possibility of ZES should be highly suspected. Patients with a family history of multiple endocrine neoplasia type 1 (MEN1), or any of the endocrinopathies associated with MEN1, that are presenting with multiple peptic ulcers should also be suspected of having ZES since approximately 25% of patients with ZES have MEN1. MEN1 is an autosomal dominant disorder characterized by pancreatic endocrine tumors, pituitary adenomas, and hyperparathyroidism. The PPIs are used as the therapies of choice in the treatment of ZES, although very high doses are sometimes required to reduce the acid hypersecretion sufficiently. Recently, gastroesophageal reflux disease (GERD) has become the most important acid-related clinical disorder. The pathogenesis of GERD involves acid in the wrong anatomical location, not excess acid production. Numerous treatments for GERD have been attempted but surgery is the most effective. Aside from surgery, the use of PPIs is the most used drugs for treatment of GERD.

The pancreas is composed primarily of 2 distinct types of secretory cells, endocrine and exocrine. The endocrine cells secrete a variety of hormones such as glucagon and insulin which have been discussed in several of the metabolic biochemistry chapters as well as in Chapters 46, 46, and 49. The exocrine pancreas is involved in the secretion of numerous enzymes (Table 43-3), electrolytes, and other substances involved in digestion. The exocrine pancreas has ducts that are arranged in clusters called acini (singular acinus). Pancreatic digestive secretions are expelled into the lumen of the acinus, and then accumulate

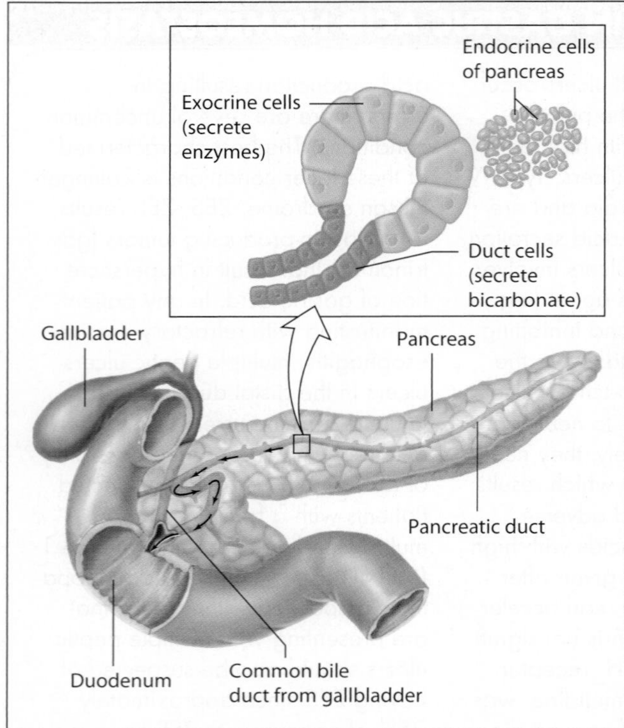

FIGURE 43-4: Structure of the pancreas. Used with permission from Widmaier EP, Raff H, Strang KT. *Vander's Human Physiology: The Mechanisms of Body Function.* 11th ed. New York: McGraw-Hill; 2008).

in intralobular ducts that drain into the main pancreatic duct. The main pancreatic duct (pancreatic duct of Wirsung) joins the common bile duct coming from the gallbladder forming the ampulla of Vater. The ampulla is connected to the duodenal papilla through which the pancreatic juice, also containing bile, enters the small intestine.

In addition to enzymes described in Table 43-3, the pancreas also secretes various cations, anions, water, and bicarbonate ion into the small intestine. Together with the pancreatic enzymes, the secretions constitute what is referred to as pancreatic juice. The cells of the pancreas tasked with electrolyte (eg, bicarbonate) secretion are called duct cells. Pancreatic bicarbonate is critical to neutralizing the gastric acid entering the small intestine from the stomach. The production and secretion of pancreatic bicarbonate is essentially the same as for the process described for gastric acid secretion by parietal cells. Like parietal cell bicarbonate production, pancreatic bicarbonate is dependent on the enzyme carbonic anhydrase. The content of bicarbonate in pancreatic juice (around 115 mEq/L) is approximately 5-times higher than what is normally present in plasma. This high concentration of bicarbonate makes the pH of pancreatic juice around 8.0.

Exocrine glands of the pancreas also contain cells termed goblet cells. Goblet cells are tasked with the production and secretion of mucus into the pancreatic juice. Goblet cells are found nearest the distal end of the pancreatic ducts and they can constitute as much as 25% of the epithelial cells at the distal end of the main pancreatic duct. Pancreatic mucus provides lubrication to the ducts as well as mechanical protection. In addition, the mucins (high-molecular-weight glycoproteins, see Chapter 39) present in pancreatic mucus serve an immunologic function by binding pathogens and interacting with immune cells.

Control of the secretory function of the acinar and duct cells of the pancreas is exerted via nervous and humoral mechanisms. The primary neural stimulus for pancreatic cell secretion of enzymes and bicarbonate is ACh released from postganglionic parasympathetic nerve endings. The primary hormonal triggers for acinar cell secretion are gastrin, cholecystokinin (CCK), and secretin. Gastrin is secreted by gastric G cells whereas, CCK is secreted by duodenal enteroendocrine I cells and secretin by S cells. All 3 hormones are secreted in response to the ingestion of food.

Cholecystokinin and ACh are the most important regulators of acinar protein secretion. Secretin is the

High-Yield Concept

Lysophosphatidylcholine (LPC, lyso-PC) is a bioactive pro-inflammatory lipid generated by the action of $sPLA_2$. In cases of acute pancreatitis it is believed that pancreatic $sPLA_2$ is inappropriately activated within the pancreatic ducts resulting in inflammation in the tissue. In acute pancreatitis the leakage of pancreatic enzymes into the blood increases. Measurement of plasma levels of pancreatic lipase and α-amylase can be of diagnostic value in cases of suspected pancreatitis.

TABLE 43-3: Pancreatic Digestive Enzymes

Enzyme	*Activator*	*Comments*
Pancreatic α-amylase	Chloride Ion	Activity is the same as salivary α-amylase
Trypsinogen	Enteropeptidase (also called enterokinase); embedded in duodenal mucosa	Cleaves proteins and peptides on the *C*-terminal side of Arg and Lys residues
Chymotrypsinogen	Trypsin	Cleaves proteins and peptides on the *C*-terminal side of aromatic amino acids, primarily Tyr, Pro, Trp
Procarboxypeptidase A (A1 and A2)	Trypsin	Cleaves proteins and peptides on the *C*-terminal side of aromatic and aliphatic amino acids
Procarboxypeptidase B	Trypsin	Cleaves proteins and peptides on the *C*-terminal side of aliphatic amino acids
Proelastase	Trypsin	Cleaves proteins and peptides on the *C*-terminal side of basic amino acids
Carboxyl ester lipase, CEL (cholesterol esterase or sterol ester hydrolase)		Hydrolyzes cholesterol esters
Pancreatic lipase		Hydrolyzes triglycerides to fatty acids and mono- and diacylglycerides; requires bile salt emulsified lipid droplets
Colipase	Trypsin	Required at lipid-water interface for pancreatic lipase to function
Secreted Phospholipase A_2 ($sPLA_2$)	Trypsin	Hydrolyzes the *sn*2 position in phospholipids such as PE, PC, PI, PS releasing lysophospholipid (LPL) and a free fatty acid; at least *11* $sPLA_2$ genes; pancreatic enzyme is encoded by the *PLA2G1B* gene
Ribonuclease		Hydrolyzes RNAs to free nucleotides
Deoxyribonuclease		Hydrolyzes DNA to free nucleotides

most important regulator of pancreatic duct cell secretion of bicarbonate. The action of CCK on acinar cells exhibits a biphasic response in that induced secretion occurs at a particular dose of hormone but secretion is inhibited at higher doses. The CCK_A receptor has the highest affinity for CCK and this receptor exists in both low affinity and high affinity states in acinar cells. Low concentrations of CCK activate the high affinity state receptor which induces acinar cell secretion, whereas high concentrations of CCK activate the low affinity state receptor leading to inhibition of secretion. ACh activates acinar cell secretion by binding to muscarinic (M3) receptors.

As indicated earlier, the hormone secretin is involved in the response to acidification of the contents of the intestines. When the pH of intestinal fluid falls below around 4.5, S cells of the duodenum release secretin. At the level of the stomach secretin inhibits gastric acid production by inhibiting the release of gastrin and GIP. At the level of the pancreas, secretin stimulates pancreatic duct cells to secrete bicarbonate which when released into the duodenum increases the pH.

Intestine

The intestines comprise a long hollow organ that runs from the stomach to the anus. The intestines are divided into three major anatomical and functional segments termed the small intestine, the large intestine, and the rectum. The small intestine is further divided into three functionally distinct segments. These segments, from the stomach to the large intestines are the duodenum, jejunum, and ileum. The small intestines are around 20 ft in length with an average diameter of 1 in. The large intestine, which is commonly referred to as the colon, is also subdivided into distinct segments. Beginning with the segment attached to the ileum these segments are the cecum, ascending colon, transverse colon, descending colon, and sigmoid colon. The large intestines are around 5 ft in length with an average diameter of 3 in.

Similar to the layers of the stomach, the intestines are layered from inside the lumen to out with glandular epithelium and muscularis mucosa (together comprising the mucosal layer), submucosa, muscularis externa (only 2 layers whereas the stomach has 3), and lastly the serosa (Figure 43-5). The muscularis externa, which is composed of both longitudinal and circular smooth muscles, provides the continuous peristalsis of the intestines that promotes the movement of digested food along the length of the gut to the rectum and the movement of digested material out of and along the gut.

The primary function of the intestines is the digestion of food and the absorption of nutrients. Almost all of the nutrients in food, the amino acids, sugars, fats, and vitamins, are absorbed through the small intestines. The duodenum is the segment of the small intestine that secretes the pancreatic digestive enzymes and bicarbonate, and bile via the ampulla of Vater. The primary secretory products of the duodenum are cholecystokinin, secretin, and GIP. Absorption of nutrients is the primary function of the jejunum, while the ileum is responsible for absorption of vitamin B_{12} and bile salts.

The primary function of the large intestines is the resorption of water from food wastes, thus creating fecal matter (the stool). The stool is then stored in the large intestines until it reaches the rectum where nerve impulses then stimulate the urge to defecate. In addition to water, the large intestines reabsorb sodium and any nutrients that may have escaped primary digestion in the ileum. The large intestine is also the site where gut bacteria (microbiota) are found. The importance of gut bacteria to human physiology is significant (see below), but in the context of digestion these microorganisms produce some vitamins and important nutrients and they digest molecules that cannot be degraded by human enzymes. Bacterial metabolism also accounts for the production of gases within the intestines.

Within the small intestine, the mucosal layer contains large numbers of invaginations termed villi. In addition, there are microvilli which dramatically increase the surface area of the small intestines and are the areas of the mucosal epithelium where nutrients are absorbed. In addition to the villi and microvilli, the small intestine contains numerous glands formed by pocket-like invaginations in the epithelium called crypts (crypts of Lieberkühn). Along the entire length of the intestinal glandular epithelium are goblet cells that produce mucus, which lubricates the intestines as well as protects the tissue from digestive enzymes. The other major cell types in intestinal crypts and villi are the enterocytes and the enteroendocrine cells (I, K, and L). Enterocytes are the cell

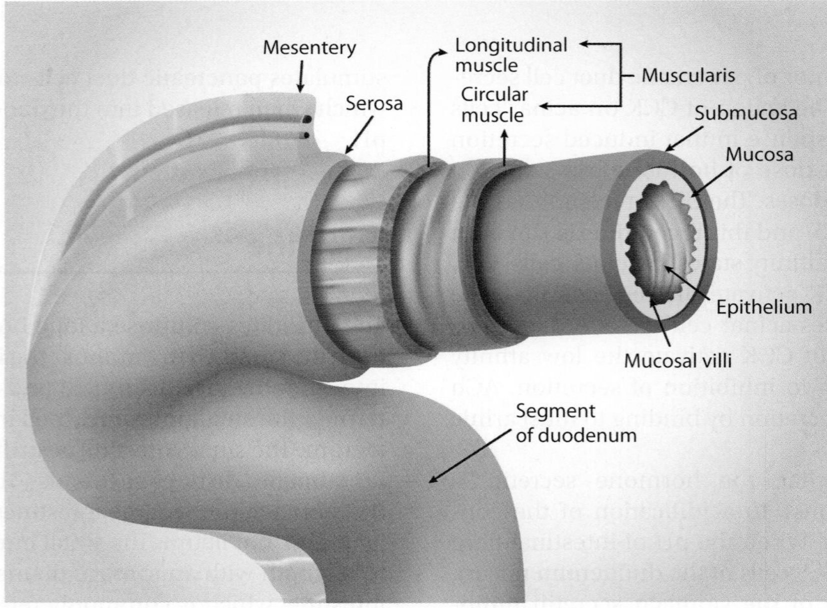

FIGURE 43-5: Macroscopic view of a section of the duodenum. Reproduced with permission of themedicalbiochemistrypage, LLC.

types that absorb the nutrients in the gut. These cells also harbor the digestive enzymes that continue to digest food as it is being absorbed. Enterocytes contain a number of enzymes that are important for digestion, but these enzymes remain associated with the brush-border membranes and are not released into the lumen of the gut. These enzymes include enteropeptidase, disaccharidases, aminopeptidases, dipeptidases, nucleotidases, and nucleosidases.

Gallbladder

The gallbladder is a small organ lying just beneath the liver between the costal margin and the lateral margin of the rectus abdominis muscle. The organ is divided into 3 sections called the fundus, body, and neck. The neck of the gallbladder tapers where it connects to the biliary tree via the cystic duct. The cystic duct then joins the common hepatic duct forming the common bile duct. The gallbladder is the storage site for bile acids that were produced from cholesterol by the liver (Chapter 27). The consumption of food, particularly lipid- and protein-rich foods, stimulates the release of CCK from duodenal enteroendocrine I cells which then enters the circulation and binds to receptors on the gallbladder. The binding of CCK to gallbladder cells induces pulsatile secretion of bile into the common bile duct which then meets with the pancreatic duct at the ampulla of Vater where they are secreted into the duodenum. Bile salts are involved in the emulsification of lipids in the intestines aiding their digestion by the various pancreatic and duodenal lipases. Unused bile salts are returned to the gallbladder through the distal ileum and the portal circulation.

Gut hormones and digestive processes

The gastrointestinal system secretes numerous hormones and neuroendocrine molecules that are critical to the overall processes of digestion as indicated earlier. However, many of these same factors play important roles in the regulation of appetite and overall feeding behaviors. As a consequence of these activities many of the gut peptides and hormones and their receptors are targets for therapeutic intervention in obesity and diabetes. Many of the activities of the gut peptides and hormones are discussed in detail in Chapter 44 and only briefly outlined here in Table 43-4.

Nervous System and Digestion

Digestion involves neural signals from the CNS and from within the gastrointestinal tract itself. The primary neural connection from the internal organs (viscera) to the CNS and back involves the vagus nerve. The vagus nerve is also called the pneumogastric nerve and is also anatomically cranial nerve X. Within the brain the dorsal nucleus of the vagus nerve sends parasympathetic outputs to the viscera, especially the intestines. The vagal nerve is composed of both afferent and efferent fibers with 80% to 90% being afferents to the brain and 10% to 20% being efferent connections that are preganglionic and make connections with postganglionic neurons of the enteric nervous system. The vagal afferent connections innervate parietal and neuroendocrine cells within the gut.

Nerve connections between the viscera and the brain also involve parasympathetic and sympathetic connections. The parasympathetic nervous system is primarily responsible for the stimulation of digestive activities that occur when the body is at rest and involves cholinergic inhibitory signals. The sympathetic nervous system mobilizes the metabolic resources of the body in response to stress such as is typical of the "fight-or-flight" response. The sympathetic nervous system is principally a noradrenergic responsive excitatory system.

Localized to the gut there is also the enteric nervous system. This system of nerve fibers functions autonomously all along the gut and also receives considerable input from the autonomic nervous system. The enteric nervous system comprises many thousands of small ganglia that reside within the walls of the esophagus, stomach, small and large intestines, pancreas, gallbladder, and biliary tree. The enteric nervous system can, and in fact it does, act completely independent of the brain and spinal cord. Interactions between the enteric nerves and the CNS involve the vagus nerve (comprising parasympathetic inputs) and prevertebral ganglia (comprising sympathetic inputs).

The functions of the enteric nervous system are to integrate information about the overall status of the gastrointestinal tract, and thereby provide outputs to control gut motility, fluid exchange, and local blood flow. The smooth muscles of the intestines that control peristalsis are responsive to both excitatory and inhibitory signals from the enteric nervous system.

TABLE 43-4: Gastrointestinal Peptides in Digestion and Feeding Behavior

Peptide	*Source(s)*	*Major Activities*
Cholecystokinin, CCK	Duodenal enteroendocrine I cells	Stimulates gallbladder contraction and bile flow increases secretion of digestive enzymes from pancreas, vagal nerves in the gut express CCK1 (CCK_A) receptors
Gastrin	Stomach antrum and duodenal enteroendocrine G cells	Stimulates gastric acid secretion from parietal cells and pepsinogen secretion from chief cells
Ghrelin	X/A-like enteroendocrine cells of the stomach oxyntic glands, minor synthesis in small intestine, pancreatic ε-cells, and hypothalamus	Regulates gastric secretions and gastric emptying, increases desire for food intake
Glucagon-like peptide 1, GLP-1	Enteroendocrine L cells of ileum	Inhibits gastric emptying, modulates pancreatic insulin and glucagon secretion
Glucose-dependent insulinotropic peptide, GIP	Enteroendocrine K cells of the duodenum and proximal jejunum	Inhibits secretion of gastric acid
Oxyntomodulin, OXM	Enteroendocrine L cells of ileum	Inhibits gastric acid secretion similar to GLP-1 action, induces satiety
Pancreatic polypeptide, PP	Pancreatic F cells and colon and rectum	Inhibits pancreatic bicarbonate and protein secretion
Peptide tyrosine tyrosine, PYY	Enteroendocrine L cells of ileum	Reduces gut motility and delays gastric emptying, inhibits gallbladder contractions and pancreatic secretions, induces satiety
Secretin	Enteroendocrine S cells of the duodenum and jejunum	Primary stimulants for pancreatic bicarbonate secretion, inhibits gastric secretions, stimulates PP secretion
Somatostatin	Stomach antrum enteroendocrine D cells, δ-cells of the pancreas, also produced in hypothalamus	Inhibits release of gastrin, also inhibits release and action of numerous gut peptides

The excitatory neurons release ACh while the inhibitory neurons release nitric oxide, vasoactive intestinal peptide (VIP), and ATP.

The enteric nervous system regulates fluid fluxes within the gastrointestinal system with the largest fluxes taking place across the small intestinal epithelium. Water moves between the lumen of the gut organs (intestines, pancreas, and gallbladder) and body fluid compartments. The absorption of water is accompanied by an inward flux of nutrients and sodium via the activation of co-transporter proteins. Along with water and sodium uptake is the outward flow of chloride and bicarbonate. Enteric control of local blood flow to the mucosa is exerted via enteric vasodilator neurons. This controls mucosal blood flow so that balance is maintained between the nutritive needs of the mucosa and the fluid exchange between the vasculature and the gut lumen.

Food Energy

When considering the amount of energy contained in various types of food components (eg, fat, protein, carbohydrate), it is most important to understand that not all of the available energy can be delivered to the human body. This is due to several factors related to loss during digestive processes, incomplete absorption of nutrients, and there may also be nondigestible constituents in some foods. Inadequate overall nutrient intake can lead to significant pathology (see Clinical Box 43-2). The absolute energy available in foods can be calculated by burning in a bomb calorimeter but this process reveals available energy in nondigestible fiber as well. Initial studies of conventional food energy were carried out in the late 19th century by the American chemist Wilbur Atwater

CLINICAL BOX 43-2: NUTRITIONAL DEFICIT DISORDERS

Marasmus and Kwashiorkor represent 2 extremes of nutritional deficit in humans. Marasmus (derived from the Greek word for decay) is a form of severe malnutrition characterized by overall energy deficiency. Kwashiorkor is a form of malnutrition due to a deficiency in protein but with sufficient caloric intake. Marasmus can occur in both children and adults, whereas Kwashiorkor is only seen in children. Marasmus results from a severe deficiency of nearly all nutrients, especially protein and carbohydrates. A typical child with marasmus looks emaciated and has a body weight less than 60% of that expected for the age. Marasmus is commonly seen in children living in poverty primarily in tropical and subtropical parts of the world, particularly in countries where the diet consists mainly of corn, rice, and beans. Treatment of marasmus is normally divided into 2 phases. The initial acute phase of treatment involves restoring electrolyte balance, treating infections, and reversing the hypoglycemia and hypothermia. This is followed by refeeding and ensuring that sufficient caloric and nutrient intake is maintained to enable catch-up growth in order to restore a healthy normal body mass. Kwashiorkor is an acute form of childhood protein-energy malnutrition characterized by edema causing the typical bulging stomach seen in affected children. Kwashiorkor also results in irritability, anorexia, skin ulcers, and hepatomegaly due to fatty infiltration. The hepatomegaly also contributes to the protuberant abdomen in these children. Kwashiorkor is common in areas of famine or poor food supply. Kwashiorkor usually occurs when a baby is weaned from protein-rich breast milk and switched to protein-poor foods. This weaning usually occurs due to the birth of another child. Treatment of Kwashiorkor involves careful administration of protein with the use of carbohydrate and fat for the majority of caloric needs of the child. This is due to the fact that the administration of too much protein will lead to increased hepatic urea cycle activity. Since the liver is already compromised due to the fatty infiltration, the metabolism of protein can exacerbate the damage and lead to liver failure and death.

but involved the complete burning of dried food in a bomb calorimeter.

The conventional assessment of energy value of a food takes into account the factors such as loss during digestion and absorption, and thus indicates the value of the food to the body as a fuel (Table 43-5). The energy content of various food components is reported on product labels as either kilojoules/gram (kJ/g) or kilocalories/gram (kcal/g). Fat is the most energy-dense macronutrient, followed by alcohol, protein, and carbohydrate.

Dietary fiber is not digested in the small intestines, and therefore imparts limited to no caloric content to the human diet. Dietary fiber is also called roughage and consists of both soluble and insoluble components. Soluble fibers are so called because they dissolve in water. These are easily fermented by intestinal bacteria and are referred to as prebiotics. Insoluble fiber can be fermented by intestinal bacteria and so can also be considered prebiotic. The advantage of insoluble fiber is that it absorbs water (particularly bulking fiber) as it transits the intestines softening the stool and thus, easing defecation. The fermentation of fiber by intestinal bacteria is known to be of physiological benefit since some of the products are absorbed and utilized for metabolic purposes such as the organic acids, acetate, propionate, and butyrate (see below).

TABLE 43-5: Standard Energy Composition of Various Food Components

Component	*Energy (kJ/g)*	*Energy (kcal/g)*
Fat	37	9
Alcohol	29	7
Protein	17	4
Carbohydrate	17	4
Organic acids	13	3
Sugar alcohols (sweeteners)	10	2.4
Fiber	8	2

Carbohydrate Digestion and Absorption

Dietary carbohydrates enter the body in complex forms, such as mono-, di-, and polysaccharides with the primary polysaccharides being plant starch (amylose and amylopectin) and animal glycogen. The carbohydrate polymer cellulose is also consumed but not digested.

TABLE 43-6: Carbohydrate Digestive Enzymes

Enzyme	*Substrate(s)*	*Products*
Salivary and pancreatic α-amylases	α(1→4) glycosidic linkages in polysaccharides	Di- and trisaccharides and shortened polysaccharides
Maltase	Maltose: glucose disaccharide in α(1→4) glycosidic linkage	Glucose
Sucrase-isomaltase	Sucrose and isomaltose	Glucose and fructose
β-Galactosidase complex (lactase + glucosylceramidase)	Lactose, ceramides	Glucose and galactose
Trehalase	Trehalose: glucose disaccharide in α(1→1) glycosidic linkage	Glucose

The first step in the metabolism of digestible carbohydrate is the conversion of the higher polymers to simpler, soluble forms that can be transported across the intestinal wall and delivered to the tissues (Table 43-6). The breakdown of polymeric sugars begins in the mouth. Saliva has a slightly acidic pH of 6.8 and contains salivary amylase that begins the digestion of carbohydrates. The action of salivary amylase is limited to the area of the mouth and the esophagus as it is virtually inactivated by the much stronger acid pH of the stomach.

The main polymeric carbohydrate digesting enzyme of the small intestine is α-amylase. This enzyme is secreted by the pancreas and has the same activity as salivary α-amylase, producing disaccharides and trisaccharides. The latter are converted to monosaccharides by intestinal saccharides, including maltases that hydrolyze di- and trisaccharides, and the more specific disaccharidases: sucrase-isomaltase, lactase (β-galactosidase), and trehalase.

The net result of the action of the various digestive enzymes is the almost complete conversion of digestible carbohydrate to its constituent monosaccharides. The resultant glucose and other simple carbohydrates are transported across the intestinal wall to the hepatic portal vein and then to liver parenchymal cells and other tissues. Intestinal absorption of carbohydrates occurs via passive diffusion, facilitated diffusion, and active transport (Figure 43-6). There are 2 intestinal transporters for glucose uptake from the lumen of the gut. One is sodium Na^+-dependent (sodium-glucose transporter 1 [SGLT1]), while the other is Na^+-independent (glucose transporter 2 [GLUT2]). SGLT1 is the major transporter of glucose from the lumen of the small intestine. Although GLUT2 does indeed transport glucose into intestinal enterocytes, this only occurs in response to glucose-mediated translocation of intracellular vesicle-associated GLUT2. Thus even in the absence of GLUT2 (such as is the case in individuals with Fanconi-Bickel

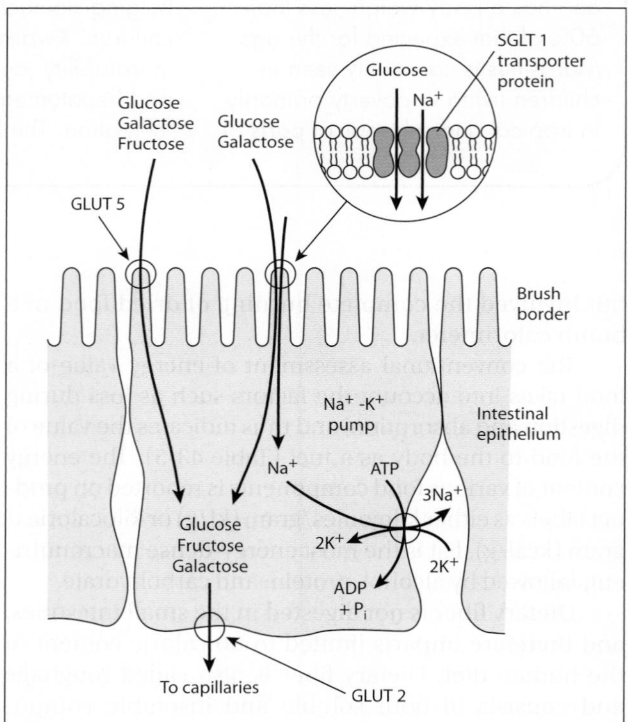

FIGURE 43-6: Transport of glucose, fructose, and galactose across the intestinal epithelium. The SGLT1 transporter is coupled to the Na^+-K^+ pump, allowing glucose and galactose to be transported against their concentration gradients. The GLUT5 Na^+-independent facilitative transporter allows fructose, as well as glucose and galactose, to be transported down their concentration gradients. Exit from the cell for all sugars is via the GLUT2 facilitative transporter. Murray RK, Bender DA, Botham KM, Kennelly PJ, Rodwell VW, Weil PA. *Harper's Illustrated Biochemistry*. 29th ed. New York: McGraw-Hill; 2012.

disease), intestinal uptake of dietary glucose is unimpaired. Galactose is also absorbed from the gut via the action of SGLT1. Fructose is absorbed from the intestine via GLUT5 uptake. Indeed, GLUT5 has a much higher affinity for fructose than for glucose.

Glucose uptake from the lumen of the gut and transepithelial transport to the portal circulation had been shown to occur via action of 2 distinct glucose transporters. First, glucose is taken up from the intestinal lumen through the action of the sodium-dependent glucose transporter 1 (SGLT1), then it is transported into the portal blood via the action of the facilitated glucose transporter GLUT2 present in the basolateral membrane. Evidence has also indicated that GLUT2 present in the apical (luminal) membrane of enterocytes was involved in glucose uptake. However, GLUT2 is not present in the apical membrane in the absence of a glucose load. The mechanism of GLUT2 presentation in the apical membrane involves a glucose-induced translocation of GLUT2 to this membrane. Thus, glucose uptake by the small intestine enhances additional uptake by promoting presentation of an additional transporter in the apical membrane.

Protein Digestion and Peptide and Amino Acid Absorption

The digestion of dietary protein begins in the stomach and continues within the lumen of the duodenum. Within the small intestines there are 2 principal pancreatic enzymes involved in protein digestion; these are trypsin, and chymotrypsin. Several additional pancreatic peptidases play a lesser role in peptide digestion and include elastase and the carboxypeptidases (see Table 42-3).

The initial enzyme involved in protein digestion is gastric pepsin. The zymogen, pepsinogen, is secreted from chief cells in the stomach in response to the action of gastrin and to vagal nerve release of ACh. In fact there are at least 8 isozymes of pepsinogen divided into 2 immunohistochemically distinct groups. Pepsinogens are activated to pepsins by stomach acid which alters their conformation freeing the normally inhibited catalytic domain. Once activated, pepsins will cleave 44 amino acids from pepsinogens generating more active pepsins. Pepsins hydrolyze peptide bonds on the *C*-terminal side of aromatic and hydrophobic amino acids. Approximately 20% of overall protein digestion is accomplished via the actions of pepsins. Due to the acidic pH optimum for the action of pepsins, these enzymes are inhibited when the chime passes from the stomach and is mixed with alkaline pancreatic juices in the duodenum.

The remainder of protein digestion occurs within the duodenum and jejunum of the small intestine. Digestion here is primarily the result of the actions of trypsin and chymotrypsin, and to a lesser extent by elastase and carboxypeptidases A and B, all of which are secreted by the pancreas. See Table 43-3 for the activities of these hydrolases. Trypsin is generated via the action of enteropeptidase action on pancreatic trypsinogen. Enteropeptidase is an enzyme secreted by cells of the crypts of Lieberkühn and resides in the brush-border membranes of duodenal mucosal cells. Trypsin then cleaves more trypsinogen to trypsin, as well as chymotrypsinogen, proelastase, and procarboxypeptidases to their active forms.

Following digestion, free amino acids, as well as peptides (2-6 amino acids in length) are absorbed by enterocytes of the proximal jejunum. Some absorption also occurs in the duodenum and a minor amount in the ileum. Although there is little nutritional significance to whole protein absorption, some undigested dietary protein does get absorbed by intestinal enterocytes. Of significance is the fact that endogenous proteins, such as intestinal hormones and peptides, are absorbed intact. This uptake occurs primarily within the large intestines.

The absorption of amino acids requires an active transport process that is dependent upon either Na^+ or H^+ cotransport. There are several amino acid transporters encompassing 7 distinct transport systems which are further grouped into 3 broad categories. There are the neutral amino acid (monoamino monocarboxylic) transporters, the dibasic (and cysteine) amino acid transporters, and the acidic (dicarboxylic) amino acid transporters. All of these transporters are members of the solute carrier (SLC) family of transporters (see Chapter 7). In all, a total of 36 amino acid transporters are expressed in humans, not all of which are found in the intestines.

Intestinal uptake of peptides involves H^+ cotransporters which are also members of the SLC family. The most abundant peptide transporter is PepT1 (SLC15A1), but there are 3 additional peptide transporters within the SLC15 subfamily. Within intestinal enterocytes the absorbed peptides are hydrolyzed to free amino acids via cytoplasmic peptidases. The free amino acids are then transported across the apical membranes of enterocytes and enter the portal circulation. Patients with Hartnup disorder, due to defective neutral amino acid transport (see Clinical Box 30-1), can remain asymptomatic on a high-protein diet due to peptide absorption via PepT1.

Lipid Digestion and Absorption

The predominant form of dietary lipid in the human diet is triglyceride (TG or TAG). Gastrointestinal lipid digestion consists of several sequential steps

High-Yield Concept

The role of colipase in pancreatic lipase function is to anchor the lipase to the surface of an emulsified lipid droplet and to prevent it from being removed by bile salts. This latter effect of bile salts results in inhibition of pancreatic lipase activity.

that include physicochemical and enzymatic events. The physicochemical processes of lipid digestion involve the formation of large micelle aggregates or emulsion particles that consist of water and water-insoluble substrates. Within the stomach and the small intestines, the peristaltic actions of these organs aids in the emulsification of lipids. Bile acids secreted into the duodenum are also important for lipid emulsification. The emulsified lipid droplets consist of a hydrophobic core containing the majority of the triglycerides, esterified cholesterol, and fat-soluble vitamins. These droplets are surrounded by an amphipathic surface monolayer of phospholipids, free cholesterol, and a few triglycerides. Lipolysis occurs at the lipid-water interface of these particles. Efficient lipid digestion requires the formation of finely dispersed emulsions that have an interface composition favorable for the anchoring of lipases. The overall rate of intestinal lipolysis is, therefore, proportional to the available surface area of the fine emulsions. The enzymes involved in intestinal lipid digestion include gastric lipase and the pancreatic enzymes including pancreatic lipase ($sPLA_2$), carboxyl ester lipase (CEL), as well as other acylglycerol hydrolases and phospholipases (Figure 43-7).

One of the first enzymes involved in the digestion of dietary lipids is lingual lipase which is secreted by serous (von Ebner) glands of the tongue. Lingual lipase remains inactive, however, until it reaches the acidic environment of the stomach where this lipase hydrolyzes medium- and long-chain triglycerides. Within the stomach a second lipase, gastric lipase, is secreted by chief cells in the mucosa of the fundus of the stomach. Gastric lipase hydrolyzes primarily short- and medium-chain fatty acid linkages on the *sn*3 position of triglycerides. The liberated medium-chain fatty acids can be absorbed directly in the stomach. Secretion of gastric lipase is stimulated by both hormonal and cholinergic mechanisms that involve gastrin, CCK, and ACh. Lingual lipase and gastric lipase comprise the 2 acidic lipases. These lipases, unlike the alkaline lipases such as pancreatic lipase, are not dependent upon bile acids or colipase for maximal hydrolytic activity. Both of these acidic lipases account for up to 30% of total lipid hydrolysis that occurs during the digestive process. Gastric lipase is responsible for the bulk of the acidic lipase activity in the gut. In the neonate, acidic lipases account for as much as 50% of total lipid digestion. Both lingual and gastric lipases are essential for the digestion of milk fat in the newborn because, unlike pancreatic lipase, they are able to penetrate fat globules in milk and initiate the digestive process.

After passing from the stomach the digestion of fat continues in the duodenum with the synergetic action of gastric lipase and colipase-dependent pancreatic lipase. Colipase is secreted by the pancreas in an inactive form, procolipase, and then activated in the intestinal lumen by trypsin.

Lipid digestion converts dietary fats into more polar derivatives with a higher degree of interaction with water facilitating their absorption by duodenal enterocytes. Triglycerides are converted to free fatty acids and glycerol via

High-Yield Concept

Most monogenic forms of diabetes, termed maturity-onset type diabetes of the young (MODY), are due to mutations in genes involved in pancreatic cell function (see Chapter 47). However, a rare form of MODY (termed MODY8) that is characterized by dominantly inherited childhood-onset pancreatic exocrine dysfunction and diabetes has been shown to be due to mutations in the CEL gene. Notably, this gene is not transcribed in pancreatic β-cells but is only expressed in the acinar cells of the pancreas and in lactating mammary gland cells. The cause of the pancreatic dysfunction in MODY8 is due to aggregation of the mutant CEL protein and the formation of amyloidotic deposits that are toxic to the pancreas resulting in an associated loss of β-cell function.

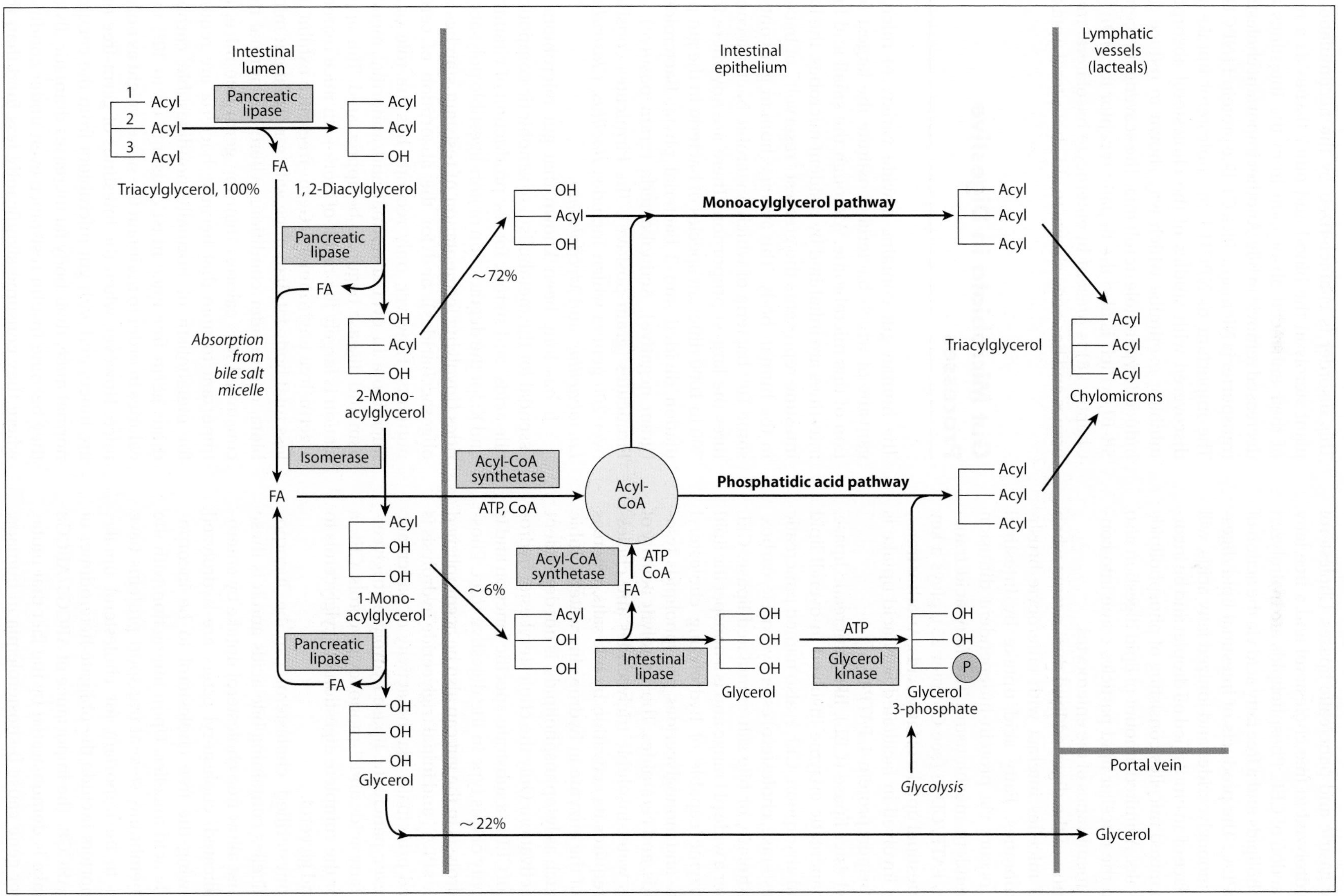

FIGURE 43-7: Digestion and absorption of triacylglycerols. The values given for percentage uptake may vary widely but indicate the relative importance of the 3 routes shown. Murray RK, Bender DA, Botham KM, Kennelly PJ, Rodwell VW, Weil PA. *Harper's Illustrated Biochemistry*. 29th ed. New York: McGraw-Hill; 2012.

the action of gastric and pancreatic lipases. Cholesterol esters are hydrolyzed to free cholesterol and a free fatty acid via the action of CEL. Phospholipids are hydrolyzed to lysophospholipids and a free fatty acid via the action of pancreatic $sPLA_2$. The products of intestinal lipid digestion, mainly monoglycerides and ionized fatty acids, will leave the surface of an emulsified oil droplet and be incorporated into mixed micelles consisting of phospholipids and/or bile salts. A limited amount of lipid digestion also occurs when the micellar lipid particles come into contact with the membranes of the enterocytes.

Absorption of the digested lipid then occurs when these mixed micelles interact with enterocyte brush-border membranes. Fatty acid uptake by intestinal enterocytes occurs via protein-independent diffusion protein-dependent mechanisms. The fatty acid transport protein, FATP/CD36 (see Chapter 25), plays a key role in the intestinal uptake of fatty acids. Another transport protein involved in facilitated fatty acid uptake is fatty acid transport protein 4, FATP4.

Carboxyl ester lipase (CEL), like pancreatic lipase, is a major pancreatic enzyme involved in overall lipid digestion and absorption. CEL is also named pancreatic cholesterol esterase, cholesterol ester hydrolase, carboxylic ester hydrolase, or bile salt–stimulated lipase. CEL functions over a wide pH range and is a nonspecific lipid digesting enzyme capable of hydrolyzing cholesteryl esters, tri-, di- and monoglycerides, phospholipids, lysophospholipids, and ceramides. The hydrolytic activity of CEL towards water-insoluble triglycerides and cholesteryl esters requires its activation by bile salts, whereas the activity of the enzyme in hydrolyzing water soluble substrates, such as lysophospholipids, is not dependent on bile salt activation. Only the cholesteryl ester hydrolytic activity of CEL is a substrate-specific function and is the only activity of this type in the digestive tract. Phospholipid hydrolysis in the gut can also be accomplished by pancreatic $sPLA_2$, and initial triglyceride hydrolysis is accomplished principally via the activity of pancreatic lipase. However, pancreatic lipase hydrolyses triglycerides only to fatty acids and 2-monoacylglycerols. CEL is important for the complete digestion of acylglycerols to fatty acids and glycerol.

Only nonesterified cholesterol can be incorporated into micelles containing bile acids and it is these complexes that allow free cholesterol uptake by enterocytes. As indicated, cholesteryl esters are hydrolyzed by CEL allowing the free cholesterol to be incorporated into bile acid micelles. Upon interaction with the enterocyte membrane, several transport proteins have been shown to be important for cholesterol uptake. These transporters include the obligate heterodimer of ABCG5 and ABCG8. The importance of ABCG5/ABCG8 in sterol uptake is demonstrated by the fact that mutations in either gene cause β-sitosterolemia in humans. This disorder is characterized by the accumulation of plant sterols in the blood and other tissues as a result of their enhanced absorption from the intestines and decreased removal in bile. Another important cholesterol transporter is Niemann-Pick C1-like protein 1 (NPC1L1). The important of NPC1L1 in cholesterol uptake was discovered with studies of the cholesterol absorption inhibitor ezetimibe which was shown to reduce diet-induced hypercholesterolemia. The scavenger receptor, SR-BI, which is also the hepatic receptor for HDL (see Chapter 28) is present in enterocyte basolateral membranes and has been shown to aid cholesterol uptake.

Gut Microbiota in Digestive Processes

The human gut contains a wide variety of microorganisms of which bacteria constitute the largest fraction of this microbiome. Although the small and large intestines are inhabited by resident microbes, the large intestine represents the greatest “reservoir” of bacteria in the human body. The average human gut contains some 10^{14} bacteria of which anaerobic bacteria constitutes the largest proportion. There are anywhere from 500 to 1000 different species of bacteria in the gut population divided into 3 bacterial phyla: Bacteroidetes (gram negative), Actinobacteria (gram positive), and Firmicutes (gram positive). The Firmicutes consist of over 200 genera which includes *Bacillus*, *Clostridium*, *Lactobacillus*, and *Mycoplasma*.

It has long been known that gut microbiota are essential for the metabolism of xenobiotic compounds, bile acids, and sterols; for the production of vitamins B and K; for the degradation of nondigestible polysaccharides (involving fermentation of resistant starches and oligosaccharides); and for the absorption of certain nutrients. However, only recently has the role of gut microbiota in overall normal and abnormal metabolism and disease begun to be appreciated. This appreciation is largely the result of work with mice reared in a germ-free environment. Germ-free mice exhibit 40% less total body fat than mice with a normal gut microbiota, even under conditions where the normal mice consumed less calories than the germ-free mice. It is important to note that because bacteria are required for metabolism of normally nondigestible carbohydrate, germ-free mice must consume up to 30% more calories in order to maintain the same weight as normal mice. However, when the intestines of germ-free mice are inoculated with gut microbiota from the cecum of normal mice, their body fat increases dramatically and they become insulin resistance even under conditions where they consume significantly less food than their germ-free littermates. This role of gut microbiota in the development of obesity and diabetes is discussed in Chapter 45.

Humans require gut microbiota in order to utilize normally nondigestible carbohydrate and the result of bacterial fermentation of these sugars is significant to overall health. The types of carbohydrate that humans cannot digest without gut bacteria are certain starches, fiber, oligosaccharides, and sugars that the body failed to digest and absorb. A typical example is the disaccharide lactose in the case of lactose intolerant individuals. The metabolic significance of bacterial digestion of carbohydrate is that they ferment these molecules into short-chain fatty acids (SCFAs). This fermentation process is referred to as saccharolytic fermentation and the major by-products are acetic acid, propionic acid, and butyric acid. These SCFAs are absorbed and utilized as sources of energy by certain host cells. For example, acetic acid is used by skeletal muscle, propionic acid by the liver, and butyric acid by gut cells. The SCFAs also stimulate intestinal epithelial cell growth and regulate their proliferation and differentiation. Bacterially produced SCFAs are also important for the absorption of dietary minerals such as sodium, calcium, magnesium, and iron. Some SCFAs are transported into enterocytes in exchange for H^+ and thereby help to maintain pH equilibrium within the gut and intestines.

Gut bacteria are also important in the control of the secretion of gastrointestinal hormones that function in digestion and appetite control. Consumption of the prebiotic, oligofructose, increases the level of GLP-1 secretion from enteroendocrine L cells as well as resulting in increased L-cell proliferation. Oligofructose represents a subgroup of the plant fructose polymer called inulin. Inulin and oligofructose are not digested in the small intestines, so have no caloric value but they stimulate the growth of certain types of gut bacteria. The roles of GLP-1 in metabolism are discussed in detail in Chapter 44.

In addition, consuming oligofructose results in increased L-cell proliferation in the proximal colon and this contributes to a higher level of GLP-1 release. Consumption of oligofructose has also been shown to protect against weight gain, reduces fat accumulation, reduces serum triglyceride accumulation, and promotes satiety, all of which are the result of changes in the composition of gut microbiota.

Gut microbiota are also essential for the appropriate development of a mature mucosal immune system. The mucosal immune system is distributed throughout the entire length of the gastrointestinal tract as well as other mucosal surfaces. Within the intestines, intact proteins can be taken up by specialized cells called M cells. These cells overly Peyer patches which are follicles of lymphoid tissue residing in the lamina propria layer of the intestine. The intact proteins are transported across the M cell basolateral membranes into the immunocompetent cells in the Peyer patch, resulting in the initiation of an immune response. This process is continuous and represents an important immune surveillance function of the gut. The role of gut microbiota in this process is evidenced from the fact that under conditions where increased levels of Firmicutes are present, there is a higher level of inflammatory signaling in the gut and the addition of antibiotics can help suppress this phenomenon. Conversely, increased levels of Bacteroidetes bacteria result in suppression of inflammatory signaling within the gut.

Just as differences in the levels of various gut bacteria are associated with alterations in intestinal immune functions, changes in gut bacteria are also associated with metabolic disruption as well as disease states. For example, obese individuals are known to harbor a different gut microbial composition than lean age and sex matched individuals. Several studies have suggested that an increased Firmicute:Bacteroidetes ratio is one of the key signatures of obesity and that this ratio can be modulated by a weight reduction diet. Several diseases have been shown to be associated with dysregulation of the gut microbiome, which includes diabetes, the metabolic syndrome, certain food allergies, asthma, Crohn disease, cardiovascular disease, and colon cancer. Because of the well-demonstrated effects of altered gut microbiomes on metabolism and disease, manipulation of gut microbiota through the use of diet, prebiotics, probiotics, and antibiotics is currently being studied for the treatment of obesity and diabetes as well as several other disorders.

High-Yield Concept

Prebiotics are any substance that cannot be digested by humans but can be fermented by gut bacteria, thereby promoting their growth and activity. Probiotics are any live bacteria consumed in food.

REVIEW QUESTIONS

1. A 57-year-old man is being examined by his physician due to complaints of frequent gnawing and burning pain in the middle and upper stomach occurring between meals and most acutely at night. Additional symptoms reported by the patient include heartburn, black stools, and on occasion seeing that his vomit looks like coffee grounds. You suspect the patient is suffering from a peptic ulcer. A defect in which of the following cells in the gastrointestinal tract would most likely be expected given this diagnosis?

A. chief
B. enterochromaffin-like (ECL)
C. enteroendocrine L cells
D. gastric mucus cells
E. parietal

Answer E: Peptic ulcers are painful sores occurring in the lining of the stomach or in the proximal duodenum. One of the most common causes of peptic ulcers is excessive gastric acid secretion from the parietal (oxyntic) cells of the stomach. On rare occasions this excess acid production is due to gastrinomas (Zollinger-Ellison syndrome) of the acid secreting parietal cells.

2. You are carrying out in vitro experiments that are designed to test the efficacy of novel compounds in the treatment of gastroesophageal reflux disease (GERD). You are testing the various compounds on gastric parietal cells in culture. You discover that one of the compounds exerts a significant inhibition of hydrogen ion (H^+) secretion from the cells. This compound most likely mimics the effects of which of the following natural peptides?

A. cholecystokinin
B. gastrin
C. gastrin-releasing peptide
D. GLP-1
E. somatostatin

Answer E: Somatostatin is secreted by enteroendocrine D cells of the stomach and duodenum, δ-cells of the pancreas, and also by the hypothalamus. In the pancreas, somatostatin acts as a paracrine inhibitor of other pancreatic hormones. In the gut, somatostatin is involved in the inhibition of gastric acid secretion. Somatostatin binds to a GPCR called the somatostatin receptor 1 (encoded by the *SSTR1* gene) that is coupled to a G_i-type G-protein that inhibits adenylate cyclase. The effect of somatostatin binding to *SSTR1* is an antagonism of the gastric acid secreting effects of histamine. Somatostatin can also interfere with the gastric effects of histamine by blocking histamine release from enterochromaffin-like cells (ECL) in the gastric mucosa.

3. You are tending to a 27-year-old woman whose chief complaint is that she can no longer taste sweetness in food, particularly fruits. You suspect that she may have a defect or disease of her tongue but physical examination as well as a small tissue biopsy show no anomalies. You order an assay of her saliva because you suspect she may have a defect in the secretion of which of the following enzymes?

A. α-amylase
B. haptocorrin
C. lingual lipase
D. lysozyme
E. mucin

Answer A: The action of α-amylase, on plant starches, releases glucose into the mouth. Glucose is sweet tasting which enhances the flavor of the food making it much more palatable and rewarding.

4. You are treating a 38-year-old man with complaints of near constant burning pain in his upper stomach which gets worse when he lies down at night. He informs you that his stools are black and that he frequently vomits up blood. You diagnose your patient as suffering from severe GI ulcerations and you suspect they are caused by Zollinger-Ellison syndrome. However, a gastric biopsy shows no apparent gastrinomas. Abnormal activity in the secretory function of which of the following cell types would most likely be associated with the symptoms in this patient?

A. chief
B. enterochromaffin-like (ECL)
C. enteroendocrine I
D. gastric mucus
E. parietal

Answer B: The principal stimulants for acid secretion are histamine, gastrin, and acetylcholine (ACh) released from postganglionic enteric neurons. Histamine is thought to be the primary stimulus. Histamine is released from enterochromaffin-like (ECL) cells in response to gastrin binding to these cells in fundal glands of the upper stomach. The released histamine then binds to H_2 receptors on parietal cells inducing a signaling cascade that results in the transport of the H^+/K^+-ATPase (proton pump) from the cytoplasm to the apical plasma membrane of the parietal cell. Excessive release of histamine would, therefore, result in excessive secretion of gastric acid leading to ulceration of the stomach mucosal lining.

5. A 63-year-old man is being seen by his physician as a follow-up to gastric surgery for the treatment of a severe duodenal ulcers. This patient has the ulcers removed by surgical resection of the proximal portion of the duodenum to the distal end of the corpus of the stomach. The patient has been prescribed a proton pump inhibitor (PPI) because the surgery required removal of the region of the stomach that contains cells involved in the negative regulation of acid secretion. Which of the following represents these antrum located cells?
A. chief
B. D
C. enterochromaffin-like (ECL)
D. G
E. parietal

Answer B: The antrum of the stomach is also referred to as the pyloric gland area. The pyloric glands contain cells that secrete gastrin (G cells) and somatostatin (D cells). Somatostatin exerts a tonic paracrine inhibition of gastrin secretion from G cells, thereby controlling overall gastric acid secretion by parietal cells of the fundus and corpus of the stomach. Somatostatin can also interfere with gastric acid secretion exerted by the action of histamine. Somatostatin blocks histamine release from enterochromaffin-like cells (ECL) in the gastric mucosa.

6. Acetylcholine (ACh) directly stimulates parietal cell secretion of gastric acid by binding to muscarinic receptors of the M3 family present on these cells. Acetylcholine can also indirectly influence gastric acid secretion by activating M2 and M4 receptors present on which of the following cell types?
A. enterochromaffin-like (ECL)
B. enteroendocrine I
C. D
D. G
E. goblet

Answer C: Vagal nerve endings contain acetylcholine (ACh) which, when released, binds to M3 muscarinic-type receptors on parietal cells directly stimulating acid production and secretion. Acetylcholine can also indirectly stimulate gastric acid secretion by inhibiting the release of somatostatin through activation of M2 and M4 muscarinic receptors on D cells.

7. A 45-year-old woman has come to her physician with complaints of abdominal pain, loss of appetite, fatigue, diarrhea, cramping, and bloating. Further history reveals that in addition to the frequent diarrhea, her stools are often bloody. Her physician suspects colitis and orders a colonoscopy which shows colonic mucosal erythema, ulcers, and bleeding. The symptoms of colitis seen in this patient are most likely due to a defect in the secretory properties of which of the following cell types?
A. chief
B. enterochromaffin-like (ECL)
C. enteroendocrine
D. goblet
E. parietal

Answer D: Goblet cells are columnar epithelia cells found in the outer mucosal layer of the intestines. Goblet cells synthesize the secretory mucin glycoproteins, as well as several other bioactive molecules that form the highly viscous extracellular layer. The mucus layer of the intestines, particularly of the colon, interacts with, and protects the epithelial layer from gut bacteria. Defective mucus layers results in increased bacterial adhesion to the surface epithelium, increased intestinal permeability, and enhanced susceptibility to colitis. In addition, changes in mucin production and mucin glycan structures are known to occur in cancers of the intestine.

8. You are treating a 43-year-old woman who complains that her stools have recently acquired a foul smell and have an oily consistency. Ultrasonic examination reveals no apparent abnormalities in the gallbladder or pancreas. Biopsy of the main pancreatic duct also shows no overt pathology. Analysis of pancreatic juice isolated during the biopsy would most likely show a reduction or loss in the presence of which of the following enzymes, accounting for the change in stool in this patient?
A. α-amylase
B. carboxyl ester lipase
C. carboxypeptidase A
D. chymotrypsinogen
E. lipase

Answer E: Pancreatic lipase is the primary lipase that hydrolyzes dietary triglycerides in the small intestines. The action of alkaline pancreatic juice results in inhibition of the activity of the acid lipases (lingual and gastric) that begin the process of triglyceride hydrolysis in the stomach. Loss of pancreatic lipase secretion would, therefore, result in incomplete digestion of dietary fats preventing their absorption and leading to increased fat content of the stools.

9. As a physician on a mission to treat patients in sub-Saharan Africa you encounter numerous children with a common cluster of signs and symptoms. These include protuberant abdomens, generalized edema, loss of muscle mass, lethargy, irritability, and fatigue. Given the constellation of symptoms in your patients, your normal course of treatment would most likely include which of the following?

A. high concentration of total protein and/or essential amino acids
B. minimal amount of protein initially
C. only carbohydrates
D. only essential fatty acids
E. total caloric increase including protein, carbohydrate, and fat

Answer B: The children you are treating are suffering from kwashiorkor which is a form of malnutrition due to a deficiency in protein but with sufficient caloric intake. Kwashiorkor is an acute form of childhood protein-energy malnutrition characterized by edema causing the typical bulging stomach seen in affected children. Kwashiorkor also results in irritability, anorexia, skin ulcers, and hepatomegaly due to fatty infiltration. The hepatomegaly also contributes to the protuberant abdomen in these children. Treatment of Kwashiorkor involves careful administration of protein with the use of carbohydrate and fat for the majority of caloric needs of the child. This is due to the fact that the administration of too much protein will lead to increased hepatic urea cycle activity. Since the liver is already compromised due to the fatty infiltration, the metabolism of protein can exacerbate the damage and lead to liver failure and death.

10. As a physician on a mission to treat patients in sub-Saharan Africa you encounter numerous children with a common cluster of signs and symptoms. These include chronic diarrhea, dizziness, fatigue, delayed wound healing, and muscle wasting. Given the constellation of symptoms in your patients, your normal course of treatment would most likely include which of the following?

A. high concentration of total protein and/or essential amino acids
B. minimal amount of protein initially
C. only carbohydrates
D. only essential fatty acids
E. total caloric increase including protein, carbohydrate, and fat

Answer E: The children you are treating are suffering from marasmus. Marasmus is a form of severe malnutrition caused by a deficiency of nearly all nutrients, especially protein and carbohydrates. A typical child with marasmus looks emaciated and has a body weight less than 60% of that expected for the age. Treatment of marasmus is normally divided into 2 phases. The initial acute phase of treatment involves restoring electrolyte balance, treating infections, and reversing the hypoglycemia and hypothermia. This is followed by refeeding and ensuring that sufficient caloric and nutrient intake is maintained to enable catch-up growth in order to restore a healthy normal body mass.

11. You are studying the gastric secretions of a patient with a rare form of nutritional malabsorption. You discover that the defect is due to a near complete loss of secretion of pepsinogen into the stomach in response to food intake. These observations could be explained by a defect in which type of gastrointestinal secretory cell?

A. chief
B. enteroendocrine I
C. enteroendocrine L
D. oxyntic
E. vagal nerve

Answer A: A gastric chief cell is a cell in the stomach that releases pepsinogen. Pepsinogen is activated into the digestive enzyme pepsin when it comes in contact with acid produced by gastric parietal cells.

12. Which of the following hormones is responsible for the stimulation of bile secretions from the gallbladder?

A. cholecystokinin (CCK)
B. gastrin
C. gastrin-releasing hormone
D. glucagon-like peptide-1 (GLP-1)
E. protein tyrosine tyrosine (PYY)

Answer A: Cholecystokinin (CCK) is secreted from intestinal enteroendocrine I cells predominantly in the duodenum and jejunum. Upon binding its receptors in the gut CCK induces contractions of the gallbladder and release of pancreatic enzymes and also inhibits gastric emptying.

13. Which of the following statements relates to the role of salivary production of mucin?

A. activates lysozyme to initiate protein degradation
B. decreases the pH of the stomach contents to prevent excess denaturation of digestive enzymes
C. hydrolyzes complex carbohydrates so that they are substrates for salivary maltase
D. increases the pH of the saliva to denature proteins in the food
E. increases the viscosity of saliva to aid in swallowing

Answer E: Mucins are glycoproteins that in combination with mucopolysaccharides mix with water to form a lubricant for ease of swallowing.

14. A 14-year-old boy presents with weight loss and diarrhea. His tongue becomes sore and blistery after eating oatmeal or rye bread, which leads to the diagnosis of celiac disease. The boy and his parents are advised to be sensitive to symptoms of tetany and paresthesias since they can occur as a consequence of malabsorption of which of the following?

A. calcium
B. carbohydrates
C. fat
D. iron
E. water

Answer A: In patients with celiac disease the protein gluten—found in bread, oats, and many other foods containing wheat, barley, or rye—triggers an autoimmune response that causes damage to the small intestine leading to widespread manifestations of malabsorption. Calcium is difficult to absorb, so patients frequently experience symptoms of hypocalcemia such as muscle cramping, tetanic contractions, numbness, and tingling sensations. For sensory and motor nerves, calcium is a critical second messenger involved in normal cell function, neural transmission, and cell membrane stability. The nerves respond to a lack of calcium with hyperexcitability.

15. A patient presented with an acute abdomen including fever, marked abdominal distension, acidosis, and leukocytosis. Laparoscopy revealed that large parts of the small intestine were necrotic, and as a consequence the entire ileum of the patient was resected. It is expected that very soon after the surgery the patient will have considerable problems resulting from the malabsorption of which of the following?

A. bile acids
B. iron
C. protein
D. sodium
E. vitamin B_{12}

Answer A: After a meal about 90 percent of the bile acids and bile salts are absorbed from the lower ileum by way of active transport. They are directed to the liver, from where they can be released again via bile into the intestine. This enterohepatic circulation of bile acids between intestine and liver is physiologically very important for normal absorption of fat and fat-soluble vitamins, and if distorted, will lead to gastrointestinal and other symptoms.

16. You are examining digestive enzymes and their processes of activation. You have isolated a mutant form of one particular enzyme and find that it remains inactive in a mixture of digestive juices. The wild-type enzyme is normally activated by hydrolysis on the *C*-terminal side of Arg and Lys residues and you determine that the mutant enzyme contains Ser residues at these critical positions. Which of the following digestive enzymes is most likely responsible for activation of the wild-type enzyme in your studies?

A. aminopeptidase
B. carboxypeptidase
C. chymotrypsin
D. enteropeptidase
E. lysozyme

Answer D: Trypsin is a pancreatic digestive enzyme derived from proteolytic cleavage of the precursor protein trypsinogen. Enteropeptidase is produced by cells of the duodenum. It is secreted from intestinal glands called the crypts of Lieberkühn following the entry of ingested food passing from the stomach. Enteropeptidase converts trypsinogen into its active form trypsin. Trypsin cleaves its target substrates on the *C*-terminal side of Arg and Lys residues.

17. A 54-year-old alcoholic man is admitted to the emergency room with an 8-hour history of severe epigastric pain. He reports that the pain radiates to his back and is more intense when he lies down. Physical examination reveals tachycardia, hypotension, and low-grade fever consistent with the early stage of shock. Which of the following serum measurements would be most useful in providing a diagnosis of his condition?

A. amylase
B. aspartate aminotransferase, AST
C. bilirubin
D. serum calcium
E. troponin I

Answer A: The hallmark of acute pancreatitis is abdominal pain that is initially localized to the epigastrium and later becomes diffuse. It typically radiates to the back and is frequently more intense in the supine position. Other common symptoms and signs include nausea, vomiting, and tachycardia. If the pancreatitis is severe, hypotension can occur due to extravasation of blood and fluids into peritoneal spaces and shock may ensue. Measurement of both pancreatic amylase and lipase enzyme levels are useful in the diagnosis of acute pancreatitis. Amylase levels rise early in the course of the disease, while elevation of lipase levels may not occur until 24 hours after onset of illness.

Although false positives and false negatives do occur, an elevated amylase level in conjunction with a consistent pattern of acute epigastric/abdominal pain is considered evidence of acute pancreatitis if other acute surgical conditions have been ruled out.

18. The manufacturer of energy bars makes claim that the fructose contained in their bars serves as an ideal source of energy for extreme mountain climbing and mountain biking expeditions. Which of the following statements concerning fructose reflects the basis for these claims?
   A. absorption of fructose into an intestinal epithelial cell is by facilitated transport and thus does not require energy
   B. metabolism of fructose generates more energy than glucose
   C. some fructose is already absorbed in the mouth and hence is the fastest way to get energy
   D. the presence of fructose aids in absorption of vitamin A, C, and D
   E. the presence of fructose inhibits reabsorption of glucose, which is then more readily available for muscle activity

Answer A: Carbohydrate absorption occurs at enterocytes of the proximal duodenum. Fructose absorption into the blood occurs via the facilitated transporters GLUT5 across the apical enterocyte membrane and then via GLUT2 across the basolateral membrane. Glucose and galactose on the other hand are transported into enterocytes via the actions of the sodium-dependent transporter, SGLT1. The energy for this secondary active transport is provided by the electrochemical sodium gradient that is created by Na^+/K^+-ATPases. Experimental conditions that collapse the sodium electrochemical gradient, such as with hypoxia, or poisoning of the Na^+/K^+-ATPase by ouabain, inhibit glucose, but not fructose absorption. Nevertheless, the physiological importance of saving energy under extreme conditions such as mountain climbing through the use of fructose as energy source is questionable given that intestinal fructose absorption is much slower than absorption of glucose and galactose.

19. Patients with functional dyspepsia and prominent nausea frequently experience spurts of excessive gastric acid exposure to the proximal duodenum. This results in increased pancreatic secretion, mainly through the action of which of the following substances?
   A. cholecystokinin, CCK
   B. gastrin
   C. glucagon
   D. secretin
   E. vasoactive intestinal polypeptide, VIP

Answer D: Acidification of the duodenal lumen triggers mechanisms to inhibit gastric acid production. Under low pH conditions duodenal enteroendocrine S cells release secretin which inhibits the release of gastrin from stomach antrum enteroendocrine G cells. The strongest stimulator for the release of secretin from S cells is contact with acidic chyme. Increased serum secretin levels stimulate water and alkali secretions from the pancreas and the hepatic ducts and inhibit gastrin release.

20. You are examining a 33-year-old man whose chief complaints are that he has experienced recent weight loss and that he believes is due to the fact that he feels full after eating only a small amount of food. You determine that these symptoms are manifest due to a delay in the normal rate of gastric emptying. Given these findings, which of the following hormones is most likely to be excessively active in this patient?
   A. cholecystokinin, CCK
   B. gastrin
   C. glucose-dependent insulinotropic peptide, GIP
   D. motilin
   E. pancreatic polypeptide, PP

Answer A: The major control mechanism for gastric emptying involves duodenal gastric feedback, hormonal as well as neural. The major hormone involved in the inhibition of gastric emptying is cholecystokinin (CCK), which is released by fat and protein digestion products. Therefore, a reduction in gastric emptying would result from increased or excessive CCK activity resulting in rapid onset of satiety due to a feeling of fullness.

21. A healthy adult male of average size contains approximately 11 kg of total body protein. Approximately 5 kg of this is available as a source of energy primarily from skeletal muscle. Which of the following most closely represents the total caloric contribution of this protein source during prolonged fasting?
   A. 1200 kcal
   B. 22,000 kcal
   C. 150,000 kcal
   D. 400,000 kcal

Answer B: The energy content of protein is approximately 4 kcal/g. Therefore, 5 kg of protein would have approximately 20,000 kcal of available energy upon catabolism.

22. A 37-year-old man is being seen in the emergency room because of a 3-month history of nausea, vomiting, excessive thirst, increased urination, and generalized weakness. The patient has a 2-year history of gastric discomfort and pain which he has been attempting to manage with large quantities of antacids, a bland diet, and milk. Which of the following laboratory abnormalities is most likely in this patient?

A. decreased serum creatinine concentration
B. decreased serum phosphorous concentration
C. decreased serum urea nitrogen concentration
D. increased serum calcium concentration
E. metabolic acidosis

Answer D: The patient would most likely manifest with milk-alkali syndrome resulting from taking too much calcium by mouth. Many antacids are calcium salts and treating oneself by drinking lots of milk and taking lots of calcium salt antacids results in increased blood calcium levels.

23. Digestion of starch can occur even in the absence of pancreatic secretions. Which of the following digestive enzymes could best account for this?

A. biliary amylase
B. Brunner gland amylase
C. intestinal brush border amylase
D. intestinal brush border sucrase
E. salivary amylase

Answer E: Salivary α-amylase is a major contributor to the digestions of dietary starches. Indeed, this enzyme is responsible for a significant portion of carbohydrate digestion in the mouth, esophagus, and stomach.

24. Pancreatic amylase in the intestine cleaves starch primarily into which of the following?

A. disaccharides and trisaccharides of glucose
B. fucose monomers
C. fucose 1-phosphate
D. glucose 6-phosphate
E. linear polymers of glucose

Answer A: The activity of salivary and pancreatic α-amylase is the hydrolysis of starch at $\alpha(1,4)$-glycosidic linkages. Amylase functions at random locations along the starch polymer hydrolyzing long-chain carbohydrates. The products of amylase activity on amylose are maltotriose and maltose, and those from amylopectin are maltose, glucose and limit dextrins.

25. Which of the following best explains why adults are more likely than children to have gastrointestinal distress after consuming dairy products?

A. adults are more likely to be allergic to milk proteins
B. adults have lower activity of the enzyme that digests milk fats
C. adults have lower activity of the enzyme that digests milk proteins
D. adults have lower activity of the enzyme that digests milk sugar
E. adults secrete more gastric acid in response to dairy products

Answer D: Lactose intolerance is the inability to digest lactose which is abundant in milk and, to a lesser extent, milk-derived dairy products. Lactose intolerant individuals have insufficient levels of digestive system lactase, the enzyme that catalyzes hydrolysis of lactose into glucose and galactose. Common symptoms of lactase deficiency include abdominal bloating and cramps, flatulence, diarrhea, and nausea. Most people normally cease to produce lactase, becoming lactose intolerant after weaning. Approximately 75% of adults worldwide show some decrease in lactase activity during adulthood. However, several populations have developed lactase persistence, where lactase production continues even in adulthood.

Checklist

✓ The digestion of food involves a complex series of events that begins with the sight and smell and even the thought of food which leads to the stimulation of the salivary glands in the mouth.

✓ Digestion begins in the mouth with chewing and mixing of the masticated food with saliva. Contained in saliva is amylase, as well as many other substances, which begins the process of carbohydrate digestion.

✓ Chewing and swallowing represent the only voluntary processes of digestion.

- ✓ All of the involuntary processes of digestion such as stomach and intestinal peristalsis; stomach and intestinal secretion of digestive enzymes, peptides, and hormones; gallbladder secretion of bile acids; and pancreatic secretion of digestive enzymes and bicarbonate occur via the actions of the enteric, parasympathetic, and sympathetic nervous systems.
- ✓ The enteric nervous system acts independent of, as well as in conjunction with, the parasympathetic and sympathetic nervous systems primarily via the vagal nerve.
- ✓ The swallowing of food deposits the partially digested material into the stomach where the acidic environment denatures proteins allowing them to be hydrolyzed by pepsin secreted from cells in the stomach. Lipid hydrolysis is initiated in this acidic environment by lingual lipase secreted in saliva and gastric lipase secreted in the stomach. Both of these lipases have optimum activity in acidic pH but are no longer active when the contents of the stomach enter the duodenum and encounter the alkaline pancreatic juice.
- ✓ Once the digested material, now referred to as chime, is passed from the stomach to the small intestines the full process of carbohydrate, protein, and lipid digestion is completed via the actions of the numerous pancreatic and intestinal brush-border membrane–associated enzymes.
- ✓ Within the duodenum and proximal jejunum, absorption of monosaccharides, amino acids, small peptides, monoacylglycerides, fatty acids, cholesterol, lysophospholipids, and glycerol takes place via both passive and active transport into intestinal enterocytes.
- ✓ Gut bacteria play a crucial role in the overall digestive process by fermenting nondigestible carbohydrates, metabolizing xenobiotics, producing certain vitamins, and aiding in nutrient absorption. The products of bacterial carbohydrate fermentation serve as energy sources for various tissues and they also act as growth and proliferative stimulators for intestinal epithelial cells. Gut bacteria also support the process of mucosal immune surveillance.

CHAPTER

44 Gut-Brain Interactions and Feeding Behaviors

CHAPTER OUTLINE

High-Yield Terms

Hypothalamus: brain region composed of several distinct nuclei, involved in coordinating the gastrointestinal and nervous systems to the endocrine system, major structure controlling appetite

Anorexigenic: causing appetite suppression

Orexigenic: causing increased appetite

Satiation: pertaining to the cessation of hunger

Satiety: the sensation of being full

Enteroendocrine cells: specialized endocrine cells of the gastrointestinal tract and pancreas

Incretin: any gut hormone associated with food intake-stimulation of insulin secretion from the pancreas

Oxyntic cells: parietal cells of gastric glands responsible for gastric acid secretion

Hypocretins: another name for the orexins

The Gut-Brain Connection

The brain, in particular the hypothalamus, plays highly critical roles in the regulation of energy metabolism, nutrient partitioning, and the control of feeding behaviors. The gastrointestinal tract is intimately connected to the actions of the hypothalamic-pituitary axis via the release of peptides that exert responses within the brain as well as through neuroendocrine and sensory inputs from the gut. The primary centers in the brain involved in the control of appetite are the hypothalamic-pituitary axis and the brain stem.

The consumption of food initiates a cascade of neuronal and hormonal responses within and by the gastrointestinal system that impact responses in the central nervous system. The brain initiates responses to feeding even before the ingestion of food. The very sight and smell of food stimulates exocrine and endocrine secretions in the gut as well as increasing gut motility. Ingestion of food stimulates mechanoreceptors leading to distension and propulsion to accommodate the food. As the food is propelled through the gut regions of the intestines secrete various hormones that circulate to the brain and impact hypothalamic responses as discussed in the sections later. The mechanoreceptor responses are transmitted via afferent nerve signals along the vagus nerve to the dorsal vagal complex in the medulla and terminating in the nucleus of the solitary tract (NTS, for the Latin term *nucleus tractus solitarii*). Projections from the NTS enter the visceral sensory complex of the thalamus which mediates the perception of gastrointestinal fullness and satiety. Several hormones released from the gut in response to food intake exert anorexigenic (appetite-suppressing) responses in the brain, particularly in the hypothalamus. These hormones include glucagon-like peptide-1 (GLP-1), cholecystokinin (CCK), peptide tyrosine tyrosine (PYY), pancreatic polypeptide (PP), and oxyntomodulin (OXM or OXY). A single orexigenic (appetite-stimulating) hormone, ghrelin, is known to be released by cells of the gut.

Gastrointestinal Hormones and Peptides

There are more than 30 peptides currently identified as being expressed within the digestive tract, making the gut the largest endocrine organ in the body. The regulatory peptides synthesized by the gut include hormones, peptide neurotransmitters, and growth factors. Indeed, several hormones and neurotransmitters first identified in the central nervous system and other endocrine organs have subsequently been found in endocrine cells and/or neurons of the gut (Table 44-1).

Glucagon-Like Peptide-1

The glucagon gene encodes a precursor protein identified as preproglucagon (Figure 44-1). Depending on the tissue of expression, coupled with the presence of specific proteases called prohormone convertases, preproglucagon can be processed into several different biological peptides in addition to glucagon. The glucagon-like peptide-1 (GLP-1), derived from the proglucagon protein, is a gut hormone that is referred to as an incretin.

The primary physiological responses to GLP-1 are glucose-dependent insulin secretion, inhibition of glucagon secretion and gastric acid secretion, and gastric emptying. The latter effect will lead to increased satiety with reduced food intake along with a reduced desire for food. The action of GLP-1 at the level of insulin and glucagon secretion results in significant reduction in circulating levels of glucose following nutrient intake. This activity has significance in the context of diabetes. The glucose-lowering activity of GLP-1 is highly transient as the half-life of this hormone in the circulation is less than 2 minutes. Removal of bioactive GLP-1 is a consequence of *N*-terminal proteolysis catalyzed by dipeptidyl peptidase IV (DPP4). DPP4 is also known as the lymphocyte surface antigen CD26 and has numerous activities unrelated to incretin inactivation.

High-Yield Concept

Upon nutrient ingestion GLP-1 is secreted from intestinal enteroendocrine L cells that are found predominantly in the ileum and colon with some production from these cell types in the duodenum and jejunum. Bioactive GLP-1 consists of 2 forms: GLP-1 (7-37) and GLP-1 (7-36) amide, where the latter form constitutes the majority (80%) of the circulating hormone.

TABLE 44-1: **Gastrointestinal Peptides and Hormones**[1]

Hormone	*Location*	*Major Action*
Bombesin, also called neuromedin B and gastrin-releasing peptide	Stomach, duodenum	Stimulates release of gastrin and CCK
Cholecystokinin (CCK)	Enteroendocrine I cells predominantly of the duodenum, jejunum	Stimulates gallbladder contraction and bile flow, increases secretion of digestive enzymes from pancreas, vagal nerves in the gut express CCK1 (CCKA) receptors (see text for details)
Gastrin	Made in enteroendocrine G cells of the gastric antrum and duodenum	Gastric acid and pepsin secretion; exists in 2 major forms: little gastrin (17 amino acids) and big gastrin (34 amino acids), both result from a single precursor protein of 101 amino acid; both species contain a Y residue in the C-terminal portion of the protein that may be either sulfated (gastrin II) or nonsulfated (gastrin I); both forms bind to the CCK2 (CCK_B) receptor on stomach and gut parietal cells with an affinity equal to that of CCK; the C-terminal tetrapeptide of both gastrins and CCK are identical and possess all the biological activities of both gastrin and CCK
Ghrelin	Primary site is X/A-like enteroendocrine cells of the stomach oxyntic (acid-secreting) glands, minor synthesis in intestine, pancreas, and hypothalamus	Regulation of appetite (increases desire for food intake), energy homeostasis, glucose metabolism, gastric secretion and emptying, insulin secretion (see test for details)
Glucagon-like peptide-1 (GLP-1)	Enteroendocrine L cells predominantly in the ileum and colon	Potentiates glucose-dependent insulin secretion, inhibits glucagon secretion, inhibits gastric emptying (see text for details)
Glucagon-like peptide-2 (GLP-2)	Enteroendocrine L cells predominantly in the ileum and colon	Enhances digestion and food absorption, inhibits gastric secretions, promotes intestinal mucosal growth
Glucose-dependent insulinotropic polypeptide (GIP), originally called gastric inhibitory polypeptide	Enteroendocrine K cells of the duodenum and proximal jejunum	Inhibits secretion of gastric acid, enhances insulin secretion (see text for details)
Motilin	Proximal small intestine	Initiates interdigestive intestinal motility, stimulates release of PP, stimulates gallbladder contractions
Obestatin	Primary site is stomach, minor synthesis in intestine	Derived from proghrelin protein, acts in opposition to ghrelin action on appetite (see text for details)
Oxyntomodulin	Enteroendocrine L cells predominantly in the ileum and colon	Contains all of the amino acids of glucagon; inhibits meal-stimulated gastric acid secretion similar to GLP-1 and GLP-2 action; induces satiety, decreases weight gain, and increases energy consumption; has weak affinity for GLP-1 receptor as well as the glucagon receptor, may mimic glucagon actions in liver and pancreas (see text for details)
Pancreatic polypeptide (PP)	Pancreas F cells, colon, and rectum	Inhibits pancreatic bicarbonate and protein secretion
Peptide tyrosine tyrosine (PYY)	Enteroendocrine L cells predominantly in the ileum and colon	Reduced gut motility, a delay in gastric emptying, and an inhibition of gallbladder contraction; exerts effects on satiety via actions in the hypothalamus (see text for details)
Secretin	Enteroendocrine S cells of the duodenum, jejunum	Pancreatic bicarbonate secretion, inhibits gastric secretions, stimulates PP secretion

(Continued)

TABLE 44-1: Gastrointestinal Peptides and Hormones1 (*continued*)

Hormone	*Location*	*Major Action*
Somatostatin	Made by D cells of the gut and δ-cells of the pancreas, also produced in hypothalamus and other organ systems	Inhibits release and action of numerous gut peptides, eg, CKK, OXM, PP, gastrin, secretin, motilin, GIP; also inhibits insulin and glucagon secretion from pancreas
Substance P, a member of the tachykinin family that includes neurokinin A (NKA) and neurokinin B (NKB)	Entire gastrointestinal tract	CNS function in pain (nociception), involved in vomit reflex, stimulates salivary secretions, induces vasodilation antagonists having antidepressant properties
Vasoactive intestinal peptide (VIP)	Pancreas	Smooth muscle relaxation; stimulates pancreatic bicarbonate secretion

[1]Not intended to be a complete listing of all the peptides of the gastrointestinal system.

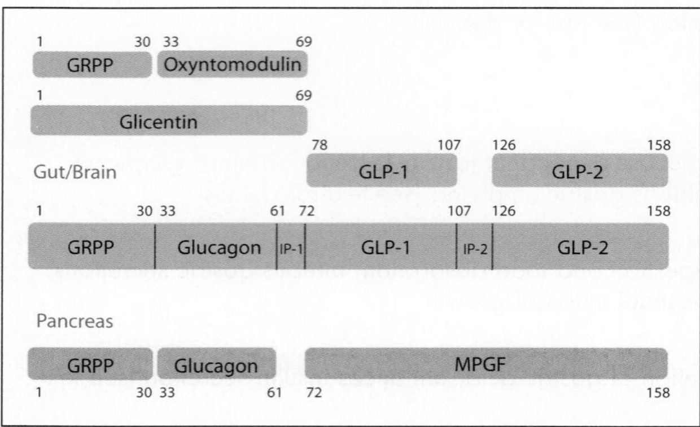

FIGURE 44-1: Structure and processing of mammalian preproglucagon. On the top half are the processing results that occur when the *GCG* gene is expressed in the gastrointestinal system and the brain. Shown on the bottom half are the processing results that occur when *GCG* gene is expressed in the pancreas. GRPP = glicentin-related pancreatic peptide. IP = intervening peptide. GLP-2 = glucagon-like peptide-2. Glicentin (composed of amino acids 1-69) is found in the small intestine but the majority is processed to GRPP and oxyntomodulin. MPGF = major proglucagon fragment comprises amino acids 72 to 158 and is found in the pancreas. Reproduced with permission of themedicalbiochemistrypage, LLC.

All of the effects of GLP-1 are mediated following activation of the GLP-1 receptor (GLP-1R). The GLP-1R is a G protein-coupled receptor (GPCR) coupled to G_s-protein activation, increased cAMP production, and activation of protein kinase A (PKA). In addition the GLP-1R is coupled to the activation of PI3K which in turn activates PKB/Akt. The other major responses to the actions of GLP-1 include pancreatic β-cell proliferation and expansion concomitant with a reduction of β-cell apoptosis. In addition, GLP-1 activity results in increased expression of the glucose transporter 2 (GLUT2) and glucokinase genes in pancreatic β-cells.

Oxyntomodulin

Oxyntomodulin (OXM) is so called given that is was originally discovered from work examining the inhibition of the activity of oxyntic glands (gastric acid secreting) of the stomach. OXM is a 37-amino acid peptide derived from the proglucagon peptide and contains the entire 29 amino acids of glucagon. Synthesis and release of OXM occurs in the enteroendocrine L cells of the distal gut. These are the same cell populations that secrete GLP-1 and PYY. The secretion of OXM occurs within 5 to 10 minutes following ingestion of food and peaks within 30 minutes. The amount of OXM that is released is directly proportional to caloric intake. In addition to stimulated release in response to food intake, OXM exhibits diurnal variation in its concentration in the blood with highest levels detected in the evening and lowest levels in the morning. Like GLP-1, OXM has demonstrated incretin activity.

A distinct OXM receptor has not been identified but the protein can bind to the GLP-1R and the glucagon receptor. Indeed, evidence indicates that the incretin and anorexigenic effects of OXM are exerted via the GLP-1R as these activities of OXM are abolished in the GLP-1R knock-out mouse. OXM exerts a protective effect on pancreatic β-cells similar to that exerted by GLP-1. Although the affinity of OXM for the GLP-1R is at least 50-fold less than that of GLP-1 itself, the ability of OXM to exert inhibition of food intake is equal to that of GLP-1.

When OXM is administered into the brain the response is suppression of the effects of circulating ghrelin. These results suggest that part of the appetite suppressing effects of OXM are mediated by reduced ghrelin as well as increased hypothalamic release of anorexigenic peptides. Of potential significance to the treatment of obesity is that when OXM is administered intravenously to human subjects there is an observed reduction (19.3%) in food intake at mealtime. Additionally significant is the fact that this reduction in desire for food intake persists over the course of 12 hours. When OXM is administered subcutaneously to overweight and obese subjects over a period of 4 weeks there is a significant reduction in body weight. Although these results prove promising for the potential for OXM in the treatment of obesity it is important to note that OXM is a target for inactivation by DPP4 just as is GLP-1.

Glucose-Dependent Insulinotropic Peptide

GIP is derived from a 153-amino acid proprotein encoded by the *GIP* gene and circulates as a biologically active 42-amino acid peptide. GIP is synthesized by enteroendocrine K cells whose locations are primarily in the duodenum and proximal jejunum. Like GLP-1, GIP is a gut hormone possessing potent glucose-dependent insulin secretion (an incretin) activity. In addition, GIP has significant effects on fat metabolism exerted at the level of adipocytes. These actions include stimulation of lipoprotein lipase (LPL) activity leading to increased uptake and incorporation of fatty acids by adipocytes. Whereas GIP exerts positive effects on pancreatic β-cell proliferation and survival similar to that shown for GLP-1, the hormone does not affect glucagon secretion nor gastric emptying. Like GLP-1, GIP is inactivated through the action of DPP4.

The GIP receptor (GIPR) is a G_s-protein coupled GPCR found on pancreatic β-cells. Stimulation of the GIPR elevates intracellular cAMP levels and also results in increased uptake of Ca^{2+} into pancreatic β-cells. Responses to GIP have been shown to be defective in T2D patients.

Cholecystokinin

Cholecystokinin (CCK) is derived via posttranslational modification of the procholecystokinin peptide. CCK was the first gut hormone to be identified as having an effect on appetite. There are several bioactive forms of CCK that are designated based upon the number of amino acids in the peptide. The 4 major forms are CCK-8, CCK-22, CCK-33, and CCK-58. The predominant form that is found in human plasma is the CCK-33 form. CCK is secreted from intestinal enteroendocrine I cells predominantly in the duodenum and jejunum. The level of CCK in the blood rises within 15 minutes of food ingestion and reaches a peak by 25 minutes. The most potent substances initiating a release of CCK from the I cells are fats and proteins. Conversely, duodenal bile acids are potent suppressors of the secretion of CCK.

CCK exerts its biological actions by binding to 2 specific GPCRs identified as CCK-1 and CCK-2. The CCK receptors are also identified as CCK_A and CCK whose designations referred to their location of prominent expression with CCK_A referring to the alimentary tract (the gut) and CCK_B referring to the brain. However, both receptors are found widely expressed in the CNS as well as the periphery.

Upon binding its receptors in the gut CCK induces contractions of the gallbladder and release of pancreatic enzymes and also inhibits gastric emptying. Within the brain, specifically the median eminence and ventromedial nucleus of the hypothalamus (VMH), CCK actions elicit behavioral responses and satiation. Central administration of CCK results in reduced food intake. Of significance to appetite control, this effect is enhanced with coadministration of leptin. The synergistic effects of CCK and leptin may be due to the fact that their receptors are colocalized to the same sensory vagal afferent neurons.

Ghrelin

Ghrelin was first discovered based upon its ability to interact with the growth hormone secretagogue (GHS) receptor and stimulate the release of growth hormone. Indeed, ghrelin was found to be the endogenous ligand for the GHS receptor. The name ghrelin is derived from **g**rowth-**h**ormone **rel**ease. The specific receptor to which ghrelin binds and activates is identified as GHSR type 1a (GHSR1a).

The ghrelin gene encodes the ghrelin preproprotein that can undergo differential processing to yield mature ghrelin peptide or obestatin. Ghrelin is produced and secreted by the X/A-like enteroendocrine cells of the stomach oxyntic (acid-secreting) glands. Because the X/A-like cells express ghrelin they are also sometimes referred to as ghrelin cells or Gr cells. X/A-like cells express the receptor for gastrin (see Table 44-1) and, therefore, it is believed that gastrin may directly stimulate ghrelin release. Smaller amounts of ghrelin are released from the small intestine and the colon. A low level of ghrelin is also produced in pancreatic ε-cells.

Due to alternative splicing and posttranslational cleavage, the 117-amino acid preproghrelin protein can be processed into ghrelin (28 amino acids corresponding to amino acids 24-51 of the preproprotein), obestatin (23 amino acids corresponding to amino acids 76-98 of the preproprotein) and des-acyl ghrelin (27 amino acids). Bioactive ghrelin is acylated on the serine at position 3 with *n*-octanoic acid. The attachment of octanoic acid to Ser3 of ghrelin is accomplished by the acyltransferase identified as ghrelin *O*-acyltransferase (GOAT; also referred to as membrane-bound *O*-acyltransferase domain-containing 4, MBOAT4). The nonacylated form of ghrelin may act as an antagonist of the acylated hormone. The des-acyl ghrelin protein is also acylated on Ser3 which is required for its activity as for full-length ghrelin.

The major effect of ghrelin is exerted within the hypothalamus at the level of the arcuate nucleus (ARC) where it stimulates the release of neuropeptide Y (NPY) and agouti-related protein (AgRP). As discussed below, the actions of NPY and AgRP enhance appetite and thus, food intake. Within the hypothalamus, ghrelin action results in activation of AMPK leading to reduced intracellular levels of long-chain fatty acids. The reduction in fatty acid levels appears to be the molecular signal leading to increased expression of NPY and AgRP. However, it is important to note that the signaling events triggered by ghrelin binding to GHSR1a are complex.

The secretion of ghrelin is the inverse of that of insulin. The primary mechanisms that are coupled to production of ghrelin are fasting, hypoglycemia, and leptin. Conversely, inhibition of ghrelin production is exerted by food intake, hyperglycemia, and obesity. The action of ghrelin at the level of increasing the release of NPY is the exact opposite to that of leptin which inhibits NPY release. Additional effects of ghrelin include inhibition of the expression of proinflammatory cytokines, modulation of exocrine and endocrine functions of the pancreas, regulation of gastric acid secretion and gastric motility, and the modulation of sleep patterns, memory and anxiety-like behavioral responses.

Obestatin

Whereas ghrelin actions result in increased appetite and food intake, obestatin action suppresses food intake. The name obestatin is derived from a contraction of obese and statin (to suppress). Release of obestatin suppresses food intake and gastric emptying activity. Like ghrelin, which is posttranslationally modified, obestatin is also modified but its modification is an amidation. The mechanism(s) by which obestatin exerts its effects is unclear since a definitive receptor has not yet been identified for this gut peptide.

Pancreatic Polypeptide

Pancreatic polypeptide (PP) was the first member of the PP-fold family (PP, PYY, and NPY) to be isolated and characterized. PP is produced and secreted by type F cells within the periphery of pancreatic islets. The stimulus for the release of PP is the ingestion of food and the level of release is proportional to the caloric intake. Increased circulating levels of PP can be detected in the blood for up to 6 hours following ingestion of food. Humoral signals that are involved in food intake-mediated secretion of PP include ghrelin, CCK, motilin, and secretin. Additionally, adrenergic stimulation secondary to either hypoglycemia or exercise results in increased release of PP. The actions of PP include delaying gastric emptying, inhibition of gallbladder contraction, and attenuation of pancreatic exocrine secretions. These gut actions of PP are associated with the mechanism referred to as the *ileal brake* which is manifest with the slowing of the passage of nutrients through the gut.

The PP-fold proteins bind to a family of receptors that were originally characterized as NPY receptors (see later). There are 4 NPY receptors in humans designated as Y1, Y2, Y4, and Y5. PP induces an anorexigenic response within the brain stem (area postremus, AP) and vagus. These responses are mediated via activation of the Y4 receptor which binds PP with highest affinity. In addition to its expression in the AP, the Y4 receptor is also expressed in regions of the hypothalamus including the ARC. Therefore, additional anorexigenic responses to PP can be induced within the hypothalamus.

PP plays an important role in the regulation of satiety. In obese individuals there is a reduced level of PP secretion in response to food intake, whereas, in anorexia nervosa there is increased PP release following consumption of food. PP may also play a role in the pathogenesis of Prader-Willi syndrome (PWS). This disorder is characterized by short stature, reduced intellect, and hyperphagia. In patients with PWS there is a reduced secretion of PP in response to food intake as well as a reduced basal level of circulating PP.

Protein Tyrosine Tyrosine

Protein tyrosine tyrosine (PYY) is another member of the PP-fold family. PYY is produced and secreted by intestinal enteroendocrine L cells of the ileum and colon. Additional gut hormones that are secreted along with PYY include GLP-1 and OXM. Secreted forms of PYY include $PYY_{1\text{-}36}$ and $PYY_{3\text{-}36}$ with $PYY_{3\text{-}36}$ being generated via the actions of DPP4. Within the central nervous system PYY is detectable in the hypothalamus, medulla, pons, and spinal cord.

The release of PYY results in reduced gut motility, delayed gastric emptying, and inhibition of gallbladder contraction. All of these actions are, like that of PP, associated with the ileal brake. CCK and gastrin are thought to mediate the rapid release of PYY in response to eating. The amount of PYY released in response to the ingestion of food is proportional to the caloric intake. PYY has a critical role in satiety. Within the CNS, PYY exerts its effects on satiety via actions in the hypothalamus, specifically the ARC. Given the role of PYY in appetite suppression it is thought that disturbances in PYY release in response to food intake may play a role in the development of obesity. Indeed, in obese humans there is a blunted PYY response following food intake compared to lean humans. Current therapeutic interventions designed to combat obesity involve studies of the efficacy of PYY at suppressing appetite.

Hypothalamic Control of Feeding Behavior

The location and organization of the hypothalamus is discussed in Chapter 49. The primary nuclei of the hypothalamus that are involved in feeding behaviors and satiety include the arcuate nucleus of the hypothalamus (ARC, also abbreviated as ARH), the dorsomedial hypothalamic nucleus (DMH or DMN), and the ventromedial hypothalamic nucleus (VMH or VMN) all of which are located in the tuberal medial area. The ARC is involved in control of feeding behavior as well as secretion of various pituitary releasing hormones, the DMH is involved in stimulating gastrointestinal activity, and the VMH is involved in satiety. Early experiments involving lesions in the hypothalamus demonstrated that the lateral hypothalamic area (LHA) is responsible for transmitting orexigenic signals and loss of this region results in starvation. The medial hypothalamic nuclei (VMH and to a lesser extent the DMH) are responsible for the sensations of satiety and lesions in these regions of the hypothalamus result in hyperphagia and obesity.

Appetite is a complex process that results from the integration of multiple signals at the hypothalamus. The hypothalamus receives neural inputs, hormonal signals such as leptin, CCK, and ghrelin, and nutrient signals such as glucose, free fatty acids, amino acids, and volatile fatty acids. Each of these elicits effects that are processed by a specific set of neurotransmitters primarily acting within the ARC (Figure 44-2). Within the ARC the orexigenic neurons express NPY and AgRP and the anorexigenic neurons express proopiomelanocortin, POMC-derived melanocortins (principally α-MSH) and cocaine and amphetamine-regulated transcript (CART). These so-called first-order neurons then act on second-order neurons. The orexigenic second-order neurons express either MCH or the orexins. The anorexigenic second-order neurons express corticotropin-releasing hormone, CRH. The net effect of the concerted action of these neuropeptide is alterations in feeding behaviors and food intake. In addition, satiety signals from the liver and gastrointestinal tract signal through the vagus nerve to the nucleus of the solitary tract (NTS, for the Latin term *nucleus tractus solitarii*). The NTS is a cluster of specialized cells within the medulla responsible for sensations of taste and visceral sensations of stretch. Activation of the NTS via the vagal nerve causes meal termination, and in combination with the hypothalamus, integrates the various signals to determine the feeding response. The activities of these neuronal pathways are also influenced by numerous factors such as nutrients, fasting, and disease to modify appetite and hence exert impacts on growth and reproduction.

Neuropeptide Y

Neuropeptide tyrosine (NPY) is a hypothalamic neuroendocrine protein that is a member of the PP family of hormones. Each of these peptide hormones contains 36 amino acids including numerous tyrosines (hence the Y nomenclature). Each of the PP family of proteins binds to a family of receptors that were originally characterized as NPY receptors designated as Y1, Y2, Y4, and Y5. Receptors Y1, Y2, and Y5 preferentially bind NPY and PYY, whereas, Y4 exhibits highest affinity for PP. The Y2 receptor is involved in anorexigenic responses whereas the Y1 and Y5 receptors have been shown to induce orexigenic responses. The Y2 receptors are referred to as inhibitory receptors with respect to the activity of NPY and they are abundantly expressed on NPY neurons in the ARC of the hypothalamus.

NPY is expressed throughout the brain with highest levels found in the ARC of the hypothalamus. NPY is one of the most potent orexigenic factors produced by the human body. Within the ARC there are 2 neuronal populations that exert opposing actions on the desire for food intake. Neurons that coexpress NPY and another neuropeptide called AgRP stimulate food intake, whereas, neurons that coexpress POMC and cocaine and amphetamine-regulated transcript (CART) suppress the desire for food intake. The Y1 and Y5 receptors mediate the bulk of the effects of NPY on the hypothalamic-pituitary-thyroid axis. Within the ventromedial nucleus (VMN) of the hypothalamus, binding of NPY to the Y1 receptor results in inhibition of neuronal function (via hyperpolarization) thereby interfering with the satiety role of the VMN. The majority of hypothalamic Y2 receptors are found on NPY-containing neurons.

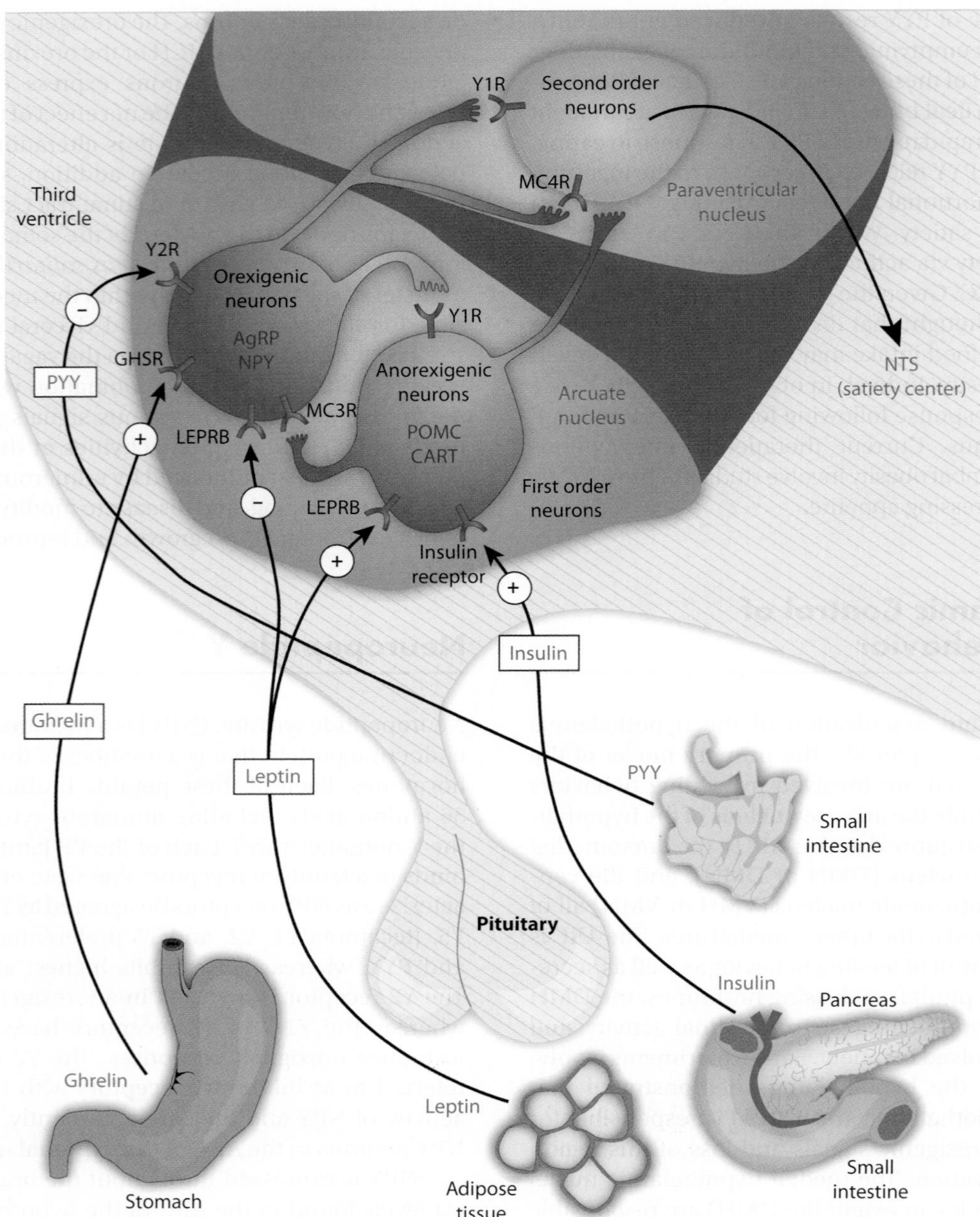

FIGURE 44-2: Hormonal circuits from the gut (stomach, small intestine, and pancreas) and fat (adipose tissue) that impact the sensations of hunger and satiety that are exerted via hypothalamic neuroendocrine pathways. Ghrelin from the stomach, leptin from adipose tissue, insulin from the pancreas, and PYY from the small intestine bind to receptors on orexigenic and/or anorexigenic neurons in the ARC of the hypothalamus. The effects of these peptide hormone-receptor interactions are release of either the orexigenic neuropeptides NPY and AgRP or the anorexigenic neuropeptides CART and the POMC-derived peptide α-MSH. These neuropeptides from the ARC travel along axons to secondary neurons in other areas of the hypothalamus such as the paraventricular nucleus (PVN). The ultimate effects of these signaling cascades are changes in the sensation of hunger and satiety in the NTS. LEPRB is the large form of the leptin receptor (see Chapter 45 for descriptions of leptin and leptin receptors). GHSR is the growth hormone secretagogue receptor to which ghrelin binds. MC3R and MC4R are melanocortin 3 receptor and melanocortin 4 receptor, respectively. Y1R and Y2R are the NPY receptors 1 and 2, respectively.

Conversely, Y2 receptor activation in the ARC results in inhibition of the actions of NPY which accounts for the anorexigenic actions associated with PP activation of Y2 receptors. Of significance to dieting and weight loss is the fact that when people lose excess weight the level of NPY increases which likely is a contributing factor to the inability of most people to keep the weight off.

NPY exerts differential orexigenic effects on food choice. NPY action causes a strong preference for carbohydrate-rich foods. NPY activity leads to reduced fatty acid oxidation while simultaneously promoting carbohydrate oxidation and fatty acid synthesis. The synthesis and release of NPY is also responsive to the particular fuel source being metabolized in the brain. Reduced hypothalamic glucose oxidation results in increased NPY release whereas fatty acid metabolism exerts no appreciable effect on NPY synthesis.

Agouti-Related Peptide

As the name implies, AgRP is a protein with sequence homology to the agouti protein which controls coat color in rodents. AgRP is expressed primarily in the ARC and is found to colocalize with neurons that also produce NPY. Although expression of AgRP is restricted to the ARC, AgRP fibers project to several brain areas as well as to multiple areas within the hypothalamus, including the paraventricular nucleus (PVN or PVH) and the perifornical lateral hypothalamus (PFLH). In addition, all of these AgRP nerve terminals contain NPY. The PVN is a region of the hypothalamus that integrates neuropeptide signals from numerous regions of the brain and hypothalamus as well as the brain stem. The PFLH is a subdomain of the lateral hypothalamic area (LHA) that is involved in arousal and food-seeking behaviors.

AgRP together with NPY represent a distinct set of ARC-expressed orexigenic peptides. AgRP is classically referred to as a member of the central melanocortin system, which in addition to AgRP comprises α-MSH (see later) and 2 melanocortin receptors identified as melanocortin receptor 3 (MC3R) and melanocortin receptor 4 (MC4R). Whereas, α-MSH is an agonist of both MC3R and MC4R, AgRP serves to antagonize the actions of α-MSH at these same receptors with highest antagonist activity on MC4R. In addition to antagonizing the effect of α-MSH at the MC3R and MC4R, AgRP suppresses the basal activity of the MC4R, thus defining AgRP as an inverse agonist.

The close functional relationship between AgRP and NPY is demonstrated by the fact that the expression of these 2 peptides is similarly modulated under identical physiological conditions such as negative energy balance or increased energy demand that occurs during food deprivation. During periods of fasting both AgRP and NPY levels rise, primarily as a result of a drop in the level of the peripheral hormones leptin (see Chapter 45) and insulin (see Chapter 46) and a rise in ghrelin. The expression of both AgRP and NPY is suppressed under conditions of positive energy balance.

Central injection of AgRP has a potent stimulatory effect on food intake which can also be seen using a MC4R antagonist. These results confirm the function of AgRP as an antagonist of α-MSH. Chronic administration of AgRP results in increased daily food intake while simultaneously decreasing oxygen consumption and the capacity of brown adipose tissue to expend energy.

There exists an antagonism between the actions of AgRP (and NPY) and the melanocortins in controlling eating and body weight. Changes in endogenous AgRP levels are opposite to those seen with the melanocortin peptides. AgRP neurons interact with POMC neurons in the ARC through the inhibitory neurotransmitter γ-aminobutyric acid (GABA). Both AgRP and NPY axons, that colocalize GABA, project onto POMC-expressing cells in the ARC. AgRP activity stimulates the release of GABA resulting in inhibition of the activity of the POMC neurons.

Leptin binds to its receptor presents on AgRP and NPY neurons and inhibits their firing resulting in reduced GABA release onto POMC neurons. This leptin-induced reduction in GABA action at POMC neurons is a disinhibition and is, in part, the mechanism by which leptin decreases feeding behaviors. Conversely, ghrelin binding its receptor activates AgRP and NPY neurons, resulting in an increase in GABA release with resultant inhibition of POMC neurons.

Melanin-Concentrating Hormone

Melanin-concentrating hormone (MCH) was originally identified as a 19-amino acid cyclic peptide that induced the lightening of the skin in fish. Subsequently the peptide was as overexpressed in response to fasting and also elevated in genetically obese mice (*ob/ob* mice). In humans MCH is expressed exclusively in the lateral hypothalamus and zona incerta (region of gray matter cells in the subthalamus below the thalamus). In humans there are 2 GPCRs that bind MCH identified as MCH1R and MCH2R. MCH1R couples to the activation of both G_q and G_i type G proteins.

Involvement of MCH in the regulation of feeding behaviors and energy homeostasis has been shown in mice where either the MCH or the *MCH1R* genes have been knocked out. Loss of MCH leads to hypophagia and lean body mass indicating that MCH is an important orexigenic hormone. In contrast, central administration of MCH results in increased food intake. Loss of the *MCH1R* gene induces hyperphagia and hyperactivity. When MCH1R antagonists are administered, there is a decrease in MCH-induced food intake. MCH1R antagonists have been shown to modulate leptin secretion and insulin release which suggests that the weight loss associated with systemic antagonist administration is due to both central and peripheral effects.

The synthesis and release of MCH is also responsive to the fuel source being metabolized in the brain. When fatty acid metabolism occurs there is no appreciable effect on MCH synthesis, however, inhibition of fatty acid oxidation results in increased MCH synthesis and release. In contrast, modulation of glucose oxidation has no effects on MCH expression.

Orexins

The orexins were identified as substances that bound to orphan GPCRs and induced an orexigenic response. The orexins constitute 2 neuroendocrine peptides derived from the same gene. These peptides are designated as orexin A and orexin B. The orexins are also referred to as the hypocretins. Orexin A corresponds to hypocretin 1 (HCRT-1) and orexin B corresponds to hypocretin 2 (HCRT-2).

The orexin preproprotein is 131 amino acids in length with the 33-amino acid orexin A peptide encoded by amino acids 33 to 65 and the 28-amino acid orexin B peptide encoded by amino acids 69 to 96. Both orexin A and orexin B peptides are *C*-terminally amidated. The *N*-terminal glutamine residue of orexin A is cyclized into a pyroglutamyl residue and the peptide contains 2 intrachain disulfide bonds. There are 2 orexin receptors identified as OX_1R and OX_2R. OX_1R exhibits an order of magnitude higher affinity for orexin A compared to orexin B whereas OX_2R has been shown to bind both peptides with equal affinity. The orexin receptors are typical GPCRs with OX_1R coupling to the G_q proteins and OX_2R coupling to both the G_q and G_i proteins.

The cell bodies of orexin expressing neurons are found in the lateral and posterior hypothalamic areas with axonal projections throughout the brain. Expression of the orexin receptors is also widely distributed throughout the central nervous system. Central injection of orexin peptides increases food consumption and wakefulness and suppresses REM sleep. The latter observations demonstrate that orexins play a causative role in the regulation of sleep-wake cycles. Indeed, loss of orexin function results in a condition in animals that mimics the sleep disorder in humans known as narcolepsy. In human narcolepsy patients there is a significant reduction in the amount of detectable orexin A and orexin B as well as an 80% to 100% reduction in the number of neurons that contain detectable prepro-orexin mRNA.

Galanin

Galanin (GAL) is a 29-amino acid peptide whose name is derived from the fact that it contains an *N*-terminal glycine residue and a *C*-terminal alanine. GAL is expressed in the gut and the brain with wide distribution throughout the hypothalamus including the PVN, the PFLH, and ARC. The expression of GAL in the hypothalamus is directly correlated to its role in energy homeostasis and the control of feeding behaviors. In addition to regulating feeding, GAL serves as a growth and prolactin-releasing factor to the lactotroph, especially in states of high estrogen exposure, is involved in learning and memory through effects in the hippocampus, and is involved in pain and seizures. Additionally, GAL exerts affective responses such as in mood disorders and anxiety. GAL exerts these myriad effects via binding to 3 distinct GPCRs identified as GALR1, GALR2, and GALR3.

Central administration of GAL elicits a strong orexigenic response with a preference for fat over protein and carbohydrates. The feeding behavior responses to GAL exposure are primarily due to binding GALR1 in the hypothalamus. GAL-induced feeding is greatly attenuated when fat is removed from the diet. The primary function of GAL when an animal is consuming a high-fat diet is to restore carbohydrate balance, through behavioral and metabolic actions, under conditions where carbohydrate intake and metabolism are suppressed.

Insulin suppresses GAL expression whereas leptin produces little or no change in basal GAL expression in the ARC and only a small suppression of GAL expression in the PVN. The differential responsiveness of GAL neurons to leptin is likely due to the low concentration of leptin receptors on GAL neurons. Administration of inhibitors of fatty acid oxidation suppresses GAL expression. Conversely, administration of inhibitors of glucose oxidation does not alter GAL expression. The ability of GAL to exert its stimulation of feeding responses may be due to its interactions with other peptide systems. The opioids are believed to have some role in mediating GAL-induced feeding, since the opioid receptor agonist naloxone attenuates the GAL feeding response. GAL may also induce feeding via an inhibition of the anorexigenic melanocortin system.

Melanocortins

The POMC-derived melanocortin peptides include α-MSH, β-MSH, γ-MSH, $ACTH^{1-24}$, and $ACTH^{1-13}$-NH_2 (desacetyl-α-MSH). The POMC-derived melanocortins belong to a family of peptides referred to as the melanocortin system (see Figure 49-3). This system includes the POMC-derived melanocortins which exhibit agonist activities, the antagonist peptide AgRP, the melanocortin receptors (MCR), and the melanocortin receptor accessory proteins (MRAPs). The MCR family of receptors consists of 5 identified members termed MC1R through MC5R.

The melanocortin system has been shown to be critical in the regulation of food intake and energy expenditure. Central administration of α-MSH, β-MSH, or $ACTH^{1-24}$ inhibits the intake of food. The actions of MSH peptides in feeding behavior are exerted primarily via peptide binding to the MC4R and to a lesser extent to the MC3R. Genetic mutations in humans that disrupt the expression and processing (this includes the proteases that process the POMC precursor) of POMC peptides and MCRs are associated with changes in energy balance and can lead to obesity and T2D. Mutations have been identified in prohormone convertase 1/3 (PC1/3) and carboxypeptidase E (CPE), as well as in the α-MSH degrading enzyme prolylcarboxypeptidase (PRCP) that are associated with energy imbalance and a propensity for obesity. In genome-wide screens for polymorphisms in genes associated with an increased risk of developing T2D the *MC4R* gene was identified (see Chapter 47). Indeed, mutations in the *MC4R* gene are the most frequent causes of severe obesity in humans.

Humans with a lack of POMC expression are unable to survive without glucocorticoid supplementation from birth. Individuals that survive have red hair, dramatically increased desire for food intake, and high propensity for obesity. Another POMC mutation that has been identified in humans resulting in obesity is a point mutation in the cleavage site between β-MSH and β-endorphin. The consequences of this mutation suggest that β-MSH may be a significant endogenous anorectic agonist that activates the MC4R.

Cocaine- and Amphetamine-Regulated Transcript

The cocaine- and amphetamine-regulated transcript (CART) peptides are neuroendocrine peptides involved in feeding behavior, drug reward systems, stress, cardiovascular functions, and bone remodeling. Expression of the *CART* gene is essentially confined to hypothalamic neuroendocrine neurons and limbic system circuits involved in reward processes. CART peptides are found in areas of the brain involved in the control of feeding behaviors including regions of the hypothalamus such as the VMN, lateral hypothalamus (LH), PVN, NTS, ARC, and the nucleus accumbens.

The human *CART* gene is transcribed into 2 alternatively spliced mRNAs that encode proCART peptides of different lengths identified as proCART1-89 and proCART1-102. However, only the proCART1-89 peptide is found in humans. The processing of proCART1-89 yields CART peptides identified as CART 42-89 and CART 49-89. A definitive CART receptor has as yet not been isolated, however, evidence suggests the CART receptor is a GPCR that activates the $G_{i/o}$ class of G proteins.

Central administration of CART peptides results in decreased food intake indicating the peptides are anorexigenic. Within the ARC of the hypothalamus CART-peptide containing neurons are surrounded by NPY expressing nerve terminals. The distribution of CART and NPY in the ARC suggests that these 2 neuropeptides may exhibit cross-talk in the regulation of feeding behavior. Food deprivation leads to decreases in the level of CART mRNA in the ARC. Conversely, when leptin is administered, the level of CART mRNA in the ARC increases.

Several human studies have also indicated that CART peptides function in appetite control. Missense mutations in the *CART* gene are associated with obesity and a single nucleotide polymorphism (SNP) was identified in the *CART* gene in several morbidly obese individuals. In addition, a polymorphism that resides approximately 156 kb upstream of the *CART* gene may be associated with obesity.

Galanin-Like Peptide

Galanin-like peptide (GALP) is a 60-amino acid peptide that is structurally related to galanin. Amino acids 9 to 21 of GALP are identical to the first 13 amino acids of GAL. The structural and sequence similarities between GALP and GAL explain the fact that GALP functions by binding with high affinity to GAL receptors. However, there are differences in affinities of the 2 peptides for the different GAL receptors. GAL binds all 3 receptor subtypes (GALR1, GALR2, and GALR3) with similar affinities, whereas, GALP binds with highest affinity to GALR3 followed by GALR2 with GALR1 binding with least affinity. Expression of GALP is almost exclusively found in the hypothalamic ARC, and GALP neurons project to the PVN but not the lateral hypothalamus.

Central injection of GALP induces an anorexigenic response. The leptin receptor is expressed on most GALP neurons and expression of GALP in the ARC is induced by leptin. In contrast, GALP expression in the ARC is significantly reduced in leptin-deficient (*ob/ob*) and leptin receptor-deficient (*db/db*) mice. Food deprivation results in reduced circulating levels of leptin and this in turn reduces the rapid entry of circulating GALP into the brain. Fasting results in a decrease in both the level of GALP mRNA as well as the number of GALP expressing neurons. Leptin administration will restore GALP expression in fasted animals as well as in leptin-deficient (*ob/ob*) mice.

Corticotropin-Releasing Factor and Related Peptides

Corticotropin-releasing factor (CRF, also known as corticotropin-releasing hormone, CRH) belongs to an interacting family of proteins that includes CRF, at least 2 different CRF receptor subtypes (CRF1 and CRF2), a CRF-binding protein (CRF-BP), and the urocortins which are endogenous CRF receptor ligands. There are 3 known urocortins identified as urocortin 1, 2, and 3 (Ucn1, Ucn2, Ucn3). CRF is a 41-amino acid peptide that is found widely expressed in the brain. CRF-expressing neurons are abundant in the hypothalamic PVN where they control the pituitary-adrenal axis regulating the release of ACTH and glucocorticoids.

CRF binds to 2 GPCRs identified as CRF1 and CRF2. In addition to binding to 2 receptors, CRF also binds to CRF-BP, which is expressed in association with CRF-expressing neurons in many brain areas including the hypothalamus. CRF-BP acts as an inhibitor of CRF action, thereby, modulating its biological actions.

Hypothalamic expression of CRF is negatively regulated by the circulating level of corticosterone such that CRF mRNA and protein levels are highest when corticosterone levels are declining. Other glucocorticoids also negatively regulate CRF expression. Diabetes leads to increased CRF expression in the PVN and this effect can be further enhanced by the administration of insulin. Expression of CRF is also stimulated in states of positive energy balance and is reduced in states of negative energy balance, such as food deprivation. Circulating nutrients also affect the level of CRF expression. When glucose levels rise, CRF levels decline with the opposite occurring when glucose levels fall. In contrast to the changes in CRF levels in response to serum glucose changes, excess fat consumption does not appear to alter CRF expression.

Central administration of CRF induces anorexigenic responses. The CRF-mediated suppression of feeding occurs along with a stimulation sympathetic nervous system activity and resting oxygen consumption which results in increased fat mobilization and oxidation and raises blood glucose while inhibiting insulin secretion. The role of CRF as an anorexigenic hormone may involve the NPY, melanocortin and CART systems, acting in a downstream fashion. The CRF neurons in the hypothalamus colocalize with both the NPY Y5 receptor and the MC4R. In addition, CRF expression in the PVN is stimulated by central administration of a melanocortin agonist but is inhibited by an MC4R antagonist. Leptin is also involved in the effects of CRF as demonstrated by the fact that the anorexigenic actions of leptin are attenuated in the presence of CRF antagonists.

REVIEW QUESTIONS

1. You are performing laser ablation experiments on laboratory animals to ascertain the effects, on feeding behaviors, of damage to certain regions of the brain. In one series of experiments it is found that loss of the targeted brain region causes the animals eat nearly continuously, no matter the time of day, nor the composition of the chow. The ablation was centered on the hypothalamus and these results strongly indicate the damage affected which of the following regions of this structure?

A. lateral hypothalamic area (LHA)
B. nucleus of the solitary tract (NTS, NST)
C. paraventricular nucleus of the hypothalamus (PVN, PVH)
D. suprachiasmatic nucleus (SCN)
E. ventromedial hypothalamus (VMH, VMN)

Answer E: The hypothalamus is involved in control of feeding behavior as well as the secretion of various pituitary releasing hormones. Specific nuclei within the hypothalamus exert different effects on appetite and the desire for food. The ventromedial hypothalamic nucleus (VMH), and to a lesser extent the dorsomedial hypothalamic nucleus (DMH) is involved in the sensation of satiety and lesions in these regions of the hypothalamus result in hyperphagia (excessive hunger) and obesity.

2. You are assessing the effects of injecting synthetic peptides into laboratory mice. You discover that injecting one of the peptides induces hyperphagia. Which of the following hormones is most likely being mimicked by the actions of the synthetic peptide?

A. cholecystokinin, CCK
B. cocaine- and amphetamine-regulated transcript, CART
C. ghrelin
D. α-melanocyte stimulating hormone, α-MSH
E. peptide tyrosine tyrosine, PYY

Answer C: Ghrelin is produced and secreted by the X/A-like enteroendocrine cells of the stomach oxyntic (acid-secreting) glands. The major effect of ghrelin is exerted within the central nervous system at the level of the arcuate nucleus where it stimulates the release of neuropeptide Y (NPY) and agouti-related protein (AgRP). The actions of NPY and AgRP enhance appetite and thus, food intake.

3. Fatty acid metabolism within the brain is not a significant pathway for the generation of ATP. However, this does not mean that fatty acid metabolism is not a useful pathway in brain. Which of the following would be expected to be found at elevated levels in brain tissues following the metabolism of free fatty acids?
A. acetate
B. alanine
C. ceramide
D. citrate
E. sphingosine

Answer C: Although β-oxidation of fatty acids represents a minor, if at all, source of the ATP pool in neurons, it is an important metabolic pathway determining the ultimate fate of fatty acids that enter the brain. As a result of fatty acid oxidation, a number of aqueous byproducts are detected in the brain such as fatty acyl-CoAs, fatty acyl-carnitines, ketone bodies, and various amino acids. Central metabolism of palmitate diverts its carbon atoms into the amino acids glutamate, glutamine, aspartate, asparagine, and GABA. In addition, numerous organic acids including citrate, malate, β-hydroxybutyrate, and acetyl-CoA result from palmitate oxidation. By far, citrate represents the largest by-product of fatty acid oxidation in the brain.

4. You are examining feeding behavior in laboratory animals in response to the addition of a test organic molecule to their chow. Following consumption of the compound you discover that the animals loose interest in food. Additional experiments demonstrate that central metabolism of palmitic acid is reduced in these animals. Given these observations you believe that the test compound is most likely inhibiting which of the following hypothalamic enzymes?
A. acetyl-CoA carboxylase
B. carnitine palmitoyltransferase I
C. fatty acid synthase
D. malonyl-CoA decarboxylase
E. medium-chain acyl-CoA dehydrogenase

Answer B: Fatty acids, specifically long-chain fatty acids via the formation of long-chain fatty acyl-CoAs, exert anorexigenic effects via the hypothalamus. Mitochondrial CPT-1 activity is involved in the central effects of fatty acids. Inhibition of hypothalamic CPT-1 leads to an increase in cytosolic long-chain acyl-CoA content and results in anorexigenic effects.

5. You are testing the effects of central administration of inhibitors of fatty acid oxidation on hypothalamic activity. Which of the following neuropeptides would you expect to see expressed at elevated levels in response to the actions of the inhibitor?
A. agouti-related peptide, AgRP
B. cocaine- and amphetamine-regulated transcript, CART
C. galanin
D. melanin-concentrating hormone, MCH
E. neuropeptide Y, NPY

Answer D: Melanin-concentrating hormone (MCH) expression is responsive to differences in fuel source availability in the brain. Pharmacological inhibition or activation of glucose metabolism exerts no effect on the expression of MCH, however, inhibition of fatty acid oxidation results in increased expression and release of the hormone.

6. The pancreatic polypeptide (PP) family of proteins binds to a family of receptors that were originally characterized as NPY receptors. There are 4 NPY receptors in humans and they are designated as Y1, Y2, Y4, and Y5. Which of the following hormone-receptor combinations is involved in exerting anorexigenic responses?
A. NPY + Y1
B. NPY + Y4
C. PP + Y4
D. PYY + Y2
E. PYY + Y4

Answer D: Receptors Y1, Y2, and Y5 preferentially bind NPY and PYY, whereas, Y4 exhibits highest affinity for PP. The Y2 receptor is involved in anorexigenic responses, whereas the Y1 and Y5 receptors have been shown to induce orexigenic responses. The Y2 receptors are thus, referred to as inhibitory receptors with respect to the activity of NPY and they are abundantly expressed on NPY neurons in the ARC of the hypothalamus.

7. Which of the following gut hormones is known to bind to one of the cholecystokinin receptors

resulting in activation of the oxyntic glands of the stomach?
A. cholecystokinin, CCK
B. gastrin
C. ghrelin
D. GLP-I
E. protein tyrosine tyrosine, PYY

Answer C: Gastrin is produced in enteroendocrine G cells of the gastric antrum and duodenum and exists in 2 forms, little gastrin (17 amino acids) and big gastrin (34 amino acids). Gastrin is responsible for inducing gastric acid production and pepsin secretion. Both forms of gastrin bind to the CCK2 (CCK_B) receptor on stomach and gut parietal cells with an affinity equal to that of CCK. Activation of the CCK_B receptor by gastrin triggers the production of gastric acid.

8. Laser ablation experiments are being performed in laboratory animals to ascertain the effects, on feeding behaviors, of damage to certain regions of the brain. In one series of experiments it is found that loss of the targeted brain region causes the animals to avoid food, no matter the time of day, nor how long they have gone without eating. The ablation was centered on the hypothalamus and these results strongly indicate the damage affected in which of the following regions of this structure?
A. lateral hypothalamic area (LHA)
B. nucleus of the solitary tract (NTS, NST)
C. paraventricular nucleus of the hypothalamus (PVN, PVH)
D. suprachiasmatic nucleus (SCN)
E. ventromedial hypothalamus (VMH, VMN)

Answer A: The hypothalamus is involved in control of feeding behavior as well as the secretion of various pituitary releasing hormones. Specific nuclei within the hypothalamus exert different effects on appetite and the desire for food. The lateral hypothalamic area (LHA) is responsible for transmitting orexigenic signals (desire for food intake) and loss of this region results in starvation.

9. A patient is diagnosed with problems in emptying the gallbladder. On a blood checkup, one hormone/peptide that is known to stimulate gallbladder contraction is inappropriately low. Which of the following hormones is most likely deficient leading to the observed symptoms?
A. cholecystokinin, CCK
B. gastrin
C. GLP-1
D. pancreatic polypeptide
E. peptide tyrosine tyrosine, PYY

Answer A: Cholecystokinin (CCK) is secreted from intestinal enteroendocrine I cells predominantly in the duodenum and jejunum. The level of CCK in the blood rises within 15 minutes of food ingestion and reaches a peak by 25 minutes. Upon binding its receptors in the gut, CCK induces contractions of the gallbladder and release of pancreatic enzymes and also inhibits gastric emptying.

10. Blocking the actions of which of the following hormones would be expected to lead to the greatest level of appetite suppression?
A. adiponectin
B. ghrelin
C. GLP-1
D. obestatin
E. peptide tyrosine tyrosine, PYY

Answer B: Ghrelin is produced and secreted by the X/A-like enteroendocrine cells of the stomach oxyntic (acid-secreting) glands. The major effect of ghrelin is exerted within the central nervous system at the level of the arcuate nucleus where it stimulates the release of neuropeptide Y (NPY) and agouti-related protein (AgRP). The actions of NPY and AgRP enhance appetite and thus, food intake.

11. Several gut-derived factors control feeding behaviors elicited by the brain. Most of these factors exert their effects by reducing the desire for food intake. The synthesis of one of these factors is stimulated by fat intake and inhibited by leptin release from adipose tissue. In addition, vagal efferents are not required for release but the activity of another gut factor is involved in its release. Which one of the following factors fits each of these statements?
A. apolipoprotein A-IV, apoA-IV
B. cholecystokinin, CCK
C. ghrelin
D. GLP-1
E. peptide tyrosine tyrosine, PYY

Answer A: Apolipoprotein A-IV (apoA-IV) is synthesized exclusively in the small intestine and the hypothalamus. Intestinal synthesis of apoA-IV increases in response to ingestion and absorption of fat and it is subsequently incorporated into chylomicrons and delivered to the circulation via the lymphatic system. Systemic apoA-IV exerts effects in the CNS involving the sensation of satiety.

12. The gut peptide ghrelin is posttranslationally modified before it is fully active. Which of the following represents the type of modification that is necessary for its biological action?

A. acetylation
B. acylation
C. methylation
D. phosphorylation
E. prenylation

Answer B: Bioactive ghrelin is acylated on the serine at position 3 with *n*-octanoic acid. The attachment of octanoic acid to Ser3 of ghrelin is accomplished by the acyltransferase identified as ghrelin *O*-acyltransferase (GOAT; also referred to as membrane-bound *O*-acyltransferase domain-containing 4, MBOAT4).

13. You are investigating the potential of a new drug to be useful in treating obesity. Specifically you are hoping that the drug either stimulates anorexigenic peptide release or inhibits orexigenic peptide release. You discover that addition of the drug to water consumed by your test animals results in inhibition of glucose oxidation within the hypothalamus. Based upon your findings what peptide would you most likely expect to see increased in these test animals?
A. agouti-related peptide, AgRP
B. cocaine- and amphetamine-regulated transcript, CART
C. galanin
D. melanin-concentrating hormone, MCH
E. neuropeptide Y, NPY

Answer E: The activation of NPY neurons in the hypothalamus exhibits fuel source specificity in that oxidation of glucose and fatty acids exert differing effects. Glucose oxidation signals ample energy supply and thus results in reduced NPY expression. On the other hand, fatty acid oxidation has limited, if any, effect on NPY release. Inhibition of glucose oxidation results in dramatically increased NPY release even in the presence of fatty acid metabolism. Thus, a compound that blocks glucose oxidation in the hypothalamus would be expected to result in a significant increase in the level of NPY expression.

14. A defect in activity of which of the following hormones has been associated with the sleep disorder known as narcolepsy?
A. agouti-related peptide, AgRP
B. cocaine- and amphetamine-regulated transcript, CART
C. galanin-like peptide, GALP
D. melanin-concentrating hormone, MCH
E. orexin A

Answer E: The orexin peptides function to increase food consumption. However, in addition to increased feeding behavior central orexin action increases wakefulness and suppresses REM sleep. These latter observations demonstrate that orexins play a causative role in the regulation of sleep-wake cycles. Indeed, loss of orexin function results in a condition in animals that mimics the sleep disorder in humans known as narcolepsy.

15. Vagal afferents are involved in the responses of the CNS to certain gastrointestinal hormones. Which of the following gut hormones exerts some of its orexigenic responses via these vagal pathways?
A. cholecystokinin, CCK
B. ghrelin
C. glucose-dependent insulinotropic peptide, GIP
D. GLP-1
E. protein tyrosine tyrosine, PYY

Answer B: Ghrelin is produced and secreted by the X/A-like enteroendocrine cells of the stomach oxyntic (acid-secreting) glands. The major effect of ghrelin is exerted within the central nervous system at the level of the arcuate nucleus where it stimulates the release of neuropeptide Y (NPY) and agouti-related protein (AgRP). The actions of NPY and AgRP enhance appetite and thus, food intake.

16. Which of the following gut hormones is responsible for the feeding phenomenon referred to as the *ileal brake*?
A. CCK
B. ghrelin
C. GIP
D. oxyntomodulin, OXM
E. protein tyrosine tyrosine, PYY

Answer E: PYY produced by and secreted from intestinal enteroendocrine L cells of the ileum and colon. The release of PYY results in reduced gut motility, a delay in gastric emptying, and an inhibition of gallbladder contraction. All of these actions are associated with the ileal brake.

17. Although the level of leptin secretion is proportional to the amount of fat in adipose tissue, obese individuals are resistant to the anorexigenic effects of the increased hormone levels. Which of the following hypothalamic hormones would be expected to have the greatest increase in expression as a consequence of obesity-induced leptin resistance?
A. cocaine- and amphetamine-regulated transcript, CART
B. galanin-like peptide, GALP
C. α-melanocyte stimulating hormone, α-MSH
D. neuropeptide Y, NPY

Answer D: Peripheral hormones that act on the ARC and thereby affect the actions of NPY (and AgRP) are leptin and ghrelin. Leptin binds to its receptor present on NPY neurons and inhibits their firing resulting in reduced GABA release onto POMC neurons. This leptin-induced reduction in GABA action at POMC neurons is a disinhibition and allows for increased release of the anorexigenic peptide, α-MSH. This is, in part, the mechanism by which leptin decreases feeding behaviors. Loss of leptin effects on NPY and POMC neurons would lead to increased orexigenic responses contributing to obesity.

18. You are studying a strain of laboratory mice that get obese even on a low-fat lab chow. In examination of the brains of these mice you find an abnormal poorly developed area of the hypothalamus. A defect in which of the following regions would most likely account for the observed obesity?

A. lateral hypothalamic area (LHA)
B. nucleus of the solitary tract (NTS, NST)
C. paraventricular nucleus of the hypothalamus (PVN, PVH)
D. suprachiasmatic nucleus (SCN)
E. ventromedial hypothalamus (VMH, VMN)

Answer E: The hypothalamus is involved in control of feeding behavior as well as the secretion of various pituitary releasing hormones. Specific nuclei within the hypothalamus exert different effects on appetite and the desire for food. The ventromedial hypothalamic nucleus (VMH), and to a lesser extent the dorsomedial hypothalamic nucleus (DMH) is involved in the sensation of satiety and lesions in these regions of the hypothalamus result in hyperphagia (excessive hunger) and obesity.

19. Which of the following brain regions sends and receives information to the visceral organs via the vagal nerve?

A. arcuate nucleus (ARC)
B. area postrema
C. nucleus of the solitary tract (NTS, NST)
D. perifornical lateral hypothalamus (PFLH)
E. ventromedial hypothalamus (VMH)

Answer C: Satiety signals from the liver and gastrointestinal tract signal through the vagus nerve to the nucleus of the solitary tract (NTS) to cause meal termination, and in combination with the hypothalamus, integrate the various signals to determine the feeding responses of the organism.

20. Which of the following hormones is expressed and released from the stomach and is involved in the stimulation of food intake?

A. cholecystokinin, CCK
B. ghrelin
C. GLP-1
D. neuropeptide Y, NPY
E. protein tyrosine tyrosine, PYY

Answer B: Ghrelin is produced and secreted by the X/A-like enteroendocrine cells of the stomach oxyntic (acid-secreting) glands. The major effect of ghrelin is exerted within the central nervous system at the level of the arcuate nucleus where it stimulates the release of neuropeptide Y (NPY) and agouti-related protein (AgRP). The actions of NPY and AgRP enhance appetite and thus, food intake.

21. Which of the following correctly reflects the consequence of insulin binding its receptor in the hypothalamus?

A. activation of melanin-concentrating hormone (MCH) release
B. activation of α-melanocyte stimulating hormone (α-MSH) release
C. activation of neuropeptide Y (NPY) release
D. inhibition of cocaine- and amphetamine-regulated transcript (CART) release
E. inhibition of galanin release

Answer B: Within the brain insulin exerts anorexigenic effects. These effects are responses to insulin binding its receptor on POMC and NPY neurons in the hypothalamus. Insulin-mediated effects include activation of POMC neurons causing release of α-MSH which exerts the anorexigenic effects, and inhibition of NPY neurons, thus blocking the orexigenic effects of NPY.

22. Genome-wide screens for gene polymorphisms associated with a predisposition to obesity have identified several loci. Which of the following hormone genes could be expected to most likely lead to an increased propensity for obesity if it were defective?

A. Agouti-related peptide, AgRP
B. cocaine- and amphetamine-regulated transcript, CART
C. neuropeptide Y, NPY
D. oxyntomodulin, OXM
E. peptide tyrosine tyrosine, PYY

Answer D: Central anorexigenic effects of OXM involve induced release of anorexigenic peptides and suppression of the orexigenic effects of circulating ghrelin. Of potential significance to the treatment of obesity, when OXM is administered intravenously to human subjects there is an observed reduction in food intake.

Additionally, when OXM is administered subcutaneously to overweight and obese subjects over a period of 4 weeks there is a significant reduction in body weight. Thus, defective OXM function would likely result in an exacerbation of the propensity to obesity.

23. Agouti-related peptide (AgRP) is an orexigenic hormone that functions to increase the desire for food intake by antagonizing the actions of which of the following anorexigenic hormones?
   A. cocaine- and amphetamine-regulated transcript, CART
   B. galanin-like peptide (GALP)
   C. GLP-1
   D. α-melanocyte stimulating hormone, α-MSH
   E. peptide tyrosine tyrosine, PYY

Answer D: AgRP together with NPY represent a distinct set of ARC-expressed orexigenic peptides. AgRP is classically referred to as a member of the central melanocortin system, which in addition to AgRP comprises α-melanocyte stimulating hormone, α-MSH (see below for description of α-MSH actions) and 2 melanocortin receptors identified as melanocortin receptor 3 (MC3R) and melanocortin receptor 4 (MC4R). Whereas, α-MSH is an agonist of both MC3R and MC4R, AgRP serves to antagonize the actions of α-MSH at these same receptors with highest antagonist activity on MC4R.

24. Patients with functional dyspepsia (disturbed indigestion) and prominent nausea frequently experience spurts of excessive acid exposure to the upper duodenum. This results in pancreatic secretion, mainly through the action of which of the following substances?
   A. cholecystokinin
   B. gastrin
   C. glucagon
   D. secretin
   E. vasoactive intestinal polypeptide

Answer D: The strongest stimulator for the release of secretin from cells in the upper small-intestinal mucosa is the contact with acidic chyme. Increased serum secretin levels stimulate water and alkali secretions from the pancreas and the hepatic ducts and inhibit gastrin release. The most potent stimulators for the release of cholecystokinin are not acid but digestion products of fat and protein. Vasoactive intestinal polypeptide does stimulate intestinal and pancreatic secretion but it acts as neurotransmitter in the enteric nervous system and is mainly released by mechanical and neuronal stimulation.

25. A 30-year-old man seeks help because he lost weight and feels full after eating only a small amount of food. He is diagnosed with a delay in gastric emptying. Which of the following hormones has at physiological levels the strongest effect in inhibiting gastric emptying?
   A. cholecystokinin
   B. gastrin
   C. glucose-dependent insulinotropic peptide
   D. motilin
   E. pancreatic polypeptide

Answer A: The major control mechanism for gastric emptying involves duodenal gastric feedback, hormonal as well as neural. The major hormone involved in the inhibition of gastric emptying is cholecystokinin (CCK), which is released by fat and protein digestion products.

26. A 60-year-old woman is admitted to the hospital with a fever and severe diarrhea for the last 24 hours. Cultures of blood, cerebrospinal fluid, urine, and stool are all negative for pathogens. The profile of gut hormones reveals elevated levels of vasoactive intestinal polypeptide (VIP). An analogue of which of the following would most likely lower her VIP levels?
   A. erythromycin
   B. histamine
   C. motilin
   D. somatostatin
   E. trypsin

Answer D: Vasoactive intestinal polypeptide (VIP) is a neurotransmitter in the brain and in the parasympathetic nerves of the digestive tract. It also acts as a hormone. VIP has a secretin-like effect on the pancreas. It increases the volume of water and bicarbonate output and affects GI blood flow and motility. All this contributes to severe secretory diarrhea in the case of VIP overproduction. Somatostatin is the best choice because it has a broad range of inhibitory effects, inhibiting GI secretions, slowing GI motility, and reducing splanchnic blood flow.

Checklist

✓ Humoral and neural circuits connect the gut and the brain creating an integrated network whereby events in the gut control responses in the brain that regulate feeding behavior and energy expenditure. Activation of these circuits in the brain, in turn, regulates the activities of the gut.

✓ The gastrointestinal system is the largest endocrine organ in the human body, expressing over 30 different peptides and hormones. Many of these peptides regulate neural circuitry in the brain involved feeding behaviors.

✓ All of the peptides of the gut that function in regulation of satiation and satiety are anorexigenic except for the stomach hormone, ghrelin, which is orexigenic.

✓ The anorexigenic gut peptides include PYY, OXM, GLP-1, CCK, and apoA-IV.

✓ The hypothalamus is a major brain structure involved in coordination of feeding behaviors and appetite. Several specific nuclei have been identified within the hypothalamus that interact in the control of feeding behaviors through the synthesis and release of various anorexigenic and orexigenic peptides.

✓ The hypothalamic orexigenic peptides include NPY, AgRP, orexins, MCH, and galanin.

✓ The hypothalamic anorexigenic peptides include α-MSH, CART, galanin-like peptide, and CRF.

CHAPTER

45 Adipose Tissue and Obesity: Associated Metabolic Disturbances

CHAPTER OUTLINE

High-Yield Terms

White adipose tissue, WAT: specialized fat tissue primarily responsible for lipid storage

Brown adipose tissue, BAT: specialized fat tissue primarily responsible for adaptive thermogenesis; cells are dense with mitochondria

Adipokines: also called adipocytokines; are endocrine- and paracrine-signaling molecules secreted by adipose tissue

Leptin resistance: refers to the phenomenon of reduced anorexigenic actions of leptin in the obese state

Body mass index, BMI: a measure for relative body fat based on an individual's weight and height

Metabolic syndrome: a disorder that defines a combination of metabolic and cardiovascular risk determinants associated with obesity and insulin resistance

Nonalcoholic fatty liver disease, NAFLD: characterized by fatty infiltration of the liver in the absence of alcohol consumption

Introduction to Adipose Tissue

Adipose tissue is not merely an organ designed to passively store excess carbon in the form of fatty acids esterified to glycerol (triglycerides). Mature adipocytes synthesize and secrete numerous enzymes, growth factors, cytokines, and hormones that are involved in overall energy homeostasis. Many of the factors that influence adipogenesis are also involved in diverse processes in the body including lipid homeostasis and modulation of inflammatory responses. In addition, a number of proteins secreted by adipocytes play important roles in these same processes. In fact, recent evidence has demonstrated that many factors secreted from adipocytes are pro-inflammatory mediators and these proteins have been termed adipocytokines or adipokines. There are currently over 50 different adipokines recognized as being secreted from adipose tissue. These adipokines are implicated in the modulation of a range of physiological responses that globally includes appetite control and energy balance. Specific metabolic processes regulated by adipose tissue include lipid metabolism, glucose homeostasis, inflammation, angiogenesis, hemostasis, and blood pressure.

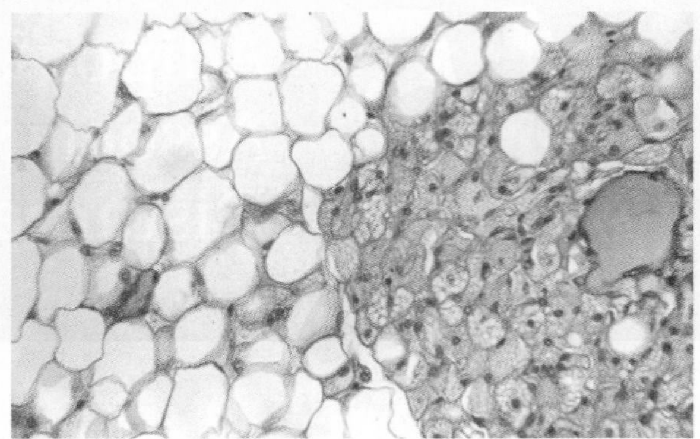

FIGURE 45-1: Histological section of adipose tissue demonstrating distinctive morphology of WAT and BAT. White adipocytes occupy the left side of the image and brown adipocytes the right side. As described below, white adipocytes are generally rounded with over 90% of the cell volume taken up by a single fat droplet. The few small mitochondria and the nucleus are compressed to the very edge of the white adipocyte. The brown adipocytes are smaller in overall size, polygonal in shape, contain several small lipid droplets, and high numbers of large mitochondria which imparts the brown color to these cells. Mescher AL. *Junqueira's Basic Histology Text and Atlas,* 13th ed. New York, NY: McGraw-Hill; 2013.

White Adipose Tissue

The major form of adipose tissue in mammals (commonly referred to as "fat") is white adipose tissue (WAT). WAT is composed of adipocytes held together by a loose connective tissue that is highly vascularized and innervated (Figure 45-1). White adipocytes are rounded cells that contain a single large fat droplet that occupies over 90% of the cell volume. The mitochondria within white adipocytes are small and few in number. The mitochondria and nucleus of the white adipocyte is squeezed into the remaining cell volume. Molecular characteristics of white adipocytes include expression of leptin but no expression of uncoupling protein 1, UCP1 (designated $UCP1^-$, $leptin^+$ adipocytes).

In addition to adipocytes, WAT contains macrophages, leukocytes, fibroblasts, adipocyte progenitor cells, and endothelial cells. The presence of the fibroblasts, macrophages, and other leukocytes along with adipocytes accounts for the vast array of proteins that are secreted from WAT under varying conditions. The highest accumulations of WAT are found in the subcutaneous regions of the body and surrounding the viscera.

Depending on its location, WAT serves specialized functions. The WAT associated with abdominal and thoracic organs (excluding the heart), the so-called visceral fat, secretes several inflammatory cytokines and is thus involved in local and systemic inflammatory processes. WAT associated with skeletal muscle secretes free fatty acids, interleukin-6 (IL-6), and tumor necrosis factor-α (TNFα) and as a consequence plays a significant role in the development of insulin resistance. Cardiac tissue associated WAT secretes numerous cytokines resulting in local inflammatory events and chemotaxis that can result in the development of atherosclerosis and systolic hypertension. Kidney associated WAT plays a role in sodium reabsorption and therefore can affect intravascular volume and hypertension.

Brown Adipose Tissue

Specialized adipose tissue that is primarily tasked with thermogenesis, especially in the neonate, is brown adipose tissue (BAT). BAT is so called because it is darkly pigmented due to the high density of mitochondria rich in cytochromes (see Figure 45-1). BAT specializes in the production of heat (adaptive thermogenesis) and lipid oxidation. Brown adipocytes are smaller in overall size compared to white adipocytes. Brown adipocytes are polygonal in shape and contain numerous large mitochondria packed with cristae. Whereas white adipocytes contain a single large fat droplet, brown adipocytes contain several small lipid droplets. Brown adipocytes are molecularly $UCP1^+$ and $leptin^-$ ($UCP1^+$, $leptin^-$ adipocytes). BAT is primarily visceral with highest concentrations around the aorta. BAT is highly vascularized and contains a very high density of noradrenergic nerve fibers.

Regulation of Adipogenesis

The process of adipocyte differentiation from a precursor preadipocyte to a fully mature adipocyte follows a precisely ordered and temporally regulated series of events. Adipocyte precursor cells emerge from mesenchymal stem cells (MSCs) that are themselves derived from the mesodermal layer of the embryo. The pluripotent MSCs receive extracellular cues that lead to the commitment to the preadipocyte lineage. Preadipocytes cannot be morphologically distinguished from their precursor MSCs but they have lost the ability to differentiate into other cell types.

The initial step in adipocyte differentiation is referred to as determination and leads to proliferating preadipocytes undergoing a growth arrest. This initial growth arrest occurs coincident with the expression of 2 key transcription factors, CCAAT/enhancer binding protein-α (C/EBPα) and peroxisome proliferator-activated receptor-γ (PPARγ). Following the induction of these 2 critical transcription factors there is a permanent period of growth arrest followed by expression of the fully differentiated adipocyte phenotype. This latter phase of adipogenesis is referred to as terminal differentiation. In the process of adipocyte differentiation PPARγ activates nearly all of the genes required. Although PPARγ and C/EBPα are the most important factors regulating adipogenesis, additional transcription factors influence the events of differentiation. Additional genes regulated by PPARγ in adipocytes are involved in lipid metabolism and/or glucose homeostasis.

Adipose Tissue Hormones and Cytokines

Adipose tissue produces and releases a vast array of protein signals including growth factors, cytokines, chemokines, acute phase proteins, complement-like factors, and adhesion molecules (Tables 45-1 and 45-2). In addition to secreted factors, adipose tissue produces several plasma membrane and nuclear receptors that can trigger changes in adipose tissue function. These include receptors for insulin, glucagon, growth hormone, adiponectin, and angiotensin II. Nuclear receptors include those for PPARγ, estrogens, androgens, vitamin D, thyroid hormone, progesterone, and glucocorticoids.

TABLE 45-1: Adipose Tissue Hormone and Cytokine Families

Functional Groups	*Member Proteins and Molecules*
Acute phase proteins	C-reactive protein (CRP), serum amyloid A3 (SAA3), plasminogen activator inhibitor-1 (PAI-1), haptoglobin
Adhesion molecules and ECM components	α_2-Macroglobulin, vascular cell adhesion molecule-1 (VCAM-1), intercellular adhesion molecule-1 (ICAM-1), collagen I, collagen III, collagen IV, collagen VI, fibronectin, matrix metalloproteinase 1 (MMP1), MMP7, MMP9, MMP10, MMP11, MMP14, MMP15, lysyl oxidase
Chemokines	Chemerin, monocyte chemotactic protein-1 (MCP-1), macrophage inhibitory protein-1 alpha (MIP-1α), regulated upon activation, normally T cell expressed and secreted (RANTES)
Complement-like factors	Adipsin, adiponectin, acylation stimulating protein (ASP)
Cytokines	IL-1β, IL-4, IL-6, IL-8, IL-10, IL-18, TNFα, macrophage migration inhibitory factor (MIF)
Growth and angiogenic factors	Fibroblast growth factors (FGFs), insulin-like growth factor-1 (IGF-1), hepatocyte growth factor (HGF), nerve growth factor (NGF), vascular endothelial cell growth factor (VEGF), transforming growth factor-β (TGF-β), angiopoietin-1, angiopoietin-2, tissue factor (TF, factor 3)
Metabolic process regulators	Adipocyte fatty acid–binding protein (aP2, FABP4), apoE, resistin, omentin, vaspin, apelin, retinol binding protein 4 (RBP4), visfatin, leptin
Other processes	COX pathway products PGE_2 and PGI_2 (prostacyclin), nitric oxide synthase pathway, renin-angiotensin system, tissue inhibitors of metalloproteinases (TIMPs)

TABLE 45-2: Adipose Tissue Hormones and Specific Functions

Factor	*Principal Source*	*Major Action*
Adiponectin; also called adipocyte complement factor 1q-related protein (ACRP30), and adipoQ	Adipocytes	See text
Adipsin; also called complement factor D	Adipocytes, liver, monocytes, macrophages	Rate limiting enzyme in complement activation
aP2, also called fatty acid binding protein 4 (FABP4)	Adipocytes, macrophages, endothelium	Involved in transport of fatty acids from lipid droplets to plasma membrane; is secreted from adipocytes and exerts hormonal function on liver to regulate hepatic glucose production
Apelin	Adipocytes, vascular stromal cells, heart	Levels increase with increased insulin, exerts positive hemodynamic effects, may regulate insulin resistance by facilitating expression of BAT uncoupling proteins (eg, UCP1, thermogenin)
Chemerin	Adipocytes, liver	Modulates expression of adipocyte genes involved in glucose and lipid homeostasis such as GLUT4 and fatty acid synthase (FAS); potent anti-inflammatory effects on macrophages expressing the chemerin receptor (chemokine-like receptor-1, CMKLR1)
C-reactive protein (CRP)	Hepatocytes, adipocytes	Is a member of the pentraxin family of calcium-dependent ligand binding proteins; assists complement interaction with foreign and damaged cells; enhances phagocytosis by macrophages; levels of expression regulated by circulating IL-6; modulates endothelial cell functions by inducing expression of various cell adhesion molecules, eg, ICAM-1, VCAM-1, and selectins; induces MCP-1 expression in endothelium; attenuates NO production by downregulating NOS expression; increase expression and activity of PAI-1
IL-6	Adipocytes, hepatocytes, activated Th2 cells, and antigen-presenting cells (APCs)	Acute phase response, β cell proliferation, thrombopoiesis, synergistic with IL-1 and TNF on T cells
Leptin	Predominantly adipocytes, mammary gland, intestine, muscle, placenta	See text
Monocyte chemotactic protein-1 (MCP-1)	Leukocytes, adipocytes	Is a chemokine defined as CCL2 (C-C motif, ligand 2); recruits monocytes, T cells, and dendritic cells to sites of infection and tissue injury
Omentin	Visceral stromal vascular cells of omental adipose tissue	The omentum is one of the peritoneal folds that connects the stomach to other abdominal tissues, enhances insulin-stimulated glucose transport, levels in the blood inversely correlated with obesity and insulin resistance
Plasminogen-activator inhibitor-1 (PAI-1)	Adipocytes, monocytes, placenta, platelets, endometrium	See Chapter 51
Resistin	Adipocytes, spleen, monocytes, macrophages, lung, kidney, bone marrow, placenta	Induces insulin resistance, levels increased in obesity, inhibits hepatic glucose uptake and glycogen synthesis, modulates endothelial cell functions, pro-inflammatory effects on smooth muscle
TNFα	Primarily activated macrophages, adipocytes	Induces expression of other autocrine growth factors, increases cellular responsiveness to growth factors and induces signaling pathways that lead to proliferation
Vaspin	visceral and Subcutaneous adipose tissue	Is a serine protease inhibitor, levels decrease with worsening diabetes

High-Yield Concept

Not all WAT secretes the same adipokines as is evident from studies of differences in adipose tissue function in various anatomical regions of the body. This is most significant when considering the clinical risks associated with increased adipose tissue mass. For example, increases in visceral WAT, even when subcutaneous fat depots are not increased, carry a greater metabolic risk for insulin resistance, diabetes, and cardiovascular disease.

Leptin

Leptin is 16-kDa peptide whose central function is the regulation of overall body weight by limiting food intake and increasing energy expenditure. However, leptin is also involved in the regulation of the neuroendocrine axis, inflammatory responses, blood pressure, and bone mass. The human leptin gene is the homolog of the mouse "obese" gene (symbol OB) that was originally identified in mice harboring a mutation resulting in a severely obese phenotype. Leptin-deficient (*ob/ob*) and leptin receptor-deficient (*db/db*) mice are obese and exhibit numerous disruptions in energy, hormonal, and immune system balance.

Leptin activates the anorexigenic axis in the arcuate nucleus (ARC) of the hypothalamus by increasing the activity of hypothalamic proopiomelanocortin (POMC) neurons and by reducing their inhibition by NPY neurons. Although it would be expected that the rising leptin levels in obesity would trigger increased anorexigenic responses in the hypothalamus, this is not the case. Elevated serum leptin results in impaired transport of leptin across the blood-brain barrier, referred to as leptin resistance.

Leptin functions by binding to its receptor which is a member of the cytokine receptor family. The leptin receptor mRNA is alternatively spliced resulting in 6 different products. The leptin receptors are named Ob-R, OB-Rb, OB-Rc, Ob-Rd, Ob-Re, and Ob-Rf. The OB-Rb mRNA encodes the long form of the leptin receptor (also called LEPR-B) and is expressed primarily in the hypothalamus but is also expressed in cells of the innate and adaptive immune systems as well as in macrophages. Activation of the receptor leads to increased PI3K and AMPK activity via activation of the Jak/STAT signaling pathway (Figure 45-2). One effect of the activation of the Jak/STAT pathway is activation of suppressor of cytokine signaling 3 (SOCS3), which then inhibits leptin signaling in a negative feedback loop. Leptin binding its receptor also results in the activation of mTOR both in the hypothalamus and in peripheral tissues. The role of leptin in the activation of mTOR function is an important factor in the ability of leptin to activate macrophages. Given that leptin levels rise in the serum of obese individuals and that leptin interaction with macrophages leads to increased macrophage inflammatory processes, it is not surprising that there is a direct correlation between leptin levels and the development of atherosclerosis.

In addition to effects on appetite exerted via central nervous system functions, leptin also exerts effects on inflammatory processes. Leptin modulates peripheral T-cell function, reduces thymocyte apoptosis, and increases thymic cellularity. These actions correlate well with observations of reduced immunologic defense when leptin levels are low. However, too much leptin is not beneficial as high concentrations can result in an abnormally strong immune response which predisposes an individual to autoimmune phenomena.

Adiponectin

Adiponectin was independently isolated by 4 different laboratories leading to different names. However,

High-Yield Concept

Levels of leptin increase in the serum in obese individuals and drop during weight loss. There is a direct correlation between the amount of body fat (WAT) an individual carries and the circulating levels of leptin.

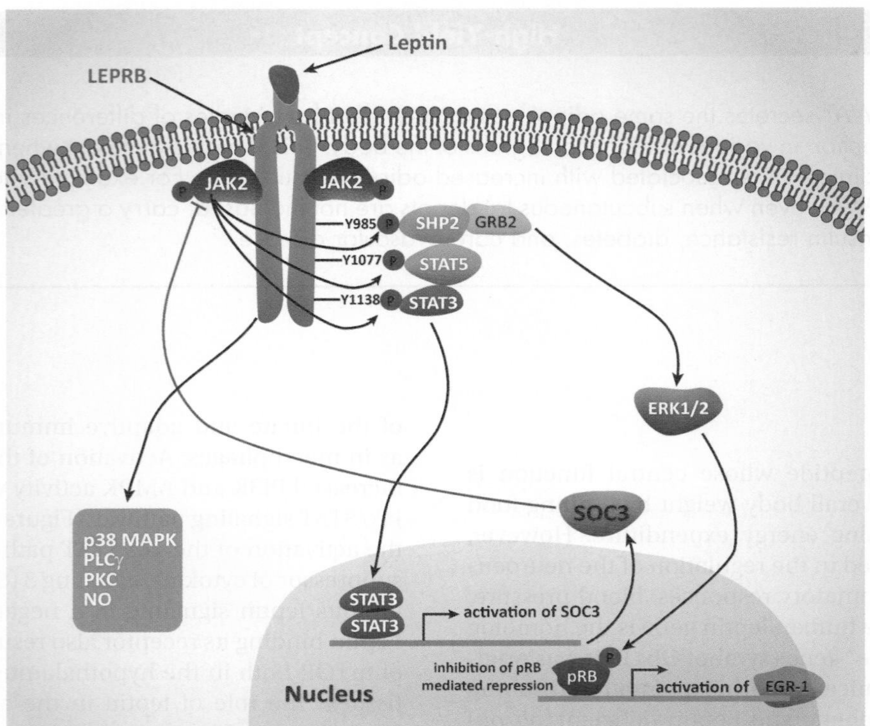

FIGURE 45-2: Leptin receptor functions: When leptin binds to its receptor (LEPR-B) the receptor undergoes a conformational change that activates the receptor-associated Jak2 tyrosine kinase. Activated Jak2 will autophosphrylate itself as well as phosphorylate the tyrosine (Y) residues in LEPR-B at positions 985, 1077, and 1138. Phosphorylated Y-985 serves as a docking site for SHP2 (SH2 domain containing protein tyrosine phosphatase, also called PTP1D). The gene that encodes SHP2 is identified as PTPN11. Phosphorylated Y-1077 serves as a docking site for STAT5 (signal transduction and activation of transcription 5). Phosphorylated Y-1138 serves as a docking site for STAT3. When SHP2, STAT5, and STAT3 bind to phosphorylated LEPR-B, they themselves are activated by Jak2-mediated phosphorylation. Activated SHP2 in turn activates GRB2 (growth factor receptor-bound protein 2) which then activates the ERK1/2 (extracellular-regulated kinase 1/2) signal pathway that results in increased transcription of the *EGR-1* (early growth response protein 1) gene. Activated STAT3 in turn activates the transcription of SOCS3 (suppressor of cytokine signaling 3). SOCS3 will then interact with Y-985 and attenuate signaling from SHP2 as well as interact with Jak2 and attenuate its tyrosine kinase activity resulting in a negative feedback loop. Reproduced with permission of themedicalbiochemistrypage, LLC.

adiponectin is considered the standard name for this adipose tissue-specific protein. Other names include adipocyte complement-related protein of 30 kDa (ACRP30) because of its homology to complement factor 1q (C1q), adipoQ, gelatin-binding protein of 28 kDa (BGP28), and adipocyte most abundant gene transcript 1 (apM1). The major biological actions of adiponectin are increases in insulin sensitivity and fatty acid oxidation.

Adiponectin contains a *C*-terminal globular domain which harbors the homology to C1q and an *N*-terminal collagen-like domain. The globular domain allows for a homotrimeric association of the protein. The association of the subunits is such that 2 trimeric globular domains interact with a single stalk of collagen domains formed from 2 trimers. Within the circulation, adiponectin exists in both a full-length form as well as a globular form that is the result of proteolytic cleavage of the full-length protein. The hormone forms complex structures such that it can be found as a trimer, hexamer, and as the high-molecular-weight oligomer. In addition to the complex structure, adiponectin is glycosylated, a modification that is essential to its activity.

Adiponectin activity is inhibited by adrenergic stimulation and glucocorticoids. Expression and release of adiponectin is stimulated by insulin and inhibited by TNF-α. Conversely, adiponectin exerts inflammatory modulation by reducing the production and activity of TNF-α and IL-6. Adiponectin levels are reduced in obese individuals and increased in patients with anorexia nervosa. In patients with Type 2 diabetes (T2D), levels of adiponectin are significantly reduced.

Adiponectin functions by interaction with specific cell-surface receptors and at least 2 receptors have been identified. AdipoR1 is expressed at highest levels in skeletal muscle and AdipoR2 in primarily expressed in the liver. Expression of adiponectin receptors is also seen in various regions of the brain. AdipoR1 is highly expressed in the medial prefrontal cortex, hippocampus, and the amygdala. AdipoR2 expression in the brain is restricted to the hippocampus and specific hypothalamic nuclei. AdipoR1 is a high-affinity receptor for globular adiponectin and has low affinity for the full-length adiponectin. In contrast, AdipoR2 has intermediate affinity for globular and full-length adiponectin. Activation of adiponectin receptors results in the phosphorylation and activation of AMPK. The adiponectin-mediated activation of AMPK results in increased glucose uptake, increased fatty acid oxidation, increased phosphorylation, and inhibition of acetyl-CoA carboxylase (ACC) in muscle. In the liver, the result is reduced glucose output as a consequence or reduced activity of gluconeogenic enzymes.

Adiponectin also plays an important role in hemostasis and inflammation by suppressing TNF-α– and IL-6–mediated inflammatory changes in endothelial cell responses and inhibiting vascular smooth muscle cell proliferation. Activation of AMPK activity in endothelial cells results in increased fatty acid oxidation and activation of endothelial NO synthase (eNOS).

Inflammatory Functions of Adipose Tissue

The significance of inflammatory responses elicited via secretion of adipose tissue–derived (WAT) cytokines relates to the fact that their production and secretion is increased in obese individuals. There is a direct link between the changes in adipose tissue function in obesity and the development of T2D and the metabolic syndrome. One key change in adipose tissue during obesity is an increase in the percentage of macrophages resident within the tissue. Macrophages are a primary source of pro-inflammatory cytokines secreted by adipose tissue.

As the level of macrophages increases in adipose tissue the level of pro-inflammatory cytokine secretion by the tissue increases. Circulating levels of both TNF-α and IL-6 increase as adipose tissue expands in obesity and these changes are directly correlated with insulin resistance and the development of T2D. Adiponectin normally exerts an important anti-inflammatory role; however, as the level of macrophage infiltration increases in obesity there is suppression of adiponectin production and secretion.

Adipose tissue-derived IL-6 accounts for approximately 30% of the circulating level of this pro-inflammatory cytokine. Visceral WAT secretes a higher percentage of the circulating IL-6 than subcutaneous WAT and this fact correlates with the negative effects of a pro-inflammatory status on the organs in obesity. As WAT density increases there is an associated increase in IL-6 secretion, which is correlated to an increase in the circulating levels of acute-phase proteins such as CRP.

In addition to the negative effects of TNF-α on adiponectin, production of the cytokine also directly decreases insulin sensitivity by inhibiting insulin receptor signaling. TNF-α also decreases endothelial nitric oxide synthase (eNOS), resulting in decreased levels of NO as well as decreased expression of mitochondrial oxidative phosphorylation genes. This leads to increased oxidative stress, accumulation of reactive oxygen species (ROS), and increased endoplasmic reticulum stress.

Lymph tissue is surrounded by pericapsular adipose tissue which increases in density with increasing obesity. This close association allows for 2-way paracrine interactions between the lymph and adipose tissues. One important interaction between lymph tissue and WAT involves leptin. Pro-inflammatory cytokine production and release from T cells is increased as a result of leptin action. Leptin effects on the vascular endothelium are also pro-inflammatory. Expression of adhesion molecules is increased by leptin binding its receptor on endothelial cells. This results in an increased ability of neutrophils and other leukocytes to adhere to the endothelium leading to increased local intravascular inflammatory processes.

Metabolic Functions of Brown Adipose Tissue

Although significant in density in newborns, adults do retain some metabolically active BAT deposits that respond to cold and sympathetic nervous system activation. Within BAT, norepinephrine interacts with all types of adrenergic receptors (α_1, α_2, and β), each of which activates distinct signaling pathways in the brown adipocyte.

Signal transduction events triggered by adrenergic stimulation of BAT result in the activation of adenylate cyclase resulting in increased cAMP production and activation of PKA. PKA phosphorylates and activates HSL leading to increased release of fatty acids. The fatty acids are taken up by the mitochondria; however, in BAT they interact with and activate the proton gradient uncoupling activity of uncoupling protein 1 (UCP1, also known as thermogenin). Uncoupling the proton gradient releases the energy of that gradient as heat. In addition to stimulating heat production in BAT, norepinephrine promotes the proliferation of brown

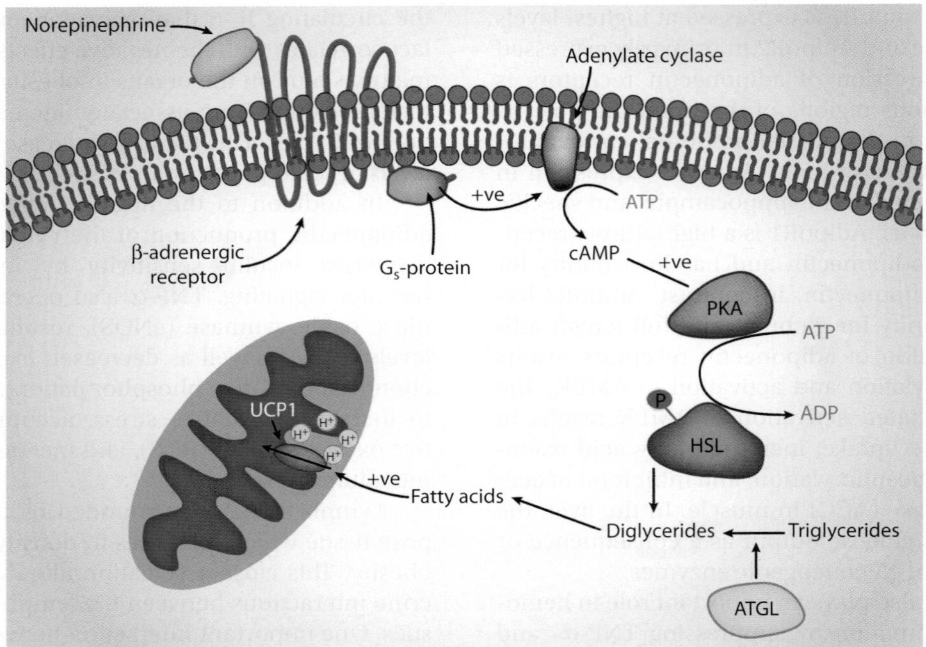

FIGURE 45-3: Hormonal mechanism of heat generation in brown fat. Norepinephrine stimulation of β-adrenergic receptors present on brown adipocytes activates adenylate cyclase resulting in increased cAMP levels and PKA activity. PKA phosphorylates and activates hormone-sensitive lipase (HSL) resulting in increased release of fatty acids. The fatty acids are transported to the mitochondria where they activate the proton gradient uncoupling activity of UCP1. This uncoupling reaction results in the generation of heat. Reproduced with permission of themedicalbiochemistrypage, LLC.

preadipocytes, promotes the differentiation of mature brown adipocytes, inhibits apoptosis of brown adipocytes, and regulates the expression of the UCP1 gene (Figure 45-3).

Similar to the endocrine role of WAT, BAT also synthesizes and secretes numerous factors. However, due to the relatively small overall size of brown fat compared to white fat the role of factors secreted from BAT serve mostly autocrine and paracrine roles. Paracrine factors synthesized by BAT include nerve growth factor (NGF), vascular endothelial cell growth factor (VEGF), angiotensinogen, and NO. The secretion of NGF occurs primarily from proliferating brown preadipocytes and in this capacity is believed to promote sympathetic innervation of the tissue which in turn permits increased norepinephrine stimulation of the cells in BAT.

Obesity

Obesity is defined as a physical condition in which an individual has a body mass index (BMI) ≥30 kg/m². The BMI is a relative measure of fat content through the relationship between an individual's weight and height. The BMI is calculated by dividing a person's weight, in kilograms, by the square of their height, in meters. The medical utility for determining a person's BMI is that this measure describes the body weight relative to height which strongly correlates with the total body fat content. It is important to note that in certain individuals, such as body builders who have large muscle mass, a high BMI does not correlate with high fat content. Most Americans measure their weight in pounds and their height in inches; it is possible to approximate ones weight from their BMI and their height in inches or their BMI from their approximate weight and their height in inches (Table 45-3). As an individual's BMI increases, there is a corresponding increase in the risk for development of diabetes, metabolic syndrome, and cardiovascular disease (Table 45-4).

Obesity is approaching epidemic proportions in the United States and many other industrialized countries. In the United States the prevalence of obesity now exceeds 30% of the population and represents the highest rate of obesity worldwide. Since 1980 the prevalence of obesity in adults in the United States has increased 2-fold. However, much more disturbing is the fact that in this same time period the rate of childhood and adolescent obesity increased 3-fold. Table 45-4 below associates a given BMI range with the risk for cardiovascular disease and atherosclerosis.

TABLE 45-3: BMI Determination From Height (Inches) and Weight (Pounds)

BMI (kg/m²)	19	20	21	22	23	24	25	26	27	28	29	30	35	40
Height (in)							**Weight (lb)**							
58	91	96	100	105	110	115	119	124	129	134	138	143	167	191
59	94	99	104	109	114	119	124	128	133	138	143	148	173	198
60	97	102	107	112	118	123	128	133	138	143	148	153	179	204
61	100	106	111	116	122	127	132	137	143	148	153	158	185	211
62	104	109	115	120	126	131	136	142	147	153	158	164	191	218
63	107	113	118	124	130	135	141	146	152	158	163	169	197	225
64	110	116	122	128	134	140	145	151	157	163	169	174	204	232
65	114	120	126	132	138	144	150	156	162	168	174	180	210	240
66	118	124	130	136	142	148	155	161	167	173	179	186	216	247
67	121	127	134	140	146	153	159	166	172	178	185	191	223	255
68	125	131	138	144	151	158	164	171	177	184	190	197	230	262
69	128	135	142	149	155	162	169	176	182	189	196	203	236	270
70	132	139	146	153	160	167	174	181	188	195	202	207	243	278
71	136	143	150	157	165	172	179	186	193	200	208	215	250	286
72	140	147	154	162	169	177	184	191	199	206	213	221	258	294
73	144	151	159	166	174	182	189	197	204	212	219	227	265	302
74	148	155	163	171	179	186	194	202	210	218	225	233	272	311
75	152	160	168	176	184	192	200	208	216	224	232	240	279	319
76	156	164	172	180	189	197	205	213	221	230	238	246	287	328

TABLE 45-4: Risks Associated With Increasing BMI

BMI	*Category*	*Waist less than or equal to 40 in. (men) or 35 in. (women)*	*Waist greater than 40 in. (men) or 35 in. (women)*
≤18.5	Underweight	N/A	N/A
18.5-24.9	Normal	N/A	N/A
25.0-29.9	Overweight	Increased risk	High risk
30.0-34.9	Obese	High risk	Very high risk
35.0-39.9	Obese	Very high risk	Very high risk
≥40	Extremely obese	Extremely high risk	Extremely high risk

High-Yield Concept

Obesity is associated with several serious and life-threatening complications resulting in significant increases in morbidity and mortality relative to lean individuals. These complications include insulin resistance (IR), T2D, nonalcoholic fatty liver disease (NAFLD; Clinical Box 45-1), atherosclerosis, degenerative disorders such as dementia, and also in many instances cancers. The combination of abdominal obesity, hyperlipidemia, IR, pro-inflammatory status, and hypertension is clinically referred to as the Metabolic Syndrome (see Chapter 48).

CLINICAL BOX 45-1: NON-ALCOHOLIC FATTY LIVER DISEASE, NAFLD

Nonalcoholic fatty liver disease (NAFLD) is the most common liver disease in the Western world. NAFLD is characterized by fatty infiltration of the liver in the absence of alcohol consumption. The mildest forms of NAFLD consists of simple steatosis (abnormal retention of lipids inside cells) and can progress to nonalcoholic steatohepatitis (NASH), which represents a deleterious hepatic inflammatory disorder characterized by advanced liver fibrosis and cirrhosis which ultimately can result in hepatocellular carcinoma and death. In the clinical environment, NAFLD is believed to account for as much as 90% of all cases of elevated liver function test enzymes in patients who do not manifest with identifiable causes of hepatic disease (eg, viral hepatitis). The abnormal deposition of fat in the liver in NAFLD comprises a complex pathophysiology. The process involves increased visceral adiposity plus insulin resistance with increased free fatty acids (FFAs) being released from adipose tissue. As there is a large increase in visceral adipose tissue in obese individuals, this contribution of adipose tissue–derived FFAs is significant to the development of NAFLD. Additional pathophysiology includes an enhanced state of hepatic oxidative stress and lipid peroxidation, decreased antioxidant defenses, early mitochondrial dysfunction, and iron accumulation. Associated with these abnormal hepatic processes is an imbalance in the secretion of adipokines and a chronic pro-inflammatory status. One of the most significant contributing factors to the development of NAFLD is insulin resistance (IR) in the liver (see Chapter 46 for the role of fatty acids in IR). Insulin resistance in the liver is associated with increased hepatic glucose output since the insulin-suppressing effects on gluconeogenesis are impaired. The increased hepatic glucose output exacerbates the hyperglycemia that is present in obesity and contributes to the IR in the periphery, ultimately resulting in progression to T2D. Peripheral IR at the level of adipose tissue and skeletal muscle results in increased circulating FFAs which make their way to the liver. In addition, the hepatic IR results in increased hepatic fatty acid synthesis which then, in conjunction with the circulating FFAs, serves as the precursors for increased triglyceride accumulation in the liver. Altered lipogenesis that occurs in the presence of hepatic and peripheral IR also contributes to the development of NAFLD. The primary transcriptional regulators of hepatic lipogenesis are SREBP-1c, ChREBP, and PPARγ. Increased activity of all 3 of these transcription factors results in an overall shift to hepatic fatty acid and triglyceride synthesis, inhibition of fatty acid oxidation, and increased glucose synthesis. Under the conditions of excess fat accumulation, there is an increase in the production of reactive oxygen species (ROS) in the liver. The increased ROS production is due to a combination of mitochondrial and peroxisomal lipid oxidation. The increased lipid peroxidation reactions result in gross morphological alterations in mitochondria and an associated impairment of electron transport exacerbating the mitochondrial dysfunction. Lipid peroxidation also induces the expression pro-inflammatory cytokines which ultimately promotes hepatic fibrosis via induction of collagen production.

Obesity and Cardiovascular Disease

Obesity is directly correlated to increased morbidity resulting primarily from hypertension and cardiovascular disease (see Chapter 48 for more details). However, since obesity is highly correlated to the development of T2D, the pathophysiological complications associated with diabetes also contribute to obesity-related mortality. As adipose tissue enlarges due to excess triglyceride accumulation, physiological changes occur that result in increased inflammatory responses in the tissue. In addition to increased pro-inflammatory events in expanding adipose, excess fat accumulation in the liver induces similar events. One consequence of the enhanced inflammatory status of the liver and adipose tissue in obesity is an associated insulin resistance (IR).

Insulin resistance induced by obesity is a major factor in the development of cardiovascular disease in obese individuals. Within the vasculature, insulin exerts vasodilator action as a result of increased nitric oxide (NO) production. This function of insulin is an important component of the ability of the hormone to enhance glucose uptake by skeletal muscle. Inactivation of endothelial cell NO production, as occurs due to IR, results in endothelial dysfunction and promotes the development of atherosclerosis (Chapter 48).

Role of Gut Bacteria in Obesity

The idea that gut bacteria can influence overall metabolism was discovered in studies using germ-free mice. Mice raised in a germ-free environment are resistant to diet-induced obesity. The primary mechanisms underlying this resistance are decreased absorption of glucose, decreased generation of short-chain fatty acids in the gut, reductions in hepatic lipogenesis, and alterations in adipose tissue metabolism that favors reduced triglyceride accumulation and increased fatty acid oxidation. When the guts of mice reared in a germ-free environment are colonized with bacteria from mice raised in a nonsterile environment, the germ-free mice amass a 60% increase in body weight and this weight gain is associated with insulin resistance. If bacteria are used from obese mice (the *ob/ob* genotype), the recipient mice have a significantly greater increase in body fat mass than in recipients that were colonized with bacteria from lean mice.

The mechanism of the weight gain in these study mice was due to increased digestion of polysaccharides resulting in higher absorption and delivery of sugars to the liver. The increased carbohydrate delivery to the liver results in increased lipogenesis. These changes in lipid profiles in the liver and adipose tissue of recolonized rodents were correlated to changes in the composition of gut microbiota such that there was a 50% reduction in the abundance of Bacteroidetes and a proportional increase in Firmicutes.

Gut microbiota are essential for the metabolism of xenobiotic compounds, production of vitamins, degradation of nondigestible polysaccharides (involving fermentation of resistant starches and oligosaccharides), and absorption of nutrients. The human gut contains a wide variety of microorganisms of which bacteria constitute the largest fraction. The average human gut contains some 10^{14} bacteria of which anaerobic bacteria constitutes the largest proportion. There are anywhere from 500 to 1000 different species of bacteria in the gut population divided into 3 bacterial phyla: Bacteroidetes (gram negative), Actinobacteria (gram positive), and Firmicutes (gram positive). The Firmicutes consist of over 200 genera which includes *Bacillus, Clostridium, Lactobacillus*, and *Mycoplasma*.

Bacteria of the Bacteroidetes phylum constitute up to 30% of the total gut flora. These bacteria are important in the digestion of otherwise nondigestible polysaccharides into monosaccharides and short-chain fatty acids (SCFAs) and also may be involved in the synthesis of vitamin K. Of significance to the relationship between gut microbiota and obesity, studies have shown that obese individuals have lower levels of Bacteroidetes and more Firmicutes than lean control subjects. When obese patients are placed either on a carbohydrate-restricted low-calorie diet or on a fat-restricted diet, their ratios of Bacteroidetes to Firmicutes approached those of lean control subjects after several months.

Given that obesity, insulin resistance, and T2D are all associated with low-grade systemic inflammation of unclear etiology, it has been proposed that one mechanism leading to this state involves inflammatory modulation by gut bacteria. Bacterial lipopolysaccharide (LPS) evokes an inflammatory response triggering the secretion of many pro-inflammatory cytokines. LPS is continuously produced by gut bacteria through the lysis of dead and dying gram-negative bacteria. LPS is also transported from the gut to peripheral tissues via interaction with chylomicrons. Since the rate of chylomicron synthesis is elevated in response to a high-fat and/or high-carbohydrate diet, there will be more LPS uptake in obese individuals due to the elevated intake of lipids and carbohydrates. The fat-induced increase in LPS uptake is referred to as metabolic endotoxemia.

Gut bacteria have also been shown to play a role in the secretion of gastrointestinal hormones that function in digestion and appetite control such as GLP-1. When animals are fed a high-fiber diet composed of nondigestible oligofructose, which can be fermented by gut bacteria, there is an increase in GLP-1 release. Oligofructose is called a prebiotic which is any substance that is nondigestible by humans but can be fermented by gut bacteria, thereby promoting their growth and activity. In addition, feeding animal oligofructose results in increased L-cell proliferation in the proximal colon and this contributes to a higher level of GLP-1 release. In humans, the consumption of oligofructose protects against weight gain, reduces fat accumulation, reduces serum triglyceride accumulation, and promotes satiety. These effects are presumably due, in part, to changes in the composition of gut microbiota.

Is There a Viral Link to Obesity?

A potential link between obesity and viral infection was initially suggested from studies that demonstrated increased body weight, increased glucose uptake, and decreased leptin secretion in animals infected with adenovirus-36 (Ad-36). Ad-36 is a virus that primarily infects humans and studies have shown that 30% of obese individuals (compared to only 11% of lean subjects) have circulating antibodies to Ad-36. The precise mechanism by which Ad-36 infection might lead to obesity is unknown. Ad-36 viral particles have been found in adipocytes and Ad-36 infection increases adipocyte differentiation from preadipocytes. It is also possible that adenoviral infection leads to increased inflammatory responses in adipose tissue, and possibly also the liver, that in turn leads to the metabolic disruptions seen to be typical of the pro-inflammatory state associated with, and resulting in, obesity.

REVIEW QUESTIONS

1. You are studying the responses of fat cells in culture to the addition of various pharmacologic compounds. You find that addition of a β-adrenergic agonist does not result in the expected change in mitochondrial proton gradients. This would indicate that there was most likely a defect in the function of which of the following?
   A. adiponectin
   B. adipose triglyceride lipase
   C. fatty acid synthase
   D. leptin
   E. UCP1

Answer E: Norepinephrine binding to brown adipocytes triggers the activation of adenylate cyclase and the production of cAMP that in turn activates PKA. PKA phosphorylates and activates hormone-sensitive lipase, HSL. Activation of HSL leads to release of free fatty acids which are taken up by the mitochondria, similarly as they would be for purposes of oxidation; however, in BAT they interact with and activate the proton gradient uncoupling activity of uncoupling protein 1 (UCP1). Uncoupling the proton gradient releases the energy of that gradient as heat.

2. Experiments have been designed to assess the effects of a novel drug on the inflammatory responses of adipose tissue in laboratory mice. Addition of the drug to the diet of the mice demonstrates a clear reduction in the production and release of pro-inflammatory cytokines from adipose tissue. This experimental drug is most likely inhibiting the action of which of the following leading to the observed results?
   A. adiponectin
   B. leptin
   C. monocyte chemotactic protein-1, MCP-1
   D. vascular cell adhesion molecule-1, VCAM-1
   E. vascular endothelial cell growth factor, VEGF

Answer C: The significance of inflammatory responses elicited via secretion of adipose tissue-derived (WAT) cytokines relates to the fact that their production and secretion is increased in obese individuals. One key change in adipose tissue that results in increased synthesis and release of pro-inflammatory adipokines is an increase in the percentage of macrophages resident within the tissue. Macrophages are a primary source of pro-inflammatory cytokines secreted by adipose tissue. The primary adipokine responsible for this infiltration is monocyte chemotactic protein-1 (MCP-1). Thus, inhibition of MCP-1 releases or function would limit increased monocyte infiltration and reduce the pro-inflammatory actions of adipose tissue.

3. The inflammatory activity of adipose tissue, particularly visceral fat, is enhanced in obese individuals. This effect of obesity is, in part, due to adipose tissue resistance to the actions of insulin. Insulin resistance in adipose tissue is reflected by a reduction in production of which of the following adipokines?
   A. adiponectin
   B. C-reactive protein, CRP
   C. monocyte chemotactic protein-1, MCP-1
   D. vascular cell adhesion molecule-1, VCAM-1
   E. vascular endothelial cell growth factor, VEGF

Answer A: Expression and release of adiponectin is stimulated by insulin; therefore, adiponectin levels are reduced in obese individuals primarily due to the loss of insulin-mediated stimulation. In patients with Type 2 diabetes, levels of adiponectin are also significantly reduced.

4. You are studying the functions associated with adiponectin by utilizing site-directed mutagenesis of an adiponectin cDNA followed by expression of the cDNA in transgenic mice. One particular mutation abolishes nearly 100% of the activity of the protein but does not affect the level of protein found in the circulation of the test mice. This mutation most likely blocks which of the following modifications that is required for adiponectin function?
   A. acetylation
   B. glycosylation
   C. phosphorylation
   D. prenylation
   E. ubiquitination

Answer B: Adiponectin contains a *C*-terminal globular domain that allows for a homotrimeric association of the protein forming the functional structure of the protein. The hormone forms complex structures such that it can be found as a trimer, hexamer, and as the high-molecular-weight oligomer. In addition to the complex structure, adiponectin is glycosylated, a modification that is essential to its activity.

5. The level of leptin that is secreted from adipose tissue increases with increasing fat deposits. Which of the following represents the major effect of leptin within the brain that is involved in overall lipid homeostasis on adipose tissue?
   A. it activates AgRP neurons in the hypothalamus
   B. it activates melanocortin neurons in the hypothalamus
   C. it activates NPY neurons in the hypothalamus
   D. it inhibits CART neurons in the brain stem
   E. it inhibits insulin-responsive neurons in the brain stem

Answer: Leptin activates the anorexigenic axis (appetite suppression) in the arcuate nucleus (ARC) of the hypothalamus by increasing the frequency of action potentials in the hypothalamic POMC neurons by depolarization through a nonspecific cation channel and by reduced inhibition by local orexigenic neuropeptide-Y (NPY) neurons.

6. Which of the following represents the least invasive means to ascertain the extent to which an individual is overweight or obese?
A. BMI
B. glucose tolerance test to measure insulin sensitivity
C. fasting lipid profile
D. fasting plasma glucose concentration
E. urine lipid content

Answer A: The BMI is a measure of the relationship between an individual's weight and height. The BMI is calculated by dividing a person's weight in kilograms by the square of their height in meters and is thus completely noninvasive and easy to determine. The medical utility for determining a person's BMI is that this measure describes the body weight relative to height and it, thus, strongly correlates with the total body fat content in adults.

7. You are treating a 38-year-old man whose chief complaint is occasional right upper quadrant pain. Analysis of blood samples shows elevated aspartate transaminase (AST) and alanine transaminase (ALT). History indicates that these same enzymes have shown elevated levels each of the past 3 years during routine blood work in conjunction with his annual physical. His history also indicates reflux esophagitis, hypertension, and hyperlipidemia. You order tests for serologic and biochemical markers for viral hepatitis and autoimmune liver disease and other metabolic liver diseases but these results are negative. The patient has gained 50 lb since the age of 18. He consumes less than 5 alcoholic beverages per week. Which of the following is the most likely diagnosis in this case?
A. cirrhosis
B. nonalcoholic fatty liver disease
C. thyrotoxicosis
D. Type 1 diabetes
E. Type 2 diabetes

Answer B: Nonalcoholic fatty liver disease (NAFLD) is the most common liver disease in the Western world. NAFLD is characterized by fatty infiltration of the liver in the absence of alcohol consumption. One of the most significant contributing factors to the development of NAFLD is insulin resistance in the liver. Additional pathophysiology includes an enhanced state of hepatic oxidative stress and lipid peroxidation, decreased antioxidant defenses, early mitochondrial dysfunction, and iron accumulation.

8. The activity of which of the following adipocyte proteins is associated with increased insulin sensitivity and fatty acid oxidation?
A. adiponectin
B. adipsin
C. leptin
D. resistin
E. vaspin

Answer A: The major biological actions of adiponectin are increases in insulin sensitivity and fatty acid oxidation.

9. You are comparing the responses of 2 strains of mice to the effects of a high-fat diet. Your observations show that one strain restricts their intake of food within a short period after accumulating a small gain in weight, whereas the other strain does not. The strain that does not limit their food intake quickly becomes obese. This latter strain of mice would most likely be shown to have a defect in the secretion of which of the following adipokines?
A. adiponectin
B. adipsin
C. leptin
D. resistin
E. vaspin

Answer C: Leptin is a peptide whose central function is the regulation of overall body weight by limiting food intake and increasing energy expenditure. Leptin exerts this effect within the brain via activation of the anorexigenic axis (appetite suppression) in the arcuate nucleus (ARC) of the hypothalamus.

10. You are carrying out experiments designed to increase energy expenditure as a therapeutic means to treat obesity. You are testing various compounds in experimental animals and find one that appears to satisfy the goals of the experiment in that mice given the compound have a significant increase in thermogenic activity in their adipose tissue. This compound is most likely activating or mimicking the activity of which of the following?
A. adiponectin
B. adipose triglyceride lipase
C. leptin
D. medium-chain acyl-CoA dehydrogenase
E. UCP1

Answer E: Uncoupling protein 1 (UCP1) is a mitochondrial protein of brown adipose tissue (BAT) involved in the process of adaptive thermogenesis.

In response to hormonal stimulation of BAT, there is an increase in fatty acid release from triglycerides. The fatty acids enter the mitochondria and activate the mitochondrial uncoupling activity of UCP1. This uncoupling releases the mitochondrial proton gradient as heat.

11. You are comparing the responses of 2 strains of mice to the effects of a high-fat diet. Your observations show that although both strains become obese on the diet, one strain has a much higher level of insulin resistance associated with the diet-induced obesity. This latter strain of mice would most likely be shown to have significantly increased levels of secretion of which of the following adipokines?
A. adiponectin
B. adipsin
C. leptin
D. resistin
E. vaspin

Answer D: Resistin is a 12-kDa protein produced by adipocytes and macrophages that induces insulin resistance. Thus the higher the level of resistin secreted, the higher the level of insulin resistance.

12. Nonalcoholic fatty liver disease (NAFLD) is characterized by fatty infiltration of the liver in the absence of alcohol consumption. This fatty infiltration in the liver is associated with increased insulin resistance. Which of the following represents the most likely target of excess hepatic fatty acids resulting in the insulin resistance associated with NAFLD?
A. glucokinase
B. PFK1
C. PFK2
D. PKA
E. PKC

Answer E: Hepatic IR is induced by the excess accumulation of FFAs. Within the hepatocyte metabolites of the FFA, re-esterification process, including long-chain acyl-CoAs and diacylglycerol (DAG), accumulate. Excess FFAs also participate in the relocation of several protein kinase C (PKC) isoforms, from the cytosol to the membrane compartment. These PKC isoforms include PKC-β2, PKC-δ, and PKC-θ. DAG is a potent activator of these PKC isoforms and the membrane-associated PKC will phosphorylate the intracellular portion of the insulin receptor on serine residues which results in impairment of insulin receptor interaction with downstream signaling proteins including insulin receptor substrate 1 (IRS1). Loss of IRS1 interaction with the receptor prevents interaction with phosphatidylinositol 3-kinase (PI3K) and its subsequent activation.

13. Which of the following, associated with obesity, is most highly correlated to the development of the metabolic syndrome?
A. elevated serum HDL
B. elevated serum total cholesterol
C. hyperglycemia
D. insulin resistance
E. proteinuria

Answer D: The hallmark feature of the metabolic syndrome is indeed insulin resistance. The hyperlipidemia typical in obese individuals leads to progressive insulin resistance, particularly in adipose tissue and skeletal muscle.

14. As the level of adipose tissue increases there is a corresponding increase in inflammatory activities associated with this tissue. Which of the following factors is the most significant to the increased pro-inflammatory activities of expanding fat mass?
A. adiponectin
B. leptin
C. monocyte chemotactic protein-1, MCP-1
D. vascular cell adhesion molecule-1, VCAM-1
E. vascular endothelial cell growth factor, VEGF

Answer C: The significance of inflammatory responses elicited via secretion of adipose tissue-derived (WAT) cytokines relates to the fact that their production and secretion is increased in obese individuals. One key change in adipose tissue that results in increased synthesis and release of pro-inflammatory adipokines is an increase in the percentage of macrophages resident within the tissue. Macrophages are a primary source of pro-inflammatory cytokines secreted by adipose tissue. The primary adipokine responsible for this infiltration is monocyte chemotactic protein-1 (MCP-1).

15. As the level of visceral fat increases there is a concomitant loss of peripheral tissue responses to insulin. Adipose tissue responses to these metabolic changes include a reduced secretion of which of the following adipokines?
A. adiponectin
B. adipsin
C. IL-6
D. leptin
E. resistin

Answer A: Expression and release of adiponectin is stimulated by insulin, therefore adiponectin levels are reduced in obese individuals primarily due to the loss of insulin-mediated stimulation. In patients with Type 2 diabetes, levels of adiponectin are also significantly reduced.

Checklist

- ✓ Adipose tissue is the major lipid storage organ in the body.
- ✓ There are 2 primary types of adipose tissue: white adipose tissue (WAT) and brown adipose tissue (BAT). WAT is primarily responsible for fatty acid storage in the form of triglycerides. BAT is primarily responsible for thermogenesis.
- ✓ WAT is composed of adipocytes held together by a loose connective tissue that is highly vascularized and innervated. White adipocytes are rounded cells that contain a single large fat droplet that occupies over 90% of the cell volume. The mitochondria within white adipocytes are small and few in number.
- ✓ BAT is composed of adipocytes that are small in size, polygonal in shape, and contain numerous large mitochondria packed with cristae. The high density of mitochondria imparts the brown color to BAT. Whereas white adipocytes contain a single large fat droplet, brown adipocytes contain several small lipid droplets.
- ✓ In addition to adipocytes, WAT contains macrophages, leukocytes, fibroblasts, adipocyte progenitor cells, and endothelial cells. The presence of the fibroblasts, macrophages, and other leukocytes along with adipocytes accounts for the vast array of proteins that are secreted from WAT under varying conditions.
- ✓ Proteins secreted from WAT regulate activities in the central nervous system that influence feeding behaviors.
- ✓ Proteins secreted from WAT modulate inflammatory responses and are directly attributable to the enhanced pro-inflammatory status present in overweight and obese individuals contributing to insulin resistance and the development of vascular disease.
- ✓ Obesity is defined as a physical condition in which an individual has a body mass index (BMI) $\geq 30 kg/m^2$.
- ✓ Obesity is associated with insulin resistance (IR), Type 2 diabetes, nonalcoholic fatty liver disease (NAFLD), atherosclerosis, degenerative disorders such as dementia, and also in many instances cancers resulting in significant increases in morbidity and mortality relative to lean individuals.
- ✓ Nonalcoholic fatty liver disease (NAFLD) is the most common liver disease in the Western world. NAFLD is characterized by fatty infiltration of the liver in the absence of alcohol consumption and is highly correlated to obesity.
- ✓ Obesity is associated with hyperlipidemia and increased fat metabolism which leads to mitochondrial dysfunction and increased reactive oxygen species (ROS) generation. Mitochondrial dysfunction leads to activation of stress responses and apoptosis which contribute to defective insulin secretion in obesity.
- ✓ The composition of the microbiota in the gut contributes to the metabolic and inflammatory disruption associated with high-fat diets and obesity. Some forms of gut bacteria are beneficial while others are detrimental to overall health. This latter fact is the basis for the use of prebiotic substances in the diet to promote the propagation of healthy gut microbiota.

CHAPTER

46 Insulin Function

CHAPTER OUTLINE

High-Yield Terms

Incretin: any gut hormone associated with food intake-stimulation of insulin secretion from the pancreas

Glucose-stimulated insulin secretion, GSIS: process of glucose uptake and metabolism by β-cells leading to increased ATP production which inhibits a potassium-dependent ATP (KATP) channel resulting in depolarization of the membrane triggering calcium influx and insulin secretory vesicle fusion with plasma membrane

ABCC8/KCNJ11: ATP-binding cassette, subfamily C, member 8 (ABCC8-encoded protein is also known as the sulfonylurea receptor, SUR) and potassium inwardly rectifying channel, subfamily J, member 11, protein components of the KATP channel of β-cells that regulates insulin secretion

TCF7L2: transcription factor 7-like 2, T-cell–specific HMG-box, involved in Wnt signal transduction, polymorphisms in this gene are the most highly correlated with potential for development of T2D

Insulin resistance, IR: a phenomenon whereby binding of insulin to its receptor results in impaired or failed propagation of normal signal transduction events

Introduction

Insulin was one of the first identified pancreatic hormones. It is secreted by the β-cells of the pancreas and directly infused, via the portal vein, to the liver where it exerts profound metabolic effects. Its major function as a pancreatic hormone is to counter the concerted action of a number of hyperglycemia-generating hormones and to maintain low blood glucose levels, particularly in response to food consumption. In addition to its role in regulating glucose homeostasis, insulin stimulates lipogenesis, diminishes lipolysis, and increases amino acid transport into cells. Because there are numerous hyperglycemic hormones, untreated disorders associated with insulin generally lead to severe hyperglycemia and shortened life span as is typically seen in poorly controlled type 2 diabetes, T2D (see Chapter 47).

Insulin also exerts activities typically associated with growth factors (Figure 46-1). Insulin is a member of a family of structurally and functionally similar molecules that includes the insulin-like growth factors (IGF-1 and IGF-2), and relaxin. The tertiary structure of all 4 molecules is similar, and all have growth-promoting activities. Insulin modulates transcription and stimulates protein translocation, cell growth, DNA synthesis, and cell replication, effects that it holds in common with the insulin-like growth factors and relaxin.

The Insulin Receptor and Signaling

All of the effects of insulin are the result of the activation of the insulin receptor. The insulin receptor belongs to the class of cell surface receptors that exhibit intrinsic tyrosine kinase activity (see Chapter 40). The insulin receptor is a heterotetramer of 2 extracellular α-subunits disulfide bonded to 2 transmembrane β-subunits (Figure 46-2).

All of the postreceptor responses initiated by insulin binding to its receptor are mediated as a consequence of the activation of several divergent and/or intersecting signal transduction pathways (see Figure 46-1).

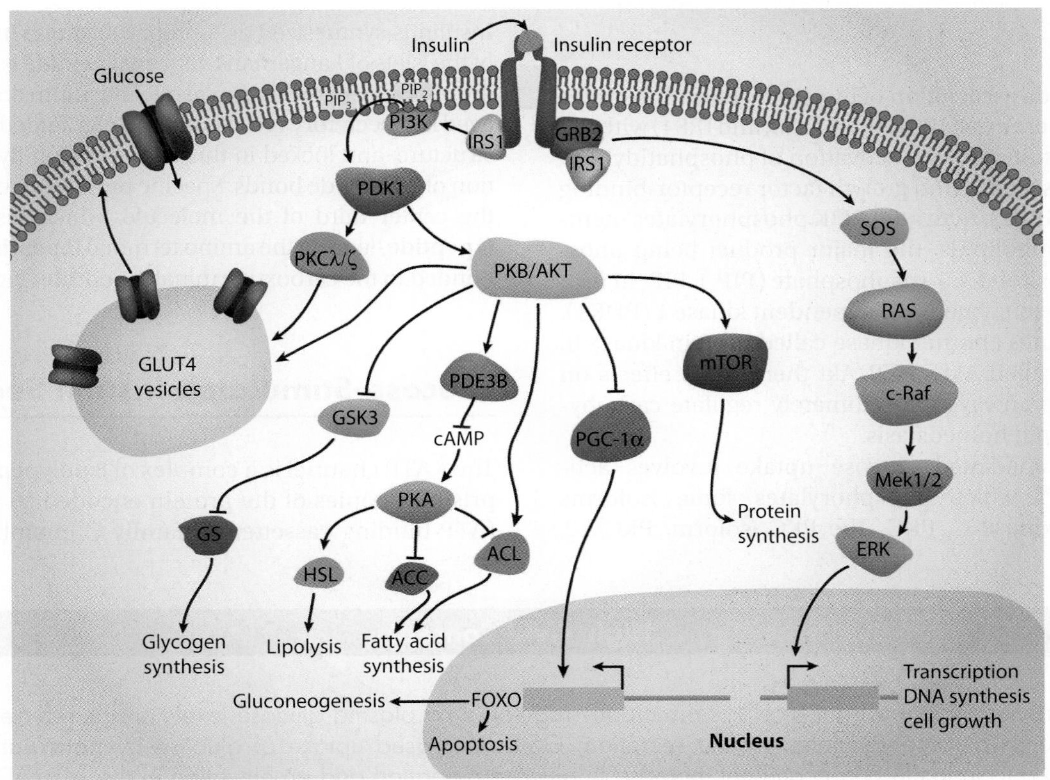

FIGURE 46-1: Multiple roles of insulin. When insulin binds to its receptor it triggers receptor autophosphorylation that in turn triggers the activation of a wide array of signal transducing proteins (highly simplified in this figure). The end results of insulin receptor activation are varied and in many cases cell-type specific but includes alterations in metabolism, ion fluxes, protein translocation, transcription rates, and growth properties of responsive cells. Protein abbreviations are described throughout the text. Reproduced with permission of themedicalbiochemistrypage, LLC.

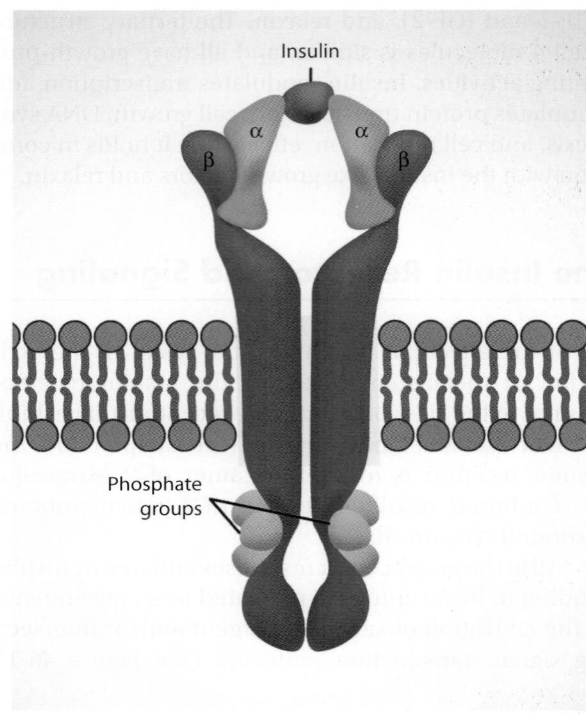

FIGURE 46-2: Structure of the insulin receptor. Reproduced with permission of themedicalbiochemistrypage, LLC.

These include association of insulin receptor substrates (of which there are 4: IRS1, IRS2, IRS3, and IRS4) with the receptor resulting in the activation of phosphatidylinositol-3 kinase, PI3K and growth factor receptor-binding protein 2 (GRB2). Activated PI3K phosphorylates membrane phospholipids, the major product being phosphatidylinositol-3,4,5-trisphosphate (PIP_3). PIP_3 in turn activates the enzyme, PIP_3-dependent kinase 1 (PDK1). PDK1 activates another kinase called protein kinase B, PKB (also called Akt). PKB/Akt then exerts effects on numerous pathways that ultimately regulate carbohydrate and lipid homeostasis.

Insulin-mediated glucose uptake involves activated PDK1 which phosphorylates some isoforms of protein kinase C, PKC. The PKC isoform, PKCλ/ζ, phosphorylates intracellular vesicles containing the glucose transporter, GLUT4, resulting in their migration to and fusion with, the plasma membrane. This results in increased glucose uptake and metabolism.

The activation of GRB2 results in signal transduction via the monomeric G-protein, RAS. Activation of RAS ultimately leads to changes in the expression of numerous genes via activation of members of the extracellular signal-regulated kinases, ERK.

In addition to its effects on enzyme activity, insulin exerts effects on the transcription of numerous genes, effects that are primarily mediated by regulated activity of sterol-regulated element-binding protein, SREBP (see Chapter 26). These transcriptional effects include (but are not limited to) increases in glucokinase, liver pyruvate kinase (LPK), lipoprotein lipase (LPL), fatty acid synthase (FAS), and acetyl-CoA carboxylase (ACC) gene expression, and decreases in glucose 6-phosphatase, fructose-1,6-bisphosphatase, and phosphoenolpyruvate carboxykinase (PEPCK) gene expression.

Functional Insulin Synthesis

Insulin is synthesized as a preprohormone in the β-cells of the islets of Langerhans. Its signal peptide is removed in the cisternae of the endoplasmic reticulum and it is packaged into secretory vesicles in the Golgi, folded to its native structure, and locked in this conformation by the formation of 2 disulfide bonds. Specific protease activity cleaves the center third of the molecule, which dissociates as **C peptide**, leaving the amino terminal **B peptide** disulfide bonded to the carboxy terminal **A peptide** (Figure 46-3).

Glucose-Stimulated Insulin Secretion

The KATP channel is a complex of 8 polypeptides comprising 4 copies of the protein encoded by the *ABCC8* (ATP-binding cassette, subfamily C, member 8) gene

High-Yield Concept

Insulin secretion from β-cells is principally regulated by plasma glucose levels and is referred to as glucose-stimulated insulin secretion, GSIS. Increased uptake of glucose by pancreatic β-cells leads to a concomitant increase in glucose oxidation and an elevation in the ATP/ADP ratio (Figure 46-4). This in turn leads to the inhibition of an ATP-sensitive potassium channel (KATP channel). The net result is a depolarization of the cell leading to Ca^{2+} influx and insulin secretion.

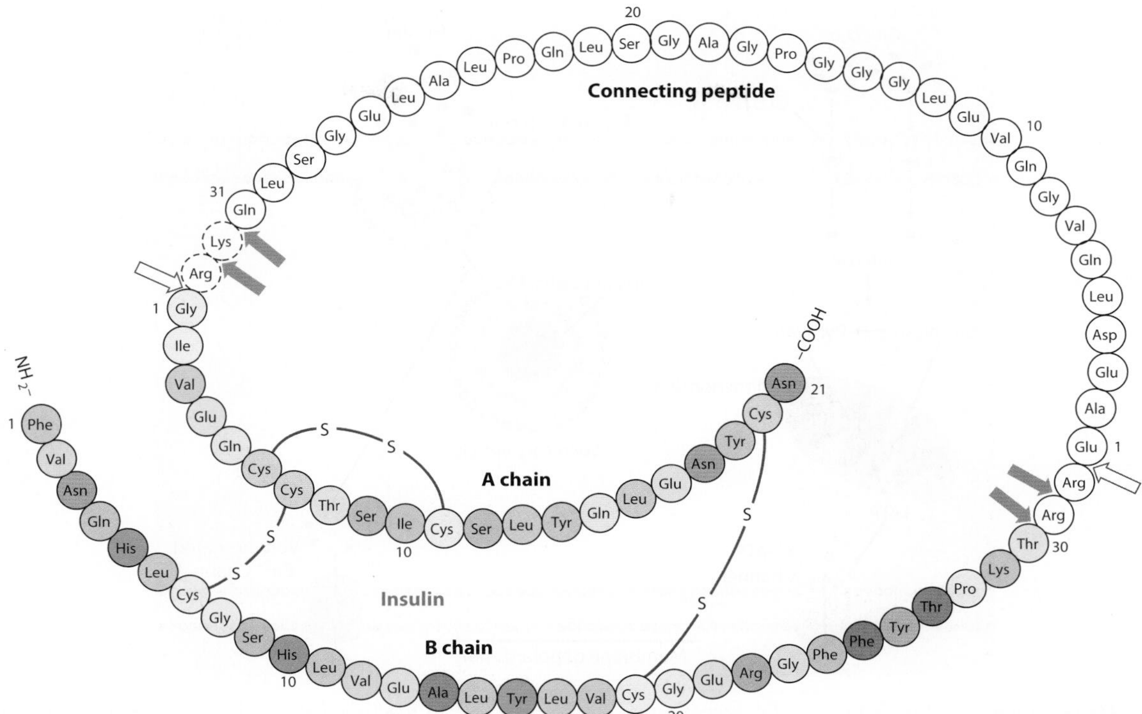

FIGURE 46-3: Structure of human proinsulin. Insulin and C-peptide molecules are connected at 2 sites by dipeptide links. An initial cleavage by a trypsin-like enzyme (open arrows) followed by several cleavages by a carboxypeptidase-like enzyme (solid arrows) results in the production of the heterodimeric (AB) insulin molecule (colored) and the C-peptide (white). Murray RK, Bender DA, Botham KM, Kennelly PJ, Rodwell VW, Weil PA. *Harper's Illustrated Biochemistry*, 29th ed. New York, NY: McGraw-Hill; 2012.

and 4 copies of the protein encoded by the *KCNJ11* (potassium inwardly rectifying channel, subfamily J, member 11; also known as Kir6.2) gene. The *ABCC8*-encoded protein is also known as the sulfonylurea receptor (SUR). The *KCNJ11*-encoded protein forms the core of the KATP channel. As might be expected, the role of KATP channels in insulin secretion presents a viable therapeutic target for treating hyperglycemia due to insulin insufficiency as is typical in type 2 diabetes.

High-Yield Concept

As opposed to the positive role of pancreatic glucose metabolism on insulin secretion, pancreatic fatty acid uptake inhibits GSIS. Increased intracellular fatty acids interfere with the nuclear localization of 2 transcription factors, FOXA2 and HNF1α, that are involved in the transcription of the glycosyltransferase GnT-4a (α-1,3-mannosyl-glycoprotein β-1,4-*N*-acetylglucosaminyltransferase, isozyme A) gene. GnT-4a, encoded by the *MGAT4A* gene, is involved in generating the core GlcNAc linkage in *N*-glycosylated proteins (see Chapter 38). *N*-glycosylation of pancreatic GLUT2 is critical for its correct membrane localization, without which there can be no glucose uptake and thus no GSIS. Of significance to diabetes is the fact that defects in the *HNF1A* gene are associated with MODY3. In addition, the transcription factor HNF1α (encoded by the *HNF1A* gene) is involved in the regulated expression of the *HNF4A*, *GLUT2*, and *LPK* genes and mutations in the *HNF4A* gene or defects in HNF4α function result in MODY1.

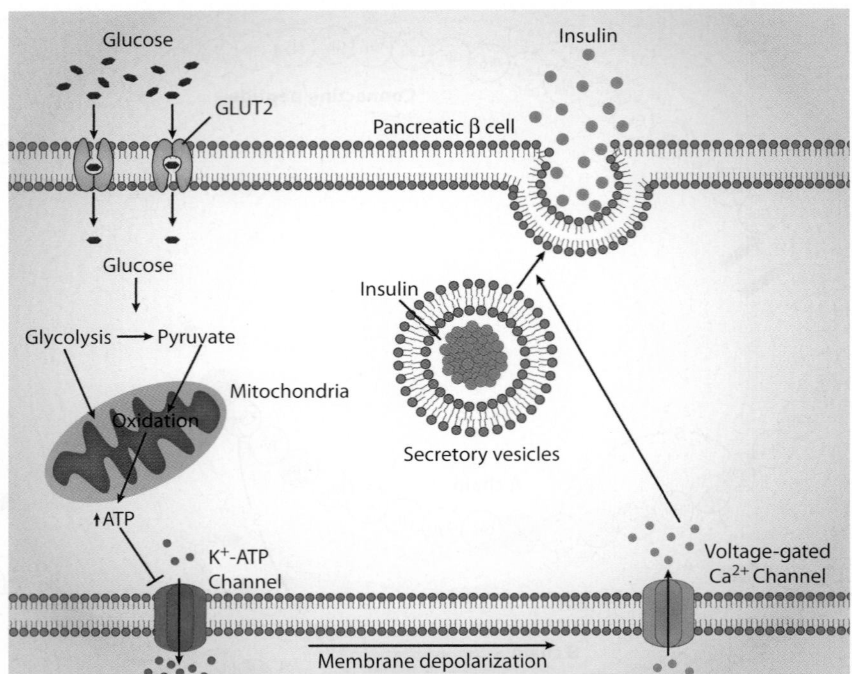

FIGURE 46-4: Glucose-stimulated insulin secretion. Glucose uptake into the β-cell is oxidized which generates ATP via mitochondrial oxidative phosphorylation. The increased ATP levels inhibit the KATP channel which leads to membrane depolarization and the opening of calcium channels. The influx of calcium triggers the fusion of insulin-containing secretory vesicles with the plasma membrane and the release of insulin to the circulation. Reproduced with permission of themedicalbiochemistrypage, LLC.

Nutrient Intake and Hormonal Control of Insulin Release

Of the many gastrointestinal hormones (see Chapter 44), 2 have significant effects on insulin secretion and glucose regulation. These hormones are GLP-1 and GIP. These 2 hormones constitute the class of molecules referred to as the *incretins*.

Details of the actions of GLP-1 and GIP are discussed in Chapter 44. Briefly, GLP-1 is derived from the product of the proglucagon gene. This gene encodes a preproprotein that is differentially cleaved dependent upon the tissue in which it is synthesized. Upon nutrient ingestion GLP-1 is secreted from intestinal enteroendocrine L cells that are found predominantly in the ileum and colon with some production from these cell types in the duodenum and jejunum.

Intestinal Wnt Signaling, GLP-1, and Insulin Secretion

There is ample evidence indicating a significant role for Wnt in the control of metabolism. Wnt action has been shown to be involved in metabolic control via its actions in both the gut and pancreas and Wnt signaling interacts with the signal transduction pathways induced by insulin. The Wnt family of growth factors was first identified by their ability to control

High-Yield Concept

Incretins are gut hormones associated with food intake-stimulation of insulin secretion from the pancreas.

High-Yield Concept

The primary physiological responses to GLP-1 are GSIS, enhanced insulin secretion, inhibition of glucagon secretion, and inhibition of gastric acid secretion and gastric emptying. The action of GLP-1 at the level of insulin and glucagon secretion results in significant reduction in circulating levels of glucose following nutrient intake. This activity has obvious significance in the context of diabetes, in particular the hyperglycemia associated with poorly controlled T2D. The glucose-lowering activity of GLP-1 is highly transient as the half-life of this hormone in the circulation is less than 2 minutes. Removal of bioactive GLP-1 is a consequence of *N*-terminal proteolysis catalyzed by dipeptidyl peptidase IV (DPP IV or DPP4).

important processes of embryonic axis determination during early development. Wnts are soluble secreted factors that exert their effects by binding to the frizzled receptors which are members of the G-protein–coupled receptor (GPCR) family. Wnt binding to frizzled results in the stabilization and activation of β-catenin. Stable β-catenin migrates to the nucleus where it activates transcription factors of the T-cell factor (TCF) family.

Wnt signaling is involved in the regulated expression of the proglucagon gene (*GCG*) in intestinal enteroendocrine L cells. Gut expression of the proglucagon gene results in the production of GLP-1 which then exerts its effects on the gut and the pancreas as described earlier. GLP-1 also exerts central effects within the brain where its actions result in increased satiety and a reduced desire for food intake.

Insulin Regulation of Carbohydrate Homeostasis

One of the major whole-body responses to the release of insulin is the modulation of glucose homeostasis. This includes stimulated uptake of glucose from the blood, primarily by adipose tissue and skeletal muscle, followed by either storage of the glucose as glycogen or the conversion of glucose carbons into fatty acids for storage in triglycerides.

In most nonhepatic tissues, insulin increases glucose uptake by increasing the number of plasma membrane glucose transporters, GLUT4. With respect to regulating the levels of blood glucose, this response to insulin is most significant in adipose tissue and skeletal muscle. In the liver and pancreatic β-cells, glucose uptake is facilitated by GLUT2 which is constitutively present in the plasma membrane.

Increases in the plasma membrane content of GLUT4 stem from an increase in the rate of recruitment of the transporters into the plasma membrane, deriving from a special pool of preformed transporters localized to vesicles in the cytoplasm (see Figure 46-1). Increased glucose uptake by liver, in response to insulin action, results from increased disposal and/or storage.

In addition to the above-described events, diminished cAMP and elevated protein phosphatase activity combine to convert glycogen phosphorylase to its inactive form and glycogen synthase to its active form, with the result that not only is glucose funneled to glycolytic products, but glycogen content is increased as well (Figure 46-5).

High-Yield Concept

The GCG promoter region contains an enhancer that harbors a canonical Wnt response element that binds the TCF transcription factor, TCF7L2. Genome-wide screens for polymorphisms associated with T2D have shown that 2 single nucleotide polymorphisms (SNPs) in the *TCF7L2* gene are the most frequently occurring SNPs associated with this disease.

High-Yield Concept

In the liver, glucose uptake is dramatically increased due to insulin-mediated increases in the activity of the enzymes glucokinase, phosphofructokinase 1 (PFK-1), and liver pyruvate kinase (LPK), the key regulatory enzymes of glycolysis. The latter effects are induced by insulin-dependent activation of phosphodiesterase (PDE) which leads to decreases in cAMP levels. Decreased cAMP results in decreased PKA activity and, as a consequence, diminished phosphorylation of LPK and phosphofructokinase 2, PFK-2. Dephosphorylation of LPK increases its activity while dephosphorylation of PFK-2 renders it active as a kinase. The kinase activity of PFK-2 converts fructose 6-phosphate into fructose 2,6-bisphosphate (F2,6BP). F2,6BP is a potent allosteric activator of the rate-limiting enzyme of glycolysis, PFK-1, and an inhibitor of the gluconeogenic enzyme, fructose-1,6-bisphosphatase (see Chapters 10 and 13). In addition, phosphatases specific for the phosphorylated forms of the glycolytic enzymes increase in activity under the influence of insulin. All these events lead to conversion of the glycolytic enzymes to their active forms and consequently a significant increase in glycolysis. In addition, glucose 6-phosphatase activity is downregulated. The net effect is an increase in the content of hepatocyte glucose and its phosphorylated derivatives, with diminished hepatic output of glucose to the blood.

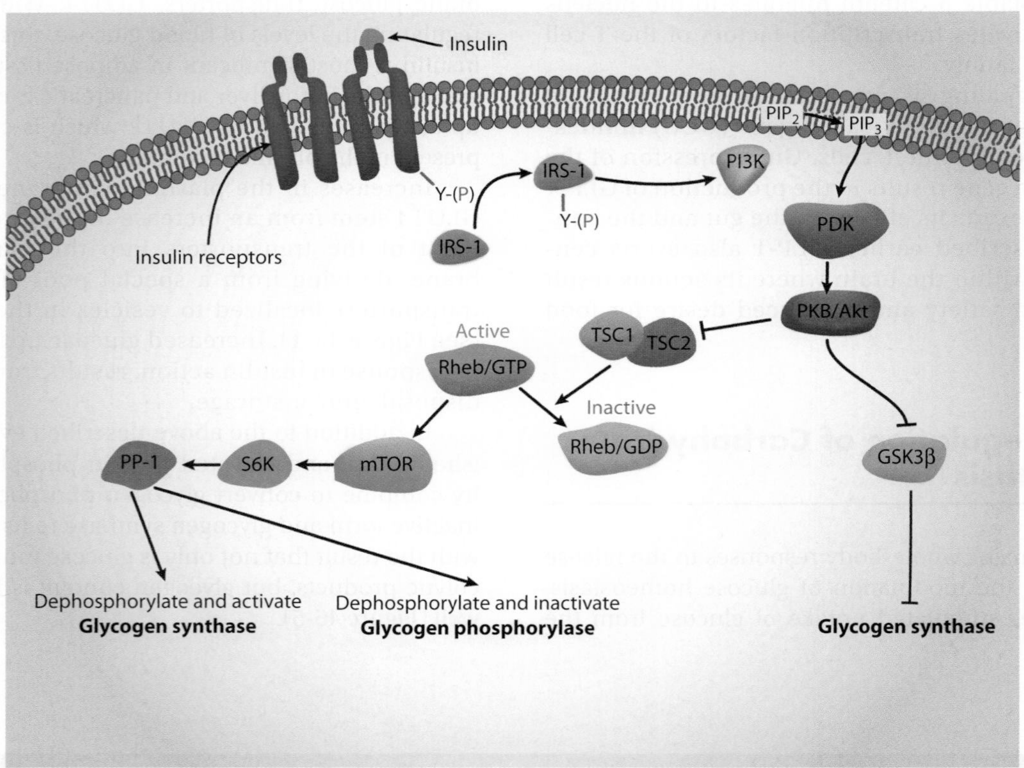

FIGURE 46-5: Insulin-mediated regulation of glycogen homeostasis. Following insulin binding to its receptor as signal transduction cascade is activated involving IRS1 and ultimately altering the activities of glycogen phosphorylase and glycogen synthase. PI3K = phosphatidylinositol-3 kinase; PIP_2 = phosphatidylinositol-4,5-bisphosphate; PIP_3 = phosphatidylinositol-3,4,5-bisphosphate; PDK1 = PIP_3-dependent protein kinase; TSC1 and TSC2 = tuberous sclerosis tumor suppressors 1 (hamartin) and 2 (tuberin); Rheb = Ras homolog enriched in brain; mTOR = mammalian target of rapamycin. PKB/Akt = protein kinase B/Akt2; GSK3 = glycogen synthase kinase 3; S6K = 70kDa ribosomal protein S6 kinase, also called p70S6K. Arrows denote either direction of flow or positive effects, T lines represent inhibitory effects.

Insulin Regulation of Lipid Homeostasis

The net effect of insulin on global metabolism is increased storage of carbon for future use as an energy source. This includes the diversion of glucose into glycogen as well as glucose and fatty acid carbons into triglycerides.

The major effects of insulin, at the level of lipid homeostasis, are activation of lipogenesis and inhibition of lipolysis. The majority of these effects are the result of insulin activation of PDE with consequent reductions in PKA-mediated phosphorylation of its substrates. Within adipocytes, decreased PKA-mediated phosphorylation of hormone-sensitive lipase (HSL) leads to reduced release of free fatty acids (FFAs) from triglycerides.

In the liver, adipose tissue, and skeletal muscle, PKA phosphorylates and inhibits the activity of ATP-citrate lyase (ACL) which is the major enzyme involved in the generation of cytoplasmic acetyl-CoA used for fatty acid and cholesterol synthesis. PKA also phosphorylates and inhibits acetyl-CoA carboxylase (ACC) which is the rate-limiting enzyme of fatty acid synthesis (see Chapter 19). Therefore, activation of PDE by insulin results in reduced PKA-mediated inhibition of ACL and ACC. Insulin-mediated activation of PKB/Akt in adipocytes results in phosphorylation and activation of ACL. Taken together, insulin-mediated increases in glycolysis and the increased activities of ACL and ACC ultimately result in increased fatty acid synthesis. Increased fatty acid synthesis leads to increased storage as triglycerides.

Insulin Function as a Growth Factor

As a growth factor, insulin modulates the transcription of numerous genes involved in cell growth and differentiation. Insulin also stimulates DNA synthesis which is required for cell proliferation. Several of the insulin-stimulated genes are involved in restricting the activation and propagation of apoptotic signals allowing for increased cell survival.

The most well-studied growth factor role for insulin is the stimulation of protein synthesis (Figure 46-6). Both translational initiation and elongation are increased in response to insulin via a cascade leading to the activation of the kinase, mammalian target of rapamycin (mTOR). Rapamycin is an immunosuppressant that gets its name from the fact that the compound was isolated from the bacterium *Streptomyces hygroscopicus* discovered on Easter Island (Rapa Nui).

mTOR is actually a component of 2 distinct multiprotein complexes termed mTORC1 and mTORC2 (mTOR complex 1 and mTOR complex 2). Activation and/or regulation of mTORC1 is involved in the control of cell proliferation, survival, metabolism, and stress responses. These events can be triggered by nutrient availability, glucose, oxygen, and numerous different types of cell surface receptor activation including insulin.

As indicated earlier, insulin action leads to an increase in the activity of PI3K which in turn phosphorylates membrane phospholipids generating PIP_3 which then activates the PDK1 which in turn phosphorylates and activates PKB/Akt. Activated PKB/Akt will phosphorylate TSC2 (tuberin) of the TSC1/TSC2 complex resulting in altered activity of the complex. The TSC1/TSC2 complex functions as a GTPase-activating protein (GAP) which increases GTP hydrolyzing activity of Rheb. The faster the GTPase action of Rheb the faster will be the reduction in Rheb activation of mTOR. When TSC1/TSC2 is phosphorylated by PKB it is less effective at stimulating the GTPase activity of Rheb and, therefore Rheb activation of mTOR will remain high in response to insulin action. In the context of protein synthesis, the activation of mTOR leads to phosphorylation and activation of p70S6K.

Both mTOR and p70S6K have been shown to phosphorylate the regulator of translation initiation, eIF-4E binding protein, 4EBP1. Phosphorylation of 4EBP1 prevents it from binding to eIF-4E. Binding of 4EBP1 to eIF-4E prevents eIF-4E from interaction with the cap structure of mRNAs which is necessary for translational initiation. Thus, the consequences of 4EBP1:eIF-4E interaction is a reduction in translation initiation. As a consequence of the concerted actions of mTOR and p70S6K, insulin results in increased initiation of protein synthesis.

Insulin also activates the kinase, PKB. Activated PKB phosphorylates and inhibits glycogen synthase kinase 3 (GSK3). One of the targets of GSK3, relative to translation, is eIF-2B. Phosphorylation of eIF-2B prevents it from performing its guanine nucleotide exchange function (GEF) in association with eIF-2. Decreased GTP for GDP exchange in eIF-2 results in reduced translational initiation. When GSK3 is inhibited in response to insulin-mediated activation of PKB, eIF-2B GEF activity remains high. High eIF-2B GEF activity means the rate of translational initiation by eIF-2 remains high so protein synthesis will be favored.

Active p70S6K also phosphorylates eEF-2 kinase (EEF2K). As the name implies, EEF2K phosphorylates eEF-2 leading to a decrease in its role in translation elongation. When phosphorylated by p70S6K, EEF2K is less active, thus eEF-2 is much more active as a consequence of insulin action. In addition, insulin

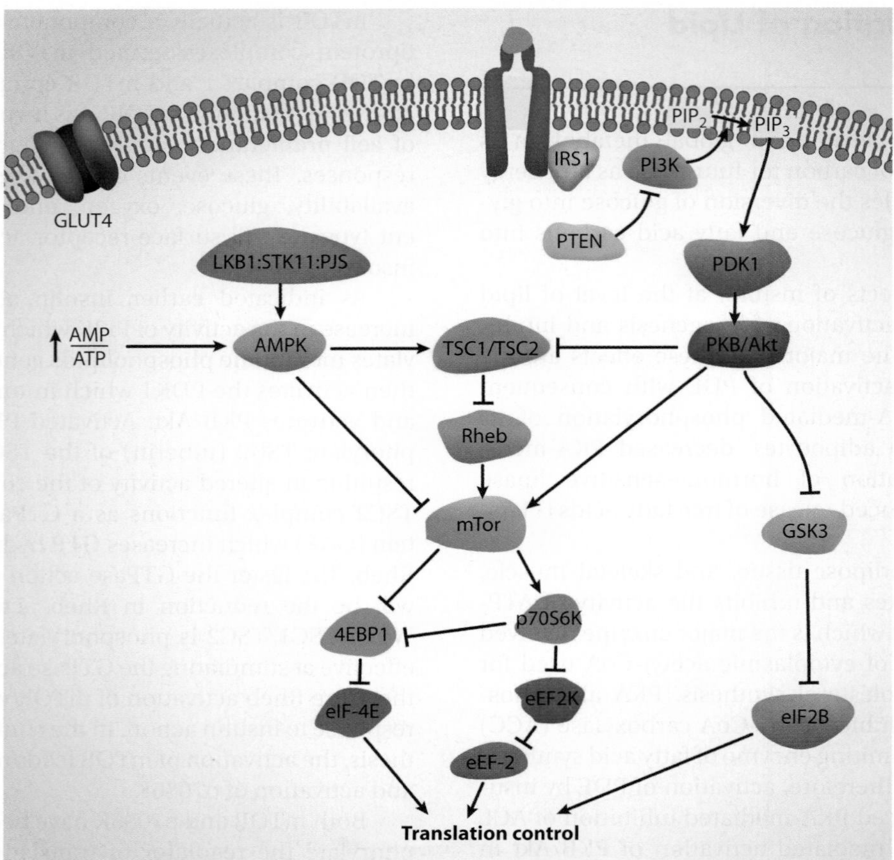

FIGURE 46-6: Insulin-mediated cascade leading to enhanced translation (not intended to be a complete description of all of the targets of insulin action that affect translation rates). Also shown is the effect of an increase in the AMP to ATP ratio which activates AMP-activated kinase, AMPK. STK11-LKB1-PJS = serine-threonine kinase 11, Peutz-Jeghers syndrome gene. IRS1 = insulin receptor substrate 1; PI3K = phosphatidylinositol-3 kinase; PIP_2 = phosphatidylinositol-4,5-bisphosphate; PTEN = phosphatase and tensin homolog deleted on chromosome 10; PDK1 = PIP_3-dependent protein kinase; TSC1 and TSC2 = tuberous sclerosis tumor suppressors 1 (hamartin) and 2 (tuberin); Rheb = Ras homolog enriched in brain; mTOR = mammalian target of rapamycin. PKB/Akt = protein kinase B; GSK3 = glycogen synthase kinase 3; 4EBP1 = eIF-4E binding protein; p70S6K = 70kDa ribosomal protein S6 kinase, also called S6K. The role of AMPK in metabolism is discussed in detail in Chapter 34. Reproduced with permission of themedicalbiochemistrypage, LLC.

action leads to a rapid dephosphorylation of eEF-2 via activation of protein phosphatase 2A (PP2A). Taken together, reduced EEF2K-mediated phosphorylation and increased eEF-2 dephosphorylation lead to increased protein synthesis.

In contrast, epinephrine diminishes insulin secretion by a cAMP-coupled regulatory path. In addition, epinephrine counters the effect of insulin in liver and peripheral tissue, where it binds to β-adrenergic receptors, induces adenylate cycles activity, increases cAMP, and activates PKA similarly to that of glucagon. The latter events induce glycogenolysis and gluconeogenesis, both of which are hyperglycemic and which thus counter insulin's effect on blood glucose levels. In addition, epinephrine influences glucose homeostasis through interaction with α-adrenergic receptors.

Lipemia in Obesity and Insulin Resistance

Obesity is of epidemic proportions in the United States and one of the most serious consequences of this disorder is the development of type 2 diabetes. Associated with obesity, and contributing to worsening of type 2 diabetes is insulin resistance (IR).

High-Yield Concept

Insulin resistance (IR) refers to the situation whereby insulin interaction with its receptor fails to elicit downstream signaling events (see Figure 46-1). Metabolically and clinically the most detrimental effects of IR are due to disruption in insulin-mediated control of glucose and lipid homeostasis in the primary insulin-responsive tissues: liver, skeletal muscle, and adipose tissue.

IR is a characteristic feature found associated with most cases of type 2 diabetes. In addition, IR is the hallmark feature of the metabolic syndrome, MetS (see Chapter 48). IR can occur for a number of reasons; however, the most prevalent cause is the hyperlipidemic and proinflammatory states associated with obesity (see Chapter 45). Excess free fatty acids (FFAs), prevalent in obesity, exert negative effects on the insulin receptor-mediated signaling pathways in adipose tissue, liver, and skeletal muscle (Figure 46-7).

Hepatic IR is induced by the excess accumulation of FFAs. Within the hepatocyte, metabolites of the FFA re-esterification process, including long-chain acyl-CoAs and diacylglycerol (DAG), accumulate. Excess FFAs also participate in the relocation of several protein kinase C (PKC) isoforms, from the cytosol to the membrane compartment. These PKC isoforms include PKC-β2, PKC-δ, and PKC-θ. DAG is a potent activator of these PKC isoforms and the membrane-associated PKCs will phosphorylate the intracellular portion of

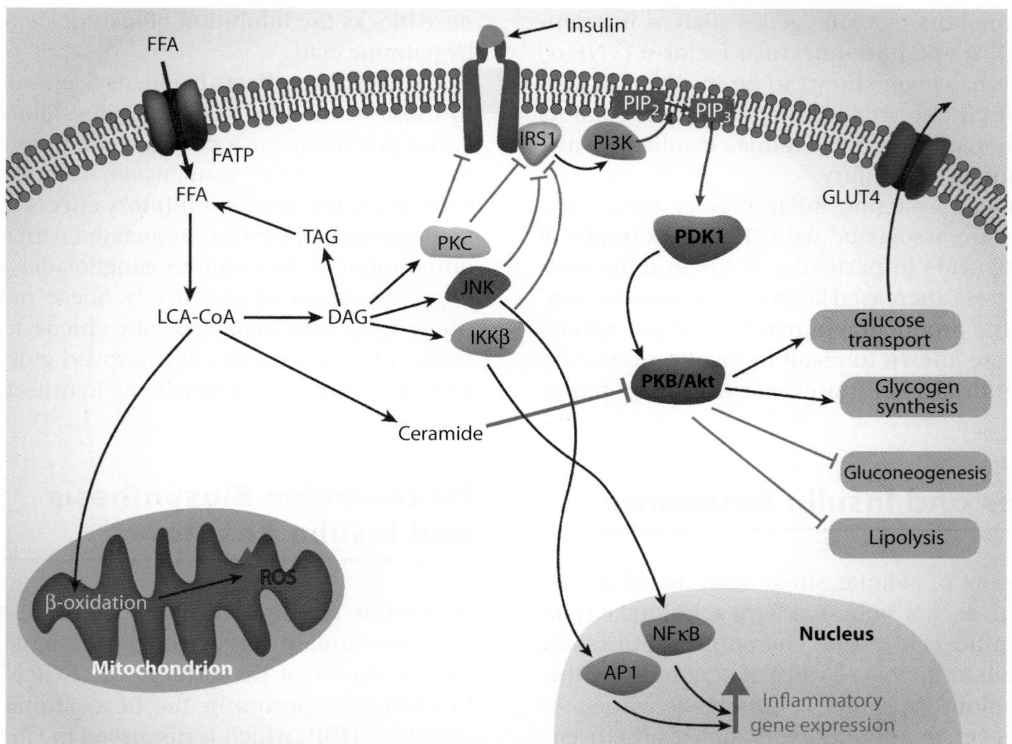

FIGURE 46-7: Model for how excess free fatty acids (FFAs) lead to insulin resistance and enhanced inflammatory responses in cells such as liver and adipose tissue. Only the major pathways regulated by insulin relative to glucose and lipid homeostasis are shown. Black arrows represent positive actions and red T lines represent inhibitory actions. JNK = Jun *N*-terminal kinase; PKC = protein kinase C; IKKβ = inhibitor of nuclear factor kappa B kinase β; ROS = reactive oxygen species; PI3K = phosphatidylinositol-3 kinase; DAG = diacylglycerol; TAG = triacylglycerols; LCA-CoA = long-chain acyl-CoAs; NFκB = nuclear factor kappa B. Akt is also known as protein kinase B (PKB). Reproduced with permission of themedicalbiochemistrypage, LLC.

the insulin receptor on serine residues which results in impairment of insulin receptor interaction with downstream signaling proteins including insulin receptor substrate 1 (IRS1) and IRS2. Loss of IRS1 and IRS2 interaction with the receptor prevents interaction with PI3K and its subsequent activation. In addition to serine phosphorylation of the insulin receptor, various PKCs have been shown to phosphorylate IRS1 and IRS2 further impairing the ability of these proteins to associate with the insulin receptor.

The FFA-induced downregulation of insulin signaling pathways results in activation of several kinases involved in stress responses. These kinases include Jun *N*-terminal kinase (JNK), inhibitor of nuclear factor kappa B kinase β (IKKβ), and suppressors of cytokine signaling 3 (SOCS-3). Like PKC, JNK activity is also regulated by FFAs and is an important contributor to the development of IR.

Activation of IKKβ (which is required for the activation of nuclear factor kappa B, NFκB) may have the most pronounced effect on inflammatory responses in the liver and adipose tissue. NFκB is the most important transcription factor activating the expression of numerous proinflammatory cytokine genes such as interleukin-1 (IL-1), IL-6, and tumor necrosis factor-α (TNF-α) each of which has been shown to be involved in promoting IR. NFκB-dependent inflammatory mediators produced in hepatocytes act to reduce insulin sensitivity and to promote liver injury.

An enhanced systemic inflammatory status and cellular stress are associated with IR. Excess intake of saturated fatty acids in particular, leads to mitochondrial and ER stress. Increased fat oxidation in mitochondria leads to the production of reactive oxygen species (ROS) which are known to result in insulin resistance. Both mitochondrial and ER stress can trigger apoptosis.

Ceramides and Insulin Resistance

Various inducers of cellular stress such as inflammatory activation, excess saturated fatty acid intake (particularly palmitic acid), and chemotherapeutics are known to result in increased rates of ceramide synthesis. Accumulation of cellular ceramides is associated with the pathogenesis of obesity, diabetes, atherosclerosis, and cardiomyopathy. Palmitic acid (C16:0) is the most abundant saturated fatty acid in the circulation and is a required precursor for ceramide synthesis (see Figure 21-2).

As shown in Figure 46-7, ceramides (as well as glucosylceramides) antagonize insulin-stimulated glucose uptake and metabolism. Animal studies have shown that pharmacological inhibition of ceramide or glucosylceramide biosynthesis leads to increased peripheral insulin sensitivity while at the same time reducing the severity of pathologies associated with IR including diabetes, atherosclerosis, hepatic steatosis, and/or cardiomyopathy.

Ceramides interfere with insulin receptor signaling, in part, by blocking the receptors' ability to activate the downstream effector kinase, PKB/Akt. Ceramides also inhibit insulin-stimulated glucose uptake by blocking PDK1-mediated enhancement of GLUT4 vesicle migration to the plasma membrane (see Figure 46-1). Overexpression of PKB/Akt in cell culture negates the effects of ceramides on insulin signal transduction. Ceramides block the translocation of PKB/Akt to the plasma membrane where it needs to be in order to respond to insulin receptor signaling. Another mechanism by which ceramides impact the activity of PKB/Akt is by activating protein phosphatase 2A (PP2A) to dephosphorylate the kinase.

Treatment of cells with acid ceramidase inhibitors results in increased endogenous ceramide levels while simultaneously blocking insulin-mediated activation of PKB/Akt. Conversely, overexpression of acid ceramidase blocks the inhibition of insulin signaling induced by palmitic acid.

The cellular effects of glucosylceramide are similar to those exerted by the ceramides. Glucosylceramide is the precursor for a complex family of gangliosides; for example, the G_{M2} ganglioside. Adipocytes are highly sensitive to the insulin inhibitory effects of glucosylated sphingolipids. Obesity is associated with adipose tissue enrichment in the complex gangliosides, G_{M2}, G_{M1}, and G_{D1a}. Treatment of genetically obese or diet-induced obese mice with highly specific glucosylceramide synthase inhibitors results in improved glucose tolerance and increased insulin sensitivity in muscle and liver.

Hexosamine Biosynthesis and Insulin Resistance

Numerous proteins involved in insulin signaling and the downstream targets of these signaling cascades can be modified by addition of *O*-GlcNAc. Synthesis of *O*-GlcNAc occurs in the hexosamine biosynthesis pathway (HBP) which is discussed in Chapter 38. With respect to insulin receptor signaling proteins, IRS1, PI3K, PKB/Akt, PDK1, and GSK3β are all known to be *O*-GlcNAcylated. These modifications have all been observed in adipocytes. Insulin-stimulated glucose uptake into adipocytes, in response to insulin, can therefore, significantly modify the flux through the HBP. Inhibition of the rate-limiting enzyme of the HBP, GFAT, prevents hyperglycemia-induced insulin resistance.

It is clear that adipocytes play a major regulatory role in HBP-mediated whole-body insulin resistance.

Insulin-mediated PI3K and PKB/Akt activation also stimulates glycogen synthesis mediated via the activation of glycogen synthase (GS). Regulation of GS activity involves a PKB/Akt-mediated inhibition of GSK3β which normally phosphorylates and inhibits GS. The insulin-stimulated increase in glycogen synthesis decreases the pool of glucose entering the HBP, thereby restricting flux through this pathway. Additionally, GS is a known *O*-GlcNAcylated protein and it is more resistant to dephosphorylation by protein phosphatase 1 (PP-1) under conditions of excess HBP flux.

REVIEW QUESTIONS

1. A 19-year-old man is brought to the emergency room unconscious and unresponsive. There are no visible signs of trauma or head injury. The attending physician orders blood work and administration of an IV bolus of glucose. The patient regains consciousness but remains unclear of how or why he passed out. History indicates the patient is not diabetic and does not take insulin shots. However, the physician suspects the patient passed out due to insulin-induced hypoglycemia. Analysis of the patient's blood for which of the following would best confirm the physician's suspicions?

A. C peptide
B. epinephrine
C. glucagon
D. glucose
E. ketones

Answer A: Insulin is synthesized as a preprohormone. Its signal peptide is removed in the cisternae of the endoplasmic reticulum and it is packaged into secretory vesicles in the Golgi, folded to its native structure, and locked in this conformation by the formation of 2 disulfide bonds. Specific protease activity cleaves the center third of the molecule, which dissociates as C peptide, leaving the amino terminal B peptide disulfide bonded to the carboxy terminal A peptide. The C peptide is released along with functional insulin. In a patient in an insulin-induced coma due to injected synthetic insulin there would not be any C peptide in their blood. The presence of elevated levels of plasma C peptide in an unconscious patient could indicate an insulinoma resulting in inappropriate release of insulin leading to unexpected hypoglycemia.

2. You are testing the effects, on insulin function, to the addition of an unknown substance to adipocytes in culture. In the presence or absence of the compound you find that insulin binds to the adipocytes with equal affinity. Insulin alone results in a 5-fold increase in the rate of glucose uptake, above the basal rate. However, following addition of your test compound the rate of glucose uptake in response to insulin is only 0.5-fold above the basal rate. Your compound is actively taken up by the adipocytes and thus is likely exerting its effects intracellularly. Which of the following substances is your test compound most likely mimicking in this cell culture system?

A. ceramide
B. glucuronate
C. glucosamine
D. glucose
E. phosphatidic acid

Answer A: The ability of ceramides to interfere with insulin receptor signaling is the result of blocking the receptors' ability to activate the downstream effector kinase, PKB/Akt. Experiments in cell culture, involving both adipocytes and skeletal muscle cells, have shown that ceramides inhibit insulin-stimulated glucose uptake by blocking translocation of GLUT4 to the plasma membrane as well as interfering with glycogen synthesis. That blockade of PKB/Akt activation is central to the effects of ceramides can be demonstrated by constitutive overexpression of the kinase which negates the effects of ceramides.

3. Addition of which of the following compounds would be expected to result in the greatest increase in insulin resistance in adipocytes in culture under conditions of hyperglycemia and hyperinsulinemia?

A. fructose
B. galactose
C. glucosamine
D. glycine
E. sialic acid

Answer C: The hexosamine biosynthesis pathway (HBP) plays a critical role in the development of insulin resistance. Impairment in insulin-stimulated glucose uptake, under hyperglycemic and hyperinsulinemic conditions involves the HBP. Inhibition of GFAT activity, the rate-limiting enzyme in the HBP, is normally observed in hyperglycemic and hyperinsulinemic conditions due to feedback inhibition by the product of the HBP, UDP-GlcNAc. However, if cells are treated with glucosamine, which enters the HBP after the GFAT catalyzed reaction, there is greater reduction in insulin-mediated glucose uptake compared to the hyperglycemic condition alone.

4. Type 1 diabetics frequently experience ketoacidosis. Administration of insulin decreases the serum concentration of ketone bodies in these patients via which of the following mechanisms?
A. decreasing formation of ketone bodies in skeletal muscle
B. decreasing lipolysis in adipose tissue
C. increasing hepatic activity of carnitine acyltransferase
D. increasing hepatic levels of acetyl-CoA
E. increasing hepatic oxidation of ketone bodies

Answer B: Insulin action at the level of adipose tissue leads to decreased lipolysis and increased lipogenesis. When insulin binds its receptor on adipocytes it triggers activation of PDE which hydrolyzes cAMP leading to reduced levels of active PKA. Less PKA means less phosphorylation and activation of HSL. This results in less free fatty acid release so that there will be less substrate for the production of ketones by the liver.

5. A 13-year-old adolescent boy with type 1 diabetes has a serum glucose concentration is 540 mg/dL. Several hours following IV administration of insulin, his serum glucose concentration decreases to 200 mg/dL. Which of the following mechanisms best explains the effect of the insulin signaling pathway on the GLUT4 transporter in this decrease resulting in the reduced serum glucose?
A. it activates GLUT4 by a cAMP-dependent mechanism
B. it increases GLUT4 mRNA
C. it increase the K_m of GLUT4 for glucose
D. it induces a conformational change in GLUT4
E. it promotes GLUT4 mobilization to the plasma membrane

Answer E: Insulin-mediated glucose uptake involves activation of the kinase, PDK1. Activated PDK1 phosphorylates some isoforms of protein kinase C, PKC. The PKC isoform, PKCλ/ζ, phosphorylates intracellular vesicles containing the glucose transporter, GLUT4, resulting in their migration to and fusion with, the plasma membrane. This results in increased glucose uptake and metabolism.

6. Pancreatic oxidation of glucose results in increased release of insulin. This mechanism is referred to as glucose-stimulated insulin secretion (GSIS). A defect in which of the following proteins would be expected to exert the greatest negative effect on GSIS?
A. AMPK
B. ABCC8
C. glucokinase
D. GLUT2
E. KCNJ11

Answer C: Glucose uptake into pancreatic β-cells involves the constitutive transporter GLUT2 which essentially transports glucose via a concentration gradient. Once inside the cell, in order to be metabolized, glucose has to be phosphorylated by glucokinase. This not only primes the glucose for oxidation but also traps it inside the β-cell. Lack of glucokinase would result in no oxidation of glucose so there would be no alteration in the ATP/ADP ratio which is important in the process of GSIS.

7. Recent evidence has identified an enzyme involved in the modification of GLUT2 in pancreatic β-cells that is critically important for glucose-stimulated insulin secretion (GSIS). Which of the following represents this modification necessary for GLUT2 action?
A. acetylation
B. acylation
C. glycosylation
D. methylation
E. phosphorylation

Answer C: The glycosyltransferase GnT-4a, encoded by the *MGAT4A* gene, is involved in generating the core GlcNAc linkage in *N*-glycosylated proteins. *N*-glycosylation of pancreatic GLUT2 is critical for its correct membrane localization, without which there can be no glucose uptake and thus, no GSIS.

8. Insulin action results in the increased expression of several genes as well as the decreased expression of others. One consequence of these global gene expression changes is increased fatty acid synthesis due, in part, to the inhibition of expression of which of the following genes?
A. *CYP7A1* (cholesterol 7α-hydroxylase)
B. glucokinase
C. liver pyruvate kinase (*LPK*)
D. *PEPCK*
E. *PDK4* (pyruvate dehydrogenase kinase 4)

Answer E: The pyruvate dehydrogenase kinases (PDK1-PDK4) regulate the activity of the PDHc. Phosphorylation of the PDHc by PDK4 results in a lower rate of pyruvate oxidation. Reduced pyruvate oxidation lowers the pool of acetyl-CoA which is required as the substrate for fatty acid and cholesterol synthesis.

Since insulin action reduces the expression of PDK4 there will be less inhibition of the PDHc and thus, more acetyl-CoA for fatty acid synthesis.

9. Insulin, being a growth factor, increases the rate of protein synthesis, in part, by increasing the activity of the kinase mTOR. Activation of mTOR in response to insulin receptor stimulation requires inhibition of which of the following upstream signaling molecules?

A. AMPK
B. GSK3
C. PKB/Akt
D. PI3K
E. TSC1/TSC2

Answer E: Insulin action leads to an increase in the activity of PI3K which in turn phosphorylates membrane phospholipids generating PIP_3 which then activates PDK1 which in turn phosphorylates and activates PKB/Akt. Activated PKB/Akt will phosphorylate TSC2 (tuberin) of the TSC1/TSC2 complex resulting in altered activity of the complex. The TSC1/TSC2 complex functions as a GTPase-activating protein (GAP) which increases GTP hydrolyzing activity of Rheb. The faster the GTPase action of Rheb the faster will be the reduction in Rheb activation of mTOR. When TSC1/TSC2 is phosphorylated by PKB it is less effective at stimulating the GTPase activity of Rheb and, therefore Rheb activation of mTOR will remain high in response to insulin action.

10. Which of the following represents a major target tissue for the action of insulin reflecting its ability to regulate circulating levels of blood glucose?

A. brain
B. heart
C. kidney
D. skeletal muscle
E. testis

Answer D: The primary targets of insulin action, at the level of glucose homeostasis, are adipose tissue and skeletal muscle. Both of these tissues express GLUT4 which is stimulated to migrate to the plasma membrane in response to insulin action resulting in increased glucose disposal from the blood. Since the overall cellular mass of skeletal muscle is so large, in relation to all other tissues, insulin-mediated glucose uptake into this tissue represents one of the major glucose-lowering effects of the hormone.

11. Activation of insulin receptors by binding of insulin results in numerous changes in the activity of other signaling proteins. Some of these changes are increases in activity, some are decreases. Of the following enzymes, which one has an increased level of activity after insulin binds its receptor?

A. GSK3
B. glycogen synthase
C. glycogen phosphorylase
D. PKA
E. protein phosphatase inhibitor 1 (PPI-1)

Answer B: One of the effects of insulin is the activation of phosphodiesterase (PDE) which leads to decreases in cAMP levels. Decreased cAMP results in decreased PKA activity and, as a consequence, diminished phosphorylation of its substrates. PKA normally phosphorylates and activates PPI-1 which then inhibits protein phosphatase-1 (PP-1) activity. Diminished PKA and elevated protein phosphatase activity in response to insulin combine to convert glycogen phosphorylase to its inactive form and glycogen synthase to its active form, with the result that not only is glucose funneled to glycolytic products, but glycogen content is increased as well.

12. The incretins are hormones that are released in response to the consumption of food. Which of the following represents one of the major effects of incretin release from intestinal epithelial cells?

A. activation of gastric emptying ensuring release of ingested food
B. enhancement in adipocyte triacylglycerol synthesis
C. enhancement of insulin secretion from the pancreas
D. repression of pancreatic cell proliferation
E. stimulation of gastric acid secretion to aid in digestion

Answer C: The incretins are molecules associated with food intake-stimulation of insulin secretion from the pancreas. Two of the many gastrointestinal hormones have significant effects on insulin secretion and glucose regulation. These hormones are glucagon-like peptide-1 (GLP-1) and glucose-dependent insulinotropic peptide (GIP). Both of these gut hormones represent the incretins.

13. Insulin receptor activation results in an increase in the flux of glucose into glycogen in skeletal muscle. A defect in which of the following proteins involved in glycogen homeostasis would be expected to result in the greatest deficit in insulin-mediated glycogenesis in these cells?

A. glucose 6-phosphatase
B. glycogen synthase-phosphorylase kinase
C. glycogen phosphorylase
D. protein phosphatase inhibitor 1 (PPI-1)
E. protein targeting glycogen (PTG)

Answer E: One of the many effects of insulin on cells is to increase glucose uptake and storage into glycogen. Glucose uptake (eg, in skeletal muscle) is mediated by insulin-induced mobilization of glucose transporters (GLUT4) to the cell surface. The glucose is then incorporated into glycogen because of insulin's effects on glycogen homeostatic enzymes. These effects are an increase in glycogen synthase and a decrease in glycogen phosphorylase activities. Increased glycogen synthesis is affected by activation of phosphate removal from 3 key enzymes via the action of protein phosphatase 1 (PP-1). These key enzymes are phosphorylase, phosphorylase kinase, and glycogen synthase. Dephosphorylation of the first 2 enzymes reduces their activity, while dephosphorylation of the latter increases its activity leading to increased glucose storage. In order for this regulatory process to be carried out quickly and effectively a subunit of PP-1 *collects* all of the regulated enzymes into a mutisubunit complex. This subunit is called protein targeting glycogen, PTG. Therefore, a defect in PTG function would reduce or eliminate the ability of insulin action to target glycogen homeostasis.

14. Although the major metabolic effect of insulin is to promote fuel storage following meals, this hormone also has growth factor activity. One of the growth-promoting responses to insulin action is an increase in the rate of translation. Which of the following proteins of translation is a target of insulin-mediated action, the consequence of which is a reduced level of phosphorylation and thus increased activity?
A. 4EBP
B. eEF-2
C. eIF-2
D. eIF-2B
E. eRF

Answer D: With respect to insulin effects on translation, these signaling cascades ultimately affect the activity of 2 kinases, mTOR and glycogen synthase kinase 3β (GSK3β). GSK3β normally phosphorylates the translation initiation factor eIF-2B, which is responsible for the exchange of GDP for GTP bound to eIF-2. This nucleotide exchange reaction is essential to reactivate eIF-2 during each round of translation. When phosphorylated eIF-2B is much slower at catalyzing the exchange, the effect of insulin in this cascade is to activate the kinase PKB/Akt which in turn phosphorylates GSK3β. When GSK3β is phosphorylated it can no longer phosphorylate eIF-2B, thus in response to insulin the nucleotide exchange action of eIF-2B is high leading to increased translation.

15. Based on your understanding of the role of insulin in the body, expression of which of the following enzymes would be expected to be reduced as a consequence of the actions of insulin?
A. acetyl-CoA carboxylase
B. hepatic glucokinase
C. lipoprotein lipase
D. PEP carboxykinase
E. pyruvate kinase

Answer D: Insulin action leads to the regulated expression of a number of genes encoding metabolic enzymes. Some of these regulatory events are positive and some are negative on gene expression. PEPCK expression is reduced in response to insulin action. Additionally, expression of fructose-1,6-bisphosphatase and glucose 6-phosphatase is reduced as a result of insulin action. Conversely, insulin action leads increased expression of acetyl-CoA carboxylase, hepatic glucokinase, lipoprotein lipase, and pyruvate kinase.

16. Which of the following activities, relating to glucose homeostasis, is directly attributable to the actions of glucagon-like peptide-1 (GLP-1)?
A. decreased fatty acid release from adipose tissue
B. decreased glucagon release from the pancreas
C. increased transit of carbohydrates through the intestines
D. stimulated degradation of hepatic glycogen stores
E. unmasking of GLUT4 transporters in skeletal muscle

Answer B: The primary physiological responses to GLP-1 are glucose-dependent insulin secretion, inhibition of glucagon secretion, and inhibition of gastric acid secretion and gastric emptying. In addition, GLP-1 activity results in increased expression of the glucose transporter 2 (GLUT2) and glucokinase genes in pancreatic cells. The action of GLP-1 at the level of insulin and glucagon secretion results in significant reduction in circulating levels of glucose following nutrient intake.

17. You are studying adipocytes isolated via biopsy from a 12-year-old male patient who exhibits chronic hyperglycemia but with normal circulating levels of insulin. Your studies of these cells demonstrate that the density of insulin receptors is similar to adipocytes from control volunteers, binding kinetics are also identical, and the receptors become autophosphorylated in response to insulin binding. Given these observations it is most likely that there is a defect in which of the following insulin signal transduction proteins leading to the observed hyperglycemia in the subject?
A. glycogen synthase kinase 3, GSK3
B. mammalian target of rapamycin, mTOR

C. phosphodiesterase, PDE
D. PIP_3-dependent protein kinase, PDK1
E. protein kinase B (PKB/Akt)

Answer D: One of the major functions of insulin is to stimulate the uptake of glucose from the blood. This is accomplished primarily by adipose tissue and skeletal muscle responses to insulin binding its receptor. The response, at the level of glucose uptake, is the stimulation of GLUT4-containing membrane vesicle migration to the plasma membrane. The hyperglycemia observed in this patient, given normal upstream insulin responses, could most likely be explained by a reduction in GLUT4 transfer to the plasma membrane of cells of these 2 major insulin-responsive tissues. The migration of GLUT4 vesicles is triggered by activation of PDK1 which in turn activates PKC isoforms (PKCλ and PKCζ) which phosphorylate proteins in the vesicular trafficking system.

18. In a comparison study of 2 related cell lines you find that one responds normally to insulin while the other has an impaired response. You discover that both cell lines bind insulin with equal affinity but that the impaired response is manifest in an inability to recruit the insulin receptor substrate 1 (IRS1) protein to the receptor. This would most likely be due to which of the following?
A. decreased activation of the tyrosine phosphatase activity of the receptor preventing removal of phosphate from the IRS1 docking site
B. inability of the receptor to phosphorylate the G-protein, RAS
C. loss of activation of PLCβ in response to insulin-binding receptor
D. serine phosphorylation of the insulin receptor preventing IRS1 from binding
E. tyrosine phosphorylation of the insulin receptor leading to the loss of the IRS1 binding site

Answer D: All of the postreceptor responses initiated by insulin binding to its receptor are mediated as a consequence of the activation of several signal transduction pathways that require autophosphorylation of tyrosine residues in the intracellular portion of the insulin receptor. These tyrosine phosphates are docking sites for proteins, such as IRS1, involved in insulin signaling. Serine phosphorylation of the insulin receptor, as well as IRS1, interferes with the ability of IRS1 to bind to the receptor resulting in reduced signaling in response to insulin receptor interaction.

19. Exogenous peripherally injected insulin differs from endogenously secreted insulin in a number of aspects, including which of the following?
A. achieves a higher concentration in the periphery than in the liver, contrary to endogenous insulin
B. contains C peptide, which is missing from secreted endogenous insulin
C. is able to bypass insulin resistance observed with endogenous insulin
D. is always extracted from animal sources and therefore is less effective due to sequence differences and anti-insulin antibodies
E. is in the form of proinsulin, whereas endogenous insulin has had C peptide removed

Answer A: The concentration of exogenous insulin is higher at the site of injection in the periphery, compared to its concentration in the liver. On the other hand, endogenous insulin is higher concentrated in the liver than in the periphery. Insulin is normally secreted by the endocrine pancreas into the portal venous drainage. Thus, it passes through the liver before being seen by the periphery. A certain fraction of insulin is extracted by the liver, so that the concentration of insulin seen by the liver is normally higher than that seen by the periphery. This discrepancy between exogenous and endogenous insulin might contribute to the problems experienced by diabetics such as hypertension and cardiovascular disease.

20. A 14-year-old adolescent girl with a 2-year history of type 1 diabetes is brought to the ER 1 hour after awakening from sleep at 2:30 AM in a cold sweat, tremulous and confused. She normally self-administers 4 injections of insulin daily, and the last injection was administered before she went to bed. Measurement of her blood glucose concentration indicates it is 40 mg/dL. Following an injection of glucagon, her serum glucose concentration increases to 175 mg/dL, and she shows clinical improvement. The beneficial effect of glucagon in this patient results from which of the following actions of this hormone in the liver?
A. adenylate cyclase stimulation
B. guanylate cyclase stimulation
C. intranuclear binding of hormone receptor to DNA
D. serine/threonine kinase activation
E. tyrosine kinase activation

Answer A: When glucagon binds to its receptor on hepatocytes it triggers the activation of a G-protein that in turn activates adenylate cyclase. The activation of adenylate cyclase results in increased production of cAMP which then activates PKA. Activated PKA results in phosphorylation of numerous substrates in the hepatocyte that dramatically increases glycogen breakdown and the activation of the gluconeogenic pathway. Both of these events lead to increased glucose release from the liver accounting for the observed increase in blood glucose.

21. Which of the following metabolic processes is promoted by insulin?
- **A.** catabolism of muscle protein
- **B.** fatty acid oxidation
- **C.** gluconeogenesis
- **D.** glycogenesis
- **E.** lipolysis

Answer D: The primary hormonal effects of insulin are the conversion of carbon energy into storage molecules. These actions include the incorporation of glucose into glycogen and the activation of lipogenesis pathways to increase the synthesis of triglycerides. Catabolic processes are inhibited in response to insulin actions.

22. You are examining the responses of adipocytes in culture to the addition of various peptide hormones. You find that after the addition of one hormone in your study there is an increase in glucose uptake from the media. Which of the following is the most likely initial event triggered by the addition of the test hormone, leading to the observed effects?
- **A.** activation of adenylate cyclase by the receptor
- **B.** autophosphorylation of threonine residues in the receptor
- **C.** interaction of the receptor with a signal cascade protein
- **D.** interaction of the receptor with the glucose transporter
- **E.** translocation of the hormone receptor complex to the nucleus

Answer C: The test hormone in this study is most likely to be insulin. All of the postreceptor responses initiated by insulin binding to its receptor are mediated as a consequence of the activation of several signal transduction pathways. One of the responses of adipocytes to insulin is the association of GRB2 with IRS1. This association activates GRB2 which in turn activates the G-protein, RAS.

23. Insulin is synthesized in the β-cells of the pancreas as a proinsulin molecule. In order for this proinsulin to be biologically active, which of the following posttranslational modifications of the hormone is required?
- **A.** acetylation of the α-amino group
- **B.** binding of zinc ions
- **C.** cleavage of peptide bonds
- **D.** oxidation of sulfhydryl groups
- **E.** phosphorylation of tyrosine residues

Answer C: Insulin is synthesized as a preprohormone in the β-cells of the islets of Langerhans. Its signal peptide is removed in the cisternae of the endoplasmic reticulum and it is packaged into secretory vesicles in the Golgi, folded to its native structure, and locked in this conformation by the formation of 2 disulfide bonds. Specific protease activity cleaves the center third of the molecule, which dissociates as C peptide, leaving the amino terminal B peptide disulfide bonded to the carboxy terminal A peptide.

24. You are carrying out experiments to examine insulin-stimulated glucose uptake in isolated skeletal muscle cells. You know that insulin first binds to its receptor on the plasma membrane of these cells triggering an increase in phosphatidylinositol-3 kinase (PI3K) activity. The net effect of increased PI3K activity is insertion of subcellular membranes containing GLUT4 protein into the plasma membrane. Which of the following is the most likely first intracellular step in this signaling cascade?
- **A.** activation of PI3K
- **B.** activation of phospholipase Cβ (PLCβ)
- **C.** autophosphorylation of the receptor tyrosine kinase
- **D.** phosphorylation of insulin receptor substrate 1 (IRS1)
- **E.** phosphorylation of mitogen-activated protein kinase (MAPK)

Answer C: All of the postreceptor responses initiated by insulin binding to its receptor are mediated as a consequence of the activation of several signal transduction pathways. These signal transduction cascades involve the activation of several different kinases, such as PI3K, that phosphorylate their substrates in response to activation from upstream factors in the insulin signaling cascade. In order for these events to occur, the intrinsic tyrosine kinase activity of the insulin receptor must be activated which results in autophosphorylation of the receptor. The tyrosine phosphorylated receptor then serves as a docking site for proteins that, in turn, activate PI3K activity.

25. You are studying the responses of myocytes in culture to the addition of insulin. Normally in myocytes when insulin binds, several proteins are phosphorylated by kinases. You discover that several target proteins are not appropriately modified in your cells. Which of the following is most likely not occurring in your cell culture in response to insulin thereby, explaining the lack of target protein phosphorylation?
- **A.** action of a G-protein in the plasma membrane
- **B.** release of Ca^{2+} from the endoplasmic reticulum
- **C.** release of diacylglycerol from phosphatidylinositol
- **D.** translocation of the glucose transporter to the plasma membrane
- **E.** tyrosine kinase activity of the insulin receptor

Answer E: All of the postreceptor responses initiated by insulin binding to its receptor are mediated as a consequence of the activation of several signal transduction pathways. These signal transduction cascades involve the activation of several different kinases that phosphorylate their substrates in response to activation from upstream factors in the insulin signaling cascade. In order for these events to occur, the intrinsic tyrosine kinase activity of the insulin receptor must be activated which results in autophosphorylation of the receptor. Lack of receptor phosphorylation will prevent signaling proteins from binding to the receptor and, therefore, they cannot be activated and as a result all downstream kinase activity will be impaired.

Checklist

- ✓ Insulin is the most significant hypoglycemia-inducing hormone in the body.
- ✓ Insulin is produced in the β-cells of the islets of Langerhans in the pancreas. Bioactive insulin is processed from a preproprotein by proteolytic digestion into a function peptide composed of an A peptide and a B peptide held together by disulfide bonds. The central portion of the proinsulin protein is called the C peptide and is not part of the functional hormone, but is released from secretory vesicles along with functional insulin.
- ✓ Secretion of insulin is stimulated primarily in response to increases in plasma glucose levels due, in part, to increased glucose oxidation within pancreatic β-cells, a process that results in increased ATP leading to inhibition of a potassium channel causing depolarization of the cell, an associated influx of calcium and insulin vesicle fusion with the plasma membrane. This is referred to as glucose-stimulated insulin secretion, GSIS.
- ✓ Gut hormones, called incretins, released in response to food intake, influence the glucose-mediated secretion of insulin.
- ✓ Increased intake of fatty acids impairs pancreatic GSIS and contributes to the etiology of obesity-induced diabetes.
- ✓ Insulin exerts activities associated with typical hormones as well as those exerted by typical growth factors. All of these dual activities are activated in response to insulin binding to its cell surface receptor. Cell-type specific responses to insulin are the result of the differential expression of signaling proteins downstream of the insulin receptor.
- ✓ The insulin receptor is a member of the class of receptors with intrinsic enzymatic activity, specifically the receptor tyrosine kinases (RTK). The insulin receptor is unique in this class in that it is a heterotetrameric receptor composed of 2 membrane-spanning β-subunits and 2 extracellular α-subunits disulfide bonded to the β-subunits.
- ✓ As a hormone, insulin stimulates glucose uptake and storage as glycogen or oxidation to acetyl-CoA for conversion to fatty acids for storage in the form of triglyceride. Insulin actions also inhibit lipolysis and stimulate lipogenesis.
- ✓ As a growth factor insulin stimulates protein synthesis, transcription profiles of numerous genes, DNA synthesis, and the inhibition of apoptosis.
- ✓ Defects in insulin-mediated signal transduction events are the basis for insulin resistance, IR. Excess free fatty acids and their metabolic intermediates are the primary culprits in the development of IR.
- ✓ IR is the precipitating event in the development of type 2 diabetes, T2D.

CHAPTER 47 Diabetes Mellitus

CHAPTER OUTLINE

High-Yield Terms

Polyuria: excessive urine output as is typical in most forms of diabetes

Polyphagia: excessive hunger typically associated with Type 1 diabetes

Polydipsia: excessive thirst as is often associated with diabetes

Oral glucose tolerance test, OGTT: a test to measure the plasma responses to intake of a bolus of glucose; used to determine insulin function and the potential for diabetes

Type 1 diabetes, T1D: insulin-dependent diabetes mellitus (IDDM); insulin-deficient form diabetes most often manifesting in children as a result of autoimmune destruction of the β-cells of the pancreas

Diabetic ketoacidosis, DKA: a potentially life-threatening condition of excess ketone production by the liver in response to uncontrolled fatty acid release from adipose tissue resulting from excess glucagon secretion

Type 2 diabetes, T2D: noninsulin-dependent diabetes mellitus (NIDDM); a form of the disease associated with peripheral insulin resistance progressing to loss of insulin production

Gestational diabetes mellitus, GDM: a specific form of diabetes mellitus characterized by glucose intolerance first appearing during pregnancy

Maturity-onset type diabetes of the young, MODY: a class of T2D caused by inherited or somatic mutations in any of several genes involved in pancreatic function

Neonatal diabetes: hyperglycemia resulting from dysfunction in insulin action within the first 6 months of life and thus, not Type 1 diabetes

HbA_{1c}: designates the glycosylated form of adult hemoglobin; is a measure of the level of glucose in the plasma

Diabetes Defined

Diabetes is any disorder characterized by excessive urinary output. The most common form of diabetes is **diabetes mellitus**, a metabolic disorder in which there is an inability to completely dispose of glucose due to disturbances in insulin function resulting in glucosuria and hyperglycemia. Additional symptoms of diabetes mellitus include polydipsia (excessive thirst), polyuria (excessive urine output), polyphagia (excessive hunger), and lipemia.

Two primary criteria are used to clinically establish an individual as suffering from diabetes mellitus. One is a fasting plasma glucose (FPG) level in excess of 126 mg/dL (7 mmol/L) where normal levels should be less than 100 mg/dL (5.6 mmol/L). The second is defined by the results of a glucose tolerance test where having plasma glucose levels in excess of 200 mg/dL (11 mmol/L) at 2 time points during an oral glucose tolerance test (OGTT), one of which must be within 2 hours of ingestion of glucose (Figure 47-1).

The earlier a person is diagnosed with diabetes (principally type 2), the better chance the person has of staving off the primary negative consequences which are renal failure, blindness and limb amputations due to circulatory problems. The American Diabetes Association recommends that physicians consider patients to be prediabetic if their FPG is above 100 mg/dL but less than 125 mg/dL and whose glucose levels are at least 140 mg/dL but less than 200 mg/dL following an oral glucose tolerance test (OGTT).

Types of Diabetes Mellitus

Diabetes mellitus is a heterogeneous clinical disorder with numerous causes. Two main classifications of diabetes mellitus exist, **idiopathic** and **secondary**. Idiopathic diabetes is divided into 2 main types: insulin dependent and noninsulin-dependent. Insulin-dependent diabetes mellitus (IDDM) is more commonly referred to as **Type 1 diabetes, T1D**. Noninsulin-dependent diabetes mellitus (NIDDM) is more commonly referred to as **Type 2 diabetes, T2D.**

Gestational diabetes mellitus (GDM) is considered a specific form of diabetes mellitus. It is characterized by glucose intolerance first appearing during pregnancy. Insulin resistance normally increases during pregnancy but most women respond to this with a compensatory increase in insulin secretion. A failure of this response is what causes gestational diabetes. Gestational diabetes most often manifests during the third trimester. Women who experience GDM are at higher risk for future development of typical Type 2 diabetes.

Another form of diabetes is **diabetes insipidus,** which is the result of a deficiency of antidiuretic hormone (ADH, also referred to as vasopressin or arginine

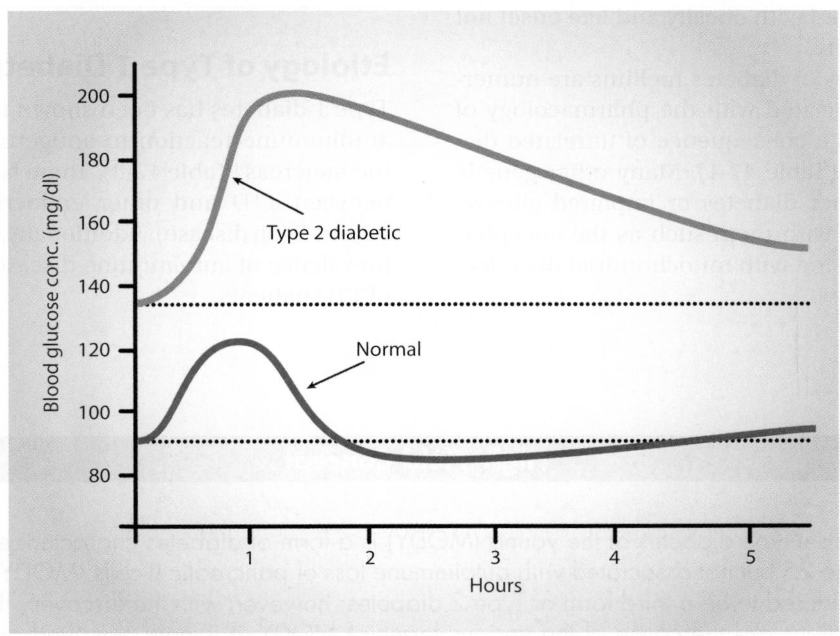

FIGURE 47-1: Glucose tolerance curve for a normal person and one with noninsulin-dependent diabetes mellitus (NIDDM, Type 2 diabetes). The dotted lines indicate the boundaries for the range of glucose concentration expected in a normal individual. Reproduced with permission of themedicalbiochemistrypage, LLC.

High-Yield Concept

There is a strong correlation between obesity and the onset of Type 2 diabetes with its associated insulin resistance. Due to the rise in childhood obesity, many children are developing Type 2 diabetes at an alarming rate. Although there is a strong correlation, it is important to recognize that obesity alone does not always lead to insulin resistance as some individuals who are obese do not experience insulin resistance and, conversely, some individuals who manifest insulin resistance are not obese. These latter observations point to the added role of genetics in the acquisition of insulin resistance.

vasopressin, AVP). The major symptom of diabetes insipidus (excessive output of dilute urine) results from an inability of the kidneys to reabsorb water.

Type 1 diabetes most often manifests in childhood (archaically called juvenile onset diabetes) and is the result of an autoimmune destruction of the β-cells of the pancreas. This form of diabetes is defined by the development of potentially fatal ketoacidosis in the absence of insulin therapy.

Type 2 diabetes is characterized by persistent hyperglycemia but rarely leads to ketoacidosis. Type 2 diabetes generally manifests after age 40 and, therefore, has the obsolete name of adult onset-type diabetes. Type 2 diabetes can result from genetic defects that cause either insulin resistance or insulin deficiency or both. There are 2 main forms of Type 2 diabetes defined as late onset associated with obesity and late onset not associated with obesity.

Secondary causes of diabetes mellitus are numerous and can be associated with the pharmacology of certain drugs and as a consequence of unrelated diseases and disorders (Table 47-1). Many other genetic syndromes have either diabetes or impaired glucose tolerance associated with them such as the encephalomyopathies associated with mitochondrial disorders (see Chapter 17).

Maturity-Onset Type Diabetes in the Young

All cases of MODY are associated with some level of impaired β-cell function characterized by defective GSIS (glucose-stimulated insulin secretion). Patients may also exhibit insulin resistance and late β-cell failure. Evidence indicates that mutations in 10-12 different genes have been correlated with the development of MODY (Table 47-2).

Type 1 Diabetes: Insulin-Dependent Diabetes Mellitus

Etiology of Type 1 Diabetes

Type 1 diabetes has been shown to be the result of an autoimmune reaction to antigens of the islet cells of the pancreas (Table 47-3). There is a strong association between T1D and other endocrine autoimmunities (eg, Addison disease). Additionally, there is an increased prevalence of autoimmune disease in family members of T1D patients.

High-Yield Concept

Maturity-onset type diabetes of the young (MODY) is a form of diabetes characterized by onset prior to age 25 but not associated with autoimmune loss of pancreatic β-cells. MODY was previously considered to be a third form of Type 2 diabetes; however, with the discovery that specific gene mutations are the cause of the various forms of MODY, it is now classified as a specific type of diabetes.

TABLE 47-1: Diseases/disorders Resulting in Secondary Diabetes	
Pancreatic disease	Pancreatectomy leads to the clearest example of secondary diabetes. Cystic fibrosis and pancreatitis can also lead to destruction of the pancreas
Endocrine disease	Some tumors can produce counter-regulatory hormones that oppose the action of insulin or inhibit insulin secretion. These counter-regulatory hormones are glucagon, epinephrine, growth hormone, and cortisol
Glucagonomas	Pancreatic cancers that secrete glucagon
Pheochromocytomas	Adrenal medullary tumors that secrete excess epinephrine
Cushing syndrome (see Clinical Box 50-2)	Most often due to excess ACTH secretion from a pituitary adenoma, results in excess cortisol secretion from adrenal glands
Acromegaly	Resulting from excess growth hormone production
Donohue syndrome	Also called Leprechaunism, impaired insulin receptor function, 3 common clinical features are hyperinsulinemia, acanthosis nigricans, and hyperandrogenism (the latter being observed only in females)
Rabson-Mendenhall syndrome	Mutations in insulin receptor gene, same 3 common clinical features seen in Donohue syndrome

TABLE 47-2: Forms of MODY

Type	*Gene*	*Encoded Protein*	*Comments*
MODY1	HNF4A	Hepatocyte nuclear factor-4α, HNF-4α	Also called transcription factor-14 (TCF14); expression of HNF-4α is associated with the growth and normal functioning of the pancreas; genes regulated by HNF-4α include *HNF1A*, *PPARA*, insulin, glucose-6-phosphatase, *GLUT2*, *L-PK* which is also expressed in the pancreas, glyceraldehyde-3-phosphate dehydrogenase (*G3PDH*), aldolase B and uncoupling protein 2, *UCP2*
MODY2	GCK	Glucokinase	Because the enzyme is responsive to glucose uptake it is often referred to as the pancreatic glucose sensor
MODY3	HNF1A	Hepatocyte nuclear factor-1α, HNF-1α	Also called transcription factor-1 (TCF1); is involved in a regulatory loop with HNF-4α controlling many genes involved in pancreatic and liver function such as the *GLUT2* and *L-PK*
MODY4	PDX1	Pancreas duodenum homeobox-1	A homeodomain-containing transcription factor; also called insulin promoter factor-1 (IPF-1); involved in pancreatic precursor determination in cells of the developing gut; major activator of insulin gene transcription in mature pancreas
MODY5	HNF1B	Hepatocyte nuclear factor-1β, HNF-1β	Also called transcription factor-2 (TCF2); is a critical regulator of a transcriptional network that controls the specification, growth, and differentiation of the embryonic pancreas; mutations in HNF-1β are associated with pancreatic hypoplasia, defective kidney development and genital malformations
MODY6	NEU-ROD1	Neurogenic differentiation 1, NeuroD1	A basic helix-loop-helix (bHLH) type transcription factor first identified as a neural fate-inducing gene; regulates insulin gene transcription
MODY7	KLF11	Krupple-like factor 11, KLF11	a zinc-finger transcription factor involved in activation at the insulin promoter; is a TGF-β-inducible transcription factor
MODY8	CEL	Carboxyl-ester lipase, CEL	Involved in dietary lipid metabolism (see Chapter 43); frameshift deletions in the variable number tandem repeats (VNTR) of the *CEL* gene are associated with pancreatic exocrine and β-cell dysfunction
MODY9	PAX4	Paired box 4, PAX4	A paired box domain-containing transcription factor; involved in the differentiation of endoderm-derived endocrine pancreas
MODY10	INS	Insulin	This form of MODY is associated with heterozygosity for missense mutations in the *INS* gene
MODY11	BLK	B-lymphocyte specific tyrosine kinase, BLK	Polymorphisms in BLK are associated with a higher prevalence of obesity and diabetes than with other MODY loci

TABLE 47-3: Most Common Autoantibodies Detected in Type 1 Diabetics

Autoantibodies	*Comments*
Islet cell cytoplasmic antibodies, ICCAs	These are the primary antibodies found in 90% of T1D patients; presence of ICCA is a highly accurate predictor of future development of T1D; ICCAs are not specific for β-cells antigens but the autoimmune attack appears to selectively destroy β-cells; titer of the ICCA tends to decline over time
Islet cell surface antibodies, ICSAs	Found in up to 80% of T1D patients; titer of ICSA declines over time; some patients with T2D have been identified that are ICSA positive
Glutamic acid decarboxylase, GAD	Found in up to 80% of T1D patients; titer of anti-GAD declines over time; 2 GAD genes, *GAD1* and *GAD2*; *GAD1* encodes GAD67, *GAD2* encodes GAD65 (reflects protein MW); *GAD1* and *GAD2* genes expressed in the brain, *GAD2* expression also in pancreas; presence of anti-GAD antibodies (both anti-GAD65 and anti-GAD67) is a strong predictor of the future development of T1D
Anti-insulin antibodies, IAAs	detectable in around 40% of children with T1D

Pathophysiology of Type 1 Diabetes

The autoimmune destruction of pancreatic β-cells in T1D leads to a deficiency of insulin secretion. It is this loss of insulin secretion that leads to the metabolic derangements associated with T1D.

The resultant inappropriately elevated glucagon level exacerbates the metabolic defects due to insulin deficiency. The most pronounced example of this metabolic disruption is that patients with T1D rapidly develop diabetic ketoacidosis in the absence of insulin administration. Particularly problematic for long-term T1D patients is an impaired ability to secrete glucagon in response to hypoglycemia. This leads to potentially fatal hypoglycemia in response to insulin treatment in these patients.

Although insulin deficiency is the primary defect in T1D, in patients with poorly controlled T1D there is also a defect in the ability of target tissues to respond to the administration of insulin. There are multiple biochemical mechanisms that account for this impairment. Deficiency in insulin leads to elevated levels of free fatty acids in the plasma as a result of uncontrolled lipolysis in adipose tissue. Free fatty acids suppress glucose metabolism in peripheral tissues such as skeletal muscle. This impairs the action of insulin in these tissues, that is, the promotion of glucose utilization. Additionally, insulin deficiency decreases the expression of a number of genes necessary for target tissues to respond normally to insulin such as glucokinase in liver and the GLUT4 class of glucose transporters in adipose tissue and skeletal muscle. The major metabolic derangements which result from insulin deficiency in T1D are impaired glucose, lipid, and protein metabolism (Figure 47-2).

Glucose metabolism

Uncontrolled T1D leads to increased hepatic glucose output. Excess glucagon stimulates hepatic glycogen breakdown and gluconeogenesis resulting in intracellular glucose levels exceeding the metabolic capacity of the liver so it is released to the blood. In addition, the level of hepatic glucokinase is regulated by insulin. Therefore, a reduced rate of glucose phosphorylation in hepatocytes leads to increased glucose delivery to the blood.

The insulin deficiency simultaneously impairs nonhepatic tissue utilization of glucose, primarily adipose tissue and skeletal muscle, resulting in hyperglycemia. Other enzymes involved in anabolic metabolism of glucose are affected by insulin primarily through induced

High-Yield Concept

In addition to the loss of insulin secretion, the function of pancreatic α-cells is also abnormal resulting in excessive secretion of glucagon in T1D patients. Normally, hyperglycemia leads to reduced glucagon secretion. However, in patients with T1D, glucagon secretion is not suppressed by hyperglycemia.

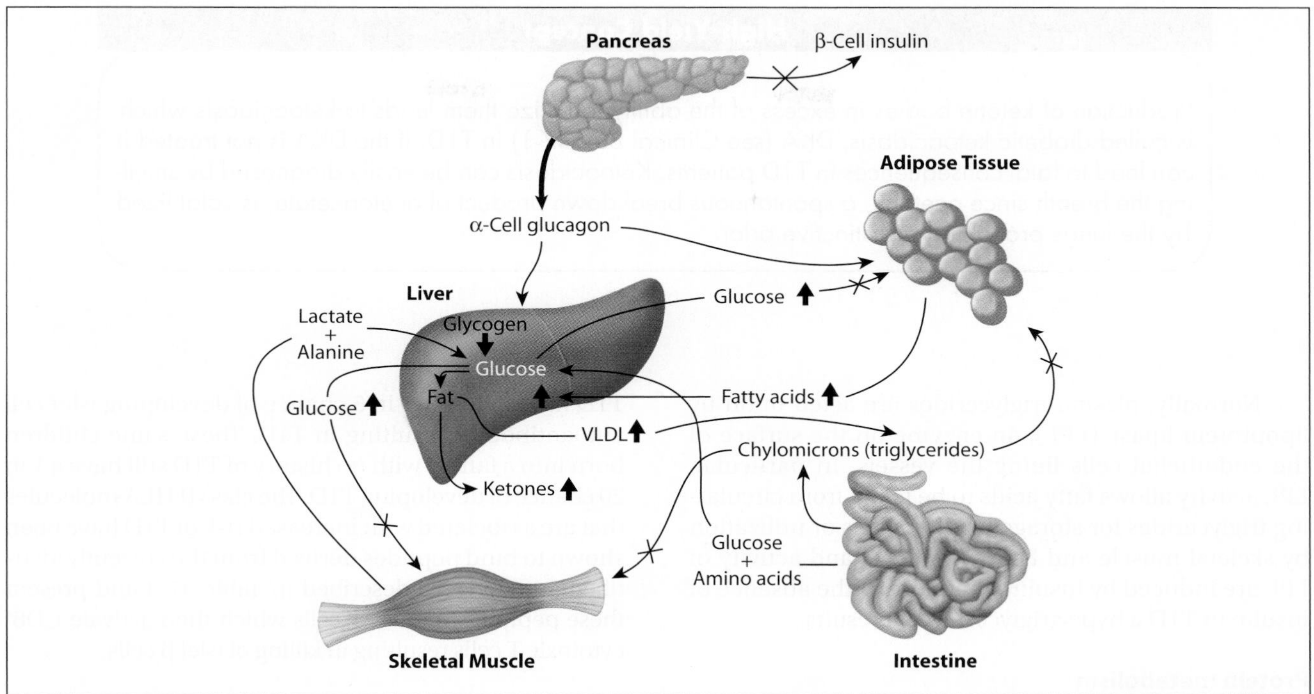

FIGURE 47-2: Metabolic disruptions occurring in T1D. The major metabolic disturbances associated with T1D are the result of the loss of insulin and uncontrolled increases in glucagon secretion from the pancreas. Glucagon stimulates triglyceride hydrolysis in adipose tissue and increases glycogen breakdown and gluconeogenesis in the liver. The glucose released from the liver is not taken up by adipose tissue or muscle due to loss of insulin-mediated GLUT4 migration to the plasma membrane. Lipid homeostasis in the liver is shifted to oxidation resulting in elevated ketone production. Whatever triglyceride that is incorporated into very-low-density lipoprotein (VLDL) in the liver and in chylomicrons from the gut cannot be taken up by adipose tissue due to the enhanced lipolysis occurring in this tissue. Skeletal muscle alanine and lactate contribute to glucose production by the liver exacerbating the hyperglycemia resulting from impaired insulin responses. Reproduced with permission of themedicalbiochemistrypage, LLC.

covalent modifications. The combination of increased hepatic glucose production and reduced peripheral tissues metabolism leads to elevated plasma glucose levels. When the capacity of the kidneys to absorb glucose is surpassed, **glucosuria** ensues. Glucose is an osmotic diuretic and an increase in renal loss of glucose is accompanied by loss of water and electrolytes, termed **polyuria**. The result of the loss of water (and overall volume) leads to the hyperactivation of the thirst mechanism (**polydipsia**). The negative caloric balance which results from the glucosuria and tissue catabolism leads to an increase in appetite and food intake (**polyphagia**).

Lipid metabolism

One major role of insulin is to stimulate the storage of food energy following the consumption of a meal. This energy storage is in the form of glycogen in hepatocytes and skeletal muscle. Additionally, insulin stimulates hepatocytes to synthesize triglycerides and storage of triglycerides in adipose tissue. Adipocyte tissue storage of triglycerides is normally favored due to insulin-mediated inhibition of lipolysis. In uncontrolled T1D there is a rapid mobilization of triglycerides due to excess glucagon release from the pancreas leading to increased levels of plasma free fatty acids (FFAs). The FFAs are taken up by numerous tissues, including the liver, and metabolized to provide energy.

Normally, the levels of malonyl-CoA are high in the presence of insulin. These high levels of malonyl-CoA inhibit carnitine palmitoyltransferase I, the enzyme required for the transport of fatty acyl-CoAs into the mitochondria where they are subjected to oxidation for energy production. Thus, in the absence of insulin, malonyl-CoA levels fall and transport of fatty acyl-CoAs into the mitochondria increases. Mitochondrial oxidation of fatty acids generates acetyl-CoA, which can be further oxidized in the TCA cycle. In hepatocytes the majority of the acetyl-CoA is metabolized into the ketone bodies (see Chapter 25). These ketone bodies leave the liver and are used for energy production by the brain, heart, and skeletal muscle. In T1D, the increased availability of free fatty acids exacerbates the reduced uptake and utilization of glucose by adipose tissue and skeletal muscle, furthering the ensuing hyperglycemia.

High-Yield Concept

Production of ketone bodies in excess of the ability to utilize them leads to ketoacidosis which is called diabetic ketoacidosis, DKA (see Clinical Box 47-1) in T1D. If the DKA is not treated it can lead to fatal consequences in T1D patients. Ketoacidosis can be easily diagnosed by smelling the breath since acetone, a spontaneous breakdown product of acetoacetate, is volatilized by the lungs producing a distinctive odor.

Normally, plasma triglycerides are acted upon by lipoprotein lipase (LPL), an enzyme on the surface of the endothelial cells lining the vessels. In particular, LPL activity allows fatty acids to be taken from circulating triglycerides for storage in adipocytes or utilization by skeletal muscle and heart. The level and activity of LPL are induced by insulin, therefore in the absence of insulin in T1D a hypertriglyceridemia results.

Protein metabolism

Insulin regulates the synthesis of many genes, either positively or negatively that then affect overall metabolism. Insulin has a global effect on protein metabolism, increasing the rate of protein synthesis and decreasing the rate of protein degradation. Thus, insulin deficiency will lead to increased catabolism of protein. The increased rate of proteolysis leads to elevated concentrations in plasma amino acids, particularly alanine and glutamine. These amino acids serve as precursors for hepatic, intestinal, and renal gluconeogenesis. In liver, the increased gluconeogenesis further contributes to the hyperglycemia seen in T1D (Clinical Box 47-1).

The Immunology of Type 1 Diabetes

The majority of genetic loci associated with the development of Type 1 diabetes (T1D) map to the human leukocyte antigen (HLA) class II proteins which are encoded for by genes in the major histocompatibility complex (MHC). This is not to say that all genetic associations in T1D are due to mutations in HLA genes as more than 40 additional T1D susceptibility loci have been identified that are not HLA genes.

The most frequently observed non-HLA genes associated with T1D are the insulin (INS), protein tyrosine phosphatase, nonreceptor type 22 (PTPN22), cytotoxic T-lymphocyte–associated protein 4 (CTLA4), interleukin-2 receptor-α (IL2RA), and interferon-induced with helicase C domain 1 (*IFIH1*) genes. Polymorphisms in the INS gene account for approximately 10% of genetic susceptibilities to T1D.

Children with the high-risk HLA alleles DR3/4–DRQ or DR4/DR4 and who have a family history of T1D have a nearly 1 in 5 chance of developing islet cell autoantibodies resulting in T1D. These same children born into a family with no history of T1D still have a 1 in 20 chance of developing T1D. The class II HLA molecules that are associated with increased risk of T1D have been shown to bind peptides derived from the currently identified autoantigens described in Table 47-3 and present these peptides to $CD4^+$ T cells which then activate $CD8^+$ cytotoxic T cells resulting in killing of islet β cells.

Type 2 Diabetes: Noninsulin-Dependent Diabetes Mellitus

Etiology of Type 2 Diabetes

Type 2 diabetes refers to the common form of idiopathic diabetes mellitus. Type 2 diabetes is generally characterized by late onset (hence the archaic term of adult-onset diabetes) and a lack of ketoacidosis. Type 2 diabetes is not an autoimmune disorder; however, there are strong genetic correlations to the susceptibility to this form of diabetes. Obesity is a major risk factor that predisposes one to T2D. Genetic studies have demonstrated a link between genes responsible for obesity and those that cause diabetes mellitus.

Pathophysiology of Type 2 Diabetes

Insulin resistance (IR) is suggested to be the primary cause of T2D. However, because a moderate degree of IR is not sufficient to cause T2D others contend that insulin deficiency is the primary cause. Patients with T2D who do not control their glucose levels through proper diet and exercise will eventually see a reduction or loss of insulin production and will, therefore, eventually require insulin injections to control their disease.

The major clinical complications of T2D are the result of persistent hyperglycemia which leads to numerous pathophysiological consequences (Figure 47-3). As the

High-Yield Concept

The highest risk populations for the development of T1D are children born with the HLA DR3/4–DQ8 serotype allele which accounts for almost 50% of all children who develop antibodies against pancreatic islet cells and thus develop T1D by the age of 5.

CLINICAL BOX 47-1: DIABETIC KETOACIDOSIS

The most severe and life-threatening complication of poorly controlled Type 1 diabetes is diabetic ketoacidosis (DKA). DKA is characterized by metabolic acidosis, hyperglycemia, and hyperketonemia. Diagnosis of DKA is accomplished by detection of hyperketonemia and metabolic acidosis (as measured by the anion gap) in the presence of hyperglycemia. The anion gap refers to the difference between the concentration of cations other than sodium and the concentration of anions other than chloride and bicarbonate. The anion gap, therefore, represents an artificial assessment of the unmeasured ions in plasma. Calculation of the anion gap involves sodium (Na^+), chloride (Cl^-), and bicarbonate (HCO_3^-) measurements and it is defined as $[Na^+ - (Cl^- + HCO_3^-)]$, where the sodium and chloride concentrations are measured in mEq/L and the bicarbonate concentration in mmol/L. The anion gap will increase when the concentration of plasma K^+, Ca^{2+}, or Mg^{2+} is decreased, when organic ions such as lactate are increased (or foreign anions accumulate), or when the concentration or charge of plasma proteins increases. Normal anion gap is between 8 and 12 mEq/L and a higher number is diagnostic of metabolic acidosis. Rapid and aggressive treatment is necessary as the metabolic acidosis will result in cerebral edema and coma eventually leading to death. The hyperketonemia in DKA is the result of insulin deficiency and unregulated glucagon secretion from α-cells of the pancreas. Circulating glucagon stimulates the adipose tissue to release fatty acids stored in triglycerides. The free fatty acids enter the circulation and are taken up primarily by the liver where they undergo fatty acid oxidation to acetyl-CoA. Normally, acetyl-CoA is completely oxidized to CO_2 and water in the TCA cycle. However, the level of fatty acid oxidation is in excess of the livers' ability to fully oxidize the excess acetyl-CoA and, thus, the compound is diverted into the ketogenesis pathway. The ketones (ketone bodies) are β-hydroxybutyrate and acetoacetate with β-hydroxybutyrate being the most abundant. Acetoacetate will spontaneously (nonenzymatic) decarboxylate to acetone. Acetone is volatile and is released from the lungs giving the characteristic sweet smell to the breath of someone with hyperketonemia. The ketones are released into the circulation and because they are acidic lower the pH of the blood resulting in metabolic acidosis. Insulin deficiency also causes increased triglyceride and protein metabolism in skeletal muscle. This leads to increased release of glycerol (from triglyceride metabolism) and alanine (from protein metabolism) to the circulation. These substances then enter the liver where they are used as substrates for gluconeogenesis, which is enhanced in the absence of insulin and the elevated glucagon. The increased rate of glucose production in the liver coupled with the glucagon-mediated inhibition of glucose storage into glycogen results in the increased glucose release from the liver and consequent hyperglycemia. The resultant hyperglycemia produces an osmotic diuresis that leads to loss of water and electrolytes in the urine. The ketones are also excreted in the urine, and this results in an obligatory loss of Na+ and K^+. The loss in K^+ is large, sometimes exceeding 300 mEq/L/24 h. Initial serum K^+ is typically normal or elevated because of the extracellular migration of K^+ in response to the metabolic acidosis. The level of K^+ will fall further during treatment as insulin therapy drives K^+ into cells. If serum K^+ is not monitored and replaced as needed (see below), life-threatening hypokalemia may develop. Each case of DKA must be treated on an individual basis. Table 47-4 shows a general scheme for diagnosis and treatment of DKA.

TABLE 47-4: Assessment and Treatment of Diabetic Ketoacidosis

Initial Assessment of DKA	Blood glucose >250 mg/dL Arterial pH <7.3 Serum bicarbonate <15 mEq/L Urinary ketones ≥3+ and/or serum ketones are positive
Monitoring	Vital signs every hour Serum glucose every hour and as needed Blood gas pH every 2 h (use arterial for 1st measurement then can use venous) Electrolytes every 1-2 h Urine ketones on each void Fluid input and output continuously Magnesium and phosphorous immediately and then every 1-2 h
Fluid management	Start normal saline at 1 L/h or 15-20 mL/kg/h initially Determine hydration status, goal being to replace 50% of estimated volume loss in the 1st 4 h, then remainder over next 8-12 h Infuse normal saline 125-500 mL/h, rate dependent on hydration status Once serum Na+ is corrected, infuse ½ normal saline at 4-14 mL/kg/h When serum glucose reaches 250 mg/dL, change fluid to D5W ½ normal saline at same rate
Insulin management	Discontinue all oral diabetic medications and previous insulin orders Give regular insulin **IV** bolus of 10 units Start insulin infusion usually at a rate of 0.15 unit/kg Insulin administration goal is to reduce serum glucose 50-70 mg/dL/h When serum glucose is ≤150 mg/dL, then can switch to adult SQ insulin with basal insulin
Potassium management	If serum K^+ is <3.3, give 40 mEq/h until it is >3.3 If serum K^+ is >3.3 but <5, give 20-30 mEq/L of IV fluids to keep serum K^+ between 4 and 5 mEq/L If serum K^+ is ≥5, do not give K^+ but check serum levels every 2 h When replacing K^+ both potassium chloride and potassium phosphate can be used Hold K^+ replacement if patient urine output is <30 mL/h
Bicarbonate management	Assess need for bicarbonate by arterial pH measurement If pH <6.9, give 100 mEq sodium bicarbonate in 1 L D5W and infuse at 200 mL/hr If pH is 6.9-7 give 50 mEq sodium bicarbonate in 1 L D5W and infuse at 200 mL/h If pH >7, do not give bicarbonate Continue sodium bicarbonate administration until pH is >7 Monitor serum K^+

glucose level rises in the blood, the blood becomes more viscous which makes circulation in the small capillaries difficult. The reduced circulation results in progressive vascular complications leading to diabetic retinopathy (referred to as diabetic blindness), peripheral neuropathy (resulting in numbness in the extremities and tingling in fingers and toes), poor wound healing, renal failure, and erectile dysfunction. In addition to these major clinical complications, the body reacts by increasing the level of glucose excretion by the kidneys leading to frequent urination (polyuria). As the glucose is excreted there is a concomitant loss of water to maintain normal osmolarity

High-Yield Concept

Unlike patients with T1D, those with T2D have detectable levels of circulating insulin. On the basis of oral glucose tolerance testing the essential elements of T2D can be divided into 4 distinct groups; those with normal glucose tolerance, chemical diabetes (called impaired glucose tolerance), diabetes with minimal fasting hyperglycemia (FPG <140 mg/dL), and diabetes in association with overt fasting hyperglycemia (FPG >140 mg/dL). Most patients with T2D will first exhibit normal to high insulin secretion but have impaired peripheral tissue responses, primarily reduced adipose tissue and skeletal muscle glucose disposal.

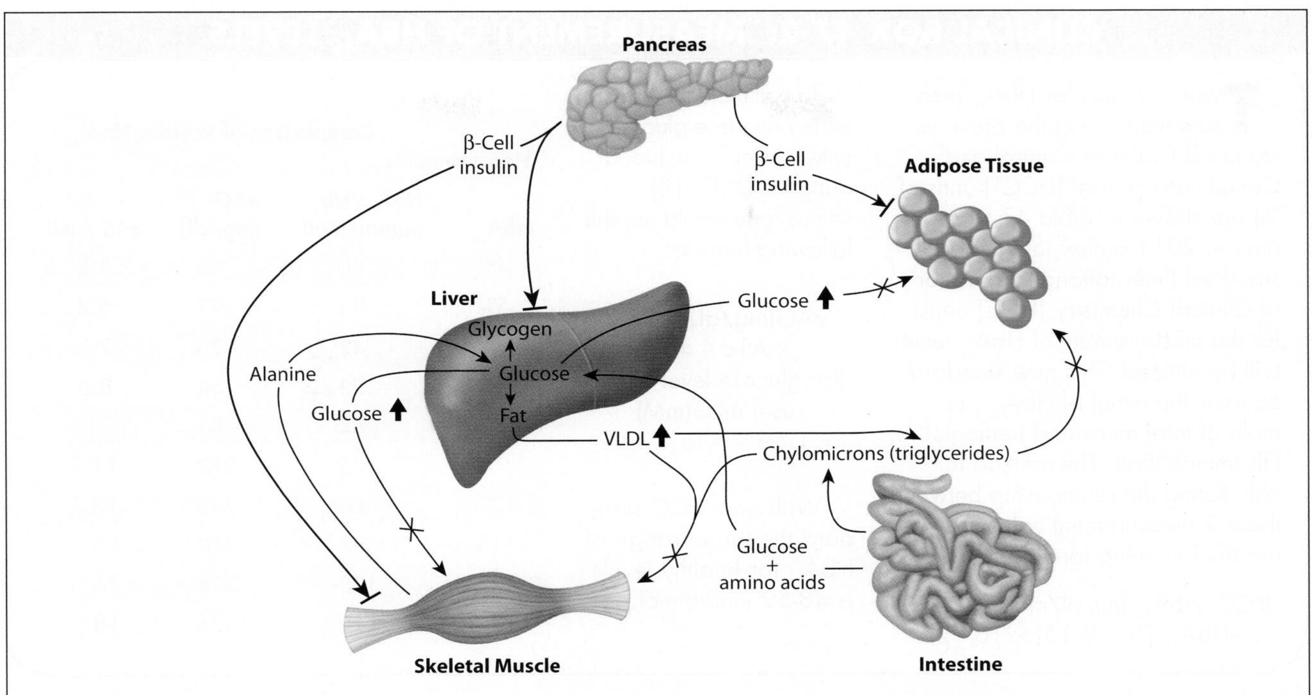

FIGURE 47-3: Metabolic disruptions occurring in T2D. The major metabolic disturbances associated with T2D are the result of impaired peripheral tissue responses to insulin, primarily the liver, skeletal muscle, and adipose tissue. The bars at the ends of the insulin arrows denote the failure of the hormone to activate normal signaling in these tissues. The insulin resistance results in elevated glucose and VLDL output by the liver; this coupled to impaired glucose uptake by skeletal muscle and adipose tissue results in hyperglycemia and hyperlipidemia. Reproduced with permission of themedicalbiochemistrypage, LLC.

of the urine. The water loss leads to excessive thirst called polydypsia.

As pointed out, persistent hyperglycemia is the major physiological complication associated with T2D. Indeed, the development of hypoglycemia inducing drugs is the major pharmacological focus of T2D therapies.

Since hemoglobin is present in red blood cells and these cells have a limited life span of 120 days in the circulation, measurement of HbA_{1c} levels is a relatively accurate measure of the amount of glucose in the blood and the length of time the level has been elevated.

Genetics of Type 2 Diabetes

Development of T2D is the result of multifactorial influences that include lifestyle, environment, and genetics. The disease arises when insulin resistance–induced compensatory insulin secretion is exhausted. A high-caloric diet, coupled with a sedentary lifestyle, is the major contributing factors in the development of the insulin resistance and pancreatic β-cell dysfunction. However, a predisposing genetic background has long been suspected in playing a contributing role in the development of T2D.

Using genome-wide association studies (GWAS), the first major susceptibility locus for T2D was identified in 1996. This locus was designated NIDDM1. The first gene identified in the NIDDM1 locus with polymorphisms correlated to T2D susceptibility was calpain 10 (*CAPN10*). Calpain 10 is a calcium-activated neutral protease that is likely to have a critical role in the survival of pancreatic β-cells. Genetic variants in *CAPN10* may alter insulin secretion or insulin action

High-Yield Concept

Assessment of therapeutic efficacy in the treatment of the hyperglycemia in T2D is accomplished by routine measurement of the circulating levels of glycosylated hemoglobin, designated as the level of HbA_{1c}, often designated as just A1c (Clinical Box 47-2). HbA1 is the major form of adult hemoglobin in the blood and the "c" refers to the glycosylated form of the protein.

CLINICAL BOX 47-2: MEASUREMENT OF HBA_{1C} LEVELS

Typical values for HbA_{1c} measurement (using the previous standard Diabetes Control and Complications Trial [DCCT] units of %) are shown in Table 47-5. Beginning in 2011 a new international standard (International Federation of Clinical Chemistry [IFCC[units) for the measurement of HbA_{1c} levels will be utilized. This new standard equates the mmol of HbA_{1c} per mole of total measured hemoglobin, Hb (mmol/mol). The method for calculating the relationship between these 2 measurement values is to use the following formula:

$$\text{IFCC–HbA}_{1c}\ (\text{mmol/mol}) = [\text{DCCT–HbA}_{1c}\ (\%) - 2.15] \times 10.929$$

To calculate the estimated average glucose (eAG) level in the blood using the DCCT (%) values, one would use the following formula:

$$\text{eAG(mg/dL)} = 28.7 \times \text{A1c} - 46.7$$

(for glucose level in mM use: $\text{eAG(mM)} = 1.59 \times \text{A1c} - 2.59$

With new IFCC standard the target range of HbA_{1c} for healthy levels is 48-59 mmol/mol.

TABLE 47-5: Comparison of Various HbA_{1c} Measurements

HbA_{1c}	HbA_{1c}/Hb (mmol/mol)	eAG (mg/dL)	eAG (mM)
4%	20	68	3.8
5%	31	97	5.4
6%	42	125	7
7%	53	154	8.5
8%	64	183	10
9%	75	212	11.7
10%	86	240	13.3
11%	97	270	15
12%	108	298	16.5
13%	119	326	18

as well as the production of glucose by the liver. Recent studies indicate that *CAPN10* may have a critical role in the survival of pancreatic β-cells.

More recent GWAS screens for single nucleotide polymorphisms (SNPs) associated with T2D have identified several new candidate genes (Table 47-6). The transcription factor *TCF7L2* (transcription factor 7-like 2, T-cell specific HMG-box) is involved in the signaling pathways initiated by the Wnt family of secreted growth factors (see Chapter 46). Two SNPs identified in the *TCF7L2* gene are the most highly correlated polymorphisms with T2D.

Neonatal Diabetes

Neonatal diabetes can be transient or permanent. If an infant suffers from the transient form they are at increased risk for developing full-blown diabetes later in life. The permanent form of the disease is termed permanent neonatal diabetes mellitus (PNDM). PNDM is a rare event occurring with a frequency of approximately 2 cases per 100,000 births. Definitive determination of PNDM requires early gene screening as soon as symptoms manifest. Very low birth weight is highly correlated to PNDM and is associated with fetal lack of insulin. The most prominent of symptoms is the onset of hyperglycemia within the first 6 months after birth. Affected infants do not secrete insulin in response to glucose or glucagon but will secrete insulin in response to sulfonylurea administration. Many infants will exhibit similar neurological abnormalities, including developmental delay, muscle weakness, and epilepsy. In patients manifesting with neurological abnormalities, there are often associated dysmorphic features, including prominent metopic suture, a downturned mouth, bilateral ptosis, and limb contractures.

Genetic evidence demonstrates that PNDM is the result of single-gene defects. The disorder can be inherited, although it is most often the result of a sporadic mutation in one of the parental gametes. At least 12 genes have been identified as being associated with the development of PNDM. The most commonly mutated genes are the potassium inwardly-rectifying channel, subfamily J, member 11 (*KCNJ11*), ATP-binding cassette transporter, subfamily C, member 8 (*ABCC8*), and insulin (*INS*) genes.

Mitochondrial Dysfunction in Obesity and T2D

Chapter 17 discusses the normal biogenesis of mitochondria and the gene defects associated with the mitochondrial encephalomyopathies.

Mitochondrial dysfunction results in increased production of reactive oxygen species (ROS), which activates

TABLE 47-6: Polymorphic Genes Associated With Increased Risk for Type 2 Diabetes[1]

Gene Name	*Gene Symbol*	*Gene Function/Comments*	*Disease Mechanism*
Calpain 10	*CAPN10*	See text	Glucose transport
Fat mass- and obesity-associated gene	*FTO*	Catalyzes the iron- and 2-oxoglutarate-dependent demethylation of 3-methylthymine in single-stranded DNA, with concomitant production of succinate, formaldehyde, and CO_2	Obesity
Insulin degrading enzyme	*IDE*	Is an extracellular thiol metalloprotease with preference for insulin, also degrades amyloid-β protein; the *IDE* gene resides within the same chromosomal locus as HHEX	β-Cell dysfunction
Potassium inwardly-rectifying channel, subfamily J, member 11	*KCNJ11*	Forms the core of the ATP-sensitive potassium (KATP) channel involved in insulin secretion, protein is also called Kir6.2	β-Cell dysfunction
Melanocortin 4 receptor	*MC4R*	Is a single exon (intronless) gene, mutations in this gene are the most frequent genetic cause of severe obesity, receptor binds α-melanocyte stimulating hormone (α-MSH)	Obesity
Peroxisome proliferator-activated receptor-γ (PPARg)	*PPARG*	Transcriptional coactivator with retinoid X receptors (RXRs), master regulator of adipogenesis, activation of adipocytes leads to increased fat storage and secretion of insulin-sensitizing adipocytokines such as adiponectin	Insulin sensitivity
Solute carrier family 30 (zinc transporter), member 8	*SCL30A8*	Permits cellular efflux of zinc	β-Cell dysfunction
Transcription factor 7-like 2 (T-cell specific HMG-box)	*TCF7L2*	See text	β-Cell dysfunction, impaired insulin secretion

[1] Not intended to be a complete presentation of all T2D-associated polymorphisms.

High-Yield Concept

Neonatal diabetes refers to a circumstance in which hyperglycemia results from dysfunction in insulin action within the first 6 months of life. The etiology of diabetes in the first year of life is different from that of the autoimmune forms of T1D more classically diagnosed when children are older.

High-Yield Concept

Mitochondrial dysfunction, particularly as it relates to the processes of oxidative phosphorylation (oxphos), is contributory to the development of encephalomyopathy, mitochondrial myopathy, and several age-related disorders that include neurodegenerative diseases, the metabolic syndrome, and diabetes. Indeed, with respect to diabetes, several mitochondrial diseases manifest with diabetic complications such as mitochondrial myopathy, encephalopathy, lactic acidosis, and stroke-like episodes (MELAS) and maternally inherited diabetes and deafness (MIDD).

stress responses leading to increased activity of MAPK and JNK. Both of these serine/threonine kinases phosphorylate IRS1 and IRS2 resulting in decreased signaling downstream of the insulin receptor such as activation of PI3K. Inhibition of PI3K results in reduced glucose uptake in skeletal muscle and adipose tissue due to impaired mobilization of GLUT4 vesicles to the plasma membrane.

Mitochondrial dysfunction also results in a reduction in the level of enzymes involved in β-oxidation leading to increases in intramyocellular lipid content. Indeed, skeletal muscle metabolism of lipids is impaired in T2D. An increased delivery of fatty acids to skeletal muscle, as well as diminished mitochondrial oxidation, results in increased intracellular content of fatty acid metabolites such as diacylglycerol (DAG), fatty acyl-CoAs, and ceramides. These metabolites of fatty acids are all known to induce the activity of protein kinase C isoforms (PKCβ and PKCδ) that phosphorylate IRS1 and IRS2 on serine residues resulting in impaired insulin signaling downstream of the insulin receptor (see Figure 46-7).

Skeletal muscle consumes large amounts of serum glucose, therefore mitochondrial dysfunction in this tissue will have the greatest impact on glucose disposal. However, adipose tissue also plays an important role in glucose homeostasis and mitochondrial dysfunction in this tissue also results in impaired glucose homeostasis contributing to the hyperglycemia in T2D. Adipose tissue secretes a number of proteins classified as adipokines (see Chapter 45). Adiponectin promotes insulin sensitivity in insulin-responsive tissues, such as skeletal muscle. Enhanced adipocyte mitochondrial biogenesis results in increased adiponectin release from adipose tissue. Conversely, expression of adiponectin expression is decreased in adipocytes with mitochondrial dysfunction.

Given that impaired mitochondrial function is clearly associated with obesity and T2D, it is not surprising that there is great interest in the use of pharmacological agents to augment mitochondrial function in the treatment of these disorders. Of significance is the fact that the thiazolidinedione (TZD) class of drug, used to treat the hyperglycemia of T2D (see the next section), activate PPARγ which in turn increases the level of activity of PGC-1α which is a major regulator of mitochondrial biogenesis. Antioxidants have also been shown to enhance mitochondrial function by reducing the production of ROS. Resveratrol (found in grape skins and red wine) is a potent antioxidant whose activity is, in part, due to its ability to activate the deacetylase SIRT1. Activated SIRT1 deacetylates PGC-1α resulting in increased transcriptional activity and, thus, enhanced mitochondrial biogenesis.

Therapeutic Intervention for Hyperglycemia

Many, if not all, of the vascular consequences of insulin resistance are due to the persistent hyperglycemia seen in T2D. For this reason, a major goal of therapeutic intervention in T2D is to reduce circulating glucose levels. There are many pharmacological strategies to accomplish these goals (Table 47-7).

Diabetes Therapies on the Horizon

Several novel targets have been identified as potential treatments for T2D. These include the hepatic-derived fibroblast growth factor 21 (FGF21), the renal sodium-glucose transporter-2 (SGLT2), the NAD$^+$-dependent deacetylase SIRT1 or sirtuin 1, and the lipid-binding G-protein–coupled receptor GPR119.

FGF21 Agonists: Expression of FGF21 is significantly elevated under conditions of a high-fat, low-carbohydrate ketogenic diet. Additionally, reductions in FGF21 expression are associated with lipemia, reduced ketogenesis, and a resultant fatty liver. Administration of FGF21 to diabetic animals results in reduction in the levels of fasting glucose and serum lipids. These observations suggest that FGF21 plays a key role in regulating the expression of genes involved in hepatic lipid homeostasis and that activation of FGF21 activity could prove to be a significant tool in the treatment of the disrupted metabolic status in diabetic individuals.

SGLT2 Antagonists: A new class of orally administered compounds that targets renal glucose transport and inducers of glucosuria are currently being tested for efficacy in treating T2D. In the kidney, glucose is filtered at the glomerulus and then reabsorbed via active transport in the proximal convoluted tubule. Two sodium-glucose cotransporters (SGLT1 and SGLT2) are responsible for this renal glucose reabsorption. SGLT1 is expressed in other tissues and accounts for approximately 10% of the renal glucose reabsorption. SGLT2 is expressed exclusively in the S1 segment of the proximal tubule and is responsible for 90% of the renal glucose reabsorption (Figure 47-4). The drug, dapagliflozin, exhibits a high degree of selectivity for SGLT2 inhibition (1000 times greater than on SGLT1) and its use is associated with a dose-dependent reduction in serum glucose and hemoglobin A_{1c} levels.

SIRT1 Activators: SIRT1 or sirtuin 1 is the homolog of the yeast (*Saccharomyces cerevisiae*) *Sir2* gene (Sir refers to **S**ilent mating type **I**nformation **R**egulator).

TABLE 47-7: **Current Hypoglycemia-Inducing Drugs used in the Treatment of T2D**

Drug class	*Primary Target*	*Comments*
Thiazolidinediones, TZDs	PPARγ	Includes rosiglitazone (Avandia) and pioglitazone (Actos); agonists of PPARγ; net effect of TZDs is a potentiation of the actions of insulin in liver, adipose tissue, and skeletal muscle, increased peripheral glucose disposal and a decrease in glucose output by the liver; TZDs stimulate expression and release of adiponectin (see Chapter 45); mutations in PPARG correlate to familial insulin resistance
Mimetics, inhibitors	GLP-1 or DPP4	GLP-1 inhibits pancreatic glucagon secretion and enhances GSIS; GLP-1 is rapidly degraded by dipeptidylpeptidase IV (DPP4); GLP-1 mimetics and DPP4 inhibitors induce dramatic reductions in plasma glucose concentrations; GLP-1 mimetics include exenatide (βYETTA), which is derived from the lizard salivary peptide (exendin-4) which activates the GLP-1 receptor; liraglutide (Victoza) is another GLP-1 mimetic; DDP4 inhibitors include sitagliptin (Januvia), vildagliptin (Glavus), and saxagliptin (Onglyza)
Biguanides		Enhance insulin-mediated suppression of hepatic glucose production and insulin-stimulated glucose uptake by skeletal muscle; metformin (Glucophage) is the most widely prescribed insulin-sensitizing drug in current clinical use; because the major site of action for metformin is the liver. its use can be contraindicated in patients with liver dysfunction; improves insulin sensitivity by increasing insulin receptor tyrosine kinase activity, enhancing glycogen synthesis and increasing recruitment and transport of GLUT4 transporters to the plasma membrane; metformin also has a mild inhibitory effect on complex I of oxidative phosphorylation, has antioxidant properties, and activates both glucose-6-phosphate dehydrogenase and AMPK; metformin is highly recommended to reduce the incidence as well as the potential for polycystic ovarian syndrome, PCOS
Sulfonylureas	SUR protein (encoded by *ABCC8* gene), component of pancreatic KATP	Referred to as endogenous insulin secretagogues because they induce the pancreatic release of endogenous insulin; have been in use for over 50 years; tolbutamide, acetohexamide, chlorpropramide, and tolazamide were first generation in the class but are no longer routinely used; glipizide (Glucotrol), glimepiride (Amaryl), and glyburide (DiaBeta, Micronase, Glynase) are second generation drugs in class; all function by binding to and inhibiting the pancreatic KATP channel involved GSIS
Meglitinides	SUR protein (encoded by *ABCC8* gene), component of pancreatic KATP, different binding site than sulfonylureas	Nonsulfonylurea insulin secretagogues; includes repaglinide (Prandin) and nateglinide (Starlix); function by binding site on KATP distinct from the sulfonylureas
Glucosidase inhibitors	α-Glucosidase	Function by interfering with the action of the α-glucosidases present in small intestinal brush border cell membranes, thereby reducing intestinal uptake of glucose; includes acarbose (Precose) and miglitol (Glyset); function locally in the intestine and have no major systemic action; common adverse side effects of these inhibitors are abdominal bloating and discomfort, diarrhea, and flatulence

SIRT1 is a member of the sirtuin family of proteins (7 members; SIRT1 through SIRT7) shown in yeasts to regulate life-span extension, epigenetic gene silencing, and suppress recombination of ribosomal DNA (rDNA). SIRT1 is an NAD$^+$-dependent deacetylase that modulates the activities of proteins that are in pathways downstream of the beneficial effects of calorie restriction. Principal pathways involved in glucose homeostasis and insulin sensitivity are affected by SIRT1 activity. In skeletal muscle, a major site of insulin-induced glucose uptake, SIRT1 and AMPK work in concert to increase the rate of fatty acid oxidation in periods of decreased nutrient availability. The plant-derived compound, resveratrol (a polyphenolic compound), is a known activator of SIRT1 function and several drugs based upon the structure of resveratrol are currently being tested as SIRT1 activators. Compounds that activate SIRT1 improve insulin sensitivity in adipose tissue, liver, and skeletal muscle resulting in lower plasma glucose.

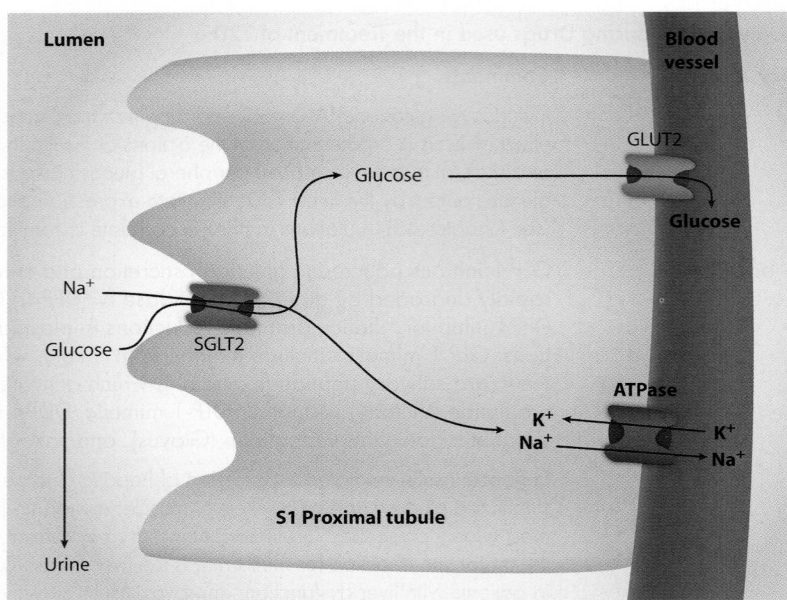

FIGURE 47-4: Diagrammatic representation of the reuptake of glucose in the S1 segment of the proximal tubule of the kidney by the Na^+-glucose cotransporter SGLT2. Following reuptake the glucose is transported back into the blood via the action of GLUT2 transporters. The Na^+ that is reabsorbed with the glucose is transported into the blood via a (Na^+-K^+)-ATPase. Reproduced with permission of themedicalbiochemistrypage, LLC.

GPR119 Agonists: The fatty acid–sensing receptor, GPR119, is a G_s-type G-coupled receptor. GPR119 is expressed at the highest levels in the pancreas and fetal liver. GPR119 binds long-chain fatty acids including various lipid amides and retinoic acid. Oleoylethanolamide (OEA) (see Chapter 23) most likely represents the endogenous ligand for GPR119. Administration of OEA causes a significant reduction in food intake and body weight gain. These effects of OEA are the result of the activation of the nuclear receptor PPARα, increased expression of fatty acid translocase, and modification of feeding behavior and motor activity. Activation of GPR119 in the pancreas is correlated with enhanced GSIS, whereas activation of GPR119 in the gut results in increased secretion of GLP-1 and GIP. These observations indicate that GPR119 activation is associated with a dual mechanism of reducing blood glucose: acting directly through pancreatic β-cells to promote GSIS, and in the gut via the stimulation of GLP1 and GIP secretion, both of which increase insulin release from the pancreas in response to food intake. Currently several small molecule agonists of GPR119 in clinical trials are being tested for their efficacy in treating T2D as well as for their efficacy in treating obesity.

REVIEW QUESTIONS

1. As a hypothetical approach to treating the hyperglycemia associated with Type 2 diabetes, a drug firm proposes to develop an inhibitor of liver glycogen phosphorylase. What is the biochemical rationale for this approach to inducing hypoglycemia?
   - A. hepatic fatty acid oxidation will decrease leading to reduced energy production needed for gluconeogenesis
   - B. hepatocytes will have a reduced capacity to store glucose following meals
   - C. liver glucose output will be reduced early during fasting
   - D. the resultant increase in glycogen storage will inhibit glucose uptake by the liver leading to increased utilization in skeletal muscle
   - E. there will be an increase in hepatic gluconeogenesis

Answer C: During early fasting, as the level of glucose in the blood falls, the pancreas releases glucagon into the circulation to counter this drop. The major site of glucagon action is the liver. There it induces the activity of the glycogen phosphorylase leading to an increase in glucose release from glycogen stores. Thus, an inhibition of glycogen phsphorylase would limit the ability of the liver to provide glucose to the blood. Negatively affecting the activity of glycogen phosphorylase would not significantly affect the rate of hepatic fatty acid oxidation, skeletal muscle glucose usage, nor hepatic gluconeogenesis.

2. In Type 1 diabetes there is an associated hyperlipidemia. The best explanation for this is that the level of an enzyme important for fat homeostasis is reduced. Which of the following is this enzyme?
A. acyl-CoA dehydrogenase (eg, MCAD)
B. carnitine palmitoyltransferase I
C. glucose 6-phosphatase
D. hepatic lipase
E. lipoprotein lipase

Answer E: One of the effects of insulin is to increase the level of lipoprotein lipase (LPL) expression in endothelial cells. The lack of normal levels of circulating insulin in Type 1 diabetics results in impaired regulation of LPL levels. Reduced LPL contributes to the hyperlipidemia associated with T1D.

3. Obesity, genetic profile, and aging all contribute to the development of Type 2 diabetes. Of the following, which is the most important additive factor for these 3 conditions in the development of Type 2 diabetes?
A. elevated hepatic ketogenesis
B. elevated pancreatic glucagon secretion
C. impaired renal clearance of glucose
D. increased adipose tissue activity leading to hyperlipidemia
E. muscle resistance to insulin

Answer E: The influence of obesity, genetic profile, and age on overall metabolism is most significant at the level of skeletal muscle sensitivity to the actions of insulin. Due to the overall mass of skeletal muscle in the body, the uptake of glucose by this tissue, and consequently its role in blood glucose homeostasis, is a significant factor in insulin responses. Progressive loss of skeletal muscle sensitivity to insulin leads to increased rates of visceral cell lipolysis and pancreatic β-cell compensation. Eventually, the pancreas can no longer continue compensating for impaired insulin responses and pancreatic β-cell decompensation occurs, further exacerbating the problem. The disrupted insulin response leads to increased hepatic gluconeogenesis, which further increases circulating glucose levels. The overall outcome of these responses is development of progressively worsening Type 2 diabetes.

4. The sulfonylurea class of drugs used to treat Type 2 diabetes function by which of the following mechanisms?
A. activating the PPARγ class of factors leading to increased hepatic glucose metabolism
B. binding to and blocking pancreatic K^+ channels leading to increased insulin secretion
C. interfering with carbohydrate digestion, thus reducing glucose intake
D. restricting hepatic glucose output, thereby reducing the hyperglycemia
E. stimulating pancreatic glucose metabolism leading to increased insulin secretion

Answer B: The sulfonylurea drugs function by binding to and inhibiting the pancreatic ATP-dependent K^+ channel (KATP) that is responsible for glucose-mediated insulin secretion. The normal pancreatic response to increased blood glucose is an increased uptake by β-cells with concomitant oxidation. The increase in glucose oxidation leads to an elevation in the ATP:ADP ratio. This in turn leads to an inhibition of the KATP channel. The net result is a depolarization of the cell leading to Ca^{2+} influx and insulin secretion.

5. Numerous pharmacological agents are currently being used in the clinic as a means to reduce the hyperglycemia associated with Type 2 diabetes. Which of the following class of compounds exerts a portion of their effects by activating the metabolic master regulator, AMPK?
A. biguanides (eg, Metformin)
B. α-glucosidase inhibitors (eg, Precose)
C. GLP-1 mimetics (eg, Byetta)
D. meglitinides (eg, Prandin)
E. sulfonylureas (eg, Glipizide)

Answer A: Metformin exerts part of its effects by modulating mitochondrial activities. Metformin has a mild inhibitory effect on complex I of oxidative phosphorylation, has antioxidant properties, and activates both glucose-6-phosphate dehydrogenase, G6PDH and AMPK. The importance of AMPK in the actions of metformin stems from the role of AMPK in the regulation of both lipid and carbohydrate metabolism. The activation of AMPK by metformin is likely related to the inhibitory effects of the drug on complex I of oxidative phosphorylation. This would lead to a reduction in ATP production and, therefore, an increase in the level of AMP and as a result activation of AMPK.

6. The Randle hypothesis was proposed to explain the acquisition of insulin resistance associated with central adiposity. Which of the following statements best reflects the basis of the Randle hypothesis?
A. an increase in adipocyte volume due to increased lipid storage causes adipocytes to lose their responsiveness to insulin
B. increased circulating free fatty acids in obese individuals impair the ability of insulin to stimulate skeletal muscle cell glucose uptake

C. long-term hyperlipidemia leads to permanent elevation in pancreatic insulin secretion that ultimately causes downregulation of insulin receptors
D. the high level of circulating free fatty acids stimulates the liver to shut off gluconeogenesis that then impairs pancreatic sensing of the need for insulin release
E. the hyperglycemia prevalent in obese individuals activates insulin release from the pancreas leading to increased adipocyte lipolysis

Answer B: The Randle hypothesis states that elevations in circulating free fatty acids (FFAs) interfere with insulin action in liver and skeletal muscle. Increased FFA uptake and metabolism by the liver results in an increased production of acetyl-CoA. All of the acetyl-CoA cannot be oxidized completely in the TCA cycle. The elevated acetyl-CoA levels result in inhibition of pyruvate dehydrogenase resulting in increased citrate transport to the cytosol. Increased cytosolic citrate inhibits 6-phosphofructokinase-1 (PFK1) resulting in reduced glucose oxidation and an increase in glucose-6-phosphate levels. Increases in glucose 6-phosphate lead to inhibition of skeletal muscle hexokinase resulting in reduced glucose utilization. In addition, the elevated plasma FFAs impair insulin receptor tyrosine phosphorylation of IRS1 resulting in defects in insulin-mediated signaling events in target cells, primarily skeletal muscle. Loss of insulin signaling in skeletal muscle prevents glucose transporter (GLUT4) mobilization to the cell surface with a resultant block to glucose uptake. The overall consequences of a high-fat diet are a progressive impairment in hepatic glucose homeostasis, impairment of insulin-mediated glucose uptake by skeletal muscle, and pancreatic β-cell decompensation. The latter leads to reduced insulin secretion and, thus, further impairment of the role of insulin in regulation of blood glucose.

7. Patients with poorly controlled diabetes have elevated levels of blood glucose. One severe consequence of the hyperglycemia is an increase in glucose attachment to serum proteins. Which of the following proteins, when glycosylated, is an excellent measure of the length of time someone has sufferred from an episode of hyperglycemia?
A. albumin
B. cholesterol
C. fatty acids
D. hemoglobin
E. transferrin

Answer D: Assessment of therapeutic management of the hyperglycemia in T2D is accomplished by routine measurement of the circulating levels of glycosylated hemoglobin, designated as the level of HbA_{1c}, often designated as just A_{1C}. Since hemoglobin is present in red blood cells and these cells have a limited life span of 120 days in the circulation, measurement of HbA_{1c} levels is a relatively accurate measure of the amount of glucose in the blood and the length of time the level has been elevated.

8. Type 1 diabetes is most often characterized by which of the following?
A. decreased glucagon secretion leading to hyperlipidemia
B. decreased insulin receptor response to insulin binding
C. elevated fatty acid oxidation leading to ketonemia
D. elevated insulin secretion leading to severe hypoglycemia
E. impaired glucagon-dependent inhibition of glycolysis leading to hyperglycemia

Answer C: The most frequent consequence of poorly controlled T1D is ketoacidosis, referred to as diabetic ketoacidosis, DKA. The hyperketonemia in DKA is the result of insulin deficiency and unregulated glucagon secretion from α-cells of the pancreas. Circulating glucagon stimulates the adipose tissue to release fatty acids which are taken up and oxidized, primarily by the liver. Under these conditions, the level of fatty acid oxidation is in excess of the livers' ability to fully oxidize the excess acetyl-CoA and, thus, the compound is diverted into ketones synthesis. The ketones are released into the circulation and because they are acidic lower the pH of the blood resulting in metabolic acidosis.

9. An investigational diabetes treatment involving a hypoglycemia-inducing drug has been developed. This drug is designed to inhibit dipeptidylpeptidase IV (DPP4) activity and has been shown to decrease plasma glucose concentration and pancreatic glucagon secretion. DPP4 hydrolyzes which of the following hormones such that its inhibition results in the observed effects?
A. glucagon
B. glucagon-like peptide-1 (GLP-1)
C. glucose-dependent insulinotropic peptide (GIP)
D. insulin
E. prohormone convertase-2/3

Answer B: GLP-1 stimulates postprandial insulin secretion and has also been shown to stimulate proliferation and inhibit apoptosis of pancreatic β-cells. GLP-1 also inhibits glucagon release from pancreatic α-cells, inhibits gastric emptying, and reduces food intake. DPP4 is involved in the degradation of GLP-1, thus DPP4 inhibitors act to prevent inactivation of and prolong the duration of action of GLP-1.

10. Which of the following would be evident in Type 1 diabetes?

A. decreased glucagon secretion leading to hyperlipidemia.
B. decreased insulin receptor response to insulin binding.
C. elevated glucagon secretion leading to hyperlipidemia.
D. elevated insulin secretion leading to severe hypoglycemia.
E. impaired glucagon-dependent inhibition of glycolysis leading to hyperglycemia

Answer C: In addition to the loss of insulin secretion by β-cells of the pancreas in T1D, the function of α-cells is also abnormal. There is excessive secretion of glucagon in T1D patients. Normally, hyperglycemia leads to reduced glucagon secretion. However, in patients with T1D, glucagon secretion is not suppressed by hyperglycemia. The resultant inappropriately elevated glucagon levels exacerbate the metabolic defects due to insulin deficiency.

11. Type 2 diabetes can best be characterized as which of the following?

A. adequate insulin secretion coupled to impaired postreceptor responses
B. being caused by autoimmune destruction of pancreatic β-cells
C. correlated to disruptions in glucagon secretion
D. lack of insulin receptors on hepatocyte
E. resulting in frequent episodes of ketoacidosis

Answer A: Unlike patients with T1D, those with T2D have detectable levels of circulating insulin but these individuals are resistant to the peripheral actions of insulin. In the progression from impaired glucose tolerance to full-blown T2D, the level of insulin secretion declines indicating that patients with T2D eventually have decreased insulin secretion. Additional studies have subsequently demonstrated that both insulin resistance and insulin deficiency is common in the average T2D patient.

12. Type 1 diabetes is highly associated with the inheritance of specific alleles of genes in the MHC cluster as well as other unrelated loci. Which of the following polymorphic alleles is most highly associated with the potential for the development of Type 1 diabetes?

A. a VNTR in the 5′ region of the insulin gene
B. glutamic acid decarboxylase 2 (GAD2)
C. HLA-B27
D. HLA-DQ
E. HLA-DR3

Answer E: The highest risk populations for the development of T1D are children born with the HLA DR3/4–DQ8 serotype allele which accounts for almost 50% of all children who develop antibodies against pancreatic islet cells and thus develop T1D by the age of 5.

13. The occurrence of type 2 diabetes (T2D) in adolescent females can lead to the development of polycystic ovarian syndrome (PCOS). PCOS is the result of follicular atresis and ovulatory dysfunction brought about by a hyper-androgenic microenvironment in the ovary. Which of the following statements reflects the underlying cause of the hyperandrogenic state in females with T2D?

A. hyperinsulinemia, associated with T2D, reduces the level of sex hormone-binding globulin leading to increased free testosterone.
B. T2D in adolescents is primarily the result of obesity and the associated disruption in fatty acid metabolism negatively affects adrenal estrogen production.
C. the increased level of circulating lipid in T2D patients competes for steroid binding to sex hormone–binding globulin resulting in a reduced transport of estrogen within the ovary.
D. the persistent hyperglycemia associated with T2D causes increased levels of glycosylated hemoglobin, which interferes with the need for increased ovarian vascularization at puberty

Answer A: In adolescent females with Type 2 diabetes, the use of metformin is highly recommended to reduce the incidence as well as the potential for polycystic ovarian syndrome, PCOS. PCOS is brought on by the hyperinsulinemia of Type 2 diabetes. Insulin effects on the ovary drive conversion of progesterone to testosterone and a reduction in serum hormone–binding globulin (SHBG). Taken together, the effects of hyperinsulinemia lead to a hyperandrogenic state in the ovary, resulting in follicular atresis and ovulatory dysfunction.

14. Metformin is one of the most prescribed hypoglycemia-inducing drugs in the treatment of Type 2 diabetes. One of the effects of metformin is a reduction in adipose tissue lipolysis which is affected via the activation of AMP-activated kinase (AMPK). Which of the following actions of AMPK explains the adipose tissue benefits of metformin?

A. activation of acetyl-CoA carboxylase
B. activation of fatty acid synthase

C. inhibition of hormone sensitive lipase
D. inhibition of mammalian target of rapamycin, mTOR
E. inhibition of 6-phosphofructokinase 2, PFK2

Answer D: AMP-activated protein kinase (AMPK) was first discovered as an activity that inhibited preparations of acetyl-CoA carboxylase (ACC) and HMG-CoA reductase (HMGR) and was induced by AMP. AMPK induces a cascade of events within cells in response to the ever-changing energy charge of the cell. Once activated, AMPK-mediated phosphorylation events switch cells from active ATP consumption (eg, fatty acid and cholesterol biosynthesis) to active ATP production (eg, fatty acid and glucose oxidation). Other important activities attributable to AMPK are regulation of insulin synthesis and secretion in pancreatic islet β-cells. Activation of AMPK results in the phosphorylation and inhibition of mTOR and as a result, all of the downstream effects of that kinase.

15. Hemoglobin is nonenzymatically glycosylated as glucose enters erythrocytes. Because erythrocytes routinely die and are replaced, the level of glycosylated hemoglobin is a good measure of the length of time glucose levels were elevated. Diabetic patients are most familiar with this process because they routinely measure for which of the following?
A. HbA_{1c}
B. HbA_2
C. HbC
D. HbG
E. HbS

Answer A: HbA_1 is the major form of adult hemoglobin in the blood and the "c" refers to the glycosylated form of the protein. Since hemoglobin is present in red blood cells and these cells have a limited life span of 120 days in the circulation, measurement of HbA_{1c} levels is a relatively accurate measure of the amount of glucose in the blood and the length of time the level has been elevated.

16. In Type 1 diabetes, the increased production of ketone bodies is primarily a result of which of the following?
A. a substantially increased rate of fatty acid oxidation by hepatocytes
B. an increase in the rate of the citric acid cycle
C. decreased cyclic AMP levels in adipocytes which causes accelerated fatty acid release
D. elevated acetyl-CoA levels in skeletal muscle driving ketone body synthesis
E. increased hepatic glucose release from glycogen driving acetyl-CoA production

Answer A: The most frequent consequence of poorly controlled T1D is ketoacidosis, referred to as diabetic ketoacidosis, DKA. The hyperketonemia in DKA is the result of insulin deficiency and unregulated glucagon secretion from α-cells of the pancreas. Circulating glucagon stimulates the adipose tissue to release fatty acids which are taken up and oxidized, primarily by the liver. Under these conditions, the level of fatty acid oxidation is in excess of the livers' ability to fully oxidize the excess acetyl-CoA and, thus the compound is diverted into ketones synthesis. The ketones are released into the circulation and because they are acidic, lower the pH of the blood resulting in metabolic acidosis.

17. You are carrying out studies with a drug to potentially treat the hyperglycemia of Type 2 diabetes. Your studies find that in cell culture this drug induces the activity of peroxisome proliferator-activated receptor-γ (PPARγ). These results indicate that your experimental drug is most likely related to which of the following class of hypoglycemia-inducing drugs already in clinical use?
A. biguanides
B. meglitinides
C. sulfonylureas
D. thiazolidinediones

Answer D: The thoiazolidinediones function as agonists for PPARγ.

18. The drug metformin is an effective treatment for the hyperglycemia associated with diabetes. One of the major sites of action for metformin is the liver and its use is ideal for obese patients and for younger Type 2 diabetics with normal liver function. Given that the drug lowers circulating levels of glucose, which of the following hepatic enzymes is most likely activated as a consequence of metformin administration?
A. AMP-activated protein kinase (AMPK)
B. glycogen phosphorylase
C. 6-Phosphofructo-1-kinase (PFK-1)
D. phosphoenolpyruvate carboxykinase (PEPCK)
E. PKA

Answer A: Metformin exerts part of its effects by modulating mitochondrial activities. Metformin has a mild inhibitory effect on complex I of oxidative phosphorylation, has antioxidant properties, and activates both glucose-6-phosphate dehydrogenase (G6PDH) and AMPK. The importance of AMPK in the actions of metformin stems from the role of AMPK in the regulation of both lipid and carbohydrate metabolism. The activation of AMPK by metformin is likely related to the inhibitory effects of the drug on complex I of oxidative phosphorylation. This would lead to a reduction in ATP production and, therefore, an increase in the level of AMP and as a result activation of AMPK.

19. Maturity-onset diabetes in the young (MODY) is characterized by onset prior to age 25. A defect in which of the following genes is known to result in the specific form of MODY called MODY2?

A. glucose 6-phosphatase
B. glucokinase
C. glycogen phosphorylase
D. hepatocyte nuclear factor-1α (HNF1α)
E. insulin promoter factor-1 (IPF-1)

Answer B: All cases of MODY have shown impaired β-cell function. Patients may also exhibit insulin resistance and late β-cell failure. MODY2 results from defects in pancreatic glucokinase.

20. Obesity is associated with hyperlipidemia resulting in an increased deliver of fatty acid to most tissues including the pancreas. Excess fatty acid oxidation in β-cells of the pancreas results in increased reactive oxygen species (ROS) production. The increased ROS production ultimately contributes to β-cell apoptosis and the need for exogenous insulin in poorly controlled Type 2 diabetes. The deleterious effects of ROS within the pancreas are amplified due to limited expression of which of the following?

A. caspase 9
B. catalase
C. glutathione peroxidase
D peroxiredoxin
E superoxide dismutase

Answer B: The oxidation of fatty acids results in the generation of ROS both via mitochondrial and peroxisomal pathways. When fatty acid levels rise significantly, as in obesity, peroxisomal oxidation of fatty acids increases. The initial enzyme in peroxisomal fatty acid oxidation generates H_2O_2. The primary antioxidant enzyme tasked with removal of H_2O_2 is catalase. Pancreatic β-cells are highly susceptible to the damaging effects of H_2O_2 due to a significantly reduced level of expression of catalase compared to other tissue.

21. A 54-year-old insulin-dependent diabetic notes that her insulin requirements have gone up dramatically in the past year (from 50 U to nearly 200 U of recombinant human insulin) and her blood glucose is still poorly controlled. A possible explanation for the worsening of her diabetes includes which of the following?

A. a high titer of anti-insulin antibodies
B. an improved diet
C. an improved exercise program
D. progression of macrovascular disease
E. weight loss

Answer A: The patient clearly has an increase in her state of insulin resistance. Given the magnitude of her increased insulin requirements, she most likely developed a high titer of anti-insulin antibodies that are preventing the injected insulin from lowering blood glucose effectively.

22. A patient with untreated diabetes mellitus is admitted to the hospital for treatment. Laboratory findings include a blood pH below 7.2. Which of the following is likely to directly result from this level of acidemia?

A. arteriolar constriction
B. decreased catabolism
C. hyperkalemia
D. hypoventilation
E. insulin sensitivity

Answer C: Acidemia is the presence of excess H^+ ions in blood, which tends to create a rise in the extracellular potassium concentration. The rule of thumb for an inorganic acid that causes the acidity is that a decrease in pH of 0.1 unit leads to a rise in plasma potassium of 0.6 mEq/L. The effect of an organic acid is a lot less. The mechanism responsible for the relationship between pH and extracellular potassium concentration is not completely understood. One effect is that the intracellular acidosis inhibits K^+ influx by reducing the activity of the Na^+-K^+-pump. An exchange of extracellular H^+ for intracellular K^+ might also contribute.

23. A 53-year-old man is being treated for hypertension and diabetes. His medications include insulin and propranolol. He presents at his physician's office complaining of muscle weakness. Blood tests reveal hyperkalemia (elevated serum potassium) as well as elevated BUN (blood urea nitrogen). Propranolol is gradually eliminated and his insulin dosage is adjusted. His serum potassium normalizes and his muscle weakness is alleviated. What probably caused his muscle weakness?

A. high potassium–mediated block of acetylcholine receptors
B. high potassium–mediated block of skeletal muscle calcium channels
C. motor neuron hyperpolarization
D. skeletal muscle depolarization with resultant Na-channel inactivation
E. skeletal muscle hyperpolarization with resultant Na-channel blockade

Answer D: Elevated serum potassium levels cause membrane depolarization with a resulting Na-channel inactivation. Fibers are thus less able to fire action potentials, leading to impaired excitation contraction coupling, with muscle weakness. Hyperkalemia in this patient is probably due to multiple factors. Since insulin promotes potassium uptake into cells, too low an insulin dosage in the diabetic can lead to hyperkalemia. In addition, propranolol can cause a shift of potassium from cell to blood. Finally, the elevated BUN indicates some renal failure, and failing kidneys cannot efficiently excrete potassium into the urine.

24. One of your diabetic patients has a blood glucose level of 200 mg/dL. Surprisingly, a dipstick test is negative for urinary glucose. How could this finding be explained?

A. dipstick tests are more sensitive for reducing sugars other than glucose
B. the patient has defective tubular glucose transporters
C. the patient has diabetes insipidus
D. the patient has significantly reduced glomerular filtration rate (GFR)
E. the patient is in a state of antidiuresis

Answer D: Glucose excretion by the kidneys depends on the glomerular filtration and tubular reabsorption rates. Glucose first appears in the urine when the capacity of the glucose transporters in the proximal tubuli cells is exceeded. This usually occurs at plasma glucose levels higher than 180 mg/dL. Patients with longstanding diabetes mellitus often have decreased renal function and reduced GFR. Under these circumstances the threshold (ie, plasma level) for excretion of glucose is higher than in a healthy person.

25. A 14-year-old adolescent girl presenting with polyuria is subsequently diagnosed with Type I diabetes mellitus. The polyuria results from an osmotic diuresis that involves primarily which part of the renal tubule?

A. collecting duct
B. glomerulus
C. juxtaglomerular apparatus
D. proximal tubule
E. thick ascending limb of the loop of Henle

Answer D: The proximal tubule reabsorbs the majority (about two-thirds) of filtered salt and water. Both the luminal salt concentration and the luminal osmolality remain constant (and equal to plasma values) along the entire length of the proximal tubule. Water and salt are reabsorbed proportionally because the water is dependent on and coupled with the active reabsorption of Na^+. The water permeability of the proximal tubule is high, and therefore a significant transepithelial osmotic gradient is not possible. Sodium is actively transported, mainly by basolateral sodium pumps, into the lateral intercellular spaces; water follows. Increased glucose filtration in diabetes will osmotically prevent water reabsorption at this site.

26. Laboratory results for a patient with uncontrolled Type I diabetes reveal hyperglycemia (634 mg/dL) and hypertriglyceridemia (498 mg/dL). Which of the following represents the most likely cause of the hypertriglyceridemia in this patient?

A. absence of hormone-sensitive lipase
B. decreased lipoprotein lipase activity
C. deficiency in apoprotein C-II
D. deficiency in LDL receptors
E. increased hepatic triglyceride synthesis

Answer B: The triacylglyceride components of VLDL and chylomicron are hydrolyzed to free fatty acids and glycerol in the capillaries of tissues such as liver, adipose tissue, and skeletal muscle by the actions of lipoprotein lipase (LPL) and hepatic triglyceride lipase (HTGL). Insulin exerts numerous effects on overall metabolic homeostasis. One of the effects of insulin that relate to the symptoms in this patient is the regulation of the expression of LPL on the surface of endothelial cells. Since Type 1 diabetics do not synthesize insulin they do not properly regulate the level of LPL which contributes to hypertriglyceridemia in these individuals.

27. A 48-year-old woman moved to a new area and is being seen for a routine physical examination as a new patient in a general medicine clinic. Her present medical history is significant for a 30-lb weight excess and an 8-year history of noninsulin-dependent diabetes mellitus, which she reports has been fairly well controlled with oral agents and a strict diet regimen. However, she is now anxious about her condition and admits to recently developing poor and irregular eating habits, and occasionally missing a medication dosage due to the high stress level surrounding her recent move. The most accurate estimation of this patient's recent glucose control would be which of the following?

A. fasting insulin and C-peptide levels
B. glucose tolerance test
C. glycated hemoglobin level
D. random serum glucose
E. urine ketone body level

Answer C: When present in high concentration, glucose can react nonenzymatically with protein amino groups to form an unstable intermediate, or Schiff base, which subsequently undergoes an internal rearrangement to form a stable glycated protein. The glycation of the amino acids valine and lysine on the β chain of hemoglobin A results in the formation of hemoglobin A_{1c} (HbA_{1c}), or glycated hemoglobin. Because red blood cells circulate for an average of 90 to 120 days, assaying HbA_{1c} provides an index of a diabetic patient's glucose control over the preceding 3 to 4 months. Although normal values vary between laboratories, on average nondiabetic subjects have HbA_{1c} levels roughly between 4% and 6%.

28. A 22-year-old man has come to see his physician because he feels thirsty all the time, has to urinate frequently, and is most concerned about his weight loss. Blood work demonstrates that his glucose levels are elevated and he has a slight increase in ketones. His physician makes a diagnosis of Type 1 diabetes. Which of the following additional abnormalities is most likely to be present prior to initiation of treatment?

A. decreased concentration of fructose 2,6-bisphosphate in the liver
B. decreased gluconeogenesis from alanine
C. decreased renal threshold for glucose
D. increased concentration of GLUT4 transporters in skeletal muscle
E. increased intestinal gluconeogenesis from muscle glutamine

Answer A: Associated with insulin deficiency in Type 1 diabetes is uncontrolled glucagon secretion. In the absence of injected insulin, these patients will experience exacerbated responses to the increased glucagon. Glucagon action in the liver includes activation of PKA. One of the targets of PKA is PFK2. When PFK2 is phosphorylated it hydrolyzes the potent PFK1 activator, fructose-2,6-bisphosphate (F2,6BP) resulting in reduced levels of F2,6BP and reduced activity of PFK1.

29. A 27-year-old woman has Type 1 diabetes. Shortly after eating lunch she measures her blood glucose with a glucose meter and finds that it is 340 mg/dL. She administers herself a dose of short-acting insulin. After this injection, which of the following is most likely to be increased in the liver of this woman?

A. cAMP
B. glucose-6-phosphatase activity
C. phosphofructokinase-1 (PFK1) activity
D. phoshorylation of pyruvate kinase
E. protein kinase A (PKA) activity

Answer C: One of the effects of insulin in cells, such as hepatocytes, is the induction of phosphodiesterase, PDE. PDE hydrolyzes cAMP which will lead to reduced activation of PKA. One of the targets of PKA is PFK2. When PFK2 is phosphorylated it hydrolyzes the potent PFK1 activator, fructose-2,6-bisphosphate (F2,6BP), resulting in reduced activity of PFK1. Conversely, in the presence of insulin PFK2 is not phosphorylated and under these conditions the enzyme synthesizes F2,6BP which results in significant increases in the activity of PFK1.

30. An unconscious 20-year-old man is brought to the ER by his frat brothers. They indicate that he had consumed several beers prior to passing out and their concern was their inability to rouse him. His best friend reports that he is Type 1 diabetic and that he injected himself with insulin about 7 hours earlier. Physical examination indicates a distinct odor of ketone on his breath. Laboratory studies demonstrate that he has an increased ketone body concentration and an increased ratio of β-hydroxybutyrate to acetoacetate in his blood. His liver cells are most likely to show which of the following ratios?

A. decreased $NADH:NAD^+$
B. decreased $NADPH:NADP^+$
C. increased $NADH:NAD^+$
D. increased $NADPH:NADP^+$
E. increased pyruvate:lactate

Answer C: Associated with insulin deficiency in Type 1 diabetes is uncontrolled glucagon secretion. In the absence of injected insulin these patients will experience exacerbated responses to the increased glucagon. This includes increased fatty acid oxidation rates in the liver and the production of ketones. The increased rate of fatty acid oxidation results in an increase in the NADH to NAD^+ level in the cell.

31. Patients with poorly controlled Type 1 diabetes exhibit elevated plasma glucose concentration. The increases result in part because, in the absence of insulin, there is a lack of induction of glucokinase in which of the following organs?

A. brain
B. kidney
C. intestine
D. liver
E. pancreas

Answer D: Insulin action involves the regulation of the activities of numerous enzymes as well as the expression of the genes encoding many of the same enzymes. One of the hepatic genes regulated by insulin is glucokinase. Reduced expression of glucokinase lowers the ability of the liver to phosphorylate and utilize glucose, thus contributing to the hyperglycemia in the absence of proper insulin administration in Type 1 diabetics.

32. You are treating a 17-year-old adolescent girl patient with Type 1 diabetes who has not been properly and regularly injecting herself with insulin. Given your understanding of her underlying metabolic dysregulation in this disease you expect her liver to undergo an increased rate of gluconeogenesis. This metabolic process is the result of secretion of which of the following hormones?

A. aldosterone
B. glucagon
C. insulin-like growth factor-II
D. somatostatin
E. thyroid hormone

Answer B: Associated with insulin deficiency in Type 1 diabetes is uncontrolled glucagon secretion. In the absence of injected insulin in this patient, she will have exacerbated responses to the increased glucagon. These responses will include increased hepatic gluconeogenesis.

33. As the attending physician in the ER you are treating a 29-year-old woman brought in by her husband. He tells you that she has complained of breathing difficulty and has been nauseous and vomiting for the past 4 hours. He also reports that she has been using insulin for the past 8 years to treat her Type 1 diabetes. She indicates that she has not given herself an injection of insulin for the past 24 hours. Her pulse is 100/min, and respirations are 30/min. Physical examination indicates lethargy, dehydration, and deep respirations. Blood work show hyperglycemia and metabolic acidosis. Which of the following best describes the current activity of the metabolic pathways in this woman liver?

	Gluconeogenesis	Glycogen Synthesis	Fatty Acid Oxidation	Glycolysis
A.	increased	increased	increased	decreased
B.	increased	increased	decreased	decreased
C.	increased	decreased	increased	decreased
D.	decreased	increased	increased	increased
E.	decreased	decreased	decreased	decreased

Answer C: Associated with insulin deficiency in Type 1 diabetes is uncontrolled glucagon secretion. In the absence of injected insulin in this patient, she will have exacerbated responses to the increased glucagon. These responses will include increased hepatic gluconeogenesis and increased glycogen breakdown. In addition, the rate of glucose oxidation will be reduced and fatty acid oxidation will be increased. All of these effects are exerted via glucagon-mediated increases in the activity of PKA.

34. You are performing comparative tests on 2 individuals. Analysis of their blood indicates that they both have elevated levels of ketone bodies. One test subject has been on an extended fast while the other is a patient who poorly controls her Type 1 diabetes. Which of the following is a common factor that is responsible for ketosis in both of these individuals?

A. depletion of pentose phosphate pathway intermediates
B. increased availability of acetyl-CoA
C. inhibition of fatty acid oxidation
D. inhibition of gluconeogenesis
E. inhibition of glycogenolysis

Answer B: Type 1 diabetes is not only associated with loss of insulin secretion but also abnormal secretion of glucagon. An individual on a fast would have reduced levels of blood glucose and the compensation for this would be increased secretion of glucagon to stimulate gluconeogenesis in the liver. Associated with increased glucagon secretion is activation of adipose tissue lipolysis. The released fatty acids are taken up primarily by the liver where they are oxidized to acetyl-CoA. In both the T1D patient and the fasting individual this increased production of acetyl-CoA will lead to increased ketone synthesis.

35. You are the physician treating a 14-year-old adolescent girl who has been poorly controlling her Type 1 diabetes. Blood analysis indicates that she has increased levels of hemoglobin A_{1c}. Which of the following best explains this increase?

A. glucose competes with other sugars for glycosylation of hemoglobin
B. hemoglobin is glycosylated in erythrocyte Golgi complexes
C. hemoglobin is nonenzymatically glycosylated when serum glucose concentrations are increased
D. an increased serum glucose concentration inhibits erythrocyte degradation by spleen cells
E. an increased serum glucose concentration inhibits lysosomal degradation of hemoglobin

Answer C: The hyperglycemia that will result from poor control of T1D results in increased circulating levels of glycosylated hemoglobin, designated as the level of HbA_{1c}, often designated as just A_{1C}. HbA_1 is the major form of adult hemoglobin in the blood and the "c" refers to the glycosylated form of the protein.

36. You are treating a 43-year-old man with a BMI of 37. Blood tests demonstrate that he is euglycemic and has an above normal level of insulin in his blood. Which of the following best explains these findings?
- A. defective glycogen synthase
- B. defective glycolysis enzyme
- C. low dietary intake of sugar
- D. pancreatic β-cell dysfunction
- E. tissue resistance to insulin

Answer E: Given the patient's BMI, he is likely to be obese and manifesting symptoms associated with Type 2 diabetes. The euglycemia in the face of increased levels of plasma insulin indicates that his pancreas is responding to the increased blood glucose but that his peripheral tissues are unresponsive to the circulating insulin.

37. An 11-year-old boy with Type 1 diabetes is brought to the ER 1 hour after awakening from sleep at midnight in a cold sweat. He is confused and poorly responsive. He is normally given 4 injections of insulin daily, and the last injection was administered by his mother before he went to bed. Measurement of his blood glucose concentration indicates it is 37 mg/dL. Following an injection of glucagon, his serum glucose concentration increases to 145 mg/dL, and he shows clinical improvement. The beneficial effect of glucagon in this patient results from which of the following actions of this hormone in the liver?
- A. adenylate cyclase stimulation
- B. guanylate cyclase stimulation
- C. intranuclear binding of hormone receptor to DNA
- D. serine/threonine kinase activation
- E. tyrosine kinase activation

Answer A: When glucagon binds to its receptor on hepatocytes it triggers the activation of a G-protein that in turn activates adenylate cyclase. The activation of adenylate cyclase results in increased production of cAMP which then activates PKA. Activated PKA results in phosphorylation of numerous substrates in the hepatocyte that dramatically increases glycogen breakdown and the activation of the gluconeogenic pathway. Both of these events lead to increased glucose release from the liver accounting for the observed increase in blood glucose.

38. Patients who do not maintain correct diet and exercise regimens will most often exhibit which of the following consequences of their increased serum glucose concentration?
- A. decreased degradation of hemoglobin A
- B. increased synthesis of immature erythrocytes
- C. insulin binding to hemoglobin A in the erythrocyte membrane
- D. nonenzymatic glycosylation of hemoglobin A in erythrocytes
- E. serum glucagon levels exceeding twice the normal levels

Answer D: The hyperglycemia commonly associated with T2D results in increased circulating levels of glycosylated hemoglobin, designated as the level of HbA_{1c}, often designated as just A_{1C}. HbA_1 is the major form of adult hemoglobin in the blood and the "c" refers to the glycosylated form of the protein.

39. Type 2 diabetics retain some level of pancreatic function. This fact explains why they rarely manifest which of the following symptoms that is typical in Type 1 diabetics?
- A. glucose intolerance
- B. hyperglycemia
- C. ketoacidosis
- D. obesity
- E. polyuria

Answer C: The most frequent consequence of poorly controlled T1D is ketoacidosis, referred to as diabetic ketoacidosis, DKA. The hyperketonemia in DKA is the result of insulin deficiency and unregulated glucagon secretion from α-cells of the pancreas. Since T2D patients have normal pancreatic α-cell function, they do not secrete excess glucagon and, therefore, rarely exhibit ketonemia.

40. You are treating a patient who recently underwent a total pancreatectomy due to pancreatic cancer. Your patient will require exogenous insulin for the same reasons as an individual with Type 1 diabetes. However, a diabetic patient will require more insulin than your pancreatectomy patient because the diabetic patient also has which of the following characteristics?
- A. hyperglucagonemia in addition to insulin deficiency
- B. insulin resistance
- C. postreceptor defects
- D. production of insulin with abnormal structure
- E. receptor-mediated increases in glucagon release

Answer A: In addition to the loss of insulin secretion typical of T1D, there is abnormal function of pancreatic α-cells. There is excessive secretion of glucagon in T1D patients. Normally, hyperglycemia leads to reduced glucagon secretion. However, in patients with T1D, glucagon secretion is not suppressed by hyperglycemia. The resultant inappropriately elevated glucagon level exacerbates the metabolic defects due to insulin deficiency.

41. A few of the more severe complications of Type 2 of diabetes are neuropathy and retinopathy. Many of the associated pathologies of diabetes arise as a result of which of the following nonenzymatic modifications of various proteins?

A. acetylation
B. glucuronidation
C. glycosylation
D. hydroxylation
E. oxidation

Answer C: The hyperglycemia commonly associated with T2D can be assessed by routine measurement of the circulating levels of glycosylated hemoglobin, designated as the level of HbA_{1c}, often designated as just A_{1C}. HbA_1 is the major form of adult hemoglobin in the blood and the "c" refers to the glycosylated form of the protein. Since hemoglobin is present in red blood cells and these cells have a limited life span of 120 days in the circulation, measurement of HbA_{1c} levels is a relatively accurate measure of the amount of glucose in the blood and the length of time the level has been elevated.

Checklist

- ✓ Diabetes mellitus is a metabolic disorder primarily associated with deregulated glucose homeostasis.
- ✓ There are 2 major types of diabetes: Type 1 and Type 2. Type 1 diabetes is associated with loss of the insulin producing cells of the pancreas and usually manifests in childhood. Type 2 diabetes is associated with a progression from peripheral tissue resistance to normal levels of insulin to eventual loss of insulin production and usually manifest later in life.
- ✓ Type 1 diabetes is characterized by frequent episodes of potentially life-threatening ketoacidosis due, in part, to abnormal regulation of pancreatic glucagon secretion.
- ✓ Due to abnormal glucagon secretion and lack of insulin secretion in Type 1 diabetes, the primary metabolic disruptions are in carbohydrate, lipid, and protein homeostasis.
- ✓ Type 2 diabetes is most frequently associated with obesity and it is the hyperlipidemia typically seen in obesity that plays a major role in peripheral resistance to the actions of insulin. Due to rising juvenile diabetes rates, Type 2 diabetes is appearing now with much higher frequency in children and young adult.
- ✓ Several related forms of diabetes are the result of defects in genes responsible for normal pancreatic function and these disorders are referred to as the maturity-onset type diabetes of the young, MODY.
- ✓ Several diseases are associated with disruptions in insulin secretion, and/or insulin actions resulting in what are referred to as secondary diabetes.
- ✓ Gestational diabetes (GDM) is a special situation whereby glucose intolerance is first apparent during pregnancy. Women who experience GDM are likely to develop Type 2 diabetes later in life.
- ✓ Neonatal diabetes refers to a circumstance in which hyperglycemia results from dysfunction in insulin action within the first 6 months of life and presents a potentially life-threatening condition.

✓ Type 1 diabetes is highly associated with polymorphisms in genes of the major histocompatibility cluster (MHC).

✓ Numerous genetic polymorphisms have been associated with an increased risk for the development of Type 2 diabetes. One of the most significant is the *TCF7L2* gene.

✓ The hyperglycemia associated with diabetes can be assessed by the measurement of glycosylated hemoglobin, identified as HbA_{1c} (A_{1c}). The efficacy of Type 2 diabetes drugs is reflected, in part, by the degree to which they can lower and control A_{1c} levels.

✓ Mitochondrial dysfunction occurs in the context of diabetes due, in part, to the hyperlipidemia associated with the obesity precipitating the disease. Excess fatty acid oxidation leads to increased production of reactive oxygen species (ROS). Increased ROS production activates stress responses that negatively affect the ability of the insulin receptor to initiate downstream effects. The net effect is a progression of the peripheral resistance to insulin seen in Type 2 diabetes.

✓ Numerous classes of drug have been developed to exert hypoglycemia inducing effects as a means to treat the hyperglycemia associated with Type 2 diabetes.

CHAPTER

48 Cardiovascular Disease: The Metabolic Syndrome and Atherosclerosis

CHAPTER OUTLINE

High-Yield Terms

Artery: blood vessels that carry blood away from the heart

Vein: blood vessels that carry blood toward the heart

Capillary: are the smallest vessels and constitute the vessels of the microcirculation

Atherogenic: relating to the processes of initiating, increasing, and/or accelerating atherogenesis

Atheroma: represents result of the accumulation of leukocytes (mostly macrophages), lipids, and debris causing swelling of the arterial wall

Metabolic syndrome: a disorder that defines a combination of metabolic and cardiovascular risk determinants that leads to coronary artery disease (CAD)

Atherosclerosis: refers to the condition in which wall of larger arteries and veins thickens as a result of the accumulation of fatty material, cells, and extracellular matrix components

The Cardiovascular System

The cardiovascular system, also referred to as the circulatory system, is comprised of the heart and the blood vessels (Figure 48-1). The heart has 2 separate sides and each side has 2 chambers. The upper chamber on each side of the heart is called an atrium and the bottom chamber on each side is called a ventricle. The ventricles are the chambers that pump the blood with each contraction. One side of the heart (left ventricle) is designed to propel the oxygenated blood into the systemic circulation. Within the tissues the erythrocytes and the blood exchange O_2 for the CO_2 generated through metabolic processes. The other side of the heart (right ventricle) is designed to propel deoxygenated blood into the pulmonary circulation where the blood becomes oxygenated in the alveoli of the lungs. Within the lungs the CO_2 is expelled during respiration and the erythrocyte hemoglobin becomes fully oxygenated once again.

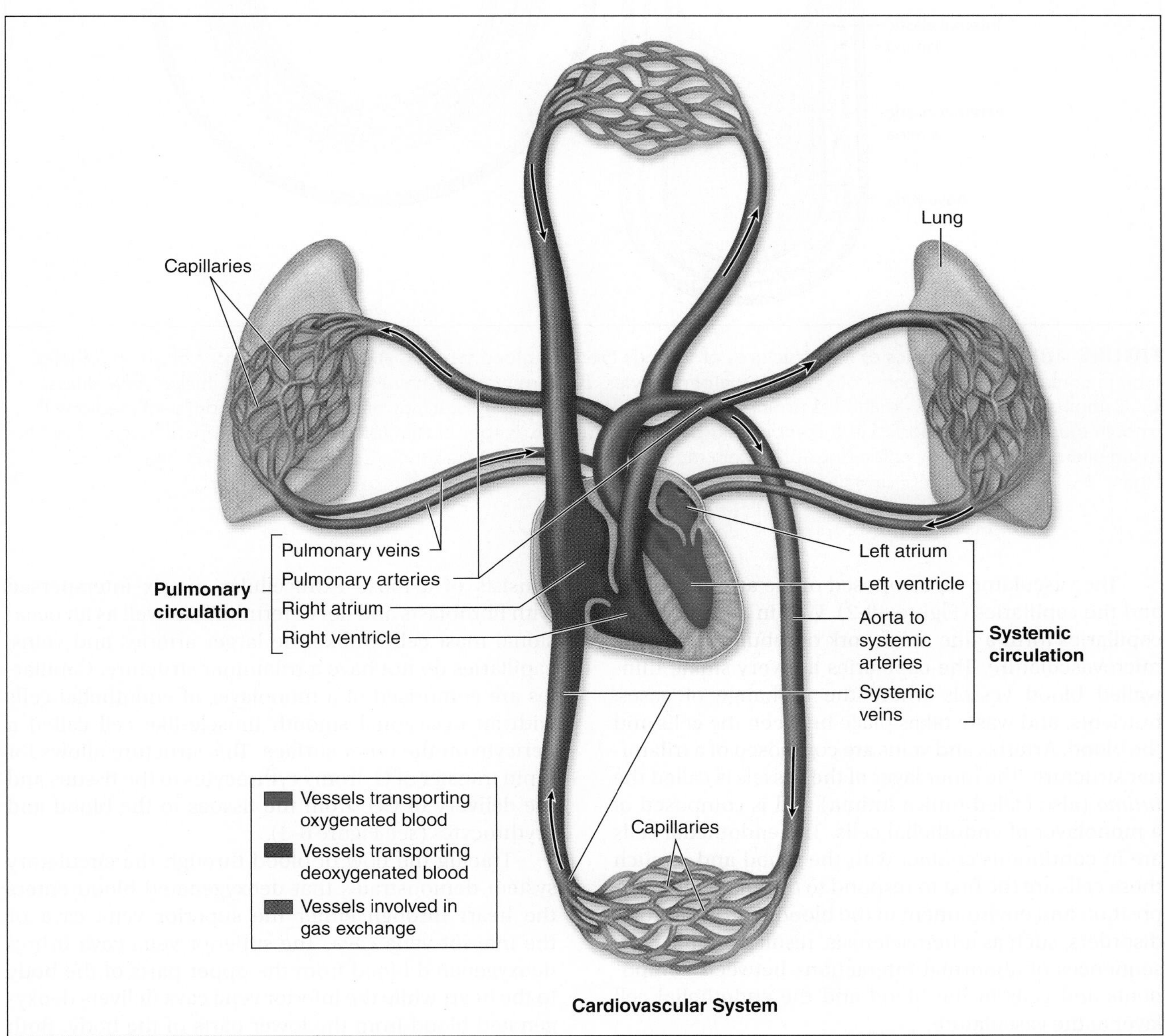

FIGURE 48-1: Diagram of the cardiovascular system. Mescher AL. Junqueira's Basic Histology Text and Atlas, 13th ed. New York, NY: McGraw-Hill; 2013.

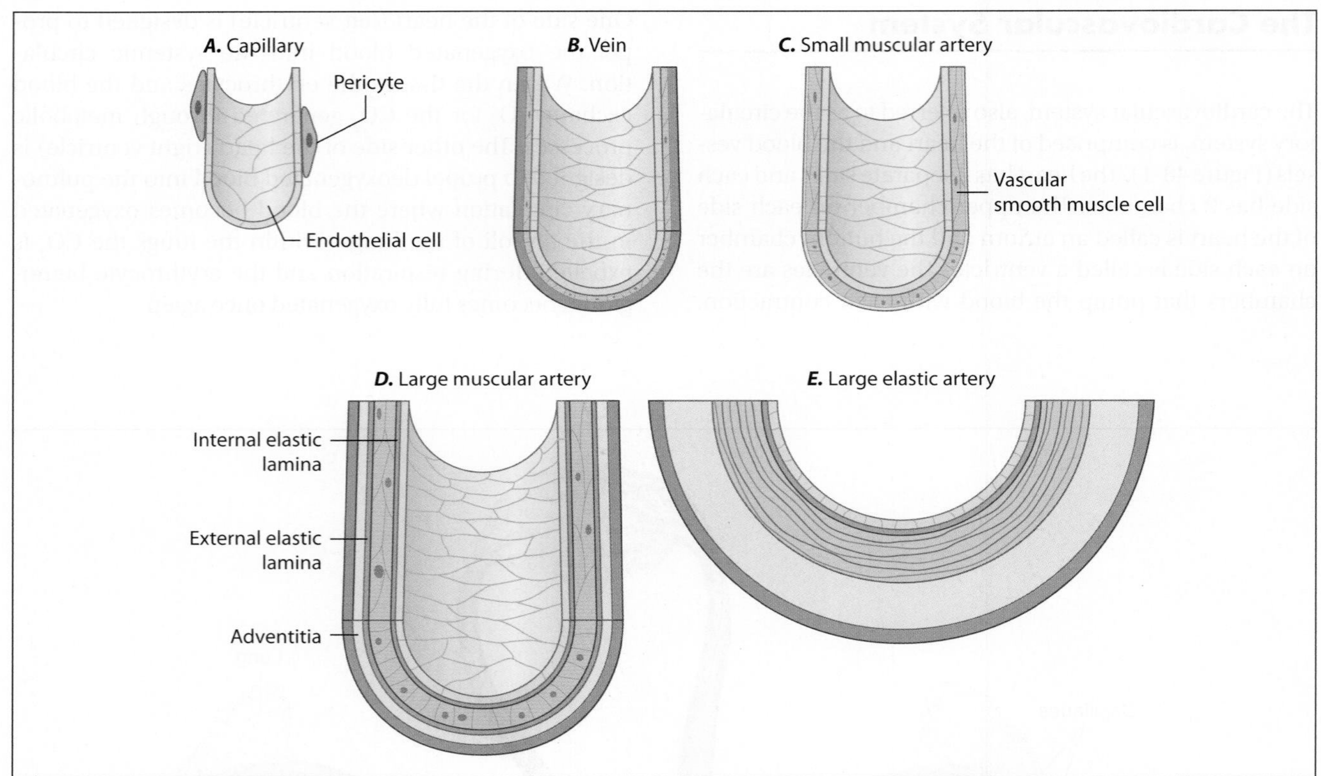

FIGURE 48-2: Schematics of the structures of various types of blood vessels. ***A.*** Capillaries consist of an endothelial tube in contact with a discontinuous population of pericytes. ***B.*** Veins typically have thin medias and thicker adventitias. ***C.*** A small muscular artery features a prominent tunica media. ***D.*** Larger muscular arteries have a prominent media with smooth muscle cells embedded in a complex extracellular matrix. ***E.*** Larger elastic arteries have cylindrical layers of elastic tissue alternating with concentric rings of smooth muscle cells. Loscalzo JL. Harrison's Cardiovascular Medicine, 2nd ed., Figure 1-1, New York: McGraw-Hill; 2013.

The vasculature is composed of the arteries, veins, and the capillaries (Figure 48-2). Within all tissues the capillaries form a fine meshwork of tubules called the microvasculature. The capillaries are very small, thin-walled blood vessels where the exchange of gases, nutrients, and waste takes place between the cells and the blood. Arteries and veins are composed of a trilaminar structure. The inner layer of the vessels is called the *intima* (also called tunica intima) and is composed of a monolayer of endothelial cells. The endothelial cells are in continuous contact with the blood and as such these cells are the first to respond to the changing composition and environment of the blood. Cardiovascular disorders, such as atherosclerosis, result from the consequences of abnormal interactions between components and cells in the blood and the endothelial cell layer of the vasculature.

The middle layer of the vessels is called the *media* (also called tunica media) and is composed of layers of smooth muscle cells. The outermost layer is called the *adventitia* (tunica adventitia or tunica externa) which consists of a loose extracellular matrix interspersed with fibroblasts and nerve terminals as well as an occasional mast cell. Unlike the larger arteries and veins, capillaries do not have a trilaminar structure. Capillaries are comprised of a monolayer of endothelial cells with an occasional smooth muscle-like cell called a pericyte on the outer surface. This structure allows for rapid transfer of O_2 from erythrocytes to the tissues and the delivery of CO_2 from the tissues to the blood and erythrocytes (see Figure 6-3).

Tracing the flow of blood through the circulatory system demonstrates that deoxygenated blood enters the heart through either the superior vena cava or the inferior vena cava. The superior vena cava brings deoxygenated blood from the upper parts of the body to the heart while the inferior vena cava delivers deoxygenated blood from the lower parts of the body. Both of these large veins deliver the deoxygenated blood to the right atrium and then to the right ventricle where it is propelled via the pulmonary artery out to the lungs. Once oxygenated, the blood returns to the heart via the pulmonary vein where it enters the left atrium, followed by the left ventricle and finally it is propelled out of the heart into the aorta. From the aorta the blood flows to the many arteries of the body and is distributed to the tissues to deliver the oxygen.

Endothelial Cells

The endothelial cell produces many endogenous substances that play important roles in the regulation of its barrier and transport functions as well as its role in vascular tone and blood flow. Two of the more important molecules secreted by endothelial cells are prostacyclin (PCI_2: an eicosanoid, see Chapter 22) and nitric oxide (NO), both of which induce vasodilation. Defective endothelial cell production of NO underlies the excessive vasoconstriction seen in many pathological conditions such as atherosclerosis. NO also plays an important role in the regulation of blood coagulation by limiting platelet adhesion to the endothelium thereby, limiting platelet activation which is critical to the onset of blood coagulation (see Chapter 51).

Endothelial cells also play important roles in the regulation of intravascular and tissue inflammatory processes. Normally, the endothelial cell surface does not allow for direct contact of white blood cells (leukocytes) such as monocytes and neutrophils. However, when endothelial cells are activated by proinflammatory cytokines released from leukocytes during injury or infection, or due to the release of bacterial products, they express a number of leukocyte adhesion molecules allowing monocytes and neutrophils to adhere. Adherence of these leukocytes establishes a local proinflammatory state. Adherent monocytes invade the intimal layer where they become macrophages and can continue to secrete factors that prolong the inflammatory state as well as to induce the underlying smooth cells to become activated. The release of proinflammatory cytokines increases the local production of reactive oxygen species (ROS) that leads to increased rates peroxidation of lipids in circulating lipoproteins, particularly low-density lipoprotein (LDL). This generates oxidized LDL (oxLDL) which, at sites of macrophage invasion, results in increased oxLDL uptake by the macrophages. The macrophages become infiltrated with fat converting them to foam cells which secret high levels of proinflammatory cytokines. This process then becomes progressive and in an individual with high circulating lipid content, such as in obesity and type 2 diabetes, the end result is severe coronary artery disease (CAD, also referred to as cardiovascular disease, CVD) and atherosclerosis. The proinflammatory state and the hyperlipidemia are 2 of the underlying causes of the metabolic syndrome (MetS).

Insulin Action and Endothelial Functions

The metabolic functions of insulin are primarily reflective of its role in glucose and lipid homeostasis in skeletal muscle, adipose tissue, and liver. However, insulin also exerts important functions in other nonclassical insulin target tissues such as the brain, pancreas, and the vascular endothelium. The ability of insulin to exert vasodilator action in the vascular endothelium as a result of increased NO production is an important component of the ability of this hormone to enhance glucose uptake by skeletal muscle. The insulin-mediated signaling pathway that triggers production of NO in vascular endothelium involves the same signaling proteins (PI3K, PKD, and Akt/PKB) that are components of metabolic regulatory pathways induced by insulin (see Chapter 46). Therefore, it is understandable why the same disruptions to insulin signaling that lead to insulin resistance result in endothelial dysfunction.

The production of NO in endothelial cells is the result of the activation of endothelial nitric oxide synthase (eNOS). The production and actions of NO and the various NOS enzymes involved are discussed in more detail in Chapter 31. With respect to insulin action, the activation of endothelial PKB leads to phosphorylation and activation of eNOS and thus increased NO production.

High-Yield Concept

Endothelial cells form the critical interface (barrier) between cells, macromolecules, and ions in the blood and the tissues. The failure of endothelial cells to carry out their highly selective barrier functions is an underlying cause of many cardiovascular disorders including pulmonary edema, hypertension, and most detrimental to survival, atherosclerosis.

High-Yield Concept

In addition to modulating vascular tone by activating signaling events in the underlying vascular smooth muscle cells, endothelial cell-derived NO reduces the production of proinflammatory cytokines, reduces leukocyte and monocyte recruitment and adhesion to the endothelium, inhibits the proliferation of vascular smooth muscle cells, inhibits apoptosis, and attenuates platelet aggregation.

Inactivation of endothelial cell NO production, as occurs due to insulin resistance, results in endothelial dysfunction and promotes the development of atherosclerosis. Elevated levels of circulating free fatty acids lead to impaired insulin signaling via the PI3K-PDK-PKB pathway in vascular endothelial cells.

Insulin exerts its mitogenic, growth-promoting, and differentiation effects via a signaling pathway that involves mitogen-activated protein kinase (MAPK) which is distinct from the PI3K-PDK-PKB pathway. The MAPK-induced pathway does not play a role in the production of NO by insulin. However, this MAPK-induced pathway plays a significant role in the development of atherosclerosis in the insulin resistant state. When insulin signaling via PI3K-PDK-PKB is impaired, the MAPK signaling pathway in endothelial cells is enhanced. In the endothelium MAPK activation by insulin results in increased expression of endothelin-1 (ET-1), plasminogen activator inhibitor type-1 (PAI-1), and the adhesion molecules intercellular adhesion molecule-1 (ICAM-1), vascular cell adhesion molecule-1 (VCAM-1), and E-selectin. ET-1 is a potent vasoconstrictor and contributes to endothelial cell dysfunction in the presence of insulin resistance. The increased expression of numerous cell adhesion molecules accelerates the adherence to the endothelium of proinflammatory leukocytes which in turn contributes to the development of atherosclerosis. Therefore, the molecules beneficial to vascular endothelial health that are induced by insulin (eg, NO) are reduced in the insulin resistant state and those that are proatherogenic (eg, ET-1, PAI-1) are increased.

Introduction to the Metabolic Syndrome

The hallmark feature of MetS is insulin resistance. Several other clinical abnormalities are also associated with MetS, including nonalcoholic fatty liver disease (NAFLD), atherosclerosis, oxidative stress, and polycystic ovary syndrome (PCOS). Although obesity, ectopic fat accumulation, and an inflammatory status are central to the pathology of MetS, not all obese individuals develop MetS and not all individuals with MetS are obese. These observations indicate that MetS has a multifactorial etiology that involves a series of complex interactions between a particular individual's dietary habits, hormonal status, and genetic background (Figure 48-3). Increasing evidence indicates that the risk of MetS can be developmentally induced. Epidemiological studies in humans and animal models of MetS demonstrate an association between poor nutrition during fetal development and an increased risk of adult cardiovascular disease.

Given the complexities of the factors contributing to MetS, numerous health groups in various countries have defined the disorder with slightly different criteria. Some health organizations believe that insulin resistance is the single most important predictor for future development of type 2 diabetes and cardiovascular disease. For this reason MetS is sometimes also called the insulin resistance syndrome. In addition, there are significant differences in ethnic predisposition to

High-Yield Concept

The metabolic syndrome, MetS (also once referred to as syndrome X), is a disorder that defines a combination of metabolic and cardiovascular risk determinants. These risk factors include insulin resistance, hyperinsulinemia, central adiposity (obesity associated with excess fat deposits around the waist), dyslipidemia, glucose intolerance, hypertension, proinflammatory status, procoagulation together with impaired fibrinolysis, and microalbuminemia.

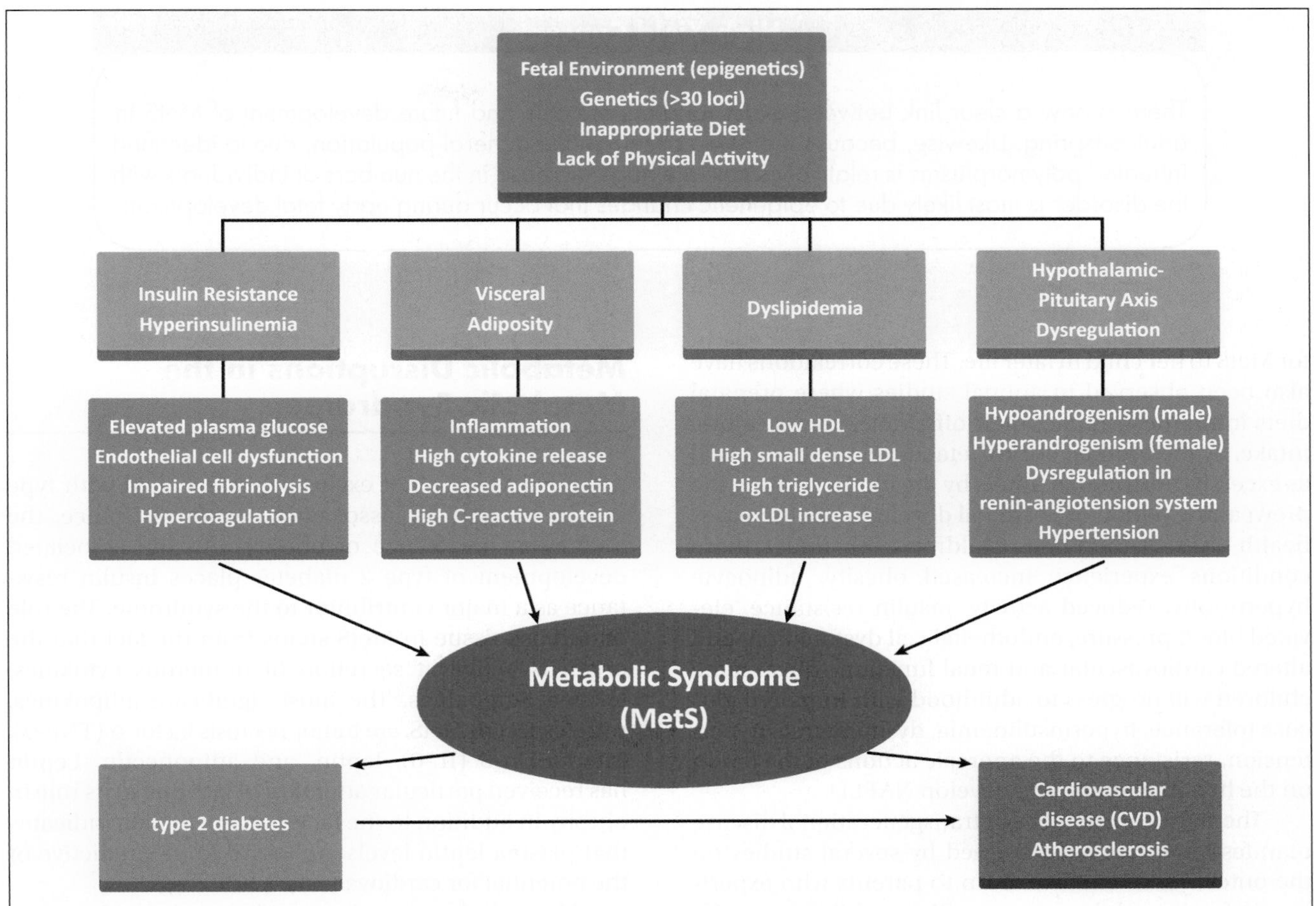

FIGURE 48-3: Concept map of the multifactorial interactions resulting in metabolic syndrome. Multiple interacting risk factors lead to global metabolic disruptions typified by insulin resistance, hyperlipidemia, and intravascular proinflammatory status. Progression of the metabolic disturbances in MetS ultimately leads to full-blown type 2 diabetes and eventually the development of cardiovascular diseases (CVD) such as atherosclerosis. Reproduced with permission of themedicalbiochemistrypage, LLC.

the effects of the dysfunctions of MetS that some criteria must be assessed with this in mind. Of particular note is the use of waist circumference as an indicator of obesity. Certain criteria have been established by the American Heart Association and the National Heart, Lung and Blood Institute as defining the metabolic syndrome (Table 48-1).

Genetic Factors in the Metabolic Syndrome

Numerous epidemiological studies have implicated developmental origins in the progression to the metabolic syndrome. There appears to be a clear correlation between poor nutritional status of the mother during fetal development and the potential for increased risk

TABLE 48-1: Criteria Established to Define the Metabolic Syndrome

Defining Criteria	*Parameters of Criteria*
Elevated fasting blood glucose	≥100 mg/dL (≥5.6 mmol/L)
Increased waist circumference	≥102 cm (≥40 in) in men ≥88 cm (≥35 in) in women
Elevated triglycerides	≥150 mg/dL (≥1.7 mmol/L)
Reduced HDL cholesterol (HDLc)	<40 mg/dL (<1.03 mmol/L) in men <50 mg/dL (<1.3 mmol/L) in women
Elevated blood pressure	≥130 mm Hg systolic or ≥85 mm Hg diastolic

High-Yield Concept

There is now a clear link between maternal dietary status and future development of MetS in adult offspring. Likewise, because the risks of MetS in the general population, due to identified inherited polymorphisms is relatively small, the huge increase in the numbers of individuals with the disorder is most likely due to epigenetic changes that occur during early fetal development.

for MetS to her child in later life. These correlations have also been observed in animal studies where prenatal diets in mothers impact their offspring. Excess caloric intake, by the mother, during fetal development as well as excessive nutritional intake by the mother during the preweaning period of postnatal development increases health risks in the child. Children born under these conditions experience increased obesity, adipocyte hypertrophy, reduced activity, insulin resistance, elevated blood pressure, endothelial cell dysfunction, and altered cardiovascular and renal function. These same children will progress to adulthood with impaired glucose tolerance, hyperinsulinemia, dyslipidemia, hypertension, resistance to the anorexic actions of the leptin on the hypothalamus, and develop NAFLD.

The role of epigenetics in transgenerational disease manifestation has been defined by several studies on the outcomes of children born to parents who experienced famine while pregnant. These children are far more likely to develop diabetes, obesity, and cardiovascular disease than children from parents of similar backgrounds who were not nutritionally deprived. Of striking significance is that the second-generation children (grandchildren of the starved mothers) were more likely to be born with low birth weight regardless of the nutritional status of their mothers. The potential for diet and nutrition to effect epigenetic changes in offspring on multiple generations has been conclusively demonstrated in animal models. In mice, the lack of adequate fetal nutrition results in a reduction in the methylation status of the promoter regions of several transcriptional regulators. Hypomethylation of genes is most often associated with increased transcriptional activation. One transcriptional regulator of key metabolic significance whose promoter has been found to be hypomethylated in offspring of nutritionally deprived mothers is peroxisome proliferator–activated receptor-α (PPARα). PPARα is highly expressed in the liver, skeletal muscle, heart, and kidney. Its function in the liver is to induce hepatic peroxisomal fatty acid oxidation during periods of fasting. Expression of PPARα is also seen in macrophage foam cells and vascular endothelium. Its role in these cells is the activation of anti-inflammatory and antiatherogenic effects.

Metabolic Disruptions in the Metabolic Syndrome

Although MetS is not exclusively associated with type 2 diabetes and the associated insulin resistance, the increasing prevalence of obesity and the associated development of type 2 diabetes places insulin resistance as a major contributor to the syndrome. The role of adipose tissue in MetS stems from the fact that the organ is active at secretion of numerous cytokines, termed adipokines. The most significant adipokines, with respect to MetS, are tumor necrosis factor-α (TNF-α), interleukin-6 (IL-6), leptin, and adiponectin. Leptin has received particular attention of late due to its role in obesity in addition to the fact that recent data indicates that plasma leptin levels are found to be predictive of the potential for cardiovascular pathology.

Many clinicians and researchers believe that insulin resistance underlies the cardiovascular pathologies of MetS. One primary reason for this is the role of insulin in fat homeostasis. A major role of insulin is to induce the storage of fuel. This can be as fat (triglycerides, TG) in adipose tissue or as carbohydrate in the form of glycogen in liver and skeletal muscle. The effect of insulin resistance at the level of fat homeostasis is an increase in circulating TG, referred to as dyslipidemia. Due to insulin resistance there is an increase in the delivery of peripheral fatty acids to the liver which in turn drives hepatic TG synthesis. These TG are then packaged very-low-density lipoprotein (VLDL) which are returned to the circulation. In the context of obesity and diabetes, the proinflammatory state of the vasculature leads to increased ROS production and subsequently oxLDL. As indicated earlier, the uptake of oxLDL by macrophages leads to foam cell production which are highly proinflammatory cells resident in the intimal layer of the vasculature.

An additional role of insulin resistance in the overall cardiac pathology associated with MetS relates to the normal role of insulin in platelet function. In platelets, insulin action leads to an increase in endothelial nitric oxide synthase (eNOS) activity that is due to its phosphorylation by AMPK. Activation of NO production in platelets leads to a decrease in thrombin-induced aggregation, thereby, limiting the procoagulant effects of platelet activation. This response of platelets to insulin function clearly indicates why disruption in insulin action is a major contributing factor in the development of hypertension, atherosclerosis, and MetS.

Taken together, the insulin resistance and its associated negative effects on metabolism, the increased levels of circulating TG, the reduced levels of high-density lipoproteins (HDLs), and hypertension, all contribute to the progression of atherosclerosis. With associated coagulation and fibrinolysis pathologies, the cardiovascular events of MetS can be devastating. Since many of these pathologies can be reversed with proper diet and exercise, lifestyle choices are critical to the development of MetS as well as to the treatment of the disorder.

Obesity and the Metabolic Syndrome

Evidence indicates that over 50% of obese adolescents go on to develop MetS. Also, given the high correlation between insulin resistance and development of MetS, it is not at all surprising that there is a strong link between obesity and MetS. Insulin resistance (identified as type 2 diabetes) is 5 to 6 times more common in individuals with a body mass index (BMI) greater than 30 kg/m^2 than in individuals of normal weight.

Although the precise mechanism(s) by which obesity leads to the development of MetS is not fully understood, there are many overlapping pathways of metabolism that are disrupted in obesity that can be identified as important in the progression to MetS. Not the least of which is the role that obesity, in particular visceral obesity, plays in the progression to insulin resistance, the hallmark of MetS.

Testing for the Metabolic Syndrome

A number of clinical laboratory tests have been developed over the years and today are used to screen and/or diagnosis MetS or one of its many pathophysiological entities (Table 48-2). The results of these tests aid physicians in diagnosis, management, and preventative maintenance of MetS.

Treatment of the Metabolic Syndrome

The treatment of MetS is multifactorial. One therapy may be able to treat more than one pathophysiological process; for example, increased exercise and/or dietary alteration. The primary therapy for MetS consists of weight loss, exercise, and smoking cessation. These 3 changes can lead to decreased blood pressure, increased insulin sensitivity, decreased triglyceride and LDL levels, and elevated HDL levels. Medications such as statins and niacin are also used to decrease circulating lipid levels (see Chapter 26).

Atherosclerosis

Atherosclerosis is defined as a progressive disease characterized by the accumulation of cells, primarily leukocytes, lipids, and fibrous elements in susceptible zones

TABLE 48-2: Diagnostic Tests for Diagnosis and Screening for MetS

Specific Test
Lipid panel with reflex to direct (measured) LDL
VLDL calculation
High-sensitivity C-reactive protein (CRP)
Oral glucose tolerance test
Fasting glucose with estimated average glucose (eAG)
Hemoglobin A_{1c} (HbA_{1c}) levels
Insulin level
C-peptide level
Microalbumin level
Thrombophilia testing

High-Yield Concept

Although, as indicated above, there are many examples of individuals who are obese but do not manifest MetS there is still a very strong correlation between obesity and increased risk for development of MetS. In addition, the incidence of MetS increases with the severity of obesity.

in the large and medium arteries. Atherosclerosis is in essence a proinflammatory condition where there is enhanced leukocyte infiltration into the vascular endothelium and an associated increase in secretion of proinflammatory cytokines which sets up a feed-forward process that builds upon itself (Table 48-3).

Multiple risk factors and an array of different stimuli, such as hypercholesterolemia, hypertension, insulin resistance, and even smoking, lead to a pathological activation of the endothelial lining of the vessel wall. The activation of endothelial cells by these pathological stimuli results in the attraction monocytes into the intima layer. Once in the intima, monocytes differentiate into macrophages and attempt to clear the cholesterol that has accumulated in this layer. Monocyte chemotactic protein-1 (MCP-1, also called monocyte chemoattractant protein-1) is the major chemokine-triggering migration of monocytes into the intima at sites of lesion formation. Macrophage colony-stimulating factor (M-CSF) contributes to the differentiation of monocytes into macrophages in this environment. Once macrophages take up cholesterol in the intima they secrete factors that attract other immune cells and promote a phenotypic switching of the underlying smooth muscle cells.

Obesity results in elevated levels of circulating lipids as well as dramatic expansion of adipose tissue. One of the principal adipose tissue proinflammatory cytokines, whose expression is increased in obesity, and which plays a critical role in the development of atherosclerosis, is TNF-α. Increased secretion of TNF-α, as well as IL-1β, leads to increased expression of various cell adhesion molecules on the surface of vascular endothelial cells. These adhesion molecules include E-selectin (also called endothelial-leukocyte adhesion molecule-1, ELAM-1), vascular cell adhesion molecule-1 (VCAM-1), and intercellular adhesion molecule-1 (ICAM-1). The presentation of these adhesion molecules allows leukocytes, such as monocytes and neutrophils, to adhere to the endothelium perpetuating the local release of proinflammatory cytokines. Expanding adipose tissue secretes ever increasing amounts of TNF-α as well as other proatherogenic factors such as plasminogen activator inhibitor type-1 (PAI-1, see Chapter 51).

The increased levels of PAI-1 inhibit the ability of plasminogen to be converted to plasmin which is required to dissolve fibrin clots that will be generated as a result of the enhanced local inflammatory processes. As the disease progresses, atherosclerotic plaque formation occurs and expands (Figure 48-4). Plaques can become large enough to result in vessel occlusion or to the release of a fibrous clot which can travel to the heart or the lungs resulting in potentially fatal embolisms.

TABLE 48-3: Proinflammatory Cytokines and Cell Surface Receptor Expression in Atherosclerosis

Molecule: Cell Source	*Functions*
Monocyte chemotactic protein-1, MCP-1 (CCL2): activated endothelial cell	Major monocyte chemokine inducing infiltration into intimal layer
Interleukin-1β, IL-1β: activated endothelial cell	Increases endothelial cell adhesion molecule expression
Interleukin-1β, IL-1β: macrophage	Enhances proinflammatory state of macrophages, induces smooth muscle cell proliferation and migration
Interleukin-8, IL-8 (CXCL8): activated endothelial cell	Major neutrophil chemokine inducing migration of neutrophils to endothelial surface
Vascular cell adhesion molecule-1, VCAM-1: activated endothelial cells	Mediates adhesion of monocytes and lymphocytes to endothelial surface, only expressed on proliferating endothelial cells
Intercellular adhesion molecule-1, ICAM-1: activated endothelial cell	Is a ligand for lymphocyte function-associated (LFA) antigens, induces lymphocyte adhesion to endothelium
E-selectin: activated endothelial cell	Major leukocyte adhesion molecule of inflammation activated endothelial cells
P-selectin: activated endothelial cells	Induces adhesion of leukocytes and platelets to the endothelial surface
Tumor necrosis factor-α, TNF-α: macrophage	Major proinflammatory cytokine of macrophages, induces activation of endothelial cells, induces activation and migration of smooth muscle cells
Interleukin-6, IL-6: macrophage	Exhibits both pro- and anti-inflammatory properties depending on signal intensity, thus ambivalent role in atherosclerosis

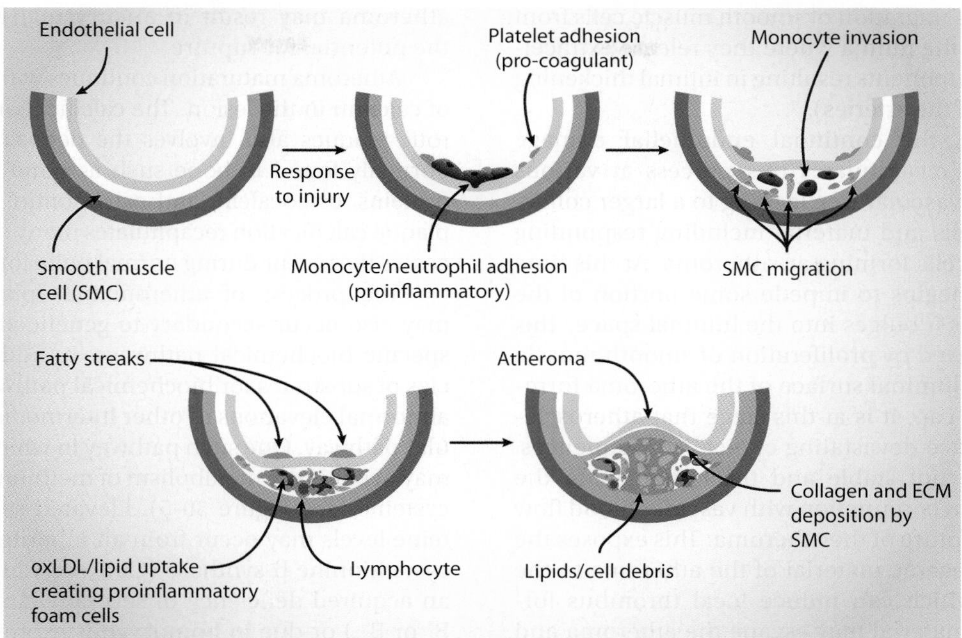

FIGURE 48-4: Evolution of an atherosclerotic plaque. Under conditions of hyperlipidemia, hypertension, a proinflammatory state, and bacterial or viral product release, the endothelial cell layer expresses leukocyte adhesion molecules that allow monocytes and neutrophils to adhere. Monocytes invade the intimal layer where they become macrophages while neutrophils secrete proinflammatory cytokines perpetuating the inflammatory state. The proinflammatory and hyperlipidemic state (commonly associated with obesity) results in lipid peroxidation, which in LDL forms oxLDL. The oxLDL binds to receptors on macrophages and are then phagocytosed which eventually converts the macrophages into foam cells. Foam cells secrete high levels of proinflammatory cytokines leading to perpetuation of the process. In addition, they express higher levels of oxLDL receptors resulting in increased uptake. Foam cells also secrete factors that stimulate smooth muscle cell (SMC) growth and migration. Activated SMC secretes extracellular matrix components resulting in stiffening of the arterial wall. Eventually, the buildup of foam cells, activated SMC, and lipid can result in rupture of the plaque resulting in hypercoagulation and production of potentially lethal occlusive thrombi. Reproduced with permission of themedicalbiochemistrypage, LLC.

Atherosclerosis is most commonly a disorder secondary to another pathophysiological process. It is the end result of a multistep process that begins with insult to the vascular endothelium. Many processes have been shown to increase vascular endothelial damage with MetS being one of the most common. Normally, endothelial cells are nonthrombogenic but in response to damage, these cells release thrombogenic (procoagulant) components. Damage to endothelial cells occurs in the wake of bacterial/viral infection such as sepsis, inflammation, turbulent flow at vascular branch points as occurs in hypertension, and in hyperlipidemic states. All of these effects on the endothelium increase tissue damage and leads to the production of ROS. Once damage to the endothelial surface occurs 2 different responses are induced both leading to a common result, the fatty streak or atherosclerotic plaque. First, on the luminal side of the endothelial injury, adhesion molecules are expressed and the permeability of the vessel wall increases allowing lipids and monocytes to cross the endothelial cell layer from the blood stream into the vascular wall. LDL is oxidized (oxLDL) and phagocytosed by macrophages via binding to the FAT/CD36 receptor (see Chapter 28) resulting in the production of foam cells. The second response is from the smooth muscle of the vascular wall itself. Endothelial

High-Yield Concept

The generation of an intravascular proinflammatory status is the major mechanism for the cardiovascular risks associated with obesity.

injury increases migration of smooth muscle cells from the media into the intima where they release extracellular matrix components resulting in intimal thickening ("hardening" of the arteries).

Over time, the continual endothelial damage reinforces and recapitulates this process at various sites along the vascular tree leading to a larger collection of lipid cells and material including responding inflammatory cells forming an atheroma. At this time the atheroma begins to impede some portion of the vascular flow as it bulges into the luminal space. This change is followed by proliferation of smooth muscle cells along the luminal surface of the atheroma forming the fibrous cap. It is at this stage that atherosclerosis can produce devastating clinical consequences. Atheromas are not stable and the bulging into the luminal space in conjunction with vascular blood flow can result in rupture of the atheroma. This exposes the highly thrombogenic material of the atheroma to the bloodstream which can induce local thrombus formation. Lipid material may escape the atheroma and travel downstream (atheroembolization) resulting in a thrombotic occlusion. Blood may leak into the atheroma, expanding it to where it occludes the vascular lumen. Finally, weakening of the native wall by the atheroma may result in aneurysmal formation with the potential for rupture.

Atheroma maturation continues with the deposition of calcium in the lesion. The calcification of atherosclerotic plaques also involves the deposition of proteins normally found in bone such as bone morphogenetic proteins, osteocalcin, and osteopontin. The process of plaque calcification recapitulates many of the same processes that occur during normal bone formation.

The process of atheromatous plaque formation may also occur secondary to genetic abnormalities in specific biochemical pathways. In addition, deficiencies of substrates for biochemical pathways can lead to abnormal elevations in other intermediates in a particular pathway. One such pathway in which these defects may occur is the metabolism of methionine and homocysteine (see Figure 30-5). Elevated serum homocysteine levels may occur from an inherited deficiency of cystathionine β-synthase (CBS, see Clinical Box 30-3), an acquired deficiency of several vitamins (folic acid, B_6 or B_{12}) or due to homozygous expression of a thermolabile form of methylenetetrahydrofolate reductase (MTHFR). Homocysteinemia (and homocystinuria) is associated with an increased risk of thrombosis, cardiovascular disease, and stroke.

REVIEW QUESTIONS

1. You are examining the characteristics of monocyte transmigration through a monolayer of endothelial cells in a culture system. Your studies reveal that the addition of an experimental compound induces a significant increase in the rate of monocyte transmigration. This compound most likely induced the expression of which in the monolayer of endothelial cells?

A. E-selectin
B. endothelial-leukocyte adhesion molecule-1, ELAM-1
C. Intercellular adhesion molecule-1, ICAM-1
D. monocyte chemotactic protein-1, MCP-1
E. vascular cell adhesion molecule-1, VCAM-1

Answer D: Monocyte chemotactic protein-1, MCP-1 (also known as chemokine C-C motif ligand 2, CCL2) is expressed by endothelial cells in response to inflammatory activation, injury, or infection. MCP-1 is the major monocyte chemoattractant inducing migration of monocytes to the site of endothelial cell activation. Once recruited to these sites the monocytes invade the underlying intimal layer where they differentiate into macrophages. Once in the intima these macrophages phagocytose oxLDL and other lipids and cellular debris becoming foam cells which further activates their proinflammatory state. The secretion of factors such as TNF-α and IL-1β by foam cells induces smooth muscle cell proliferation and their migration into the intima.

2. During a routine examination of a 58-year-old male patient, blood work indicates a significant elevation in the level of homocysteine. Elevated levels of homocysteine in the blood have been shown to correlate with cardiovascular dysfunction and thus, it is imperative to determine the cause of this patient's homocysteine levels. Analysis for activity of which of the following enzymes is likely to show a defect resulting in the elevation in serum homocysteine in this patient?

A. cystathionine β-synthase
B. dihydrofolate reductase
C. dihydropteridine reductase
D. methionine adenosyltransferase
E. methionine synthase

Answer A: Homocystinurias/homocystinemias represent a family of inherited disorders resulting from defects in several of the genes involved in the conversion of methionine to cysteine. The most common causes of homocystinuria are defects in the cystathionine β-synthase (*CBS*) gene. Common symptoms of homocystinuria are dislocated optic lenses, osteoporosis, lengthening and thinning of the long bones, and an increased risk of abnormal blood clotting (thromboembolism). Some instances of genetic homocystinuria respond favorably to pyridoxine therapy, suggesting that in these cases the defect in CBS is a decreased affinity for the cofactor, pyridoxal phosphate.

3. You are examining a 63-year-old woman who has come to you complaining of headache, light-headedness, and facial swelling. Upon physical examination of the patient you suspect she may have restricted blood flow in a major artery or vein so you order a routine angiography. The results of the angiography indicate a reduction in blood flow entering the right side of the heart. Where is the most likely location of the restriction to blood flow?

A. common iliac artery
B. external carotid artery
C. pulmonary artery
D. superior vena cava
E. thoracic aorta

Answer D: The superior vena cava is a large diameter vein that carries deoxygenated blood from the upper half of the body to the heart's right atrium. The patient is likely suffering from superior vena cava syndrome which results from direct obstruction of the vein usually due to a malignancy such as bronchogenic carcinoma. Common symptoms of the disorder are shortness of breath, facial and upper limb edema, cough, light-headedness, and headache.

4. You are carrying out a routine follow-up examination a 59-year-old asymptomatic man. He jogs a little bit everyday and plays golf. His LDL in the past was 177 mg/dL. He has a history of hypertension, and there is a history of premature heart disease in his family. A stress test is normal to stage 6. He is on a statin, an antihypertensive, and low-dose aspirin. Physical examination demonstrates he is 6 ft 2 in tall and weighs 220 lb with a waist circumference of 41 in and his BMI is 28 kg/m^2. His blood pressure, on this treatment, is 150/88 mm Hg; his cholesterol is 220 mg/dL, LDL is 140 mg/dL, HDL is 36 mg/dL, triglycerides are 220 mg/dL, and his fasting blood glucose is 120 mg/dL. Because he is doing so well, he stops his statin and low-dose aspirin. Decreased activity in which of the following would be apparent in this patient given his change in medication?

A. adiponectin
B. monocyte chemotactic protein-1, MCP-1
C. nitric oxide synthase, NOS
D. plasminogen activator inhibitor-1, PAI-1
E. prostaglandin E_2, PGE_2

Answer C: Part of the cardiovascular benefits of aspirin is related to its dose-dependent differential effects on inflammatory events. Only at low doses (eg, 81 mg) will aspirin elicit its most important anti-inflammatory benefits. The low-dose anti-inflammatory effects of aspirin are due to its ability to trigger the synthesis of the lipoxins (see Chapter 24) which are anti-inflammatory and proresolving metabolites of arachidonic acid. One of the major effects of lipoxin production is the activation of endothelial nitric oxide synthase (eNOS). The induction of NO by aspirin is correlated, in a dose-dependent manner, with a reduction in leukocyte accumulation at sites of inflammation. The induced production of NO by aspirin plays a significant role in the protective effects of aspirin on the cardiovascular system.

5. Which of the following represents a fibrous clot present in the circulation due to being sheared from a fixed clot somewhere else in the body?

A. embolus
B. hemangioma
C. plaque
D. thrombus
E. thrombophlebitis

Answer A: An embolus is any detached, intravascular mass (most often a clot) carried by the circulation, which is capable of clogging arterial capillary beds at a site distant from its point of origin.

6. A 46-year-old man is being evaluated by his physician in the course of a routine physical examination for his new job. He denies any complaints at present, nor any recent history of illness or injury. His last physical examination was over 10 years ago for a job-related injury to his knee. He has no allergies, takes no prescription medications, but takes acetaminophen occasionally for his "aches and pains." Family history is significant for his mother and brother having heart disease, hypertension, and obesity. His mother has had 2 myocardial infarctions, and his older brother takes oral medication for type 2 diabetes. He carries a significant amount of central fat, his waist is 44 in, and his calculated BMI is 36 kg/m^2. The working diagnoses of obesity and hypertension are attributed to the patient's history and is suggestive of the metabolic syndrome. Testing for which of the following would be most beneficial to ensure proper diagnosis and treatment in this patient?

A. creatine phosphokinase levels in the serum
B. creatinine clearance rate
C. fasting serum cholesterol level
D. liver enzyme levels in the serum
E. serum insulin levels

Answer E: The metabolic syndrome, MetS is a disorder that defines a combination of metabolic and cardiovascular risk determinants. These risk factors include insulin resistance, hyperinsulinemia, central adiposity (obesity associated with excess fat deposits around the waist), dyslipidemia, glucose intolerance, hypertension, proinflammatory status, and microalbuminemia. The hallmark feature of MetS is indeed insulin resistance which can be assessed by the presence of hyperinsulinemia, especially in the presence of hyperglycemia.

7. You are examining a 62-year-old female patient during a routine physical. The examination shows the patient is 5 ft 4 in tall, weighs 150 lb, has a waist circumference of 38 in, and a calculated BMI of 26 kg/m^2. Her blood pressure is 128/80 mm Hg and blood analysis indicates elevated fasting plasma glucose and hypertriglyceridemia. The physical examination and blood work indicate your patient is likely manifesting symptoms of the metabolic syndrome. Which of the following would be a useful test to confirm this initial diagnosis?

A. bile excretion rate
B. C-reactive protein (CRP) levels
C. creatine phosphokinase level in the serum
D. creatinine clearance rate
E. serum aspartate aminotransferase level

Answer B: The metabolic syndrome, MetS is a disorder that defines a combination of metabolic and cardiovascular risk determinants. These risk factors include insulin resistance, hyperinsulinemia, central adiposity (obesity associated with excess fat deposits around the waist), dyslipidemia, glucose intolerance, hypertension, and a proinflammatory status. C-reactive protein is synthesized in the liver in response to proinflammatory cytokine release from macrophages and adipose tissue. The protein is a member of the acute phase proteins which are proteins whose levels increase in the blood in response to inflammation. Thus, measurement of CRP levels is excellent indicator of a proinflammatory status as is typical in the metabolic syndrome.

8. You are carrying out a routine examination of a 54-year-old white male patient with a past medical history of hypertension. He has no complaints other than some dyspnea on exertion, which has been long-standing. Current medications include a thiazide diuretic and aspirin. He does not get much physical activity during the day. Physical examination indicates he is 5 ft 11 in tall, weighs 210 lb, has a waist circumference of 40.5 in, and a calculated BMI of 29 kg/m^2. His blood pressure is 135/80 mm Hg sitting and 130/80 mm Hg standing. The rest of his physical examination is unremarkable. Blood work indicates total cholesterol of 230 mg/dL, HDL 38 mg/dL, LDL 152 mg/dL, triglycerides 200 mg/dL, and fasting plasma glucose 120 mg/dL. Based on these observations and test results this patient is the greatest risk for which of the following?

A. esophageal reflux disease
B. gallstones
C. insulin resistance
D. liver failure
E. renal failure

Answer C: Insulin resistance (IR) refers to the situation whereby insulin interaction with its receptor fails to elicit downstream signaling events. Metabolically and clinically the most detrimental effects of IR are due to disruption in insulin-mediated control of glucose and lipid homeostasis in the primary insulin-responsive tissues: liver, skeletal muscle, and adipose tissue. IR is a characteristic feature found associated with obesity resulting in type 2 diabetes. In addition, IR is the hallmark feature of the metabolic syndrome (MetS). IR can occur for a number of reasons however, the most prevalent cause is the hyperlipidemic and proinflammatory states associated with obesity.

9. You are treating a 48-year-old white woman who is clearly manifesting signs and symptoms of the metabolic syndrome, MetS. Given the correlation between MetS and coronary artery disease (CAD), treatment to increase expression of which of the following would be most beneficial to treating intravascular inflammation associated with MetS in this patient?

A. endothelial-leukocyte adhesion molecule-1, E-selectin
B. monocyte chemotactic protein-1, MCP-1
C. nitric oxide, NO
D. tumor necrosis factor-α, TNF-α
E. vascular endothelial growth factor, VEGF

Answer C: Increased levels of nitric oxide (NO) production by endothelial cells are an important component in intravascular integrity, vascular tone, and the regulation of coagulation. In addition to modulating vascular tone by activating signaling events in the underlying vascular smooth muscle cells, endothelial cell-derived NO reduces the production of proinflammatory cytokines, reduces leukocyte and monocyte recruitment and adhesion to the endothelium, inhibits the proliferation of vascular smooth muscle cells, inhibits apoptosis, and attenuates platelet aggregation. In addition, events initiated by NO that are important for blood coagulation include inhibition of platelet aggregation and adhesion and inhibition of neutrophil adhesion to platelets and to the vascular endothelium.

10. A 62-year-old woman has had atrial fibrillation since experiencing a myocardial infarction 7 months prior. Two weeks ago she was hospitalized following a car accident in which she suffered a compound fracture of her left femur and several severe contusions. She now returns to the emergency room with right flank pain, hematuria, and left-sided paralysis. These newly developing problems are most likely the result of which of the following?

A. air embolism from the compound fracture
B. bone marrow embolus from the fractured femur
C. fat embolism from the fractured femur
D. systemic thromboemboli from the left atrium
E. venous thromboemboli from the deep leg veins

Answer D: Atrial fibrillation produces turbulence which is conducive to the formation of thrombi which can then embolize throughout the systemic circulation. In this patient the right flank pain and hematuria and left-sided paralysis suggest that thromboemboli traveled to the right kidney and the brain, respectively.

Checklist

✓ The cardiovascular system is responsible for the flow of oxygenated blood from the lungs to the tissues and the return of deoxygenated blood from the tissues to the lungs. The system comprises the heart, the arteries, and the veins. Exposure of the cardiovascular system to toxins, excess metabolic components, and other "irritants" induces an intravascular proinflammatory state ultimately leading to debilitating disease and dysfunction within the vasculature.

✓ Endothelial cells line the arteries, veins, and capillaries and represent one of the primary regulatory cells in the vasculature. These cells form a critical interface between cells and macromolecules in the blood and the cells of the tissues. The failure of endothelial functions is an underlying cause of many cardiovascular disorders including pulmonary edema, hypertension, and atherosclerosis.

✓ Smooth muscle cells (SMC) underlie the intimal layer of the vessels and provide the elasticity necessary for changes in local pressures allowing for normal blood flow. Normally SMCs are not active at growth or migration, but when stimulated by activated endothelial cells and intimal resident macrophages these cells become activated, migrate into the intima, and secrete extracellular matrix components resulting in loss of vessel patency.

✓ Insulin plays a critical role in vascular integrity and loss of insulin sensitivity at the level of the endothelium is a significant factor in the development of atherosclerosis. The role of insulin in endothelial integrity is principally due to its ability to induce the activity of endothelial nitric oxide synthase, eNOS. The production of NO by endothelial cells modulates vascular tone, reduces the production of proinflammatory cytokines, reduces leukocyte and monocyte recruitment and adhesion to the endothelium, inhibits the proliferation of vascular smooth muscle cells, inhibits apoptosis, and attenuates platelet aggregation.

✓ The metabolic syndrome is characterized as a disorder that defines a combination of metabolic and cardiovascular risk determinants. These risk factors include insulin resistance, hyperinsulinemia, central adiposity, dyslipidemia, glucose intolerance, hypertension, proinflammatory status, and microalbuminemia with the hallmark feature being insulin resistance.

✓ Atherosclerosis represents a debilitating condition in which the vessel wall (primarily large arteries and veins) thickens during an intravascular proinflammatory state. The thickening is due to the accumulation of macrophages within the intimal layer, fatty materials such as LDL and triglycerides. The lipemia characteristic of obesity and the resulting insulin resistance are significant contributors to the risk and development of atherosclerosis.

CHAPTER

49 Peptide Hormones

CHAPTER OUTLINE

High-Yield Terms

Endocrine glands: secrete chemicals or hormones into the circulation

Exocrine glands: excretes chemicals or hormones via ducts

Paracrine: refers to any substance secreted by one cell which acts on cells next to or in close proximity to the source

Autocrine: refers to any substance secreted by one cell which acts on the secreting cell itself

Cretinism: a condition of severely stunted physical and mental growth due to untreated congenital deficiency of thyroid hormones

Thyrotoxicosis: the condition resulting from hyperthyroidism leading to excess production and release of thyroid hormoness

Basics of Peptide Hormone Structure and Function

The integration of metabolic and hemostatic functions is carried out by the nervous system, the immune system, and the endocrine system. The endocrine system is composed of a number of tissues that secrete their products, endocrine hormones, into the circulatory system; from there they are disseminated throughout the body, regulating the function of distant tissues and maintaining homeostasis. In a separate but related system, exocrine tissues secrete their products into ducts and then to the outside of the body or to the intestinal tract. Classically, endocrine hormones are considered to be derived from amino acids, peptides (Table 49-1), or sterols (Chapter 50) and to act at sites distant from their tissue of origin. However, some secreted substances act at a distance (classical endocrines), close to the cells that secrete them (paracrine), or directly on the cell that secreted them (autocrine).

Hormones are normally present in the plasma and interstitial tissue at concentrations in the range of 10^{-7} M to 10^{-10} M. Because of these very low physiological concentrations, sensitive protein receptors have evolved in target tissues to sense the presence of very low concentrations of ligands. In addition, systemic feedback mechanisms have evolved to regulate the production and activity of endocrine hormones.

Once a hormone is secreted by an endocrine tissue, it generally binds to a specific plasma protein carrier, with the complex being disseminated to distant tissues. Plasma carrier proteins exist for all classes of endocrine hormones. Carrier proteins for peptide

TABLE 49-1: Major Peptide Hormones

Hormone	*Structure*	*Functions*
	Skeletal Muscle Hormones	
Irisin	22-kDa proteolytic fragment of the transmembrane protein FNDC5 (fibronectin type III domain–containing protein 5)	See text
	Pituitary Hormones	
Adrenocorticotropic hormone (ACTH) also called corticotropin	Anterior pituitary peptide derived from POMC; polypeptide = 39 amino acids	See text
Follicle-stimulating hormone (FSH)	Anterior pituitary peptides; 2 proteins: α is 96 amino acids; β is 120	See text
Growth hormone (GH, or somatotropin)	Anterior pituitary peptide; protein of 191 amino acids	See text
Lipotropin (LPH)	Anterior pituitary peptides derived from POMC; β polypeptide = 93 amino acids; γ polypeptide = 60 amino acids	Increases fatty acid release from Adipocytes
Luteinizing hormone (LH); human chorionic gonadotropin (hCG) is similar and produced in placenta	Anterior pituitary peptides; 2 proteins: α is 96 amino acids; β is 121	See text
Melanocyte-stimulating hormones (MSH)	Anterior pituitary peptides derived from POMC; α polypeptide = 13 amino acids; β polypeptide = 18 amino acids; γ polypeptide = 12 amino acids	See Chapter 44
Oxytocin	Posterior pituitary peptide; polypeptide of 9 amino acids CYIQNCPLG (C's are disulfide bonded)	See text
Prolactin (PRL)	Anterior pituitary peptide; protein of 197 amino acids	See text
Thyroid-stimulating hormone, TSH (thyrotropin)	Anterior pituitary peptides; 2 proteins: α is 96 amino acids; β is 112	Acts on thyroid follicle cells to stimulate throid hormone synthesis
Vasopressin (antidiuretic hormone, ADH)	Posterior pituitary peptide; polypeptide of 9 amino acids CYFQNCPRG (C's are disulfide bonded)	See text

(continued)

TABLE 49-1: Major Peptide Hormones (*continued*)		
Hormone	***Structure***	***Functions***
	Hypothalamic Hormones and Peptides	
Corticotropin-releasing factor (CRF or CRH)	Protein of 41 amino acids	Acts on corticotrope to release ACTH and β-endorphin (lipotropin)
Gonadotropin-releasing factor (GnRF or GnRH)	Polypeptide of 10 amino acids	Acts on gonadotrope to release LH and FSH
Growth hormone-releasing factor (GRF or GRH)	Protein of 40 and 44 amino acids	Stimulates GH secretion
Melanin-concentrating hormone, MCH	19-amino-acid cyclic peptide	See Chapter 44
Neuropeptide Y (NPY)	36 amino acids, 5 receptors termed Y receptors	See Chapter 44
Orexins	2 peptides from single preproprotein; orexin A is 33 amino acids, orexin B is 28 amino acids	See Chapter 44
Prolactin-releasing factor (PRF)	This may be TRH	Acts on lactotrope to release prolactin
Prolactin-release inhibiting factor (PIF or PIH)	Is the neurotransmitter dopamine	Acts on lactotrope to inhibit prolactin release
Somatostatin (SIF; also called growth hormone-release inhibiting factor, GIF)	Polypeptide of 14 and 28 amino acids	Inhibits GH and TSH secretion
Thyrotropin-releasing factor (TRH or TRF)	Peptide of 3 amino acids: EHP	Stimulates TSH and prolactin secretion
	Thyroid Hormones	
Thyroxine and triiodothyronine	Iodinated dityrosine derivatives	Responds to TSH and stimulates oxidations in many cells
Calcitonin	Protein of 32 amino acids	See text
Calcitonin gene-related peptide (CGRP)	Protein of 37 amino acids, product of the calcitonin gene derived by alternative splicing of the precursor mRNA in the brain	Acts as a vasodilator
	Parathyroid Hormone	
Parathyroid hormone(PTH)	Protein of 84 amino acids	See text
	Adipose Tissue Hormones	
See Chapter 45		
	Hormones and Peptides of the Gut	
See Chapter 44		
	Pancreatic Polypeptide (Polypeptide Fold) Family	
Amphiregulin	2 peptides: 78 amino acid truncated form and 84 amino acid form with 6 additional *N*-terminal amino acids	Homology to EGF and binds to the EGF receptor (EGFR)
Pancreatic polypeptide (PP)	36 amino acids	See Chapter 44
Peptide tyrosine tyrosine (PYY)	36 amino acids	See Chapter 44
Neuropeptide Y (NPY)	36 amino acids, 5 receptors termed Y receptors	See Chapter 44

(*continued*)

TABLE 49-1: Major Peptide Hormones (*continued*)

Hormone	*Structure*	*Functions*
	Pancreatic Hormones	
Amylin	37 amino acids, intrachain disulfide bonded	See text
Glucagon	polypeptide of 29 amino acids	See text
Insulin	Disulfide bonded dipeptide of 21 and 30 amino acids	See Chapter 46
Pancreatic polypeptide (PP)	Polypeptide of 36 amino acids	See Chapter 44
Somatostatin	14 amino acid version	Inhibition of glucagon and somatotropin release
	Placental Hormones	
Chorionic gonadotropin	2 proteins: α is 96 amino acids; β is 147	Activity similar to LH
Chorionic somatomammotropin, also called placental lactogen	Protein of 191 amino acids	Acts like prolactin and GH
Relaxin	2 proteins of 22 and 32 amino acids	Produced in ovarian corpus luteum, inhibits myometrial contractions, secretion increases during gestation
	Gonadal Hormones	
Inhibins A and B	1 protein (α is 134 amino acids; β is 115 and 116 amino acids)	Inhibition of FSH secretion
	Adrenal Medullary Hormones	
Epinephrine (adrenalin)	Derived from tyrosine	Classic "fight-or-flight" response, increases glycogenolysis, lipid mobilization, smooth muscle contraction, cardiac function, binds to all classes of catecholamine receptors (α- and β-adrenergic)
Norepinephrine (noradrenalin)	Derived from tyrosine	Classic "fight-or-flight" response, lipid mobilization, arteriole contraction, also acts as neurotransmitter in the CNS, released from noradrenergic neurons, binds all catecholamine receptors except β_2-adrenergic
	Liver Hormones	
Angiotensin II	Polypeptide of 8 amino acids derived from angiotensinogen (present in the α_2-globulin fraction of plasma)	See text
	Cardiac Hormones	
Atrial natriuretic peptide (ANP)	Several active peptides cleaved from a 126-amino-acid precursor	See text

hormones prevent hormone destruction by plasma proteases. Carriers for steroid and thyroid hormones allow these very hydrophobic substances to be present in the plasma at concentrations several hundred-fold greater than their solubility in water would permit. Carriers for small, hydrophilic amino acid-derived hormones prevent their filtration through the renal glomerulus, greatly prolonging their circulating half-life.

Many amino acid and peptide hormones are elaborated by neural tissue, with ultimate impact on the entire system. The hypothalamic-releasing hormones (archaically called releasing factors) represent the archetype family of neutrally derived peptide hormones. Releasing hormones are synthesized in neural cell bodies of the hypothalamus and secreted at the axon terminals into the portal hypophyseal circulation, which directly bathes the anterior pituitary (see below). The pituitary hormones are carried via the systemic circulation to target tissues throughout the body. At the target tissues they generate unique biological activities.

Receptors for Peptide Hormones

With the exception of the thyroid hormone receptors, the receptors for amino acid–derived and peptide hormones are located in the plasma membrane. Receptor structure for amino acid and peptide hormones is varied and includes single transmembrane-spanning receptors, G-protein–coupled receptors (GPCRs), and multisubunit receptors.

Upon hormone binding signals are transduced to the interior of the cell, where second messengers and phosphorylated proteins generate appropriate metabolic responses. The main second messengers are cAMP, Ca^{2+}, inositol triphosphate (IP_3), and diacylglycerol (DAG). The generation of cAMP occurs via activation of GPCRs whose associated G-proteins (G_s) activate adenylate cyclase generating cAMP and the subsequent activation of PKA.

Peptide hormone GPCRs also couple to G-protein (G_q) activation of phospholipase C-β (PLCβ), which then hydrolyzes membrane phosphatidylinositol 4,5-bisphosphate (PIP_2) to produce 2 messengers: IP_3, which is soluble in the cytosol, and DAG, which remains in the membrane phase. Cytosolic IP_3 binds to sites on the ER, opening Ca^{2+} channels and allowing stored Ca^{2+} to flood the cytosol. There it activates numerous enzymes, many by activating their calmodulin or calmodulin-like subunits. DAG has 2 roles: it binds and activates protein kinase C (PKC), and it opens Ca^{2+} channels in the plasma membrane, reinforcing the effect of IP_3. Like PKA, PKC phosphorylates serine and threonine residues of many proteins, thus modulating their catalytic activity.

Only one receptor class, that for the natriuretic peptides (eg, atrial natriuretic peptide, ANP: also sometimes called atrial natriuretic factor, ANF) has been shown to be coupled to the production of intracellular cGMP. The receptors for the natriuretic factors are integral plasma membrane proteins, whose intracellular domains catalyze the formation of cGMP following ligand binding. Intracellular cGMP activates a protein kinase G (PKG), which phosphorylates and modulates enzyme activity, leading to the biological effects of the natriuretic factors.

The Hypothalamic-Pituitary Axis

The hypothalamus is located below the thalamus and just above the brain stem and is composed of several domains (nuclei) that perform a variety of functions. The hypothalamus forms the ventral portion of the region of the brain called the diencephalon. Anatomically the hypothalamus is divided into 3 broad domains termed the posterior, tuberal, and anterior regions. Each of these 3 regions is further subdivided into medial and lateral areas. The various nuclei of the hypothalamus constitute the functional domains of the various hypothalamic areas. One important function of the hypothalamus is to link the central nervous system to the endocrine system via the pituitary gland (also termed the hypophysis). The hypothalamus is involved in the control of certain metabolic processes as well as other functions of the autonomic nervous system. The hypothalamus synthesizes and secretes a variety of neurohormones, referred to as hypothalamic-releasing hormones (or factors), that act upon the pituitary to direct the release of the various pituitary hormones (Figure 49-1).

The pituitary gland has 2 lobes called the posterior and anterior lobes. Each lobe secretes peptide hormones that exert numerous effects on the body. The posterior pituitary excretes the 2 hormones, oxytocin and vasopressin. The anterior pituitary secretes 6 hormones: (1) adrenocortiocotropic hormone (ACTH, also called corticotropin), (2) thyroid-stimulating hormone (TSH), (3) follicle-stimulating hormone (FSH), (4) luteinizing hormone (LH), (5) growth hormone (GH), and (6) prolactin (PRL). The hormone ACTH is derived from a large precursor protein identified as proopiomelanocortin (POMC). The secretion of the anterior pituitary hormones is under control of the hypothalamus, hence the description of the system as the hypothalamic-pituitary axis. The secretion of the hormones ACTH, TSH, FSH, LH, and GH are stimulated by signals

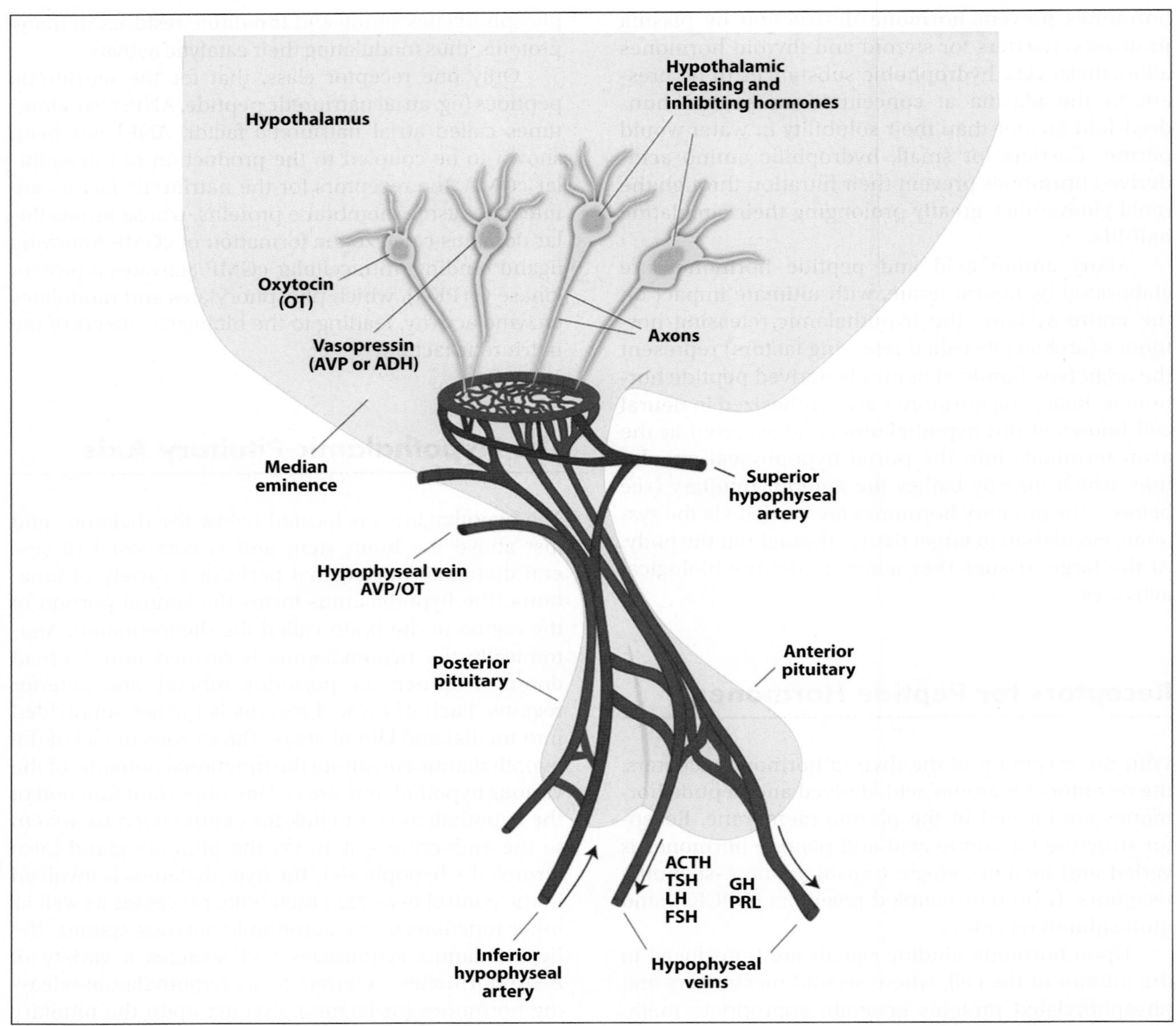

FIGURE 49-1: Diagrammatic representation of the interactions between the hypothalamus and the pituitary. The hypothalamic releasing and inhibiting hormones exert their effects on the release of anterior pituitary hormones. Oxytocin and vasopressin (antidiuretic hormone) are released directly from hypothalamic axons that terminate in the posterior pituitary, and the hormones are secreted from there directly into the systemic circulation. Reproduced with permission of themedicalbiochemistrypage, LLC.

High-Yield Concept

The cell types that synthesize and secrete the various anterior pituitary hormones are specialized secretory cells. The cells that secrete ACTH are called corticotropes (or corticotrophs). The cells that secrete thyroid-stimulating hormone are called thyrotropes (or thyrotrophs). The cells that secrete follicle-stimulating hormone and luteinizing hormone are called gonadotropes (or gonadotrophs). The cells that secrete prolactin are called lactotropes (or lactotrophs). The cells that secrete growth hormone are called somatotropes (or somatotrophs).

from the hypothalamus, whereas PRL secretion is inhibited by hypothalamic signals.

The secretion of anterior pituitary hormones results in response to hypophysiotropic hormones that are carried in the portal hypophysial vessels from the hypothalamus to the pituitary. These hypothalamic hormones are commonly referred to as releasing or inhibiting hormones. There are 7 hypothalamic releasing and inhibiting hormones: (1) corticotropin-releasing hormone (CRH), (2) thyrotropin-releasing hormone (TRH), (3) gonadotropin-releasing hormone (GnRH), (4) luteinizing hormone–releasing hormone (LHRH), (5) growth hormone–releasing hormone (GRH or GHRH), (6) growth hormone release–inhibiting hormone (GIH, more commonly called somatostatin), and (7) prolactin release–inhibiting hormone (is in fact the catecholamine, dopamine). Hypothalamic extracts also contain a prolactin-releasing substance (sometimes referred to as prolactin-releasing hormone, PRH). Several peptides found in the hypothalamus (eg, TRH) can stimulate prolactin secretion, so it is as yet unclear whether PRH is the physiologic prolactin-releasing substance. GnRH has been shown to stimulate the release of both FSH and LH and as a consequence the term GnRH is more appropriately used than LHRH.

The hypothalamic-releasing and -inhibiting hormones are secreted from the median eminence of the hypothalamus. The GnRH-secreting neurons are primarily in the medial preoptic area of the hypothalamus. The somatostatin-secreting neurons reside in the periventricular nuclei. The TRH-secreting and CRH-secreting neurons are found in the medial parts of the periventricular nuclei. The GRH-secreting neurons reside in the arcuate nuclei, which is the same region that contains dopamine-secreting neurons. Most of the receptors for the hypophysiotropic hormones are GPCRs.

Additional important hypothalamic peptides include the orexins, melanin-concentrating hormone (MCH), members of the pancreatic polypeptide (PP) family, cocaine- and amphetamine-regulated transcript (CART) peptide, Agouti-related peptide (AgRP), galanin (GAL), and galanin-like peptide (GALP). The functions of each of these peptides are discussed in Chapter 44.

Vasopressin and Oxytocin

The principal hormones of the posterior pituitary are the nonapeptides oxytocin and vasopressin. Vasopressin is also called arginine vasopressin (AVP) or antidiuretic hormone (ADH). The amino acid sequences of vasopressin and oxytocin differ by only 2 amino acids. Both of these hormones are synthesized as prohormones in neural cell bodies of the hypothalamus and mature as they pass down axons in association with carrier proteins termed neurophysins. The axons terminate in the posterior pituitary, and the hormones are secreted directly into the systemic circulation. The neurophysins themselves are derived from the oxytocin and vasopressin preproproteins. The oxytocin preproprotein contains neurophysin I and the vasopressin preproprotein contains neurophysin II.

Vasopressin is also known as antidiuretic hormone (ADH), because it is the main regulator of body fluid osmolarity. The designation arginine vasopressin (AVP) is used when discussing vasopressins from different mammals as marsupials and pigs produce a vasopressin peptide where the arginine is replaced by a lysine and is thus, referred to as lysine vasopressin. The secretion of vasopressin is regulated in the hypothalamus by osmoreceptors which sense water and Na^+ concentration and stimulate increased vasopressin secretion when plasma osmolarity increases. The secreted vasopressin increases the reabsorption rate of water in kidney tubule cells, causing the excretion of urine that is concentrated in Na^+ and thus yielding a net drop in osmolarity of body fluids.

Vasopressin binds plasma membrane receptors which activate signaling events through G-proteins coupled to the cAMP second messenger system or through the PLCβ pathway. There are 3 kinds of vasopressin receptors designated V_{1A}, V_{1B} (also called V_3), and V_2. The V_{1A} (gene symbol = *AVPR1A*) and V_{1B} (gene symbol = *AVPR1B*) receptors signal via hydrolysis of PIP_2 resulting in increased intracellular Ca^{2+} concentration. The V_2 receptors activate adenylate cyclase and result in increased cAMP levels. V_1 receptors are found in blood vessels and vasopressin binding triggers vascular contraction resulting in increased blood pressure. The V_2 receptors are

High-Yield Concept

Vasopressin deficiency leads to production of large volumes of watery urine and to polydipsia. These symptoms are diagnostic of a condition known as diabetes insipidus. Diabetes insipidus has numerous causes that include effects on both the pituitary and kidneys.

found primarily in the collecting ducts of the kidneys and are responsible for triggering vasopressin-mediated water retention, thereby affecting osmolarity. Mutations in the gene encoding the V_2 receptor (gene symbol = AVPR2) are responsible for X-linked nephrogenic diabetes insipidus.

Oxytocin is produced in the magnocellular neurosecretory cells of the hypothalamus and then stored in axon terminals of the anterior pituitary. While stored in the pituitary, oxytocin is bound to neurophysin I in Herring bodies. Secretion of oxytocin is stimulated by electrical activity of the oxytocin cells of the hypothalamus. The actions of oxytocin are elicited via the interaction of the hormone with high affinity receptors. The oxytocin receptor is a GPCR whose affinity for ligand is dependent upon Mg^{2+} and cholesterol, both of which act as positive allosteric regulators. Oxytocin secretion in nursing women is stimulated by direct neural feedback obtained by stimulation of the nipple during suckling. This response to oxytocin is referred to as the "let-down response." Its physiological effects include the contraction of mammary gland myoepithelial cells, which induces the ejection of milk from mammary glands. The other primary action of oxytocin is the stimulation of uterine smooth muscle contraction leading to childbirth.

In males the circulating levels of oxytocin increase at the time of ejaculation. It is believed that the increase in oxytocin levels causes increased contraction of the smooth muscle cells of the vas deferens, thereby propelling the sperm toward the urethra.

The Gonadotropins

The glycoprotein hormones are the most chemically complex family of the peptide hormones and include TSH and the gonadotropins, FSH, LH, and hCG. All members of the family are highly glycosylated. Each of the glycoprotein hormones is an (α:β) heterodimer, with the α-subunit being identical in all members of the family. The biological activity of the hormone is determined by the β-subunit, which is not active in the absence of the α-subunit. The α-subunit gene is identified as chorionic gonadotropin, alpha: CGA. All members of the glycoprotein hormone family transduce their intracellular effects via GPCRs coupled to adenylate cyclase activation. The gonadotropins bind to cells in the ovaries and testes, stimulating the production of the steroid sex hormones estrogen, testosterone (T), and dihydrotestosterone (DHT).

FSH and LH

The synthesis and release of FSH and LH is controlled by the action of the hypothalamic-releasing factor, GnRH. The function of GnRH is to induce an episodic release of both FSH and LH that determines the onset of puberty and ovulation in females. GnRH binds to its receptor on gonadotropes and initiates a signaling cascade that results in the release of FSH and LH.

The control of the hypothalamic-pituitary axis at the level of FSH and LH is controlled by several additional proteins including follistatin, activin, and leptin. Follistatin is a protein that binds to and inhibits proteins of the transforming growth factor-β family (TGFβ) of which activin is a member. Therefore, follistatin inhibits the activity of activin on promoting FSH synthesis and release.

In females, FSH stimulates follicular development and estrogen synthesis by granulosa cells of the ovary. In males, FSH promotes testicular growth and within the Sertoli cells of the testes it enhances the synthesis and secretion of T and DHT. In females, LH induces thecal cells of the ovary to synthesize estrogens and progesterone and promotes estradiol secretion. The surge in LH release that occurs in midmenstrual cycle is the responsible signal for ovulation. Continuous LH secretion stimulates the corpus luteum to produce progesterone. In males, LH binds to Leydig cells of the testes to induce the secretion of T.

hCG

Human chorionic gonadotropin (hCG) is produced only during pregnancy. The actions of hCG are exerted on luteal cells of the ovary. Initially the developing embryo synthesizes and secretes hCG. Following implantation the cells of the syncytiotrophoblast produce and secrete hCG. The production of hCG increases markedly after implantation; its appearance in the plasma and urine is one of the earliest signals of pregnancy and the basis of many pregnancy tests. The role of hCG during pregnancy is to prevent disintegration of the corpus luteum so as to maintain the synthesis of progesterone by this tissue.

Thyroid-Stimulating Hormone

Secretion of TSH is stimulated by thyrotropin-releasing hormone (TRH) from the hypothalamus (Figure 49-2). TRH, a tripeptide, is synthesized by neurons in the supraoptic and supraventricular nuclei of the hypothalamus and stored in the median eminence. TRH is transported to the anterior pituitary via the pituitary portal circulation and binds to a specific receptor located on thyroid-stimulating hormone (TSH) and prolactin-secreting cells. Binding of TRH to its receptor activates a typical PLCγ-mediated signaling cascade. The TRH-induced signaling leads to TSH secretion as well as increased

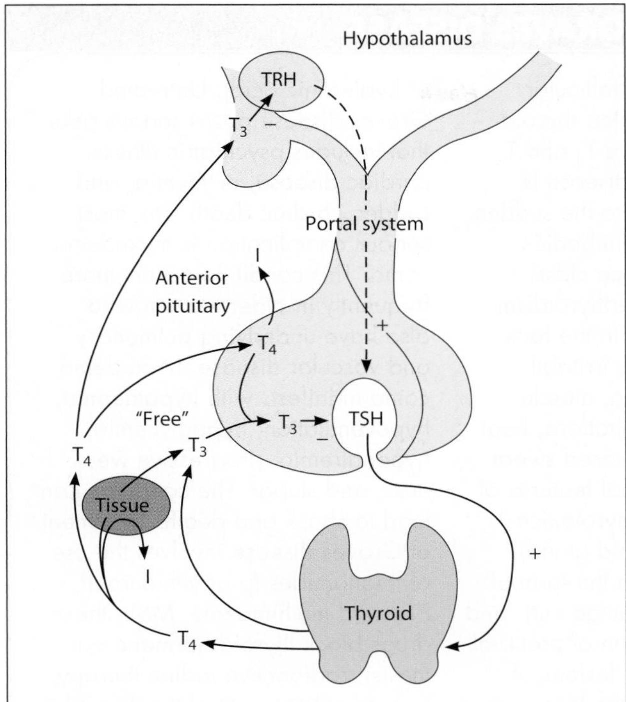

FIGURE 49-2: The hypothalamic-hypophysial-thyroidal axis. TRH produced in the hypothalamus reaches the thyrotrophs in the anterior pituitary by the hypothalamo-hypophysial portal system and stimulates the synthesis and release of TSH. In both the hypothalamus and the pituitary, it is primarily T_3 that inhibits TRH and TSH secretion, respectively. T_4 undergoes monodeiodination to T_3 in neural and pituitary as well as in peripheral tissues. Gardner DG, Shoback D. Greenspan's Basic and Clinical Endocrinology, 9th ed., Figure 7-15, New York: McGraw-Hill; 2011.

TSH transcription and posttranslational glycosylation. The TRH-mediated release of TSH is pulsatile with peak secretion being exerted between midnight and 4 AM.

The synthesis and release of TSH is controlled by two principal pathways. The first is exerted by the level of triiodothyronine (T_3; see Chapter 50) within thyrotropic cells which regulates TSH expression, translation, and release. The second mode of regulation is that exerted by TRH. While in the circulation TSH binds to receptors on the basal membrane of thyroid follicles triggering a signaling cascade that results in increased secretion of the thyroid hormones, T_3, and thyroxine (T_4). TSH-binding to its receptor also results in increased TSH synthesis and thyroid cell growth. TSH causes an increase in the synthesis of a major thyroid hormone precursor, thyroglobulin. Thyroglobulin is glycosylated and contains more than 115 tyrosine residues, which become iodinated and are used to synthesize T_3 and T_4 (see Chapter 50).

Numerous congenital and acquired forms of hypothyroidism and hyperthyroidism are the result of alterations in the expression, processing, and function of the TSH receptor (TSHR). The most common TSHR disorder resulting in hyperthyroidism (thyrotoxicosis) is Graves disease (Clinical Box 49-1).

When hypothyroidism is evident in conjunction with sufficient iodine intake, it is either autoimmune disease (Hashimoto thyroiditis) or the consequences of treatments for hyperthyroidism that are the cause. In the embryo, thyroid hormone is necessary for normal development and hypothyroidism in the embryo is responsible for cretinism, which is characterized by multiple congenital defects and mental retardation. Because the neurological consequences of congenital hypothyroidism are severe, neonatal screening for thyroid hormone levels at birth is routine. Most infants born with congenital hypothyroidism appear normal at birth. However, if left untreated the symptoms will include a thick protruding tongue, poor feeding, prolonged jaundice (which exacerbates the neurological impairment), hypotonia (recognized as "floppy baby syndrome"), episodes of choking, and delayed bone maturation resulting in short stature.

The Proopiomelanocortin Family

POMC is expressed in both the anterior and intermediate lobes of the pituitary gland. The primary protein product of the POMC gene is a 285-amino-acid precursor that can undergo differential processing to yield at least 8 peptides, dependent upon the location of synthesis and the stimulus leading to their production.

High-Yield Concept

Graves disease represents the most common form of hyperparathyroidism. At the other end of the spectrum are disorders that lead to hypothyroidism. Deficiency in iodine is the most common cause of hypothyroidism worldwide. Indeed the practice of producing iodized table salt was to stem the occurrence of hypothyroidism.

CLINICAL BOX 49-1: GRAVES DISEASE

Graves disease is the most common cause of hyperthyroidism in the developed world representing 50% to 80% of all cases. In the United States, Graves disease also represents the most common autoimmune disease. Graves disease occurs at highest frequency in women, individuals with other autoimmune disorders, and smokers. The disease results from an autoimmune defect in genetically susceptible individuals resulting in thyroid hormone excess (thyrotoxicosis) and thyroid gland hyperplasia. These individuals produce thyroid-stimulating autoantibodies (TSAb; also called thyroid-stimulating immunoglobulins, TSIs), which bind to and activate the TSH receptor (TSHR). TSAbs bind to the TSHR and mimic the TSH stimulation of thyroid follicular cells. The hyperactivated thyroid then secretes excessive T_3 and T_4. The onset of Graves disease is most often acute due to the sudden production of TSHR antibodies. Patients will experience classical symptoms of hyperthyroidism including weight loss in the face of increased appetite, irritability, insomnia, diarrhea, muscle weakness, heart palpitations, heat intolerance, and increased sweat production. The clinical features of Graves disease are thyrotoxicosis, goiter (enlarged thyroid gland), an ophthalmopathy in the form of exophthalmos (eyes bulge out), and dermopathy in the form of pretibial myxedema (localized lesions of the skin, primarily in the lower legs, resulting from the deposition of hyaluronic acid). Untreated Graves disease poses serious risks that includes psychiatric illness, cardiac disease, arrthymia, and sudden cardiac death. The most serious complication is myxedema coma. This condition occurs more frequently in older women who also have underlying pulmonary and vascular disease. Myxedema coma manifests with hypothermia, hypoventilation, hypoglycemia, hyponatremia, progressive weakness, and stupor. The condition can lead to shock and death. Treatment of Graves disease involves the use of thionamides (propylthiouracil, PTU and methimazole, MMI: these drugs block thyroid hormone synthesis), radioactive iodine therapy, or surgical removal of the thyroid gland.

POMC is produced in the pituitary, the ARC of the hypothalamus, the nucleus of the solitary tract (NTS), as well as in several peripheral tissues such as the skin and reproductive organs. Within the brain, neurons that respond to POMC-derived peptides (termed POMCm neurons) are critical in the regulation of overall energy balance via the melanocortin peptides, primarily α-MSH (see Chapter 44).

The processing of POMC involves glycosylations, acetylations, and extensive proteolytic cleavage at sites shown to contain regions of basic protein sequence (Figure 49-3). The proteases that recognize these cleavage sites are tissue-specific, so, for example, the physiologically active product of the anterior pituitary is ACTH.

Adrenocorticotropic Hormone

Adrenocorticotropic hormone (ACTH) is the main physiologically active product of the actions of the hypothalamic-releasing hormone (CRH) on the anterior pituitary. Although CRH is the primary stimulus for ACTH release, other hormones also exert effects on ACTH release. CRH stimulates a pulsatile secretion of ACTH with peak levels seen before waking and declining as the day progresses. Negative feedback on ACTH secretion is exerted by cortisol at both the hypothalamic and anterior pituitary levels. Thus, the primary product of the systemic actions of ACTH regulates the further actions of this corticotropic hormone. Additional factors that influence ACTH secretion include physical, emotional, and chemical stresses. These stressors include pain, cold exposure, acute hypoglycemia, trauma, depression, and surgery. The stress-mediated increases in ACTH secretion are the result of the actions of vasopressin and CRH.

The biological role of ACTH is to stimulate the production of adrenal cortex steroids, principally the glucocorticoids, cortisol, and costicosterone. ACTH also stimulates the adrenal cortex to produce the mineralocorticoid, aldosterone, as well as the androgen, androstenedione. ACTH exerts its effects on the adrenal cortex by binding to a specific receptor that is a member of the melanocortin receptor family, melanocortin-2 receptor (MC2R). The main cortical cell response to ACTH is increased activity of CYP11A1 (also called P450-linked side chain-cleaving enzyme, P450ssc, 20,22-desmolase, or cholesterol desmolase), which converts cholesterol to pregnenolone during steroid hormone synthesis (Chapter 50).

Secondary adrenal insufficiency occurs in patients with deficiencies in pituitary ACTH production or secretion. Whereas, primary adrenal insufficiency (adrenal hypoplasia) is characteristic of Addison disease (see

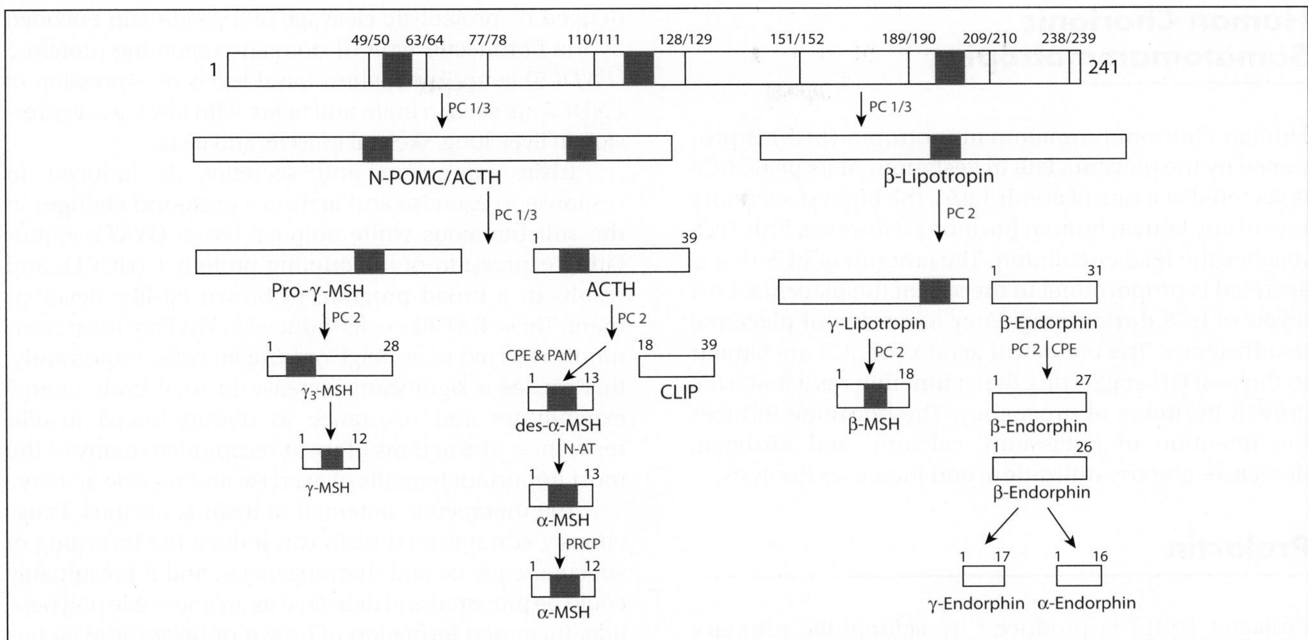

FIGURE 49-3: Processing of the POMC precursor protein. Cleavage sites consist of the sequences, Arg-Lys, Lys-Arg, or Lys-Lys. Enzymes responsible for processing of POMC peptides include prohormone convertase 1/3 (PC1/3), prohormone convertase 2 (PC2), carboxypeptidase E (CPE), peptidyl α-amidating monooxygenase (PAM), N-acetyltrasferase (N-AT), and prolylcarboxypeptidase (PRCP). Adrenocorticotropic hormone (ACTH) and β-lipotropin are products generated in the corticotrophic cells of the anterior pituitary under the control of corticotrophin-releasing hormone (CRH). Alpha-melanocyte–stimulating hormone (α-MSH), corticotropin-like intermediate lobe peptide (CLIP), γ-lipotropin, and β-endorphin are products generated in the intermediate lobe of the pituitary under the control of dopamine. α-, β- and γ-MSH are collectively referred to as melanotropin or intermedin. The blue-shaded boxes represent the heptapeptide sequence that constitutes the MSH core. Reproduced with permission of themedicalbiochemistrypage, LLC.

Clinical Box 50-1), which was originally diagnosed as the result of lesions in the adrenal glands caused by tuberculosis. Secondary adrenal insufficiency is characterized by weakness, fatigue, nausea, vomiting, and anorexia. On the opposite side of the abnormal ACTH spectrum are the adrenal hyperplasias. These include the congenital adrenal hyperplasias (CAH; see Chapter 50) and Cushing syndrome (see Clinical Box 50-2).

Growth Hormone

Growth hormone (GH), human chorionic somatomammotropin, hCS (also called human placental lactogen, hPL), and prolactin (PRL) comprise the growth hormone family. All have about 200 amino acids, 2 disulfide bonds, and no glycosylation. Although each has special receptors and unique characteristics to their activity, they all possess growth-promoting and lactogenic activity.

Mature GH is synthesized in acidophilic pituitary somatotropes as a single polypeptide chain. Because of alternate RNA splicing, a small amount of a somewhat smaller molecular form is also secreted. Expression of GH occurs only in the pituitary. The growth-promoting effects of GH are due to induced secretion of insulin-like growth factor 1 (IGF-1). The metbolic effects of GH include the promotion of gluconeogenesis and amino acid uptake by cells, and it induces the breakdown of tissue lipids which provides the energy needed to support the stimulated protein synthesis induced by increased amino acid uptake.

There are a number of genetic deficiencies associated with GH. GH-deficient dwarfs lack the ability to synthesize or secrete GH, and these short-statured individuals respond well to GH therapy. Pygmies lack the IGF-1 response to GH but not its metabolic effects. Laron dwarfs have normal or excess plasma GH, but lack liver GH receptors and have low levels of circulating IGF-1. The defect in these individuals is clearly related to an inability to respond to GH by the production of IGF-1. The production of excessive amounts of GH before epiphyseal closure of the long bones leads to gigantism, and when GH becomes excessive after epiphyseal closure, acral bone growth leads to the characteristic features of acromegaly.

Human Chorionic Somatomammotropin

Human chorionic somatomammotropin (hCS) is produced by the placenta late in gestation. At its peak, hCS is secreted at a rate of about 1 g/d, the highest secretory rate of any known human hormone. However, little hCS reaches the fetal circulation. The amount of hCS that is secreted is proportional to the size of the placenta. Low levels of hCS during pregnancy are a sign of placental insufficiency. The biological actions of hCS are similar to those of GH suggesting that it functions as a maternal growth hormone of pregnancy. The hormone induces the retention of potassium, calcium, and nitrogen; decreases glucose utilization; and increases lipolysis.

Prolactin

Prolactin (PRL) is produced by acidophilic pituitary lactotropes. Prolactin is known to bind zinc (Zn^{2+}) and the binding of this metal stabilizes prolactin in the secretory pathway. Prolactin is the lone tropic hormone of the pituitary that is routinely under negative control by prolactin release–inhibiting hormone (PIH or PIF), which is now known to be dopamine. Decreased hypophyseal dopamine production, or damage to the hypophyseal stalk, leads to rapid upregulation of PRL secretion. Prolactin does not appear to play a role in normal gonadal function, yet hyperprolactinemia in humans results in hypogonadism.

Prolactin secretion increases during pregnancy and promotes breast development in preparation for the production of milk and lactation. During pregnancy the increased production of estrogen enhances breast development, but it also suppresses the effects of prolactin on lactation. Following parturition, estrogen (as well as progesterone) levels fall allowing lactation to occur. This is to ensure that lactation is not induced until the baby is born.

Irisin: Exercise-Induced Skeletal Muscle Hormone

Irisin, named after the Greek Goddess Iris, messenger of the Olympian Gods, was discovered in studies aimed at defining mechanisms by which exercise results in improvement in metabolic status in obesity and Type 2 diabetes (T2D). Exercise has been shown to increase whole body energy expenditure in excess of the calories that are required for the actual work performed. The role of exercise in improving metabolic status in tissues other than skeletal muscle suggested that a protein was secreted from exercising muscle and acting on tissues such as adipose tissue and liver. This secreted protein is irisin and it derived by proteolytic cleavage of a proprotein encoded by the fibronectin type III domain-containing protein 5 (*FNDC5*) gene. The highest basal levels of expression of FNDC5 are seen in brain and heart, with low basal expression in liver, lung, skeletal muscle, and testis.

Irisin expression and secretion is induced in response to exercise and activates profound changes in the subcutaneous white adipose tissue (WAT), stimulating expression of uncoupling protein 1 (UCP1), and results in a broad program of brown fat-like development. These BAT-like cells induced in WAT are most commonly referred to as beige or brite fat cells. Importantly, this causes a significant increase in total body energy expenditure and resistance to obesity-linked insulin resistance. The actions of irisin recapitulate many of the most important benefits of exercise and muscle activity.

The therapeutic potential of irisin is obvious. Exogenously administered irisin can induce the browning of subcutaneous fat and thermogenesis, and it presumably could be prepared and delivered as an injectable polypeptide. Increased formation of brown or beige/brite fat has been shown to have antiobesity and antidiabetic effects.

Natriuretic Hormones

Natriuresis refers to enhanced urinary excretion of sodium. This can occur in certain disease states and through the action of diuretic drugs. At least 3 natriuretic hormones have been identified. Atrial natriuretic peptide (ANP) was the first cardiac natriuretic hormone identified. This hormone is secreted by cardiac muscle when sodium chloride intake is increased and when the volume of the extracellular fluid expands. A brain natriuretic peptide (BNP) has been identified and found in human heart and blood (but not human brain). Human BNP is also referred to as ventricular natriuretic factor but is still identified as BNP. In humans, a third natriuretic peptide (CNP) is present in the brain but not in the heart.

The action of ANP is to cause natriuresis presumably by increasing glomerular filtration rate (its exact mechanism of action remains unclear). ANP induces relaxation of the mesangial cells of the glomeruli and thus may increase the surface area of these cells so that filtration is increased. Alternatively, ANP might act on tubule cells to increase sodium excretion. Other effects of ANP include reducing blood pressure, decreasing the responsiveness of adrenal glomerulosa cells to stimuli that results in aldosterone production and secretion, inhibition of secretion of vasopressin, and decrease in vascular smooth muscle cell responses to vasoconstrictive agents. These latter actions of ANP are counter to the effects of angiotensin II. ANP also lowers renin secretion by the kidneys, thus lowering circulating angiotensin II levels.

Three different ANP receptors have been identified: ANPR-A, ANPR-B, and ANPR-C. Both ANPR-A and ANPR-B proteins span the plasma membrane and their intracellular domains possess intrinsic guanylate cyclase activity. When ANP binds there is an increase in guanylate cyclase activity leading to production of cyclic GMP (cGMP), which serves as the second messenger for ANP (or BNP and CNP) signaling.

Renin-Angiotensin System

The renin-angiotensin system is responsible for regulation of blood pressure. The intrarenal baroreceptor system is a key mechanism for regulating renin secretion. A drop in pressure results in the release of renin from the juxtaglomerular cells of the kidney. Renin secretion is also regulated by the rate of Na^+ and Cl^- transport across the macula densa. The higher the rate of transport of these ions, the lower the rate of renin secretion. The only function for renin is to cleave a 10-amino-acid peptide from the *N*-terminal end of angiotensinogen (Figure 49-4). This decapeptide is called angiotensin I. Angiotensin I is then cleaved by the action of angiotensin-converting enzyme (ACE) removing two amino acids from the *C*-terminal end of angiotensin I generating the bioactive hormone, angiotensin II.

Angiotensin II is one of the most potent naturally occurring vasoconstrictors. The vasoconstrictive action of angiotensin II is primarily exerted on the arterioles and leads to a rise in both systolic and diastolic blood pressure. It is this action of angiotensin II on blood pressure that led to the development of a class of drugs called the ACE inhibitors for use as antihypertensive drugs. As the name implies, ACE inhibitors prevent ACE from converting angiotensin I to angiotensin II.

In individuals that are depleted of sodium or who have liver disease (eg, cirrhosis), the pressive actions of angiotensin II are greatly reduced. These conditions lead to increased circulating levels of angiotensin II, which in turn leads to a downregulation in the numbers of angiotensin II receptors on smooth muscle cells. As a consequence, administration of exogenous angiotensin II to these individuals has little effect.

Other physiological responses to angiotensin II include induction of adrenal cortex synthesis and secretion of aldosterone. Angiotensin II also acts on the brain leading to increased blood pressure,

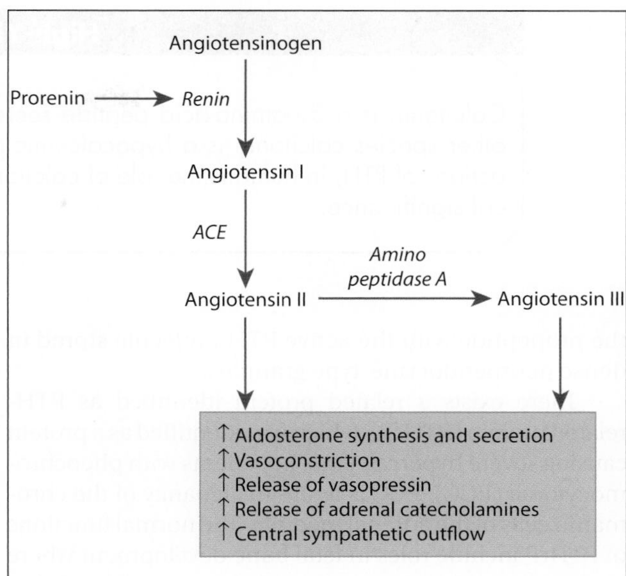

FIGURE 49-4: Steps in the production of angiotensin peptides by the renin-angiotensin system (ACE, angiotensin-converting enzyme).

vasopressin and ACTH secretion, and increased water intake. Angiotensin II affects the contractility of the mesangial cells of the kidney, leading to decreased glomerular filtration rate. One additional effect of angiotensin II is to potentiate the release of norepinephrine.

Two distinct types of angiotensin II receptor have been identified, AT_1 and AT_2. The AT_1 receptor is a GPCR coupled to G_q-protein that activates PLCβ. Although the AT_2 receptors are serpentine in structure, they do not appear to be coupled to activation of G-proteins.

Parathyroid Hormone (PTH)

Parathyroid hormone (PTH) is synthesized and secreted by chief cells of the parathyroid glands in response to systemic Ca^{2+} levels. There are 4 parathyroid glands that lie adjacent to the thyroid gland and consist of 2 superior glands and 2 inferior glands. As PTH is synthesized it is processed through the ER and Golgi apparatus where first the signal peptide is removed and then

High-Yield Concept

Among the drugs most widely employed to lower blood pressure are the angiotensin-converting enzyme (ACE) inhibitors. These compounds are potent competitive inhibitors of the enzyme that converts angiotensin I to the physiologically active angiotensins II and III.

High-Yield Concept

Calcitonin is a 32-amino-acid peptide secreted by C cells of the thyroid gland. Although in other species calcitonin is a hypocalcemic peptide that exerts its effects by antagonizing the actions of PTH, in humans the role of calcitonin in calcium homeostasis is of limited physiological significance.

the propeptide with the active PTH molecule stored in dense neuroendocrine-type granules.

There exists a related protein identified as PTH-related protein (PTHrP), which was identified as a protein causing severe hypercalcemia in patients with pheochromocytoma (PCC). PCC is a rare malignancy of the chromaffin cells of the adrenal medulla. The normal functions of PTHrP include roles in fetal bone development where it suppresses the maturation of chondrocytes so that the onset of hypertrophic differentiation during endochondral bone growth is delayed. In addition, PTHrP exhibits antiproliferative effects in adults by regulating epidermal and hair follicle cell growth as well as inhibiting angiogenesis.

The synthesis and secretion of PTH from chief cells is constitutive, but Ca^{2+} regulates the level of PTH in chief cells (and thus its secretion) by increasing the rate of PTH proteolysis when plasma Ca^{2+} levels rise and by decreasing the proteolysis of PTH when Ca^{2+} levels fall. The role of PTH is to regulate Ca^{2+} concentration in extracellular fluids. The feedback loop that regulates PTH secretion involves the parathyroid gland, Ca^{2+}, and the its target tissues

There are 2 receptors that recognize PTH identified as the PTH-1 and PTH-2 receptors (PTH1R and PTH2R). Both receptors are related to a small subfamily of peptide hormone receptors that include the receptors for ACTH, calcitonin, vasoactive intestinal peptide (VIP), and secretin. The PTH receptors are GPCRs coupled to G_s-proteins that activate adenylate cyclase as well as G_q-proteins that activate PLCβ. The PTH1R is activated by both PTH and PTHrP, whereas the PTH2R is activated only by PTH.

The response to PTH is complex but in all tissues it leads to increases in Ca^{2+} levels in extracellular fluids. PTH induces the dissolution of bone by stimulating osteoclast activity, which leads to elevated plasma Ca^{2+} and phosphate. In the kidney, PTH reduces renal Ca^{2+} clearance by stimulating its reabsorption; at the same time, PTH reduces the reabsorption of phosphate and thereby increases its clearance. Finally, PTH acts on the liver, kidney, and intestine to stimulate the production of the steroid hormone 1,25-dihydroxycholecalciferol (calcitriol), which is responsible for Ca^{2+} absorption in the intestine.

Although the primary function of PTH is to respond to reduced circulating Ca^{2+} levels and a portion of its action results in resorption of bone Ca^{2+}, the use of recombinant PTH has proven beneficial in the treatment of osteoporosis. PTH increases bone turnover (resorption), but it also increases the formation of new bone and the latter effect on bone is more pronounced than resorption. Intermittent infusion of recombinant PTH (Forteo) results in new bone formation and has shown efficacy in the treatment of the bone loss associated with osteoporosis. This PTH-induced phenomenon occurs as a result of the laying down of a protein matrix and mineralization that occurs not only in the previous existing matrix, but in the new matrix that is formed.

Calcitonin Family

There are 2 calcitonin genes identified as α (*CALCA*) and β (*CALCB*). Transcription of the *CALCA* gene yields 2 different mRNAs as a result of alternative splicing. The 2 mRNAs are translated into 2 distinctly different proteins with distinct biological activities. These 2 proteins are calcitonin and the neuropeptide calcitonin gene-related protein (CGRP, also identified as α-CGRP). The *CALCB* gene encodes β-CGRP (also identified as CGRP-2) mRNA which is translated into CGRP in the central nervous system. The CGRP produced from the *CALCB* gene exhibits cardiovascular effects and neurotransmitter functions and may serve a role in early development. The calcitonin receptor (CTR) is closely related to the PTH and the secretin receptors which together, as described above for PTH, form a distinct subfamily of GPCRs.

In humans, the major benefits of calcitonin are its use in the treatment of osteoporosis and to suppress bone resorption in Paget disease. Paget disease (osteitis deformans) is a disorder of bone remodeling that results in accelerated rates of bone turnover and disruption of normal bone architecture. The naturally occurring calcitonins vary in amino acid sequence between species. The salmon calcitonin is 10 to 100 times more potent than mammalian calcitonins in lowering serum calcium levels and because of this activity it is used

High-Yield Concept

Skeletal muscle cells do not respond to glucagon due to the lack of glucagon receptors on these cells.

therapeutically such as in the treatment of Paget disease. The other medically significant fact related to calcitonin is its use as a biomarker for sporadic and inherited forms of medullary cancers.

In addition to calcitonin and CGRP, the calcitonin family of peptides includes amylin, adrenomedullin (AM), and adrenomedullin 2 (AM2, also known as intermedin). These peptides all interact with receptor complexes that contain the calcitonin receptor at their cores. The 2 GPCRs which are receptors for these peptides are the CTR and the calcitonin receptor-like receptor (CLR, also known as CRLR). CTR and CLR can form complexes with members of the membrane protein family called the receptor activity-modifying proteins (RAMPs), which consists of RAMP1, RAMP2, and RAMP3 in humans. RAMPs regulate receptor pharmacology, receptor signaling, and receptor trafficking. RAMP association with CTR or with CLR generates multiple distinct receptor subtypes with different specificities for the calcitonin peptide family. CLR together with RAMP1 forms the CGRP receptor. In contrast, 2 AM receptors are formed by CLR and RAMP2 or RAMP3, respectively. Interaction of each of the 3 RAMPs with CTR form the amylin receptors described below.

Pancreatic Hormones

The pancreas is composed of endocrine and exocrine glands. The exocrine glands are composed of the digestive enzyme–secreting cells (see Chapter 43). The endocrine glands are called islets of Langerhans and these glands are composed of at least 5 cell types (Table 49-2).

TABLE 49-2: Secretory Products of Islets of Langerhans Cells in the Pancreas

Cell Type	*Substances Secreted*
α-cell	Proglucagon, glucagon, ghrelin
β-cell	Insulin, amylin, proinsulin, C peptide, GABA
δ-cell	Somatostain-14
ε-cell	Ghrelin
PP cell (F cell)	Pancreatic polypeptide

The primary function of the pancreatic endocrine hormones, insulin, glucagon, amylin, and somatostatin is the regulation of whole-body energy metabolism, principally by regulating the concentration and activity of numerous enzymes involved in catabolism and anabolism of the major cell energy supplies. The details of insulin functions are discussed in Chapter 46.

Glucagon

Glucagon is a 29-amino-acid hormone synthesized by the α-cells of the islets of Langerhans as a very much larger proglucagon molecule (see Figure 44-1). The principal effect of glucagon is on the liver, which is the first tissue perfused by blood-containing pancreatic secretions. The role of glucagon is well established. It binds to plasma membrane receptors and is coupled through G-proteins to adenylate cyclase. The resultant increases in cAMP and PKA reverse all of the effects that insulin has on liver. Glucagon-mediated activation of PKA also leads to a marked elevation of circulating glucose, with the glucose being derived from liver gluconeogenesis and liver glycogenolysis.

Glucagon also binds to receptors in adipose tissue resulting in increased activation of hormone-sensitive lipase (HSL) resulting in increased release of stored fatty acids. The released fatty acids enter the circulation, are bound by albumin, and transported to various tissues for oxidation. In the liver, the oxidation of fatty acids is necessary to provide the energy needed for gluconeogenesis which is activated in liver in response to glucagon.

Somatostatin

Somatostatin is secreted by enteroendocrine D cells of the stomach and duodenum, δ-cells of the pancreas, and is also secreted by the hypothalamus. There are 2 forms of somatostatin identified as SS-28 and SS-14. Both forms have identical *C*-terminal sequences. The SS-28 form is the predominant form within the gut. In neural tissue somatostatin inhibits GH secretion, while in the pancreas it acts as a paracrine inhibitor of other pancreatic hormones. It has been speculated that somatostatin secretion responds principally to blood glucose levels, increasing as blood glucose levels rise and thus leading to downregulation of glucagon secretion. In the gut, somatostatin is involved in the inhibition of gastric acid secretion.

Somatostatin binds to GPCRs called the somatostatin receptors of which there are 5 identified as SSTR1-SSTR5. All 5 receptors are coupled to a G_i-type G-protein that inhibits adenylate cyclase. Somatostatin binding to SSTR1 present on pancreatic β-cells results in inhibition of insulin secretion. Binding to SSTR2 on α-cells results in increased release of glucagon. The effect of somatostatin binding to SSTR1 in the gut is an antagonism of the gastric acid secreting effects of histamine. Somatostatin can also interfere with the gastric effects of histamine by blocking histamine release from enterochromaffin-like cells (ECL) in the gastric mucosa.

Amylin

Amylin is a 37-amino-acid peptide that is secreted from β-cells of the pancreas simultaneously with insulin in response to nutrient intake. Amylin has also been called islet amyloid polypeptide (IAPP). Approximately 60% of amylin peptide present in the plasma is glycosylated. The functional significance of the glycosylation is currently unknown and when assayed in vitro the glycosylated peptide is biologically inactive. The primary actions attributable to amylin secretion are reduction in the rate of gastric emptying, suppression of food intake, and suppression of postmeal glucagon secretion. Collectively these 3 actions compliment the plasma glucose regulating actions of insulin. The anorexigenic actions of amylin are most likely mediated within the CNS via neurons in the area postrema. The plasma half-life of amylin is quite short being less than 15 minutes. A stable analog of amylin called pramlintide (Symlin) is used as an adjunct to insulin treatment for T1D and T2D. Patients who use pramlintide show a modest degree of weight loss. Current trials are being undertaken to establish the efficacy of pramlintide in the treatment of obesity in patients without diabetes.

Amylin exerts its effect via interaction with 3 distinct GPCR complexes. These complexes all contain the calcitonin receptor (CTR) as a core protein and either one of 3 receptor activity-modifying proteins (RAMPs): RAMP1, RAMP2, or RAMP3. The specific amylin receptors result from the dimerization of various splice variants of the calcitonin receptor (CTRa or CTRb) with either RAMP1, RAMP2, and RAMP3. These receptors are commonly referred to as AMY_1, AMY_2, and AMY_3 with either an a or b in the subscript designating which CTR splice variant of the calcitonin receptor is in the complex. Amylin receptors are expressed in the nucleus accumbens, the dorsal raphe, and the area postrema in the hind brain. Within the area postrema, the key second messenger system associated with the amylin receptors appears to be cGMP.

REVIEW QUESTIONS

1. You are attending to your 51-year-old female patient who has come to you complaining that she is losing weight, yet is continuously hungry and eating more than usual. She also reports that she is experiencing irritability, insomnia, diarrhea, muscle weakness, heart palpitations, and intolerance to heat. You suspect your patient is suffering from Graves disease. Assay for which of the following in her blood would most likely confirm your diagnosis?

A. decreased growth hormone
B. decreased vasopressin
C. elevated insulin
D. insulin receptor autoantibodies
E. thyroid hormone receptor autoantibodies

Answer E: Graves disease is the most common autoimmune disease, affecting 0.5% of the population in the United States, and represents 50% to 80% of cases of hyperthyroidism. The disorder occurs more commonly in women, smokers, and patients with other autoimmune diseases. Graves hyperthyroidism results from the production of autoantibodies that bind to and activate the thyroid-stimulating hormone (TSH) receptor on the surface of thyroid follicular cells. This activation stimulates follicular cell growth, causing diffuse thyroid enlargement and increased production of thyroid hormones.

2. A 67-year-old postmenopausal woman is being examined by her physician due to back pain, an apparent loss of height, and the inability to stand erect. Her physician orders a spinal x-ray which shows vertebral thinning typical of osteoporosis. Which of the following hormones would be the most useful in attempting to treat this patient's condition?

A. ACTH
B. growth hormone
C. parathyroid hormone
D. thyroid hormone
E. vitamin D

Answer C: Although the primary function of PTH is to respond to reduced circulating Ca^{2+} levels and a portion of its action results in resorption of bone Ca^{2+}, the use of recombinant PTH has proven beneficial in the treatment of osteoporosis. PTH increases bone turnover (resorption) but it also increases the formation of new bone and the latter effect on bone is more pronounced than resorption. Intermittent infusion of recombinant PTH results in new bone formation and has shown efficacy in the treatment of the bone loss associated with osteoporosis.

3. You are treating a 27-year-old male patient for recent onset of hypertension. The patient reports that he has not consumed any alcohol nor does he use any medications or illegal drugs. Analysis of serum electrolytes indicates a reduced level of potassium. You suspect the patient is experiencing a disruption in the normal responses to vascular volume. A blood test to assay for an increase in which of the following hormones would be useful in the diagnosis of the cause of the hypertension in this patient?

A. atrial natriuretic peptide
B. oxytocin
C. parathyroid hormone
D. renin
E. thyroid-stimulating hormone

Answer D: The renin-angiotensin system is responsible for regulation of blood pressure. The intrarenal baroreceptor system is a key mechanism for regulating renin secretion. A drop in pressure results in the release of renin from the juxtaglomerular cells of the kidneys. Renin cleaves a 10-amino-acid peptide from the *N*-terminal end of angiotensinogen-generating angiotensin I. Angiotensin I is then cleaved by the action of angiotensin-converting enzyme (ACE) generating the bioactive hormone, angiotensin II. Increased production of renin would, therefore, lead to inappropriate generation of angiotensin II and an associated hypertension.

4. You are an experimental endocrinologist studying the effects of a peptide analog on the functions of the kidney. When you administer the analog to laboratory mice you are able to measure a significant increase in urinary excretion of sodium. Which of the following known peptides exerts effects most similar to your peptide analog?

A. atrial natriuretic peptide
B. calcitonin
C. irisin
D. oxytocin
E. renin

Answer A: Natriuresis refers to enhanced urinary excretion of sodium. Atrial natriuretic peptide (ANP) was the first cardiac natriuretic hormone identified. This hormone is secreted by cardiac muscle when sodium chloride intake is increased and when the volume of the extracellular fluid expands. Although the precise mode of action of ANP to increase sodium excretion has not been characterized, it is known that ANP induces relaxation of the mesangial cells of the glomeruli and thus may increase the surface area of these cells so that filtration is increased. Alternatively, ANP might act on tubule cells to increase sodium excretion.

5. You are treating a 63-year-old postmenopausal woman who has complained that she no longer has the ability to stand erect without pain. She also reports that she suffered a minor ulna fracture when she accidently bumped into the door frame entering her bathroom. An x-ray of her spine demonstrates vertebral thinning typical of osteoporosis. In the absence of recombinant parathyroid therapy, which of the following hormones would be most useful in treating this woman's condition?

A. ACTH
B. calcitonin
C. corticotropin-releasing hormone
D. growth hormone
E. thyroid stimulating hormone

Answer B: Calcitonin is a hypocalcemic peptide that exerts its effects in numerous species by antagonizing the effects of PTH. In humans, however, the role of calcitonin in calcium homeostasis is of limited physiological significance. In humans, the major benefits of calcitonin are its use in the treatment of osteoporosis and to suppress bone resorption in Paget disease.

6. A hormone of the hypothalamic-pituitary-gonadal axis is known to stimulate follicular development and estrogen synthesis by granulosa cells of the ovary of female. In males, this same hormone promotes testicular growth and it enhances the synthesis and secretion of testosterone and dihydrotestosterone by Sertoli cells. Which of the following is the hormone exerting these actions?

A. follicle-stimulating hormone
B. gonadotropin-releasing hormone
C. growth hormone
D. luteinizing hormone
E. prolactin-releasing hormone

Answer A: In females, FSH stimulates follicular development and estrogen synthesis by granulosa cells of the ovary. In males, FSH promotes testicular growth and within the Sertoli cells of the testes it enhances the synthesis and secretion of T and DHT.

7. You are treating a 37-year-old woman who complains of an extreme thirst. She gets the greatest

relief from consuming large quantities of ice water or by sucking on ice cubes. She reports that she also has to frequently urinate. You suspect she may be suffering from diabetes mellitus but assay for urine glucose shows that it is not elevated. Indeed the patient's urine is quite dilute. A deficiency in which of the following hormones is the most likely cause of the symptoms in this woman?
 A. ACTH
 B. follicle-stimulating hormone
 C. renin
 D. thyroid-stimulating hormone
 E. vasopressin

Answer E: The secretion of vasopressin is regulated in the hypothalamus by osmoreceptors, which sense water and Na^+ concentration and stimulate increased vasopressin secretion when plasma osmolarity increases. The secreted vasopressin increases the reabsorption rate of water in kidney tubule cells, causing the excretion of urine that is concentrated in Na^+ and thus yielding a net drop in osmolarity of body fluids. Vasopressin deficiency leads to production of large volumes of watery urine and to polydipsia. These symptoms are diagnostic of diabetes insipidus.

8. As the level of visceral fat increases, there is a concomitant loss of peripheral tissue responses to insulin. Adipose tissue responses to these metabolic changes include a reduced secretion of which of the following adipokines?
 A. adiponectin
 B. adipsin
 C. IL-6
 D. leptin
 E. resistin

Answer A: Expression and release of adiponectin is stimulated by insulin and inhibited by TNF-α. Levels of adiponectin are reduced in obese individuals and increased in patients with anorexia nervosa. There are sex-related differences in adiponectin levels as well similar to that seen for leptin where age and weight matched males have lower levels than females. In patients with type 2 diabetes, levels of adiponectin are significantly reduced.

9. Blocking the actions of which of the following hormones would be expected to lead to the greatest level of appetite suppression?
 A. adiponectin
 B. ghrelin
 C. GLP-1
 D. obestatin
 E. peptide tyrosine tyrosine, PYY

Answer B: Ghrelin is produced and secreted by the X/A-like enteroendocrine cells of the stomach oxyntic (acid secreting) glands. The major effect of ghrelin is exerted within the central nervous system at the level of the arcuate nucleus where it stimulates the release of neuropeptide Y (NPY) and agouti-related protein (AgRP). The actions of NPY and AgRP enhance appetite and, thus, food intake.

10. You are treating a patient exhibiting hypotension who also manifests with signs of hepatic failure. The hypotension associated with liver failure most closely reflects an imbalance in which of the following hormone systems?
 A. ACTH
 B. aldosterone
 C. corticotropin-releasing hormone (CRH)
 D. cortisol
 E. renin-angiotensin

Answer E: The renin-angiotensin system is responsible for regulation of blood pressure. The intrarenal baroreceptor system is a key mechanism for regulating renin secretion. A drop in pressure results in the release of renin from the juxtaglomerular cells of the kidneys. The only function for renin is to cleave a 10-amino-acid peptide from the *N*-terminal end of angiotensinogen-generating angiotensin I. Angiotensin I is then cleaved by angiotensin converting enzyme yielding angiotensin II. Angiotensinogen is produced by and secreted from hepatocytes. In individuals that are depleted of sodium or who have liver disease (eg, cirrhosis), the pressive actions of angiotensin II are greatly reduced.

11. Interference with the action of angiotensin-converting enzyme (ACE) is an effective means at reducing elevations in blood pressure. The circulating concentration of which of the following hormones would be affected as a consequence of the use of ACE inhibitors?
 A. ACTH
 B. aldosterone
 C. corticotrophin-releasing hormone, CRH
 D. estradiol
 E. gonadotropin-releasing hormone, GnRH

Answer B: Angiotensin-converting enzyme (ACE) is responsible for the cleavage of 2 amino acids from angiotensin I, generating angiotensin II. Angiotensin II is a peptide hormone of the rennin-angiotensin system responsible for regulation of blood pressure. The intra-renal baroreceptor system is a key mechanism for regulating renin secretion. A drop in pressure results in the release of renin from the juxtaglomerular cells of the kidneys. Renin secretion is also regulated by the rate of

Na^+ and Cl^- transport across the macula densa. The higher the rate of transport of these ions, the lower is the rate of renin secretion. The only function for renin is to cleave a 10-amino-acid peptide from the *N*-terminal end of angiotensinogen yielding angiotensin I. ACE action then generates angiotensin II, one of the most potent naturally occurring vasoconstrictors. In addition to the vascular effects, other physiological responses to angiotensin II include induction of adrenal cortex synthesis and secretion of aldosterone. Release of aldosterone leads to further Na^+ retention by the kidneys with the consequences being an additional pressive effect on the vasculature. Thus, the use of ACE inhibitors would not only reduce the production of angiotensin II but also aldosterone.

12. Which of the following peptide hormones is released in response to stimulation of pituitary gonadotropes?

A. ACTH
B. follicle-stimulating hormone
C. growth hormone
D. prolactin
E. thyroid-stimulating hormone

Answer B: Hypothalamic gonadotropin-releasing hormone (GnRH) binds to receptors on pituitary gonadotropes and induces the release of follicle-stimulating hormone.

13. Which of the following is the hypophyseotropic hormone that regulates the activity of the lactotrophs of the anterior pituitary?

A. corticotrophin-releasing hormone, CRH
B. gonadotropin-releasing hormone, GnRH
C. growth hormone-releasing hormone, GRH
D. prolactin-releasing factor, PRF
E. thyrotropin-releasing hormone, TRH

Answer D: The lactotrophs of the anterior pituitary secrete prolactin in response to the action of prolactin releasing factor, PRF.

14. In renal insufficiency, calcium absorption is reduced and leads to increased bone resorption, a condition referred to as renal osteodystrophy. Treatment with which of the following can assist in the amelioration of the symptoms of this condition?

A. antidiuretic hormone
B. calcitonin
C. calcitriol
D. growth hormone
E. parathyroid hormone

Answer C: Calcitriol [1,25-$(OH)_2$-D] is the hormonally active form of vitamin D and functions in concert with PTH and calcitonin to regulate serum calcium and phosphorous levels. The major function of calcitriol is the induction of synthesis of an intestinal calcium-binding protein, calbinden, which facilitates intestinal absorption of calcium. Oral administration of calcitriol will increase intestinal calcium uptake, but the hormone does not enter the peripheral circulation in significant amounts. Therefore, patients with renal osteodystrophy may need intravenous administration of calcitriol.

15. A 17-year-old adolescent boy who reports to his physician that he is incapable of obtaining an erection is also quite embarrassed by the apparent enlargement of his breasts (gynecomastia). These symptoms, when present in males, are associated with an excessive production of which of the following hormones?

A. corticotropin-releasing hormone
B. gonadotropin-releasing hormone
C. growth hormone
D. melanocyte-stimulating hormone
E. prolactin

Answer E: Prolactin is necessary for initiation and maintenance of lactation. Physiologic levels act only on breast tissue primed by female sex hormones. Endocrine dysfunction leading to excessive prolactin production is associated with breast enlargement and impotence in males.

16. Acromegaly is characterized by protruding jaw; enlargement of the nose, hands, feet, and skull; and a thickening of the skin. This disorder is the result of excessive production of which of the following hormones?

A. corticotropin-releasing hormone
B. gonadotropin-releasing hormone
C. growth hormone
D. insulin-like growth factor II
E. thyroid-stimulating hormone

Answer C: Acromegaly results when there is an excess production of growth hormone after epiphysial closure and cessation of long bone growth.

17. A patient is diagnosed with problems in emptying the gallbladder. On a blood checkup, one hormone/peptide that is known to stimulate gallbladder contraction is inappropriately low. Which of the following hormones is most likely deficient leading to the observed symptoms?

A. cholecystokinin
B. gastrin
C. GLP-1

D. pancreatic polypeptide
E. peptide tyrosine tyrosine (PYY)

Answer A: Cholecystokinin (CCK) is secreted from enteroendocrine I cells, predominantly of the duodenum, jejunum, following the consumption of food. The primary digestive effects of CCK are to stimulate gallbladder contraction and bile flow and increase secretion of digestive enzymes from the pancreas.

18. The pancreas play an important role in the control of blood glucose by its secretion of insulin and glucagon. The release of insulin and glucagon is inhibited by somatostatin, which is also secreted by the pancreas. Which of the following cells of the pancreas secrete somatostatin?
A. acinar cells
B. α-cells
C. β-cells
D. δ-cells
E. F cells

Answer D: Delta cells of the islet of Langerhans in the pancreas secrete somatostatin-14, a 14-amino-acid peptide, that inhibits the release of insulin and glucagon.

19. A well-nourished 21-year-old woman presents with hypocalcemia. Her blood concentration of parathyroid hormone (PTH) is 150 pg/mL (normal 10-65 pg/mL). Her blood concentration of 1,25-dihydroxycholecalciferol is normal. Her BUN is normal. She is treated with a synthetic version of human PTH, and her blood calcium concentration normalizes. Which of the following is most likely causing her hypocalcemia?
A. decrease in total number of PTH receptors in kidney
B. deficiency of 1-α-hydroxylase activity in kidney
C. hepatocellular defect
D. secretion of an inactive PTH hormone molecule
E. severe vitamin D deficiency

Answer D: PTH promotes calcium reabsorption from distal tubules of the nephron. A high PTH value is the body's normal response to a low level of calcium in the blood. The facts that the woman responds normally to synthetic human PTH and that her BUN is normal exclude kidney failure as a cause of her hypocalcemia and make the release of an inactive PTH the best choice.

20. Which of the following refers to peptide hormones whose actions are exerted on cells adjacent to their site of synthesis but not on the cell of synthesis?
A. autocrine
B. chemokine
C. exocrine
D. paracrine

Answer D: Hormones that are synthesized in one cell and released into the surroundings to act on adjacent cells are referred to as paracrine hormones.

21. A motor vehicle accident caused complete pituitary stalk transection. Secretion of all pituitary hormones is lost except for one, whose blood level actually increases. Which one of the following pituitary hormones is distinctive in that its primary control is by inhibition rather than stimulation by the hypothalamus?
A. gonadotropin-releasing hormone
B. growth hormone
C. prolactin
D. proopiomelanocortin, POMC
E. thyroid-stimulating hormone

Answer C: The primary control over prolactin secretion is inhibition by hypothalamic dopamine; all other anterior pituitary hormones are primarily controlled by hypothalamic hormone stimulation. Hence, with stalk transection, loss of connection of the hypothalamus to the pituitary is associated with decreased secretion of all pituitary hormones except prolactin, whose secretion increases in the absence of dopamine.

22. A 39-year-old woman reports headaches, weakness and fatigue, and frequent urination over the past several weeks. Physical examination reveals diastolic hypertension. Laboratory findings include hypokalemia and reduced renin levels. Which of the following is the most likely cause of these various findings?
A. Conn syndrome
B. diabetes insipidus
C. diabetes mellitus
D. pheochromocytoma
E. polycystic renal disease

Answer A: Primary aldosteronism caused by an aldosterone-secreting adrenal neoplasm is known as Conn syndrome. Excess aldosterone production leads to increased sodium retention and reciprocal potassium depletion in the renal distal tubule; polyuria results from impairment in urinary concentrating ability. Increased sodium reabsorption and associated extracellular fluid expansion lead to diastolic hypertension and suppression of the renin-angiotensin pathway. Muscle weakness and fatigue are a consequence of hypokalemia, which may be severe in some cases.

23. A 55-year-old male presents with headache and visual field changes. He is 6½ ft tall and has a puffy face. His skin on hands and feet is thickened, and compared to a picture of him at age 30, his nose, ears and jaw seem larger. His teeth are separated (diastema). He seems to sweat more and complains of bad sleep. Which of the following would provide the greatest therapeutic benefit in this patient?

A. GHRH
B. growth hormone
C. insulin
D. somatostatin
E. thyroid hormones

Answer D: The symptoms are consistent with acromegaly. It is a rare disease resulting from chronic exposure to growth hormone in adulthood and presents with elevated serum growth hormone levels and elevated serum IGF-1 levels. One treatment option for acromegaly is medication with somatostatin analogues. These synthetic forms have a longer half-life than the normal polypeptide hormone, which is also called somatotropin release–inhibiting factor (SRIF).

24. Altered plasma renin levels can occur in both normal and pathologic conditions. Which of the following states is associated with a decrease in plasma renin levels?

A. heart failure
B. primary aldosteronism
C. renal artery stenosis
D. salt restriction
E. upright posture

Answer B: Most patients with primary aldosteronism (Conn syndrome) have an adrenal adenoma. The increased plasma aldosterone concentration leads to increased renal Na^+ reabsorption, which results in plasma volume expansion. The increase in plasma volume suppresses renin release from the juxtaglomerular apparatus and these patients usually have low plasma renin levels. Secondary aldosteronism is due to elevated renin levels and may be caused by heart failure or renal artery stenosis.

25. A person has an elevated plasma osmolality and reduced plasma antidiuretic hormone (ADH) level and excretes a large volume of osmotically dilute urine. The urine contains no glucose. What is the most likely explanation for this situation?

A. congestive heart failure
B. nephrogenic diabetes insipidus
C. neurogenic diabetes insipidus
D. primary polydipsia
E. uncontrolled diabetes mellitus

Answer C: Normally an elevated plasma osmolarity will stimulate increased antidiuretic hormone secretion and cause increased renal water reabsorption which should lower the elevated plasma osmolarity. Since in this case antidiuretic hormone is reduced in the face of elevated osmolarity and the kidney is not reabsorbing water, it is clear that neurogenic diabetes insipidus is present.

26. Although most cases of hypertension are "essential," meaning the underlying disorder is unknown, about 10% of cases are "secondary hypertension" due to a specific, usually treatable cause. Which of the following conditions can lead to secondary hypertension?

A. adrenal insufficiency
B. estrogen deficiency
C. hyperparathyroidism
D. renal artery stenosis
E. volume depletion

Answer D: A fixed lesion of the renal artery results in impaired perfusion. When the kidney is poorly perfused, it increases renin secretion, which increases blood pressure as a means to improve renal blood flow. Under conditions of renal artery stenosis, the appropriate treatment is surgical correction of the arterial lesion.

27. Renin is released from the kidneys in response to a drop in blood pressure. The function of renin is to generate angiotensin I, which is accomplishes by which of the following mechanisms?

A. interaction with a steroid receptor in the cell nucleus
B. proteolysis of antidiuretic hormone (ADH, vasopressin)
C. proteolytic cleavage of the precursor in blood
D. stabilization of angiotensin I mRNA
E. transcriptional activation of the angiotensin I gene

Answer C: The intrarenal baroreceptor system is a key mechanism for regulating renin secretion. A drop in pressure results in the release of renin from the juxtaglomerular cells of the kidneys. The only function for renin is to cleave a 10-amino-acid peptide from the *N*-terminal end of angiotensinogen circulating in the blood. This proteolytic reaction generates angiotensin I.

28. Parathyroid hormone regulates the concentration of the most potent vitamin D metabolite by increasing which of the following conversion?

A. cholecalciferol to 24,25-dihydroxycholecalciferol

B. cholecalciferol to 25-hydroxycholecalciferol
C. 7-dehydrocholesterol to cholecalciferol
D. ergosterol to ergocalciferol
E. 25-hydroxycholecalciferol to 1,25-dihydroxycholecalciferol

Answer E: Parathyroid hormone (PTH) is synthesized and secreted by chief cells of the parathyroid glands in response to reductions in systemic Ca^{2+} levels. The release of PTH triggers an overall increase in serum calcium by both stimulating bone resorption and vitamin D–mediated uptake from the gut. The role of PTH in the hormonal function vitamin D is to enhance the expression of the enzyme responsible for the conversion of 25-hydroxycalciferol to calcitriol. This enzyme is 25-hydroxyvitamin D_3 1-α-hydroxylase present in the proximal convoluted tubules of the kidneys and in bone.

29. You are treating a 54-year-old man with extreme abdominal pain. Ultrasonic examination shows enlargement of the pancreas with lobular structures clearly visible. Biopsy of the tissue indicates the patient has a glucagonoma. Which of the following laboratory findings would also be expected in this patient?
A. decreased (<6%) hemoglobin A_{1c}
B. decreased serum concentration of free fatty acids
C. hypoinsulinemia
D. increased (350-400 mg/dL) serum glucose concentration
E. increased serum concentration of amylin

Answer D: A glucagonoma is a tumor associated with the α-cells of the pancreas that secrete glucagon. Enhanced secretion of glucagon would lead to an increase in hepatic gluconeogenesis and glycogen breakdown. The glucose would then be transported to the blood (resulting in hyperglycemia) preferentially over being oxidized due to the glucagon-mediated inhibition of the glycolytic enzyme, PFK1.

30. Administration of which of the following hormones is most likely to produce a positive nitrogen balance?
A. aldosterone
B. cortisol
C. epinephrine
D. glucagon
E. insulin

Answer E: Positive nitrogen balance refers to the situation where the rate of nitrogen incorporation into macromolecules exceeds the nitrogen excretion rate in an individual. Positive nitrogen balance is most often associated with increased protein synthesis. One of the major growth factor effects of insulin is increased protein synthesis which would most likely be associated with positive nitrogen balance.

31. You are studying the effects of atrial natriuretic factor (ANF) in an experimental animal model. You find that addition of ANP to these animals results in increased activity of a guanylate cyclase. Which of the following is most likely to result from the increased cGMP concentrations in this animal?
A. activation of protein kinase activity
B. hydrolysis of GTP in the GTP-G protein complex
C. increased formation of phosphorylated protein kinase A
D. increased intracellular cAMP concentrations
E. stabilization of the ANF receptor

Answer A: Production of cGMP, similar to the effects of cAMP production, results in the activation of a specific protein kinase. In the case of cGMP the serine/threonine kinase is cGMP-dependent protein kinase, PKG.

Checklist

✓ The endocrine system is composed of a number of tissues that secrete their products, endocrine hormones, into the circulatory system; from there they are disseminated throughout the body, regulating the function of distant tissues and maintaining homeostasis.

✓ Peptide hormones constitute the largest class of endocrine system molecules.

✓ Peptide hormones of the endocrine system can function in the classical sense which involves secretion from one cell type followed by dissemination via the blood to distance responsive cells. Peptide hormones can also exert highly local effects termed paracrine hormones, or they can even act on the secreting cell itself, termed autocrine hormones.

✓ Peptide hormones can be quite small encompassing only a few amino acids to several hundred.

✓ All peptide hormones exert their biological effects by binding to cell surface plasma membrane receptors. The peptide hormone receptors are most often members of the GPCR family, but also include members of the single transmembrane family of receptors.

✓ Some of the most important whole body homeostatic regulating peptide hormones are produced and secreted by the hypothalamic-pituitary axis.

✓ Most peptide hormones are produced from a single gene. A critically relevant exception to this is the proopiomelanocortin (POMC) gene which produces a propeptide of 241 amino acids that, depending on the source of synthesis, can be processed into several different peptides, each with distinct biological functions.

CHAPTER

50 Steroid and Thyroid Hormones

CHAPTER OUTLINE

High-Yield Terms

Androstanes: any 19-carbon steroid hormone, such as testosterone or androsterone, which controls the development and maintenance of male secondary sex characteristics

Estranes: any 18-carbon steroid hormone, such as estradiol and estrone, produced chiefly by the ovaries and responsible for promoting estrus and the development and maintenance of female secondary sex characteristics

Pregnanes: any 21-carbon steroid hormone, such as progesterone, responsible for changes associated with luteal phase of the menstrual cycle, differentiation factor for mammary glands

Cytochrome P450, CYP: any of a large number of enzymes produced from the cytochrome P450 genes, are involved in the synthesis and metabolism of various molecules and chemicals

Glucocorticoids: any of the group of corticosteroids predominantly involved in carbohydrate metabolism

Mineralocorticoids: steroid hormones characterized by their influence on salt and water balance

Hormone response elements, HREs: specific nucleotide sequences, residing upstream of steroid target genes, that are bound by steroid hormone receptors

The Steroid Hormones

The steroid hormones are all derived from cholesterol. The conversion of C_{27} cholesterol to the 18-, 19-, and 21-carbon steroid hormones (designated by the nomenclature C with a subscript number indicating the number of carbon atoms, eg, C_{19} for androstanes) involves the rate-limiting, irreversible cleavage of a 6-carbon residue from cholesterol, producing pregnenolone (C_{21}).

Common names of the steroid hormones are widely recognized, but systematic nomenclature is gaining acceptance and familiarity. Steroids with 21 carbon atoms are known systematically as pregnanes, whereas those containing 18 and 19 carbon atoms are known as estranges and androstanes, respectively. The important mammalian steroid hormones are shown in Table 50-1 along with the structure of the precursor, pregnenolone.

All the steroid hormones exert their action by passing through the plasma membrane and binding to intracellular receptors. The mechanism of action of the thyroid hormones is similar; they interact with intracellular receptors. Both the steroid and thyroid hormone-receptor complexes exert their action by binding to specific nucleotide sequences in the DNA of responsive genes. These DNA sequences are identified as hormone response elements, HREs. The interaction of steroid-receptor complexes with DNA leads to altered rates of transcription of the associated genes.

Steroid Hormone Biosynthesis

The particular steroid hormone class synthesized by a given cell type depends upon its complement of peptide hormone receptors, its response to peptide hormone stimulation, and its genetically expressed complement of enzymes. Luteinizing Hormone (LH) stimulates the synthesis of progesterone and testosterone. Follicle-stimulating hormone (FSH) stimulates the synthesis of estradiol. Adrenocorticotropic hormone (ACTH) stimulates the synthesis of the glucocorticoids, principally cortisol. Angiotensin II stimulates the production of aldosterone.

Many of the enzymes of steroid hormone biosynthesis are members of the cytochrome P450 family of enzymes and they have common, preferred, and official nomenclatures. These enzymes are most correctly identified by the CYP acronym and include the family number, subfamily letter, and polypeptide number. Many of these enzymes are still identified by their historically common names or by the P450 nomenclature which includes a number designating the site of action of the particular enzyme (Table 50-2).

The first reaction in converting cholesterol to C_{18}, C_{19}, and C_{21} steroids involves the cleavage of a 6-carbon group from cholesterol-generating pregnenolone. This reaction is the principal committing and rate-limiting step in steroid biosynthesis. The enzyme system that catalyzes the cleavage reaction is historically referred to as desmolase. This enzyme is a cytochrome P450 enzyme and is also called P450-linked side chain cleaving enzyme (P450ssc) or more correctly CYP11A1. Other names include 20,22-desmolase or cholesterol desmolase. CYP11A1 is present in the mitochondria of steroid-producing cells, but not in significant quantities in other cells. In order for cholesterol to be converted to pregnenolone in the adrenal cortex it must be transported into the mitochondria where CYP11A1 resides. This transport process is mediated by steroidogenic acute regulatory protein (StAR). This transport process is the rate-limiting step in steroidogenesis.

Mitochondrial CYP11A1 is a complex enzyme system consisting of the cytochrome P450 and adrenodoxin (a P450 reductant). The activity of each of these components is increased by 2 principal PKA-dependent processes. First PKA phosphorylates a cholesteryl-ester esterase resulting in increased concentrations of cholesterol, the substrate for CYP11A1. Second, long-term regulation is effected at the level the *CYP11A1* gene which contains a cAMP regulatory element (CRE) that binds cAMP resulting in increased transcription.

Steroids of the Adrenal Cortex

The adrenal cortex is responsible for production of 3 major classes of steroid hormones: glucocorticoids, which regulate carbohydrate metabolism; mineralocorticoids, which regulate the levels of sodium and potassium; and androgens, whose actions are similar to that of steroids produced by the male gonads. The adrenal cortex is composed of 3 main tissue regions: zona glomerulosa, zona fasciculata, and zona reticularis. Although the pathway to pregnenolone synthesis is the same in all zones of the cortex, the zones are histologically and enzymatically distinct, with the exact steroid hormone product dependent on the enzymes present in the cells of each zone (Figure 50-1).

Zona glomerulosa cells lack CYP17A1 that converts pregnenolone and progesterone to their C_{17} hydroxylated analogs. CYP17A1 is a single microsomal enzyme that has 2 steroid biosynthetic activities: 17α-hydroxylase which

TABLE 50-1: Structures of the Mammalian Steroid Hormones

Pregnenolone	produced directly from cholesterol, the precursor molecule for all C_{18}, C_{19}, and C_{21} steroids
Progesterone	a progestogen, produced directly from pregnenolone and secreted from the *corpus luteum*, responsible for changes associated with luteal phase of the menstrual cycle, differentiation factor for mammary glands
Aldosterone	the principal mineralocorticoid, produced from progesterone in the *zona glomerulosa* of adrenal cortex, raises blood pressure and fluid volume, increases Na^+ uptake
Testosterone	an androgen, male sex hormone synthesized in the testes, responsible for secondary male sex characteristics, produced from progesterone
Estradiol	an estrogen, principal female sex hormone, produced in the ovary, responsible for secondary female sex characteristics
Cortisol	dominant glucocorticoid in humans, synthesized from progesterone in the *zona fasciculata* of the adrenal cortex, involved in stress adaptation, elevates blood pressure and Na^+ uptake, numerous effects on the immune system

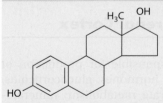

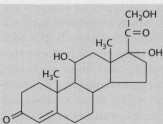

TABLE 50-2: **Primary Activities Required for Steroid Hormone Synthesis**

Common name(s)	*Gene*	*Activities*	*Primary site of expression*
Steroidogenic acute regulatory protein	*StAR*	Mediates mitochondrial import of cholesterol	All steroidogenic tissues except placenta and brain
Desmolase, P450ssc	*CYP11A1*	Cholesterol-20,23-desmolase	Steroidogenic tissues
3β-Hydroxysteroid dehydrogenase type 1	*HSD3B2*	3β-Hydroxysteroid dehydrogenase	Steroidogenic tissues
P450c11	*CYP11B1*	11β-Hydroxylase	Only in zona fasciculata and zona reticularis of adrenal cortex
P450c17	*CYP17A1*	Two activities: 17α-hydroxylase and 17,20-lyase	Steroidogenic tissues
P450c21	*CYP21A2*	21-Hydroxylase	All zones of adrenal cortex
Aldosterone synthase	*CYP11B2*	18α-Hydroxylase	Exclusive to zona glomerulosa of adrenal cortex
Estrogen synthetase	*CYP19A1*	Aromatase	Gonads, brain, adrenals, adipose tissue, bone
17β-Hydroxysteroid dehydrogenase type 3	*HSD17B3*	17-Ketoreductase	Steroidogenic tissues
Sulfotransferase	*SULT2A1*	Sulfotransferase	Liver, adrenals
5α-Reductase type 2	*SRD5A2*	5α-Reductase	Steroidogenic tissues

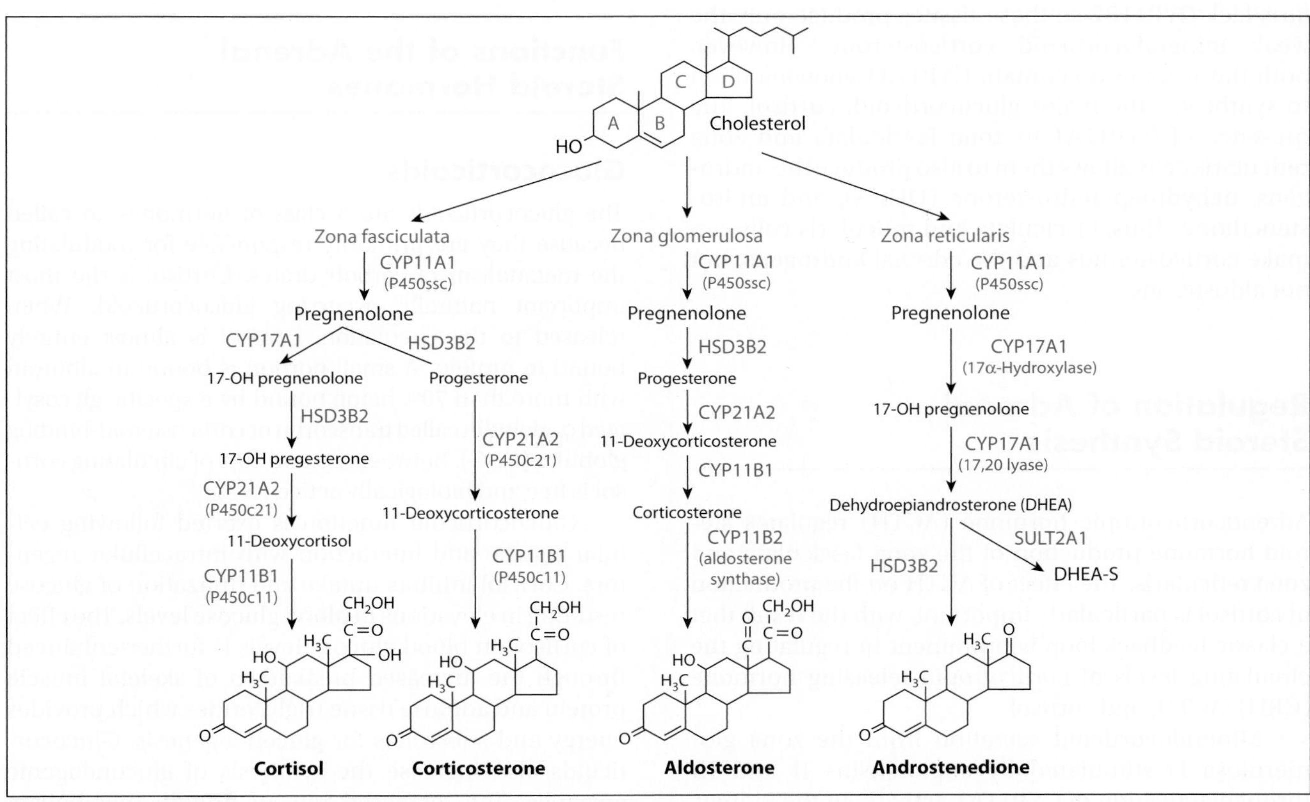

FIGURE 50-1: Synthesis of the various adrenal steroid hormones from cholesterol. Only the terminal hormone structures are included. 3β-DH and $\Delta^{4,5}$-isomerase are the 2 activities of 3β-hydroxysteroid dehydrogenase type 1 (gene symbol *HSD3B2*), P450c11 is 11β-hydroxylase (CYP11B1), P450c17 is CYP17A1. CYP17A1 is a single microsomal enzyme that has 2 steroid biosynthetic activities: 17α-hydroxylase which converts pregnenolone to 17-hydroxypregnenolone (17-OH pregnenolone) and 17,20-lyase which converts 17-OH pregnenolone to DHEA. P450c21 is 21-hydroxylase (CYP21A2, also identified as CYP21 or CYP21B). Aldosterone synthase is also known as 18α-hydroxylase (CYP11B2). The gene symbol for sulfotransferase is *SULT2A1*. Reproduced with permission of themedicalbiochemistrypage, LLC.

converts pregnenolone to 17-hydroxypregnenolone (17-OH pregnenolone) and 17,20-lyase which converts 17-OH pregnenolone to DHEA. Since zona glomerulosa cells lack CYP17A1, the pathways to the glucocorticoids (deoxycortisol and cortisol) and the androgens (dehydroepiandrosterone [DHEA] and androstenedione) are blocked in these cells. The next reaction of glomerulosa cell steroidogenesis is the conversion of pregnenolone to progesterone. This reaction requires the 2 enzyme activities of HSD3B2: the 3β-hydroxysteroid dehydrogenase and $\Delta^{4,5}$-isomerase activities.

Zona glomerulosa cells are unique in the adrenal cortex in that they express the enzyme responsible for converting corticosterone to aldosterone, the principal and most potent mineralocorticoid. This enzyme is CYP11B2 (18α-hydroxylase or P450c18) which is historically called aldosterone synthase. The result is that the zona glomerulosa is mainly responsible for the conversion of cholesterol to the weak mineralocorticoid, corticosterone, and the principal mineralocorticoid, aldosterone.

Cells of the zona fasciculata and zona reticularis lack CYP11B2 so these tissues produce only the weak mineralocorticoid corticosterone. However, both these zones do contain CYP17A1 allowing them to synthesize the major glucocorticoid, cortisol. The presence of CYP17A1 in zona fasciculata and zona reticularis cells allows them to also produce the androgens, dehydroepiandrosterone (DHEA), and androstenedione. Thus, fasciculata and reticularis cells can make corticosteroids and the adrenal androgens, but not aldosterone.

Regulation of Adrenal Steroid Synthesis

Adrenocorticotropic hormone (ACTH) regulates steroid hormone production of the zona fasciculata and zona reticularis. The effect of ACTH on the production of cortisol is particularly important, with the result that a classic feedback loop is prominent in regulating the circulating levels of corticotropin-releasing hormone (CRH), ACTH, and cortisol.

Mineralocorticoid secretion from the zona glomerulosa is stimulated by angiotensins II and III through activation of CYP11A1 activity. In the kidney, aldosterone regulates sodium retention by stimulating expression of mRNA for the Na^+/K^+-ATPase responsible for the reaccumulation of sodium from the urine. The interplay between renin from the kidney and plasma angiotensinogen is important in regulating plasma aldosterone levels, sodium and potassium levels, and ultimately blood pressure. This feedback loop is closed by potassium, which is a potent stimulator of aldosterone secretion. Changes in plasma potassium of as little as 0.1 mM can cause wide fluctuations (±50%) in plasma levels of aldosterone. Potassium increases aldosterone secretion by depolarizing the plasma membrane of zona glomerulosa cells and opening a voltage-gated calcium channel, with a resultant increase in cytoplasmic calcium and the stimulation of calcium-dependent processes.

Although fasciculata and reticularis cells each have the capability of synthesizing androgens and glucocorticoids, the main pathway normally followed is that leading to glucocorticoid production. However, when genetic defects occur in the 3 enzyme complexes leading to glucocorticoid production, large amounts of the androgen, dehydroepiandrosterone (DHEA), are produced resulting in hirsutism and other masculinizing changes in secondary sex characteristics.

Functions of the Adrenal Steroid Hormones

Glucocorticoids

The glucocorticoids are a class of hormones so called because they are primarily responsible for modulating the metabolism of carbohydrates. Cortisol is the most important naturally occurring glucocorticoid. When released to the circulation, cortisol is almost entirely bound to protein. A small portion is bound to albumin with more than 70% being bound by a specific glycosylated α-globulin called transcortin or corticosteroid-binding globulin (CBG). Between 5% and 10% of circulating cortisol is free and biologically active.

Glucocorticoid function is exerted following cellular uptake and interaction with intracellular receptors. Cortisol inhibits uptake and utilization of glucose resulting in elevations in blood glucose levels. The effect of cortisol on blood glucose levels is further enhanced through the increased breakdown of skeletal muscle protein and adipose tissue triglycerides which provides energy and substrates for gluconeogenesis. Glucocorticoids also increase the synthesis of gluconeogenic enzymes. The increased rate of protein metabolism leads to increased urinary nitrogen excretion and the induction of urea cycle enzymes. Glucocorticoids also inhibit vitamin D–mediated intestinal calcium uptake, retard the rate of wound healing, and interfere with the rate of linear growth.

In addition to the metabolic effects of the glucocorticoids, these hormones are immunosuppressive and anti-inflammatory. The anti-inflammatory activity of the glucocorticoids is exerted, in part, through inhibition of phospholipase A_2 (PLA_2) activity with a consequent reduction in the release of arachidonic acid from membrane phospholipids (see Chapter 22). It is the anti-inflammatory activity of glucocorticoids that warrants the use of related drugs such as prednisone, in the acute treatment of inflammatory disorders.

Mineralocorticoids

The major circulating mineralocorticoid is aldosterone. As the name implies, the mineralocorticoids control the excretion of electrolytes. This occurs primarily through actions on the kidneys but also in the colon and sweat glands. The principal effect of aldosterone is to enhance sodium reabsorption in the cortical collecting duct of the kidneys. However, the action of aldosterone is exerted on sweat glands, stomach, and salivary glands to the same effect, that is, sodium reabsorption. This action is accompanied by the retention of chloride and water resulting in the expansion of extracellular volume. Aldosterone also enhances the excretion of potassium and hydrogen ions from the medullary collecting duct of the kidneys.

Androgens

The androgens, androstenedione and DHEA, circulate bound primarily to sex hormone–binding globulin (SHBG). Although some of the circulating androgen is metabolized in the liver, the majority of interconversion occurs in the gonads, skin, and adipose tissue. DHEA is rapidly converted to the sulfated form, DHEA-S, in the liver and adrenal cortex. The primary biologically active metabolites of the androgens are testosterone and dihydrotestosterone which function by binding intracellular receptors, thereby effecting changes in gene expression leading to the manifestation of the secondary sex characteristics.

Defects in Adrenal Steroidogenesis

Defective synthesis of the steroid hormones produced by the adrenal cortex can have profound effects on human development and homeostasis. Addison disease (Clinical Box 50-1) represents a disorder characterized by adrenal insufficiency that was first identified in a patient who presented with chronic adrenal insufficiency resulting from progressive lesions of the adrenal glands caused by tuberculosis. In addition to diseases that result from the total absence of adrenocortical function, there are syndromes that result from hypersecretion of adrenocortical hormones. Disorders that manifest with adrenocortical hyperplasia are referred to as Cushing syndrome (Clinical Box 50-2).

The CAHs are a group of inherited disorders that result from loss-of-function mutations in one of several genes involved in adrenal steroid hormone synthesis. In the virilizing forms of CAH the mutations result in impairment of cortisol production and the consequent accumulation of steroid intermediates proximal to the defective enzyme. The majority of CAH cases (90% to 95%) are the result of defects in CYP21A2 with a frequency of between 1 in 5000 and 1 in 15,000 (Clinical Box 50-3). However, defects in several additional genes result in the various other forms of CAH including CYP11B1, HSD3B2, and CYP19A1.

Gonadal Steroid Hormones

Although many steroids are produced by the testes and the ovaries, the 2 most important are testosterone and estradiol. These compounds are under tight biosynthetic control, with short and long negative feedback loops that regulate the secretion of follicle-stimulating hormone (FSH) and luteinizing hormone (LH) by the pituitary and gonadotropin-releasing hormone (GnRH) by the hypothalamus. Low levels of circulating sex hormone reduce feedback inhibition on GnRH synthesis (the long loop), leading to elevated FSH and LH.

High-Yield Concept

Despite the characterizations of adrenal insufficiency and adrenal hyperplasia, there remained uncertainty about the relationship between adrenocortical hyperfunction and virilism (premature development of male secondary sex characteristics) referred to as adrenogenital syndromes. These adrenogenital syndromes are now more commonly referred to as congenital adrenal hyperplasias (CAHs).

CLINICAL BOX 50-1: ADDISON DISEASE

Primary adrenal insufficiency is characterized by inadequate secretion of glucocorticoids and mineralocorticoids as a result of impaired function or destruction of the adrenal cortex. The disorder was originally associated with tuberculosis and referred to as Addison disease. Currently, 70% to 90% of cases of Addison disease are the result of autoimmune adrenalitis and frequently manifests in patients with other immunological and autoimmune disorders. Addison disease frequency is higher in females than males and is usually diagnosed between 30 and 50 years of age. The loss of cortisol and aldosterone synthesis and release from the adrenal cortex results in increased secretion of ACTH from pituitary corticotropes. This distinguishes primary adrenal insufficiency from secondary which is the result of ACTH deficiency. The characteristic clinical presentation of acute primary adrenal insufficiency includes orthostatic hypotension, agitation, confusion, circulatory collapse, abdominal pain, and fever. The clinical findings in chronic primary adrenal insufficiency include a longer history of malaise, fatigue, anorexia, weight loss, and joint and back pain. Darkening of the skin, especially in the sun-exposed areas, is a hallmark sign of primary adrenal insufficiency. Patients may also crave salt and develop unusual food preferences. Biochemical features for both presentations include hyponatremia, hypoglycemia, hyperkalemia, unexplained eosinophilia, and mild prerenal azotemia. Biochemical testing is needed to confirm the diagnosis of adrenal insufficiency. The disorder can be excluded by serum cortisol levels of more than 19 mg/dL (524 nmol/L) and is likely if the value is less than 3 mg/dL (83 nmol/L). Measurement of urine-free cortisol is not a useful diagnostic test. Measurement of plasma ACTH helps to determine if the disorder is primary (values above the normal range) or secondary (low values). Hypokalemia and elevated plasma renin activity identify mineralocorticoid deficiency which aids in the discrimination of primary adrenal insufficiency. Treatment of Addison disease involves physiological replacement of the deficient glucocorticoid and mineralocorticoid hormones. Patients with acute adrenal insufficiency should receive fluid resuscitation and medical care as appropriate, in addition to supraphysiological doses of hydrocortisone given intravenously. For chronic therapy, oral hydrocortisone provides glucocorticoid replacement that can be easily titrated and given as divided doses during the day to grossly recapitulate the normal diurnal pattern of cortisol secretion. Oral fludrocortisone replaces mineralocorticoids.

CLINICAL BOX 50-2: CUSHING SYNDROME

Cushing syndrome describes the clinical consequences of chronic exposure to excess glucocorticoid irrespective of the underlying cause. Endogenous causes of Cushing syndrome are rare and include a cortisol-producing adrenal tumor, excess secretion of ACTH from a pituitary tumor (Cushing disease), or an ectopic ACTH-producing tumor (ectopic Cushing syndrome). Cushing syndrome is most commonly associated with prolonged administration of supraphysiological glucocorticoid treatment (including tablets, inhalers, nasal sprays, and skin creams) and is referred to as iatrogenic Cushing syndrome. Cushing syndrome may mimic common conditions such as obesity, poorly controlled diabetes, and hypertension, which progress over time and often coexist in patients with metabolic syndrome. Untreated Cushing syndrome is associated with high rates of mortality predominantly from cardiovascular events (congestive cardiac failure or myocardial infarction) or infection. Cushing syndrome affects the musculature (causing myopathy and congestive cardiac failure), the bones (causing early osteoporosis), reproductive function (causing menstrual irregularity and infertility), and leads to mood disturbance. As a consequence, a delay in proper diagnosis can result in irreversible organ damage. The characteristic features of Cushing syndrome are psychiatric disturbances (depression, mania, and psychoses), central obesity, hypertension, diabetes, moon-shaped face, thin fragile skin, easy bruising, and purple striae (stretch marks). In addition, Cushing syndrome patients manifest with gonadal dysfunction that is characteristic of hyperandrogenism with excess body and facial hair (hirsutism) and acne. The most common symptoms that lead to a diagnosis of Cushing syndrome are weight gain, depression, subjective muscle weakness, and headache. Since these latter symptoms are not in and of themselves diagnostic of Cushing syndrome it is important to assess for any possible use of exogenous glucocorticoids, especially inhalers and skin creams. Management of Cushing syndrome depends on the underlying cause. Surgical resection of the pituitary, adrenal, or ACTH-producing tumor is the primary treatment of choice and is often curative. If the disease is secondary to exogenous glucocorticoid treatment then titration of the steroid dose as soon as clinically possible is indicated.

CLINICAL BOX 50-3: CONGENITAL ADRENAL HYPERPLASIAS

Congenital adrenal hyperplasia resulting from deficiencies in the *CYP21A2* gene represent the most commonly occurring forms (>95%) of the disease. There are two *CYP21* genes but one is a pseudogene (CYP21P). The active *CYP21* gene is identified as CYP21A2, CYP21, CYP21B, and 21-hydroxylase. Older nomenclature identifies the *CYP21P* gene as the 21-hydroxylase A gene (or *CYP21A1*) and *CYP21A2* as the 21-hydroxylase B gene. All 21-hydroxylase activity is synthesized from the mRNA encoded by the *CYP21A2* gene. The majority of the mutations in *CYP21A2* that result in CAH have been identified and the severity of the disorder can be correlated to specific mutations and the consequent effect of the mutation on enzyme activity. Deficiencies in CYP21A2 result in decreased secretion and plasma concentration of cortisol. The reduced levels of cortisol result in a reduction in the negative feedback exerted by this hormone on the hypothalamic-pituitary axis. The reduced negative feedback leads to increased secretion of corticotropin-releasing hormone (CRH) and ACTH. The resultant high plasma concentrations of ACTH are responsible for the adrenocortical hyperplasia characteristic of this disorder. CAH resulting from CYP21A2 deficiencies is divided into 3 distinct clinical forms. The most severe enzyme impairment mutations result in the *salt-losing form*. Females with this form of the disease present at birth due to ambiguity in the external genitalia. Males with the salt-losing form present with acute adrenal crisis shortly after birth or in early infancy. Females who present with no acute adrenal crisis and only mild masculinization of the external genitalia and males who present with virilism early in life are considered to be suffering from the *simple virilizing form* of CAH. The final clinical form of CAH manifests only in females at puberty or shortly thereafter with symptoms of mild excess androgen development resulting in hirsutism, amenorrhea, and infertility. This form of the disorder is referred to as the attenuated form or the late onset or nonclassic form.

Salt-losing form: In the salt-losing form of this disorder the degree of loss of enzyme activity is severe to complete. As a result of the level of enzyme deficiency the synthesis of cortisol is negligible. Because CYP21A2 is also needed for the synthesis of aldosterone, which is a major hormone involved in Na^+ retention by the kidney, there is excessive salt loss leading to hyponatremic dehydration which can be fatal if not treated. Although there is some aldosterone made, the level of salt loss exceeds the ability of the adrenal cortex to make sufficient aldosterone to compensate. The net result is an acute adrenal crisis. The near-complete, or complete, loss in cortisol production results in maximal activity of the CRH-ACTH axis leading to maximal adrenal androgen secretion with the result being masculinization of the female genitalia. The first sign of CAH due to CYP21A2 deficiency is, in fact, the ambiguous female genitalia in neonates. The masculinization can be so extreme as to result in the fusion of the labia and the formation of a penile urethra. Diagnosis of the salt-losing form of this disorder is made in females born with masculinized genitalia, who are of normal 46,XX karyotype, with marked elevation in plasma 17α-hydroxyprogesterone and androstenedione, as well as serum chemistry showing hyponatremia, hypochloremia, and hyperkalemic acidosis.

Simple virilizing form: In the simple virilizing form of the disorder the deficiency in CYP21A2 is not complete or as severe as in the salt-losing form. As a result the adrenal cortex can compensate for salt loss with increased aldosterone synthesis and release. In addition, the increased ACTH release result in normal plasma cortisol levels and thus, there is no glucocorticoid deficit. However, as in the salt-losing form the CRH-ACTH axis is hyperactive leading to excessive adrenal androgen synthesis with consequent masculinization of the female genitalia.

Attenuated form: As the name of this form of disease implies, patients with the attenuated form exhibit only mild reductions in CYP21A2 activity. Symptoms associated with this form of the disorder manifest in females at puberty. There are no signs of masculinization of the genitalia in females with this form of the disease. Although females have relatively normal breast development, the androgen excess results in excessive body hair (hirsutism), amenorrhea, and the development of small ovarian cysts.

The latter peptide hormones bind to gonadal tissue and stimulate CYP11A1 activity, resulting in sex hormone production.

The biosynthetic pathway to sex hormones in male and female gonadal tissue includes the production of the androgens, androstenedione, and dehydroepiandrosterone. Testes and ovaries contain an additional enzyme, 17β-hydroxysteroid dehydrogenase (HSD17B3), that enables androgens to be converted to testosterone.

In males, LH binds to Leydig cells, stimulating production of the principal Leydig cell hormone, testosterone. Testosterone is secreted to the plasma and also carried to Sertoli cells by androgen-binding protein (ABP). In Sertoli cells the Δ4 double bond of testosterone is reduced, producing dihydrotestosterone. Testosterone and dihydrotestosterone are carried in the plasma, and delivered to target tissue, by a specific gonadal-steroid binding globulin (GBG). In a number of target tissues, testosterone can be converted to dihydrotestosterone (DHT). DHT is the most potent of the male steroid hormones, with an activity that is 10 times that of testosterone. Because of its relatively lower potency, testosterone is sometimes considered to be a prohormone (Figure 50-2).

Testosterone is also produced by Sertoli cells, but in these cells it is regulated by FSH. In addition, FSH stimulates Sertoli cells to secrete androgen-binding protein (ABP), which transports testosterone and DHT from Leydig cells to sites of spermatogenesis. There, testosterone acts to stimulate protein synthesis and sperm development.

In females, LH binds to thecal cells of the ovary, where it stimulates the synthesis of androstenedione and testosterone. An additional enzyme complex known as aromatase (CYP19A1, also called estrogen synthetase) is responsible for the final conversion of the latter 2 molecules into the estrogens. Aromatase is a complex enzyme present in the ER of the ovary and in numerous other tissues in both males and females. Its action involves hydroxylations and dehydrations that culminate in aromatization of the A ring of the androgens (Figure 50-3).

Aromatase activity is also found in granulosa cells, but in these cells the activity is stimulated by FSH. Normally, thecal cell androgens produced in response to LH diffuse to granulosa cells, where granulosa cell aromatase converts these androgens to estrogens. As granulosa cells mature they develop competent large numbers of LH receptors in the plasma membrane

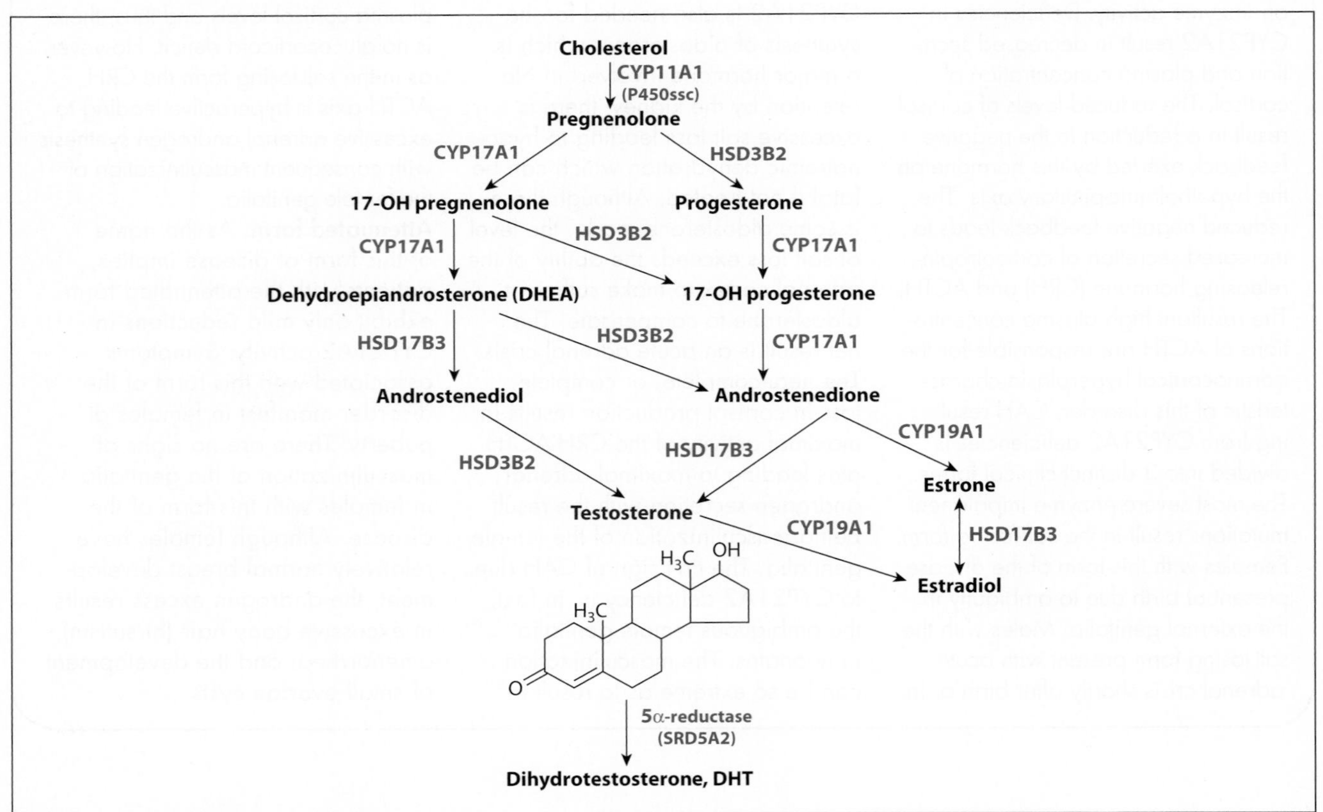

FIGURE 50-2: Synthesis of the male sex hormones in Leydig cells of the testis. P450ssc, 3β-DH, and P450c17 are the same enzymes as those needed for adrenal steroid hormone synthesis. 17,20-lyase is the same activity of CYP17A1 described earlier for adrenal hormone synthesis. Aromatase (also called estrogen synthetase) is CYP19A1. 17-Ketoreductase is also called 17β-hydroxysteroid dehydrogenase type 3 (gene symbol *HSD17B3*). The full name for 5α-reductase is 5α-reductase type 2 (gene symbol *SRD5A2*).

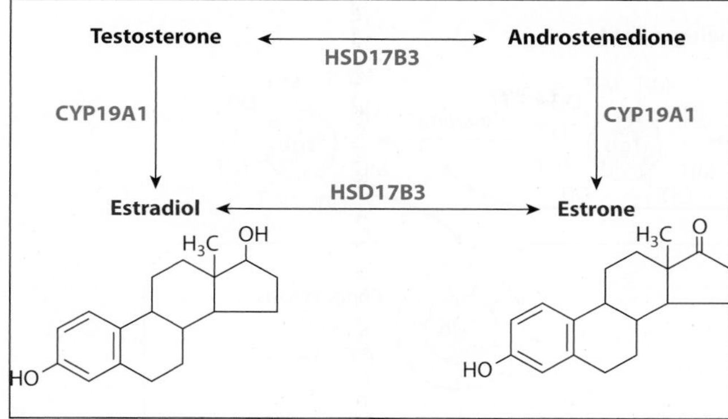

FIGURE 50-3: Synthesis of the major female sex hormones in the ovary. Synthesis of testosterone and androstenedione from cholesterol occurs by the same pathways as indicated for synthesis of the male sex hormones. Aromatase (also called estrogen synthetase) is CYP19A1. Reproduced with permission of themedicalbiochemistrypage, LLC.

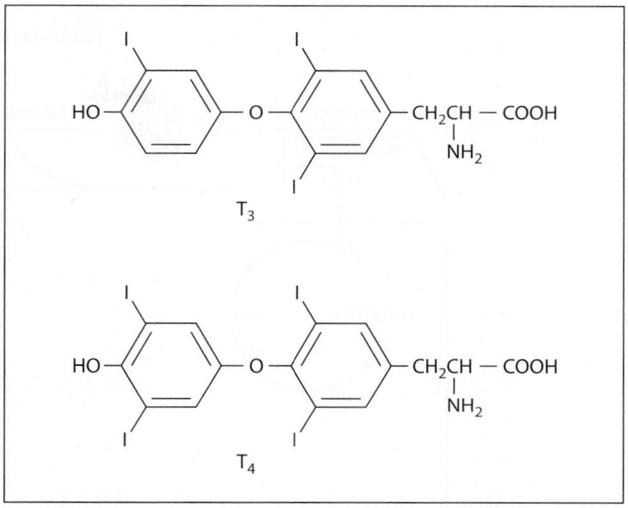

FIGURE 50-4: Structures of T_3 and T_4.

and become increasingly responsive to LH, increasing the quantity of estrogen produced from these cells. Granulosa cell estrogens are largely, if not all, secreted into follicular fluid. Thecal cell estrogens are secreted largely into the circulation, where they are delivered to target tissue by the same globulin (GBG) used to transport testosterone.

Thyroid Hormones

The thyroid hormones are triiodothyronine (T_3) and thyroxine (T_4) (Figure 50-4). These hormones are derived from the thyroid hormone precursor, thyroglobulin. Thyroglobulin is glycosylated and contains more than 115 tyrosine residues, which become iodinated and are used for the synthesis of both T_3 and T_4. Thyroglobulin is exocytosed through the apical membrane into the closed lumen of thyroid follicles, where it accumulates as the major protein of the thyroid and where maturation takes place. Briefly, a Na^+/K^+-ATPase–driven pump concentrates iodide (I^-) in thyroid cells, and the iodide is transported to the follicle lumen. There it is oxidized to I^+ by a thyroperoxidase found only in thyroid tissue. The addition of I^+ to tyrosine residues of thyroglobulin is catalyzed by the same enzyme, leading to the production of thyroglobulin containing monoiodotyrosyl (MIT) and diiodotyrosyl (DIT) residues. The thyronines, T_3 and T_4, are formed by combining MIT and DIT residues on thyroglobulin (Figure 50-4).

Mature, iodinated thyroglobulin is taken up in vesicles by thyrocytes and fuses with lysosomes. Lysosomal proteases degrade thyroglobulin releasing amino acids and T_3 and T_4, which are secreted into the circulation. These compounds are very hydrophobic and require a carrier protein for delivery to target tissues. In the plasma, T_3 and T_4 are bound to a carrier glycoprotein known as thyroxin-binding globulin and are disseminated throughout the body in this form. The synthesis and release of the thyronines requires that there be a continuous process of iodination and deiodination of thyroglobulin (Figure 50-5).

A feedback loop that regulates T_3 and T_4 production is a single short negative loop, with the T_3 and T_4 being responsible for downregulating pituitary thyroid-stimulating hormone (TSH) secretion. Meanwhile, continuously secreted hypothalamic thyrotropin-releasing hormone (TRH) is responsible for upregulating TSH production. The TSH actually secreted by thyrotropes is

High-Yield Concept

T_3 is the most active thyroid hormone and is responsible for normal development, differentiation, and metabolic balance.

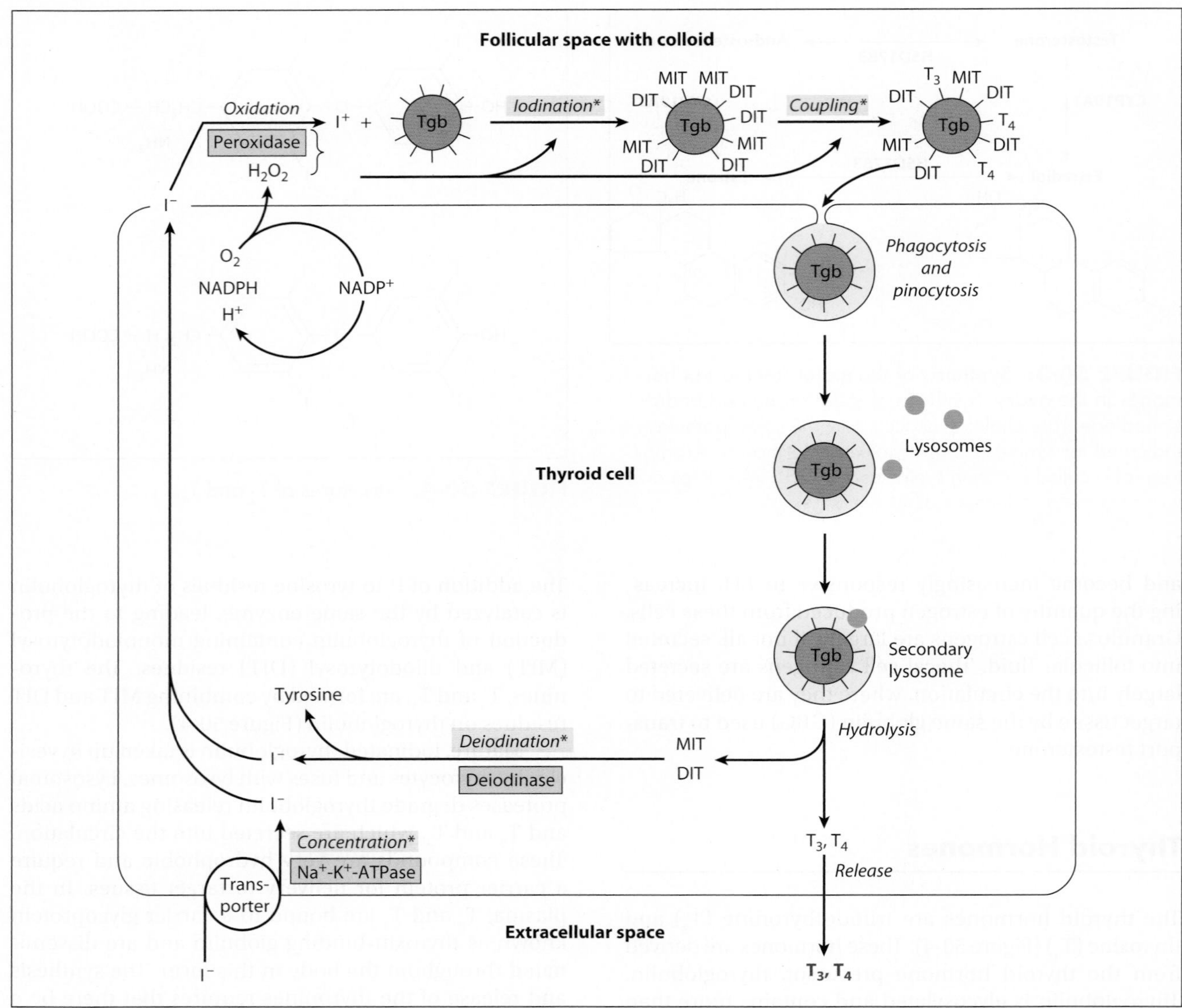

FIGURE 50-5: Model of iodide metabolism in the thyroid follicle. A follicular cell is shown facing the follicular lumen (top) and the extracellular space (bottom). Iodide enters the thyroid primarily through a transporter (bottom left). Thyroid hormone synthesis occurs in the follicular space through a series of reactions, many of which are peroxidase-mediated. Thyroid hormones, stored in the colloid in the follicular space, are released from thyroglobulin by hydrolysis inside the thyroid cell. (DIT, diiodotyrosine; MIT, monoiodotyrosine; Tgb, thyroglobulin; T3, triiodothyronine; T4, tetraiodothyronine.) Asterisks indicate steps or processes where inherited enzyme deficiencies cause congenital goiter and often result in hypothyroidism. Murray RK, Bender DA, Botham KM, Kennelly PJ, Rodwell VW, Weil PA. *Harper's Illustrated Biochemistry*. 29th ed. New York, NY: McGraw-Hill; 2012.

the net result of the negative effects of T_3 and T_4 and the positive effect of TRH (see Figure 49-2).

T_3 exerts these effects at the level of gene expression and at the level of metabolic regulation. Transcriptional regulation is exerted by T_3 binding to receptors of the nuclear receptor family (see Chapter 40). Humans express 2 thyroid hormone receptors (TR), identified as TRα and TRβ, from 2 distinct genes. Each gene also generates at least 2 splice variants (TRα1 and TRα2, TRβ1 and TRβ2).

Thyroid hormones increase hepatic gluconeogenesis and glycogen breakdown. This can lead to exacerbation of hyperglycemia in type 2 diabetes (T2D) especially in conditions of hyperthyroidism. Additional hepatic effects of T_3 are increased cholesterol metabolism. Within skeletal muscle T_3 increases protein

High-Yield Concept

Hypothyroidism refers to the clinical syndrome resulting from deficiency in the thyroid hormones. The general manifestation of hypothyroidism is a reduced level of metabolic processes. Hyperthyroidism, commonly called thyrotoxicosis, refers to the clinical syndrome resulting when tissues are exposed to high levels of the thyroid hormones.

turnover as well as increasing the speed of muscle contraction and relaxation. T_3 stimulates the activity of Na^+-K^+-ATPases in all tissues except the brain, spleen, and testis. This action results in increased oxygen consumption and the generation of heat. The increased demand for oxygen results in increased erythropoiesis. Within the erythrocyte, T_3 also increases the production of 2,3-BPG allowing for increased O_2 dissociation from hemoglobin. Metabolic effects of T_3 are also exerted at the level of the actions of the catecholamines. The number of β-adrenergic receptors is increased in heart, skeletal muscle, and adipose tissue in response to the actions of T_3. Indeed, most of the clinical consequences of thyrotoxicosis (Graves disease, see Clinical Box 49-1) are due to increased catecholamine sensitivity.

Hypo- and Hyperthyroidism

The syndrome is associated with a generalized acceleration in metabolic processes. In most cases, thyrotoxicosis is the result of hyperthyroidism resulting from dysregulation of TSH activity and for this reason is discussed in relation to the most common form of thyrotoxicosis, Graves disease (see Clinical Box 49-1).

Hypothyroidism is classified as primary, secondary, or tertiary (Table 50-3). Primary hypothyroidism is the most common and is due to thyroid failure. Secondary is the result of pituitary TSH deficiency. Tertiary is due to hypothalamic deficiency in TRH. Hypothyroidism can also result from peripheral resistance to the actions of the thyroid hormones. The most common form of hypothyroidism is Hashimoto thyroiditis (autoimmune thyroiditis). The most serious complication associated with untreated end-stage hypothyroidism is myxedema coma. This condition occurs more frequently in older females who also have underlying pulmonary and vascular disease. Myxedema coma manifests with hypothermia, hypoventilation, hypoglycemia, hyponatremia, progressive weakness, and stupor. The condition can lead to shock and death.

TABLE 50-3: **Etiology of hypothyroidism**
Primary:
1. Hashimoto thyroiditis:
a. With goiter
b. "Idiopathic" thyroid atrophy, presumably end-stage autoimmune thyroid disease, following either Hashimoto thyroiditis or Graves disease
c. Neonatal hypothyroidism due to placental transmission of TSH-R blocking antibodies
2. Radioactive iodine therapy for Graves disease
3. Subtotal thyroidectomy for Graves disease, nodular goiter, or thyroid cancer
4. Excessive iodide intake (kelp, radiocontrast dyes)
5. Subacute thyroiditis (usually transient)
6. Iodide deficiency (rare in North America)
7. Inborn errors of thyroid hormone synthesis
8. Drugs
a. Lithium
b. Interferon-alfa
c. Amiodarone
Secondary: Hypopituitarism due to pituitary adenoma, pituitary ablative therapy, or pituitary destruction
Tertiary: Hypothalamic dysfunction (rare)
Peripheral resistance to the action of thyroid hormone

Gardner DG, Shoback D. Greenspan's Basic and Clinical Endocrinology, 9th ed., Table 7-6, New York: McGraw-Hill; 2011.

Steroid and Thyroid Hormone Receptors

Steroid and thyroid hormone receptors are ligand-activated proteins that directly regulate transcription of target genes. Unlike peptide hormone receptors, steroid hormone receptors are found in the cytosol and the nucleus. The steroid and thyroid hormone receptor superfamily of proteins includes not only the receptors for steroid hormones (androgen receptor, AR; progesterone receptor, PR; estrogen receptor, ER), but also for thyroid hormone (TR), vitamin D (VDR), retinoic acid (RAR), mineralocorticoids (MR), and glucocorticoids (GR). This large class of receptors is known as the nuclear receptors.

The nuclear receptors all contain a ligand-binding domain (LBD), a DNA-binding domain (DBD), and 2 activation function domains (AF-1 and AF-2). The secondary structure of the steroid hormone DBD forms a unique type of zinc finger that coordinates a zinc atom with only 4 cysteine residues and no histidine. When these receptors bind ligand they undergo a conformational change that renders them activated to recognize and bind to specific nucleotide sequences. These specific nucleotide sequences in the DNA are referred to as hormone-response elements (HREs). When ligand-receptor complexes interact with DNA they alter the transcriptional level. Details of the nuclear receptors are discussed in Chapter 40.

REVIEW QUESTIONS

1. A 45-year-old woman was being regularly reviewed in primary and secondary care because of a 5-year history of type 2 diabetes that had required early insulin treatment, refractory hypertension, and subsequent chronic kidney disease. She had previously described other symptoms, including weight gain, bruising, flushes, and low mood, all of which had been attributed to obesity and menopause. She was not taking any glucocorticoids. After presenting to her local emergency department with a Colles' fracture after a low impact fall, she was referred to the endocrinology department for suspected Cushing syndrome. Analysis for which of the following would be most useful in confirming the initial diagnosis?

A. decreased plasma levels of thyroid-stimulating hormone
B. increased levels of plasma ACTH
C. increased urine T_3
D. reduced free plasma testosterone
E. reduced urine cortisol

Answer B: The primary symptoms of Cushing syndrome result from the tissues being exposed to high levels of cortisol for too long. The most common cause of Cushing syndrome is a pituitary adenoma that secretes excess amounts of ACTH. ACTH stimulates the adrenal cortex to synthesize the glucocorticoids, primarily cortisol. Therefore, measurement of elevated plasma ACTH levels can indicate Cushing syndrome. Because ACTH induces cortisol production one would expect to see elevated urinary cortisol in addition to the elevated plasma ACTH.

2. A 27-year-old woman presented to the ER complaining of nausea and vomiting for 1 week. She also reported 8 months of progressively worsening fatigue. The patient was previously very active as a ballet student, but for the past 8 months she stopped participating in ballet because of lack of energy and poor concentration. One week prior to admission, she developed nausea and had several episodes of vomiting which provoked her visit to the ER. She also reported a poor appetite for months and had lost 10 lb. Physical examination showed dryness and darkening of the skin in several areas. She repeatedly denied purposefully restricting food intake or binging and purging behaviors. There was no abdominal pain, diarrhea, fevers, dysuria, or headache. As the attending physician you suspect this patient is exhibiting signs of Addison disease. Testing for which of the following would be most useful in your diagnosis?

A. decreased plasma estrogen
B. decreased urinary cortisol
C. increased plasma ACTH
D. increased plasma aldosterone
E. increased plasma cortisol

Answer B: Addison disease is characterized by general malaise and debility, irritability of the stomach, and hyperpigmentation. The disease results from a primary failure of the adrenal cortex to synthesize and secrete glucocorticoid (cortisol) and mineralocorticoid (aldosterone) hormones. Currently, 70% to 90% of cases of Addison disease are the result of autoimmune adrenalitis and frequently manifests in patients with other immunological and autoimmune disorders. Addison disease frequency is higher in females than males and is usually diagnosed between 30 and 50 years of age.

3. A 45-year-old woman is being examined by her physician because she is concerned about her weight gain, fatigue, muscle weakness, and thinning hair. Physical examination shows a "buffalo hump," facial hirsutism, and red striae in abdominal and underarm areas. She indicates that she is not on any medication and there is no significant past history or family history. Laboratory studies show an elevated fasting blood glucose (11 mmol/L: 198 mg/dL) and a 24-hour urinary cortisol of 2276 nmol/24 h. These signs and symptoms are most likely the result of which of the following?

A. Addison disease
B. Cushing syndrome
C. Graves disease

D. hyperthyroidism
E. pituitary adenoma

Answer B: Cushing syndrome describes the clinical consequences of chronic exposure to excess glucocorticoid irrespective of the underlying cause. Cushing syndrome may mimic common conditions such as obesity, poorly controlled diabetes, and hypertension, which progress over time and often coexist in patients with metabolic syndrome. The characteristic features of Cushing syndrome are psychiatric disturbances (depression, mania, and psychoses), central obesity, hypertension, diabetes, moon-shaped face, thin fragile skin, easy bruising, and purple striae (stretch marks). In addition, Cushing syndrome patients manifest with gonadal dysfunction that is characteristic of hyperandrogenism with excess body and facial hair (hirsutism) and acne. The most common symptoms that lead to a diagnosis of Cushing syndrome are weight gain, depression, subjective muscle weakness, and headache.

4. A 63-year-old woman presented with increasing darkening of the skin, dizziness, easy fatigability, nausea with occasional vomiting, and progressive weight loss over 8 months prior to presentation. Physical examination showed a pulse of 106 bpm, supine blood pressure was 100/60 mm Hg and 70/40 mm Hg on sitting. She could not stand on account of severe postural dizziness. Radiological diagnostic tests included an abdominal ultrasound showing normal liver, spleen, pancreas, and pelvic organs. However, the left kidney was not outlined. A CT scan of the abdomen showed a nonenhancing oval-shaped left suprarenal mass with calcification. The signs and symptom in this patient are most likely the result of which of the following?
A. Addison disease
B. Cushing syndrome
C. Graves disease
D. hyperthyroidism
E. pituitary adenoma

Answer A: Addison disease is characterized by general malaise and debility, irritability of the stomach, and hyperpigmentation. The disease results from a primary failure of the adrenal cortex to synthesize and secrete glucocorticoid (cortisol) and mineralocorticoid (aldosterone) hormones. One of the most common causes of Addison disease is an adrenocortical adenoma which in this case is evident from the CT scan showing a suprarenal mass.

5. Which of the following processes is induced in males in response to the synthesis and release of follicle-stimulating hormone (FSH)?
A. FSH is a female-specific hormone and thus does not exert effects in males
B. growth arrest of spermatogonia to ensure their proper level of maturation
C. stimulation of adrenal steroidogenesis
D. stimulation of spermatogenesis
E. testosterone production and secretion

Answer D: FSH promotes testicular growth and spermatogenesis. Within the Sertoli cells of the testes it enhances the synthesis and secretion of the steroid hormones, testosterone and dihydrotestosterone.

6. Congenital adrenal hyperplasia, resulting from 21-hydroxylase (CYP21A2) deficiencies, is divided into 3 distinct clinical forms. The most severe enzyme-impairing mutations result in the salt-losing form. Females with this form of the disease present at birth due to ambiguity in the external genitalia. The physiological effect of salt losing is due to which of the following hormone defects?
A. cortisol production is negligible resulting in increased ACTH release from the pituitary
B. cortisol production is negligible due to loss of ACTH control of hypothalamic responses
C. the adrenal cortex compensates for loss of CYP21A2 by producing excess aldosterone
D. the adrenal cortex compensates for loss of CYP21A2 by producing no androstenedione
E. there is an associated dysregulation of androgen synthesis which normally controls aldosterone synthesis

Answer A: The biological role of ACTH is to stimulate the production of adrenal cortex steroids, principally the glucocorticoids cortisol and corticosterone. ACTH also stimulates the adrenal cortex to produce the mineralocorticoid, aldosterone as well as the androgen, and androstenedione. Negative feedback on ACTH secretion is exerted by cortisol at both the hypothalamic and anterior pituitary levels. Loss of cortisol production results in unregulated and excess secretion of ACTH leading to increased androgen production resulting in the masculinizing effect seen in 21-hydroxylase deficiency.

7. Which of the following is true with respect to the actions of the mineralocorticoids?
A. decrease carbohydrate metabolism
B. increase appearance of the secondary sex characteristics
C. increase synthesis of androgens
D. regulate aldosterone secretion
E. regulate sodium retention by the kidneys

Answer E: The principal mineralocorticoid, produced by zona glomerulosa cells of the adrenals, is aldosterone. Synthesis of aldosterone is primarily controlled by the rennin-angiotensin system and is thus involved in control of blood pressure. Aldosterone causes sodium reabsorption by the kidneys which in turn regulates water balance and leads to increases in blood pressure by increasing fluid volume.

8. A 32-year-old woman is diagnosed with hypertension, hypernatremia, hypokalemia, and alkalosis. Measurements of plasma glucocorticoid levels show them to be within the normal range; however, renin and angiotensin II levels are suppressed. Ultrasound indicates the possible existence of an adrenal cortical mass. These symptoms are likely due to excess production of which of the following hormones?
A. aldosterone
B. androstenedione
C. dehydroepiandrosterone (DHEA)
D. estradiol
E. testosterone

Answer A: The principal mineralocorticoid, produced by zona glomerulosa cells of the adrenals, is aldosterone. Synthesis of aldosterone is primarily controlled by the rennin-angiotensin system and is thus involved in control of blood pressure. Reduced or inhibited function in the renin-angiotensin system will lead to excess aldosterone release from the adrenals. Aldosterone causes sodium reabsorption by the kidneys which in turn regulates water balance and leads to increases in blood pressure by increasing fluid volume manifest with the hypertension and hypernatremia evident in this patient.

9. Steroid hormones interact with specific receptors within target cells. The steroid-receptor complexes then regulate the rate of which of the following intracellular processes?
A. posttranscriptional processing of specific mRNAs
B. posttranslational processing of specific proteins
C. replication of DNA
D. transcription of specific genes
E. translation of specific mRNAs

Answer D: Steroid hormones are lipophilic and hence freely penetrate the plasma membrane of all cells. Within target cells, steroid hormones interact with specific receptors. These receptor proteins are composed of 2 domains: a hormone-binding domain and a DNA-binding domain. Following hormone-receptor interaction the complex is activated and enters the nucleus. The DNA-binding domain of the receptor interacts with specific nucleotide sequences termed hormone response elements (HREs). The binding of steroid-receptor complexes to HREs results in an altered rate of transcription of the associated gene(s). The effects of steroid-receptor complexes on specific target genes can be either stimulatory or inhibitory with respect to the rate of transcription.

10. A baby girl is born with ambiguous genitalia and diagnosed with severe classical congenital deficiency of adrenal 21-hydroxylase enzyme. Without any treatment, which of the following would you expect in the girl's future?
A. delayed puberty
B. hypernatremia
C. hypopigmentation
D. salt-wasting crises
E. tall stature

Answer D: Because CYP21A2 is also needed for the synthesis of aldosterone, which is a major hormone involved in Na^+ retention by the kidney, there is excessive salt loss leading to hyponatremic dehydration which can be fatal if not treated. Although there is some aldosterone made, the level of salt loss exceeds the ability of the adrenal cortex to make sufficient aldosterone to compensate. The net result is an acute adrenal crisis.

11. High-dose glucocorticoid therapy for treatment of rheumatoid arthritis remains highly controversial. It is widely agreed that it is highly effective in controlling acute rheumatoid inflammation, but it may also result in significant adverse effects. Complications of high-dose glucocorticoid therapy include which of the following?
A. excessive growth in children and acromegaly in adults
B. hyperkalemia
C. hyponatremia
D. suppression of the hypothalamic-pituitary-adrenal axis
E. volume depletion

Answer D: High-dose exogenous glucocorticoids suppress the adrenal neuroendocrine axis. Patients treated for longer than 2 weeks need to be tapered off glucocorticoids slowly to avoid adrenal insufficiency. Other complications of high-dose glucocorticoids include growth suppression in children and volume overload. Hyperkalemia and hyponatremia are observed in adrenal insufficiency due to loss of mineralocorticoid effects and are not relevant to glucocorticoid therapy.

12. A 4-year-old child with signs of precocious (early-onset) puberty is brought to a clinic for evaluation and found to have a congenital deficiency of 21-hydroxylase. Feedback inhibition of the pituitary gland is lost and excess ACTH is secreted. As a result, which of the following happens?

A. adrenal cortical atrophy occurs
B. adrenal medullary hypertrophy occurs
C. excess cortisol is released
D. precursors to cortisol synthesis increase
E. serum cholesterol falls dramatically

Answer D: In the adrenogenital syndrome the failure to make cortisol due to lack of the adrenal enzyme 21-hydroxylase results in an inability to provide negative feedback suppression of ACTH production. As a result, the adrenal glands are under constant stimulation to maximize steroidogenesis. Substrates that cannot reach cortisol flow down other pathways and by mass action drive the massive overproduction of androgens, which can also be peripherally aromatized to estrogens.

13. A 35-year-old weightlifter who has been injecting testosterone for muscle mass augmentation is evaluated for sterility and found to have an extremely low sperm count. Which of the following is an effect of testosterone and contributes to the mentioned sterility?

A. activation of inhibin
B. feedback activation of leptin
C. feedback inhibition of GnRH
D. inhibition of seminal prostaglandins
E. lowered core temperature

Answer C: Testosterone directly inhibits the secretion of GnRH from the hypothalamus, which affects secretion of LH and FSH and consequently secretion of testosterone. To initiate spermatogenesis, both FSH and testosterone are necessary. To maintain spermatogenesis after puberty, extremely high concentrations of testosterone seem to be required. Systemically administered testosterone does not raise the androgen level in the testes to as great a degree and it additionally inhibits LH secretion. Consequently, the net effect is generally a decrease in sperm count.

14. A 40-year-old woman complains of chronic fatigue, aching muscles, and general weakness. Physical examination reveals a modest weight gain, dry skin, and slow reflexes. Laboratory findings include TSH: >10 mU/L (normal range 0.5-5 mU/L), free T_4: low to normal. Which of the following is the most likely explanation?

A. hyperthyroidism due to autoimmune thyroid disease
B. hyperthyroidism due to iodine excess
C. hyperthyroidism secondary to a hypothalamic-pituitary defect
D. hypothyroidism due to autoimmune thyroid disease
E. hypothyroidism secondary to a hypothalamic-pituitary defect

Answer D: The described symptoms are typical for hypothyroidism. A primary thyroid gland deficiency leads to low T_4 levels and high TSH levels. The most common cause of thyroid gland failure is called autoimmune thyroiditis or Hashimoto thyroiditis. It develops slowly due to persistent inflammation of the thyroid caused by the patient's own immune system. Middle-aged women are most commonly affected. The measurement of elevated TSH levels in blood is of high diagnostic value since it helps determine even minor degrees of hypothyroidism. Correct diagnosis is critical because treatment usually continues for life, and stopping of the treatment and reevaluating the original diagnosis is often difficult.

15. A newly wed 23-year-old woman and her 28-year-old husband are evaluated for infertility. They have been unable to conceive a child despite regular intercourse for the past 12 months. The first step of this couple's infertility workup is to determine whether ovulation occurs regularly. Which of the following hormones is directly responsible for ovulation?

A. estradiol
B. estriol
C. follicle-stimulating hormone (FSH)
D. inhibin
E. luteinizing hormone (LH)

Answer E: Although the early maturation of an ovarian follicle depends on the presence of FSH, ovulation is induced by a surge of LH. Although estrogens usually have a negative feedback effect on LH and FSH secretion, the LH surge seems to be a response to elevated estrogen levels. In concert with FSH, LH induces rapid follicular swelling. LH also acts directly on the granulosa cells, causing them to decrease estrogen production, as well as initiating production of small amounts of progesterone. These changes lead to ovulation.

16. A baby girl is born with ambiguous genitalia and diagnosed with severe classical congenital deficiency of adrenal 21-hydroxylase enzyme. Without any treatment, which of the following would you expect in the girl's future?

A. delayed puberty
B. hypernatremia

C. hypopigmentation
D. salt-wasting crises
E. tall stature

Answer D: CYP21A2 (21-hydroxylase) deficiency is the most common enzyme defect in the adrenal gland. In one form of the disorder, called the "salt-wasting" form, aldosterone synthesis is impaired. This is due to the fact that progesterone cannot be converted to 11-deoxycorticosterone, an intermediate on the adrenal mineralocorticoid pathway toward aldosterone. The lack of aldosterone leads to a lack of sodium reabsorption by the distal renal tubules and hence to low serum sodium concentrations. If untreated, hyponatremic dehydration, hyperkalemia, and metabolic acidosis develop. By the second or third week of life, continuous dehydration, worsened by vomiting, leads to circulatory collapse, termed salt-wasting crisis. The lack of 21-hydroxylase also leads to a decrease of cortisol synthesis. This is due to the fact that 17α-hydroxyprogesterone cannot be converted to 11-deoxycortisol, the precursor of cortisol. By feedback regulation, low serum cortisol concentration results in increased production of ACTH. Increased ACTH leads to adrenal gland hyperstimulation and increased production of adrenal androgens, which results in precocious puberty. In the moderate form of classical 21-hydroxlyase deficiency, virilization before puberty is the most prevalent symptom.

17. Cushing syndrome is characterized by rapid weight gain, particularly of the trunk and face with sparing of the limbs (central obesity). Another common sign is the growth of fat pads along the collar bone and on the back of the neck (buffalo hump) and a round face often referred to as a "moon face" and excessive "sweating." This disorder results from overproduction of which of the following hormones?
A. ACTH
B. aldosterone
C. growth hormone
D. progesterone
E. thyrotropin-releasing hormone (TRH)

Answer A: Cushing syndrome most often results from pituitary corticotrope adenomas resulting in excess ACTH production and secretion. The characteristic features of Cushing syndrome are psychiatric disturbances (depression, mania, and psychoses), central obesity, hypertension, diabetes, moon-shaped face, thin fragile skin, easy bruising, and purple striae (stretch marks). In addition, Cushing syndrome patients manifest with gonadal dysfunction that is characteristic of hyperandrogenism with excess body and facial hair (hirsutism) and acne.

18. You are treating a 37-year-old female patient whose signs and symptoms lead you to suspect she is suffering from an endocrine disorder. You order a series of tests to aid in your diagnosis. A basic metabolic panel showed elevated sodium of 111 mmol/L (normal range 135-145), potassium 4.5 mmol/L, chloride 78 mmol/L, bicarbonate 23 mmol/L, glucose 85 mg/dL, and creatinine 0.7 mg/dL. Further testing showed serum osmolality at 234 mOsm/kg (normal range 275-295) and urine sodium less than 20 mmol/L consistent with severe hypovolemic hyponatremia. A random cortisol level was less than 0.2 μg/dL. The plasma ACTH level was elevated at 882 pg/dL (normal range 5-27). These test results most likely indicate the patient is suffering from which of the following disorders?
A. Addison disease
B. Cushing syndrome
C. Graves disease
D. hyperthyroidism
E. pituitary adenoma

Answer A: Addison disease results from a primary failure of the adrenal cortex to synthesize and secrete glucocorticoid (cortisol) and mineralocorticoid (aldosterone) hormones resulting in metabolic disturbances. Electrolytes (sodium, potassium, chloride, and carbon dioxide) are measured to help detect and evaluate the severity of an existing electrolyte imbalance characteristic of Addison disease. With Addison disease, the sodium, chloride, and carbon dioxide levels are often low, while the potassium level may be very high. If the adrenal gland is either not functioning normally or not being stimulated by ACTH, then cortisol levels will be consistently low.

19. You are treating a 29-year-old woman who came to you complaining of a 3-month history of increased sweating and palpitations with weight loss of 15 lb. Physical examination shows she is nervous and agitated with an obvious, diffuse, nontender, smooth enlargement of her thyroid, over which a bruit could be heard. She had a fine tremor of her fingers and a resting pulse rate of 150/min. Laboratory studies indicate the elevated serum T_3 of 4.8 nmol/L (normal: 0.8-2.4) and a T_4 of 48 nmol/L (normal: 9-23). Measurement of her thyroid-stimulating hormone showed that it was low normal, 0.4 mU/L (normal 0.4-5 mU/L). The signs and symptoms exhibited by your patient most likely indicate she is suffering from which of the following?
A. Addison disease
B. Cushing syndrome
C. Graves disease

D. hyperthyroidism
E. pituitary adenoma

Answer C: Graves disease is the most common autoimmune disease, affecting 0.5% of the population in the United States, and represents 50% to 80% of cases of hyperthyroidism. The disorder occurs more commonly in women, smokers and patients with other autoimmune diseases. Graves hyperthyroidism results from the production of autoantibodies that bind to and activate the thyroid-stimulating hormone (TSH) receptor on the surface of thyroid follicular cells. This activation stimulates follicular cell growth, causing diffuse thyroid enlargement and increased production of thyroid hormones referred to as thyrotoxicosis.

20. Cells of the zona fasciculata of the adrenal cortex do not synthesize the potent mineralocorticoids because they lack expression of which of the following enzymes?
A. CYP11B1, 11β-hydroxylase
B. CYP11B2, aldosterone synthase
C. CYP17A1, 17α-hydroxylase, and 17,20-lyase
D. CYP19A1, aromatase
E. CYP21A2, 21-hydroxylase

Answer B: Cells of the zona fasciculata and zona reticularis do not express aldosterone synthase (CYP11B2; 18α-hydroxylase; P450c18) that converts corticosterone to aldosterone, and thus these tissues produce only the weak mineralocorticoid corticosterone.

21. You are treating a patient whose symptoms lead you to suspect that he is suffering from Cushing syndrome. Testing for which of the following would aid in your diagnosis in this patient?
A. decreased plasma T_3
B. decreased urinary cortisol
C. elevated plasma ACTH
D. elevated plasma growth hormone
E. elevated urinary testosterone

Answer C: Cushing syndrome most often results from pituitary corticotrope adenomas resulting in excess ACTH production and secretion. The excess ACTH results in increased glucocorticoid production by the adrenal glands resulting in elevated cortisol release.

22. You are treating a patient whose symptoms lead you to suspect that she is suffering from Addison disease. Testing for which of the following would aid in your diagnosis in this patient?
A. decreased plasma glucose
B. decreased plasma potassium
C. decreased plasma sodium
D. elevated plasma bicarbonate
E. elevated urinary cortisol

Answer C: Addison disease results from a primary failure of the adrenal cortex to synthesize and secrete glucocorticoid (cortisol) and mineralocorticoid (aldosterone) hormones resulting in metabolic disturbances. Electrolytes (sodium, potassium, chloride, and bicarbonate) are measured to help detect and evaluate the severity of an existing electrolyte imbalance characteristic of Addison disease. With Addison disease, the sodium, chloride, and bicarbonate levels are often low, while the potassium level may be very high. If the adrenal gland is either not functioning normally or not being stimulated by ACTH, then cortisol levels will be consistently low.

23. A 2-month-old infant girl with a history of persistent physiological jaundice following birth is now reported by her parents to sleep excessively and display little activity. Physical examination reveals abnormal deep tendon reflexes, hypothermia, and muscular hypotonia. Based on this information, which of the following would be the best therapy for her condition?
A. antibiotics
B. growth hormone
C. thiamine
D. thyroxine
E. vitamin D

Answer D: This infant has cretinism, a condition caused by a neonatal lack of thyroxine. Thyroid agenesis, iodine deficiency, ingestion of goitrogens, and hereditary enzymatic deficiencies may all result in a relative lack of biologically active thyroxine. Affected children may display lethargy, jaundice, hypothermia, muscular hypotonia, and mental retardation. Medicinal replacement of thyroxine is therapeutic. The mental retardation may not be reversible, however, unless treated early.

24. During a routine physical examination, a 16-year-old adolescent boy is found to have only minimal secondary sexual development, gynecomastia, and a tall, eunuchoid habitus. A chromosomal determination on this individual would most likely reveal which of the following?
A. 45, XO
B. 45, YO
C. 46, XX
D. 46, XY
E. 47, XXY

Answer E: The physical description of this boy is that of Klinefelter syndrome. This condition is not usually diagnosed until after puberty when the secondary sexual characteristics do not develop normally. Most of these individuals are 47, XXY but some may have additional X or Y chromosomes.

25. A 38-year-old woman has experienced the gradual onset of a goiter. Serum T_4 and T_3 are within the reference range and thyroid-stimulating hormone (TSH) is slightly increased. Serum antithyroid peroxidase (antimicrosomal) antibodies are detected but there are no TSH receptor antibodies. Which of the following is the most likely diagnosis?
A. chronic autoimmune thyroiditis
B. Graves disease
C. primary atrophy of the thyroid
D. Riedel struma
E. subacute thyroiditis

Answer A: Patients with chronic autoimmune thyroiditis or Hashimoto disease may demonstrate several different serum thyroid autoantibodies, but these vary from patient to patient. Thyroid peroxidase antibodies are found in roughly 85% of patients with Hashimoto disease, about 40% of patients with Graves disease, and in less than 15% of patients with other thyroid disorders. The absence of TSH receptor antibodies rules out Graves disease, making Hashimoto disease the most likely diagnosis.

26. All steroid hormone receptors share several structural similarities including the DNA-binding domain. The DNA-binding domain of the steroid hormones is known as which of the following?
A. cI repressor
B. Cro dimer operator complex
C. kinase
D. phosphotyrosine
E. zinc finger

Answer E: The DNA-binding domain of steroid hormones consists of 2 nonrepetitive globular motifs where zinc is coordinated with 4 cysteine residues. This secondary and tertiary structure is distinct from that of the more classic zinc fingers which also include histidines in the coordination of the zinc atom. In the steroid hormone receptor the domain is called a type II zinc finger.

27. A 20-year-old man with type 2 diabetes awakens at 3:00 AM after 5 hours of sleep feeling queasy and light-headed. He tests his serum glucose and finds that it is 49 mg/dL. In response to his hypoglycemia, cortisol is secreted by the adrenal cortex and induces the synthesis of which of the following enzymes in the adrenal medulla?
A. acetyl-CoA carboxylase
B. homocysteine methyltransferase
C. methionine adenosyltransferase
D. methylmalonyl-CoA racemase
E. phenylethanolamine *N*-methyltransferase, PNMT

Answer E: Phenylethanolamine *N*-methyltransferase (PNMT) is an adrenal medullary enzyme whose activity is induced by cortisol. PNMT catalyzes the conversion of norepinephrine to epinephrine (see Chapter 31). The increased synthesis and release of epinephrine will trigger fatty acid release from adipose tissue and gluconeogenesis and glycogen breakdown in the liver. The released fatty acids are oxidized in the liver for ATP production necessary for gluconeogenesis to proceed.

28. Glucocorticoids enhance the expression of specific genes by binding to glucocorticoid receptors, resulting in which of the following?
A. activation of GTP-binding protein
B. activation of MYC
C. activation of receptor tyrosine kinase
D. binding of the receptor-steroid complex to DNA
E. formation of a JUN-FOS (AP1) complex

Answer D: Glucocorticoids are members of the steroid or thyroid family of molecules that function by binding to intracellular receptors. Upon ligand binding the steroid hormone receptors migrate to the nucleus where the DNA-binding domain in the receptor binds to specific sequences in target genes.

29. Receptors for all of the members of the steroid hormone family share which of the following features?
A. calcium-mediated intracellular effects
B. GTP-binding proteins
C. mitochondrial membrane association
D. plasma membrane association
E. zinc-containing DNA-binding domains

Answer E: The DNA-binding domain of steroid hormones consists of 2 nonrepetitive globular motifs where zinc is coordinated with 4 cysteine residues. This secondary and tertiary structure is distinct from that of the more classic zinc fingers which also include histidines in the coordination of the zinc atom. In the steroid hormone receptor the domain is called a type II zinc finger.

30. The synthetic glucocorticoid, dexamethasone, binds to, and activates the glucocorticoid receptor. Which of the following activities of the glucocorticoid receptor is the most likely even after dexamethasone is eliminated from the body?
A. catalyzes formation of stable tyrosine-phosphate bonds
B. competes with β-arrestin for binding to adrenergic receptors

C. couples to G-proteins with low intrinsic GTPase activity
D. depletes cellular stores of glutathione
E. induces proteins that remain functional after the drug is eliminated

Answer E: Glucocorticoids are members of the steroid or thyroid family of molecules that function by binding to intracellular receptors. Upon ligand binding the steroid hormone receptors migrate to the nucleus where the DNA-binding domain in the receptor binds to specific sequences in target genes. Activation of target genes results in increased expression of the proteins encoded by the responsive genes and some of these proteins may exhibit a prolonged half-life such that they will be present after the initial stimulus (dexamethasone) is removed.

31. A 47-day-old newborn has ambiguous genitalia. Serum sodium concentration is 120 mEq/L and serum potassium concentration is 7 mEq/L. Chromosome analysis shows a 46,XX karyotype. This infant most likely has a defect in the synthesis of which of the following hormones?
A. ACTH
B. cortisol
C. estradiol
D. progesterone
E. testosterone

Answer B: CYP21A2 (21-hydroxylase) deficiency is the most common enzyme defect in the adrenal gland. In one form of the disorder, called the "salt-wasting" form, aldosterone synthesis is impaired. The lack of 21-hydroxylase leads to a decrease of cortisol synthesis. This is due to the fact that 17α-hydroxyprogesterone cannot be converted to 11-deoxycortisol, the precursor of cortisol. By feedback regulation, low serum cortisol concentration results in increased production of ACTH. Increased ACTH leads to adrenal gland hyperstimulation and increased production of adrenal androgens, which results in precocious puberty. Females with this form of the disease present at birth due to ambiguity in the external genitalia.

32. A full-term newborn has ambiguous genitalia. Ultrasonographic examination shows a uterus and bilateral uterine tubes. Chromosomal analysis shows a 46,XX karyotype. Which of the following most likely occurred during development?
A. decreased 5α-reductase activity in cells of the genital tubercle
B. deficient activity of 21-hydroxylase in cells of the adrenal cortex
C. failure of formation of the urogenital folds
D. increased atresia of primordial follicles
E. increased numbers of Sertoli cells

Answer B: CYP21A2 (21-hydroxylase) deficiency is the most common enzyme defect in the adrenal gland. The lack of 21-hydroxylase leads to decreased cortisol synthesis. By feedback regulation, low serum cortisol concentration results in increased production of ACTH. Increased ACTH leads to adrenal gland hyperstimulation and increased production of adrenal androgens during fetal development which results abnormal gonadal development. Females with this form of the disease present at birth due to ambiguity in the external genitalia.

33. After cortisol interacts with its receptor, which of the following events is most likely occur?
A. activation of adenylate cyclase by the receptor
B. autophosphorylation of tyrosine residues in the receptor
C. endocytosis of the hormone-receptor complex
D. interaction of the receptor with a G-protein
E. translocation of the hormone-receptor complex to the nucleus

Answer E: Cortisol is a glucocorticoid. The glucocorticoids are members of the steroid or thyroid family of molecules that function by binding to intracellular receptors. Upon ligand binding the steroid hormone receptors migrate to the nucleus where the DNA-binding domain in the receptor binds to specific sequences in target genes.

Checklist

✓ All steroid hormones are derived from cholesterol and contain 18-, 19-, or 21-carbon atoms.

✓ The thyroid hormones are iodinated derivatives of the amino acid tyrosine.

- ✓ The steroid hormones can be grouped into the adrenal cortical steroids and the gonadal steroids.
- ✓ The major adrenal cortical steroids are the glucocorticoids, the mineralocorticoids, and the androgens. Each of these hormones is synthesized in one of 3 specialized zones of the adrenal cortex called the zona glomerulosa, zona reticularis, and zona fasciculata.
- ✓ Synthesis of the adrenal steroids is under the control of the hypothalamic-pituitary axis with specific anterior pituitary hormones exerting influence on adrenal steroidogenesis, primarily controlled by ACTH.
- ✓ Glucocorticoids, primarily cortisol, exert a feedback regulation on the rate and level of their synthesis by inhibiting ACTH release from the pituitary.
- ✓ Synthesis of the mineralocorticoids is also influenced by the renin-angiotensin system of the kidneys and liver.
- ✓ Defects in several of the adrenal steroid biosynthesizing enzymes as well as defects in hypothalamic-pituitary function result in potential severe and life-threatening disorders.
- ✓ The synthesis of gonadal steroid hormones is also controlled by the hypothalamic-pituitary axis, primarily involving pituitary follicle-stimulating hormone and luteinizing hormone.
- ✓ The steroid and thyroid superfamily of hormones, which also includes vitamin D and retinoic acid, all bind to intracellular receptors. These receptors all contain a ligand-binding domain, a DNA-binding domain, and transcription regulatory domains. Binding ligand promotes migration of the complex to the nucleus and binding to specific sequences (hormone response elements) in target genes.

CHAPTER

51 Hemostasis: Blood Coagulation

CHAPTER OUTLINE

High-Yield Terms

Hemostasis: refers to the process of blood clotting and then the subsequent dissolution of the clot following repair of the injured tissue

Intrinsic pathway: pathway of coagulation initiated in response to contact of blood with a negatively charged surface; primarily represents a pathophysiological reaction

Extrinsic pathway: pathway of coagulation initiated in response to release of tissue factor in response to vascular injury; represents the normal physiological pathway of coagulation

Platelets: also called thrombocytes; are small, disk-shaped nonnucleated fragments released from megakaryocytes involved in initiating hemostasis

Platelet glycoproteins: refers to several types of platelet surface receptors (eg, GPIIb-GPIIIa) involved in the processes of platelet activation and aggregation

Kallikrein: any of several serine proteases that cleave kininogens to form kinins; includes plasma and tissue kallikreins

Kinin: any of a group of vasoactive polypeptides (eg, bradykinin) formed by kallikrein-catalyzed cleavage of kininogens causing vasodilation and altering vascular permeability

Tenase complex: the complex of calcium ions and factors VIIIa, IXa, and X on the surface of activated platelets

Prothrombinase complex: a complex composed of platelet phospholipids, calcium ions, factors Va and Xa, and prothrombin

Thrombus: refers to the blood clot which is the final product of the blood coagulation

von Willebrand factor, vWF: a complex multimeric glycoprotein that is produced by and stored in the α-granules of platelets and found associated with subendothelial connective tissue.

Factor V Leiden: an inherited disorder of blood clotting resulting from a variant factor V that causes a hypercoagulability disorder

Partial thromboplastin time (PTT): assay for defects in activities of the intrinsic pathway of coagulation

Prothrombin time (PT): assay for defects in activities of the extrinsic pathway of coagulation

Events of Hemostasis

The ability of the body to control the flow of blood following vascular injury is paramount to continued survival. The process of blood clotting and then the subsequent dissolution of the clot following repair of the injured tissue is termed hemostasis. Hemostasis proceeds through a series of 4 coordinated events required to respond to the loss of vascular integrity.

1. The initial phase of the process is vascular constriction. This limits the flow of blood to the area of injury.
2. Activation of platelets is absolutely required for hemostasis to proceed. Platelets become activated by thrombin and aggregate at the site of injury, forming a temporary, loose platelet plug. Platelets clump by binding to collagen that becomes exposed following rupture of the endothelial lining of vessels. Upon activation, platelets release contents of their granules that are critical for the coagulation cascade. In addition to induced secretion, activated platelets change their shape to accommodate the formation of the plug.
3. To ensure stability of the initially loose platelet plug, a fibrin mesh (also called the clot) forms and entraps the plug. If the plug contains only platelets and fibrin, it is termed a **white thrombus**; if red blood cells are present, it is called a **red thrombus.**
4. Finally, the clot must be dissolved in order for normal blood flow to resume following tissue repair. The dissolution of the clot occurs through the action of plasmin.

Two pathways lead to the formation of a fibrin clot: the intrinsic and extrinsic pathways (Figure 51-1). Although they are initiated by distinct mechanisms, the 2 converge on a common pathway that leads to clot formation. Both pathways are complex and involve numerous different proteins termed clotting factors (Tables 51-1 and 51-2). Fibrin clot formation in response to tissue injury is the most clinically relevant event of hemostasis under normal physiological conditions. This process is the result of the activation of the extrinsic pathway. The intrinsic pathway has low significance under normal physiological conditions. Most significant clinically is the activation of the intrinsic pathway by contact of the vessel wall with bacteria, lipoprotein particles, and other charged molecules.

Platelet Activation and von Willebrand Factor (vWF)

Hemostasis requires that platelets adhere to exposed collagen, release the contents of their granules, and aggregate (Figure 51-2). Interaction of platelets with exposed collagen involves at least 2 collagen glycoprotein receptors identified as GPIa-IIa and GPVI. The GPIa-IIa receptor is a member for the integrin family of proteins and is, therefore, also identified as integrin $\alpha_2\beta_1$. The GPVI receptor recognizes type III collagen.

Following binding to collagen the adhesion of platelets to the endothelial cell surface is mediated by von Willebrand factor (vWF). von Willebrand factor is a complex multimeric glycoprotein that is produced by and stored in the α-granules of platelets. It is also synthesized by megakaryocytes and found associated with subendothelial connective tissue. The function of vWF is to act as a bridge between a specific glycoprotein complex on the surface of platelets (GPIb-GPIX-GPV) and collagen fibrils. The GPIb part of the complex is composed of 2 proteins, GPIbα and GPIbβ, encoded by separate genes. Platelets also contain another collagen receptor.

Inherited deficiencies of vWF are the causes of von Willebrand disease, vWD (see Clinical Box 51-1). The importance of the interaction between vWF and the GPIb-GPIX-GPV complex of platelets is demonstrated by the inheritance of bleeding disorders caused by defects in 3 of the 4 proteins of the complex, the most common of which is Bernard-Soulier

High-Yield Concept

In addition to its role as a bridge between platelets and exposed collagen on endothelial surfaces, vWF binds to and stabilizes coagulation factor VIII. Binding of factor VIII by vWF is required for normal survival of factor VIII in the circulation.

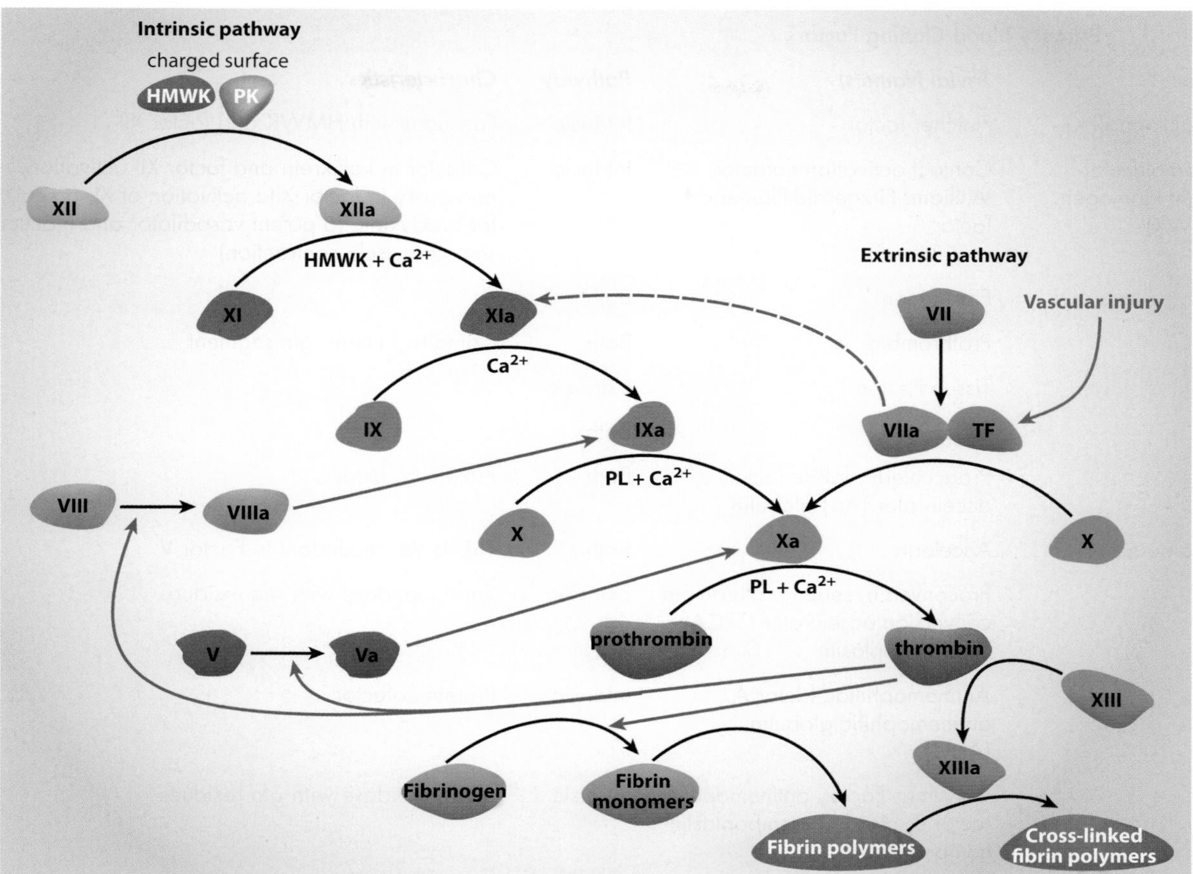

FIGURE 51-1: The clotting cascades. The intrinsic cascade (which has less in vivo significance in normal physiological circumstances than the extrinsic cascade) is initiated when contact is made between blood and exposed negatively charged surfaces. The extrinsic pathway is initiated upon vascular injury which leads to exposure of tissue factor, TF (also identified as factor III), a subendothelial cell-surface glycoprotein that binds phospholipid. The green dotted arrow represents a point of crossover between the extrinsic and intrinsic pathways. The two pathways converge at the activation of factors X to Xa. Factor Xa has a role in the further activation of factors VII to VIIa as depicted by the green arrow. Active factor Xa hydrolyzes and activates prothrombin to thrombin. Thrombin can then activate factors XI, VIII, and V, furthering the cascade. Ultimately the role of thrombin is to convert fribrinogen to fibrin and to activate factors XIII to XIIIa. Factor XIIIa (also termed transglutaminase) cross-links fibrin polymers solidifying the clot. HMWK, high-molecular-weight kininogen; PK, prekallikrein; PL, phospholipid.

syndrome (also called giant platelet syndrome; see Clinical Box 51-2).

Once adherent to the endothelium, further activation of platelets involves binding of thrombin as well as several factors released from platelet granules such as ADP and TXA_2 (see Figure 51-2). Platelets contain 3 types of granules termed dense, alpha, and lysosomal. Dense granules contain serotonin, calcium ions, and ADP. Alpha granules contain fibronectin; vWF; coagulation factors I, V, and IX; protein S; high-molecular-weight kininogen (HMWK); platelet factor-4 (PF-4); thrombospondin-1; and plasminogen activator inhibitor-1 (PAI-1). Lysosomal granules contain acid hydrolases, β-galactosidase, and β-glucuronidase.

Thrombin binds to a class of GPCR on platelets called the protease activated receptors (PARs), specifically PAR-1, -3 and -4 (Figure 51-3). PARs utilize a unique mechanism to convert the result of extracellular proteolytic cleavage into an intracellular signaling event. PARs carry their own ligand which remains inactive until protease cleavage, such as by thrombin, "unmasks" the ligand. Following thrombin cleavage the unmasked ligand is still a part of the intact PAR but is now capable of interacting with the ligand-binding

TABLE 51-1: Primary Blood-Clotting Factors

Factor	*Trivial Name(s)*	*Pathway*	*Characteristics*
Prekallikrein (PK)	Fletcher factor	Intrinsic	Functions with HMWK and factor XII
High-molecular-weight kininogen (HMWK)	Contact activation cofactor; Williams-Fitzgerald-Flaujeac factor	Intrinsic	Cofactor in kallikrein and factor XII activation, necessary in factor XIIa activation of XI, precursor for bradykinin (a potent vasodilator and inducer of smooth muscle contraction)
I	Fibrinogen	Both	
II	Prothrombin	Both	Contains N-term. *gla* segment
III	Tissue Factor	Extrinsic	
IV	Calcium	Both	
V	Proaccelerin, labile factor, accelerator (Ac-) globulin	Both	Protein cofactor
VI (same as Va)	Accelerin	Both	This is Va, redundant to Factor V
VII	Proconvertin, serum prothrombin conversion accelerator (SPCA), cothromboplastin	Extrinsic	Endopeptidase with *gla* residues
VIII	Antihemophiliac factor A, antihemophilic globulin (AHG)	Intrinsic	Protein cofactor
IX	Christmas Factor, antihemophilic factor B, plasma thromboplastin component (PTC)	Intrinsic	Endopeptidase with *gla* residues
X	Stuart-Prower Factor	Both	Endopeptidase with *gla* residues
XI	Plasma thromboplastin antecedent (PTA)	Intrinsic	Endopeptidase
XII	Hageman factor	Intrinsic	Endopeptidase
XIII	Protransglutaminase, fibrin-stabilizing factor (FSF), fibrinoligase	Both	Transpeptidase

domain of the PAR resulting in the activation of numerous signaling cascades. Because the activation of PARs requires proteolytic cleavage the activation process is irreversible.

Platelet activation by collagen and thrombin leads to activation of members of the PLC family resulting in increased IP_3 and DAG production and the consequent signal cascades induced by these second messengers. The activation-stimulated release of ADP from platelet granules triggers ADP-mediated receptor activation of PLA_2. Active PLA_2 hydrolyzes membrane phospholipids releasing arachidonic acid. The arachidonic acid serves as a substrate for production and release of thromboxane A_2 (TXA_2). TXA_2 is a potent vasoconstrictor and inducer of platelet aggregation that functions by binding to receptors that function through the PLC pathway.

The calcium that is released from the ER in response to IP_3 binding activates myosin light chain kinase (MLCK). Activated MLCK phosphorylates the light chain of myosin which then interacts with actin, resulting in altered platelet morphology and motility. This altered mobility allows enhanced adhesion and the shape change aids in the aggregation of platelets.

One of the most important substituents of platelet granules is ADP. The released ADP binds to members of the purinergic receptor family, specifically $P2Y_1$ and $P2Y_{12}$, the consequences of which are further stimulation of platelets. The important role of ADP in platelet activation can be appreciated from the use of ADP

TABLE 51-2: Functional Classification of Clotting Factors

Zymogens of Serine Proteases	***Activities***
Factor XII	Binds to exposed collagen at site of vessel wall injury, activated by HMWK and kallikrein
Factor XI	Activated by factor XIIa
Factor IX	Activated by factor XIa in presence of Ca^{2+}
Factor VII	Activated by thrombin in presence of Ca^{2+}
Factor X	Activated on surface of activated platelets by tenase complex and by factor VIIa in presence of tissue factor and Ca^{2+}
Factor II	Activated on surface of activated platelets by prothrombinase complex
Cofactors	***Activities***
Factor VIII	Activated by thrombin; factor VIIIa is a cofactor in the activation of factor X by factor IXa
Factor V	Activated by thrombin; factor Va is a cofactor in the activation of prothrombin by factor Xa
Factor III (tissue factor)	A subendothelial cell-surface glycoprotein that acts as a cofactor for factor VII
Fibrinogen	***Activity***
Factor I	Cleaved by thrombin to form fibrin clot
Transglutaminase	***Activity***
Factor XIII	Activated by thrombin in presence of Ca^{2+}; stabilizes fibrin clot by covalent cross-linking
Regulatory/Other Proteins	***Activities***
von Willebrand factor	Associated with subendothelial connective tissue; serves as a bridge between platelet glycoprotein GPIb/IX and collagen
Protein C	Activated to protein Ca by thrombin bound to thrombomodulin; then degrades factors VIIIa and Va
Protein S	Acts as a cofactor of protein C; both proteins contain *gla* residues
Thrombomodulin	Protein on the surface of endothelial cells; binds thrombin, which then activates protein C
Antithrombin III	Most important coagulation inhibitor, controls activities of thrombin and factors IXa, Xa, XIa, and XIIa

receptor antagonists (eg, clopidogrel), in the control of thrombosis (see below). ADP also modifies the platelet membranes leading to exposure of platelet glycoprotein receptor complex GPIIb-GPIIIa. GPIIb-GPIIIa constitutes a receptor for vWF and fibrinogen, resulting in fibrinogen-induced platelet aggregation. The GPIIb-GPIIIa complex is also a member of the integrin family; therefore, it is also called integrin αIIb-β_3. The importance of the GPIIb-GPIIIa in platelet activation and coagulation is demonstrated by the fact that bleeding disorders result from inherited defects in this glycoprotein complex. The most commonly inherited platelet dysfunction is Glanzmann thrombasthenia, which results from defects in the GPIIb protein of this complex (see Clinical Box 51-3). In addition, the importance of this complex is the anticoagulant function of antibodies to this receptor (eg, abciximab: see below).

The Kallikrein-Kinin System in the Intrinsic Pathway

Activation of the intrinsic pathway of coagulation, in part, involves the contribution of the kallikrein-kinin system. This system comprises a complex of proteins

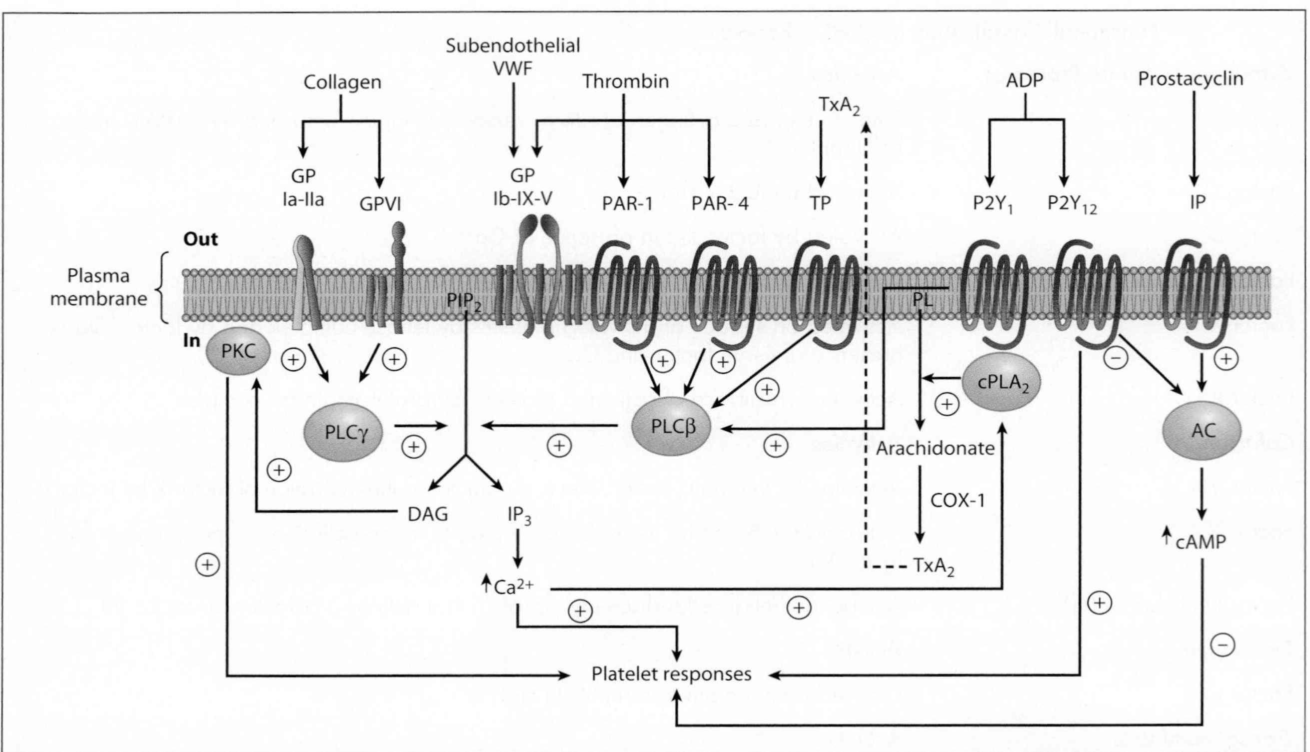

FIGURE 51-2: Diagrammatic representation of platelet activation by collagen, thrombin, thromboxane A_2, and ADP, and inhibition by prostacyclin. The external environment, the plasma membrane, and the inside of a platelet are depicted from top to bottom. Platelet responses include, depending on the agonist, change of platelet shape, release of the contents of the storage granules, and aggregation. (AC, adenylyl cyclase; cAMP, cyclic AMP; COX-1, cyclooxgenase-1; $cPLA_2$, cytosolic phospholipase A_2; DAG, 1,2-diacylglycerol; GP, glycoprotein; IP, prostacyclin receptor; IP_3, inositol 1,4,5-trisphosphate; $P2Y_1$, $P2Y_{12}$, purinoceptors; PAR, protease activated receptor; PIP_2, phosphatidylinositol 4,5-bisphosphate; PKC, protein kinase C; PL, phospholipid; PLCβ, phospholipase Cβ; PLCγ, phospholipase Cγ; TP, thromboxane A_2 receptor; TxA_2, thromboxane A_2; VWF, von Willebrand factor.) The G proteins that are involved are not shown. Murray RK, Bender DA, Botham KM, Kennelly PJ, Rodwell VW, Weil PA. *Harper's Illustrated Biochemistry.* 29th ed. New York: McGraw-Hill; 2012.

that when activated leads to the release of vasoactive kinins. The kinins are released from both high-molecular-weight kininogen (HMWK) and low-molecular-weight kininogen (LMWK) as a result of activation of either tissue kallikrein or plasma kallikrein. The kinins are involved in many physiological and pathological processes including regulation of blood pressure and flow (via modulation of the renin-angiotensin pathway), blood coagulation, cellular proliferation and growth, angiogenesis, apoptosis, and inflammation. Kinin action on endothelial cells leads to vasodilation, increased vascular permeability, release of tissue plasminogen activator (tPA), production of nitric oxide (NO), and the mobilization of arachidonic acid, primarily resulting in prostacyclin (PGI_2) production by endothelial cells. With respect to hemostasis, the most important kinin is bradykinin which is released from HMWK. Bradykinin is a 9-amino-acid vasoactive peptide that induces vasodilation and increases vascular permeability.

These 2 kallikreins are serine proteases whose major substrates are HMWK (plasma kallikrein) and LMWK (tissue kallikrein). HMWK is considered an α-globulin and is composed of 6 functional domains. The protein circulates in the plasma as single-chain polypeptide. The heavy chain contains domains 1, 2, and 3 and the light chain comprises domains 5 and 6. The heavy and light chains are linked together through domain 4 which also contains the bradykinin sequence. Domain 1 contains a low-affinity calcium-binding site. Domains 2 and 3 inhibit cysteine proteases. Domain 3 also has platelet and endothelial cell–binding activity. Domain 5 has sequences for heparin binding and antiangiogenic properties. The binding of HMWK to negatively charged surfaces occurs through a histidine

CLINICAL BOX 51-1: vON WILLEBRAND DISEASE

Von Willebrand disease (vWD) is caused by deficiencies in the gene-encoding von Willebrand factor (vWF). vWD is the most commonly occurring bleeding disorder with clinically significant forms affecting approximately 1 in 1000 individuals. However, abnormalities in vWF have been estimated to occur with a frequency of 1 in 100 persons, thus a relatively small fraction of persons harboring mutations in vWF are actually symptomatic. There are both dominant and recessive forms of vWD. The characteristic feature of vWD is bleeding from mucocutaneous sites (typical skin and mucous membranes) rather than from deep tissues and joints. vWF is involved in 2 important reactions of blood coagulation. The first is the interaction of vWF with specific receptors on the surface of platelets and the subendothelial connective tissue. This interaction allows platelets to adhere to areas of vascular injury. The second role of vWF is to bind to and stabilize factor VIII allowing factor VIII to survive in the blood. As a consequence of these roles for vWF, deficiencies result in defective platelet adhesion and to secondary deficiencies in factor VIII. Since factor VIII deficiency results in hemophilia A, it is not surprising that vWF deficiencies can manifest with clinical symptoms that appear to be hemophilia A. The most common form of the vWD (type 1) is an autosomal dominant disorder resulting from quantitative deficiency in vWF. Recessive inheritance of a virtual lack of vWF protein characterizes the clinically severe form of the disease called type 3 vWD. The inheritance of qualitative defects in vWF (dysfunctional protein) is characteristic of type 2 vWD. The type 2 category is further subdivided into 4 variants that are based upon the functional characteristics of the mutant protein. In type 2A vWD the residual vWF has reduced function. In type 2B vWD the mutant vWF has an increased affinity for the GPIb protein of the platelet GPIb-IX-V complex. In type 2M vWD there is the presence of normal vWF multimeric complexes, but they exhibit reduced platelet-dependent function. In type 2N vWD there are factor VIII deficiencies that are the result of mutations in vWF that does not bind to factor VIII. In patients with type 1 and type 3 vWD the severity of the disease is related to the degree of functional deficiency in vWF. Clinically, type 1 and type 3 vWD patients can manifest from insignificant problems to life-threatening complications. Patients with type 2 vWD may exhibit symptoms whose severity may be greater than would be expected based upon a knowledge of the functional defect. Symptoms of vWD often present shortly after birth. The common symptoms are easy bruising, bleeding from the gums, cutaneous hematomas, and prolonged bleeding from cuts and abrasions. Individuals with severe forms of vWD can have bleeding complications because they either lack sufficient vWF to promote platelet adhesion at the site of vascular injury or they are factor VIII deficient due to the lack of the stabilizing action of vWF on factor VIII. Therefore, the therapeutic response to vWD requires an understanding of these distinct functions of vWF. Mucocutaneous and postsurgical bleeding can be treated by raising the level of factor VIII. In order to address the platelet adhesion deficit in vWD, it is necessary to increase the level of functional vWF. This can be accomplished using fresh frozen plasma or cryoprecipitates. The limitation to these approaches is that a large volume of frozen plasma is needed to deliver sufficient amount of vWF and cryoprecipitates are known to be associated with possible disease transmission. Platelet transfusions can be helpful in some patients with vWD, especially those who are refractory to factor VIII-vWF concentrates.

High-Yield Concept

In the presence of Ca^{2+}, factor XIa activates factor IX to factor IXa. Active factor IXa cleaves factor X leading to its activation to factor Xa. The activation of factor Xa requires assemblage of the tenase complex (Ca^{2+} and factors VIIIa, IXa, and X) on the surface of activated platelets.

CLINICAL BOX 51-2: BERNARD-SOULIER SYNDROME

Bernard-Soulier syndrome (BSS) is the second most common inherited bleeding disorder that results as a consequence of defects in platelet function. It is characterized by, among other symptoms, the presence of giant platelets. Hence the disorder is also known as giant platelet syndrome. In addition to the presence of giant platelets, patients experience a prolonged bleeding time. Although platelets from these individuals will aggregate in response to the presence of epinephrine, collagen, and/or ADP, they will not aggregate in the presence of ristocetin. Ristocetin is an antibiotic isolated from *Amycolatopsis lurida* which was formerly used to treat staphylococcal infections. Ristocetin induces binding of vWF to platelet GPIb-IX-V and as a consequence of this activity the compound is used in a diagnostic assay for vWD. Bernard-Soulier syndrome is an autosomal recessive disorder in which most patients have either a decrease or absence in 3 of the 4 proteins of the platelet GPIb-IX-V complex. At least 18 different molecular defects have been identified resulting in Bernard-Soulier syndrome. Mutations in GPIbα result in type A BSS, mutations in GPIbβ result in type B BSS, and mutations in GPIX result in type C BSS. At least 6 missense mutations in the GPIX gene have been identified in BSS patients. No known mutations in GPV are associated with BSS. The clinical manifestations of BSS are similar to those in patients with dysfunctional platelets. These symptoms include mucocutaneous bleeding, gastrointestinal hemorrhage, and purpuric skin bleeding (bleeding from purplish patches on the skin). In female patients there is the additional complication of menorrhagia. Evaluation of BSS is done by analysis of platelet number and size. All patients will have some level of and platelets that are from 3 to 20 times normal size. Bleeding times are increased in BSS but the distinguishing abnormality is the failure of platelet aggregation (agglutination) in the presence of ristocetin. This aggregation defect cannot be corrected by the addition of normal plasma. Treatment of bleeding in BSS is accomplished by local application of pressure, topical thrombin, and platelet transfusion. In female patients hormonal management of menses is important.

CLINICAL BOX 51-3: GLANZMANN THROMBASTHENIA

Glanzmann thrombasthenia (weak platelets) represents a heterogenous group of bleeding disorders. The hallmark of the disease is the failure of platelets to bind fibrinogen and aggregate in the presence of a variety of physiological agonist such as ADP, thrombin, epinephrine, or collagen. Glanzmann thrombasthenia is an autosomal recessive bleeding disorder in which the underlying defect in all patients is an abnormality in the genes encoding either the GPIIb (αIIb) or GPIIIa (β3) proteins of the GPIIb-GPIIIa complex. The platelet GPIIb-GPIIIa complex is the most abundant platelet receptor representing approximately 15% of the total protein on the surface of platelets. Although Glanzmann thrombasthenia is a rare disorder, it is the most recognized inherited disorder of platelet function. The molecular abnormalities causing Glanzmann thrombasthenia range from major gene deletions and inversions to single point mutations. These mutations have been grouped according to the biochemical consequences and include transcriptional and protein functional defects. Among the functional defects there are protein stability mutants, glycoprotein complex maturation mutants, and ligand-binding mutants. The clinical manifestations of Glanzmann thrombasthenia are significant mucocutaneous bleeding that is evidenced at an early age. Lifelong repeated bleeding occurs at sites of minor trauma such as the gums (gingival) and the nose (epistaxis). In females heavy bleeding during menstruation may require therapeutic intervention. Severe intracranial or gastrointestinal hemorrhage can occur spontaneously (ie, unprovoked by injury) and is a significant cause of mortality in 5% to 10% of Glanzmann thrombasthenia patients. Treatment of the disorder is limited to local measures such as the application of pressure. Platelet transfusion may be useful but only on a limited basis as resistance will develop to the infused platelets.

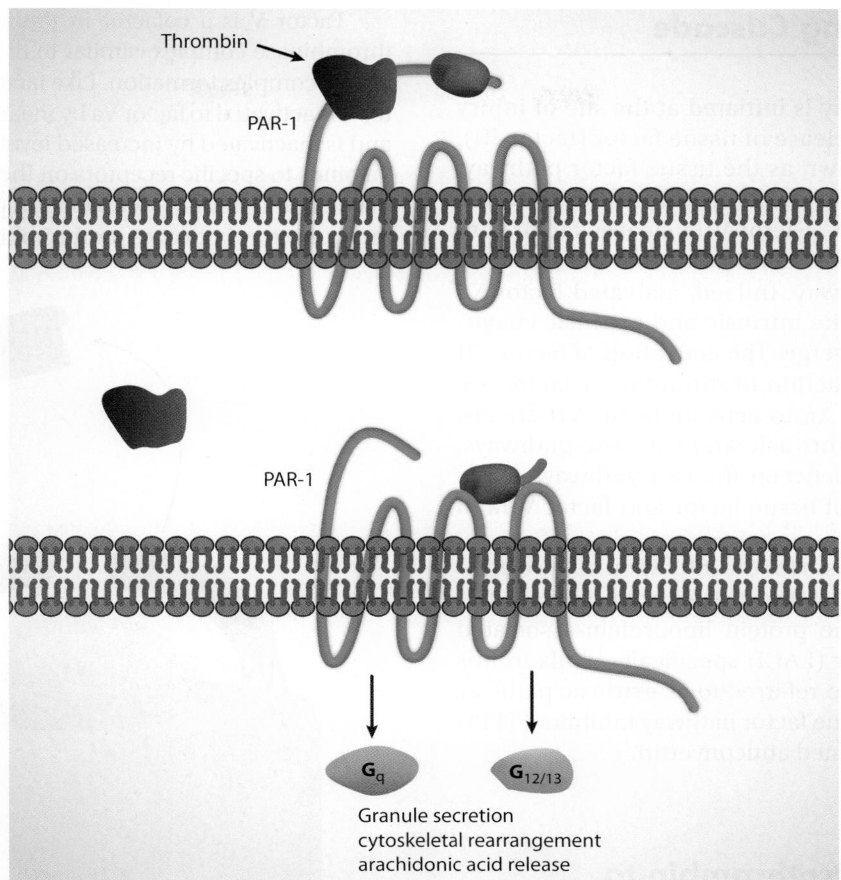

FIGURE 51-3: Mechanism of activation of protease-activated receptor 1 (PAR-1) by thrombin. Reproduced with permission of themedicalbiochemistrypage, LLC.

region of the light chain which is in domain 5. Domain 6 contains the prekallikrein and factor XI-binding sites. By being able to bind to charged surfaces via domain 5 and simultaneously binding factor XI and prekallikrein via domain 6, HMWK can serve as the cofactor in activation of the intrinsic pathway which is referred to as contact activation.

The plasma kinin forming system is composed of factor XII, and XI, prekallikrein, and HMWK. Factor XII, prekallikrein, and HMWK reversibly bind to endothelial cells, platelets, and granulocytes. When plasma makes contact with a negatively charged surface factor XII binds and is autoactivated to factor XIIa (the "a" signifies the activated factor). Factor XIIa then activates prekallikrein to kallikrein and kallikrein cleaves HMWK releasing bradykinin. There is also reciprocal activation of factor XII by kallikrein resulting in amplification of the system. Several physiologic substances serve as the charged surface to which the contact system binds. These substances include phospholipids, hematin (hydroxide of heme), fatty acids, sodium urate crystals, protoporphyrin, sulfatides, heparins, chondroitin sulfates, articular cartilage, endotoxin, L-homocysteine, and amyloid β-protein. Contact activation also occurs via lipoproteins, principally oxidized LDL (oxLDL). This is the basis of the role of hyperlipidemia in the promotion of a prothrombotic state and the development of atherosclerosis (see Chapter 48).

One of the responses of platelets to activation is the presentation of phosphatidylserine (PS) and phosphatidylinositol (PI) on their surfaces. The exposure of these phospholipids allows the tenase complex to form. The role of factor VIII in this process is to act as a receptor, in the form of factor VIIIa, for factors IXa and X. The activation of factor VIII to factor VIIIa (the actual receptor) occurs in the presence of minute quantities of thrombin. As the concentration of thrombin increases, factor VIIIa is ultimately cleaved by thrombin and inactivated. This dual action of thrombin, upon factor VIII, acts to limit the extent of tenase complex formation and thus the extent of the coagulation cascade.

Extrinsic Clotting Cascade

The extrinsic pathway is initiated at the site of injury in response to the release of tissue factor (factor III), and thus is also known as the tissue factor pathway. Tissue factor is a cofactor in the factor VIIa-catalyzed activation of factor X. Factor VIIa cleaves factor X to factor Xa in a manner identical to that of factor IXa of the intrinsic pathway. Indeed, activated factor Xa is the site at which the intrinsic and extrinsic coagulation cascades converge. The activation of factor VII occurs through the action of thrombin or factor Xa. The ability of factor Xa to activate factor VII creates a link between the intrinsic and extrinsic pathways. An additional link between the two pathways exists through the ability of tissue factor and factor VIIa to activate factor IX.

A major mechanism for the inhibition of the extrinsic pathway occurs at the tissue factor-factor VIIa-Ca^{2+}-Xa complex. The protein lipoprotein-associated coagulation inhibitor (LACI) specifically binds to this complex. LACI is also referred to as extrinsic pathway inhibitor (EPI) or tissue factor pathway inhibitor (TFPI) and was formerly named anticonvertin.

Activation of Prothrombin to Thrombin

The common point in both pathways is the activation of factor X to factor Xa. Factor Xa activates prothrombin (factor II) to thrombin (factor IIa). Thrombin, in turn, converts fibrinogen to fibrin (see Figure 51-1).

Factor V is a cofactor in the formation of the prothrombinase complex, similar to the role of factor VIII in tenase complex formation. Like factor VIII activation, factor V is activated to factor Va by means of minute amounts and is inactivated by increased levels of thrombin. Factor Va binds to specific receptors on the surfaces of activated platelets and forms a complex with prothrombin and factor Xa. Factor Xa cleaves prothrombin to thrombin.

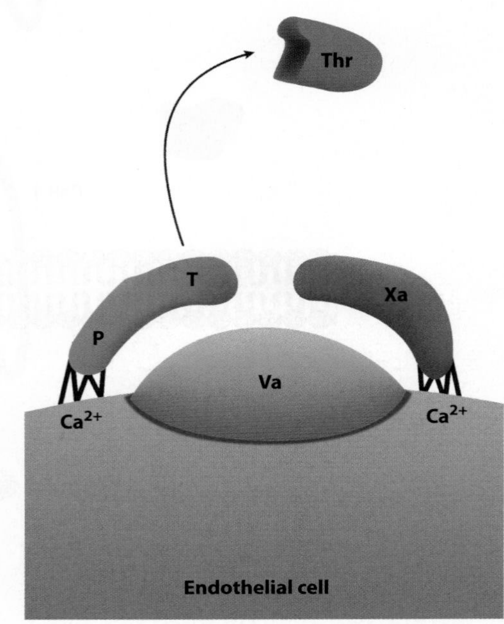

FIGURE 51-4: Formation of the prothrombinase complex and release of active thrombin. Prothrombin (PT) binds to the complex of calcium ion, active factor V (Va), and active factor X (Xa) which then leads to the catalytic release of active thrombin. Reproduced with permission of themedicalbiochemistrypage, LLC.

High-Yield Concept

The formation of a complex between factor VIIa and tissue factor is believed to be a principal step in the overall clotting cascade. Evidence for this stems from the fact that persons with hereditary deficiencies in the components of the contact phase of the intrinsic pathway do not exhibit clotting problems.

High-Yield Concept

The activation of thrombin occurs on the surface of activated platelets and requires formation of a **prothrombinase complex** (Figure 51-4). This complex is composed of platelet phospholipids, Ca^{2+}, factors Va and Xa, and prothrombin.

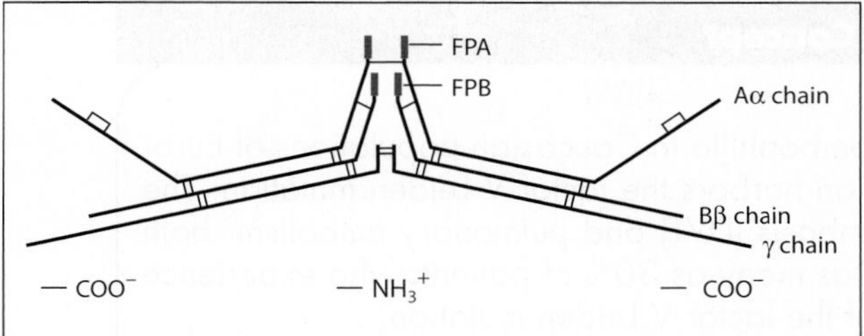

FIGURE 51-5: Diagrammatic representation (not to scale) of fibrinogen showing pairs of Aα, Bβ, and γ chains linked by disulfide bonds. (FPA, fibrinopeptide A; FPB, fibrinopeptide B.) Murray RK, Bender DA, Botham KM, Kennelly PJ, Rodwell VW, Weil PA. *Harper's Illustrated Biochemistry*. 29th ed. New York: McGraw-Hill; 2012.

Thrombin Activation of Fibrin Clot Formation

The major role of thrombin in hemostasis is the catalytic digestion of fibrinogen to fibrin. Fibrinogen (factor I) consists of 3 pairs of polypeptides $([A\alpha][B\beta][\gamma])_2$. The 6 chains are covalently linked near their *N*-terminals through disulfide bonds (Figure 51-5). The A and B portions of the Aα and Bβ chains comprise the **fibrinopeptides** A and B, respectively. Thrombin hydrolyses fibrinogen between the fibrinopeptide and the **a** and **b** portions of the protein releasing the fibrinopeptides.

The release of the fibrinopeptides generates fibrin monomers with a subunit structure $(\alpha\beta\gamma)_2$. These monomers spontaneously aggregate in a regular array, forming a somewhat weak fibrin clot. In addition to fibrin activation, thrombin converts factor XIII to factor XIIIa, a highly specific transglutaminase that introduces cross-links between the fibrin monomers generating an insoluble fibrin clot (Figure 51-6).

Thrombin also activates thrombin-activatable fibrinolysis inhibitor (TAFI), thereby modulating the rate of fibrin clot dissolution (fibrinolysis). TAFI is also known as carboxypeptidase U (CPU) whose activity leads to removal of *C*-terminal lysines from partially degraded fibrin. This leads to an impairment of plasminogen activation, thereby reducing the rate of fibrinolysis.

Control of Thrombin Levels

There are 2 principal mechanisms by which thrombin activity is regulated. The predominant mechanism is the regulated conversion of prothrombin to thrombin. The activation of thrombin is also regulated by specific thrombin inhibitors. Antithrombin III is the most important since it can also inhibit the activities of factors IXa, Xa, XIa, and XIIa; plasmin; and kallikrein. The activity of antithrombin III is potentiated in the presence of heparin. Heparin binds to a specific site on antithrombin III, producing an altered conformation of the protein, and

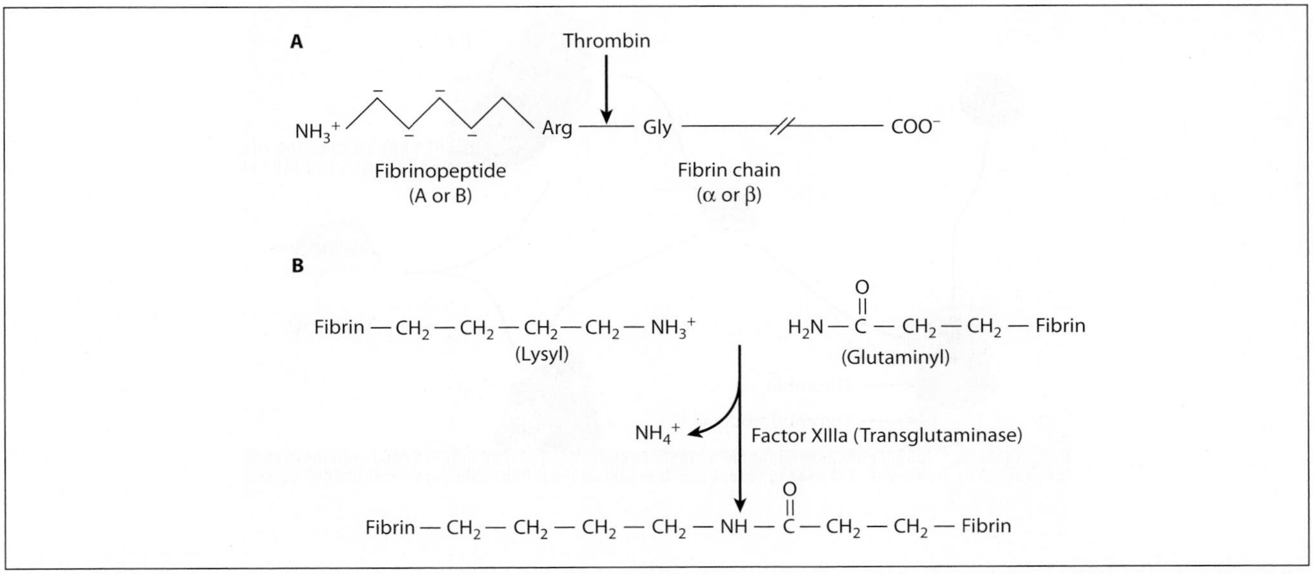

A

Thrombin

NH_3^+ — Arg ↓ Gly —//— COO^-

Fibrinopeptide (A or B) — Fibrin chain (α or β)

B

$\text{Fibrin}-CH_2-CH_2-CH_2-CH_2-NH_3^+$ (Lysyl) + $H_2N-\overset{O}{\overset{\|}{C}}-CH_2-CH_2-\text{Fibrin}$ (Glutaminyl)

↓ Factor XIIIa (Transglutaminase), NH_4^+ released

$\text{Fibrin}-CH_2-CH_2-CH_2-CH_2-NH-\overset{O}{\overset{\|}{C}}-CH_2-CH_2-\text{Fibrin}$

FIGURE 51-6: Formation of a fibrin clot. (A) Thrombin-induced cleavage of Arg-Gly bonds of the Aα and Bβ chains of fibrinogen to produce fibrinopeptides (left-hand side) and the α and β chains of fibrin monomer (right-hand side). (B) Cross-linking of fibrin molecules by activated factor XIII (factor XIIIa). Murray RK, Bender DA, Botham KM, Kennelly PJ, Rodwell VW, Weil PA. *Harper's Illustrated Biochemistry*. 29th ed. New York: McGraw-Hill; 2012.

High-Yield Concept

Factor V Leiden is the most common inherited thrombophilia in Caucasian populations of European descent. Overall, 5% of the world population harbors the factor V Leiden mutation. The symptoms of factor V Leiden are deep vein thrombosis (DVT) and pulmonary embolism, both of which can be fatal. In fact, it is estimated that as many as 30% of patients who experience DVT and/or pulmonary embolisms are carriers of the factor V Leiden mutation.

the new conformation has a higher affinity for thrombin as well as its other substrates. This effect of heparin is the basis for its clinical use as an anticoagulant. The naturally occurring heparin activator of antithrombin III is present as heparan and heparan sulfate on the surface of vessel endothelial cells. It is this feature that controls the activation of the intrinsic coagulation cascade.

Protein C: Control of Coagulation and Intravascular Inflammation

Protein C (PC) is a trypsin-like serine protease that serves as a major regulator of the coagulation process. Protein S (PS) serves as a cofactor for the functions of activated protein C (abbreviated aPC, and also APC).

In addition to its role in the formation of a fibrin clot, thrombin plays an important regulatory role in the overall coagulation process via the activation of protein C. Thrombin combines with thrombomodulin present on endothelial cell surfaces forming a complex that converts protein C to protein Ca (Figure 51-7). The cofactor protein S and protein Ca degrade factors Va and VIIIa, thereby limiting the activity of these two factors in the coagulation cascade.

The importance of aPC in controlling Va activity can be seen in the hypercoagulopathy (thrombophilia) referred to as factor V Leiden. This thrombophilia is caused by a mutation in the factor V gene resulting in a protein that is not effectively degraded by aPC.

Loss of protein C results in massive and usually lethal thrombotic complications in infants with homozygous PC deficiency. In individuals who are

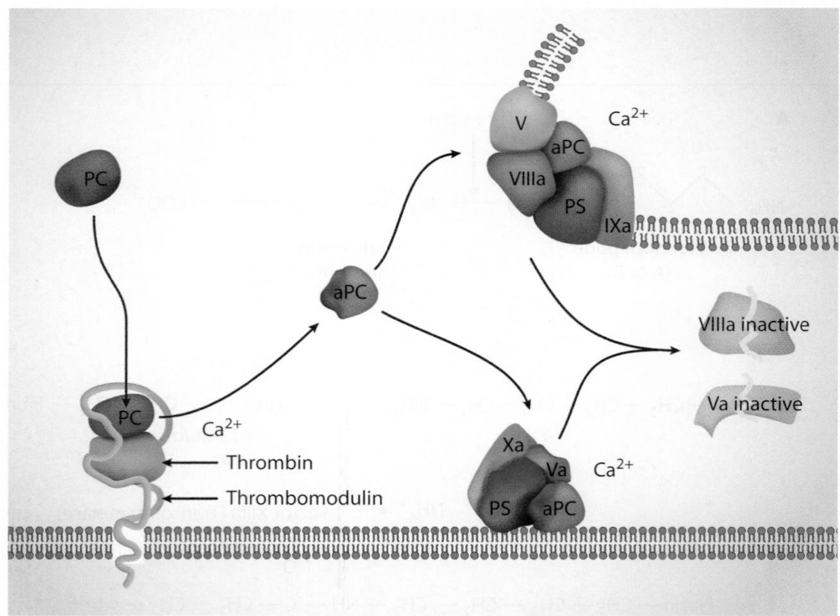

FIGURE 51-7: Role of thrombomodulin in thrombin activation of protein C (PC). Thrombomodulin is an endothelial cell surface glycoprotein that binds thrombin and protein C. The "capture" of thrombin and protein C allows thrombin to activate protein C. Active protein C (APC) then interacts with its cofactor protein S (PS) and cleaves active factors VIII (VIIIa) and V (Va) into inactive forms, thereby terminating their role in coagulation. Reproduced with permission of themedicalbiochemistrypage, LLC.

heterozygous for PC deficiencies, there is an increased risk for venous thrombosis.

Although the role of aPC in the termination of coagulation is extremely important, it also serves many additional functions that alter the inflammatory processes occurring in the vasculature. Activated PC binds to the endothelial protein C receptor (EPCR) and leads to the activation of PAR-1 which elicits cytoprotective and anti-inflammatory responses within endothelial cells. The EPCR is also found on monocytes, neutrophils, fibroblasts, and keratinocytes. The cytoprotective effects of aPC include protection of the endothelial cell barrier and induction of antiapoptotic signaling pathways as well as expression of eNOS. Additional endothelial responses to aPC include inhibition of the expression and actions of the potent pro-inflammatory transcription factor NFκB. The suppression of NFκB action results in down regulation of the synthesis of endothelial pro-inflammatory cytokines and the cell adhesion molecules. The anti-inflammatory and cytoprotective effects of aPC were the basis for the development of the antisepsis drug dotrecogin alpha (subsequently removed from the market).

Dissolution of Fibrin Clots

Degradation of fibrin clots is the function of plasmin, a serine protease that circulates as the inactive proenzyme, plasminogen. Any free-circulating plasmin is rapidly inhibited by α_2-antiplasmin. Plasminogen binds to both fibrinogen and fibrin allowing it to be incorporated into a clot as it is formed. Tissue plasminogen activator (tPA) and, to a lesser degree, urokinase are serine proteases which convert plasminogen to plasmin. Inactive tPA is released from vascular endothelial cells following injury; it binds to fibrin and is consequently activated. Urokinase is produced as the precursor, prourokinase, by epithelial cells lining excretory ducts. The role of urokinase is to activate the dissolution of fibrin clots that may be deposited in these ducts. The level of active tPA is controlled by binding to specific inhibitory proteins. At least 4 distinct inhibitors have been identified, of which plasminogen activator-inhibitor type 1 (PAI-1) and type 2 (PAI-2) are of greatest physiological significance.

Active tPA cleaves plasminogen to plasmin which then digests the fibrin (Figure 51-8). The soluble degradation product no longer contains the binding sites for plasmin or plasminogen leading to their release. The released plasminogen and plasmin are rapidly inactivated primarily by α_2-antiplamin (Clinical Box 51-4).

Coagulation disorders

Disorders in coagulation can result from defects in any of the processes of platelet adherence and activation or with any of the proteins required for coagulation. Tissue factor (factor III) is the only coagulation factor for which a congenital defect has not been identified. Coagulation disorders can result in hypercoagulation (referred to as the coagulopathies) or in an inability to coagulate. The most common coagulopathy is Factor V Leiden. The hemophilias (Clinical Box 51-5) are probably the best known coagulation disorders. However, the most common cause of defective coagulation is von Willebrand disease, vWD (Clinical Box 51-1). Deficiency in factor XI confers an injury-related bleeding tendency that was initially termed hemophilia C.

Deficiency in antithrombin III results in another type of coagulopathy. This disorder is seen in approximately 2% of patients with venous thromboembolic disease. Deficiencies result from mutations that affect synthesis or stability of antithrombin III or from mutations that affect the protease and/or heparin binding sites of the protein. Clinical manifestations of antithrombin III deficiency include DVT and pulmonary embolism. Thrombosis may occur spontaneously or in association with surgery, trauma, or pregnancy. Treatment of acute episodes of thrombosis is by infusion of heparin (for 5-7 days) followed by oral anticoagulant therapy.

Several cardiovascular risk factors are associated with abnormalities in fibrinogen. As a result of the acute-phase response or through other poorly understood mechanisms, elevated plasma fibrinogen levels

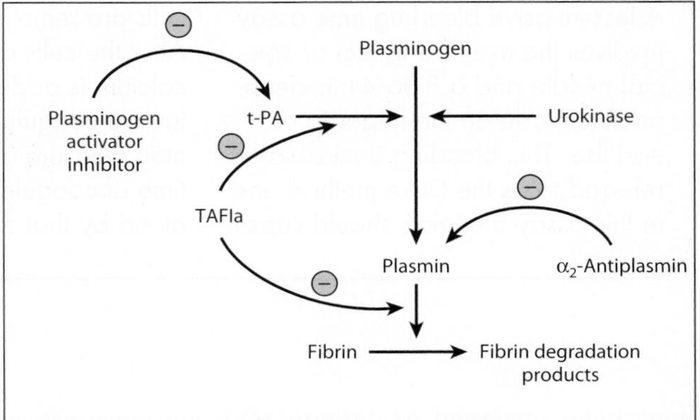

FIGURE 51-8: Initiation of fibrinolysis by the activation of plasmin. Scheme of sites of action of tissue plasminogen activator (t-PA), urokinase, plasminogen activator inhibitor, α_2-antiplasmin, and thrombin-activatable fibrinolysis inhibitor (TAFIa) (the last 3 proteins exert inhibitory actions). Murray RK, Bender DA, Botham KM, Kennelly PJ, Rodwell VW, Weil PA. *Harper's Illustrated Biochemistry.* 29th ed. New York: McGraw-Hill; 2012.

CLINICAL BOX 51-4: BLOOD COAGULATION TESTS AND INTERPRETATIONS

The primary test for determination of coagulation activity are bleeding time, prothrombin time (PT), partial thromboplastin time (PTT), and activated partial thromboplastin time (aPTT).

Bleeding time assays are used to evaluate the vascular and platelet responses that are associated with hemostasis. The bleeding time is a frequent assay performed on preoperative patients to ensure there is an adequate response to vessel injury prior to surgery. As indicated above, the rapid responses to vascular injury (occurring within seconds) are vessel constriction and platelet adhesion to the vessel wall. The Ivy method for determining the bleeding time involves the use of a blood pressure cuff (sphygmomanometer) which is placed on the forearm and inflated to 40 mm Hg. A superficial incision is then made on the forearm and the time it takes for bleeding to stop is recorded. With the Ivy method bleeding should stop within 1 to 9 minutes. Any bleeding time greater than 15 minutes would be indicative of a defect in the initial responses of vessels and platelets to vascular injury. A less-invasive bleeding time assay involves the use of a lancet or special needle and a 3- to 4-mm-deep prick is made on the fingertip or earlobe. This bleeding time assay is referred to as the Duke method and in this assay bleeding should cease within 1 to 3 minutes. The bleeding time is affected (prolonged) by any defect in platelet function, by vascular disorders, and in von Willebrand disease but is not affected by other coagulation factors. Disorders that are commonly associated with an increased bleeding time include thrombocytopenia, disseminated intravascular coagulation (DIC), Bernard-Soulier syndrome, and Glanzmann thrombasthenia. Abnormal bleeding times are also found in patients with Cushing syndrome, severe liver disease, leukemia, and bone marrow failure.

The **prothrombin time (PT)** is an assay designed to screen for defects in fibrinogen, prothrombin, and factors V, VII, and X and thus measures activities of the extrinsic pathway of coagulation. When any of these factors is deficient then the PT is prolonged. A normal PT is 11.0 to 12.5 seconds. A PT greater than 20 seconds is indicative of coagulation deficit. The PT is measured using plasma after the blood cells are removed. A blood sample is collected in a tube containing citrate or EDTA to chelate any calcium and thus inhibit coagulation and then the cells are removed by centrifugation. After the cells are removed excess calcium is added to the plasma to initiate coagulation. The most common measure of PT is to divide the time of coagulation of a patients' blood by that of a known standard and this value is referred to as the international normalized ratio (INR). Normal INR values range from 0.8 to 1.2. PT is used to determine the correct dosage of the warfarin class of anticoagulation drugs (eg, Coumadin), for the presence of liver disease or damage, and to evaluate vitamin K status.

The **partial thromboplastin time (PTT)** is used to assay for defects in the intrinsic pathway of coagulation. The PTT assay has been modified by the addition of activators that shorten the normal clotting time and this form of the assay is referred to as the activated partial thromboplastin time (aPTT). The PTT is normally prescribed in patients with unexplained bleeding or clotting. The assay will evaluate the function of fibrinogen, prothrombin, and factors V, VIII, IX, X, XI, and XII. A defect in any of these factors will result in a prolonged PTT (or aPTT). A normal PTT is 60 to 70 seconds, whereas for the aPTT the normal range is 30 to 40 seconds. The PTT is a standard assay used to assess the efficacy of heparin anticoagulant therapy. Prolonged PTTs are associated with acquired or congenital bleeding disorders associated with coagulation factor deficiency, vitamin K deficiency, liver disease, DIC, von Willebrand disease, leukemia, hemophilia, and heparin administration.

have been observed in patients with coronary artery disease, diabetes, hypertension, peripheral artery disease, hyperlipoproteinemia, and hypertriglyceridemia. In addition, pregnancy, menopause, hypercholesterolemia, use of oral contraceptives, and smoking lead to increased plasma fibrinogen levels. Although rare, there are inherited disorders in fibrinogen. These disorders include afibrinogenemia (a complete lack of fibrinogen), hypofibrinogenemia (reduced levels of fibrinogen), and dysfibrinogenemia (presence of dysfunctional fibrinogen).

Factor XIII is a tetramer of 2 different peptides, A and B (forming A_2B_2). Hereditary deficiencies occur resulting in the absence of either subunit. Clinical manifestation of factor XIII deficiency is delayed bleeding, although primary hemostasis is normal. Deficiency leads to neonatal umbilical cord bleeding, intracranial hemorrhage, and soft tissue hematomas.

CLINICAL BOX 51-5: THE HEMOPHILIAS

Hemophilia A is referred to as classic hemophilia and was first recognized in the second century AD. The disease is an X-linked bleeding disorder caused by defects in the gene-encoding factor VIII (F8 gene). Multiple mutations have been identified in the F8 gene leading to hemophilia A. Patients with hemophilia A suffer from joint and muscle hemorrhage, easy bruising, and prolonged bleeding time from wounds. Almost all patients with hemophilia A have normal platelet function, so the bleeding from minor cuts or abrasions is generally not severe. Hemophilia A can be divided into severe or moderate disease. Approximately 50% to 60% of hemophilia A patients suffer from the severe form of the disease and have less than 1% normal factor VIII activity. Patients with moderate hemophilia A have from 1% to 20% of normal factor VIII. Because hemophilia A is an X-linked disease, almost all patients are male and the occurrence worldwide is 1 in 5000 male births. It is possible that an affected female can result from the mating of an affected male with a carrier female, but the Mendelian frequency for such a situation is approximately 1 in 50 million female births. A more common mechanism for presentation of hemophilia A in females is the process of X chromosome inactivation, which could lead to inactivation of the X chromosome that harbors the wild-type factor VIII gene. The frequency and severity of the bleeding in hemophilia A patients is inversely correlated to the level of residual factor VIII protein circulating in the blood. The weight bearing joints are the ones most affected in the disease and include the hips, knees, ankles, and elbows. If the bleeding in the joints is left untreated it will lead to severe swelling and pain, joint stiffness, and inflammation. Blood in the synovial fluid of the joints is highly irritating, causing synovial overgrowth and a tendency to cause additional bleeding from the vascular tissues of the joint. The bleeding results in the deposition of iron in chondrocytes with the consequences being the development of degenerative arthritis. Muscle bleeding, like joint bleeding, is most prevalent in large load-bearing muscle groups such as in the thigh, calf, buttocks, and posterior abdominal wall. Since all of these untoward clinical symptoms are the result of a lack of factor VIII in the blood, replacement of factor VIII by intravenous infusion of recombinant protein completely normalizes the blood coagulation processes.

Hemophilia B, also known as factor IX deficiency or Christmas disease, is an X-linked bleeding disorder caused by defects in the gene-encoding factor IX (F9 gene). Factor IX is also known as the Christmas factor, hence the association of hemophilia B with the term Christmas disease. Activation of factor IX to factor IXa requires the cofactor, factor VIII. Multiple mutations in the F9 gene have been identified leading to hemophilia B. Hemophilia B results in a bleeding disorder that is clinically indistinguishable from the more common hemophilia A. Hemophilia B occurs in approximately 1 in 30,000 male births. The major symptom of hemophilia B is spontaneous bleeding into the joints and the soft tissues of the body. The disease exhibits three levels of manifestation. The severe disease results in patients with less than 1% of normal factor IX protein in the circulation, moderate disease results from 1% to 5% of normal factor IX protein, and mild disease is found when patients have 6% to 30% of normal factor IX. The most common clinical symptom of hemophilia B that requires therapeutic intervention is soft tissue hemorrhage and hemarthroses (bleeding in the joints). The leading cause of morbidity and mortality in hemophilia B patients is intracranial hemorrhage. Severely affected patients are usually diagnosed before age 1. The most effective treatment for hemophilia B patients is the administration of recombinant factor IX.

Pharmacological Intervention in Bleeding

Coumarin drugs (based on the chemical benzopyrone) such as warfarin as well as heparin and heparan sulfate are useful as anticoagulants. Heparin is useful as an anticoagulant because it binds to, and activates, antithrombin III which then inhibits the serine proteases of the coagulation cascade. Heparin is abundant in granules of the mast cells that line the vasculature. In response to injury, the heparin is released and inhibits coagulation. The coumarin drugs inhibit coagulation by inhibiting the vitamin K-dependent γ-carboxylation reactions necessary to the function of thrombin, and factors VII, IX, and X as well as proteins C and S. Because functional coagulation factors are present at the outset of coumarin administration, it takes several days for their maximum effect to be realized. For this reason, heparin is normally administered first followed by warfarin or warfarin-related drugs.

The plasminogen activators also are useful for controlling coagulation. Because tPA is highly selective for the degradation of fibrin in clots, it is extremely useful in restoring the patency of the coronary arteries following thrombosis, in particular during the short period following myocardial infarct. Streptokinase (an enzyme from the Streptococci bacterium) is another plasminogen activator useful from a therapeutic standpoint. However, it is less selective than tPA, being able to activate circulating plasminogen as well as that bound to a fibrin clot.

Aspirin is an important inhibitor of platelet activation. By virtue of inhibiting the activity of COX, aspirin reduces the production of TXA_2 by platelets. Aspirin also reduces endothelial cell production of prostacyclin (PGI_2), an inhibitor of platelet aggregation and a vasodilator. Localized to the site of coagulation is a balance between the levels of platelet derived TXA_2 and endothelial cell derived PGI_2. This allows for platelet aggregation and clot formation but preventing excessive accumulation of the clot, thus maintaining blood flow around the site of the clot. Endothelial cells regenerate active COX faster than platelets because mature platelets cannot synthesize the enzyme, requiring new platelets to enter the circulation (platelet half-life is approximately 4 days). Therefore, PGI_2 synthesis is greater than that of TXA_2. The net effect of aspirin is more in favor of endothelial cell-mediated inhibition of the coagulation cascade. This reflects one of the significant cardiovascular benefits to low dose administration of aspirin.

Newer classes of anticoagulation drugs are being developed that function by inhibiting the activation of platelets and their subsequent aggregation. The drug clopidogrel is an irreversible inhibitor of the ADP receptor on platelet membranes. When ADP binds to platelets they are activated and aggregate leading to amplification of the coagulation response. Clopidogrel is prescribed for the treatment of peripheral vascular and cerebrovascular disease as well as coronary artery disease to prevent the formation of thrombotic plaques.

Another target of pharmacological intervention in coagulation involving platelets is the role of GPIIb-GPIIIa in fibrinogen-induced platelet aggregation. The GPIIb-GPIIIa antagonists more completely inhibit platelet aggregation than do aspirin or clopidogrel. The current family of these drugs includes **ReoPro** (abciximab), a monoclonal antibody, **Integrilin** (eptifibatide: a cyclic hexapeptide derived from a protein found in the venom of the southeastern pygmy rattlesnake), and **Aggrastat** (tirofiban: a synthetic organic nonpeptide molecule).

REVIEW QUESTIONS

1. You are examining a 9-year-old boy who is brought in by his parents for unexplained bleeding problems from birth. He experiences easy bruising, bleeding from the gums, and frequent epitaxis. His parents were first cousins, but they showed no bleeding problems. Hemostatic analysis of the boy's blood showed dramatically prolonged plasma prothrombin clotting time. Given the limited data in this case, a defect/deficiency in which of the following is most likely in this patient?

A. factor VIII
B. factor XI
C. factor XIII
D. fibrinogen
E. high-molecular-weight kininogen, HMWK

Answer D: Defects associated with factors of the pathways of blood coagulation can also be assessed with specific assays. The prothrombin time (PT) is an assay designed to screen for defects in fibrinogen, prothrombin, and factors V, VII, and X and thus measures activities of the extrinsic pathway of coagulation. When any of these factors is deficient then the PT is prolonged. A normal PT is 11.0 to 12.5 seconds. A PT greater than 20 seconds is indicative of coagulation deficit.

2. You are tending to a 5-year-old boy with a suspected case of congenital deficiency in coagulation. He had bled from the umbilical and circumcision sites during his first week of life. He experiences frequent ecchymoses and hematomas within 12 to 24 hours after trauma. His parents are first cousins, but there is no family history of bleeding disorders. A bleeding disorder workup was initiated and the results indicated that PT, PTT, fibrinogen, platelet aggregation studies, and von Willebrand factor were normal. The patient's plasma was incubated with thrombin and Ca^{2+} and the resultant clot dissolved in the presence of urea. Given these findings, which of the following is most likely defective/deficient in this patient?

A. factor VII
B. factor VIII
C. factor XIII
D. tissue factor pathway inhibitor, TFPI
E. prothrombin

Answer C: Factor XIII is also known as fibrin-stabilizing factor or fibrinoligase. Factor XIII is converted to its active form (XIIIa) by thrombin in the presence of Ca^{2+}. The reaction catalyzed by factor XIIIa is the formation of γ-glutamyl-ε-lysine bonds between fibrin monomers.

Deficiency in factor XIII is characterized by delayed bleeding even though primary hemostasis is normal. Typical symptoms include neonatal bleeding from the umbilical cord, intracranial hemorrhage, soft tissue hematomas, recurrent spontaneous miscarriage, and abnormal wound healing. Umbilical cord bleeding after birth occurs in over 90% of afflicted individuals. Presumptive diagnosis of factor XIII deficiency is made with a clot solubility screening test and confirmation was accomplished by demonstrating the absence of factor XIII by latex agglutination.

3. A 66-year-old Caucasian man of Italian decent was admitted to the hospital for a grade III draining ulceration and underlying osteomyelitis of the left fifth metatarsal head. Past medical history was significant for Type 1 diabetes. Past surgical history was significant for a resection of an infected tibial sesamoid of the right foot. Prior to treatment of the ulceration routine clotting tests were performed and showed significantly prolonged activated partial thromboplastin (aPTT) time (69.5 second; normal 30-40 second), while prothrombin time (PT) was normal. Given these findings, which of the following factors of coagulation is most likely to be defective in this patient?
A. factor VII
B. factor XI
C. prekallikrein
D. tissue factor
E. tissue factor pathway inhibitor, TFPI

Answer B: The partial thromboplastin time (PTT) is used to assay for defects in the intrinsic pathway of coagulation. The PTT assay has been modified by the addition of activators that shorten the normal clotting time and this form of the assay is referred to as the activated partial thromboplastin time (aPTT). The PTT is normally prescribed in patients with unexplained bleeding or clotting. The assay will evaluate the function of fibrinogen, prothrombin, and factors V, VIII, IX, X, XI, and XII. A defect in any of these factors will result in a prolonged PTT (or aPTT). A normal PTT is 60 to 70 seconds, whereas for the aPTT the normal range is 30 to 40 seconds. The PTT is a standard assay used to assess the efficacy of heparin anticoagulant therapy. Prolonged PTTs are associated with acquired or congenital bleeding disorders associated with coagulation factor deficiency, vitamin K deficiency, liver disease, DIC, von Willebrand disease, leukemia, hemophilia, and heparin administration.

4. You are examining the processes of blood coagulation utilizing in vitro assays involving the addition of potential inhibitory compounds. In your control assay the rate of fibrin clot formation, following addition of whole blood, takes 16 seconds. The addition of your compound results in fibrin clot formation in 3 seconds. Given the observed results, which of the following proteins is most likely targeted for inhibition by the test compound?
A. factor V
B. factor XIII
C. fibrinogen
D. protein C
E. thrombin

Answer : Protein C (PC) is a trypsin-like serine protease that serves as a major regulator of the coagulation process. Thrombin cleavage of PC removes the activation peptide generating aPC. When activated through cleavage by thrombin, aPC cleaves both factor Va and factor VIIIa into inactive enzymes. This results in the termination of the role of VIIIa as the scaffold for the formation of the tenase complex and Va as a cofactor in the conversion of prothrombin to thrombin in the prothrombinase complex. The net effect, at the level of coagulation, of the activation of PC is termination of further increases in thrombin production and a halt to further fibrin clot formation. A lack of aPC activity would be apparent if fibrin clotting was accelerated due to lack of inhibition of factors Va and VIIIa.

5. Although the role of aPC in the termination of coagulation is extremely important, it also serves many additional functions that alter the inflammatory processes occurring in the vasculature. The anti-inflammatory functions of aPC are, in part, due to the activation of which of the following?
A. antithrombin III
B. protease activated receptor-1, PAR-1
C. thrombin
D. thrombomodulin
E. tissue plasminogen activator, tPA

Answer B: Activated PC binds to the endothelial protein C receptor (EPCR) and leads to the activation of PAR-1 which elicits cytoprotective and anti-inflammatory responses within endothelial cells. The cytoprotective effects elicited via aPC activation of PAR-1 include protection of the endothelial cell barrier and induction of antiapoptotic signaling pathways as well as expression of eNOS. Additional endothelial responses to aPC activation of PAR-1 occur via inhibition of the expression and actions of the potent pro-inflammatory transcription factor NFκB. The suppression of NFκB action results in downregulation of the synthesis of endothelial pro-inflammatory cytokines such as IL-6 and IL-8, the chemokine MCP-1 (monocyte chemoattractant protein-1), and the cell adhesion molecule ICAM-1 (intercellular adhesion molecule-1).

6. A 3-year-old boy was brought to the ER by his mother for oozing blood from his mouth following a fall nearly 6 hours ago. History indicates that the child tends to bleed for prolonged periods from his immunization sites, but there is no history of bruising or hematomas. There was no known family history of bleeding disorders. Physical examination shows no petechia, bruises, or joint swelling. Hemostatic tests resulted in a PT of 11.3 second (normal 11-12.5 second) and an aPTT of 59.7 second (normal 30-40 second). Given these test results and the signs and symptoms in this child, which of the following disorders is most likely causing his bleeding?

A. afibrinogenemia
B. antithrombin III deficiency
C. factor XI deficiency
D. hemophilia A
E. von Willebrand disease

Answer E: von Willebrand disease (vWD) results from defects in von Willebrand factor (vWF). The disorder is characterized by bleeding from mucocutaneous sites (typical skin and mucous membranes) rather than from deep tissues and joints. vWF is involved in 2 important reactions of blood coagulation. The first is the interaction of vWF with specific receptors on the surface of platelets and the subendothelial connective tissue. This interaction allows platelets to adhere to areas of vascular injury. The second role of vWF is to bind to and stabilize factor VIII allowing factor VIII to survive in the blood. As a consequence of these roles for vWF, deficiencies result in defective platelet adhesion and to secondary deficiencies in factor VIII. Since factor VIII deficiency results in hemophilia A, vWF deficiencies can manifest with clinical symptoms that appear to be hemophilia A.

7. You are treating a patient manifesting with a hypercoagulopathy evident by frequent deep vein thrombosis (DVTs) and pulmonary emboli. This patient most likely suffers from which of the following disorders?

A. antithrombin III deficiency
B. Bernard-Soulier syndrome
C. factor V Leiden
D. hemophilia A
E. von Willebrand disease

Answer C: The hypercoagulopathy (thrombophilia) referred to as factor V Leiden is caused by a mutation in the factor V gene resulting in a protein that is not effectively degraded by aPC. Factor V Leiden is the most common inherited thrombophilia in Caucasian populations of European descent. Overall, 5% of the world population harbors the factor V Leiden mutation. The symptoms of factor V Leiden are deep vein thrombosis (DVT) and pulmonary embolism, both of which can be fatal. In fact, it is estimated that in as many as 30% of patients who experience DVT and/or pulmonary embolisms are carriers of the factor V Leiden mutation.

8. A deficiency in which of the following blood coagulation factors could most likely be suspected in a patient exhibiting a prolonged aPTT time?

A. factor VII
B. factor XIII
C. factor IX
D. protein C
E. tissue factor pathway inhibitor, TFPI

Answer C: The partial thromboplastin time (PTT) is used to assay for defects in the intrinsic pathway of coagulation. The PTT assay has been modified by the addition of activators that shorten the normal clotting time and this form of the assay is referred to as the activated partial thromboplastin time (aPTT). The assay will evaluate the function of fibrinogen, prothrombin, and factors V, VIII, IX, X, XI, and XII. A defect in any of these factors will result in a prolonged PTT (or aPTT).

9. The mother of a 4-year-old boy brings her son to his pediatrician for a repeated episodes of easy bruising and epistaxis. Blood work reveals a prolonged PTT, a normal PT, and a prolonged bleeding time. Platelet count is 285,000/uL. Based on these laboratory findings, what is the most likely diagnosis?

A. disseminated intravascular coagulation
B. hemophilia B
C. primary fibrinolysis
D. vitamin K deficiency
E. von Willebrand disease

Answer E: Partial thromboplastin time (PTT), prothrombin time (PT), bleeding time, and platelet count are key laboratory tests used to differentiate between bleeding disorders. PTT measures plasma clotting time to assess the integrity of the intrinsic coagulation pathway (factors XII, XI, IX, VIII, X, V; prothrombin; and fibrinogen). PT measures plasma clotting time to assess the integrity of the extrinsic pathway (factors VII, V, X; prothrombin; and fibrinogen). Bleeding time measures the time needed for a standard skin puncture to stop bleeding and assesses platelet ability to form a hemostatic plug. von Willebrand disease results from deficiencies in both factor VIII and in von Willebrand factor (vWF), which combine to form a circulating complex. Synthesized by endothelial cells, vWF is important in the facilitation of platelet adhesion to subendothelial collagen. As a constituent in the factor VIII-vWF circulating complex, it serves to stabilize factor VIII and significantly increase its half-life; thus, a deficiency in vWF will cause a secondary decrease in factor VIII levels. von Willebrand disease demonstrates autosomal dominant inheritance and is believed to be one of the most common inherited bleeding disorders. Patients show bleeding after minor trauma, with the most common sites including skin (easy bruising) and mucous membranes (epistaxis). Coagulation tests reveal a prolonged PTT, a normal PT, and a prolonged bleeding time with normal platelet count.

10. A 47-year-old fireman is admitted to the emergency room for extensive burns received while battling a fire. A few hours after admission, he develops pregangrenous changes in multiple digits of hands, his left foot, and his nose. A short time later, he experiences bleeding from his mucous membranes and IV site, as well as the development of multiple petechiae. Which of the following is the major initiating mechanism of this clinical scenario?

A. antithrombin III deficiency
B. multiple air emboli
C. release of thromboplastin
D. supervening infection
E. tissue hypoxemia

Answer C: This patient is exhibiting the typical findings of disseminated intravascular coagulation. This is initiated by the release of tissue factor or thromboplastic substance (either exogenous, eg, amniotic fluid, or endogenous, eg, tissue damage as in this case) into the circulation. This activated the coagulation cascade, resulting in the formation of multiple thrombi that can block the microcirculation and produce ischemia and necrosis in vulnerable tissues. As thrombus formation continues, platelets and clotting factors can be exhausted, allowing hemorrhage to occur. The ischemic changes and hemorrhage are both apparent in this patient. Given the history and timing of this case, trauma leading to the release of tissue factor is more likely. However, endothelial injury may also initiate disseminated intravascular coagulation (DIC) by the release of tissue factor.

11. A 6-year-old boy has a long history of a hereditary bleeding disorder characterized by spontaneous nontraumatic hemorrhages into joint spaces, skeletal muscle, and mucous membranes. Laboratory studies reveal a normal prothrombin time, elevated partial thromboplastin time, very low factor VIII, normal factor X, normal factor XI, and normal platelet aggregation studies with ristocetin. Which of the following is the most likely diagnosis?

A. Christmas disease
B. hemophilia A
C. hemophilia B
D. Rosenthal syndrome
E. von Willebrand disease

Answer B: Hemophilia A is a genetic disorder characterized by very low levels of factor VIII, elevated partial thromboplastin time, normal prothrombin time, normal platelet aggregation with ristocetin, and spontaneous hemorrhages into joints, soft tissues, and mucosal surfaces.

12. A 26-year-old woman complains of the acute onset of anuria, purpura, and mental confusion. Her peripheral blood film displays marked thrombocytopenia and abundant schistocytes. Laboratory studies reveal elevations of bilirubin, creatinine, and lactose dehydrogenase. A skin biopsy shows numerous intravascular thrombi within the dermal microvasculature. What is the most likely diagnosis?

A. acute idiopathic thrombocytopenia purpura
B. Bernard-Soulier syndrome
C. Glanzmann thrombasthenia
D. May-Hegglin anomaly
E. thrombotic thrombocytopenic purpura

Answer E: Thrombotic thrombocytopenic purpura is an acute microangiopathic hemolytic anemia. The clinical picture usually includes mental alterations, anuria, mucosal bleeding, and purpura. An abnormal platelet aggregating substance is the likely initiating event.

13. You are tending to a patient with a high tendency to bleeding. He bruises easily and has bleeding from his gums. Analysis of coagulation factors in his blood shows normal levels of factor V but low levels of factor VIII. Injection of factor VIII provides only minimal benefit and you find that the injected protein is rapidly degraded. Using a platelet aggregation test you find that combination of your patients serum with normal platelets results in only 20% of the platelet aggregation seen with both samples from a normal individual. Based on these findings you determine that your patient is deficient in which of the following factors of coagulation?

A. factor X
B. factor XII
C. fibrinogen
D. thrombin
E. von Willebrand factor

Answer E: von Willebrand disease (vWD) results from defects in von Willebrand factor (vWF). The disorder is characterized by bleeding from mucocutaneous sites (typical skin and mucous membranes) rather than from deep tissues and joints. vWF is involved in two important reactions of blood coagulation. The first is the interaction of vWF with specific receptors on the surface of platelets and the subendothelial connective tissue. This interaction allows platelets to adhere to areas of vascular injury. The second role of vWF is to bind to and stabilize factor VIII allowing factor VIII to survive in the blood. As a consequence of these roles for vWF, deficiencies result in defective platelet adhesion and to secondary deficiencies in factor VIII. Since factor VIII deficiency results in hemophilia A, vWF deficiencies can manifest with clinical symptoms that appear to be hemophilia A.

14. Which of the following represents a critical role of thrombin in the promotion of coagulation?

A. activation of protein C
B. activation of thrombin-activatable fibrinolysis inhibitor, TAFI
C. cleavage, leading to activation, of PAR-1
D. cleavage of factor X to Xa
E. cleavage of factor XIII to XIIIa

Answer E: Thrombin not only promotes the formation of a stable clot but its actions also lead to self-limiting of the extent of the coagulation process. The formation of a stable fibrin clot is a critical role of thrombin in the promotion of coagulation. Thrombin-mediated release of the fibrinopeptides generates fibrin monomers that spontaneously aggregate in a regular array, forming a somewhat weak fibrin clot. In addition to fibrin activation, thrombin converts factor XIII to factor XIIIa, a highly specific transglutaminase that introduces cross-links composed of covalent bonds between the amide nitrogen of glutamines and ε-amino group of lysines in the fibrin monomers forming a stable clot.

15. Which of the following is the final step in the coagulation cascade, leading to clot formation?

A. conversion of thrombin to prothrombin
B. plasmin catalyzed degradation of fibrin fibers
C. polymerization of prothrombin
D. release of tissue factor
E. thrombin catalyzed conversion of fibrinogen to fibrin

Answer E: Thrombin-mediated release of the fibrinopeptides generates fibrin monomers that spontaneously aggregate in a regular array, forming a somewhat weak fibrin clot. In addition to fibrin activation, thrombin converts factor XIII to factor XIIIa, a highly specific transglutaminase that introduces cross-links composed of covalent bonds between the amide nitrogen of glutamines and ε-amino group of lysines in the fibrin monomers forming a stable clot.

16. ReoPro (abciximab) is a member of a class of anticoagulant drugs that function by inhibiting the role of platelets in hemostasis. Which of the following protein complexes is the target of ReoPro action?

A. GPIa-GPIIa
B. GPIb-GPIX-GPV
C. GPIIb-GPIIIa
D. prothrombinase complex
E. tenase complex

Answer C: Abciximab is a GPIIb-GPIIIa antagonist, which is an anticoagulant drug that inhibits platelet aggregation regardless of the agonist. Therefore, abciximab more completely inhibits platelet aggregation than does aspirin or clopidogrel.

17. Accumulating evidence indicates that the nonsteroidal anti-inflammatory (NSAID) aspirin is effective in the control of numerous chronic conditions such as atherosclerosis. The principal cardiovascular benefit from aspirin is due to its ability to reduce the incidence and severity of thrombotic episodes. The anticoagulant effect of aspirin occurs through its ability to inhibit which of the following activities?

A. cyclooxygenase
B. fibrin cross-linking by factor XIIIa
C. phospholipase A_2
D. thrombin binding to activated platelets
E. von Willebrand factor

Answer A: Aspirin is an important inhibitor of platelet activation. By virtue of inhibiting the activity of cyclooxygenase, aspirin reduces the production of TXA_2 by platelets. Aspirin also reduces endothelial cell production of prostacyclin (PGI_2), an inhibitor of platelet aggregation and a vasodilator. Localized to the site of coagulation is a balance between the levels of platelet derived TXA_2 and endothelial cell derived PGI_2. This allows for platelet aggregation and clot formation but preventing excessive accumulation of the clot, thus maintaining blood flow around the site of the clot. Endothelial cells regenerate active cyclooxygenase faster than platelets because mature platelets cannot synthesize the enzyme, requiring new platelets to enter the circulation (platelet half-life is approximately 4 days). Therefore, PGI_2 synthesis is greater than that of TXA_2. The net effect of aspirin is more in favor of endothelial cell-mediated inhibition of the coagulation cascade.

18. Which of the following proteins of the coagulation cascade forms an active complex with tissue factor to initiate the extrinsic clotting cascade?

A. factor VII
B. factor VIII
C. factor IX

D. fibrinogen
E. protein S

Answer A: The extrinsic pathway is initiated at the site of injury in response to the release of tissue factor (factor III) and thus, is also known as the tissue factor pathway. Tissue factor is a cofactor in the factor VIIa-catalyzed activation of factor X.

19. Hemophilia B results from a deficiency in which of the following proteins?
A. factor VIII
B. factor IX
C. fibrinogen
D. thrombin
E. von Willebrand factor

Answer B: Hemophilia B results from deficiencies in factor IX. The prevalence of hemophilia B is approximately one-tenth that of hemophilia A. All patients with hemophilia B have prolonged coagulation time and decreased factor IX clotting activity. Like hemophilia A, there are severe, moderate, and mild forms of hemophilia B and reflect the factor IX activity in plasma.

20. Hemophilia A results from a deficiency in which of the following proteins?
A. factor VIII
B. factor IX
C. fibrinogen
D. thrombin
E. von Willebrand factor

Answer A: Hemophilia A is classic hemophilia. It is an X-linked disorder resulting from a deficiency in factor VIII. There are severe, moderate, and mild forms of hemophilia A that reflect the level of active factor VIII in the plasma.

21. Which of the following factors of blood coagulation is the major inhibitor of the extrinsic clotting cascade?
A. antithrombin III
B. high-molecular-weight kininogen (HMWK)
C. lipoprotein-associated coagulation factor (LACI)
D. α_2-macroglobulin
E. protein S

Answer C: A major mechanism for the inhibition of the extrinsic pathway occurs at the tissue factor-factor VIIa-Ca^{2+}-Xa complex. The protein, lipoprotein-associated coagulation inhibitor (LACI) specifically binds to this complex. LACI is also referred to as extrinsic pathway inhibitor (EPI) or tissue factor pathway inhibitor (TFP)I and was formerly named anticonvertin.

22. The conversion of fibrinogen to fibrin is catalyzed by which of the following?
A. antithrombin III
B. heparin
C. plasmin
D. prothrombin
E. thrombin

Answer E: Active thrombin hydrolyses fibrinogen at 4 arg-gly (R-G) bonds between the fibrinopeptide and the a and b portions of the protein. Thrombin-mediated release of the fibrinopeptides generates fibrin monomers which spontaneously aggregate in a regular array, forming a somewhat weak fibrin clot.

23. Patients who exhibit a prolonged mucocutaneous bleeding time with a normal coagulation time, clot retraction, and platelet count and have reduced levels of the coagulation factor VIII have a deficiency in which protein involved in hemostasis?
A. factor IX
B. fibrinogen
C. thrombin
D. tissue factor
E. von Willebrand factor

Answer E: von Willebrand disease (vWD) results from defects in von Willebrand factor (vWF). The disorder is characterized by bleeding from mucocutaneous sites (typical skin and mucous membranes) rather than from deep tissues and joints. vWF is involved in 2 important reactions of blood coagulation, one of which is to bind to and stabilize factor VIII allowing factor VIII to survive in the blood. Deficiencies in vWF can, therefore, result in deficiencies in factor VIII.

24. Presentation of the platelet membrane protein complex, GPIIb-GPIIIa, which binds with von Willebrand factor, is necessary for which of the following?
A. activation of PKC leading to phosphorylation of myosin light chain and platelet morphology changes
B. cleavage and activation of high-molecular-weight kininogen
C. inducing platelet cross-linking
D. release of thrombin from platelet granules
E. stimulation of endothelial and smooth muscle cell interaction resulting in vasoconstriction

Answer C: Activated platelets release the contents of their granules. Contained in the dense granules is ADP. The release of ADP further stimulates platelets increasing the overall activation cascade. ADP also modifies the platelet membranes leading to exposure platelet glycoprotein receptor complex: GPIIb-GPIIIa.

GPIIb-GPIIIa constitutes a receptor for vWF and fibrinogen, resulting in fibrinogen-induced platelet aggregation.

25. Which of the following is the final step in the coagulation cascade, leading to clot formation?
A. conversion of thrombin to prothrombin
B. plasmin-catalyzed degradation of fibrin fibers
C. polymerization of prothrombin
D. release of tissue factor
E. thrombin-catalyzed conversion of fibrinogen to fibrin

Answer E: Thrombin is a plasma protease that converts fibrinogen to fibrin. Once formed, fibrin polymerizes with other fibrin monomers to form large, insoluble fibrin fibers. A clot consists of a meshwork of fibrin fibers. Tissue factor is involved in coagulation, but it participates in the initial step in the extrinsic pathway.

26. A deficiency in which of the following factors of hemostasis, whose symptoms generally do not appear prior to age 15, would manifest with recurrent deep vein thrombosis, pulmonary embolism, and cerebral vein thrombosis?
A. antithrombin III
B. factor VIII
C. fibrinogen
D. protein C
E. von Willebrand factor

Answer A: Antithrombin III is the most important since it can also inhibit the activities of factors IXa, Xa, XIa, and XIIa. The activity of antithrombin III is potentiated in the presence of heparin by the following means: heparin binds to a specific site on antithrombin III, producing an altered conformation of the protein, and the new conformation has a higher affinity for thrombin as well as its other substrates. This effect of heparin is the basis for its clinical use as an anticoagulant. The naturally occurring heparin activator of antithrombin III is present as heparan and heparan sulfate on the surface of vessel endothelial cells. It is this feature that controls the activation of the intrinsic coagulation cascade. Thrombin activity is also inhibited by α_2-macroglobulin, heparin cofactor II, and α_1-antitrypsin. The characteristic features of antithrombin deficiency are deep vein and cerebral vein thrombosis and pulmonary embolism. The thromboembolic events associated with a deficiency in antithrombin are rarely seen in individuals younger than 15 years of age. The reason for this is suggested to be due to the high levels of α_2-macroglobulin present in childhood.

27. Which of the following factors is present only in the intrinsic pathway of blood coagulation?
A. factor I (fibrinogen)
B. factor II (prothrombin)
C. factor V
D. factor VIII
E. factor X

Answer D: Clotting factors that are unique to the intrinsic pathway include factors VIII, IX, XI, and XII. The activation of factor X represents the point of convergence of the intrinsic and extrinsic pathways. Factors required for clotting that are activated subsequent to activation of factor X are all part of the common pathway. The defect in hemophilia A is a deficiency in factor VIII, or the antihemophilic factor. This factor acts at the last step of the intrinsic pathway. Factor VIII, which is activated by minute amounts of thrombin, acts in concert with activated factor IX, a proteolytic enzyme, to activate factor X.

28. Heparin is a rapidly acting, potent anticoagulant that has many important clinical uses. Which of the following is an action of heparin?
A. activates antithrombin III
B. activates prothrombin
C. decreases prothrombin time
D. inhibits calcium action
E. promotes vitamin K activity

Answer A: Thrombin is a critical enzyme in the coagulation cascade. It not only can activate factors VIII and V, it also acts on fibrinogen to form fibrin. Thrombin is essential for clot formation. Antithrombin III modulates the coagulation cascade, serving to inhibit thrombin activity. Heparin acts as an anticoagulant because it accelerates the action of antithrombin III.

29. Platelet aggregation requires the interaction of fibrinogen with a receptor on activated platelets. Which of the following is the most likely composition of this receptor?
A. factor XII (Hageman factor)
B. GPIb-GPIX-GPV
C. GPIIb-GPIIIa
D. thrombin
E. von Willebrand factor

Answer C: Activation of platelets leads to exposure platelet glycoprotein receptor complex: GPIIb-GPIIIa. GPIIb-GPIIIa constitutes a receptor for vWF and fibrinogen, resulting in fibrinogen-induced platelet aggregation.

30. Activated platelets stimulate vasoconstriction through the production of which of the following?
A. leukotriene C_4
B. platelet-activating factor (PAF)

C. prostacyclin (PGI_2)
D. prostaglandin E_2 (PGE_2)
E. thromboxane A_2 (TXA_2)

Answer E: When platelets bind to exposed collagen, there results an activation of phospholipase A_2 (PLA_2), which then hydrolyzes membrane phospholipids, leading to liberation of arachidonic acid. The arachidonic acid release leads to an increase in the production and subsequent release of thromboxane A_2 (TXA_2), which is a potent vasoconstrictor and inducer of platelet aggregation.

Checklist

✓ Hemostasis is the process of blood clotting and then the subsequent dissolution of the clot following repair of the injured tissue. This involves platelets, interaction of blood with vessel walls, and numerous coagulation factors, many of which are synthesized as proenzymes (serine protease zymogens) in the liver.

✓ Blood coagulation requires a coordinated series of 4 events that begins with vasoconstriction to slow the loss of blood, then platelets adhere to the collage exposed at the site of injury leading to activation and aggregation, coagulation factor cascade is initiated terminating with the formation of a cross-linked fibrin clot, when the damage is repaired the clot must be dissolved returning the vessel to normal function.

✓ Effective and efficient hemostasis requires that platelets adhere to the exposed ECM at the site of vessel injury. The adherence of platelets results in their activation leading to the release of platelet granule contents and platelet aggregation.

✓ Platelet adhesion requires exposed collagen as well as the subendothelial glycoprotein, von Willebrand factor.

✓ There are 2 primary coagulation cascades that are initiated under distinctly different circumstance but that converge by activation of factor X. The intrinsic pathway of coagulation is initiated in response to contact of blood with a negatively charged surface and primarily represents a pathophysiological reaction. The extrinsic pathway is initiated in response to release of tissue factor in response to vascular injury and represents the normal physiological pathway of coagulation.

✓ For clotting to come to completion, the clotting cascades converge on the activation of factor X which then activates thrombin. Thrombin hydrolyzes fibrinogen and the resulting fibrinopeptides aggregate. Thrombin also activates factor XIII which catalyzes cross-linking of the fibrin monomers.

✓ Regulation of the clotting cascades is also initiated by thrombin such that thrombin serves not only to ensure a clot forms but also ensures that the clotting process does not become excessive. Thrombin regulates the extent of coagulation by activating protein C, which then hydrolyzes and inhibits the activities of factor VIII and factor V.

✓ Clot dissolution following tissue repair is catalyzed by plasmin. Plasmin is released from plasminogen via the action of tissue plasminogen activator (tPA) or urokinase.

✓ Numerous bleeding disorders and hypercoagulation disorders result from defects in the processes of hemostasis including platelet function and clotting cascade factors. Deficiencies in von Willebrand factor are the leading cause of bleeding disorders. Hemophilia A and B are the most widely recognized bleeding disorders.

✓ Numerous pharmacological agents are used to control the rate of coagulation including those that interfere with platelet function and those that interfere with clotting factor processing or function.

CHAPTER

52 Cancer Biology

CHAPTER OUTLINE

Cancer Defined
Genetic Alterations and Cancer
Types of Cancer
Aerobic Glycolysis and Cancer
Metastases
Viruses and Cancer
Classifications of Proto-Oncogenes
Proto-oncogenes and Inherited Cancer Syndromes
Tumor Suppressors
Epigenetics: DNA Methylation and Tumor Suppressors
Breast Cancers
Gastrointestinal Cancers
Hematopoietic and Lymphoid Cancers

High-Yield Terms

Carcinogen: any substance, such as a chemical, or any type of radiation that is directly involved in causing cancer

Neoplasm: any abnormal mass of tissue, medically synonymous with the term tumor

Malignancy: medically describes any condition that becomes progressively more severe, with respect to cancers the term characterizes invasiveness and the tendency to metastasize

Metastasis: refers to the spread of cancer from a site of origin to a new organ or another part of the body

Proto-oncogene: any normal gene that can become an oncogene due to gene mutation or abnormal expression

Oncogene: any gene that has the potential to cause cancer, in tumor cells, these genes are often mutated or expressed at high levels

Tumor suppressor: any gene that prevents the unregulated growth of cells, loss of function of this class of gene can result in cancer, also called antioncogene

Cancer Defined

Cancers, in the broadest terms, are a wide array of diseases typified by unregulated cell growth. The medical and biological term is *neoplasm* and defines an abnormal tissue that grows more rapidly than normal and continues to grow and proliferate in the absence of the originating growth signal. Neoplasms are transformed cells that can also harbor the characteristics of immortality. Transformation is a multistep process which results in the generation of the neoplastic cells. Immortalization refers to cells with unlimited life span but is not directly associated with aberrant growth or malignancy. Neoplasms can be benign or malignant. In the strictest sense, malignancy is defined as the ability to generate invasive tumors when cells are transplanted in vivo. However, medically this is not a useful definition due to the time required for the assessment of this capability. Therefore, it is more appropriate to define a malignant tumor, or mass, by its potential to worsen, to invade the surrounding tissues, and to exhibit the potential for metastases. *Metastasis* is the ability of cells from a tumor to break away from the original mass and spread to another location in the body. Although these terms broadly define all cancers, different types of cancers from different tissues exhibit a wide range of altered characteristics (Figure 52-1).

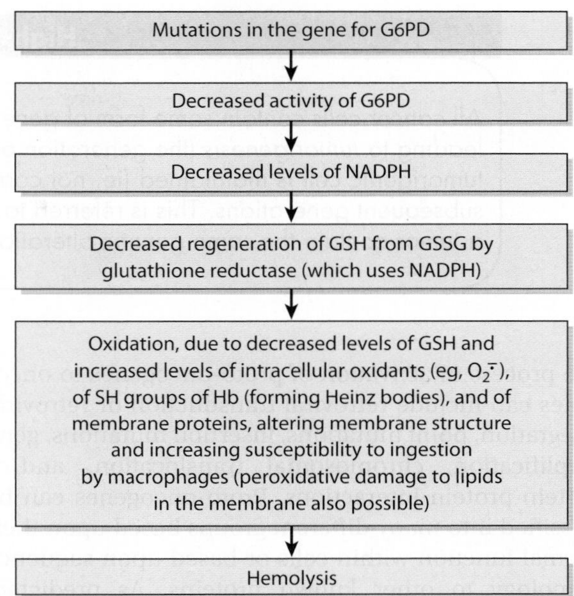

FIGURE 52-1: Some biochemical and genetic changes occurring in human cancer cells. Many changes are observed in cancer cells with many of the most significant diagrammed here. The roles of mutations in activating oncogenes and inactivating tumor suppressor genes are discussed in the text. Abnormalities of cell cycling and of chromosome structure, including aneuploidy, are common. Alterations of microRNA molecules that regulate gene activities have been reported, and the relationship of stem cells to cancer cells is a very active area of research. Telomerase activity is often detectable in cancer cells. Tumors sometimes synthesize certain fetal antigens, which may be measurable in the blood. Changes in plasma membrane constituents (eg, alteration of the sugar chains of various glycoproteins—some of which are cell adhesion molecules—and glycolipids) have been detected in many studies, and may be of importance in relation to decreased cell adhesion and metastasis. Various molecules can pass out of cancer cells and can be detected in the blood as tumor biomarkers. Angiogenic factors and various proteinases are also released by some tumors. Many changes in metabolism have been observed; for example, cancer cells often exhibit a high rate of aerobic glycolysis. (CAM, cell adhesion molecule; ECM, extracellular matrix.) Murray RK, Bender DA, Botham KM, Kennelly PJ, Rodwell VW, Weil PA. *Harper's Illustrated Biochemistry*, 29th ed. New York, NY: McGraw-Hill; 2012.

Genetic Alterations and Cancer

The genetic damage present in a cancer cell can arise either spontaneously or the mutation can be inherited. Inherited mutations are classified as familial cancers such that the inheritance of the mutation predisposes an individual to cancer. This of course does not always mean that an individual acquiring an inherited mutation will develop cancer just that the individual has an increased likelihood relative to an individual who does not possess the mutant gene. Spontaneous mutations resulting in cancer are most often the result of exposure to some form of carcinogen. Carcinogens can be chemicals, radiant energies (such as ultraviolet or gamma irradiation), or oncogenic viruses. Chemical and radiant energy generally result in DNA damage that exceeds the capability of a cell to repair and thus, the damage is propagated in the resultant daughter cells. Often, individuals who harbor existing mutations in DNA repair process genes are highly susceptible to cancers caused by these types of carcinogens.

The genetic damage found in cancer cells is of 2 types referred to as dominant or recessive. Dominant mutations are associated with genes defined as *proto-oncogenes*. The distinction between the terms proto-oncogene and oncogene relates to the activity of the protein product of the gene. A proto-oncogene is a gene whose protein product has the capacity to induce cellular transformation provided it sustains some genetic insult. An oncogene is a gene that has sustained some genetic damage and, therefore, produces a protein capable of cellular transformation.

High-Yield Concept

All cancer cells contain some form of genetic damage that appears to be the responsible event leading to *tumorigenesis* (the generation of cancer). The genetic damage present in a parental tumorigenic cell is maintained (ie, not correctable) such that it is a heritable trait of all cells of subsequent generations. This is referred to as clonal expansion such that all subsequent cells of a tumor contain the same genetic alteration that was present in the originating cell.

The process of activation of proto-oncogenes to oncogenes can include retroviral transduction or retroviral integration, point mutations, insertion mutations, gene amplification, chromosomal translocation, and/or protein-protein interactions. Proto-oncogenes can be classified into many different groups based upon their normal function within cells or based upon sequence homology to other known proteins. As predicted, proto-oncogenes have been identified at all levels of the various signal transduction cascades that control cell growth, proliferation and differentiation. Proto-oncogenes that were originally identified as resident in transforming retroviruses were initially designated with the letter **c**—indicative of the cellular origin as opposed to **v**—to signify original identification in retroviruses. Recessive mutations are associated with genes referred to as *tumor suppressors*, growth suppressors, recessive oncogenes, or antioncogenes.

Types of Cancer

Sarcomas are cancers derived from transformed cells with a mesenchymal origin. These cancers include those affecting bone, muscle, connective tissue, fat, and the vasculature. Although hematopoietic cells (the cells of blood) are derived from mesenchymal stem cells and thus, hematopoietic cancers (leukemias and lymphomas) are strictly defined as sarcomas, they are more commonly separated into the separate category of liquid cancers.

Carcinomas are cancers derived from transformed epithelial cells that originate from the endoderm or ectoderm layer of the developing embryo. These cells are found in the lining of the mouth, throat, stomach and intestines, the mammary ducts, the pancreas, the prostate gland, and the lungs. Carcinomas represent the most common types of cancers in humans and can be divided into several distinct variants defined by histology (Table 52-1).

Aerobic Glycolysis and Cancer

Overall metabolism in cancer cells is accelerated relative to normal differentiated cells of the same tissue. This is due, in part, to the expression of growth-promoting genes. Cancer cells can accommodate high rates of metabolism because they are changed in such a way as to allow rapid influx of nutrients, often without the need for the extracellular signals (eg, hormones) required of normal cells. Within the blood, the carbohydrate glucose and the amino acid glutamine, account for the vast majority of metabolic carbon and nitrogen.

In cancer cells (as well as many proliferating cells) the fate of glucose depends not only on the proliferative state of the cell but also on the activities of the specific glycolytic enzymes that are expressed. Cancer cells only express the PKM2 form of pyruvate kinase but at low levels. Low PKM2 activity, in conjunction with increased glucose uptake and oxidation, facilitates the diversion of glucose carbons

High-Yield Concept

The majority of the known proto-oncogenes in the human genome have been identified by either of 2 means: as the transforming genes (oncogenes) of transforming retroviruses or through transfection of DNA from tumor cell lines into nontransformed cell lines and screening for resultant tumorigenesis.

High-Yield Concept

Human cancers can be divided into 2 broad categories with one representing solid tumors and the second the liquid cancers. Solid cancers are the sarcomas and carcinomas. The liquid cancers are the blood-borne cancers, the hematopoietic cancers.

TABLE 52-1: Histologically Defined Types of Carcinoma

Carcinoma	*Characteristics*
Adenocarcinoma	Originates in glandular tissues, the cancerous cells do not need to be part of a gland but they exhibit secretory properties
Adenosquamous carcinoma	Mixed tumor containing both adenocarcinoma and squamous cell carcinoma cell types
Anaplastic carcinoma	A heterogeneous group of high-grade carcinomas whose cells lack distinct histological or cytological evidence of the more specifically differentiated neoplasms
Large cell carcinoma	Large, rounded, or overtly polygonal-shaped cells with abundant cytoplasm, most commonly found in lung cancers
Small cell carcinoma	Small, round, primitive-appearing cells with little evident cytoplasm, commonly found in lung cancers, also called oat-cell carcinomas
Squamous cell carcinoma	Derived from the most superficial epithelial layers, consist of flat, scale-like cells called squamous epithelial cells

into the biomass needed for cancer cells to continue to grow at high rates. Also, in cells expressing PKM2 there is increased phosphorylation of the upstream glycolytic enzyme phosphoglycerate mutase (PGAM1) which increases its mutase activity. The phosphate donor is phosphoenolpyruvate (PEP) which is the substrate for pyruvate kinase. Phosphate transfer from PEP to PGAM1 yields pyruvate without concomitant generation of ATP (see Figure 10-5). This alternate pathway allows for a high rate of glycolysis that is needed to support the anabolic metabolism observed in many proliferating cells. Targeting PKM2 for the treatment of cancers has shown promise since recent work has demonstrated that small molecule PKM2-specific activators reduce the incorporation of glucose into lactate and lipids and result in decreased pools of nucleotide, amino acid, and lipid precursors accounting for the suppression of tumorigenesis observed with these drugs.

Metastases

A significant factor leading to mortality associated with cancer is the spread of the cancer from the site of its origination to another, or many other, locations. The process of cancer spreading is clinically referred to as metastasis. A simplified view of metastasis is diagrammed in Figure 52-2. In order for a cancer cell

High-Yield Concept

The rate of glycolysis is elevated in all cancer cells and in 1924 Otto Warburg made an observation that cancer cells metabolism glucose in a manner that was distinct from the glycolytic process occurring in normal cells. Warburg discovered that, unlike most normal tissues, cancer cells tended to "ferment" glucose into lactate even in the presence of sufficient oxygen to support mitochondrial oxidative phosphorylation. This observation became known as the Warburg effect (see Clinical Box 10-1).

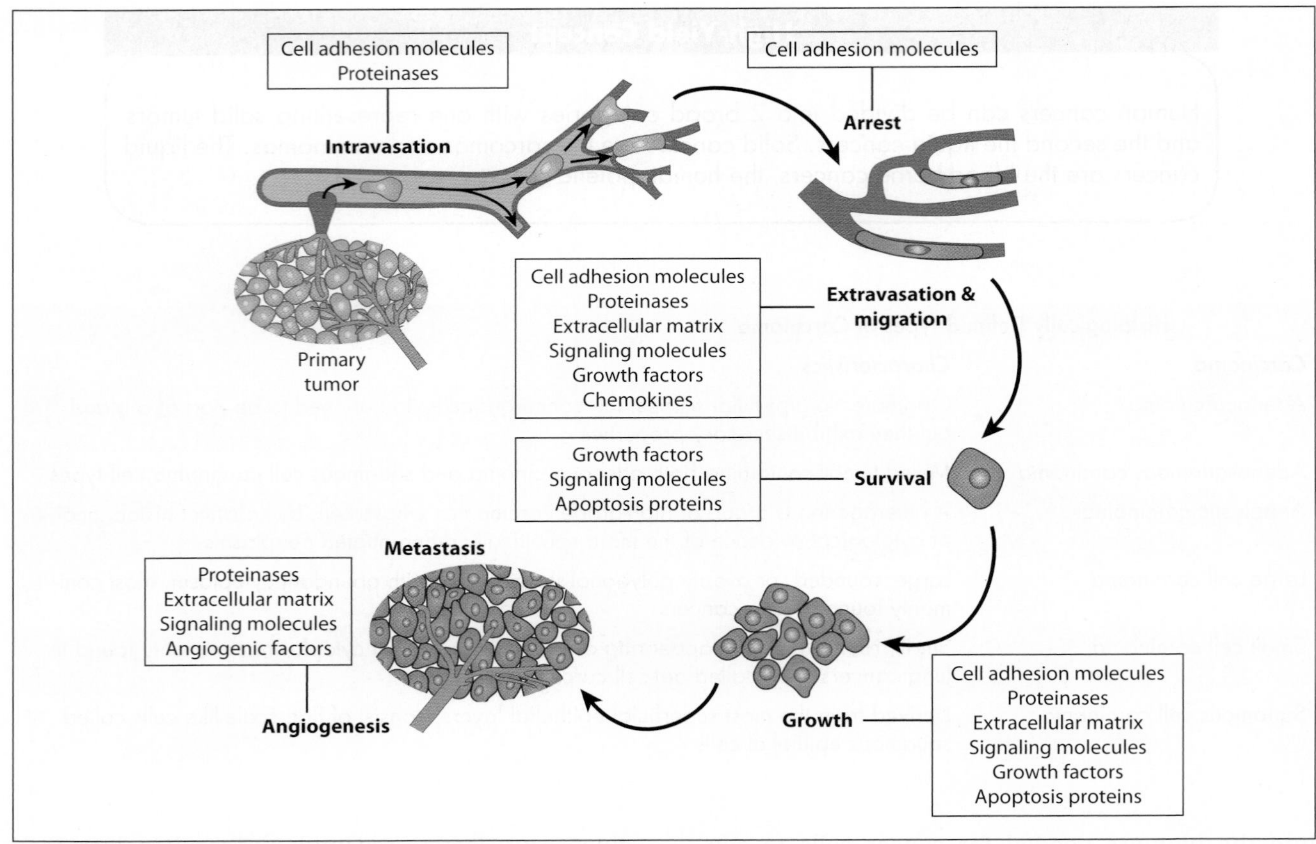

FIGURE 52-2: Simplified scheme of metastasis. Schematic representation of the sequence of steps in metastasis, indicating some of the factors believed to be involved. Murray RK, Bender DA, Botham KM, Kennelly PJ, Rodwell VW, Weil PA. *Harper's Illustrated Biochemistry*, 29th ed. New York, NY: McGraw-Hill; 2012.

to metastasize it must first break away from the primary tumor and enter the blood stream. Many of the required processes of metastasis are outlined in Table 52-2. The process by which the cell enters the blood is called *intravasation*. The cell can then migrate to a new location usually where its migration is arrested in a small capillary. There the cell migrates into the local extracellular matrix (ECM) and begins to grow and divide. The process of migration into the ECM is referred to as *extravasation*. In order for a new tumor to form there must be an adequate blood supply to the site and this is accomplished via the secretion of angiogenic factors. Angiogenesis is the process of new vessel synthesis and this process is a current target of several anticancer therapies. One of the growth factors involved in stimulating angiogenesis is vascular endothelial growth factor (VEGF). The monoclonal antibody drug Avastin (bevacizumab) targets VEGF and in so doing prevents the growth of new vessels in various types of cancers.

In order for a cancer cell to break away, it must be released from the ECM of the primary tumor. Two mechanisms are involved in this process. One is a reduction in the expression of cell adhesion molecules. One cell adhesion molecule, particularly associated with metastatic cancers is E-cadherin. Cadherins are a class of calcium-dependent adhesion molecule. Reduction or loss of E-cadherin is highly correlated to the metastatic potential of several types of cancers. In particular, prostate cancers with reduced levels of E-cadherin are much more virulent than similar cancers with normal E-cadherin levels. Indeed, because of this association between E-cadherin levels and metastatic potential, E-cadherin is often considered to be a tumor suppressor. The other mechanism required for cancer cells to metastasize is that the ECM of the tumor must be locally degraded. One of the most important class of enzymes involved in ECM remodeling is the matrix metalloproteinases (MMPs). Many metastatic cancers express elevated levels of MMPs, particularly MMP-2 and MMP-9, leading to degradation of the basement membrane and ECM allowing the cells to escape to the blood.

TABLE 52-2: Some Important Points Regarding Metastasis
• An epithelial-mesenchymal cell transition is often found in cancers, allowing increased movement of potentially metastatic cells.
• Metastasis is relatively inefficient (only about 1:10,000 tumor cells may have the genetic potential to colonize).
• Metastatic cells must evade various cells of the immune system to survive.
• Changes in cell surface molecules (eg, CAMs and others) are involved.
• Increased proteinase activity (eg, of MMP-2 and MMP-9) facilitates invasion.
• The existence of metastasis enhancer and suppressor genes has been shown.
• Some cancer cells metastasize preferentially to specific organs.
• Metastasis gene signatures may be detected by gene microarray analysis; they can be of prognostic value.

Abbreviations: CAM, cell adhesion molecule; MMP, metalloproteinase.
Murray RK, Bender DA, Botham KM, Kennelly PJ, Rodwell VW, Weil PA. *Harper's Illustrated Biochemistry,* 29th ed. New York, NY: McGraw-Hill; 2012.

TABLE 52-3: Some Viruses That Cause or Are Associated With Human Cancers

Virus	*Genome*	*Cancer*
Epstein-Barr virus	DNA	Burkitt's lymphoma, nasopharyngeal cancer, B cell lymphoma
Hepatitis B	DNA	Hepatocellular carcinoma
Hepatitis C	RNA	Hepatocellular carcinoma
Human herpesvirus type I	DNA	Kaposi's sarcoma
Human papilloma viruses (certain types)	DNA	Cancer of the cervix
Human T-cell leukemia virus type 1	RNA	Adult T-cell leukemia

Note: It has been estimated that virus-linked human cancers are responsible for ~15% of total cancer incidence.
Murray RK, Bender DA, Botham KM, Kennelly PJ, Rodwell VW, Weil PA. *Harper's Illustrated Biochemistry,* 29th ed. New York, NY: McGraw-Hill; 2012.

Viruses and Cancer

Tumor cells can arise by the carcinogenic actions of specific tumor viruses (Table 52-3). Tumor viruses are of 2 distinct types. There are viruses with DNA genomes (eg, papilloma and adenoviruses) and those with RNA genomes called the retroviruses. It should be noted that not all DNA or RNA viruses cause cancer in animals, for example the influenza (Orthomyxoviridae family) and measles (Paramyxoviridae family) viruses, which are RNA viruses, are not tumor viruses.

Tumor-causing retroviruses are common in chickens, mice, and cats but rare in humans. The human T-cell leukemia viruses (HTLVs) and human immunodeficiency virus (HIV) are the most notable examples of RNA tumor viruses in humans. The HTLV belong to the Oncoviridae family of viruses and HIV belongs to the Lentiviridae family. Another human RNA virus that causes cancer is the hepatitis C virus (HCV) which belongs to the Flaviviridae family of viruses.

Retroviruses can induce the transformed state within the cells they infect by 2 mechanisms. Both of these mechanisms are related to the life cycle of these viruses. When a retrovirus infects a cell its RNA genome is converted into DNA by the viral encoded RNA-dependent DNA polymerase (reverse transcriptase). The DNA then integrates into the genome of the host cell where it can remain, being copied as the host genome is duplicated during the process of cellular division. Contained within the sequences at the ends of the retroviral genome are powerful transcriptional promoter sequences termed long terminal repeats (LTRs). The LTRs promote the transcription of the viral DNA leading to the production of new virus particles.

At some frequency the integration process leads to rearrangement of the viral genome and the consequent incorporation of a portion of the host genome into the viral genome. This process is termed transduction. Occasionally this transduction process leads to the virus acquiring a gene from the host that is normally involved in cellular growth control. Because of the alteration of the host gene during the transduction process as well as the gene being transcribed at a higher rate due to its association with the retroviral LTRs the transduced gene confers a growth advantage to subsequent infected cells. The end result of this process is unrestricted cellular proliferation leading to tumorigenesis. The transduced genes are termed oncogenes. The normal cellular gene in its unmodified, nontransduced form is termed a proto-oncogene.

The second mechanism by which retroviruses can transform cells relates to the powerful transcription promoting effect of the LTRs. When a retrovirus genome integrates into a host genome it does so randomly. At some frequency this integration process leads to the placement of the LTRs close to a gene that encodes a growth-regulating protein. If the protein is expressed at an abnormally elevated level it can result in cellular transformation. This is termed retroviral integration-induced transformation. It has been shown that HIV induces certain forms of cancers in infected individuals by this integration-induced transformation process.

Cellular transformation by DNA tumor viruses, in most cases, has been shown to be the result of protein-protein interaction. Proteins encoded by the DNA tumor viruses, termed tumor antigens or T antigens, can interact with cellular proteins. This interaction effectively sequesters the cellular proteins away from their normal functional locations within the cell. The predominant types of proteins that are sequestered by viral T antigens have been shown to be of the tumor suppressor type. It is the loss of their normal suppressor functions that results in cellular transformation.

Classifications of Proto-Oncogenes

Given the complexity of inducing and regulating cellular growth, proliferation and differentiation, it was suspected for many years that genetic damage to genes encoding growth factors, growth factor receptors, and/or the proteins of the various signal transduction cascades would lead to cellular transformation. This suspicion has proven true with the identification of numerous genes, whose products function in cellular signaling, that are involved in some way in the genesis of the tumorigenic state (Table 52-4).

Proto-Oncogenes and Inherited Cancer Syndromes

Hereditary cancer syndromes have their origin in random genetic mutations that occur in the germ cells and, thus are passed on in the germ line of an individual with typical mendelian patterns of inheritance. Specific hereditary susceptibility syndromes have been characterized that increase the risk of malignancies of the breast, ovary, colon, endometrium, and endocrine organs (Table 52-5). The most prevalent hereditary cancer syndromes are hereditary nonpolyposis colorectal cancer (HNPCC), familial adenomatous polyposis (FAP, Clinical Box 52-3), hereditary breast and ovarian cancer (HBOC), and multiple endocrine neoplasia type 2 (MEN2). The identification of hereditary cancer susceptibility syndromes, at the level of the gene, has significant medical implications. One major benefit of being able to test for cancer susceptibility genes is that individuals in high-risk families, who did not themselves inherit the susceptibility gene, can avoid unnecessary medical interventions.

Tumor Suppressors

Tumor suppressor genes are genes that regulate the growth of cells and when these genes are functioning properly, they can prevent and inhibit the growth of tumors. Tumor suppressor genes were first identified by making cell hybrids between tumor and normal cells. On some occasions a chromosome from the normal cell reverted the transformed phenotype of the tumor cell. When a tumor suppressor gene is altered, for example due to sustaining a mutation, the protein product of the gene may lose the ability to properly controlling cell growth. Under these conditions the cell can grow and proliferate in an uncontrolled way leading to development of cancer. Several familial cancers have been shown to be associated with the loss of function of a tumor suppressor gene (Table 52-6). There are 3 main classifications of tumor suppressor genes. These include genes that encode proteins that tell cells to stop growing and dividing. Another class encodes proteins responsible for repairing DNA damage prior to allowing cells to complete the cell cycle. The third class encodes proteins that are involved in regulating cell death processes, called apoptosis.

Epigenetics: DNA Methylation and Tumor Suppressors

The term epigenetics is used to define the mechanism by which changes in the pattern of inherited gene expression occur in the absence of alterations or changes in the nucleotide composition of a given gene. This is simply defined as the phenotypic consequences that can be observed due to alterations "on" the genes and not by alterations "to" the genes. Several different types of epigenetic events have been identified and include DNA methylation and histone modifications (see Chapter 35). DNA methylation is likely to be the most important epigenetic event controlling and maintaining the pattern of gene expression during development.

Whereas, epigenesis plays a vital role in the regulation, control, and maintenance of gene expression leading to the many differentiation states of cells in an organism, recent evidence has identified a linkage between epigenetic processes and disease.

TABLE 52-4: Various Proto-Oncogene Classifications and Cancer[1]	
Class	***Examples, Comments***
Growth factors	*SIS* gene (the v-sis gene is the oncogene in simian sarcoma virus), encodes the PDGF-B chain, v-sis was the first oncogene to be identified as having homology to a known cellular gene int-2 gene (named for the fact that it is a common site of integration of mouse mammary tumor virus) encodes an FGF-related growth factor
Receptor tyrosine kinase	Many receptor tyrosine kinases have been shown to have oncogenic potential *FMS* ("fims") gene encodes the colony-stimulating factor-1 (CSF-1) receptor and was first identified as a retroviral oncogene *FLG* ("flag") gene, named because it has homology to the *FMS* gene, hence fms-like gene, encodes a form of the fibroblast growth factor (FGF) receptor. Epidermal growth factor receptor (EGFR, also called HER1 for human EGF receptor 1) is amplified in numerous cancers, in particular in squamous cell carcinomas. *NEU* ("new") gene was identified as an EGF receptor-related gene in an ethylnitrosourea-induced neuroblastoma, also identified as HER2 (human EGF receptor 2), is the target of the anticancer drug Herceptin (trastuzumab).
Nonreceptor tyrosine kinases	SRC was the first identified oncogene; it is the archetypal protein tyrosine kinase. ABL (first identified in the Abelson murine leukemia virus) is frequently rearranged in chronic myelogenous leukemias (CMLs), the majority of rearrangements involve a reciprocal translocation between the ABL chromosome (9) and chromosome 22 near a locus termed the breakpoint cluster region (BCR), the result is a constitutively active ABL tyrosine kinase domain fused to the BCR coding region forming what is referred to as the BCR-ABL fusion protein, this translocation is called the Philadelphia chromosome (Ph^+), BCR-ABL is the target of the anticancer drug Gleevec (imatinib mesylate).
G-protein–coupled receptors (GPCR)	*MAS* gene in mammary carcinoma is the angiotensin receptor.
G-proteins	Three different homologs of the *RAS* gene (RAS, H-RAS, and N-RAS), each of which was identified in a different type of tumor cell, with *RAS* being one of the most frequently disrupted genes in colorectal carcinomas.
Serine/threonine kinases	*RAF* gene is involved in the signaling pathway of most receptor tyrosine kinases. *MOS* gene (originally identified in the Moloney murine sarcoma virus) is normally expressed in germ cells and functions during oocyte maturation.
Nuclear receptors and transcription factors	Many genes altered in cancer encode transcription factors. *MYC* gene was originally identified in the avian myelocytomatosis virus, disrupted human *MYC* found in numerous hematopoietic cancers. *FOS* gene was identified as the transforming gene in the Finkel-Biskis-Jinkins (FBJ) murine osteogenic sarcoma virus, interacts with a second proto-oncogenic protein, JUN, to form a transcriptional regulatory complex.

[1]only a few representative examples of each class included.

Most significant is the link between epigenesis at the level of DNA methylation and cancer. Alterations in DNA methylation have been suggested to be a contributing factor in nearly half of all human cancers. In most cases the higher the level of DNA methylation the more transcriptionally repressed is the methylated gene. The best characterized epigenetic "lesions" in malignant cells are the promoter CpG island hypermethylations that lead to transcriptional repression of tumor suppressor genes. These changes have been observed in numerous cancers and were first fully characterized in retinoblastomas (the *RB* gene), breast cancers (the *BRCA1* gene), renal

TABLE 52-5: Hereditary Cancer Syndromes Caused by Dominant Genes

Syndrome	*Cloned Gene*	*Function*	*Chromosomal Location*	*Tumor Types*
Ataxia telangiectasia (AT)	*ATM* (AT mutated): 4 complementation groups: ATA, ATC, ATD, and ATE are associated with mutations in the *ATM* gene	Gene product encodes a kinase, one substrate is p53	11q22.3	Lymphoma, cerebellar ataxia, immunodeficiency
Beckwith-Wiedemann syndrome (BWS)	BWS caused by changes in a 1-Mb region that encompasses at least 15 genes: *CDKN1C* (also called p57[KIP2]) is likely responsible for the cancers	CDKN1C is a cyclin-dependent kinase inhibitor, cell cycle regulator	11p15.5	Genomic imprinting disorder resulting in Wilms tumor, adrenocortical cancer, hepatoblastoma
Bloom syndrome	*BLM*	DNA helicase RecQ protein-like-3	15q26.1	Solid tumors, immunodeficiency
Fanconi anemia, 13 complementation groups	*FANCA*, B, C, D1, D2, E, F, G, I, J, L, M, N *FANCA*, C, E, F, G, and L form nuclear multiprotein complex *FANCD1* = *BRCA2* *FANCN* = *PALB2* which is a nuclear-binding partner for *BRCA2*	Components of DNA repair machinery	FANCA=16q24.3 FANCC=9q22.3 FANCD2=3p25.3 FANCE=11p15	Acute myeloid leukemia (AML), pancytopenia, chromosomal instability
Hereditary papillary renal cancer (HPRC)	*MET*: originally identified in a human osteogenic cell line treated with *N*-methyl-*N*-nitro-*N*-nitrosoguanidine	Transmembrane receptor for hepatocyte growth factor (HGF)	7q31	Renal papillary cancer
Hereditary prostate cancer, numerous loci: HPC1 (PRCA1), HPCX, MXI1, KAI1, PCAP	*HPC1* and *PRCA1* are same designation, ribonuclease L (RNaseL) maps to this locus	RNaseL involved in mRNA degradation	1q24-q25	Prostate cancer
Multiple endocrine neoplasia type 2	*MEN2*, also known as RET (meaning rearranged during transfection)	Transmembrane receptor tyrosine kinase for glial-derived neurotrophic factor (GDNF)	10q11.2	Medullary thyroid cancer, type 2A pheochromocytoma, mucosal hartoma
Xeroderma pigmentosum (XP), 8 complementation groups	*XPA*, B, C, D, E, F, G, and variant XP (*XPV*)	DNA repair helicases, nucleotide excision repair	XPA = 9q22.3 XPC = 3p25 XPD = 19q13.2-q13.3 XPE=11p12-p11 XPF = 16p13.3-p13.13	Skin cancer

TABLE 52-6: Properties of a Few Important Tumor Suppressor Genes

Syndrome	*Cloned Gene*	*Function*	*Chromosomal Location*	*Tumor Types*
Cowden syndrome	*PTEN* = phosphatase and tensin homolog	Phosphoinositide 3-phosphatase, protein tyrosine phosphatase	10q23.3	Breast cancer, thyroid cancer, head and neck squamous carcinomas
Deleted in colorectal carcinoma	*DCC*	Transmembrane receptor involved in axonal guidance via netrins	18q21.3	Colorectal cancer
Deleted in pancreatic carcinoma 4	*DPC4* also known as *SMAD4*	Regulation of TGF-β/BMP signal transduction	18q21.1	Pancreatic carcinoma, colon cancer
Familial adenomatous polyposis	*APC*	Signaling through adhesion molecules to nucleus	5q21	Colon cancer
Familial breast cancer	*BRCA1*	See Table 52-7	17q21	Breast and ovarian cancer
Familial breast cancer	*BRCA2*	See Table 52-7	13q12.3	Breast and ovarian cancer
Familial melanoma	*CDKN2A* = cyclin-dependent kinase inhibitor 2A gene produces 2 proteins: p16INK4 and p14ARF	p16INK4 inhibits cell-cycle kinases CDK4 and CDK6; p14ARF binds the p53 stabilizing protein MDM2	9p21	Melanoma, pancreatic cancer, others
Familial retinoblastoma	*RB1*	See Clinical Box 52-1	13q14	Retinoblastoma, osteogenic sarcoma
Gorlin syndrome: nevoid basal cell carcinoma syndrome (NBCCS)	PTCH protein = patched	Transmembrane receptor for sonic hedgehog (shh), involved in early development through repression of action of smoothened	9q22.3	Basal cell skin cancer
Hereditary nonpolyposis colorectal cancer type 1: HNPCC1; also known as Lynch syndrome	*MSH2*	DNA mismatch repair	2p22-p21	Colorectal cancer
Hereditary nonpolyposis colorectal cancer type 2: HNPCC2	*MLH1*	DNA mismatch repair	3p21.3	Colorectal cancer
Li-Fraumeni syndrome	*p53*	See Clinical Box 52-2	17p13	Brain tumors, sarcomas, leukemia, breast cancer
Multiple endocrine neoplasia type 1	*MEN1*	Intrastrand DNA crosslink repair	11q13	Parathyroid and pituitary adenomas, islet cell tumors, carcinoid
Neurofibromatosis type 1	NF1 = tumor suppressor protein = neurofibromin 1	Catalysis of RAS inactivation	17q11.2	Neurofibromas, sarcomas, gliomas
Neurofibromatosis type 2	NF2 protein = merlin, also called neurofibromin 2	Linkage of cell membrane to cytoskeleton	22q12.2	Schwann cell tumors, astrocytomas, meningiomas, ependymomas

(*Continued*)

TABLE 52-6: Properties of a Few Important Tumor Suppressor Genes (*Continued*)

Syndrome	*Cloned Gene*	*Function*	*Chromosomal Location*	*Tumor Types*
Peutz-Jeghers syndrome (PJS)	STK11 protein = serine-threonine kinase 11 was also known as LKB1	Phosphorylates and activates AMP-activated kinase (AMPK), AMPK involved in stress responses, lipid and glucose metabolism	19p13.3	Hyperpigmentation, multiple hamartomatous polyps, colorectal, breast and ovarian cancers
Tuberous sclerosis 1	TSC1 protein = hamartin	Forms complex with TSC2 protein, inhibits signaling to downstream effectors of mTOR	9q34	Seizures, mental retardation, facial angiofibromas
Tuberous sclerosis 2	TSC2 protein = tuberin	See TSC1	16p13.3	Benign growths (hamartomas) in many tissues, astrocytomas, rhabdomyosarcomas
von Hippel-Lindau syndrome	*VHL*	Regulation of transcription elongation	3p26-p25	Renal cancers, hemangioblastomas, pheochromocytoma
Wilms tumor	*WT1*	Transcriptional regulation	11p13	Pediatric kidney cancer, nephroblastoma

CLINICAL BOX 52-1: RETINOBLOASTOMA

Retinoblastoma (RB) is a rare type of eye cancer that forms in immature cells of the retina and most often manifest in early childhood prior to the age of 5. Diagnosis of retinoblastoma after the age of 6 is extremely rare due to the terminal differentiation of retinal epithelial cells. In most children with retinoblastoma, the disease affects only one eye. However, in about 30% of children with retinoblastoma the cancer develops in both eyes. The most common first sign of retinoblastoma is a visible whiteness in the pupil referred to as leukocoria. This is also called amaurotic cat's eye reflex. Additional symptoms of retinoblastoma include crossed eyes or eyes that do not point in the same direction (strabismus), persistent eye pain, redness, or irritation; and blindness or poor vision in the affected eye(s). Retinoblastoma is often curable when it is diagnosed early. If not treated promptly, the cancer can spread to other parts of the body leading to life-threatening metastasis. When retinoblastoma is associated with a gene mutation that occurs in all of the body's cells, it is known as germinal retinoblastoma. Individuals with this form of retinoblastoma also have an increased risk of developing several other cancers outside the eye. Specifically, they are more likely to develop a cancer of the pineal gland in the brain (pinealoma), a type of bone cancer known as osteosarcoma, cancers of soft tissues such as muscle, and an aggressive form of skin cancer called melanoma. In the familial form of this disease individuals inherit a mutant, loss-of-function allele from an affected parent. A subsequent later somatic mutational event inactivates the normal allele resulting in retinoblastoma development. This leads to an apparently dominant mode of inheritance. The requirement for an additional somatic mutational event at the unaffected allele means that penetration of the defect is not always complete. There are also sporadic forms of retinoblastoma which requires 2 independent somatic mutational events to occur and is, thus extremely rare. The gene responsible for retinoblastoma is called the retinoblastoma susceptibility gene (RB). The RB RNA encodes a 110 kDa protein (pRB) of 928 amino acids. pRB is a nuclear localized phosphoprotein. Detectable levels of pRB can be found in most proliferating cells but the protein is not detectable in any retinoblastoma cells, typical of the case for many cancers involving tumor suppressor genes. The largest percentage (30%) of retinoblastomas contains large scale deletions

CLINICAL BOX 52-1: RETINOBLOASTOMA (*Continued*)

in the RB gene. The germline mutations at RB occur predominantly during spermatogenesis as opposed to oogenesis. However, the somatic mutations occur with equal frequency at the paternal or maternal locus. In contrast, somatic mutations at RB in sporadic osteosarcomas occur preferentially at the paternal locus. This may be the result of genomic imprinting. The major function of pRB is in the regulation of cell cycle progression. Its ability to regulate the cell cycle correlates to the state of phosphorylation of pRB. Phosphorylation is maximal at the start of S phase and lowest after mitosis and entry into G_1. Stimulation of quiescent cells with mitogen induces phosphorylation of pRB, while in contrast, differentiation induces hypophosphorylation of pRB. It is, therefore, the hypophosphorylated form of pRB that suppresses cell proliferation. One of the most significant substrates for phosphorylation by the G_1 cyclin-CDK complexes that regulate progression through the cell cycle is pRB. pRB forms a complex with the E2F family of transcription factors, a result of which renders E2F inactive (Figure 52-3). When pRB is phosphorylated by G_1 cyclin-CDK complexes it is released from E2F allowing E2F to transcriptionally activate genes. In the context of the cell cycle, E2F increases the transcription of the S-phase cyclins as well as leads to increases in its own transcription. Transformation by the DNA tumor viruses, SV40, adeno, polyoma, and human papilloma, is accomplished by binding of the transforming proteins (T antigens) of these viruses to pRB when pRB is in the hypophosphorylated, proliferation inhibitory, state.

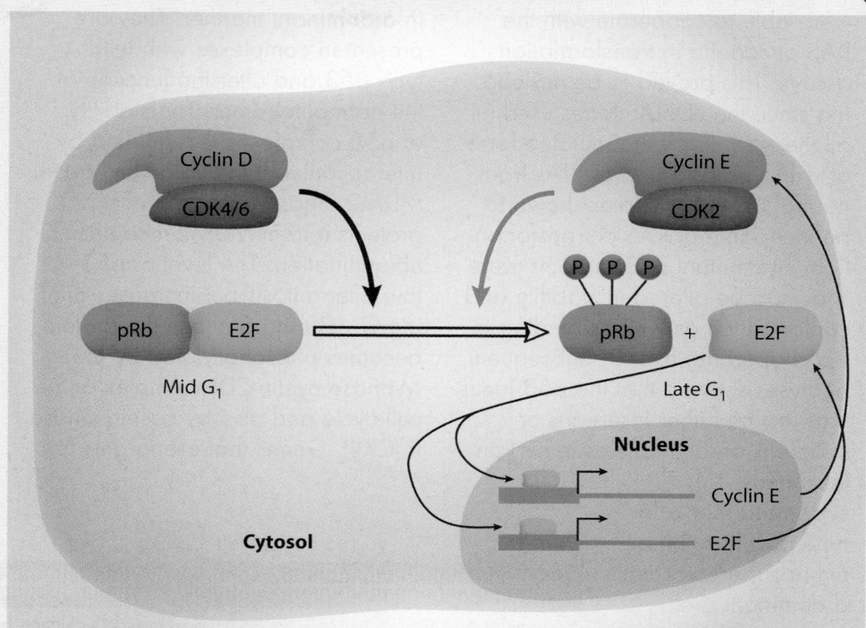

FIGURE 52-3: pRB regulation of the E2F transcription factor. When hypophosphorylated, pRB binds to E2F preventing it from migrating to the nucleus and therefore, when bound to pRB the E2F protein is incapable of activating transcription. When pRB is phosphorylated, primarily at low levels by CDK2, it releases E2F which enters the nucleus and activates its own transcription as well as the cyclin E gene. Production of cyclin E gene results in a dramatic increase in CDK2 kinase activity. This results in further phosphorylation of pRB keeping E2F in the transcriptionally active state allowing for progression into S phase of the cell cycle. Reproduced with permission of themedicalbiochemistrypage, LLC.

CLINICAL BOX 52-2: LI-FRAUMENI SYNDROME

Li-Fraumeni syndrome (LFS) is a rare autosomal dominant disorder that greatly increases the risk of developing several types of cancer, particularly in children and young adults. The disorder is named for the 2 physicians who first recognized and described the syndrome: Frederick Pei Li and Joseph F. Fraumeni, Jr. The cancers most often associated with Li-Fraumeni syndrome include breast cancer, a form of bone cancer called osteosarcoma, and cancers of soft tissues (such as muscle) called soft tissue sarcomas. Other cancers commonly seen in this syndrome include brain tumors, cancers of blood-forming tissues (leukemias), and a cancer called adrenocortical carcinoma that affects the outer layer of the adrenal glands. LFS is linked to germline mutations in the tumor suppressor gene, *p53*. The p53 protein is involved in the blocking cell cycle progression while DNA repair takes place or if the DNA damage is severe enough p53 initiates a program of apoptosis. It was first thought that p53 was a dominant oncogene since cDNA clones isolated from tumor lines

CLINICAL BOX 52-2: LI-FRAUMENI SYNDROME (*Continued*)

were able to cooperate with the RAS oncogene in transformation assays. This proved to be misleading since the cDNA clones used in all these studies were mutated forms of wild-type p53 and cDNAs from normal tissue were later shown to be incapable of RAS cotransformation. The mutant p53 proteins were shown to be altered in stability and conformation as well as binding to the chaperone, hsp70. Subsequent analyses showed that the p53 locus was lost by either insertions or deletions on both alleles in certain leukemias. This suggested that wild-type p53 may be a tumor suppressor not a dominant proto-oncogene. Direct confirmation came when it was shown that wild-type p53 could suppress transformation in oncogene cooperation assays with mutant p53 and RAS. It has now been demonstrated that mutant p53 involvement in neoplasia is more frequent than any other known tumor suppressor or dominant proto-oncogene. The protein encoded by p53 is a transcription factor whose activity is regulated by its state of phosphorylation. The p53 protein binds to target DNA sequences as a tetramer which explains the fact that mutant p53 proteins act in a dominant manner. They are present in complexes with wild type p53 and alter the function of the normal tetramer. The stability of p53 complexes is regulated by interaction with the ubiquitin ligase, MDM2. Phosphorylation of p53 protects it from MDM2-mediated ubiquitination. The level of p53 is low after mitosis but increases during G_1. During S phase the protein becomes phosphorylated by the M-phase cyclin-CDK complex of the cell cycle and also by casein kinase II (CKII). Genes that are targets for transcriptional regulation by p53 are involved in the control of cell cycle progression and the suppression of cell growth. One major cell cycle–regulating gene that is a target for p53 is the CDK inhibitory protein (CIP), $p21^{CIP}$. Activation of p53 by DNA damage-mediated phosphorylation (via the ATM kinase) results in increased expression of $p21^{CIP}$ with a resultant arrest in the G_1 and G_2 phases of the cell cycle (Figure 52-4). If the damaged DNA is unable to be repaired, p53 triggers activation of apoptosis.

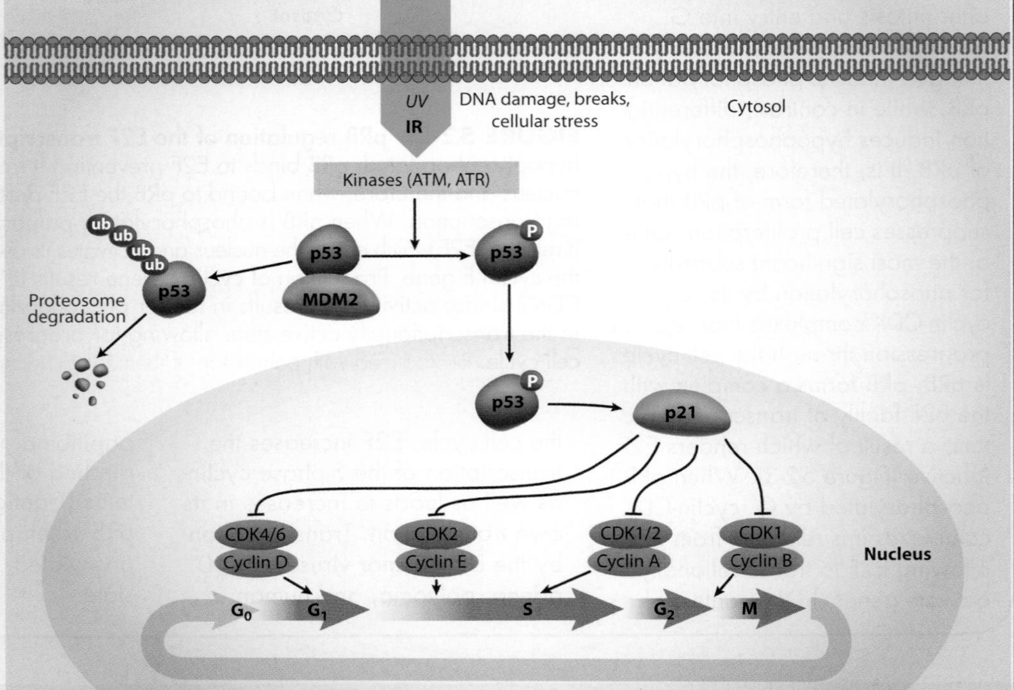

FIGURE 52-4: DNA damage induction of p53 and activation of $p21^{CIP}$. Ionizing radiation, or other causes of DNA damage, activate the ataxia-telangiectasia mutated (ATM) kinase. ATM phosphorylates p53 which stabilizes the protein and releases it from MDM2. The phosphorylated p53 then migrates to the nucleus where it activates transcription of various target genes. One target of p53 is the gene encoding CDK inhibitory protein 21, $p21^{CIP}$. Increased expression of $p21^{CIP}$ results in inhibition of G_1-S- and S-cyclin-CDK complexes ensuring that cells do not progress through S phase of the cell cycle until DNA damage is repaired. Reproduced with permission of themedicalbiochemistrypage, LLC.

carcinomas (the *VHL* gene), and numerous types of cancers involving hypermethylation of the cyclin-dependent kinase (CDK) inhibitory gene, *p16*. Hypermethylation of the *p16* gene has been observed in nearly 20% of all primary human neoplasms.

Eukaryotic cells express several related enzymes involved in DNA methylation called DNA methyltransferases (DNMTs). Maintenance of DNA methylation patterns is required following DNA replication and mitosis to ensure that the resulting daughter cells remain in the same state of differentiation as the parental cell. DNMT1 is the primary maintenance DNA methylase involved in this process. Changes in methylation patterns during development are the primary mechanisms associated with gene silencing leading to altered differentiation states of cells in the embryo. DNMT1 and DNMT3a have been shown to work in concert with one another to lead to hypermethylation of CpG islands and likely play pivotal roles in the genesis of cancers involving tumor suppressor silencing.

Breast Cancers

Breast cancers include any cancer originating from breast tissue but are most commonly seen in cells of the inner lining of milk ducts or the lobules that supply the ducts with milk. Cancers originating from milk ducts are known as ductal carcinomas, whereas, those originating from lobules are known as lobular carcinomas. Breast cancers account for almost 23% of all cancers in women worldwide. Most forms of breast cancer are spontaneous and not due to the inheritance of a specific mutant gene. The primary risk factors for breast cancer include smoking, dietary lifestyle including high-fat diets, obesity, and alcohol consumption. Although most breast (and ovarian) cancers are spontaneous, inherited mutations in several genes have been shown to be associated with an increased risk of developing these types of cancers (Table 52-7). To date 7 loci have been identified that when mutated predispose an individual to breast and ovarian cancer. These loci are BRCA1, BRCA2, ATM, CHEK2, BRIP1, PALB2, and RAD51C. Of significance is that all of these breast cancer susceptibility genes encode proteins that function in some aspect of DNA damage repair.

Gastrointestinal Cancers

The gastrointestinal (GI) system is site of more malignant tumors than any other organ system. The most common locations for GI cancers are the large intestine (colon) and the rectum (colorectal cancers) but cancers of the mouth, esophagus, stomach, and small intestines, are included when discussing overall GI cancer rates. Almost all colon cancers are adenocarcinomas that result from adenomatous polyps (Figure 52-5). Although most colon cancers arise from adenomatous polyps the majority of them do not give rise to cancer. Routine colonoscopy is designed to examine for the presence of these polyps and they can be removed during the procedure.

With respect to overall GI cancers, the differences in worldwide distribution rates can be explained almost

TABLE 52-7: Breast and Ovarian Cancer Susceptibility Genes

Gene	*Function, Role in Cancer*
ATM	**A**taxia-**t**elangiectasia **m**utated, first identified as causing ataxia telangiectasia, is a PI3K-type kinase activated by DNA damage
BRCA1	**Br**east **ca**ncer **1**, early onset, along with *BRCA2*, the first genes identified as being mutated in inherited forms of breast and ovarian cancer, both are tumor suppressors involved in DNA repair and chromosomal stability
BRCA2	**Br**east **ca**ncer **2**, early onset, is also known as Fanconi anemia complementation group D1 (*FANCD1*) gene, plays a major role in high-risk breast cancer predisposition
BRIP1	**BR**CA1 **i**nteracting **p**rotein C-terminal helicase 1, functions in double-strand DNA break repair in concert with BRCA1, is also known as Fanconi anemia complementation group J (FANCJ)
CHEK2	Cell cycle **che**ckpoint **k**inase 2. CHEK2 is a serine-threonine kinase that is activated by ATM protein in response to DNA double-strand breaks, regulates function of BRCA1 protein in DNA repair, exerts a number of critical roles in cell cycle control and apoptosis
PALB2	**Pa**rtner and **l**ocalizer of **B**RCA2, binds directly to BRCA1 and serves as the molecular scaffold in the formation of the BRCA1-PALB2-BRCA2 complex, is also known as Fanconi anemia complementation group N (FANCN)
RAD51C	A member of the RAD51 family of related proteins involved in recombinational DNA repair and meiotic recombination

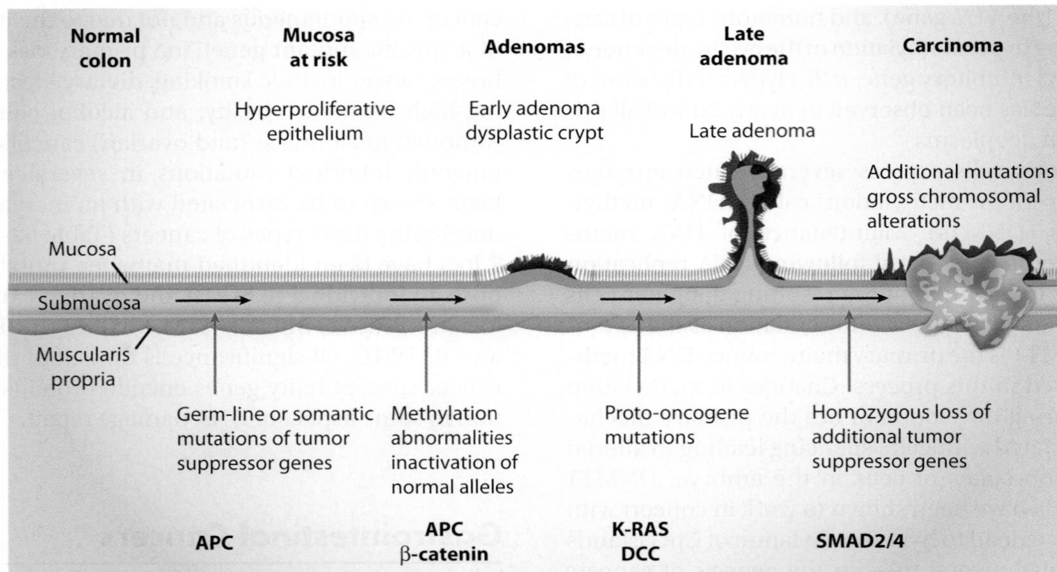

FIGURE 52-5: Progression of normal colonic mucosa to full-blown adenocarcinoma. The initial step in colorectal carcinoma is formation of an adenoma, most often associated with loss of adenomatous polyposis coli (APC) gene function. Larger adenomas and early carcinomas acquire progressively more and more mutations such as in the β-catenin and small GTPase (K-RAS) genes. This is followed by loss of chromosome 18q which disrupts SMAD2/4 function. Many additional mutations are known to be associated with this progressive development to a full blown carcinoma but are not depicted here such as in the p53 and TGFβ genes as well as gross chromosomal alterations due to microsatellite instability. Reproduced with permission of themedicalbiochemistrypage, LLC.

entirely by environmental factors. There are, however, several well-defined inherited genetic disorders that predispose an individual to colorectal carcinomas. Cancers of the upper GI, mouth, esophagus, and stomach are almost entirely due to influences of the diet. The most prevalent dietary causes of GI cancers are high fat, high calorie, and low-fiber diets, typical of what is seen in the Western-style diet. Cancers of the lower GI, the colorectal cancers, are much more often related to genetic factors including inheritance or somatic acquisition of gene mutations predisposing one to development of cancer.

Many colorectal cancers are initiated due to inheritance of mutated tumor suppressor genes or through somatic mutations in these same genes. One of the most frequently mutated tumor suppressor genes responsible for initiation of colorectal cancers in the adenomatous polyposis coli gene (*APC*). Inherited mutations in *APC* are the cause of familial adenomatous polyposis, FAP (Clinical Box 52-3). Another well characterized inherited colorectal carcinoma syndrome is hereditary nonpolyposis colorectal cancer, HNPCC. HNPCC results from inherited mutations in at least 5 different genes involved in the repair of DNA damage. Specifically, these genes are involved in DNA mismatch repair, *MMR* genes. HNPCC accounts for 5% of all cases of colorectal cancer and patients who inherit an *HNPCC* mutation have an 80% chance of developing colorectal cancer. Because *HNPCC* gene mutations are present in all cell types these individuals have increased risk of cancers in multiple other locations. In women with HNPCC, uterine (endometrial) cancers are quite common.

Hematopoietic and Lymphoid Cancers

Hematological cancers represent those cancers affecting cells of the blood and bone marrow, the myeloid cancers, as well as cancers of the lymphatic system, the lymphoid cancers. Myeloid lineage cancers include the erythroid cells, granulocytes, monocytes, megakaryocytes, and mast cells. The lymphoid lineage cancers include the lymphomas, the lymphocytic leukemias, and the myelomas. There is a close association between gross chromosomal abnormalities and the development of leukemias and lymphomas. The lymphomas account for approximately 4% of all cancers in the United States. The leukemias, account for approximately 2% to 4% of all incidences of cancer in the United States and for 3% to 5% of all cancer deaths. The leukemias are particularly devastating emotionally because they are the most common cancers in children.

The most commonly occurring types of leukemias are acute lymphoblastic leukemia (ALL), acute myelogenous leukemia (AML), chronic lymphocytic leukemia (CLL), and chronic myelogenous leukemia (CML, Clinical Box 52-4). Lymphomas account for approximately 56% of all hematological cancers and

CLINICAL BOX 52-3: FAMILIAL ADENOMATOUS POLYPOSIS COLI

Familial adenomatous polyposis (FAP) is an inherited disorder characterized by a highly elevated risk of developing colorectal carcinoma. FAP is associated with germline mutations in the adenomatous polyposis coli (*APC*) gene. Somatic mutations in *APC* are also highly correlated to the initiation of colorectal cancer in the general population. Multiple colonic polyp development, within the first decades of life, is characteristic of FAP. These polyps become malignant carcinomas and adenomas later in life. FAP adenomas appear as a result of loss-of-function mutations to the *APC* gene which characterizes the gene as a tumor suppressor. To date, more than 120 different germline and somatic mutations have been identified in the *APC* gene. The vast majority of these mutations lead to C-terminal truncation of the APC protein. The protein-coding region of the *APC* gene is extremely large encompassing 2844 amino acids. The APC protein is found associated with other proteins in the cytosol. One of these APC-associated proteins is β-catenin. The catenins are a family of proteins that interact with the cytoplasmic portion of the cadherins (cell-cell adhesion family of proteins), thus linking the cadherins to the actin cytoskeleton. Catenins are equally important in the signaling cascade initiated by the Wnt family of proteins that are involved in embryonic patterning and development of the nervous system. The Wnt proteins are secreted factors that interact with cell-surface receptors. Wnt-receptor interaction induces the activity of the cytoplasmic phosphoprotein disheveled. Activated disheveled inhibits the serine/threonine kinase glycogen synthase kinase-3β (GSK-3β). When GSK-3β is inhibited, β-catenin becomes hypophosphorylated. The hypophosphorylated form of β-catenin migrates to the nucleus and interacts with transcription factors (in particular with T-cell factor/lymphoid enhancer-binding factor-1 (TCF/LEF-1), thereby, inducing expression of various genes. The suspected role of APC in this pathway is to bind phosphorylated β-catenin. The APC-β-catenin complex stimulates the ubiquitination of β-catenin resulting in its degradation in the proteosome. Mutations which lead to a loss of APC, or to a loss of APC interaction with β-catenin, result in constitutive activation of TCF/LEF-1 and unrestricted cell growth. Within the colon this leads to development of adenomatous polyps. Subsequent mutations (see Figure 52-5) in other genes results in the eventual progression to adenocarcinoma.

CLINICAL BOX 52-4: CHRONIC MYELOGENOUS LEUKEMIA, CML

Chronic myelogenous leukemia (CML) is a cancer associated with unregulated growth of myeloid lineage cells of the bone marrow which then accumulate in the blood. The affected cells are mature granulocytes (eosinophils, basophils, and neutrophils) and granulocyte precursors. In the first stages of CML, many patients do not have any symptoms of the disease and can remain symptom-free for several years. CML is most often diagnosed between the ages of 45 and 55 with 30% of diagnosed patients being over the age of 65. CML is most often discovered through routine blood tests (a complete blood count, CBC), not due to the presentation of overt symptoms. Detection of CML through a CBC is due to the identification of increased numbers of granulocytes of all types. During the progression of CML the number of cancer cells accumulates to the point of interference with normal functions resulting in the manifestation of symptoms. These symptoms can include bleeding and bruising, anemia, fatigue, loss of weight, loss of appetite, night sweats, enlarged lymph nodes, and recurrent infections. Definitive diagnosis of CML is accomplished via the detection of a specific chromosomal translocation in metaphase cells. This translocation is referred to as the Philadelphia chromosome and its presence is denoted as Ph⁺. The Philadelphia chromosome results from a translocation between chromosomes 9 and 22 (t[9:22]). The t(9:22) translocation fuses the Abelson tyrosine kinase (ABL) on chromosome 9 with the BCR locus on chromosome 22. The *ABL* gene was first identified as an oncogene in murine leukemias. The BCR locus was originally identified as a region of frequent chromosomal breakage and thus, termed the breakpoint cluster region, BCR. The BCR-ABL fusion protein results in constitutive activation of the tyrosine kinase activity of ABL. The normal function of ABL is to regulate the activity of a number of cell cycle–regulating proteins. Loss of regulated ABL activity therefore leads to unregulated cell cycle progression leading to malignancy. The drug Gleevec (imatinib mesylate) was the first drug specifically designed to target the tyrosine kinase activity of the BCR-ABL oncoprotein and has been used with high success in the treatment of CML.

are classified as Hodgkin or non-Hodgkin lymphomas. There are 4 generalized categories of Hodgkin lymphoma all of which are characterized by the spread of the disease from one lymph node to another. Hodgkin lymphoma can be diagnosed by histological examination of the affected lymph cells. These cells have a characteristic multinucleated appearance and are called Reed-Sternberg cells (RS cells).

Non-Hodgkin lymphomas (NHLs) represent all other lymphomas that are not distinctly Hodgkin lymphomas. There are at least 16 different types of characterized NHL. Due to the continued expansion of NHL types there is a move to abandon the Hodgkin and NHL terms in the description of lymphomas. The incidence of NHL has doubled in the past 30 years and numerous reports correlate this increase to increasing exposure to polychlorinated biphenyls (PCBs). Like most hematological cancers, 80% to 90% of NHLs are associated with gross chromosomal abnormalities. The most common chromosomal aberrations are translocations between chromosomes 8 and 14 (identified as t[8:14]) and those between chromosomes 14 and 18 (t[14:18]). The t(8:14) translocation was the first chromosome abnormality to be molecularly characterized. The MYC proto-oncogene on chromosome 8 becomes fused to the immunoglobulin heavy chain enhancer region on chromosome 14 causing highly unregulated expression of the *MYC* gene resulting in abnormal cell growth and proliferation. The t(14:18) translocation disrupts the *BCL2* gene on chromosome 18 resulting in loss of BCL2-mediated regulation of apoptosis.

REVIEW QUESTIONS

1. You are treating a 47-year-old woman who has come to you with complaints of fatigue, chronic headaches, and radiating pain and fullness on her left side. A routine blood test indicates the presence of increased immature white cells (blasts), reduced platelets, and reduced leukocytes. You order a cytogenetic analysis of the blasts and the results indicate the presence of a chromosomal abnormality consistent with a t(9:22) translocation. This patient is most likely suffering from which of the following?

A. acute lymphocytic leukemia, ALL
B. acute myelogenous leukemia, AML
C. chronic myelogenous leukemia, CML
D. Hodgkin lymphoma
E. Non-Hodgkin lymphoma, NHL

Answer C: Chronic myelogenous leukemia (CML) is a cancer associated with unregulated growth of myeloid lineage cells. The affected cells are mature granulocytes (eosinophils, basophils, and neutrophils) and granulocyte precursors. CML is most often discovered through routine blood tests (a complete blood count, CBC), not due to the presentation of overt symptoms. Detection of CML through a CBC is due to the identification of increased number of granulocytes of all types. Definitive diagnosis of CML is accomplished via the detection of a specific chromosomal translocation in metaphase cells. This translocation is referred to as the Philadelphia chromosome and its presence is denoted as Ph^+. The Philadelphia chromosome results from a translocation between chromosomes 9 and 22 (t[9:22]). The t(9:22) translocation fuses the Abelson tyrosine kinase (ABL) on chromosome 9 with the BCR locus on chromosome 22. The BCR-ABL fusion protein results in constitutive activation of the tyrosine kinase activity of ABL.

2. You are treating a 37-year-old African-American man who has come to you complaining of abdominal distension, night sweats, and shortness of breath all of which have developed over the last 4 weeks. Physical examination decreased breath sounds in right lung base and a 2-cm lymph node appreciated on left inguinal region. Excision biopsy and culture of cells from the inguinal lymph node identified the presence of a chromosomal translocation between chromosomes 14 and 18. Your patient is most likely suffering from which of the following?

A. acute lymphocytic leukemia, ALL
B. acute myelogenous leukemia, AML
C. chronic myelogenous leukemia, CML
D. Hodgkin lymphoma
E. Non-Hodgkin lymphoma, NHL

Answer E: Non-Hodgkin lymphomas (NHLs) are a diverse group of blood cancers that include any kind of lymphoma except Hodgkin lymphomas. There are at least 16 different characterized types of NHL that vary significantly in their severity, from indolent to very aggressive. Many NHL cells contain gross chromosomal aberrations including translocations. The most common translocations found in NHL are the t(8:14) and the t(14:18) translocations.

3. A 27-year-old man is being examined by his physician to ascertain the cause of the bumps appearing on his skull and jaw. Close examination of the patient also shows epidermoid cysts, extra teeth, and freckle-like spots on the insides of his eyes. Family history indicates that his mother died of colorectal cancer when the patient was only 6 years old. Given the external signs apparent in this patient you recommend a colonoscopy which shows hundreds of polyps. Which of the following genes is most likely defective in this patient accounting for all of the observed symptoms?

A. *APC*
B. *NF1*
C. *p53*
D. *RB*
E. *VHL*

Answer A: Germline mutations in the adenomatous polyposis coli (*APC*) gene are responsible for familial adenomatous polyposis (FAP). Multiple colonic polyp development characterizes the disease. These polyps arise during the second and third decades of life and become malignant carcinomas and adenomas later in life. Genetic linkage analysis assigned the APC locus to 5q21. In addition to polyps in the GI tract, people with FAP often have other signs of FAP including lumps or bumps on the skull and jaw (osteomas), cysts on the skin (epidermoid cysts), dental changes (extra teeth), noncancerous tumors most often found in the abdomen (desmoid tumors), and freckle-like spots on the inside of the eye.

4. You are a genetic counselor discussing the results of a global genetic profile a 37-year-old woman had done through an online testing company. She is particularly concerned because the test flagged a mutation in a gene identified as *PALB2*. You inform her that mutations in this gene are highly correlated to a particular cancer. Which of the following is this cancer?

A. breast cancer
B. colorectal cancer
C. fibrosarcoma
D. lymphoma
E. retinoblastoma

Answer A: Several genetic loci have been shown to predispose an individual to these types of cancer. To date 7 loci have been identified that when mutated predispose an individual to breast and ovarian cancer. These loci are BRCA1, BRCA2, ATM, CHEK2, BRIP1, PALB2, and RAD51C. Of significance is that all of these breast cancer susceptibility genes encode proteins that function in some aspect of DNA damage repair. The *PALB2* gene is partner and localizer of BRCA2 and encodes a protein that interacts with BRCA2 protein in the nucleus. PALB2 binds directly to BRCA1 and serves as the molecular scaffold in the formation of the BRCA1-PALB2-BRCA2 complex.

5. You are treating a 6-year-old girl who fell off her bike and broke her arm. She appears healthy in all other respects, however, during your examination you observe that she has several large and dark café-au-lait patches on her back and upper legs. As her physician you inform her parents that she may have inherited a mutated form of a gene called *NF1*. Which of the following would this child be most likely to experience as a result of a mutation in this gene?

A. breast cancer
B. colorectal cancer
C. lymphoma
D. neurofibroma
E. retinoblastoma

Answer D: Germline mutations at the NF1 locus result in multiple abnormal melanocytes (café-au-lait spots) and benign neurofibromas. Some patients also develop benign pheochromocytomas and CNS tumors. A small percentage of patients develop neurofibrosarcomas which are likely to be Schwann cell derived. Development of benign neurofibromas versus malignant neurofibrosarcomas may be the difference between inactivation of one NF1 allele versus both alleles, respectively.

6. You are treating a 26-year-old man who presented with exudative macular edema. Ocular and systemic studies revealed the presence of retinal and central nervous system hemangioblastomas, adrenal pheochromocytoma, as well as multiple pancreatic and renal cysts. Detailed family history revealed that his father had died from cerebral vascular accident at the age of 54 and had been treated for uncontrolled blood pressure, but was not investigated for possible presence of adrenal gland tumor. This patient is most likely suffering from defective function of which of the following genes?

A. *APC*
B. *NF1*
C. *p53*
D. *RB*
E. *VHL*

Answer E: von Hippel-Lindau syndrome (VHL) results from inheritance of a mutated copy of the *VHL* gene. As a consequence of somatic mutation or loss of the normal *VHL* gene, individuals are predisposed to a wide array of tumors that include renal cell carcinomas, retinal angiomas, cerebellar hemangioblastomas, and pheochromocytomas. One characteristic feature of tumors from VHL patients is the high degree of vascularization, primarily as a result of the constitutive expression of the vascular endothelial growth factor (*VEGF*) gene.

7. A 57-year-old woman has come to her physician to determine if something is seriously wrong with her as she has been suffering from fatigue, chronic headaches, and radiating pain and fullness on her left side for the past 5 months. Her physician orders a routine blood test that indicates the presence of increased immature white cells (blasts) that also contain the Philadelphia chromosome. This leads to a diagnosis of chronic myelogenous leukemia, CML. CML results from this translocation due to abnormal regulation of which of the following genes?

A. *ABL*
B. *MYC*
C. *p53*
D. *pRB*
E. *RAS*

Answer A: Chronic myelogenous leukemia (CML) is a cancer associated with unregulated growth of myeloid lineage cells of the bone marrow which then accumulate in the blood. The affected cells are mature granulocytes (eosinophils, basophils, and neutrophils) and granulocyte precursors. Definitive diagnosis of CML is accomplished via the detection of a specific chromosomal translocation in metaphase cells. This translocation is referred to as the Philadelphia chromosome and its presence is denoted as Ph^+. The Philadelphia chromosome results from a translocation between chromosomes 9 and 22 (t[9:22]). The t(9:22) translocation fuses the Abelson tyrosine kinase (ABL) on chromosome 9 with the BCR locus on chromosome 22. The BCR-ABL fusion protein results in constitutive activation of the tyrosine kinase activity of ABL. The normal function of ABL is to regulate the activity of a number of cell cycle–regulating proteins. Loss of regulated ABL activity therefore, leads to unregulated cell cycle progression leading to malignancy.

8. Which of the following defines the term neoplasm?

A. any of the many cancers of the lymphatics or hematopoietic system
B. cells that generate invasive tumors when transplanted
C. malignant cells from carcinomas and sarcomas
D. results from the consequences of chromosomal translocations
E. tissue that grows in the absence of an initial growth-stimulating signal

Answer E: A neoplasm is defined as an abnormal mass of cells resulting from neoplasia. Neoplasia is abnormal growth and proliferation of cells occurring in the absence of normal growth-promoting factors that were initially required by the cells.

9. Which of the following defines the meaning of the term proto-oncogene?

A. always expressed in a normal cell
B. always transcription factors
C. always virally derived
D. never expressed in a normal cell
E. tightly regulated in a normal cell

Answer E: A proto-oncogene is a normal gene that can become an oncogene due to mutations or increased expression. Proto-oncogenes code for proteins that help to regulate cell growth and differentiation and therefore, these genes are under tight regulatory control.

10. Which of the following familial cancers results from a defect in the tumor suppressor gene, *p53*?

A. familial adenomatous polyposis coli (FAP)
B. Li Fraumeni syndrome
C. neurofibromatosis type 1
D. retinoblastoma
E. Wilms tumor

Answer B: Li-Fraumeni syndrome (LFS) is a rare autosomal dominant disorder that greatly increases the risk of developing several types of cancer, particularly in children and young adults. LFS is linked to germline mutations in the tumor suppressor gene, *p53*.

11. Analysis of a tumor cell line indicates that there is a dramatically increased level in the activity of the transcription factor E2F. Which of the following is the most likely explanation for this observation?

A. an increase in the expression of pRB resulting in increased binding of pRB to E2F
B. hypophosphorylation of pRB so that it can no longer interact with E2F
C. loss of expression of pRB which normally activates E2F
D. mutation in pRB that prevents its phosphorylation so that it cannot interact with the gene to which it normally binds and coactivates with E2F
E mutation in the domain of pRB to which E2F binds, the consequences of which lead to constitutive E2F activity

Answer E: Members of the E2F family of transcription factors play critical roles in regulating cell cycle transit through the G_1-S restriction point. The activity of E2F is regulated by interaction with the protein product of the retinoblastoma susceptibility tumor suppressor gene, *pRB*. Interaction of pRB and E2F occurs when pRB is in a hypophosphorylated state. Members of the cyclin-dependent kinase family of cell cycle–regulating kinases target pRB for phosphorylation. When phosphorylated, pRB dissociates from E2F allowing E2F to enter the nucleus and transcriptionally activate genes involved in DNA synthesis as well as its own transcription. Transcription of both cyclin E and CDK2 are activated by E2F. These 2 proteins form a complex that promotes progression through S phase of the cell cycle and also act to keep E2F active by adding to the phosphorylation state of pRB. Thus, any defect in the ability of pRB to bind to E2F will lead to constitutive activation of DNA synthesis leading to unrestrained proliferation.

12. Numerous cancers are caused by a genetic phenomenon termed "loss of heterozygosity," LOH. This phenomenon led to the identification of genes termed tumor suppressors, because it is the loss of their function that leads to cancer. Which of the following has been shown to result from defects in a tumor suppressor gene as a consequence of LOH?
- **A.** Creutzfeldt-Jakob disease
- **B.** Crouzon syndrome
- **C.** Huntington disease
- **D.** Li-Fraumeni syndrome
- **E.** Prader-Willi syndrome

Answer D: Li-Fraumeni syndrome is a rare inherited form of cancer that involves breast and colon carcinomas, soft tissue sarcomas, osteosarcomas, brain tumors, leukemia, and adrenocortical carcinomas. These tumors develop at an early age in LFS patients. The tumor suppressor gene found responsible for LFS is *p53*. Mutant forms of p53 are found in approximately 50% of all tumors. The normal p53 protein functions as a transcription factor that can induce either cell cycle arrest or apoptosis (programmed cell death) in response to DNA damage.

13. Mutant genes that affect several organ systems and bodily functions frequently show variable expressivity. A phenomenon referred to as phenotypic variation. The most striking example of phenotypic variability is manifest in an autosomal dominant condition characterized by the appearance of café au lait spots on the skin and cutaneous and subcutaneous neurofibromas. These symptoms are associated with which of the following?
- **A.** familial adenomatous polyposis
- **B.** familial hypercholesterolemia
- **C.** Li Fraumeni syndrome
- **D.** von Hippel-Lindau syndrome
- **E.** von Recklinghausen disease (type I neurofibromatosis)

Answer E: von Recklinghausen disease (neurofibromatosis type I), an autosomal dominant disorder, is one of the most striking disorders that exhibits variable expressivity (phenotypic variation). Symptoms can range from the benign appearance of café au lait spots to severe disfiguring cutaneous neurofibromas, sarcomas, and gliomas. This disorder is caused by disruption in the neurofibromin gene whose protein product functions in the catalysis of inactivation of the signaling protein RAS.

14. The protein encoded by the adenomatous polyposis coli (*APC*) gene is a tumor suppressor whose role is to regulate the activity of cellular signaling induced by the Wnt growth factor. Therefore, loss of APC activity is associated with unrestrained cellular proliferation. Which of the following signaling molecules is the target for APC interaction?
- **A.** β-catenin
- **B.** MYC
- **C.** p53
- **D.** pRB
- **E.** von Hippel-Lindau protein (pVHL)

Answer A: When Wnts bind to the frizzled-LRP5/6 receptor complex the intracelular proteins axin, disheveled, and GSK-3β are recruited to the receptor complex. This prevents axin from interacting with APC which in turn prevents a destructive complex, comprised of APC, axin, GSK-3β, and β-catenin (as well as several other proteins) from forming. The role of this latter complex is to induce the phosphorylation of β-catenin which results in its destruction. β-catenin has been shown to directly interact with APC and mutations in APC that lead to colon cancer result in a protein that does not bind to β-catenin. Complexes of APC and β-catenin bind to GSK-3β. APC functions as a molecular scaffold coordinating the activities of β-catenin and GSK-3β such that APC assists in the ability of GSK-3β to phosphorylate β-catenin leading to its degradation.

15. Which of the following is considered an alkylating agent and has been shown to be effective in cancer chemotherapy?
- **A.** doxorubicin
- **B.** cyclophosphamide
- **C.** methotrexate
- **D.** vinblastine
- **E.** etoposide

Answer B: Cyclophosphamide is a nitrogen mustard alkylating agent that adds an alkyl group guanine bases in DNA. The alkyl group is added to the number 7 nitrogen atom of the imidazole ring. Cyclophosphamides are used to treat cancers and autoimmune disorders. The cyclophosphamides are prodrugs that are converted in the liver to active forms that have chemotherapeutic activity.

16. The Philadelphia chromosome is the result of a translocation between chromosomes 9 and 22 leading to the generation of a chimeric tyrosine kinase gene, *BCR-ABL*. This chromosomal abnormality is associated with which of the following disorders?

A. Burkitt lymphoma
B. chronic myeloid leukemia
C. Fanconi anemia
D. Li-Fraumeni syndrome (LFS)
E. von Hippel-Lindau syndrome (VHL)

Answer B: Chronic myeloid leukemia is characterized as a pluripotent stem cell disease of the hematopoietic system that results from a consistent chromosomal translocation. This translocation is known as the Philadelphia chromosome and results from a translocation between chromosomes 9 and 22. The translocation occurs within the proto-oncogenic tyrosine kinase gene, *ABL* on chromosome 9 and the BCR locus on chromosome 22 (t9:22). The *ABL* gene was first identified as the transforming protein of Abelson murine leukemia virus. The BCR (breakpoint cluster region) locus is so named because it was a region on chromosome 22 identified in numerous chromosomal breakpoints. The result of the Philadelphia translocation is a fusion protein, BCR-ABL, that has uncontrolled tyrosine kinase activity leading to the ability to transform cells.

17. A 62-year-old woman with chronic hepatitis B infection and a 3-year history of cirrhosis presents with jaundice, increasing ascites, left upper quadrant pain, and malaise. Liver biopsy is performed after an abdominal CT scan reveals the presence of an 18-cm mass in the left lobe. Histology demonstrates abnormally thickened hepatic cords composed of moderately well-differentiated hepatocytes with an increased nuclear to cytoplasmic ratio and prominent nucleoli; many cells contain bile and eosinophilic material within the cytoplasm. Which of the following oncogenic mechanisms is most likely responsible for the initial hit underlying the changes in the patient's liver?

A. failure of immune surveillance
B. hepatic conversion of procarcinogen to a carcinogenic metabolite
C. loss of p53 tumor suppressor gene
D. spontaneous chromosomal point mutation
E. viral DNA insertion into the host genome

Answer E: This woman's history of chronic hepatitis B infection and cirrhosis greatly increase her risk for hepatocellular carcinoma. This diagnosis is confirmed by the microscopic description of the liver biopsy findings, which are classical for hepatocellular carcinoma. This tumor usually arises in a cirrhotic liver and, worldwide, hepatitis B infection is a major cause of cirrhosis. In such individuals, hepatitis virus DNA integration into host DNA can be demonstrated and is strongly suspected of having a role in the initiation of hepatocellular carcinoma. There are other factors that are also suspected of having a role but given this woman's medical history and the high prevalence of hepatocellular carcinoma in hepatitis B-positive populations viral-mediated oncogenesis is the most likely scenario.

18. A 29-year-old woman presents with weakness, fatigue, easy bruising, and nosebleeds. Analysis of her blood reveals a reciprocal translocation between chromosomes 22 and 9, and low leukocyte alkaline phosphatase levels. These findings confirm a diagnosis of which of the following?

A. acute lymphoblastic leukemia
B. Burkitt lymphoma
C. chronic myelogenous leukemia
D. follicular lymphoma
E. Hodgkin lymphoma

Answer C: Ninety percent of individuals with chronic myelogenous leukemia have an acquired Philadelphia chromosome abnormality consisting of a translocation between chromosomes 22 and 9. The translocation places the proto-oncogene ABL from chromosome 9 next to the breakpoint cluster region (BCR) on chromosome 22. The unique gene sequence BCR-ABL confers a growth advantage with subsequent clonal expansion.

19. Your patient is a 49-year-old woman who has experienced a 2-year history of recurrent burning chest pain. Your previously prescribed medications and antacids have provided her with minimal relief. No physical abnormalities are noted during this visit. You perform an upper endoscopy and take a biopsy specimen. Histological examination of the biopsy shows a microinvasive adenocarcinoma arising from intestinal metaplasia in the distal portion of the esophagus. The most likely cause of the loss of cohesion of the neoplastic epithelial cells in this lesion is a decrease in the expression of which of the following molecules?

A. E-cadherin
B. fibronectin
C. I-CAM
D. laminin
E. P-selectin

Answer A: E-cadherin is an epithelial cell adhesion molecule whose expression is often downregulated during carcinoma progression and metastatic spread of tumors. Although many other cell adhesion molecules can play a role in cancer cell migration away from a primary tumor, adenocarcinomas are epithelial in origin and thus, E-cadherin is the most likely molecule whose expression is altered in this patient.

20. You are studying the characteristics of a particular protein isolated from cells of a squamous cell carcinoma and comparing it to the same protein isolated from nonaffected cells from the same tissue. When grown in culture, the normal cells arrest in the G_0 phase of the cell cycle. Analysis of the 2 proteins demostrates that the normal protein binds to DNA, whereas, the mutated protein from the carcinoma cells does not. These findings are most characteristic of which of the following?
- **A.** growth factor receptors
- **B.** GTP-binding proteins
- **C.** nonreceptor tyrosine kinases
- **D.** oncogene proteins
- **E.** tumor suppressor gene proteins

Answer E: Tumor suppressor genes are genes that regulate the growth of cells. When these genes are functioning properly, they can prevent and inhibit the growth of tumors. When tumor suppressor genes are altered or inactivated (due to a mutation), they lose the ability to make a protein that controls cell growth. Cells can then grow uncontrolled and develop into a cancer. Tumor suppressor proteins are often nuclear localized transcription factors, such as p53, that bind to target DNA sequences.

21. Your current patient is a 49-year-old man. You just performed a partial hepatic resection to remove a solitary 7-cm mass that was discovered by ultrasound. Histological examination of the biopsied mass indicates hepatocellular carcinoma. Genetic analysis indicates a mutation of the *p53* tumor suppressor gene in an area identified as a mutational "hot spot." Which of the following agents is the most likely carcinogen causing this patient's disease?
- **A.** aflatoxin B1
- **B.** *Clonorchis sinensis*
- **C.** ethanol
- **D.** hepatitis A virus
- **E.** vinyl chloride

Answer A: Aflatoxin B1 is an aflatoxin produced by the fungi *Aspergillus flavus* and *Aspergillus parasiticus*. Aflatoxins are toxic and among the most carcinogenic substances. When aflatoxins enter the body they are metabolized by the liver where the resultant compounds are highly carcinogenic due primarily from the induction of mutations in the *p53* gene.

22. Which of the following mechanisms characterizes the usual action of most oncogenes?
- **A.** defective DNA repair
- **B.** dominant negative
- **C.** gain-of-function
- **D.** haploinsufficiency
- **E.** loss-of-function

Answer C: An oncogene is a gene that has the potential to cause cancer and results from alteration in a proto-oncogene, either mutation or altered expression. Cancer normally results due to a dominant gain-of-function mutation or gain-of-function changes in the expression of the proto-oncogene.

23. You are studying the responses of cultured intestinal epithelial cells to various types of ionizing radiation. The cells you are using contain a functional *p53* gene. Following exposure to ultraviolet light, which of the following events is most likely to occur?
- **A.** apoptosis is inhibited
- **B.** cells are prevented from entering S phase
- **C.** the concentration of p53 decreases
- **D.** replication of DNA is enhanced
- **E.** transcription of metaphase cyclins is increased

Answer B: The protein encoded by p53 is a nuclear localized phosphoprotein. The p53 protein is a transcription factor that regulates the expression of numerous genes involved in suppression of cell growth. Phosphorylation regulates the activity of p53. The level of p53 is low after mitosis but increases during G_1. During S phase the protein becomes phosphorylated by the M-phase cyclin-CDK complex of the cell cycle and also by casein kinase II (CKII). One major cell cycle–regulating gene that is a target for p53 is the CDK inhibitory protein (CIP), p21CIP. Activation of p53 results in increased expression of p21CIP with a resultant arrest in the G_1 phase of the cell cycle so they cannot begin DNA synthesis in S phase.

24. A 27-year-old man has undergone a routine colonoscopy because of his concern over a family history of colon cancer. There is no family history of any other types of cancer. During the colonoscopy a single 2-cm polyp is seen and removed. Histological examination of the polyp shows a villous adenoma. Metaphase chromosomal spread shows microsatellite instability but no translocations or deletions. This patient has most likely inherited a defect that has led to interference in which of the following processes?
- **A.** cell adhesion regulation
- **B.** DNA mismatch repair
- **C.** growth factor receptor expression

D. regulation of apoptosis
E. signal transduction

Answer B: DNA mismatch involves a series of enzymes that recognize and repair erroneous insertions, deletions, and misincorporation of bases that can arise during DNA replication and recombination, as well as repairing some forms of DNA damage. Microsatellite instability refers to a condition of genetic hypermutability that results from impaired DNA mismatch repair mechanisms.

25. A 38-year-old woman has had a biopsy taken from her cervix due to an abnormal Pap smear result. Histological analysis of the biopsy tissue shows grade 3 intraepithelial neoplasia. Additionally, the results demonstrate that the cancerous cells are widely dispersed. Altered expression of which of the following is the most likely cause of the dispersion of the neoplastic cells throughout the biopsy tissue?

A. cadherins
B. elastases
C. laminin receptors
D. matrix metalloproteinases
E. tissue inhibitors of metalloproteinases

Answer A: The cadherins are a class of calcium-dependent cell adhesion proteins that ensure cells within tissues stay bound together. Loss of cell adhesion can lead to cell migration from tissues, characteristic of metastases. One cadherin in particular, E-cadherin, has been shown to play an important role in the metastatic potential of numerous epithelial cancers. Reduced, or loss of, expression of E-cadherin is correlated with high rates of metastasis, especially in prostate cancers. Matrix metalloproteinases are involved in the degradation of the ECM and are also involved in metastases so their inhibition would lead to reduced metastatic capability.

Checklist

✓ Cancers are the result of some form of insult to the genetic makeup of a cell. These insults can, and do, include point mutations, insertions, deletions, gross chromosomal abnormalities (eg, translocations), and viral disruption of the genome.

✓ The vast majority of cancers are the result of alterations in the function of genes involved in aspects of cell signaling from growth factors, receptors, intracellular signaling molecules, and transcription factors. Additional classes of affected genes in cancer are those that regulate progression through the cell cycle.

✓ Cancers can continue to grow unrestricted due to induced loss-of-growth regulatory signals as well as the induction of unregulated nutrient intake. Solid tumors can expand because they induce the expression of factors involved in the production of new vessels (angiogenesis).

✓ With respect to nutrient intake and metabolism, all cancer cells express a particular form of the glycolytic enzyme, pyruvate kinase (specifically the PKM2 isoform), that leads to most glycolysis proceeding to lactate instead of to complete oxidation in the TCA cycle. This unique glycolytic metabolism is referred to as the Warburg effect and it allows glucose carbons to be diverted into the biomass necessary for cancer cell proliferation.

✓ The vast majority of human cancers result from genetic alterations in somatic cells. However, there are many cancers that result from germline transmission (inheritance) altered genes that predispose an individual to a particular form of cancer.

✓ Cancers are the result of changes in 2 distinct classes of gene: the dominant cancer-causing genes are referred to as oncogenes and cancer results from any gain-of-function mutation in the original proto-oncogene; the recessive cancer-causing genes are referred to as the tumor suppressors and cancer results from and loss-of-function mutation to the gene.

- ✓ Epigenetics plays a role in cancers and is most often related to changes in DNA methylation status. Many cancers have been found to result from hypermethylation of tumor suppressor genes resulting in their transcriptional silencing.
- ✓ Cancer metastasis is the process by which a tumor cell can break away from the originating tumor and migrate to a new location in the body forming new tumor sites. Metastasis requires several properties unique to cancer that include loss of cell adhesion, breakdown of the ECM, penetration into the vasculature, evasion of immune surveillance, and colonization of the new site.
- ✓ Overall, cancer is a multistep process that occurs in different pathways in different individuals even when considering the same type of cancer. This makes treatments difficult within the context of a given type of cancer in different individuals.

Index

Page numbers followed by italic *f* or *t* denote figures or tables, respectively.

D

G

H

O

P

U